# Routledge Handbook of Global Public Health in Asia

Global public health is of growing concern to most governments and populations, nowhere more so than in Asia, the world's largest and most populous continent. Whilst major advances have been made in controlling infectious diseases through public health measures as well as clinical medical treatments, the world now faces other challenges including ageing populations and the epidemic crisis of obesity and non-communicable diseases. New emerging infections continue to develop and the growing threats to health due to environmental pollution and climate change increase the need for resilience and sustainability. These threats to health are global in nature, and this Handbook will explore perspectives on current public health issues in South, Southeast and East Asia, informing global as well as regional debate.

Whilst many books cite Western examples of the development of global public health, this Handbook brings together both Western and Eastern scholarship, creating a new global public health perspective suitable to face modern challenges in promoting the population's health. This Handbook is essential reading not only for students, professionals and scholars of global public health and related fields but is also written to be accessible to those with a general interest in the health of Asia.

**Siân M. Griffiths** is Emeritus Professor and the Founding Director of the Centre for Global Health in the School of Public Health and Primary Care at the Chinese University of Hong Kong and Visiting Professor at the Institute of Global Health Innovation, Imperial College, London, UK.

**Jin Ling Tang** is Professor of Epidemiology at the School of Public Health and Primary Care and Director of the Shenzhen Institute of Public Health at the Chinese University of Hong Kong.

**Eng Kiong Yeoh** was Secretary of Health in the HKSAR until 2003 and is now Director of the School of Public Health and Primary Care at the Chinese University of Hong Kong.

'Deep insights into the complexities of health, its determinants and the wider development context in Asia have been hard to come by for students, practitioners and policy makers. This Handbook remedies this shortfall with a highly authoritative, expert account of global public health in Asia.'

*Sir Liam Donaldson, Chair in Health Policy, Imperial College, London and former Chief Mecical Officer of the UK*

'This Handbook represents a joint effort of the global community of healthcare professionals. Experts in public health and policy makers from North to South and East to West contribute their knowledge and share their experiences on various topics of global health. I pay tribute to their great efforts in this important work. I recommend this book to every medical student, practising medical practitioner, healthcare policy maker and academic in the healthcare profession.'

*Joseph J. Y. Sung, Mok Hing Yiu Professor of Medicine and Vice-Chancellor and President of the Chinese University of Hong Kong (CUHK) since 2010*

'The book is a significant contribution to our understanding of health in this most populous region of the world – a region that has seen remarkable improvements in health, especially over the past two decades. With a focus on East and Southeast Asia, it is highly recommended as an excellent source of information and analysis.'

*Richard A. Cash MD, MP, Senior Lecturer, Department of Global Health and Population, Harvard School of Public Health and Visiting Professor, Public Health Foundation of India*

'This Handbook is one of the most important readings for those interested in global public health in general and in Asia specifically. It offers fascinating insights into the many great achievements that Asian countries have made over the past decades, and the enormous challenges that those countries are facing in the years to come.'

*Shenglan Tang, Professor of Medicine and Global Health and Associate Director of Duke Global Health Institute, USA*

'With the accelerated globalization, great changes have taken place in health systems, medical technology and the disease spectrum which demand multi-discipline cooperation to explore the solutions to a series of issues brought by globalization from different perspectives. This book provides good support to learn about global health including challenges in global health and strategy as well as best practice in response to these challenges. The book can be used not only as a textbook for medical students, but also provides valuable learning material for public health professionals.'

*Yan Guo, School of Public Health, Peking University, China*

# Routledge Handbook of Global Public Health in Asia

*Edited by Siân M. Griffiths, Jin Ling Tang and Eng Kiong Yeoh*

Routledge
Taylor & Francis Group
LONDON AND NEW YORK

First published 2014
by Routledge
2 Park Square, Milton Park, Abingdon, Oxon, OX14 4RN

and by Routledge
711 Third Avenue, New York, NY 10017

*Routledge is an imprint of the Taylor & Francis Group, an informa business*



*British Library Cataloguing in Publication Data*
A catalogue record for this book is available from the British Library

*Library of Congress Cataloging in Publication Data*
Routledge handbook of global public health in Asia / edited by Siân M. Griffiths, Jin Ling Tang and Eng Kiong Yeoh.
pages cm
Includes bibliographical references and index.
1. Public health–Asia. 2. Medical policy–Asia. I. Griffiths, Siân, editor of compilation. II. Tang, Jin Ling, editor of compilation. III. Yeoh, Eng Kiong, editor of compilation.
RA525.R68 2014
362.109–dc23

2013036831

ISBN: 978-0-415-64382-5 (hbk)
ISBN: 978-1-315-81871-9 (ebk)

Typeset in Bembo
by RefineCatch Ltd, Bungay, Suffolk

MIX
Paper from responsible sources
FSC
www.fsc.org
FSC® C013056

Printed and bound in Great Britain by
TJ International Ltd, Padstow, Cornwall

# Contents

# Figures

# Tables

# Boxes

# Contributors

**Anisha Abraham** is a Consultant at the Chinese University of Hong Kong and an Honorary Associate Professor of Paediatrics at the Prince of Wales Hospital in Hong Kong.

**Syed Masud Ahmed** is a Professor at the Centre for Equity and Health Systems and the Coordinator at the Centre of Excellence for Universal Health Coverage at the James P. Grant School of Public Health at BRAC University in Dhaka, Bangladesh.

**Mohammed K. Ali** is an Assistant Professor at the Hubert Department of Global Health and Department of Epidemiology at the Rollins School of Public Health at Emory University, Atlanta, GA, USA.

**Pascale Allotey** is a Professor of Public Health and the Head of Global Public Health at the Jeffrey Cheah School of Medicine and Health Sciences at the Monash University campus in Sunway, Malaysia. She is also the Associate Director (International) of the South East Asia Community Observatory (SEACO) – a health and demographic surveillance site based in Segamat, Johor.

**Rachel M. Amiya** is a Doctoral Student at the Department of Community and Global Health at the Graduate School of Medicine at the University of Tokyo, Japan.

**Sue Atkinson** is a Professor and the Co-Chair of the Climate and Health Council, London, UK.

**Haley L. Cash** is an epidemiologist at the Ministry of Health in Palau.

**Constance Chan** was the former Controller at the Centre for Food Safety, Food and Environmental Hygiene Department from 2007 to 2012, Hong Kong.

**Emily Y. Y. Chan** is Associate Professsor at the Faculty of Medicine at the Chinese University of Hong Kong. She is Director of the Centre for Global Health at the School of Public Health and Primary Care and the Director of the Collaborating Centre for Oxford University and the Chinese University of Hong Kong for Disaster and Medical Humanitarian Response.

**Sophia S. C. Chan** was a Professor of Nursing and the Director of Research at the School of Nursing at the University of Hong Kong until October 2012. She was also a Council Member and Vice Chair at the Hong Kong Council on Smoking and Health from 2009 to 2012. She is currently the Under Secretary for Food and Health of the Hong Kong Special Administrative Region.

**Phitaya Charupoonphol** is an Associate Professor and the Dean of the Faculty of Public Health at the Mahidol University, Bangkok, Thailand.

**Patsy Y. K. Chau** is a Research Associate at the Division of Health System, Policy and Management at the Jockey Club School of Public Health and Primary Care at the Chinese University of Hong Kong.

**Julius Cheah** is a Research Officer in Global Public Health at the Jeffrey Cheah School of Medicine and Health Sciences at the Monash University campus in Sunway, Malaysia.

**Weihong Chen** is a Professor at the Key Lab of Environment and Health, School of Public Health, Tongji Medical College, Huazhong University of Science and Technology, China.

**Tung-liang Chiang** is a Postdoctoral Research Fellow at the Central Clinical School, Faculty of Medicine, Nursing and Health Sciences, Monash University, Melbourne.

**Josette Chor** is an Assistant Professor at the Jockey Club School of Public Health and Primary Care at the Faculty of Medicine at the Chinese University of Hong Kong.

**Eric P. F. Chow** is a Research Assistant at the Kirby Institute at the University of New South Wales, Sydney, Australia.

**Roger Y. Chung** is the Research Assistant Professor at the Jockey Club School of Public Health and Primary Care at the Chinese University of Hong Kong.

**Vincent C. H. Chung** is an Assistant Professor at the School of Public Health and Primary Care at the Chinese University of Hong Kong.

**Shauna Downs** is a Doctoral Candidate at the Menzies Centre for Health Policy at the University of Sydney, Australia.

**Tim Evans** is the Director of Health Nutrition and Population at the World Bank in Washington, DC. At the time of writing the chapter, he was the Dean of the James P Grant School of Public Health at BRAC University in Dhaka, Bangladesh.

**Hildy F. Fong** is Executive Director at the Center for Global Public Health at the University of California, Berkeley.

**Siân M. Griffiths** is Emeritus Professor and the Founding Director of the Centre for Global Health in the School of Public Health and Primary Care at the Chinese University of Hong Kong and Visiting Professor at the Institute of Global Health Innovation, Imperial College, London, UK.

**Jinping Guo** joined the Save the Children China Programme in 2009 as a Senior Education Project Officer.

**Maria Elena Baltazar Herrera** is a Professor and core faculty of the Asian Institute of Management and Research Director of the AIM RVR Center for Corporate Social Responsibility, in the Philippines. She is also an actuary and is the Managing Director of Solutions Incorporated, an employee benefits and actuarial consulting firm.

**Y. Y. Ho** is a Consultant of Community Medicine in Risk Assessment and Communication at the Centre for Food Safety, Food and Environmental Hygiene Department in Hong Kong.

**Tomiko Hokama** is a Professor Emeritus of Child Health and Vice President at the University of the Ryukyus in Okinawa, Japan. She is a certified Paediatrician and Specialist from the Japan Paediatric Society.

**Peter Horby** is a Senior Clinical Research Fellow at the Oxford University Clinical Research Unit in Vietnam and Associate Professor at the Long Loo School of Medicine, Singapore.

**Johnny Yu Jiang** is an Associate Professor at the Chinese Academy of Medical Sciences and Peking Union Medical College, Beijing, China.

**Linghui Jiang** has been working on maternal and child health projects in rural China for six years since she started her first job at Save the Children.

**Masamine Jimba** is a Professor and Chair of the Department of Community and Global Health at the Graduate School of Medicine at the University of Tokyo, Japan.

**Jean H. Kim** is an Associate Professor at the Jockey Club School of Public Health and Primary Care at the Chinese University of Hong Kong.

**T. H. Lam** is the Chair Professor in Community Medicine and Sir Robert Kotewall Professor in Public Health of the School of Public Health at the University of Hong Kong.

**Joseph T. F. Lau** is a Professor at the Jockey Club School of Public Health and Primary Care at the Chinese University of Hong Kong.

**S. H. Lee** was Emeritus Professor of Community Medicine at the Chinese University of Hong Kong and an Honorary Adviser at the Jockey Club School of Public Health and Primary Care at the Faculty of Medicine at the Chinese University of Hong Kong.

**Stephen Leeder** is a Professor of Public Health and Community Medicine at the Menzies Centre for Health Policy at the University of Sydney, Australia.

**Jing Hua Li** is a PhD student at the Jockey Club School of Public Health and Primary Care at the Chinese University of Hong Kong.

**Lanjuan Li** is a Professor of Infectious Diseases and the Director of the State Key Laboratory for Diagnosis and Treatment of Infectious Diseases, Zhejiang University School of Medicine, China.

**Liming Li** is a Professor of Epidemiology at the School of Public Health at the Peking University Health Science Center, Beijing, China.

**Jun Lv** is an Associate Professor at the School of Public Health at the Peking University Health Science Center, Beijing, China.

**Shan Lv** is an Assistant Professor at the National Institute of Parasitic Diseases of the Chinese Center for Disease Control and Prevention, WHO Collaborating Center on Malaria, Schistosomiasis and Filariasis in Shanghai, China.

**Ronald C. W. Ma** is a Professor at the Department of Medicine and Therapeutics at the Chinese University of Hong Kong. He is also the Immediate Past President of Diabetes Hongkong.

**Judith Mackay** is the Asian Consultancy on Tobacco Control; and Senior Advisor, World Lung Foundation.

**Pia MacRae** is the Country Director for Save the Children China programmes. She previously ran the Tropical Health and Education Trust in London.

**Manu Raj Mathur** is a Research Scientist and Assistant Professor, Public Health Foundation of India, New Delhi.

**Graeme Maugham** is the Treasurer at the Climate and Health Council and a Sustainability Manager at Peabody Trust, London, UK.

**Bryan Mercurio** is the Professor, Vice Chancellor's Outstanding Fellow of the Faculty of Law and Associate Dean (Research) at the Chinese University of Hong Kong.

**Amal K. Mitra** is a Professor of Epidemiology and Biostatistics and a Fulbright Scholar at the Department of Public Health of the University of Southern Mississippi, Hattiesburg, Mississippi, USA.

**David Molyneux** is an Emeritus Professor and Senior Professional Fellow at the Centre for Neglected Tropical Diseases at the Liverpool School of Tropical Medicine, UK.

**Jin Mou** is a Research Fellow at the Department of Family Practice at the University of British Columbia (UBC), Vancouver, Canada.

**K. M. Venkat Narayan** is the Ruth and O.C. Hubert Chair of Global Health and Professor of Epidemiology and Medicine at Emory University, Atlanta, GA, USA.

**Vural Özdemir** is an Associate Professor of Human Genetics (the Council of Higher Education, Turkey), and Vice Dean at the Faculty of Communications at Gaziantep University, Turkey. He is also an Advisor to the Gaziantep University President for International Affairs and Global Development Strategy. Additionally, he is Editor-in Chief for *OMICS: A Journal of Integrative Biology* (New York, USA).

**Kai Hong Phua** is a Professor of Health and Social Policy at the Lee Kuan Yew School of Public Policy, National University of Singapore. He worked at the Ministry of Health, Singapore, prior to teaching public health administration and health economics, and serving as Head (Health Services Research) at the Faculty of Medicine. He has consulted for international health organizations, government ministries of health and the healthcare industry throughout Asia.

**K. Srinath Reddy** is a Professor and the President of the Public Health Foundation of India, in New Delhi.

**Daniel D. Reidpath** is a Professor of Population Health and the Head of the Public Health Unit at the Jeffrey Cheah School of Medicine and Health Sciences at the Monash University campus in Sunway, Malaysia. He is also the Director of the South East Asia Community Observatory (SEACO) – a health and demographic surveillance site based in Segamat, Johor.

**Junko Saito** is a Doctoral Student at the Department of Community and Global Health at the Graduate School of Medicine at the University of Tokyo, Japan.

**Jonathan M. Samet** is a Professor and Flora L. Thornton Chair at the Department of Preventive Medicine at the Keck School of Medicine. He is also the Director of the Institute for Global Health at the University of Southern California, USA.

**Yu Mon Saw** is a Doctoral Student at the Department of Community and Global Health, Graduate School of Medicine at the University of Tokyo, Japan.

**Hongbing Shen** is the Vice President of Nanjing Medical University and the Professor of Epidemiology at the Department of Epidemiology and Biostatistics at the Nanjing Medical University, China.

**Roopa Shivashankar** is a Senior Research Associate at the Public Health Foundation of India (PHFI) and the Centre for Chronic Disease Control (CCDC) in India.

**Rosamund J. Southgate** is a British doctor training in Public Health Medicine in the UK. She is currently working with Public Health England, an agency of the UK Government Department of Health. She recently completed a Fellowship at the Chinese University of Hong Kong (CUHK)–Oxford University Centre for Disaster and Medical Humanitarian Response at CUHK and a secondment to the Western Cape Government Department of Health in Cape Town, Republic of South Africa.

**Lisa R. Staimez** is a Post-Doctoral Fellow at the Hubert Department of Global Health at Emory University. She was supported by the Molecules to Mankind Program and the Nutrition and Health Sciences Program in the Division of Biological and Biomedical Sciences at the Laney Graduate School at Emory University, Atlanta, GA, USA.

**Peter Steinmann** is a Post-Doctoral Research Fellow at the Department of Epidemiology and Public Health at the Swiss Tropical and Public Health Institute, an associated institute of the University of Basel, Switzerland.

**Robin Stott** is the Co-Chair of the Climate and Health Council, London, UK.

**Joseph J. Y. Sung** is a Mok Hing Yiu Professor of Medicine and has been the Vice Chancellor and President of the Chinese University of Hong Kong (CUHK) since 2010. In 2011, Professor Sung was elected to the Chinese Academy of Engineering (CAE) as an Academician in recognition of his contributions in the field of gastroenterology.

**Bruno F. Sunguya** is a Doctoral Student at the Department of Community and Global Health at the Graduate School of Medicine at the University of Tokyo, Japan.

**Siripen Supakankunti** is the Director at the Centre for Health Economics and a Programme Director of the MSc in Health Economics and Health Care Management at the Faculty of Economics at the Chulalongkorn University, Bangkok, Thailand.

**Jin Ling Tang** is Professor of Epidemiology at the School of Public Health and Primary Care and Director of the Shenzen Institute of Public Health at the Chinese University of Hong Kong.

**Anne Marie Thow** is a Lecturer in Health Policy at the Menzies Centre for Health Policy at the University of Sydney, Australia.

**Thomas Tsang Ho-Fai** was the Controller at the Centre for Health Protection in Hong Kong SAR Government during 2007–2012.

**Jürg Utzinger** is a Professor at the Department of Epidemiology and Public Health at the Swiss Tropical and Public Health Institute, an associated institute of the University of Basel, Switzerland.

**John Walley** is Professor of International Public Health and the Co-Research Director of the Communicable Diseases Health Service Delivery (COMDIS-HSD) research programme, Nuffield Centre for International Health and Development, University of Leeds, UK. He is a Fellow of the Faculty of Public Health UK.

**Harry Hao-Xiang Wang** is a Lecturer at the School of Public Health and Primary Care at the Faculty of Medicine at the Chinese University of Hong Kong. He is also the Post-Doctoral Research Fellow at the General Practice and Primary Care in the Institute of Health and Wellbeing at the University of Glasgow, UK.

**Jia-Ji Wang** is a Professor at the School of Public Health at the Guangzhou Medical University, China.

**Mary Beth Weber** is an Assistant Professor at the Hubert Department of Global Health at the Rollins School of Public Health at Emory University, Atlanta, GA, USA.

**Xiaolin Wei** is an Assistant Professor at the Jockey Club School of Public Health and Primary Care at the Chinese University of Hong Kong, and Honorary Senior Research Fellow at the University of Leeds. He is also a Fellow of the Faculty of Public Health.

**Andromeda H. S. Wong** is a Research Associate at the School of Public Health and Primary Care at the Chinese University of Hong Kong.

**Carmen Wong** is the Director at the Centre of Research and Promotion in Women's Health and the Assistant Professor at the Division of Family Medicine and Primary Health Care at the Jockey Club School of Public Health and Primary Care at the Chinese University of Hong Kong.

**Martin Wong** is the Director of the Jockey Club Bowel Cancer Education Centre at the Chinese University of Hong Kong. He is also the Associate Professor at the Jockey Club School of Public Health and Primary Care at the Faculty of Medicine at the Chinese University of Hong Kong.

**Mary Lai Lin Wong** is the Chief Executive Officer of the Health Travel Advisory Council at the Ministry of Health, Malaysia. She has worked in the Corporate Policy and Industry Division,

Ministry of Health and in hospital administration. She completed her PhD studies at the National University of Singapore, a Masters in Health Services Management at the University of Manchester and a BA (Hons) at the University of Malaya.

**Samuel Y. S. Wong** is a Professor and Head at the Division of Family Medicine and Primary Healthcare at the School of Public Health and Primary Care at the Chinese University of Hong Kong.

**Tze Wai Wong** is a Research Professor at the School of Public Health and Primary Care at the Chinese University of Hong Kong.

**Fan Wu** is the Director General at the Shanghai Municipal Center for Disease Control and Prevention, the People's Republic of China.

**Tangchun Wu** is a Professor at the Key Lab of Environment and Health, School of Public Health, Tongji Medical College, Huazhong University of Science and Technology, China.

**Carrie H. K. Yam** is a Research Associate at the Division of Health System, Policy and Management at the Jockey Club School of Public Health and Primary Care at the Chinese University of Hong Kong.

**Guo-Jing Yang** is a Professor at the Jiangsu Institute of Parasitic Diseases, Key Laboratory on Control Technology for Parasitic Diseases at the Ministry of Health, China.

**Ruikan Yang** is the Health Advisor of the China programme at Save the Children.

**Peiling Yap** is a Post-Doctoral Research Fellow at the Department of Epidemiology and Public Health at the Swiss Tropical and Public Health Institute, an associated institute of the University of Basel, Switzerland.

**Junko Yasuoka** is an Assistant Professor at the Department of Community and Global Health at the Graduate School of Medicine Health at the University of Tokyo, Japan.

**Eng Kiong Yeoh** was Secretary of Health in the HKSAR until 2003 and is now Director of the School of Public Health and Primary Care at the Chinese University of Hong Kong.

**Vincent T. F. Yeung** is a Consultant and the Chief of Service at the Department of Medicine and Geriatrics at Our Lady of Maryknoll Hospital, Hong Kong. He is also a Past President of Diabetes Hongkong.

**Azadeh Zabetian** is a Postdoctoral Associate at the Yale program of applied translational research, School of Medicine, Yale University, New Haven, CT, USA.

**Junfeng (Jim) Zhang** is Professor of Global and Environmental Health, Duke Global Health Institute and Nicholas School of the Environment, Duke University, Durham, NC, USA.

**Lei Zhang** is a Senior Lecturer at the Kirby Institute, University of New South Wales, Sydney, Australia.

**Xiao-Nong Zhou** is a Professor and Director of the National Institute of Parasitic Diseases of the Chinese Center for Disease Control and Prevention, and the Director of the WHO Collaborating Center on Malaria, Schistosomiasis and Filariasis in Shanghai, China.

# Foreword

The history of medicine has always been focused on diagnosis, treatment and rehabilitation of medical conditions *at a personal level*. However, due to the rapid development of information technology, the massive and unprecedented changes faced by the planet we are living on, the convenience of international travel and the globalization of the world economy, health has become a global issue.

An outbreak of the Severe Acute Respiratory Syndrome (SARS) in 2003 struck Hong Kong in a totally unprepared state. The newly emerged viral infection infected 1,755 citizens and claimed 299 lives in a calamity that lasted 100 days. The city came to a standstill and the economy faced a challenge like never before. Moreover, within one week, the deadly disease spread to different continents threatening the health of various populations and the global economy. It dawned on the world that we are far from being saved from the new microbes that come from animal reservoirs. The health authorities across nations realized that infectious diseases have no respect for borders and international collaboration was mandatory. The World Health Organization now plays an important role in orchestrating the battle against such new diseases.

Climate change and ecological imbalance have always posed major hazards to health worldwide. Air pollution, vector-borne diseases related to alterations in temperature and precipitation, water contamination and food safety create increasing problems in both developing and developed countries. Major disasters, such as earthquakes, tsunamis and flooding, carry major health impacts that cannot be overemphasized. Preparedness to face insidious changes in the environment and the sudden alterations in the earth's systems deserve more attention in health education. Once again, governmental policy, professional advice and international collaboration are called for to combat these challenges.

Medical problems related to chronic non-communicable conditions, such as diabetes, obesity, hypertension, tobacco and alcohol consumption have continued to grow over the last decades. The rising incidence of cancer is partly related to global ageing populations and partly to changes in lifestyles in our sophisticated societies. There is a great urgency to intervene in human behaviour and for modification of lifestyles in order to prevent a pandemic of metabolic disease, cardiovascular diseases and malignancies. Besides advances in science, the establishment of a cost-effective healthcare delivery system in both developed and developing countries holds the key to success in preventing further deterioration of health hazards and offering help to those who are in need.

This Handbook represents a joint effort of the global community of healthcare professionals. Experts in public health and policy makers from North to South and East to West contribute their knowledge and share their experiences on various topics of global health. I pay tribute to their great efforts in this important work. I recommend this book to every medical student, practising medical practitioner, healthcare policy maker and academic in the healthcare profession.

*Joseph J. Y. Sung MD, PhD*
*Vice Chancellor of the Chinese University of Hong Kong*

# Acknowledgements

The editors would like to thank Victoria Khroundina and Christine Ko for all their help in compiling this book.

We would like to dedicate this book to all colleagues, collaborators and students wherever they may be in the world who share our commitment to developing global health knowledge and practice, especially those who have contributed to this book. In particular we dedicate this book to our colleague and mentor Professor S. H. Lee (1933–2014).

# Part I
# Historical context and introductory concepts

# Introduction to Part I.1: historical context

*Siân M. Griffiths*

We start by using Hong Kong as a case study in historical development of public health and healthcare systems. Public health in Asia is introduced to us through the eyes of Professor S. H. Lee who was the Director of Health in Hong Kong between 1989 and 1994. An inveterate advocate of public health, Professor Lee is well known across the region – and indeed the world – not only as teacher and mentor of the Director General of the World Health Organization (WHO), Dr Margaret Chan, but as a campaigner for health promotion and public health.*

As a former British colony, Hong Kong has much in common with other countries in Asia formerly under colonial rule, both benefiting from, and disadvantaged by, their colonial legacy. Whilst many structures are robust, the process of colonial handover back to China has also created inertia in the healthcare system as new forces come into play. For example, whilst primary care services in the UK have continued to develop and have taken up a greater role in public health service delivery within an integrated model, primary care in Hong Kong remains fragmented, mainly out of pocket and the population is prone to doctor shopping rather than being steered into secondary services through the gatekeeping role of the General Practitioner (GP). The majority of public health services continue to be provided by the Department of Health through the model of maternal and child health, school health and other clinic-based services, and population-based data necessary for assessing health outcomes are not routinely collected. As such, Hong Kong is similar to many other Asian countries in that its healthcare development has been influenced by history and its development closely tied to political and socio-economic changes. As a region, Asia has the highest number of countries that rely on out-of-pocket payment for health services and as such getting sick can be a catastrophic event not only for individuals but their families.

Taking a historical perspective, Professor Lee wrote from experience about the changes he has seen and some of the important formative events in public health. For example, he describes the impact of trade on patterns of infectious disease, in particular the epidemic of bubonic plague at the end of the nineteenth century, which stimulated the development of health services for all groups in the community, including the previously excluded Chinese

* Sadly, he passed away in January 2014, before he could see his chapter in print.

locals. He describes the important scientific contribution made by Dr Yersin from the Institute of Pasteur in France and Dr Kitassato from Japan who together discovered the aetiology of plague whilst working in Hong Kong. Consequently, the importance of hygiene in the home and freedom from rats was underpinned by the public health policy of 'Keeping the House Clean'. The need for good public health systems and control of infectious diseases was further underlined by the Temple Street outbreak of cholera in the 1960s, showing once again the need for good water through sanitation and illustrating the principles elucidated by John Snow and the Broad Street pump incident in nineteenth-century London. Further illustrations of the need for robust public health systems include the response to the influx of Vietnamese refugees who flooded into Hong Kong in boats in the 1970s, and by the SARS epidemic in 2003. SARS demonstrated the global nature of infectious disease, spreading from the index case in the Kowloon hotel not only into the local community but by air travel to Vietnam, Canada and mainland China within a few days. Professor Lee, as a member of the HKSAR Inquiry team, helped formulate the response to the epidemic, which focused on better communication, building resilience, enhancing research and increasing capacity with the founding of the Centre for Health Protection.

Hong Kong, with its rapid growth and need to build health systems to accommodate increasing urban populations, is an exemplar for what is occurring in many areas of global transition, facing rapid socio-economic changes and development with increasing wealth, but also facing the difficulty of providing equitable health services in social systems that leave the market to play a significant role in healthcare provision. Culturally determined choice of services is another important part of service provision and Professor Lee describes the importance of the role of Traditional Chinese Medicine (TCM) – described later in the book in Chapter 41 – which is encouraged as part of the official policy not only in post-handover Hong Kong and in China, but across other Asian countries through the work of the WHO.

# 1

# Historical perspectives in public health

## Experiences from Hong Kong

*S. H. Lee*[1]

## Introduction

History helps us understand the policies and problems we face today. This chapter will describe the history of public health in Hong Kong over two periods. The first period will cover the early days before World War II (1840s–1940s), and the second will examine public health after the end of World War II and be further divided into three phases, with each phase having its own distinct historical events. Phase 1 covers 1945 to 1960, Phase 2 covers the 1970s and the 1980s, and Phase 3 covers the 1990s to the present.

## Early colonial medical service

Hong Kong was ceded to Britain under the Treaty of Nanjing in 1842. Lord Palmerston, the British Foreign Secretary, described Hong Kong in 1841 as 'a barren island with hardly a house upon it'. Sir Henry Pottinger, the first Governor of Hong Kong, reported in 1843 that 'the island was visited by a great deal of severe and often fatal sickness. The major infectious diseases were dysentery, cholera and malaria, commonly known as "Hong Kong Fever". Hong Kong Fever carried off 24% of garrison troops and 10% of European residents.'

The *Hong Kong Government Gazette* of May 1841 stated that the population consisted of some 7,450 fishermen and villagers. The newly arrived British traders were concentrated to build docks and warehouses on the waterfront. The construction work attracted many labourers from the Pearl River Delta.

Back then, tropical diseases were common among the British garrison force. In 1843, 24 per cent of the British garrison force and 10 per cent of the European residents had died of fever (malignant malaria), which gave Hong Kong an unwelcoming reputation for being the 'White Man's Grey Evil'.

In 1843, a government medical service was formed. In 1849, the Government Civil Hospital at Sai Ying Pun, which catered to police, civil officers and prisoners, was opened. The Chinese seldom used these services, partly because of their inability to speak English, but mainly because of their mistrust in Western medicine. With the support of Governor

MacDonald, the first hospital for the Chinese, the Tung Wah Hospital, was built in 1870. In 1893, a missionary hospital, the Nethersole Hospital, was opened.

## Early epidemics in Hong Kong prior to World War II

### *Bubonic plague*

From 1894 to 1923, Hong Kong was severely affected by the bubonic plague. In the early days of the twentieth century, many working people from China came to Hong Kong to look for jobs. They usually concentrated in the western part of the island, in a district known as Tai Ping Shan Street (see Figure 1.1). The housing conditions, and the environmental hygiene and sanitation, in that district were very poor, which facilitated the easy spread of the disease.

Historically, there had been three pandemics of plague. The first two were commonly known as the plague of Justinian and the Black Death. The third was a major pandemic that began in China's Yunnan Province in 1855. This pandemic spread to all inhabited continents and ultimately killed more than 12 million people in China and India alone.

In 1894, the bubonic plague also struck Hong Kong. The epidemic spread quickly among the overcrowded population of Tai Ping Shan. Hundreds of sick and dying patients filled the Tung Wah Hospital. After two months, the death rates dropped below epidemic rates, but the disease continued to remain endemic in Hong Kong until the late 1920s.

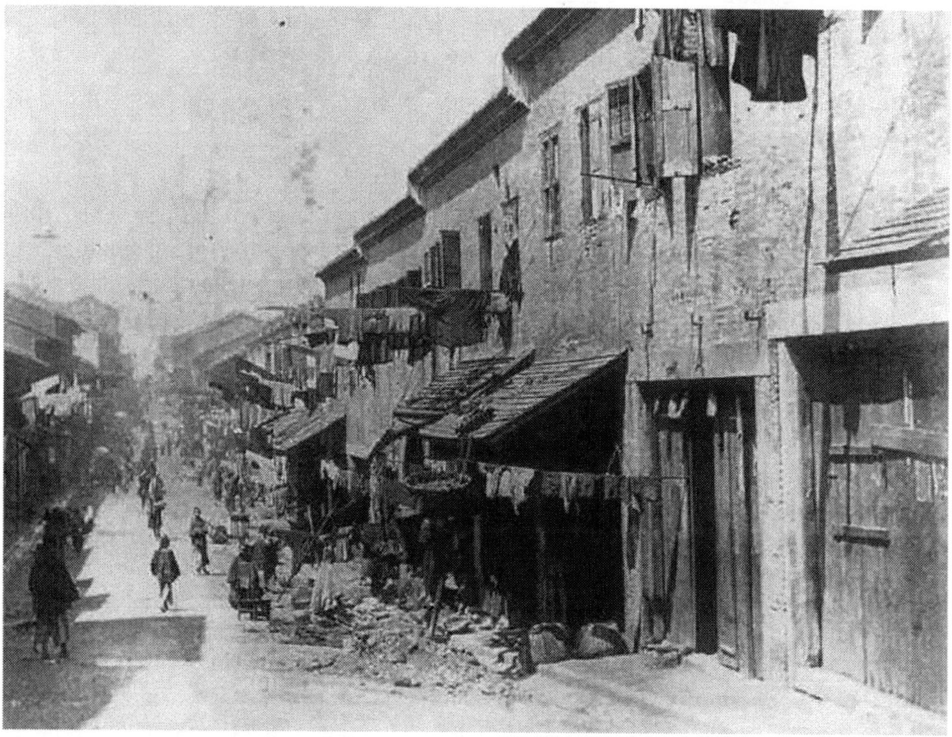

*Figure 1.1* Tai Ping Shan Street in 1880 [1]

Following the spread of the plague, the Sanitary Board organized cleansing teams which consisted of medical officers, policemen, garrison members and volunteers to launch white washing and disinfecting processes in the infected areas. The year 1894 could be described as the 'saddest and most disastrous year in history', and a commemorative plaque was erected in a park near Tai Ping Shan Street to remind people of this epidemic.

The epidemic lasted for over twenty years, with 21,867 people being affected and 20,489 dying from the disease, a high mortality rate of 93.7 per cent. The practice of quarantine started in the early phases of the epidemic. Patients were isolated in a naval ship known as *Hygeia*. But the patients did not like being kept there and wanted to go to the Tung Wah Hospital instead. Although Hong Kong suffered severely from this epidemic, an important contribution was made with the discovery of the aetiology of the plague and development of effective measures against the epidemic. Dr Yersin from the Institute of Pasteur in France and Dr Kitassato from Japan came to Hong Kong and worked together to discover the aetiology of the plague. The importance of keeping the house clean and free from rats was fully realized, and the concept of 'Keeping the House Clean' began then.

### *Smallpox*

Smallpox was also prevalent. A smallpox hospital was set up at Kennedy Town from the Tung Wah Infectious Disease Hospital. The disease remained a public health problem until the early twentieth century.[2]

## Public health after World War II

### *Phase 1 (1945–1960)*

This period saw the emergence of many infectious diseases and the expansion of public health services. The problems of refugees coming from China to Hong Kong covered two periods. The first period was in the late 1930s when many soldiers from the Nationalist army in China fled to Hong Kong during the Sino-Japanese War.

The second period was after World War II in the 1950s. In the immediate post-war period, many local residents who had fled Hong Kong because of the Japanese occupation had returned to Hong Kong. Overcrowding, poor environmental hygiene and sanitation, shortage of water supply and the spread of infectious diseases were the major public health problems at the time (see Figure 1.2).

The predominant infectious diseases were tuberculosis, cholera and common childhood infectious diseases, such as diphtheria, poliomyelitis, whooping cough and measles. The public health strategy adopted was to improve environmental hygiene, sanitation and water supply, and to develop maternal and child health services, which included, in particular, starting immunization campaigns.

This strategy was most effective, as reflected in the general improvement of the health of the population and the disappearance of many common childhood infectious diseases.

### Progress on controlling tuberculosis

Due to the development of better control measures, including anti-tuberculosis chemotherapy, BCG vaccination of newborn infants and the improved standards of living, the

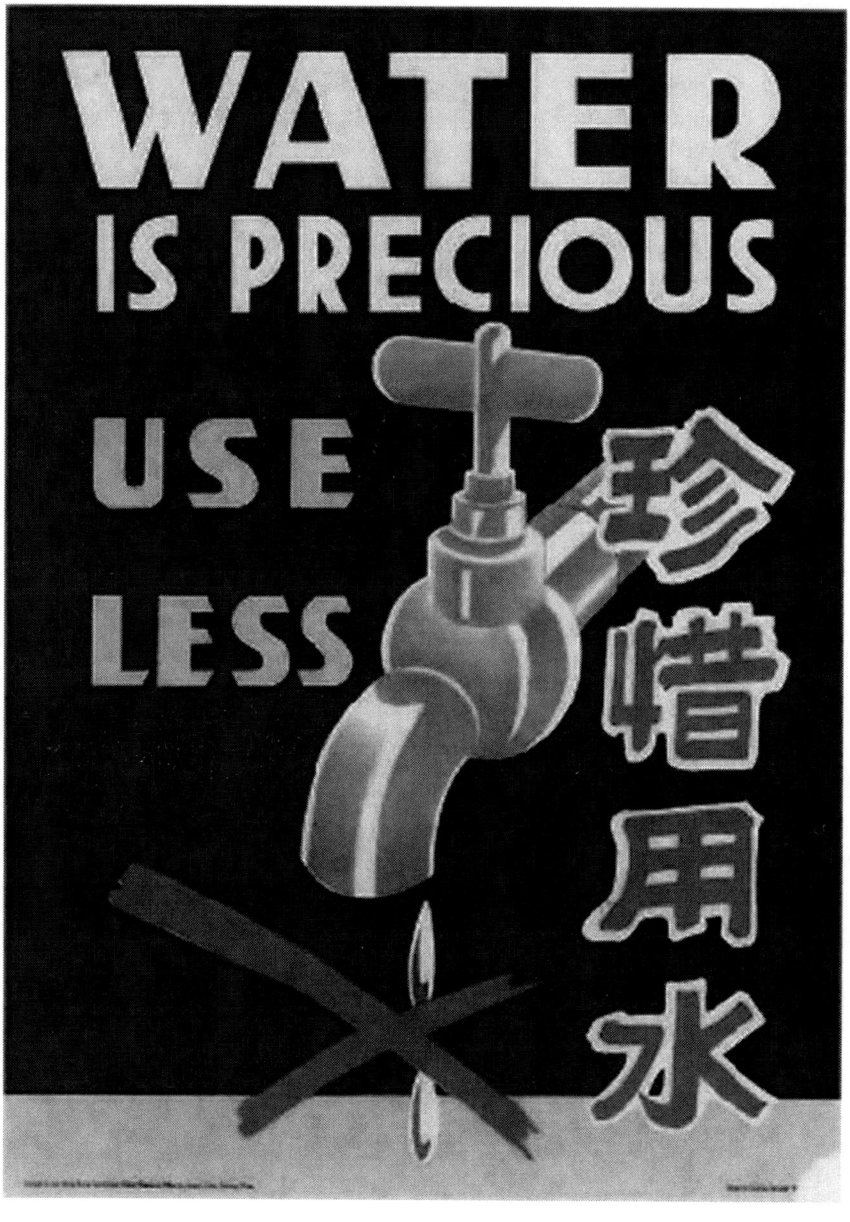


*Figure 1.2* 'Water is precious, use less' [2]

notification rate of tuberculosis in Hong Kong fell impressively after 1952. In 1952, when the incidence of the disease reached its peak, the notification rate was 697.2 per 100,000. In 2009, the rate was 74.1 per 100,000.

The fall in the notification rate was most significant during the 1950s and 1960s, but the decline was not so remarkable in the 1970s and 1980s. In terms of absolute numbers, the actual numbers of new cases has not changed very much in the last two decades, averaging about 6,000 to 8,000 notifications per year. The increase in population, particularly arising from the influx of refugees and immigrants from neighbouring areas in the past years, probably attributes to this steady figure. The death rates from tuberculosis also fell dramatically from 168.1 per 100,000 in 1952 to 2.9 in 2009.

The control and preventive measures against tuberculosis in Hong Kong consist of BCG vaccination, case finding, chemotherapy, bacteriology and research. The main achievements in the prevention and control of tuberculosis in Hong Kong are:

a. Reduction of incidence, prevalence and deaths from tuberculosis;
b. Reduction in the need for tuberculosis beds making beds available for other more urgent needs; and
c. Reduction in treatment time through the introduction of the Directly Observed Treatment Short-course (DOTS).

Despite Hong Kong's successful control of the disease, there is increasing evidence from many parts of the world that population movements and immigration from areas of high prevalence of tuberculosis to low prevalence areas can result in an increased number of cases. With an increasing movement of population from China to Hong Kong, this might result in an increase in the local tuberculosis problem as has been the case in the past. Furthermore, the tuberculosis problem has an added dimension because of its association with HIV infection and anti-TB drug resistance remains a grave concern (see Chapter 16).

For many years, a surveillance system has existed to monitor the epidemiology of the disease in Hong Kong more closely than in the past, and also to evaluate on a continuing basis the success of the service programme, particularly the efficacy of chemotherapy. Studies such as drug resistance surveys, evaluation of BCG vaccination at birth and new diagnostic methods of tuberculosis are areas that provide good opportunities for further development of tuberculosis control in future.

## Controlling cholera

The surveillance of cholera in Hong Kong is an integral part of the surveillance programme for diarrhoeal diseases. The programme comprises of:

a. A prompt reporting system consisting of a network of hospitals, clinics and laboratories in both the public and private sectors to report all laboratory suspected/confirmed cases of cholera to the health authorities;
b. An efficient laboratory service for hospitals and clinics to provide prompt diagnosis of cases of cholera;
c. Adequate facilities for the isolation and proper treatment of cases by a team of medical experts experienced in the clinical management of cholera;
d. Experienced public health personnel in the Regional Offices to undertake prompt investigation of cases of cholera and apply effective control measures to prevent the spread of infection, such as disinfection, surveillance of contacts and health education; and
e. Special surveillance measures, when indicated, e.g. for refugees and illegal immigrants entering the territory from an infected area, for persons at risk such as food and water sampling.

Like other diarrhoeal diseases, cholera is commonly transmitted by contaminated food or water. In 1854, a classical example of water transmitting cholera was the Broad Street Pump in London. In Hong Kong, a similar example was the Temple Street Well in Kowloon [3]. In the 1960s, there was severe shortage of water in Hong Kong and the supply of mains water was restricted to every fourth day for only four hours. A restaurant in Temple Street in Kowloon had illegally connected the water supply system from a well in the backyard of the restaurant to the mains water storage tank on the roof. The well water was originally used as flushing water for all toilets in the restaurant. Due to the illegal connection between the well water system and the mains water system, the drinking water in the restaurant was contaminated. A food handler incubating cholera used the toilet in the restaurant. This resulted in the occurrence of a water-borne outbreak of cholera. The affected customers all pointed to the restaurant and after closing the restaurant for disinfection, the outbreak stopped.

As far as Hong Kong is concerned, with a good health infrastructure for the detection, isolation and treatment of cases, and an efficient health organization in the application of control measures, there should be no cause for alarm. Past experience has shown that even though the disease has been introduced in to Hong Kong many times, due to adequate sewage disposal, safe water supply, health education and prompt action to contain the spread of the infection, cholera has never reached a level where it became a major public health threat in Hong Kong.

### *Phase 2 (1970s–1980s)*

During this time, chronic non-communicable diseases (NCDs) grew in importance as a public health threat, and treatment and rehabilitation services expanded. The main contributing factors included ageing of the population, changes in the socio-economic environment and changes in the lifestyles of the population.

More chronic diseases, accidents and injuries were encountered, and rising mental health problems put a heavy load on hospital and rehabilitation services. During this period, many new hospitals, specialist clinics and rehabilitation centres were opened, and old hospitals underwent reconstruction and expansion.

The introduction of new technologies also attracted attention in the allocation of resources. High priority was given to the development of secondary and tertiary levels of care and public health was relegated to low priority.

### Vietnamese boat people

During the 1970s, there was conflict between the Northern and the Southern parts of Vietnam. Many Vietnamese residents in the Southern part fled from their country from fear of the communist regime in the Northern part of Vietnam with its base at Hanoi.

When the Vietnamese refugees (known as Vietnamese boat people) first arrived near the Hong Kong territory, the boats were not allowed to enter pending the decision from the United Nations (UN) whether Hong Kong should be the 'first port of call' for the boat people from Vietnam. After confirmation was received, Hong Kong became the temporary home for thousands of Vietnamese boat people who arrived in Hong Kong by boats every day. A UN High Commissioner Office for Refugees (UNHCR) was established in Hong Kong to deal with many problems arising from the refugees.

One of the great fears that Hong Kong was facing was the risk of introduction of infectious diseases through the arrival of the boat people, in particular the threat of the plague as Vietnam was a hyper-endemic area for this disease. Thus, during the arrival of the first refugee ship, the Hong Kong government deployed a large number of members of the

Auxiliary Medical Services to undertake the screening of the boat people and the disinfection of their belongings.

### *Phase 3 (1990s–present)*

This period continues to see the increase in chronic diseases and also the emergence of new diseases, such as HIV/AIDS, H5N1 'avian flu' and 'SARS', as well as the resurgence of old diseases, such as tuberculosis and cholera. Healthcare reforms have also been on the political agenda.

## Development of medical and health services in Hong Kong

There has been a distinct difference in the development of medical and health services in Hong Kong in the period before and after World War II. When Hong Kong was a British territory, medical services for the public were provided by local charitable organizations, notably the Tung Wah Group of Hospitals and the Alice Ho Miu Ling Nethersole Hospital. The government's role at the time was only concerned with the provision of medical services for the military and naval personnel in the form of the British Military Hospital and the Royal Naval Hospital. Only in the first part of the twentieth century had the government begun to develop public hospitals, such as the Queen Mary Hospital (1937) and the Kowloon Hospital (1926).

After the end of World War II, the government fully took on the role of developing medical and health services for the public. A high-power Medical Development Advisory Committee (MDAC) was set up to be responsible for the development of medical and health facilities and health manpower development in Hong Kong.[3]

In 1989, the Department of Health was established. In the same year, the government also set up a working party to review primary health care and make recommendations for its future development. The working party's report formed the basis to expand health promotion and disease prevention as the most effective way of providing healthcare services.

The first step of healthcare reform in Hong Kong took place in April 1989. The former Medical and Health Department was split into two departments: the Department of Health, which was responsible for public health functions, and the Hospital Services Department that was temporarily set up to oversee the public hospital services pending the establishment of the Hospital Authority, which was the ultimate authority for the management of all public hospitals in Hong Kong, including government-owned hospitals and hospitals operated by non-government charitable organizations with financial subsidy from the government (subvented hospitals). In 1991, the Hospital Authority was formally established when its ordinance was enacted, and it took over the functions of the Hospital Services Department to manage all government and subvented hospitals.

The reason that this important step of healthcare reform took place was to improve the efficiency and effectiveness of operations of hospital services. From the 1970s to 1980s, government hospitals were facing heavy pressure – the wards were overcrowded, but on the other hand, there was under-utilization of beds in subvented hospitals. The morale of the hospital staff was low, and the terms of employment of the staff in government and subvented hospitals were different. The establishment of the Hospital Authority rectified all these unsatisfactory conditions and made significant improvements in the environments of all public hospitals, both former government hospitals and subvented hospitals. The Hospital Authority, unlike the Department of Health, is strictly not a government department, but the funding and policy guidance still comes from government. The Hospital Authority is still accountable to the Secretary for Food and Health but, being a non-government department, it has its flexibility to set out its vision, mission and core values to serve the public.

In 1998, the Hong Kong government invited an expert team in health economics from Harvard University to undertake a comprehensive review on the delivery of medical and health services in Hong Kong. The expert team produced a report entitled, *Improving Hong Kong's Health Care System. Why and for Whom?* [4]. The report pointed out that Hong Kong's healthcare system was too hospital based and too treatment oriented. There was compartmentalization in the provision of medical and healthcare services between the public sector and private sectors, and also between the Department of Health and the Hospital Authority. These problems undermined the effective delivery of healthcare services to meet the changing needs of the ageing population. The report also recommended setting up a medical savings account system to improve the methods of financing health care.

### *Savings account system*

Under this system, Hong Kong residents would be required to contribute to an individual saving account, called a 'MEDISAGE' account. Contributions to this account would be invested. Funds from the MEDISAGE would only be used to purchase an individual long-term care insurance policy upon retirement or disability. International experience indicates that contributions over the working life of an individual at the rate of 1 per cent of wages would suffice to pay for a single-premium insurance policy for long-term care at age 65. If a worker dies before they reach retirement age the accumulated fund in their MEDISAGE account would become part of their estate.

Following the Harvard expert team's review, there have been several healthcare reform consultation documents published by the Hong Kong government to seek the public's views on the future healthcare delivery services in Hong Kong. These include: *Lifelong Investment in Health* (2000), *Building a Healthy Tomorrow* (2005) and *Your Health, Your Life* (2008). Thus, the 1990s was a period of healthcare reform and a phase of public concern on the repeated occurrence of a number of major outbreaks of infectious diseases.

The major steps of healthcare reform as proposed by the most recent document *Your Health, Your Life* included:

a. Enhance primary care;
b. Promote public–private partnership on health care;
c. Develop electronic health record sharing;
d. Strengthen public healthcare safety net; and
e. Reform healthcare finance arrangements.

In the 2008–09 budget, the Hong Kong government reserved HK$50 billion to finance the implementation of healthcare reform. Although the road to healthcare reform is long and full of challenges, the government's commitment to share the responsibilities for healthcare reform together with the community is well demonstrated.

The healthcare system in Hong Kong in 2014 is a mixed system, consisting of both the public and private sectors. The main healthcare providers in the public sector are the Hospital Authority and the Department of Health. The Hospital Authority is responsible for the provision of hospital services, specialist clinics and general outpatient clinics, as well as rehabilitation, accident and emergency services, and the education and training of doctors, nurses and other healthcare personnel. The Department of Health is responsible for the regulation and implementation of policy, as well as the provision of maternal child health services and some clinical services, such as immunization, student health, women's health and elderly care. Under the Centre for Health Protection (CHP), it is responsible for population-wide health promotion and health education for the prevention and control of both infectious diseases and non-communicable diseases (NCDs).

Around 92 per cent of hospital beds in Hong Kong belong to the public sector, with the private sector responsible for providing the remaining 8 per cent. However, 70 per cent of primary care services are provided by general practitioners/family doctors in the private sector. The general outpatient clinics in the public sector only cover 15 per cent of the outpatient services, mainly providing care for elderly people and those with NCDs. The remaining 15 per cent is provided by Traditional Chinese Medicine (TCM) practitioners (see Chapter 41).

Much of the health care in Hong Kong is funded by the government. The healthcare policy in Hong Kong is to protect the health of the general population and to provide medical and healthcare services for the majority of the population who need subsidized care. The government has to ensure that no one is denied medical care because of lack of means.

Hong Kong's success in the development of medical and health services is owed not only to the commitment and support from the government, but also to the enormous contributions from charitable voluntary organizations and philanthropists, and tributes must be paid to them.[4]

Mention must also be made to the development of Chinese traditional medicine (see Chapter 41). In the nineteenth century, there was no legislation controlling the practice of Chinese traditional medicine. According to the Treaty of Nanjing, the culture and practice of the Chinese community had to be respected. As long as you are a Chinese, you would practise traditional Chinese medicine without the need for registration.

Before Hong Kong was returned to China, it had been discussed whether legislation should be introduced to regulate the practice of traditional Chinese medicine for the purpose of protecting people's health because several incidents of poisoning from the usage of Chinese herbal medicine had been reported. In 1989, the government set up a working party to review the practice of Traditional Chinese Medicine. In 1994, a report with recommendations to introduce legislation for the regulation of the practice of traditional Chinese medicine in Hong Kong was produced. In 1999, Chinese traditional medicine Ordinance Chapter 549 was passed, and a council on Chinese Traditional Medicine was established in the same year. There are now seventeen Traditional Chinese Medicine clinics set up by the Hospital Authority, and proper educational courses for the training of practitioners in Traditional Chinese Medicine have been established at the Baptist University, the University of Hong Kong and the Chinese University of Hong Kong.

## Establishing channels of communication with the Ministry of Health in mainland China

Every day, there are thousands of people crossing the border between Hong Kong and mainland China. As the spread of infectious diseases knows no geographical boundaries, the exchange of epidemiological information on infectious diseases with mainland China is essential in the surveillance and control of infectious diseases. With the assistance of the World Health Organization (WHO) and the support of the Health Minister in China,

Dr Chan Min Cheung, I was able to establish a platform whereby the health officials from mainland China, Hong Kong and Macau could have regular meetings, held on a rotation basis in Shenzhen, Hong Kong and Macau for the exchange of epidemiological information on the surveillance and control of infectious diseases.

In 1990, with the assistance of the Ministry of Health in China, I was able to secure support from the WHO for Hong Kong to host for the first time the Regional Committee Meeting of the WHO Western Pacific Regional Office. In 2009, Hong Kong hosted the sixtieth session of the WHO Regional Committee Meeting for the Western Pacific, the second time it has performed this role.

## Development of maternal and child health services in Hong Kong

The year 2012 was the eightieth anniversary of the development of maternal and child health services in Hong Kong. Early in the twentieth century, Hong Kong started to develop its maternal and child health as a priority to protect the health of the vulnerable group of the population: mothers and children.

Maternal and child health services covered two groups of people: women of childbearing age and children from birth to 5 years of age. The services included maternal health, ante-natal and post-natal care, child health, vaccination and family planning. The services were delivered at maternal and child health centres (MCHCs), which were well distributed throughout urban and rural areas in Hong Kong.

A typical MCHC usually consisted of a four-storey building with the general outpatient clinic on the ground floor, maternal and child health services on the first floor, a maternity home of twenty beds on the second floor and staff quarters on the third floor. The services were practically free and easily accessible.

In addition, the Hong Kong government operated a territory-wide screening programme in public and private hospitals for congenital hypothyroidism and gluces-6-phosphate dehydrogenase (G-6-PD) deficiency among newborn infants. A child assessment service was later developed to detect developmental abnormalities, such as hearing, vision and growth. A referral system to specialist clinics was also established to deal with any special problems. Because of the expansion of maternal and child health services, the services were later brought under the administration of the Family Health Services to reflect the wide range of services provided for mothers and children. For children older than 5 years, the Hong Kong government set up a Student Health Service to take care of the needs of school-age children.

The success of the development of maternal and child health services in Hong Kong could be reflected by the tremendous improvements in infant mortality rates and maternal mortality rates over the years. The infant mortality rate in 2009 was 1.7 per 1,000 registered live births. Both the maternal mortality and infant mortality rates are among the lowest in the world. The success in developing maternal and child health services in Hong Kong was mainly due to the following three factors:

1 *The services were easily accessible, practically free and well distributed throughout the territory.* Apart from the services being provided by the MCHCs, there was a home-visiting programme whereby health staff would visit the children's homes to provide services such as vaccination, especially for children living in outlying islands. If necessary, the health staff took advantage of the floating dispensary or the 'flying doctor helicopter' services to provide vaccination or primary care services to mothers and children living in the remote areas of the New Territories.

2 *The coverage of the vaccination programme for children under 5 years old is practically 100 per cent.* The common childhood infectious diseases, such as diphtheria, poliomyelitis, whooping cough and measles were either eradicated or brought under control.
3 *The dedicated health staff, including doctors and nurses in the MCHCs, who devoted their whole careers to working at the MCHCs.* The MCHC services in the early days had set up a Health Visitors School to train nurses to provide services such as counselling, health education, parents group discussions and even home visits for newborn babies. Their dedication and devotion have definitely contributed to the great success in developing maternal and child health services in Hong Kong.

## Development of public health in Hong Kong since its return to mainland China, 1997–2014

In 1997, signifying the end of colonial rule, Hong Kong was designated as the Hong Kong Special Administrative Region (HKSAR) and the Hong Kong government was addressed as the Government of the Hong Kong Special Administrative Region (the Government of HKSAR). Under the Basic Law, the HKSAR operates under the one-country, two-systems approach (see Chapter 3). In other words, Hong Kong continues its free market economy and mainland China continues its socialist system. Administratively, the Hong Kong SAR government will continue to have its own independent executive and legislative powers to administer the city.

Over the past seventeen years, the major developments in public health in Hong Kong have included:

1 *Controlling the emergence of new infectious diseases.* In 1997, the epidemic of avian influenza (H5N1) broke out in Hong Kong, lasting from May 1997 to January 1998. A total of eighteen human cases were reported and six died from the disease. The epidemic was brought under control by a large-scale culling of all chickens, including chickens from local farms and those imported from mainland China. The origin of the infection was from chickens and human cases occurred due largely to close contact with chickens, and were most prevalent in workers of chicken farms or markets. Although the epidemic was brought under control, individual human cases continued to be reported in some countries and areas in the Asia-Pacific region. The disease has now become endemic in this region.

Another new emerging infectious disease encountered was Severe Acute Respiratory Syndrome (SARS) in 2003 and the human swine influenza in 2009. In November 2002, there had been reports of an outbreak of unknown infectious disease in the neighbouring city of Guangzhou in mainland China, but details were not available to the Department of Health in Hong Kong. In February 2003, a visitor from Guangzhou came to Hong Kong. The visitor had been harbouring the infection before his arrival to Hong Kong, became ill after arrival and was admitted into a public hospital. This visitor was the primary source of spreading the infection, first in Hong Kong, and later to other cities in other parts of the world. The outbreak of SARS in Hong Kong affected 1,755 people and 300 died from the disease. About 20 per cent of the affected persons were medical and nursing staff working in hospital wards where the SARS patients were treated and six of them died due to the spread of infection. The outbreak of SARS not only impacted on the health of the population, but also had great social impact on the economic situation of the city. International tourism and public eating premises were severely affected as people were afraid of becoming infected and so stayed away from public places.

The first outbreak of human swine influenza H1N1 occurred in May 2009 when a traveller from Mexico (where the first human case was reported) came to Hong Kong. When he arrived, he had symptoms of influenza and was admitted into hospital. Laboratory investigation confirmed that he was suffering from swine influenza H1N1. The hotel where the patient stayed was isolated and all the residents and staff in that hotel were put in quarantine. At that time, the WHO announced a global warning of human swine influenza because the disease had also been reported in other countries. Later when the disease was found to have spread to other areas in Hong Kong, particularly schools, the contingency plan was changed, from an emerging outbreak containment phase to an outbreak containing phase. The quarantine measures for the hotel residents were lifted and the control was concentrated on keeping the patients at home, treating affected persons on an outpatient basis, encouraging the practice of personal hygiene and, later, the introduction of a vaccine against the human swine influenza for high risk groups, such as the elderly, chronically ill, the very young and healthcare workers.

2 *Expansion of public health services against infectious diseases.* Although SARS caused Hong Kong a great deal of human and economic loss, it also allowed it to turn threat into opportunity. After the SARS epidemic, as early as in April 2004, the Hong Kong government established the Centre for Health Protection (CHP), with the special function of dealing with the prevention and control of infectious diseases. The CHP established close collaboration with the Health Protection Agency in Colindale, London, particularly in the areas of training staff in disease control and surveillance. At the same time, the government of Hong Kong implemented the recommendations contained in the report of the Expert Committee on SARS [5] in the areas of collaboration, communication and coordination with local professionals, community and health authorities in mainland China, as well as in the area of surge capacity for infectious disease control in hospitals, laboratory facilities, and in education and training of public health workers (see Figure 1.3).

3 *Development of Schools of Public Health.* The first purposely designed School of Public Health in Hong Kong was opened at the Medical Faculty of the Chinese University of Hong Kong in 2001. The school provides a full range of postgraduate and Master's degree courses in various areas of public health. The school has attracted many overseas students from mainland China and other countries. In 2009, the first Bachelor degree course in public health was launched, attracting a large number of undergraduate students. In 2008, the functions of the School of Public Health were further expanded to include primary care and the school now has the double function of being a School of Public Health and Primary Care.

The Li Ka Shing Faculty of Medicine of the University of Hong Kong established its School of Public Health in 2009. Both schools of public health play a very important role in the education and training of public health workers and in research.

4 *Medical education conferences across the Straits, including Hong Kong.* The first medical education conference involving the universities and medical schools in China, Taiwan and Hong Kong was held in China in 1996. This was the first initiative of the universities and medical schools in these countries to establish close collaboration, cooperation and communication concerning medical education of students in these areas. There is common agreement among the educators from these areas for the need to strengthen the methods of teaching and education for medical students so they will be capable and

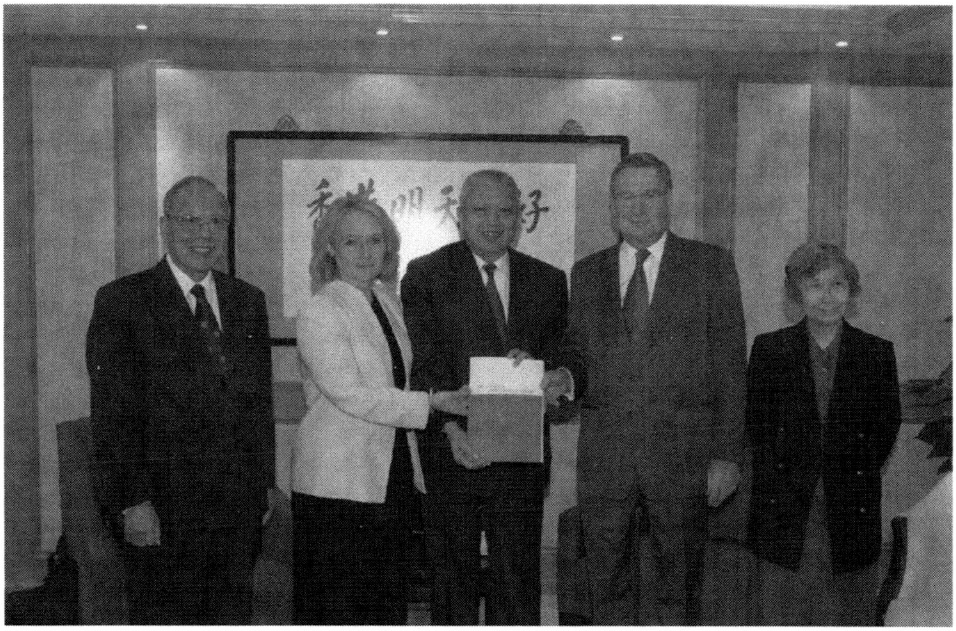

*Figure 1.3* SARS Expert Committee Report [5]

competent to meet the changing needs, and face the new challenges, in health care in this region.

Since 1996, similar conferences have been held on a rotation basis in China, Taiwan and Hong Kong on an annual or biennial basis. Up until 2012, thirteen medical education conferences had been held.

5 *Establishment of the World Association of Chinese Public Health Professionals.* In 2004, following the SARS epidemic, the World Association of Chinese Public Health Professionals was established in Hong Kong. The objective of establishing such a professional association among ethnic Chinese from different parts of the world was to establish a platform where they could share each other's experiences in public health and establish channels of communication. Many ethnic Chinese public health professionals are working in various capacities, such as in government, academic institutes and research institutes. Traditionally, the Chinese community has its own traditional beliefs and behaviours in health. It was thus a good opportunity to establish this platform of cooperation and communication among the Chinese public health professionals from different parts of the world. I am the founding President of the Association and there are three Vice-Presidents from China, Macau and the United States. The council members of the Association come from different parts of world including Canada, the United States, Europe, Australia, Taiwan and Singapore. Biennial conferences are held on a rotation basis in China and Hong Kong.

6 *Establishing closer collaboration with the World Health Organization (WHO).* Since Hong Kong's return to China, there has been much closer collaboration with the WHO. The health officials in Hong Kong are now part of the Chinese delegation attending the WHO Regional meetings in Manila and the WHO General Assembly in Geneva. In 2009, Hong Kong was the host of the WHO Regional Meeting for the Western Pacific. In 2007,

Dr Margaret Chan, former Director of Health in Hong Kong, became the Director General (DG) of the WHO in Geneva. In 2012, much to the delight and pride of the healthcare professionals in Hong Kong, Dr Margaret Chan was given another term of appointment as DG of WHO for a further five years.

7 *Healthy settings.* Since 1998, Hong Kong started a series of settings-based approaches to health promotion projects. This means carrying out health promotion activities in places where people live, work or study. The settings include schools, cities, workplaces, hospitals and university campuses. The projects are known as healthy schools, healthy cities, healthy and safe workplaces, healthy housing estates, healthy hospitals and health promoting universities. In all these activities, the spirit of partnership involving government, community, private sector, non-government organizations, families and individuals in all efforts to promote healthy lifestyles and behaviours, and improve the physical and social environment for health, is greatly emphasized. Currently, all eighteen districts in Hong Kong have established Steering Committees on Healthy Cities involving the community to promote community health. In 2004, Hong Kong joined the alliance for healthy cities in the Asia-Pacific region and, in 2007, it was the host of the first Asia-Pacific Region Conference on Healthy Universities held at the Chinese University of Hong Kong.

## Achievements of public health in Hong Kong

To summarize, Hong Kong's achievements in public health over the past two centuries covered four major areas:

1 From a single determinant of health to total determinants of health;
2 From a barren island to an international city;
3 From local public health to regional and global public health; and
4 From solely a government-led administration in public health to community mobilization at different levels in public health, such as healthy cities, healthy schools, healthy workplace, health promoting university, and healthy and safe housing estates.

## Lessons learnt

In assessing the history of public health in Hong Kong over the past two centuries, we have learnt several lessons. First, we are seeing the emergence of a number of outbreaks of new infectious diseases. Second, with the changes in lifestyles and behaviours, many socially related public health problems, such as smoking, drug abuse, obesity and mental stress, arise because of political and socio-economic factors. Third, with the ageing of the population, chronic NCDs have become the leading causes of death and ill-health in Hong Kong. With the rising cost in health care, NCDs put a heavy burden on medical and health care, and the healthcare system is under severe strain. To summarize, Hong Kong is at present facing a complex burden of diseases, including infectious diseases both new and old, chronic NCDs, mental health, and accidents and injuries.

## Future directions for public health in Hong Kong

The future directions for public health in Hong Kong should focus on the following priorities:

- More emphasis on health promotion and disease prevention;
- Developing a new approach – physical, psycho-social aspects of health;
- Take into account the total determinants of health, including economic, political and social factors;
- Multi-sectoral and multidisciplinary approaches;
- Both patient-based and community-oriented care; and
- Develop linkages with mainland China.

There should also be a recognition of the impact of globalization on public health, the need for education and training of public health professionals, the importance of research, and the necessity of building partnerships for health at national, regional and international levels (see Figure 1.4).

In view of the movement of population and the increase in volume of trade in the Pearl River Delta Region, Hong Kong can play an important role in linking the cities and areas in this region to work together to achieve the objective of 'Health for All and All for Health'.

## Acknowledgements

The contents of this chapter apart from the personal contributions of the writer himself come from a good variety of sources including annual departmental reports of the former Medical and Health Department, the Department of Health, the Hospital Authority, and other publications of professional bodies and organizations.

The chapter also contains valuable historical photographs, including from the Hong Kong Medical Science Museum. The writer would like to express his personal gratitude to all the

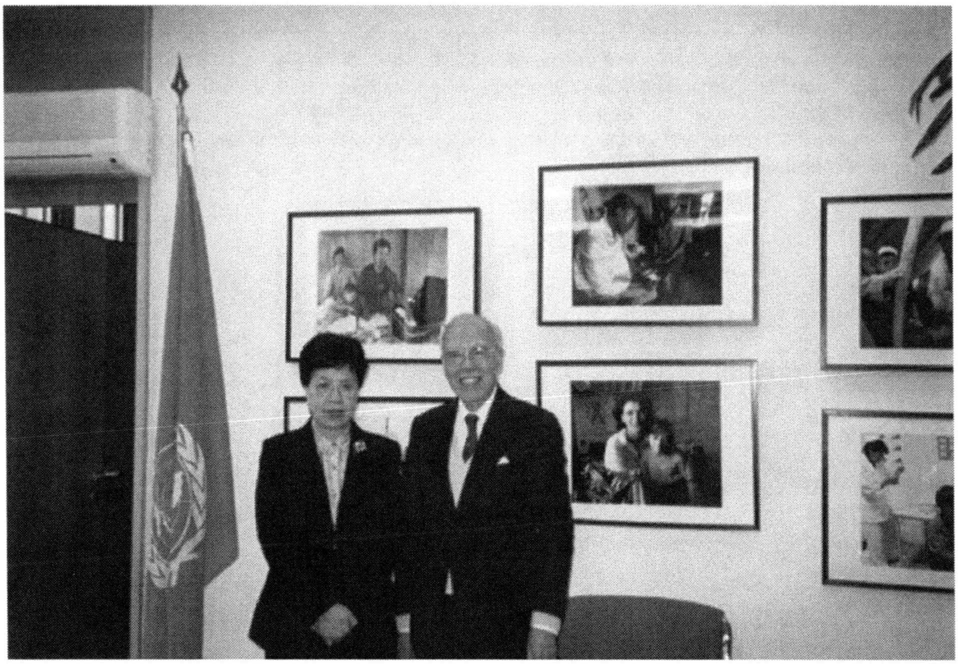

*Figure 1.4* WHO Head Office, Geneva 2007 – the author with DG Dr M. Chan [author]

contributors. All these contributions have greatly enhanced the value of this chapter on the historical perspectives of public health in Hong Kong.

Public health is a science and art of promoting health, preventing disease and prolonging life through the organized efforts of society. The achievements of public health in Hong Kong over the past owed a great deal to the contributions from the healthcare professionals, the community and the government. Tributes should be paid to all of them for their dedication and devotion in improving the health of the population in Hong Kong.

## Notes

1 Sadly Professor Lee died from a stroke in January 2014. Active to the last, he will be sorely missed for his energy and inspiration to all in public health.

2 In July 1979, I submitted a 'Declaration of Hong Kong Free from Smallpox' to the WHO; the last case of smallpox was reported in 1959.

3 I served as the Secretary of MDAC and was personally involved in the development of many hospitals and clinics in Hong Kong.

4 I would like to mention a philanthropist, Sir Shiu-kin Tang, as an example. Sir Shiu-kin Tang made generous donations to the government by building a hospital, specialist clinic and dental centre at Morrison Hill in Queen's Road, East. His contributions were not confined to medical services, as schools and welfare centres were also built with his generous donations. I assisted him in developing the medical facilities at Morrison Hill. After his death, the government named a lane in Morrison Hill, 'Shiu Kin Lane', in recognition of his generosity and tremendous contribution to medical, educational and welfare services in Hong Kong.

## References


1. Historical pictures from Hong Kong Museum of Medical Sciences Society.
2. Lee, S. H. *Prevention and Control of Communicable Diseases in Hong Kong*. Government Printer, Hong Kong, 1994.
3. Van de Linde, P. A. M, Forbes, G. I. Observations on the Spread of Cholera in Hong Kong, 1961–1963. *Bulletin of the World Health Organization* 1965; 32(4).
4. Harvard Team. *Improving Hong Kong's Health Care System: Why and for Whom?* Health and Welfare Bureau of the Government of Hong Kong SAR Government, 1999.
5. SARS Expert Committee. *SARS in Hong Kong: From Experience to Action*. Report of the SARS Expert Committee, October 2003.

# Introduction to Part I.2: introductory concepts

*Siân M. Griffiths*

## Setting the scene

Professor Lee's account of the developments in public health in Hong Kong traces the transitional changes from a barren island to global financial centre. He emphasizes the need to understand, and act on, one of the underlying themes that emerge from the contributions to this book, that of the interrelationship between poverty and health. The Millennium Development Goals (MDGs), a global strategy to eliminate world poverty, demonstrate the shared consensus of the unacceptability of poverty and disadvantage, and the need to achieve equity and greater opportunity for the 20.6 per cent of the world's population still living on less than US$1.25 a day. Improving public health is a key component of the MDGs – both directly, in the aspirations to improve child health and maternal health and combat HIV/AIDS, and also indirectly through strategies for raising educational standards, promoting gender equality and seeking environmental sustainability.

In Chapter 2, Junko Yasuoka and colleagues review the establishment of the Millennium goals and the progress made towards their achievement in Southeast Asia. We know from the work of the Commission on Social Determinants that the conditions in which we work, live and play contribute to our health, and if we are to achieve greater equity, especially for poorer countries, we need to ensure that the social determinants that influence our health are taken into account by both policy makers and by healthcare providers. The MDGs are both directly and indirectly related to health. Whilst ensuring better health care for pregnant women will contribute to improving maternal health so too will ensuring higher literacy rates amongst women. Laos is one of the poorest countries in Asia and Yasuoka *et al.* use it as a case study for examining progress made towards the MDGs. Their analysis highlights the complexity of comparisons of on- and off-track progress, which can obscure where progress has been made. They argue that, overall, the MDGs have been useful and have succeeded in improvement although analysis in East Asia shows that progress is patchy. For example, one of the major determinants of a mother's survival is whether or not the birth is attended by a skilled health professional, and Bhutan has made significant progress by increasing the skilled birth attendance rate by nearly 60 per cent (from 14.9 per cent in 1994 to 71.4 per cent in 2007). However, when it comes to access to antenatal care, another major determinant of a mother's survival, in each of the four countries (Afghanistan, Bangladesh, Lao PDR and Nepal) with the highest estimated maternal mortality ratio (MMR ≥ 300), skilled health professionals attend less than one in four births, and less than two in three births among expectant mothers who have received antenatal care at least once. Despite the failures of progress and the limitations of the MDGs, the authors argue that the MDGs have served effectively as a tool to generate discussion, focus attention and help assign accountability for leaders' pledges, and encouraged global political consensus and have acted as a focus for advocacy. However, in their critique they also point to the important lessons learnt which need to be translated into policies and targets in the post-MDG era, for example those promulgated by the UN System Task Team on the Post-2015 UN Development Agenda [1, 2, 3]. The Task Team outlines a vision for the post-2015 development agenda suggesting key dimensions of inclusive economic and social development, environmental sustainability, and peace and security.

In Chapter 3, Fong and Mou describe migration in terms of push and pull factors. The increase in migration from rural to urban areas within China has been due both to the push factors related to rural poverty, and the pull factors of better economic opportunities and quality of life achievable in the sprawling urban conurbations surrounding the urban and industrializing zones. Including migrants working within the same administrative regions but in different counties, there are approximately 200 million migrants in China, creating significant public health challenges. Discussing these challenges using the lens of public health practice in the domains of health protection, health services and health improvement, it is clear from the literature that whilst some migrant groups are at risk of socio-economic disadvantage and poorer health, others – including their families left behind – benefit from their improved economic circumstances. The overall picture is complex, dynamic and challenging for authorities providing services both in areas of inward movement and in areas where older people and children are left behind. The sheer scale of migration within China, particularly in areas such as the Pearl River Delta, requires new solutions including insurance systems to increase access and building programmes to provide Community Health Clinics to enable locally based care.

Not only are there direct employment-related health risks due to the environment in which many migrants work, but there is also lifestyle-related morbidity including mental health needs. And whilst many young people in China are moving where the work is, the population is rapidly ageing. By 2050, one-third of the population will be over 60 and for every hundred people aged 20 to 64, there will be forty-five people aged over 65, compared with about fifteen in 2010.

Japan has also faced the demographic challenges of an ageing society. As of 2010, the population of Japan was 128.06 million of which 23.1 per cent (29.29 million) were elderly (over 65 years of age). Japan has the world's highest elderly population and in their case study in Chapter 4, Hokama and Cash describe the responses by the Japanese government and by Japanese society to this growing issue. In order to effectively manage Japan's ageing population, the Japanese government has developed policies to combat the financial and social issues surrounding elderly care. Since the numbers of elderly will continue to grow, not only are there positive incentives to increase the fertility rate but also efforts to ensure a healthier old age with individualized care plans based on individual needs.

Another country with a burgeoning population is India, just overtaking China as the world's most populous country. Reddy and Mathur's analysis in Chapter 5 is that the present health profile of India reflects the mixed effects of multiple transitions (demographic, nutritional and epidemiologic) superimposed on an uneven economic development, an under-resourced health system and inadequate multi-sectoral action on the determinants of health. There are wide-ranging disparities in health indicators and India's health indicators lag behind other emerging economies such as China and Sri Lanka. The infant mortality rate (IMR) in India is three times higher than in China and four times higher than in Sri Lanka and Thailand, and 42 per cent of children under 5 years of age are undernourished, whilst 14 per cent of urban adolescents (15 million) are reported to be overweight or obese. Infectious diseases such as tuberculosis, malaria and HIV/AIDS remain major public health challenges, and at the same time non-communicable diseases (NCDs) are now the leading causes of death and disability. Clean drinking water is available only to 68.2 per cent of the people, while 53 per cent still practise open defecation in the absence of domestic toilets. Poverty, limited education and lack of women's empowerment are barriers to health, most visible in the northern and central Indian states. Reddy and Mathur describe the health system as being burdened with multiple handicaps as it faces the concomitant challenges posed by the diseases of underdevelopment and the disorders of maladapted modernity. With only 1.04 per cent of the GDP being spent on health, among the lowest in the world, the system is ready for the current reform process which not only focuses on acceptable and affordable development of universal health care but also on the creation of a public health cadre with a defined career pathway at both centre and state levels.

And whilst population demography and the distribution of disease are changing, science continues to advance and new paradigms of treatment are emerging. In his chapter on genomics and public health, Özdemir highlights the impact of 'Big Data', massive availability of information especially from genomics, and the move from a science where data collection was an essential locus of the scientific endeavour to one where data collection is automated or at least made easier and is available in digital form. He argues that the perspective of public health genetics requires us to seek new collaborative possibilities that emerge with genomics so that rather than viewing populations as a homogenous entity, public health genomics firmly recognizes the previous silent heterogeneity in population substructure. The rapid proliferation of genomics tests will impact on public health practice and as the possibilities of personalized medicine expand, public health practitioners will need to be mindful of and responsive to individual differences in the population. A population perspective will be required to optimize new genome-based technologies to improve health, focusing on prevention, the application of evidence-based multidisciplinary science and for consideration of the ethical, legal and social implications, including addressing health disparities.

The field of genomics represents the importance of research for future health and health care. In their chapter, Allotey and colleagues discuss the current state of public health research in Asia. They highlight that an important aspect of research capacity relates to the funding available. Although several countries across the region have made commitments to support health research, very few have the formal infrastructure, such as national research councils, to promote or support local investigator-driven research. The status of epidemiology and capacity in the region is mixed. The majority of publications (in English-language peer-reviewed journals) on public health research are generated from institutions and researchers in China, India, Thailand, Singapore and Bangladesh. There are gaps, for example, in the evidence base for policy – and not all countries have a strong social science input into public health research or technical expertise for advocacy. In general, the approach at the national and professional levels remains largely clinical in focus and is disease driven, although some countries, such as Thailand, consistently include the need for social justice and access for the poor in their public health research.

The need to strengthen the academic base of public health in Asia underpins Chapter 8 by Evans and Ahmed, which highlights that like many other regions in the world, Asia is facing severe shortages, skews in skill-mix and an inequitable distribution of health workers be they clinical or public health professionals. Public health education, they argue, has for too long been considered a sub-specialization of clinical medicine as opposed to a field in and of itself that requires full-time professionals in its own right, as well as making a critical contribution to the training of clinical health professionals. Faculty development is thus a critical but missing part of the public health education development agenda. The institutional landscape of educational institutions responsible for the training of public health workers in the Asian region, as in many other parts of the world, reflects the absence of clear policies and strategies for development of the public health workforce. Thus, despite the encouraging growth in the number of public health institutions in the Asian region, such as those discussed in Chapter 5, there are still many countries with a vastly inadequate institutional infrastructure relative to need, although in some places innovative ways of sourcing faculty are being found, for example by creating part-time or visiting appointments, recruitment of 'greying' professionals who have more time and interest in teaching, and accessing pedagogic resources online.

## References


1. United Nations. *Millennium Development Goals and post-2015 Development Agenda.* [Online]. Available from: http://www.un.org/en/ecosoc/about/mdg.shtml/.
2. United Nations. *We Can End Poverty 2015. MDGs Overview.* [Online]. Available from: http://www.un.org/millenniumgoals/beyond2015.shtml.
3. United Nations. Development, Policy and Analysis Division. *Preparing for the Development Agenda beyond 2015.* [Online]. Available from: http://www.un.org/en/development/desa/policy/untaskteam_undf/index.shtml.

# 2

# Achieving the Millennium Development Goals

## Relevance for low-income countries in Asia

*Junko Yasuoka, Junko Saito, Yu Mon Saw, Bruno F. Sunguya, Rachel M. Amiya and Masamine Jimba*

## Introduction

Years of debate, effort and struggle went into setting specific goals to promote the economic and social development of the world's poorest countries. Antecedents of the development framework that ultimately emerged between 2000 and 2001 can be traced back to the Universal Declaration of Human Rights in 1948, the Development Decade of the 1960s and several United Nations (UN) summits held in the second half of the twentieth century [1].

At the Millennium Summit in 2000, 189 countries, represented by 147 heads of state and government, ratified the Millennium Declaration. Six fundamental values were presented to guide international relations in the twenty-first century: freedom, equality, solidarity, tolerance, respect for nature and shared responsibility. Seven key objectives were further identified to translate these values into action: peace, security and disarmament; development and poverty eradication; protection of our common environment; human rights, democracy and good governance; protection of vulnerable people; meeting of the special needs of Africa; and strengthening of the UN [2, 3].

To follow up the Millennium Declaration, the UN secretariat consulted its members, representatives of the World Bank, the International Monetary Fund (IMF), and the Organization for Economic Cooperation and Development (OECD). The resulting roadmap was contained in the September 2001 Report of the Secretary-General to the UN General Assembly. In 2001, the conceptual content of the Millennium Declaration was translated into eight Millennium Development Goals (MDGs). All the UN member states and at least 23 other international organizations have since agreed to achieve these goals by the year 2015.

The MDGs are framed as follows:

1 Increasing incomes and reducing hunger;
2 Achieving universal primary education;
3 Eliminating gender inequality;
4 Reducing child mortality rates;

| Millennium Development Goals | |
|---|---|
| *Goal 1*<br>Eradicate extreme poverty and hunger | *Goal 2*<br>Achieve universal primary education |
| *Goal 3*<br>Promote gender equality and empower women | *Goal 4*<br>Reduce child mortality |
| *Goal 5*<br>Improve maternal health | *Goal 6*<br>Combat HIV/AIDS, malaria and other diseases |
| *Goal 7*<br>Ensure environmental sustainability | *Goal 8*<br>Global partnership for development |

*Figure 2.1* The eight Millennium Development Goals (MDGs)

5 Improving maternal health;
6 Reversing the spread of HIV/AIDS, tuberculosis, and malaria;
7 Reversing the loss of natural resources and biodiversity, and improving access to water, sanitation, and good housing; and
8 Establishing effective global partnerships [4] (see Figure 2.1).

Building upon this core agenda, several new targets have subsequently been added, including those arising from the World Summit in 2005. For example, a target of 'achieving universal access to reproductive health' was added. This target was excluded during the initial negotiation of the MDGs but eventually integrated into MDG 5 due to the efforts of the UN Population Fund (UNFPA) and several non-governmental organizations (NGOs) working in family planning and reproductive health [4–6].

This chapter provides an overview of the progress and challenges that low-income countries are facing to achieve the MDGs. First, we look at a case study from the Lao People's Democratic Republic (Lao PDR), which elucidates the meaning of being 'on track' or 'off track' in terms of achieving the MDGs. Then, we present a summary of the progress in achieving the MDGs in the South, East and Southeast Asian regions. Following this, we review the challenges experienced in these, and other, regions in working towards the MDGs and, finally, we propose a way forward as a post-2015 development agenda.

## Gauging progress on the MDGs: off track, but not derailed, in Lao PDR

Since the MDGs were first established, great efforts have been made in many low- and middle-income countries to achieve the targets set. Lao PDR is no exception. However, this landlocked nation in mainland Southeast Asia has shown the least overall progress amongst the 13 countries in the South, East and Southeast Asian regions defined as low-income economies by the World Bank in 2000. In Lao PDR, 13 out of 22 targets were defined as being 'off-track' in 2011 (see Table 2.1), although being off track did not mean an utter lack of developmental progress.

*Table 2.1* MDG progress in South, East and Southeast Asian countries

| *Goal* | | *1* | | *2* | | | *3* | | | *4* | | *5* | | | *6* | | | *7* | | | | | |
|---|---|---|---|---|---|---|---|---|---|---|---|---|---|---|---|---|---|---|---|---|---|---|---|
| | | *$1.25 per day poverty* | *Underweight children* | *Primary enrolment* | *Reaching last grade* | *Primary completion* | *Gender primary* | *Gender secondary* | *Gender tertiary* | *Under-5 mortality* | *Infant mortality* | *Maternal mortality* | *Skilled birth attendance* | *Antenatal care (≥ 1 visit)* | *HIV prevalence* | *TB incidence* | *TB prevalence* | *Forest cover* | *Protected area* | *$CO_2$ emissions* | *ODP substance consumption* | *Safe drinking water* | *Basic sanitation* |
| East Asia | DPR Korea | | ▶ | | | | | | | ■ | ■ | ■ | ● | ● | | ◀ | ● | ◀ | ● | ● | ● | ● | ◀ |
| | Mongolia | ■ | ● | ● | ■ | ▶ | ● | ● | ● | ● | ▶ | ■ | ● | ● | ▶ | ● | ● | ◀ | ● | ◀ | ● | ▶ | ■ |
| Southeast Asia | Cambodia | ▶ | ▶ | ■ | ◀ | ▶ | ▶ | ▶ | ■ | ■ | ■ | ■ | ■ | ■ | ● | ● | ● | ◀ | ● | ◀ | ● | ▶ | ■ |
| | Indonesia | ● | ■ | ● | ■ | ● | ● | ● | ● | ▶ | ■ | ■ | ▶ | ▶ | ◀ | ▶ | ● | ◀ | ● | ◀ | ● | ■ | ■ |
| | Lao PDR | ▶ | ■ | ■ | ■ | ■ | ▶ | ■ | ▶ | ▶ | ■ | ■ | ■ | ■ | ◀ | ◀ | ● | ◀ | ● | ◀ | ● | ■ | ▶ |
| | Myanmar | | ■ | | ■ | ● | ● | ● | | ■ | ■ | ■ | ■ | ■ | ● | ▶ | ● | ◀ | ● | ◀ | ● | ■ | ● |
| | Viet Nam | ● | ▶ | | ▶ | | | | | ■ | ■ | ▶ | ▶ | ▶ | ● | ● | ● | ● | ● | ◀ | ● | ● | ● |
| South Asia | Afghanistan | | ▶ | | | | ■ | ◀ | ◀ | ■ | ■ | ■ | ■ | ■ | | ▶ | ● | ▶ | ▶ | ◀ | ● | ▶ | ■ |
| | Bangladesh | ■ | ▶ | ◀ | ■ | ◀ | ● | ● | ■ | ▶ | ▶ | ■ | ■ | ■ | ▶ | ▶ | ● | ◀ | ● | ◀ | ● | ■ | ■ |
| | Bhutan | | ■ | ■ | ■ | ▶ | ● | ● | ■ | ▶ | ■ | ● | ▶ | ▶ | ◀ | ● | ● | ● | ● | ◀ | ● | ■ | ■ |
| | India | ■ | ■ | ● | ■ | ▶ | ● | ▶ | ■ | ■ | ■ | ■ | ■ | ■ | ● | ▶ | ◀ | ● | ● | ◀ | ● | ● | ■ |
| | Nepal | ■ | ■ | | ■ | ■ | ▶ | ▶ | ■ | ▶ | ■ | ■ | ■ | ■ | ● | ▶ | ◀ | ◀ | ● | ● | ● | ● | ■ |
| | Pakistan | ● | ■ | ■ | ◀ | ■ | ▶ | ▶ | ■ | ■ | ■ | ■ | ■ | ■ | ◀ | ▶ | ● | ◀ | ▶ | ◀ | ● | ■ | ■ |

● Early achiever ▶ On track ■ Slow ◀ Regressing/no progress

*Source*: [39].

Lao PDR is one of the poorest countries in Southeast Asia, with an estimated population of 5.9 million. The country has a low population density and 71 per cent live in rural areas (see Figure 2.2). It is ethnically diverse and ethnic minorities live primarily in the highlands, where health services are sparse and the road infrastructure is poor [7]. The national health system is underfunded and private health expenditure made up nearly 70 per cent of the total health expenditure in 2010 [8]. Some of the many challenges faced by Lao PDR, in common with other low- and middle-income countries, are a lack of human resources, very low utilization rates for health facilities and limited skills among health professionals [9, 10].

Lao PDR is indeed 'off track' on many of the health-related MDGs, but this does not mean the country has failed in its pursuit of health development. For example, the maternal

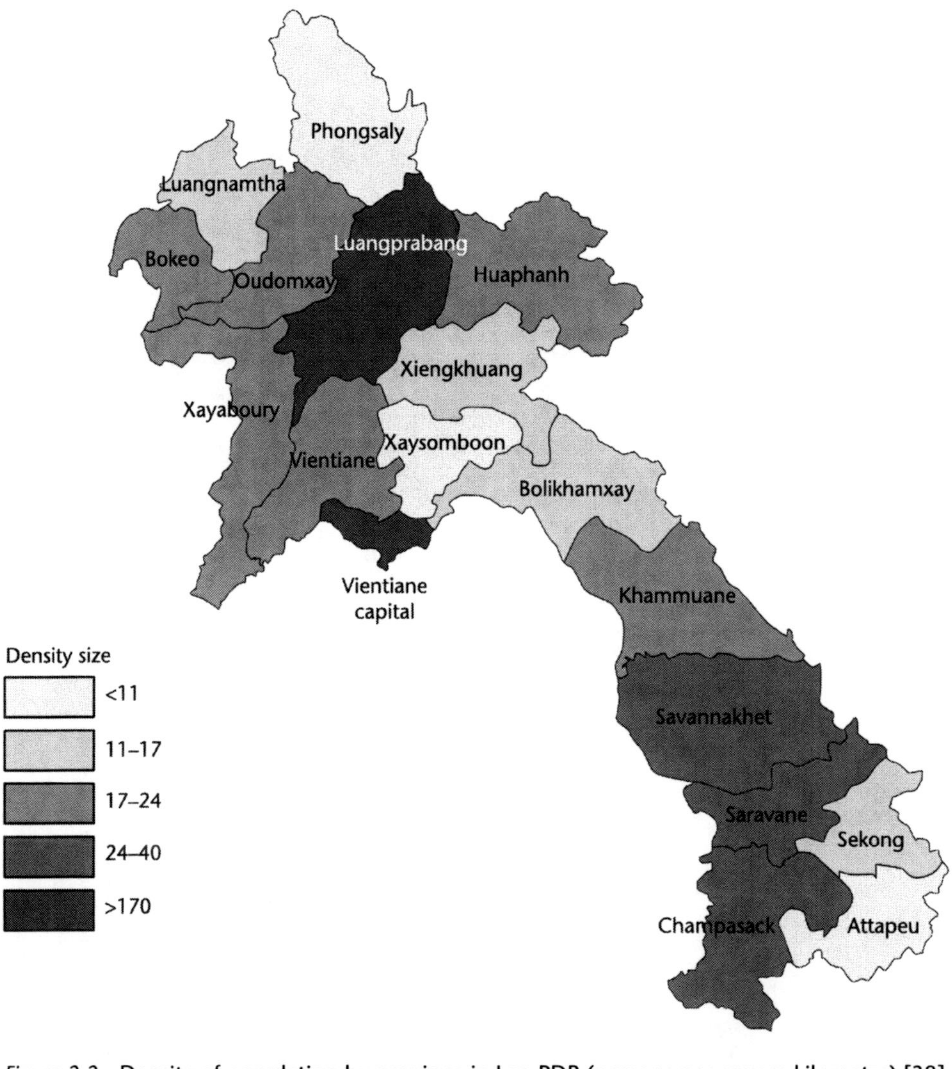


*Figure 2.2* Density of population by province in Lao PDR (persons per square kilometre) [38]

mortality ratio (MMR, deaths per 100,000 live births) dropped from 1,200 to 580 in the period between 1990 and 2008. Despite this progress, Lao PDR has been labelled as exhibiting insufficient progress towards achieving MDG 5. Meanwhile, Vietnam, designated as the best performing country for MMR reduction in the region, has been widely applauded for being 'on track', with a fall in death rates from 170 in 1990 to 56 in 2008. Thus, whilst Lao PDR showed a 51.7 per cent MMR reduction, Vietnam showed a 67 per cent reduction, and this relatively small difference defines the dividing line for 'on track' versus 'off track' status between the two countries. In the context of evaluating progress towards the MDGs, this dichotomy is somehow considered reasonable.

In addition, some of the 'one-size-fits-all' indicators simply do not fit Lao PDR [11], as demonstrated by the HIV/AIDS-related target delineated in MDG 6. Lao PDR has been labelled as a country making no progress, or even regressing, on this front. Such a poor result is, however, a reflection of a slight increasing trend in low-level HIV prevalence (from 0.1 per cent in 2001 to 0.2 per cent in 2009) among the population aged 15 to 49 years since 2001. Because of this low general prevalence, MDG 6 is not included among the six priority areas in the national strategies of Lao PDR to accelerate MDG achievement. Instead, the national target for 2015, distinct from the MDG targets, is to maintain the national HIV prevalence at less than 1 per cent [9, 12]. In this regard, the lens of the MDGs, meaningful as it may be in context, is distorting. Thus the measurement of progress should be seen within the context of the national agenda and efforts must be made to understand the gap that exists between the MDGs and the unique, tailor-made targets set by national governments.

Similarly, some international programmes related to the MDGs are donor-driven and do not always match the priorities set by a given country. The Global Fund, for example, has strongly supported reducing communicable diseases as a key objective, while Lao PDR has prioritized maternal and child health [13]. Aid agencies tend to focus on predetermined agendas designed to show swift impacts. Such strategies, however, do not always lead to sustainable outcomes, as they have typically been enacted through programmes running parallel to, rather than integrated into, the existing healthcare systems [6, 14]. In Lao PDR, for example, the HIV and TB programmes generally remain vertical and mostly weakly integrated with the general health system, such as in the separate financing, governance and planning functions for these programmes [13]. Further progress will depend largely on developing medium-term and long-term strategies that pay more attention to the development of health systems [6].

Despite being labelled as an 'off-track' country, Lao PDR has been successful in achieving several of the health-related MDGs, albeit in a qualified manner. For example, the country is 'on track' for achieving the target for reducing child mortality, but the rate achieved (54 per 1,000 live births in 2010) remains exceptionally high relative to other neighbouring middle-income countries in the region, such as Thailand and Vietnam. Moreover, both skilled birth attendance and immunization coverage rates – indicators considered key to strategies aimed at accelerating reductions in child mortality, especially in remote areas – have hovered at low levels (20.3 per cent for skilled birth attendance in 2006 and 59.0 per cent for measles immunization in 2009) [9].

In summary, failures in achieving the MDGs do not always equate to failures of development. By the same token, successes in the MDG realm do not always mean successes in development. No stigma should be attached to those countries that find themselves 'off track' because the MDGs are not always sufficient to capture the full picture of the progress underway in a country.

## Achievements of the MDGs in South, East and Southeast Asia

Although the MDG agenda does not always reflect or account for the unique development paths of individual countries, many lives have been saved or changed profoundly for the better in South, East and Southeast Asia since the establishment of the MDGs. This section focuses on thirteen case study countries (see Table 2.1) in the region defined in 2000 as low-income economies by the World Bank. Data without a corresponding citation are sourced from the UN MDG database.

### *The health-related MDGs*

Of the eight MDGs, three are specifically related to health: MDG 4 (reducing child mortality), MDG 5 (improving maternal health) and MDG 6 (combating HIV/AIDS, malaria and other diseases).

#### MDG 4 – Reduce child mortality

Steady progress has been made in reducing the under-5 mortality rate (U5MR, deaths per 1,000 live births among children younger than 5 years of age) in the developing world, and the declines have been accelerated between 2000 and 2010 (annual rate of reduction: 2.4 per cent a year) as compared to the period between 1990 and 2000 (annual rate of reduction: 1.9 per cent a year). However, progress remains insufficient to reach the global target for MDG 4. Among the thirteen countries included in the case study, only Mongolia has already achieved the target, reducing its U5MR from 107 deaths in 1990 to 32 in 2010. The remaining countries vary in their level of progress: five (Bangladesh, Bhutan, Indonesia, Lao PDR and Nepal) are 'on track' to meet the target, while the progress of the other seven lags behind. All 'on-track' countries, except for Indonesia, have made striking progress, each going from nearly 150 deaths per 1,000 live births in 1990 to around 50 in 2010. However, Afghanistan's U5MR has remained remarkably high at 149 deaths per 1,000 live births in 2010, ranking it the eleventh worst in the world.

Although child mortality rates are generally decreasing in the region, the majority of deaths are now happening at an earlier age. In the thirteen countries studied, the percentage of infant deaths (those occurring between birth and 1 year of age) has increased from 68.8 per cent in 1990 to 78.7 per cent in 2010. Furthermore, progress has been slow on reducing mortality in the neonatal period (spanning the first four weeks of life), during which 41 per cent of child deaths occur globally. This is in part due to a lack of attention to neonatal deaths through international public health policies and programmes [15]. Within the case study countries, Afghanistan and Pakistan are among the fifteen countries globally with the highest neonatal mortality rates – 39 deaths per 1,000 live births in 2009 [15].

#### MDG 5 – Improve maternal health

Globally, the MDG 5 for maternal health has shown the worst progress compared with other goals. Whilst the target is an average annual decline in MMR of 5.5 per cent over the period from 1990 to 2015, the global average decline between 1990 and 2008 has been just 2.3 per cent [16]. Among the thirteen case study countries, MDG 5 indicators still lag far behind the MDG targets, despite some significant progress. The exceptions are Bhutan and Vietnam, each of which achieved an average annual decline of more than 5.5 per cent between 1990 and 2008. On the other end of the spectrum, the most inadequate progress, with rates of decline of less than 2 per cent, has been observed in Afghanistan and the Democratic People's Republic of Korea (DPR Korea) – 1.0 per cent and 0.4 per cent, respectively [16].

Two of the major determinants of a mother's survival are whether or not the birth is attended by a skilled health professional and whether or not antenatal care is accessible. Bhutan, the only early achiever of the target for skilled birth attendance, has made significant progress by increasing the rate of professionally attended births by nearly 60 per cent (from 14.9 per cent in 1994 to 71.4 per cent in 2007). However, in each of the four countries (Afghanistan, Bangladesh, Lao PDR and Nepal) with the highest estimated MMR (MMR ≥300), skilled health professionals attend less than one in four births and less than two in three births among expectant mothers who have received antenatal care at least once.

## MDG 6 – Combat HIV/AIDS, malaria and other diseases

Since 2001, the global HIV incidence rate has declined steadily, reaching the targeted 25 per cent decline by 2009, with progress in Sub-Saharan Africa at the helm. Yet the number of people living with HIV continues to rise due to expanding antiretroviral treatment coverage. Among the case study countries, five (Cambodia, India, Myanmar, Nepal and Vietnam) have already achieved the target for HIV prevalence. However, rates of condom use at last high-risk sexual encounter among young people aged 15–24 is still quite low in some countries, including India (22 per cent among women and 37 per cent among men in 2006). Universal access to treatment for HIV/AIDS is unlikely to be achieved by 2015, though worldwide coverage has been significantly expanded. Rates of coverage remain quite variable among eleven of the thirteen countries (there are no data available for Afghanistan and DPR Korea). Cambodia has already achieved universal access, with antiretroviral therapy coverage of at least 80 per cent among the population in need, while two countries (Nepal and Pakistan) had coverage of less than 20 per cent in 2010.

Major progress has been made against malaria, too. An estimated 655,000 malaria deaths occurred in 2010, of which 91 per cent were from Africa and 86 per cent were children under 5 years of age. Globally, the estimated incidence of malaria has decreased by 17 per cent since 2000 [17]. Among the case study countries, except for Mongolia as a malaria-free country, five (Afghanistan, Bhutan, DPR Korea, Nepal and Vietnam) reported that malaria cases fell by more than half between 2000 and 2010. The remaining countries reported either little change (Cambodia, India, Indonesia and Lao PDR) or increasing case numbers (Bangladesh, Myanmar and Pakistan) [18].

In terms of other targeted infectious diseases, the burden of tuberculosis is gradually decreasing as well. Globally, the annual incidence rate has fallen to about 1 per cent and the world is 'on track' to achieve the corresponding MDG target if this trend continues. Among the case study countries, only DPR Korea and Lao PDR are exceptions to the pattern of reducing the tuberculosis incidence.

### *The other MDGs*

The remaining MDGs to be addressed herein (MDG 1, MDG 2, MDG 3 and MDG 7) are not classified as directly related to health. Nevertheless, those goals play an important role towards achieving the health-related MDGs. Among the thirteen low-income countries, five have successfully increased incomes and reduced hunger, or are on track to do so (MDG 1), while only Vietnam is on track to achieve the full primary schooling coverage target contained in MDG 2. Overall, the most significant successes have been in improving gender equity (MDG 3) and access to safe drinking water and better sanitation (MDG 7) in the thirteen case study countries.

## MDG 1 – Eradicate extreme poverty and hunger

One of the greatest MDG successes worldwide has been in poverty reduction. The global poverty rate is expected to fall below 15 per cent by 2015. With this milestone, the world will have surpassed the MDG target, which is set at a 23 per cent decline. This is despite the global economic crisis, which could well have hindered progress and, in some cases, even increased the depth of poverty [19]. However, meeting the hunger-reduction target remains a difficult prospect in many regions of the developing world. The proportion of undernourished people remained at 16 per cent between 2005 and 2007, representing approximately 837 million people worldwide, and fell by only 2 per cent since the period 1990 to 1992 [4].

Among the thirteen low-income countries in focus, only five (Cambodia, Indonesia, Lao PDR, Pakistan and Vietnam) are early achievers, or 'on track', for reducing poverty, while four (Mongolia, Bangladesh, India and Nepal) are currently 'off track'. Meeting the target for reducing the prevalence of underweight children under 5 years of age will be achieved by six countries who are early achievers or 'on track' (Afghanistan, Bangladesh, Cambodia, DPR Korea, Mongolia and Vietnam), while seven countries are 'off track' for reaching this target (Bhutan, India, Indonesia, Lao PDR, Myanmar, Nepal and Pakistan). Thus, only Cambodia and Vietnam are early achievers, or 'on track', for both poverty and hunger reduction targets in South and Southeast Asia.

## MDG 2 – Achieve universal primary education

In the developing world, the primary education net enrolment ratio (NER) is rising slowly (from 82 per cent in 1999 to 89 per cent in 2009). Among the case study countries, four have achieved an NER higher than 90 per cent (India, Indonesia, Mongolia and Vietnam). Especially notable is progress achieved in Bhutan, which increased its NER by more than 30 per cent over the period from 1999 to 2009 (from 55.9 per cent to 88.4 per cent).

In contrast, progress in increasing the ratio of pupils who complete a full course of primary education has seen less progress and is far from meeting the MDG target. On average, 72.5 out of 100 children in the eleven case study countries completed primary education, with specific rates ranging from 54.5 in Cambodia to 94.4 in Mongolia, based on available data as of 2008 (excluding Afghanistan and DPR Korea, for which available data were insufficient). The remaining challenges, along with universal primary school enrolment, are to improve the quality of primary education, improve retention of children in schools and properly adapt education for children living in conflict zones [4]. Impacts of conflict zones on achieving MDG targets may be felt both directly and indirectly. For example, poverty and hunger are caused by conflict (MDG 1). Conflict also creates barriers to accessing education that might affect MDG 2 [20].

## MDG 3 – Promote gender equality and empower women

Female education rates are improving in the developing world. In 2009, for every 100 boys, there were 96 girls enrolled in primary and secondary schools across the developing world [4]. This is a significant improvement from 1999, especially in South Asia, where the ratio has jumped from 83 to 95 girls per 100 boys in primary, and from 75 to 89 girls per 100 boys in secondary, education. The tertiary level of education, meanwhile, presents the highest ratio of female students among all levels of education, at 97 girls for every 100 boys, though there is a considerable difference across regions [4].

Twelve of the thirteen case study countries (excluding Afghanistan) have also achieved significant progress in terms of the Gender Parity Index (GPI) in primary education – especially India, where the GPI rose from 0.76 in 1991 to 0.97 in 2007. The GPI is designed to measure the ratio of girls to boys in primary, secondary and tertiary education. It is calculated by dividing the female Gross Enrolment Ratio for the given level of education by that same ratio for males. In Afghanistan, they are lagging far behind in terms of girls' access to education and are seriously 'off track' for achieving the related MDG target, with a GPI of 0.67 in 2009, but they are likely to meet the target by 2020, as the ratio has been steadily increasing since 2004 [4]. At the same time, cultural constraints must be mitigated, such as through teaching single sex classes and providing security for girls in conservative areas [19, 21, 22].

### MDG 7 – Ensure environmental sustainability

Steady progress has been made towards improving access to safe drinking water and the global MDG target of 89 per cent coverage by 2015 will be met if this trend continues. In contrast, progress towards the goal for sanitation has been much slower, especially in South Asia, where almost two-thirds of the population practises open defecation. Among the thirteen case study countries, half (Afghanistan, Cambodia, India, DPR Korea, Mongolia, Nepal and Vietnam) are 'on track' to achieve the MDG target on safe drinking water, while only three countries (Lao PDR, Myanmar and Vietnam) are 'on track' to achieve the sanitation target. Other countries are making slow progress and require greater acceleration towards development on these fronts.

## *Linking the health-related and other MDGs*

Whereas MDGs 4 to 6 are directly related to health, the other MDGs are linked to promoting health through development in various, more indirect ways. For instance, in as much as poverty remains a cause of hunger and, ultimately, undernutrition, hunger and undernutrition (MDG 1) are seen as underlying causes of many diseases [23]. To wit, food insecurity and hunger have been linked with rapid spread and progression of diseases including HIV/AIDS [24, 25]. Families suffering from such ailments have continued to fall into the vicious cycle of poverty leading to food insecurity and seguing into hunger, widening the gender equity gap (MDG 3) and affecting children's educational attainment (MDG 2).

Likewise, gender-based inequities (MDG 3) render women and their children more vulnerable to poor health. In particular, educated mothers (MDG 2) who are literate, well informed and empowered have a greater capacity to promote their children's health [23]. Along similar lines, better sanitation and safe drinking water (MDG 7) translate into fewer opportunities to acquire infections, especially among children and other high-risk groups such as people living with HIV/AIDS [9].

To improve global health in general, more global partnerships should be fostered (MDG 8). Such partnerships have been seen to have an appreciable impact on key health-related issues of global concern, including HIV/AIDS, malaria and TB (MDG 6). Through living examples of global initiatives like the Global Fund to Fight AIDS, TB and Malaria (GFATM), the Bill and Melinda Gates Foundation (BMGF), the Global Alliance for Vaccines and

Immunization (GAVI), the Clinton Foundation HIV/AIDS Initiative (CHAI), and other bilateral and multilateral organizations, more vertical programmes targeting specific health-related areas have been implemented. Given their complex interlinkages and interdependencies, the MDGs clearly cannot be implemented in isolation, but rather must be tackled through concerted multilateral, multifaceted interventions.

## Limitations of the MDGs

Challenges in fully realizing the MDG vision notwithstanding, the framework they represent has undoubtedly facilitated notable successes and real progress in the field of international development. The MDGs have served effectively as a tool to generate discussion, focus attention and help assign accountability for leaders' pledges. The goals have helped to galvanize the aid community and reverse the aid declines after the end of the Cold War. Of particular note, the United States, the European Union, Canada, Norway and other regions promised in 2002 to substantially increase aid as a result of the MDG negotiations [12]. The MDG agenda has also had notable success in encouraging global political consensus, especially in terms of providing a focus for advocacy, improving the targeting and flow of aid, and refining the monitoring of development projects [3]. At the same time, the MDGs have been marked by a variety of common limitations, as summarized below.

*Limited involvement of developing countries in formulating the MDG framework*: The involvement of developing countries was limited in the process of formulating the MDG framework [3] and only 22 per cent of the world's national parliaments formally discussed the MDGs [5, 7]. This is one of the reasons why Lao PDR ended up establishing its own target for HIV control.

*Conceptualization and execution*: The very specific nature of the MDGs generated considerable gaps in coverage and failed to realize synergies that could arise across their implementation, such as synergies between education, health, poverty and gender. In addition, several targets present a measure of goal achievement that is too narrow or that might not identify a clear means of delivery [3].

*Lack of clear ownership and leadership*: In particular, new targets such as 'achieving universal access to reproductive health', added at a later stage, have not been very successful. This is attributable not only to their complexity, but also to the limited national ownership and/or lack of engagement by national governmental organizations [3].

*Inequity*: Issues of equity arise because many of the goals seek to attain specific minimum standards, e.g. of income, education or maternal/child survival. To bring people above this threshold might realistically mean a focus on those for whom least effort is required, neglecting groups that are more difficult to reach for geographical, ethnic or other reasons [3]. For example, MDG 4, aimed at reducing the U5MR by two-thirds, can be achieved by a variety of policy interventions, some of which could actually make children from poor communities worse off. Therefore, success in achieving MDG 4 cannot always be regarded as a success in the true spirit of the Millennium Declaration [26].

*Limited accountability for failing*: The MDGs might be reasonably expected to have diminished their effectiveness due to diffused accountability for failing to meet them [27]. In fact, the weakness of the monitoring and follow-up mechanisms is widely regarded as one of the major limitations of the MDG framework. This weakness has resulted in a lack of mutual accountability on the part of national governments, international institutions and other actors to achieve the MDGs.

*Problems of design*: Several studies have pointed out that it is impossible to meet the MDGs because of how they were originally designed, rather than due to a lack of policy effort, commitment or aid [26, 28, 29]. The MDGs are poorly and arbitrarily designed to measure progress against poverty and deprivation, and their design makes relative performance look worse than it really is. For example, in the case of MDG 4 (to reduce child mortality by two-thirds), the relationship between increased mortality reduction and initial mortality has made it more unlikely that a high-mortality region like Africa would attain the proportional goal [29].

As we approach 2015, there is considerable interest in assessing the present goals and in considering the future of the development goals after 2015 [3].

## Overcoming MDG challenges in preparation for the post-MDG era

This section discusses possible pathways to achieve the health-related MDGs in preparation for the post-2015 era of development agenda setting.

To date, Asian countries have experienced varying degrees of both successes and failures in attempts to achieve the targets set for the health-related MDGs. In several countries, variations are observed by socio-economic strata and between urban and rural areas. For example in Lao PDR, MDGs present a useful global picture of development, but the interpretation of being 'on track' or 'off track' must be made very carefully. For instance, a status of 'off track' does not mean that all previous MDG-oriented interventions have categorically failed. Appreciating the history of development efforts requires the data gathered to be put to good use to assist policy making in order to move forward.

As highlighted in the thirteen case studies, the implied 'one-size-fits-all' approach constitutes an important flaw in the design of the MDG framework. For the purpose of sustainable development, any new agenda should consider each country's distinct needs, plans, levels of economic development, population size, culture, stability and overarching vision. For example, among the thirteen low-income countries in Asia, a more tailored approach is needed in regions facing special economic constraints, such as Myanmar, Lao PDR and Cambodia; in conflict and post-conflict countries, such as Afghanistan and Pakistan; and in population-dense countries, such as Indonesia, Bangladesh and India.

Achieving the health-related MDGs has generally entailed a heavy investment of capital. The push has, therefore, been especially difficult for the low-income Asian countries, largely dependent on external developmental aid such as Official Development Assistance (ODA) [30]. Countries receiving low shares of ODA funding, such as Myanmar [31], have correspondingly encountered greater obstacles in achieving the targets. Even with the somewhat meagre progress achieved, sustaining the pace is no easy proposition since it entails continued dependency on the ODA.

At the starting line of the MDG era, Asian countries naturally entered the 'race' with varied levels of economic development. Economic and development levels, in turn, determine the magnitude of health problems faced by a nation, and they also define the speed of progress to achieve the health-related MDG targets where comparisons of progress become a numbers game. Therefore, the Asian countries with comparably worse health indicators have been seen as making more progress than their counterparts. This is because it is comparatively easier to see progress for the countries that started with a higher burden of disease compared to those entering the MDG era with relatively better health indicators. Also, even with similar investments of capital, a significant reduction is naturally expected for countries with a higher burden compared to those with a low burden of a similar disease. For example, Myanmar and Cambodia showed higher levels of progress towards MDG 6 than Lao PDR, Pakistan or Afghanistan. This is primarily because Myanmar and Cambodia had comparably high burdens of HIV and TB at the outset.

Close attention must also be paid to non-communicable diseases (NCDs), which have undermined the achievement of the MDGs in many settings. It is estimated that NCDs will continue to increase in developing countries and the greatest increases will be observed in Africa. The existing links between NCDs and HIV/AIDS, tuberculosis, and child and maternal health mean that NCDs need to be tackled if the MDG targets are to be achieved and if more progress is to be made in low-income countries in the post-MDG era [32].

Even if the time frame for the unmet MDG targets were to be extended beyond 2015, sustainable development in this region is unlikely to be realized under the current terms [33]. To achieve sustained development in health, a preferable strategy would be for low-income countries in the region to embrace the Sustainable Development Goals (SDGs) agenda proposed by UN Secretary-General Ban Ki-Moon's high-level global sustainability panel, convened in the lead-up to the Rio+20 summit in June 2012 [34]. The SDGs are built upon the so-called 'triple bottom line' approach to human wellbeing, incorporating social inclusion and health as core functions of the development agenda. Though the SDGs may encompass a vision for global development, the approach in each region should be tailored to suit national interests [34]. Moreover, specific policies should be formulated to yield cost-effective interventions relevant to the time, context and internal revenue of each country, necessitating minimal dependence on the ODA. For example, countries should be encouraged to use their own health plans to design and implement policies and interventions that are feasible using their national revenues first rather than acting according to the wishes of donors, who naturally provide funds for what they personally see as important.

On a practical level, ODA has been a key ingredient in the observed successes surrounding the health-related MDGs [35]. The strides made in attaining MDGs 4 and 6, for instance, were partly due to support from donor agencies, including the United States Agency for International Development (USAID), GFATM, the Presidential Malaria Initiative and GAVI [4]. On the other hand, over-reliance on ODA has arguably weakened countries' ownership of the health and development agenda [36]. The challenge of sustaining such expensive and donor-financed projects beyond the lifespan of the MDGs warrants serious consideration and financial reforms. Thus far, ODA would appear not to represent any sort of definitive answer for a sustainable international development agenda [37].

## Conclusion

In the end, the real value of the MDGs is in the fodder they have provided for the public health and development community as a whole to continually think and act for promoting health and development in low-income countries. In this sense alone, they should be appreciated as an important stepping-stone. Such a limited framework, however, is just one element of the goals to be pursued in each country. Based on lessons learned in the MDG era, we need to rethink what 'development' means for low-income countries and to whom it is beneficial. Global aid communities may feel satisfied with the achievement of the MDGs, but if individuals in each country are still suffering from unreasonable pain or discomfort, achieving such targets is simply not enough. To go beyond this, we have to create a new paradigm of development goals – one that will truly improve the health and wellbeing of people living in underserved areas, especially in low-income countries.

## References


1. Hulme, D. The making of the millennium development goals: human development meets results-based management in an imperfect world. Manchester, UK: Brooks World Poverty Institute, 2007.
2. UN. United Nations Millennium Declaration. Resolution adopted by the UN General Assembly. A/RES/55/2. New York: United Nations, 2000.
3. Waage, J., Banerji, R., Campbell, O., Chirwa, E., Collender, G., Dieltiens, V., *et al.* The Millennium Development Goals: a cross-sectoral analysis and principles for goal setting after 2015, Lancet and London International Development Centre Commission. *Lancet* 2010, 376(9745):991–1023.
4. UN. *Millennium Development Goals Report.* New York: United Nations, 2011.
5. UNDP. Public choices, private decisions: sexual and reproductive health and the Millennium Development Goals. New York: United Nations Millennium Development Group, 2011.
6. Richard, F., Hercot, D., Ouédraogo, C., Delvaux, T., Samaké, S., van Olmen, J., *et al.* Sub-Saharan Africa and the health MDGs: the need to move beyond the 'quick impact' model. *Reproductive Health Matters* 2011, 19(38):42–55.
7. Lao Statistics Bureau. Poverty in Lao PDR. Available at: http://www.nsc.gov.la/index.php?view=article&catid=9%3Alecs&id=55%3Apovertyin-lao-pdr-2008&format=pdf&option=com_content&Itemid=80
8. WHO. Global Health Observatory Data Repository 2012. Available at: http://apps.who.int/ghodata/?vid=1901
9. UNDP. Accelerating progress towards the MDGs: innovative options for reaching the unreached. Lao People's Democratic Republic. Lao PDR: United Nations Development Program, 2010.
10. Manithip, C., Edin, K., Sihavong, A., Wahlström, R., Wessel, H. Poor quality of antenatal care services: is lack of competence and support the reason? An observational and interview study in rural areas of Lao PDR. *Midwifery* 2012, Jul.
11. Vandemoortele, J. The MDG conundrum: meeting the targets without missing the point. *Development Policy Review* 2009, 27(4):355–71.
12. UNDP. What will it take to achieve the Millennium Development Goals? – An international assessment. New York: United Nations Development Programme, 2010.
13. Mounier-Jack, S., Rudge, J. W., Phetsouvanh, R., Chanthapadith, C., Coker, R. Critical interactions between Global Fund-supported programmes and health systems: a case study in Lao People's Democratic Republic. *Health Policy Plan* 2010, 25 Suppl 1:i37–42.
14. Ali, N., Hill, C., Kennedy, A., IJsselmuiden, C. What factors influence national health research agendas in low and middle income countries? New York: Council on Health Research for Development (COHRED), 2006. Available at: http://www.cohred.org/downloads/cohred_publications/rp5.pdf
15. Oestergaard, M. Z., Inoue, M., Yoshida, S., Mahanani, W. R., Gore, F. M., Cousens, S., *et al.* Neonatal mortality levels for 193 countries in 2009 with trends since 1990: a systematic analysis of progress, projections, and priorities. *PLoS Medicine* 2011, 8(8).
16. WHO. *Trends in Maternal Mortality: 1990 to 2008.* Geneva, Switzerland: World Health Organization, 2010.
17. UN. *Millennium Development Goals Report.* New York: United Nations, 2012.
18. WHO. *World Malaria Report.* Geneva, Switzerland: World Health Organization, 2011.
19. ADB. The key indicators for Asia and the Pacific 2011. Asian Development Bank. Available at: http://www.adb.org/key-indicators/2011/main
20. Hill, P. S., Mansoor, G. F., Claudio, F. Conflict in least-developed countries: challenging the Millennium Development Goals. *Bulletin of the World Health Organization* 2010, 88(8):562.
21. Jones, A. Afghanistan on the educational road to access and equity. *Asia Pacific Journal of Education* 2007, 28(3):277–90.
22. WHO. *Dying for Change. Poor people's experience of health and ill-health.* Geneva, Switzerland: World Health Organization, 2010.
23. Rogers, R. Understanding literacy development 'lifelong and life wide'. *Reading Research Quarterly* 2011, 46(1):86–96.
24. Weiser, S. D., Young, S. L., Cohen, C. R., Kushel, M. B., Tsai, A. C., Tien, P. C., *et al.* Conceptual framework for understanding the bidirectional links between food insecurity and HIV/AIDS. *American Journal of Clinical Nutrition* 2011, 94(6):1729S–39S.

25. Miller, C. L., Bangsberg, D. R., Tuller, D. M., Senkungu, J., Kawuma, A., Frongillo, E. A., *et al.* Food insecurity and sexual risk in an HIV endemic community in Uganda. *AIDS and Behavior* 2011, 15(7):1512–19.
26. Clemens, M., Kenny, C., Moss, T. The trouble with the MDGs: confronting expectations of aid and development success. *World Development* 2007, 35(5):735–51.
27. Reidpath, D. D., Morel, C. M., Mecaskey, J. W., Allotey, P. The Millennium Development Goals fail poor children: the case for equity-adjusted measures. *PLoS Medicine* 2009, 6(4).
28. White, H., Black, R. *Millennium Development Goals: a drop in the ocean?* New York: Routledge, 2004.
29. Easterly, W. How the Millennium Development Goals are unfair to Africa. *World Development* 2009, 37(1):26–35.
30. UN. *Investing in Development: a practical plan to achieve the Millennium Development Goals.* New York: United Nations Millennium Project, 2005.
31. UNDP. *Human Development Report 2011. Equity and sustainability: a better future for all.* New York: United Nations Development Programme, 2011.
32. WHO. *Accelerating the MDGs by Addressing NCDs.* New York: World Health Organization, 2010.
33. Koehler, G., Gasper, D., Jolly, R., Simane, M. *Human Security and the Next Generation of Comprehensive Human Development Goals.* Brighton: Institute of Development Studies, 2012.
34. Sachs, J. D. From Millennium Development Goals to sustainable development goals. *Lancet* 2012, 379(9832):2206–11.
35. Feeny, S., Clarke, M. *The Millennium Development Goals and Beyond: international assistance to the Asia-Pacific.* Basingstoke: Palgrave Macmillan, 2009.
36. Feeny, S., Clarke, M. Achieving the Millennium Development Goals in the Asia Pacific region: the role of international assistance. *Asia Pacific Viewpoint* 2008, 49(2):198–212.
37. Moyo, D. *Dead Aid: why aid is not working and how there is a better way for Africa.* New York: Allen Lane, 2009.
38. National Statistics Center of the Lao PDR. Population distribution and migration. 2007. Available at: http://www.nsc.gov.la/Products/Populationcensus2005/PopulationCensus2005_chaptr2.htm
39. ESCAP/ADB/UN. Accelerating equitable achievement of the MDGs: closing gaps in health and nutrition outcomes. 2011. Available at: http://www.unescap.ord/pdd/calendar/CSN-MDG-NewDelhi-Nov-2011/MDG-Report2011-12.pdf

# 3

# Migration and health

## Lessons from China

*Hildy F. Fong and Jin Mou*

## Introduction: a brief history of migration in China

### *Pre-1978: origins of China's Household Registration System*

The Household Registration System (HRS), commonly referred to as the *hukou* system, has been China's predominant mechanism for population management since its formal inception in 1958 [1]. The foundation was laid at the time of China's 'Great Leap Forward', when the goals of its economy shifted towards the production of the heavy industries, such as energy, iron and steel. The new policies of the state led by Chairman Mao Zedong had halted agricultural production of traditional private farming and instead formed agricultural collectives which favoured industrialization. The *hukou* system was created as a social institution system that would support industrialization goals for China's economy. It controlled migration and spatial hierarchies of the population, which in turn supported an artificial balance under the conditions of a dual economy by controlling flows of resources between cities and the countryside [2].

However, this also led to a stark imbalance between agricultural and industrial sectors and, eventually, created socio-economic gaps between populations in rural and urban areas which exist to this day. Peasants were inevitably tied to the land in rural areas to support heavy industry development and their movements were restricted. As an ascribed attribute, a person's *hukou*, either agricultural (rural) or non-agricultural (urban), determined the person's access to state-funded social welfare including employment, subsidized housing, food, education, medical care and pensions [3]. The HRS was successful in halting rural influxes into Chinese cities throughout the Cultural Revolution (1966–1976) until 1978, during which policies rigorously controlled formal migration from rural to urban areas. Though urban residents were allowed to move between cities and flows from the opposite direction were allowed, migration was still severely restricted and rarely sanctioned. Transferring one's agricultural *hukou* status to non-agricultural status via higher education, serving in the army and/or membership in the Chinese Communist Party represented a rise in social status and a rare form of social mobility.

### *From 1978 to 2000: reforms and the rise of migration*

The year 1978 marked the official end of the Cultural Revolution and was a turning point for economic reform in the country. Migration policies were soon relaxed to some extent under Deng Xiaoping's new socialist market economy, as they became increasingly incompatible with China's rapid development. China's central leadership boosted agricultural production on the country's limited arable land, which created an increasing surplus of workers throughout rural areas. In response, the government adjusted to changes within the labour market by easing some *hukou* restrictions to regulate and reallocate the excess of rural workers. Additionally, development of township and village enterprises was encouraged. Population movement began to swell as people in both rural and urban areas were affected.

Migration is often analysed in terms of push and pull factors. Push factors, such as economic, social or political problems, drive people away from a place while pull factors attract migrants to a place (i.e. employment opportunities, better quality of life, etc.) [4]. Increased migration in China during the decade after the Cultural Revolution centred on factors tied to political reasons and economic growth, motivated at its core by an inherent pull of the Chinese to seek better lives. The late 1980s brought even more urbanization leading to an unprecedented wave of internal migration. As economic reform progressed, patterns emerged favouring eastern coastal development in areas such as Shanghai, Guangzhou and Shenzhen [5]. The number of peasants who left home for jobs increased sharply from less than 2 million in the early 1980s to 30 million in 1989. This swelled to 62 million in 1993 and 80 million in 1995 [6].

### *Migration in twenty-first-century China: continuing growth and implications for public health*

According to the National Population Census of China, the number of rural–urban migrants reached 88.4 million in 2000, 73 per cent of the total number of internal migrants in China. By 2004, the Chinese National Statistical Bureau estimated that 118 million rural–urban migrants are living in urban areas, representing 23.8 per cent of China's total rural working population. Consensus between the Ministry of Agriculture and the Ministry of Labour and Social Security estimate there are now approximately 120 million rural–urban migrants in the country. Including migrants working within the same administrative regions but in different counties, there are approximately 200 million [7] migrants and migrant populations are projected to reach 350 million by 2050 [8].

Migration in China has had major repercussions for the nation's public health system and also effects on the health of migrants themselves. Some of the challenges are outlined in Figure 3.1.

In this chapter, we will present an overview of the key public health challenges facing migrants in twenty-first-century China through a review of current literature and policies.

## Migrant populations in China

The International Organization for Migration (IOM) defines migration as a population movement, encompassing any kind of movement of people, whatever its length, composition or cause [4]. In China the term migrants most often refers to rural-to-urban economic migrants who move internally from rural to urban areas for work purposes. However, migrant

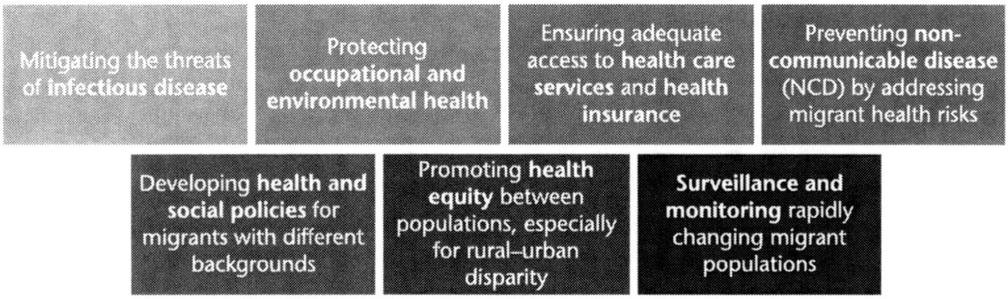


*Figure 3.1* Challenges posed by migration on the public health system in China

communities are comprised of diverse sub-populations covering many traditional and non-traditional groups who have varying patterns of mobility and socio-demographic factors. Therefore, definitions and classifications often overlap.

### *Predominant classifications of migrants: local, temporary and floating populations*

Permanent (or local) residents hold a local identification card and are permanent residents of a particular locality by birth, or by other application methods such as paying steep fees, marriage, parental reunion with children or government allocation. Migrants, both temporary and floating populations, are distinguished from local residents by whether they hold a local *hukou* identification or obtain a temporary residency.

China's temporary population refers to migrants without a *hukou* living in a locale for one month or more and who are required by the local public security departments to register with the Temporary Population Management System (TPMS) [9], and hold a temporary resident card. However, there are deficiencies in the TPMS systems and some migrants do not register to avoid registration fees or the complex process involved. Thus, population statistics based on registration may not truly reflect migration population sizes, especially in large cities.

The term the 'floating population' refers to migrants who live in a locale (classified duration is less than one month but in reality this is not always the case) and do not hold either a permanent local ID or a temporary residence card. They may not be required to have one or have voluntarily decided not to register. These 'invisible' floating populations are characteristically self-employed, unemployed or hired by informal sectors. Because of their status, floating migrants may be unable to access most state-funded social services such as public education or health insurance schemes entitled to registered individuals. Of the highly mobile floating population, many move bi-directionally, coming and going from cities according to the farming seasons, job markets, economy or family arrangements [10–11].

### *Sub-populations impacted by migration*

Migration has had significant impact on local ecologies, especially at community and family levels. Although urban–urban migration exists (often from smaller to bigger cities), rural–urban migration is mostly addressed in health literature. Literature mostly discusses those migrant workers who find non-agricultural work in urban areas in order to send financial aid to support their families back in rural areas. In 2004, 30.3 per cent of migrant workers worked in the manufacturing industry, 22.9 per cent in the construction industry, 10.4 per cent in the service industry, 6.7 per cent in hospitality services and 4.6 per cent in wholesale or business [17]. Migrant workers tend to be younger, healthier and more likely to be male and single [11]. This has changed rapidly, however, in larger cities where there are rising and nearly equal numbers of female migrant workers. Until the mid-1980s, most global migration was male-dominated but women now account for nearly half of the global migration [12]. Migrant factory workers are a sub-group of migrant workers. From a public health perspective, they have a higher risk of exposure to certain occupational and environmental health hazards [13].

There is also rural–urban movement of young migrants who do not live in their place of birth. Migrants who are children, adolescents or young adults are often labelled by Chinese sociologists as 'the new generation' [10]. Young migrants are often unregistered residents like their parents, thus they do not hold a temporary or permanent *hukou*. There are now also many children born to migrants in urban areas who are not entitled to a *hukou* in their birth city – they must by law be registered in their parents' registered locale. For these young migrants, this means full denial of legitimate access to the public education system and, in many places, health insurance. Child migrants are forced to seek education in migrant private schools and health care in the more expensive private sector or limited-cover from services in community clinics. In recent years, some more developed areas including Shenzhen have started a pilot for children's health insurance schemes that involve some of the eligible migrant children (those whose parents have been members of the social security scheme for a year or more are eligible). Similarly, progress has been seen in providing migrant children with free education in the public system in a few big cities; however, the same set of eligibility criteria applies. Child labourers are another sub-population of young migrants facing extreme social conditions.

As working adults from rural areas leave their homes for the city, they leave behind both the old and the young. Studies show that there is an estimated 20 million left-behind children in China [14]. It has also been found that parental migration is a risk factor for unhealthy behaviours amongst left-behind adolescents in rural China [15] and children often suffer negative psychosocial health consequences [16]. The left-behind ageing population is another group resulting from split households in rural areas, an increasing concern since ageing population rates are rising. In particular, China's 'one-child policy' has left a complex situation of who will take care of the ageing population. Due to self-selection, young and healthy people are more likely to migrate, leaving the weak and sick at home [11]. Migrants who become ill or fail to find work stay at home, which places an even bigger burden on rural communities. See Box 3.1 for a case study on cross-border migration.

## Migrant health challenges

Public health research on migrants in China provides a rich and complex area for topical study. Research on Chinese migrants has focused on many different perspectives, mostly highlighting the vulnerability and marginalization of migrants. However, while migrants in urban areas face some disadvantages, there is empirical evidence that studying rural–urban migrants is much more complex. Not all migrants are disadvantaged and poor – in some cases, migrants may be healthier than those left behind or are satisfied with their migration experience. The next sections address key messages from literature on migrant health using the three domains of health protection, health services and health improvement (see Figure 3.2).

## Box 3.1 Hong Kong SAR: a special case of cross-border migration

The repatriation of Hong Kong (HK) to the People's Republic of China from Great Britain in 1997 led to significant increases in migration between HK and mainland China [18]. HKSAR now follows the 'One Country, Two Systems' political system under the jurisprudence of The Basic Law. 'The Law' granted, among other things, the right of permanent residency in HK to mainland-born children with at least one parent with HK permanent residency. It also eased the right to abode in Hong Kong for adults through Certificates of Entitlements (CoE). Migrants who have entered the region for not more than seven years are called newly-arrived migrants. The Law also entitled children of mainland citizens right of abode in HKSAR if they are born in HKSAR. This catapulted the number of mainland mothers giving birth in HKSAR to secure HKSAR citizenship for their children, many of whom returned to mainland China to reside. These children, an evolving group in research, use both HKSAR and mainland health systems, and can be called cross-border migrant children [18]. Cross-border births include children born in HKSAR to two visiting mainland parents or to cross-boundary marriages of one mainland parent and one HKSAR parent.

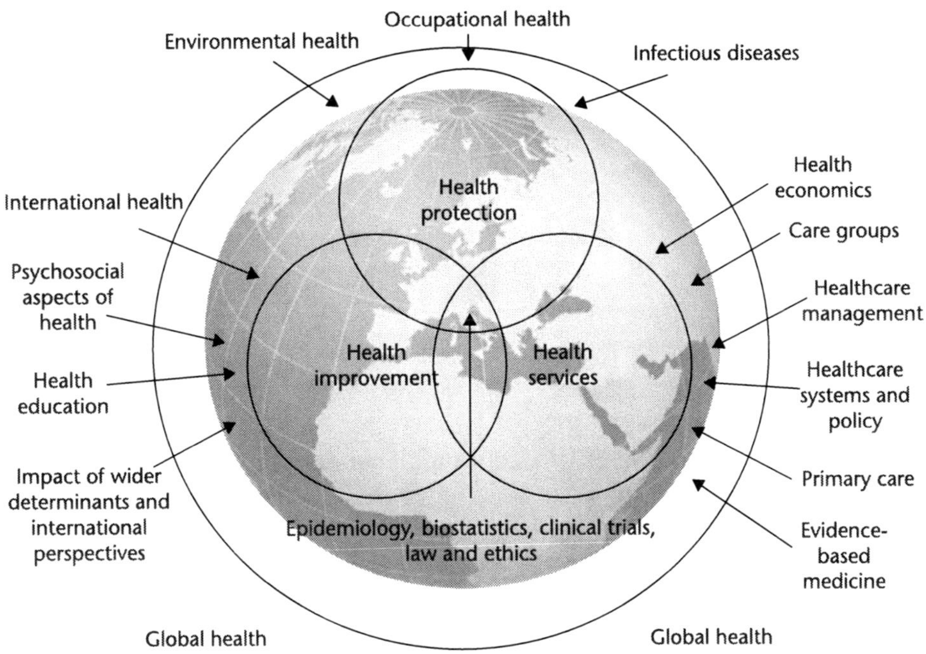


*Figure 3.2* Interrelation between the domains of health protection, health services and health improvement on a global health scale [79]

## Health protection: infectious diseases and occupational and environmental health risks

### *Infectious diseases*

The 2003 severe acute respiratory syndrome (SARS) epidemic originating in China showed how migrants are a highly mobile group at risk of both being vectors and becoming victims of an infectious disease [11]. From a health protection perspective, migrants are more vulnerable to communicable diseases such as acute respiratory infections; diarrhoeal, parasitic and sexually transmitted diseases; and tuberculosis [11]. In particular, HIV/AIDS, tuberculosis (TB) and infectious diseases preventable by childhood immunization have been challenges.

#### HIV/AIDS

In China, HIV/AIDS is a leading cause of death compared to other infectious diseases [19]. Migration has been a significant factor in the HIV risk epidemic since the 1980s when sporadic cases of HIV/AIDS surfaced amongst intravenous drug user (IDU) communities in the Yunnan Province–Myanmar border region. In the mid-1990s, the generalized epidemic grew as large numbers of migrants, infected from blood donations in the Guangdong Province, were sent back to their home provinces by health authorities. Drug users, migrant workers, sex workers and travelling business people still remain at-risk groups. Research has explored how seasonal economic migration facilitates HIV transmission across regions (see Box 3.2). Services that address screening and prevention of sexual health issues are not only essential for migrants, but migrant women in particular. This will be discussed further in a later section.

#### Tuberculosis

This is another major migrant health challenge in China and is the primary cause of death from infectious disease in adults. China has the second highest TB burden behind India and its migrant population has a particularly high risk of TB infection and transmission. Annually,

### Box 3.2 Migration and HIV/AIDS: major concerns highlighted in research

- Flourishing commercial sex industries catering to migrant workers is a growing concern in transmission to the general population.
- Higher proportions of floating migrants have had multiple sex partners.
- Migrants returning to hometowns periodically for holidays lead to STI/HIV acquired elsewhere to be spread to partners.
- Although HIV incidence and prevalence rates are not widely available [21], migrant workers have higher STD rates [20].
- Growing numbers of drug users, internal migration, high-risk behaviours and low condom use, are part of the challenge [21].

### Box 3.3 Tuberculosis challenges for migrants

- 'Migratory' nature of the migrant population increases exposure to TB.
- Marginalised working and living environments promote transmission.
- Poor financial status prevents diagnosis and treatment.
- Little knowledge and awareness of TB.
- Inadequate referral to TB dispensaries.
- Potential social stigma in the workplace.

*Source*: [32].

there have been 1.3 million new cases reported (80 per cent of TB patients are from rural areas), while there are 150,000 deaths reported each year [31]. TB control is a major challenge to China's public health and control has been relatively poor throughout the country (see Box 3.3 and Chapter 16). As well as that, poverty has been found to be strongly associated with TB incidence even after controlling for smoking and other risk factors, thus poverty schemes are a consideration for future TB policy [33].

## Childhood immunization

Access to immunization is a critical health protection issue for migrant children in China. Immunizations of vaccine-preventable infectious diseases are essential because they are a low-cost, high-impact public health intervention. Migration affects how whole populations receive and access health care and immunization rates are a simple measure for the risk of infectious diseases in a community. There has been great improvement in the immunization of children as a whole since the 1982 inception of China's Experts Advisory Committee on Immunization Programme (EACIP) [22]. Furthermore, in 2005, China's Ministry of Health supported a law requiring that the expanded immunization programme (EPI) provide immunizations for eleven diseases such as hepatitis B, tuberculosis and measles free of charge. This was expanded to twelve vaccines in 2008. Because of these incentives, immunization coverage is now much improved.

However, immunization rates of routine vaccines are still low in rural areas and large cities among migrant children [25]. Some townships and villages, governed by provincial governments, face issues such as limited vaccine supplies and budgets, and encounter difficulties reaching migrant children (see Box 3.4).

Additionally, community context and socio-economic status of the family are important factors in child vaccination status. Evidence shows that children born in rural areas, whose families are more likely to travel to big cities for work, have mothers with lower levels of knowledge, attitude and practice measures of immunization [30]. A majority of children immunized at Shenzhen Community Health Centres (CHCs) in the Guangdong Province were found to be unregistered migrant children with lower socio-economic statuses than local children. Caregivers experienced significant service inadequacies in CHCs with more migrants and poorer households attending [18], therefore the consistency of health services in CHCs serving high numbers of migrant workers should be considered. Caregivers of migrant children were more likely to find the price of immunization a disincentive,

### Box 3.4 Immunization of migrant children: evidence from research

- A study of child migrants in Beijing reported an 'alarmingly' low age-appropriate immunization coverage of migrant children in densely populated areas in the city [28], not attaining the MOH's goal of 85 per cent coverage.
- In the Henan province, coverage for children from floating populations was found to be less than 30 per cent [29].
- Migrant children of low SES are less likely to be healthier than local children due to being 'under-vaccinated' [23–24].
- Annual measles incidence in China has increased with half of the cases occurring in children of migrant workers with lower immunization coverage and lower antibody concentrations than children of non-migrants [26–27].

the education of the mother was a significant factor for immunization delay and poorer self-reported health of a caregiver was found to affect the perception of the importance of immunization as well [18].

There are also other infectious diseases that pose a threat to China's migrant population for example malaria, schistosomiais and parasitic diseases associated with rural poverty or overcrowded urban environments [14]. The increased mobility of migrants to, and from, their home cities perpetuates risks of reintroduction and transmission of disease.

## *Occupational and environmental health risks*

### Occupational health threats

Industrialization, urbanization and economic growth over the last thirty years have led to tremendous challenges for occupational health and safety (OHS) in both rural and urban China. Migrant workers in general are at a higher risk than the general population for occupational disease and injuries including silicosis (a type of pneumoconiosis), chemical poisoning and accidents caused by machinery. Over half of the migrant workers work in either manufacturing or construction industries where there is more exposure to risk and the work is mainly in the category of 'Three-D' jobs – a colloquial term that describes the often dirty, dangerous and degrading nature of migrant labour.

Workers are more at risk of harmful exposures to dust, fumes and toxic chemicals, and biological and physical hazards including noise, heat, vibration, inflammable materials and compressed air. Barriers to the healthcare system, a lack of medical insurance, weak enforcement of occupational health and safety regulations in working environments and low awareness of occupational risks contribute to the problem [34] as does the lack of occupational health services for migrant workers. Long working hours, overcrowded living conditions, inappropriate dorm facilities and poor general health are other issues. As a result, migrant workers account for approximately 80 per cent of deaths in mining, construction and chemical factories, and form a vast majority of the 700,000 annual victims of industrial accidents [35–37]. As well as that, approximately 90 per cent of patients suffering from occupational diseases are migrant workers.

In construction work, injuries are a major cause of death. Main causes include falls, collapse of structures, being struck by falling objects, electrocution and machine-related injuries. Migrants working in coal mines and other metallurgical industries in China are at a high risk for occupational lung diseases (pneumoconiosis) and mining accidents. China's fatality rates for coal mining are significantly higher than in other countries [38]. Suicides due to overwork and migration-related stress are also commonly seen, as are non-communicable diseases, such as cancer related to exposure to chemical poisoning, toxins and dangerous materials. Socio-economic conditions, such as close living quarters and exposure to other workers who travel frequently, increase exposed risk to infectious diseases such as TB, HIV/AIDS and others.

### Migration and environmental health

The correlations between environmental health and migrant health are difficult to measure. Migrants and their families are more likely to live in environments where 'Three-D' work is performed and/or live in housing conditions that escalate the magnitude of health risks. Migrants are at a higher risk of being affected by poor environmental quality including the pollution of air, water and food [14]. An example is the environmental waste recycling town in Guiyu County where millions of tons of overseas and domestic e-waste are dumped annually. In its 28 villages, nearly half of the residents are migrants and their families, and many of these migrant families are engaged in e-waste recycling operations to process e-waste [39]. This makes them at a much greater health risk of being exposed to toxic chemicals such as polychlorinated dibenzo-p-dioxins, dibenzofurans and heavy metals.

From an environmental perspective, urbanization and environmental degradation are causes of migration. Push factors of environmental degradation and displacement include administrative displacement (e.g. The Three Gorges), droughts and floods, earthquakes, resource depletion and conversion of farmland [14]. As an example, the 2002 environment-related migration and resettlement was supported by some official policies of the Chinese government. For example, a plan was implemented to displace 1.5 million people in west China over a five-year period up until 2010 [40].

## Challenges for health services

> Governments should ensure that national health systems take into account the health needs of migrant workers and make health services available to them.
>
> *(William Lacy Swing, director general, IOM)*

### *Health insurance reforms*

Health insurance for migrants is essential as insurance status has been found to be a significant factor in health utilization [41]. In China, health insurance systems are inequitably distributed amongst migrants with many of them being under-covered or uncovered by any kind of insurance in their urban destinations. This is a major challenge for China's health reforms to be addressed in the country's health service strategy. Historically, when there was a deep divide between rural and urban populations prior to the 1970s, populations in villages and communes (beginning in the 1950s) were covered by the Rural Cooperative Medical Scheme (RCMS), while workers of state-owned enterprises (SOE) and other government employees were covered by the Labour Insurance Scheme (LIS) and the Government Insurance Scheme (GIS).

In the post-reform era after 1978, 'old' systems of health have struggled to meet the needs of China's rapidly changing society. Challenges are often reflected in China's review of health and social sectors presented in recent 'Five Year Strategic Plan' policies (*Wunian Jihua*). From the early 1980s to 2003, China's health system sharply transformed into a market-oriented one, which has been criticized for decreasing health access because it has increased out-of-pocket expenditures, led to catastrophic expenses, widened rural–urban inequalities and caused a slowdown in health improvements [42]. Other issues include over-prescription of pharmaceutical drugs, lack of health workers, and an overburden in hospitals and the tertiary sector. For migrants, the healthcare system has been inadequately in tune with the dual rural–urban risks of the moving populations. Most challenging has been the transfer of migrant health insurance.

## New Rural Cooperative Medical Scheme: challenge for rural–urban migrants

In 2003, the voluntary New Rural Cooperative Medical Scheme (NRCMS/NCMS) was formally introduced to extend inpatient and outpatient coverage to rural residents. The funding schemes vary by county. By 2009, the NCMS had been successful in reaching 91.5 per cent of the rural population in 2,729 counties. The 2008 government contribution covered an average of 80 per cent of the costs while households contributed the other 20 per cent [43]. Since 2005, the Urban Resident Basic Medical Insurance scheme (URBMI) was reformed to benefit formal sector workers with basic medical insurance along with their children, the elderly, people with disabilities and other non-working urban residents. However, despite a theoretical coverage existing, the above two systems have little flexibility for migrants to transfer their health insurance if needed.

Although many rural–urban migrants are covered by the NCMS, there are barriers and policies that restrict health care for people with a rural *hukou*. The NCMS policies, which are guided by funding decisions made at county level, often require participants to use designated health facilities within the county. Also, though the NCMS pays for out-of-county care, reimbursements are much lower and what is covered is often inadequate. In 2006, a study of two large provinces that send out many migrants found that 55.2 per cent of migrants who used inpatient services received no reimbursement from the NCMS. The procedures for reimbursement were found to be long, cumbersome and unpleasant [44]. In 2010, national policies called for fewer barriers to medical insurance transfer for migrants [45]. Other concerns to be considered by policy makers include lower utilization rates of 'designated' health facilities in rural NCMS counties by migrants and the inequity of financial resources in different geographical locations. Some regions are wealthier than others and there are more resources for their populations.

## Employment-based mechanisms for migrant health coverage

Another health coverage option is emerging in many cities for migrant workers and there often exist unanimous prerequisites for valid employment before migrants can be registered into this type of scheme. Many have been successfully implemented to provide contributions that help insure migrants' direct medical costs. In urban areas throughout China, migrant worker health insurance schemes are designed based on each city's system so there is much variance. Some differences include the levels of premiums and co-payments, waiting periods, reimbursement levels, deductibles and ceilings, whether the coverage is linked to occupational injury or retirement insurance (as they are in Shanghai and Chengdu) and the designation of health facilities to be used.

For example, programmes such as the Medical Insurance System for Migrant Employees (MISM) in Shenzhen, China's first Special Economic Zone (SEZ) and the largest migrant city [46] have ambitious goals for universal coverage for all migrant workers. The insurance system developed quickly from a trial scheme in March 2005 to a programme covering more than 5.3 million migrant workers by 2011 through 700 designated health facilities. This was an 8.9 per cent increase in annual coverage [47]. Following a State Council Guideline document addressing critical migrant worker issues in 2006, health insurance reforms were also initiated in some other pioneer cities including Shanghai, Beijing and Chengdu [48]. Coverage rates ranged from 21.5 per cent in Beijing to 75 per cent in Shenzhen. Migrant health insurance schemes are supplemented with Coordinative Severe Disease Reimbursement Networks, which aim at avoiding catastrophic costs caused by severe diseases among insured migrants.

Although pioneer health insurance schemes in China's big cities are decentralized and financed through local government input, deficiencies such as a lack of a national transfer mechanism, high deductibles, low reimbursement rates, undesirable coverage, and exclusion of the unemployed and those who are employed in informal sectors are major challenges to be targeted for further policy improvement. While the dispute regarding the significance of personal medical savings accounts is pending and insurance transfer is currently rare for rural–urban migrants, the challenges of providing insurance for migrants – high physical mobility and complex patterns of migration, existence of less addressed 'invisible' populations (i.e. unemployed women, the elderly and children), fluctuating uptake rates and instability – are grey zones and may lead to catastrophic results for certain sub-populations.

Migrant children are particularly vulnerable to not being covered or being covered insufficiently by health insurance. This is due to their lower socio-economic status and because parents are often constrained by limited income and low awareness of insurance programmes [18]. Generally, there is a paucity of research on health access of migrant children in China.

### *Health service challenges*

The increasing demand and reforms to provide much broader and deeper insurance coverage have translated into more demand on healthcare resources and services. How to meet migrants' health needs on the provider side is entangled with China's complex and tough health reforms. In response, some major national strategies have been able to achieve better migrant health, improve the quality of care at lower-level facilities, and encourage quality, efficiency and equality of services through primary-care system reforms [49]. One such system is the National Essential Medicine System (NEMS), which was set up to reduce spending on drugs and out-of-pocket expenditures. In a few Chinese pioneer cities such as Shenzhen, implementation of national health reform initiatives have been successfully integrated with local health plans. Of all reforms, moving from a hospital-based towards a community-based care model has been one of the most effective.

## Role of Community Health Centres (CHCs)

CHCs have been an integral part of China's healthcare reform over the last decade. In Shenzhen, 634 CHCs employ more than 50,000 health workers – a rapid growth from less than 300 CHCs operational in 2005 [46]. The emergence and expanded existence of CHCs in many Chinese cities has had a significant impact on migrant health because of the affordability and accessibility of essential medical care at community level that CHCs provide. Zero mark-up policies and zero dispensing fee policies have broken collusion between providers and the pharmaceutical sector, thus reducing drug prices and overall healthcare costs. This growing trend has been especially helpful for migrants who are uninsured or unemployed, and the urban poor overall. For the most part, large cities in China have adopted strategies that bind migrant workers' insurance with CHCs and, as a result, CHCs are the first point of contact for migrants who are seeking health services.

Other supposed benefits of the CHC network expansion (which are likewise challenges in many places) include strengthened training for general practitioners; enhanced CHC infrastructures in migrant communities; flexible office hours aimed at migrant workers' schedules; resource allocation for Traditional Chinese Medicine integration, mental health, children and maternal health; supply of basic preventive medicine/public health packages; and vertically integrated delivery systems via new referral mechanisms regulated by insurance guidelines.

## Further challenges to healthcare services

Recent changes to the healthcare system have aimed to reduce health inequity and improve health outcomes of migrants, but the reforms have yet to be fully tested for long-term effectiveness. Based on limited evidence that evaluates the impact of recent reforms, such as medical insurance plans and primary-care centred initiatives for better migrant health outcomes and utilization, inequities still remain. There are gaps in insurance coverage, problems in monitoring and evaluating systems to ensure general health quality and barriers to sufficient health access [41]. Thus, close monitoring of the implementation throughout the healthcare system and scientific evaluations of effectiveness/performance are warranted.

Other challenges of migrant health are also issues for the whole system. These include a lack of qualified general practitioners, insufficient funding for central and western small cities and poorly incorporated medical records at different care levels [50]. Additional factors such as migrant-specific health-seeking tendencies – self-medication, and disease neglect and delay – compound the challenge of providing effective and quality healthcare services. These need to be addressed by healthcare policy makers and providers throughout the system.

Tracking migrant populations is also a challenge in China's healthcare reform. To implement national health insurance transferability, some policy makers have suggested the implementation of a unique identifier link to people's personal insurance cards that permits a separation between the registration and care utilization locations of migratory individuals. It is suggested that the current schemes, administrative institutions and networks should be integrated and interconnected, and that a citizen-based, universal, nationwide health insurance scheme is needed [51]. There are overwhelming technical barriers to establishing a nationwide electronic medical records (EMR) system [52] of linking insurance systems in different cities. Administrative and institutional barriers also exist, including unbalanced economic development, social situations (including whether it is a migrant-sending or migrant-receiving society), enforcement on employers' sponsorship, financial prosperity of each region and financial pressure to increase subsidies/benefits.

## Health improvement: focus on prevention of non-communicable diseases (NCDs)

Despite China's success over the last twenty years, changes in the urban lifestyle associated with dietary patterns, unhealthy behaviours and pollution have led to the rapid increase of NCD-related risk factors, particularly among low-income groups and migrants (of whom women, children and the left-behind are of most concern). Since migrants form the majority of China's population growth due to urbanization and because escalating health inequities persist, there are major health improvement issues facing migrant communities. Among issues to address is the promotion of healthy lifestyles to prevent rapidly rising rates of NCDs. This includes health promotion in response to risk factors for migrants at a community level and takes into account such factors as smoking, mental health illness (including depression, addiction and suicide), injury, inadequate women's health (breast cancer, maternal health, sex education, etc.) and occupational disease risks. Greater risks, compounded by reduced health access and lower awareness, highlight health improvement needs for Chinese migrants.

### *Tobacco*

Some studies on rural–urban migrants in China have shown that increased smoking prevalence and nicotine dependence are positively associated with migration. Studies have found that solitude, urban 'maladaptation' and the migratory process are significant reasons for migrants to smoke [53]. Migrant workers have been found to be more likely to smoke if they are male, earn higher incomes, and have greater mobility and whose durations of migration are longer. Few studies have been done on women, as they are generally much less likely to smoke, but exposure to female cigarette brands and marketing may increase the susceptibility to smoking among rural-to-urban migrant women [54].

However, not all studies showed increased smoking prevalence in migrants. One study found lower rates of smoking among migrant factory workers in Shenzhen compared to the general Chinese population [55]. This study, however, identified a high-risk group of male migrant factory workers who smoked heavily and consumed alcohol more frequently than others, showing that longer working hours and a lack of rest were associated with higher rates of smoking. It also found that frequent Internet use and lack of insurance were associated with lifetime smoking and with poorer mental health. Increased accumulated working time in the city increased female workers' likelihood of smoking as well. These findings point towards risk amongst migrant worker populations, supporting other studies attributing the migratory lifestyle (i.e. solitude, stress and increasing but still low-level income) with smoking initiation and heavy smoking.

Although there are no data currently available specifically on smoking-attributable mortality in China's migrant populations, China is the world leader in tobacco consumption and smoking-related deaths (lung cancer). Therefore, understanding smoking patterns of China's migrants and related factors may help to effectively provide health promotion interventions for this population. Challenges in providing effective health education to migrants may include how to address these migratory factors and focus on high-risk sub-groups. For example, it is suggested that future tobacco control programmes focus on the psychological issues facing migrants. Other solutions involve multi-level intervention through schools, workplaces and households in the migrant aggregated communities. Internet cafés, which are venues for male migrants to smoke and drink while using the Internet, may be appropriate locations for more intensive interventions.

## *Mental health*

Evidence has shown that China's rural–urban migrants suffer from lower mental health status than both local urban residents and their rural counterparts in communities from which they emigrate. There is a possible deteriorative effect of the migratory experience on mental health status among migrants, and an urgent need for etiological studies, mental health promotion and prevention efforts among this growing population. In 2010, several migrants working in one of the major contract manufacturers of China, Foxconn, committed suicide, drawing immense media and public attention. This is an extreme example of the severe mental health issues that exist among young workers, especially young second-generation factory migrant workers. However, facing an emerging public health problem as such, there is low awareness, deeply rooted stigma, professional shortage of mental health staff and poorly integrated care [56]. Provision of mental healthcare services and screening is not well developed in China and, until recently, suicide was not even included in Chinese psychiatric texts.

Development of mental health services that improve screening, diagnosis and treatment for migrant populations and other high-risk groups is urgently needed. Suicide is a leading cause of death in young people in China [57]. Some universal risk factors of suicidal ideation/attempts have been found, which point to younger females, smokers, heavy drinkers, those with family history of suicide, those with a lack of social support and those who have migrated [58]. Migration, together with poverty and deprivation, income inequality, occupational stress and social discrimination, has been found to be causally linked with mental health of Chinese youth. Depression and addressing developmental disorders are under-researched in China, but the harm of low self-esteem and unmet migrant child social and health support have proven effects on future health behaviours and risk factors.

The mental health status of left-behind children and the elderly, of which depressive symptoms and anxiety are the most frequently cited problems, also warrants further attention and intervention. In addition to policy and system change to address service provision, revision of health policy frameworks and promotion of social equity, scholars articulate that mental health literacy is an essential life skill that must be taught before the need arises.

## *Women's health*

Although there are dramatic sex ratio disparities occurring in China with many more males being born than females – 118.08 males for every 100 females in 2010, according to the China National Population and Family Planning Commission – there is still an ever-increasing number of young female migrant workers. The World Bank has reported that many women in migrant populations have low incomes and poor living conditions, such as lack of winter heating in the northern parts of the country and small living areas. Current studies amongst this sub-population have highlighted low immunity to rubella [59], higher rates of STDs (for example, chlamydia infection) [60], poor provision of maternal health (antenatal care, abortion, reproductive health) and other higher behavioural risk factors.

Analysis on maternal mortality rates in Beijing, Shanghai and Guangzhou from 2000 to 2002 showed that maternal mortality of migrant women from rural areas in big cities was significantly higher than that of city women, with many of the deaths being caused by direct obstetric reasons that would have been avoidable with proper education and/or services [61]. Other studies have substantiated that reproductive health needs of young unmarried female migrants, workers especially, are not being adequately met and they are often unable to access information and services [62, 63]. Although young female migrants are sexually active, many lack basic knowledge of contraception and reproductive health and do not use reproductive health services [63]. Unmet needs for contraception are issues and there is a need to enhance open communication on sexual health by government sources, and to increase the availability of education materials, condoms and other services.

The health issues pertaining to many migrant women can be attributed to poor sexual health education, especially amongst women from rural China moving to urban areas, as well as a lack of policies supporting migrant women's health in their urban areas. For example, the prevalence of chlamydia for Chinese migrant women was found to be triple that of rural non-migrant women [60]. Attitudes and low knowledge rates are also partially due to reasons such as the stigma that pre-marital sex is a taboo, discrimination of pregnant migrant women (which denies female migrants' legitimate leave for doctor visits) and higher biological vulnerability of certain diseases in females. Under such circumstances, maternal health services, as well as other risk prevention programmes specifically designed for migrant women and covered by insurance schemes, are urgently needed in China. Employment-based health education might be initiated to add efficiency and cultural responsiveness.

### *Culture, social stigma and the healthy migrant effects*

The study of culture and social stigma effects on migrant health in China is incredibly complex. Generally, how migrants perceive and experience health, disease and the healthcare system, has not been sufficiently studied in literature even though culture and stigma play a role in public health in practice. Migrants face different social stigmas than the rest of the general population. Stereotyping, separation, status loss, discrimination, unfair treatment and exclusion are some challenges they may encounter which may affect their mental and physical wellbeing. There are some key factors to be considered in this domain which can be seen in Figure 3.3.

*Education*: Research shows that a lack of secondary education among migrants makes them more likely to become migrant labourers. The majority of rural–urban migrants only have a junior middle school education which is a consideration for health promotion.

*Other social determinants*: Language skills and integration in new communities (including housing, employment, environment, etc.) are also factors that affect health outcomes to varying degrees. Social characteristics are major influencers on health.

*Traditional healing*: Impacts of health seeking behaviours in rural areas of origination are important. Self-medication, informal healers, traditional medicine and misconceptions of private clinic versus hospital treatment are considerations. Traditional models of medicine and healing play a tremendous role in health-related behaviours in migrants. Understanding them is crucial in developing culturally appropriate initiatives.

*Geography and duration of stay*: Geographical mobility and transitions are challenging life changes for migrants. When expected duration of stay in a given location is limited, there are disincentives for migrants to invest time and money in insurance programmes, personal health and safety measures. Conscious and unconscious trading of poor future health for present economic opportunity has been discussed.

*Figure 3.3* Ideas to consider when discussing social stigma faced by migrants

### Healthy migrant effect

Although there are numerous public health issues that stem from migration, one of the most important phenomena relates to the 'healthy migrant effect' (or the 'healthy immigrant effect' (HIE)), which has been proved by many studies. The 'healthy migrant effect' refers to lower mortality rates of first-generation permanent migrants, which is attributable to self-selection of healthy migrants, but may also be attributable to the fact that unhealthy migrants who have gone back home for health care or have become unemployed are not captured in migrant studies [64]. For example, in the Zhejiang Province of eastern China, migrant self-reported health was better and migrants were less likely to report acute illness, chronic disease and disability than permanent rural or urban residents [64].

Migration is an important factor in economic growth that may improve health, both directly and indirectly. In 2005, not only did urban migrants send home the equivalent of US$65.4 billion, but they also acted as information 'bridges' between advanced cities and less-developed rural areas.

However, studies on healthcare access and utilization indicators have mostly reported on the inequities among Chinese rural-to-urban migrants. In addition to inequities between local residents and migrants in health utilization rates, health-seeking patterns of the most vulnerable migrant groups, such as females, the unemployed, the elderly and children, are concerns in academic and policy sectors. Issues have been gradually addressed and reconstructed in the background of the current national health reforms, which focus on evolving health policies to encourage insurance schemes as well as primary-care centred services to allow better healthcare accessibility for the Chinese internal migrants.

## Response to migrant health challenges: lessons

By addressing migrants, and those most vulnerable and at-risk for disease, China is able to address public health from a stance of health equity and from a perspective of the social determinants of health. Throughout this chapter we have discussed the key public health challenges facing migrants in the domains of health protection, health services and health improvement. It is clear from the literature that some migrant groups are at risk of socio-economic disadvantage and poorer health, though further research and policy will need to be done to improve our understanding. Addressing the issue of migrants in public health in China is strategic and helpful to predict future population health issues as migrants are a reflection of current society and a group much too large to be ignored. Lessons learned from policy making for migrants are compatible with public health improvement throughout China.

### *Lessons from the health protection perspective*

From a health protection perspective, China has made great strides in addressing migrant issues, mostly in large cities where stimulating economic growth is a priority. Factors for success have included:

- Government acknowledgement of the role of migration in infectious diseases;
- Creation of policies supporting universal coverage followed by strict implementation;
- Allocation of financial resources towards migrant issues; and
- Expansion of information and surveillance systems.

Since the national health sector reform in 2000, China has developed its CDCs' network in the country to incorporate anti-epidemic stations and public health programmes [65]. The SARS epidemic in 2003 challenged China's public health infrastructure and the government significantly prioritized funding for public health. A national Internet-based communicable disease reporting system was implemented in 2004 [66].

TB policies and integration of services supported by the government have improved TB control significantly. With TB budgets increasing nearly seven-fold by 2005, China has been able to achieve the global targets for TB control [67]. However, differences in quality and access due to stakeholder motivations and resource allocation still exist between more affluent east China and poorer west China, and for migrants without health insurance [66]. HIV/AIDS policies have also improved through initiatives such as the 'Four Frees and One Care' policy, China's Comprehensive AIDS Response Programme (China CARES), improved laboratory facilities, a free national antiretroviral (ART) programme and strong international collaboration; all supported by the State Council AIDS working committee chaired by a vice premier with 29 ministers and 7 local provincial governors [67]. By the end of 2006, there were 393 national HIV sentinel surveillance sites in all 31 provinces and 370 provincial sentinel sites following national HIV surveillance protocol. Diagnosis and treatment of TB and HIV/AIDS is free for migrants in some areas, but the literature has highlighted an uneven distribution of sentinel surveillance sites, insufficient coverage and poor targeted surveillance for migrants. There is definitely still a need to further address migrants in infectious disease policies.

Since 2005, migrant children could receive free EPI immunizations throughout the country, regardless of their *hukou*. This policy has been effective in covering children nationwide and overall there has been immense improvement (e.g. eradication of wild-type poliomyelitis). The next steps will be to raise the immunization rates for some migrant children and to address cost challenges for non-EPI covered immunizations. Inequalities of coverage rates for migrant children and outbreaks of rabies and measles should be addressed by policies that focus more on behaviours, barriers to access and health service quality of CHCs. Supplementary immunization activities administer up to 2 million doses of measles vaccines each year [68]; however, catch-up campaigns may miss migrant children, especially if they are unplanned or unregistered births. Vaccination campaigns for controlling measles in migrant populations have proven successful in the Guangdong Province using comprehensive mobilization, communication with the mass media and support from government departments [69].

China has also improved its policies and laws on employer responsibilities to migrant workers in the workplace, including their safety and health protection. Such policies include the Labour Contract Law which holds employers accountable if working conditions and environment negatively impacts on the physical and mental health of the employee. The Law of the PRC on Work Safety iterates employers' obligations to reduce the risk of industrial accidents and mandates local governments to monitor workplaces [70]. At an international level, the Chinese government has ratified the International Covenant on Economic, Social and Cultural Rights and ILO Conventions, which in principle commits China's support of labour rights and worker protection. However, questions have been raised about the implementation of the laws, as well as capacity for reinforcement. Thus, monitoring and evaluation of policies from an occupational and environmental health perspective need to be of utmost importance. There is a need for complete, accurate and up-to-date data and research to facilitate policies and interventions.

Environmental health policies do not address migrants for the most part, but strides towards acknowledging environmental health have been positive. The 2008 Beijing Olympics

Air Pollution policies were successful and since then the Beijing municipal government launched 14 phases of air pollution control, which resulted in a gradual increase in the number of blue sky days each year. China recently released its first National Environment and Health Action Plan which emphasizes the need to coordinate activities across many sectors and ministries. It identifies coordinated and shared data collection and environmental monitoring as a crucial feature of future environmental health policies. Environmental sustainability was addressed in China's eleventh five-year plan, which reiterated the intention to reduce greenhouse-gas emissions per unit gross domestic [71]. However, migrants and the increased risks from environmental hazards are largely ignored in policy.

### *Lessons from the health services perspective*

From a health services perspective, migrants have benefited most from reforms when they are:

- Clear and targeted policies that address well-defined populations;
- Supported by primary care at community level; and
- Implemented innovatively to reach hard-to-track migrants.

Reforms that are clearly targeted for well-defined migrant populations, such as the expansion of migrant worker insurance schemes and building more CHCs in urban areas with many rural–urban migrants, are the most effective and are more likely to be well implemented. For example, between August 2010 and December 2011, Chongqing, one of the five national central cities in China, awarded full urban-welfare rights to 3 million migrants in its rural areas [72]. Nearby in Chengdu, the capital of the Sichuan Province, there are plans to eliminate welfare-related barriers to migration through an integration of health insurance for rural and urban residents [72, 73]. Reforms impose a big financial burden on local governments, but this region is relatively wealthy and migrants are acknowledged and well defined in regional policy. This shows that health reform policies must also be community-centred.

Besides acknowledging the needs of migrants in health service sectors, other challenges include how to ensure universal access for migrants if they move from place to place and how to provide universal implementation of quality services between different levels of government. Shenzhen made bold moves towards insuring migrant children for inpatient care and outpatient care for severe diseases. Though the city was first to implement a compulsory health insurance scheme that covers all children and juveniles despite child registration status [74], enforcement of policy may be affected due to the lack of information amongst migrants especially if their children do not go to public schools where such information is distributed. In the city, most migrant children attend private institutions because they are not registered to use local schools. The policies must target migrant populations the right way and reach them in the right places. Additionally, goals for the universal health coverage of unregistered migrant children regardless of their *hukou* should be prioritized as a national policy agenda.

Improved health innovation and technology in a highly mobile population is key in tracking migrants and providing good services. To reduce the mismatch between the migrant management system data and the real number of information about migrants, some pioneer cities like Shenzhen started to implement a new Resident Card System (RCS). Initiated in August 2008, the free-of-charge RCS is linked to migrant health insurance, occupational safety insurance and the retirement pension system, and it is anticipated it will be linked with low-rent/low-cost housing. According to statistics from the Shenzhen Public Security Bureau, the RCS covered 10.71 million migrants in the city up to December 2009. However, the RCS may face the difficulty of excluding those who move out of Shenzhen since no measure has been taken to record migrants' departure, whether their stay was long or short term [75].

### *Lessons from the health improvement perspective*

From a health improvement perspective, lessons from China suggest public health programmes can be effective if they are:

- Implemented at community level for migrants using an integrated approach;
- Culturally sensitive to migrant needs and health beliefs; and
- Supported by national policies supporting specific health priorities.

Although central government policies may allow migrants to receive care, service programmes that are not implemented at community level specifically for migrants may not reach them. Instead, migrants may turn to other informal sources of health information such as uninformed mass media or word of mouth. For example, studies have discussed the need for new strategies by the government to provide appropriate, specific, friendly and accessible services about reproductive health for unmarried young migrant women [76] because although there are services available, migrant women are not using them.

Integrated programmes and policies are also important in addressing health improvement issues. Tobacco has been discussed as a risk factor for the future health of young female migrants, and while it is necessary to have community cessation programmes, studies have stressed the importance of integrated programmes for tobacco control, which include government involvement and corporate responsibility. For example, tobacco control advocates have explored regulations to restrict packaging on, and advertisement for, female-targeted cigarette brands as these female cigarette brands have been shown to have strong associations with current smoking rates amongst female migrants (OR 5.69, 95 per cent CI 3.44 to 9.41) [54]. In 2008, joint government bodies released the Regulations on Cigarette Packaging and Labelling in the Territories of the People's Republic of China (the Labelling Regulations) [77]. However, new cigarette package design did not eventually comply with the requirements due to poor regulation. This is an example of how better implementation and monitoring of tobacco restrictions and requirements is necessary to promote healthy lifestyles. Similarly, to improve mental health among migrants, scholars have also highlighted that for programmes to be successful, they need to bridge the gaps between academic, governmental and community sectors, and migrants themselves [78].

Health improvement efforts must also be culturally sensitive to migrants' needs and health beliefs. For example, to improve the mental health of rural–urban migrants, it is vital to provide public education programmes to help them understand their mental health and provide mental health services to support this. However, how to do this effectively requires understanding of impacts of stigmatization and discrimination of these groups. It has been hypothesized that stigmatization affects social isolation and social adjustment, and that this is exacerbated by numerous demographic and psychosocial factors [78]. Therefore, to address public mental health for migrants, who represent many different narratives, interventions and services should be evidence-based and carried out cautiously. To improve women's health, understanding patterns of how health risks are distributed among sub-groups of female migrants tagged by their region of origin, migratory history and occupation is fundamental in order to build successful health promotion initiatives.

## Conclusion: moving public health forward for migrants in Asia

The geographical breadth of China and the mobility of migrants present challenges for public health. Given the complexities and wide breadth of health issues discussed in this chapter, promotion of public health in an age of migration will need to focus on the shifting patterns of migration and their effects, support populations of migrants with a focus on health equity and require efforts at all levels of society.

China's migration challenges are seen elsewhere in Asia and throughout the world. Although groups of migrants and the narratives will differ, lessons can be shared between countries to develop strategies, coordinate global health systems and adapt successful policies.

## References


1. Decree of the President of the People's Republic of China. Regulations on Household Registration in the People's Republic of China. January 9, 1958.
2. White, L.T. Deviance, modernization, rations, and household register in urban China, in Amy Auerbacher Wilson, Sidney Leonard Greenblatt, and Richard Whittingham Wilson (eds) *Deviance and Social Control in Chinese Society*, Praeger Publishers (1977), pp. 151–172.
3. Perry, E. J., and Selden, M. (eds) (2003). *Chinese Society: Change, conflict, and resistance*. London: RoutledgeCurzon.
4. International Organization of Migration. *Key Migration Terms*. Retrieved from: http://www.iom.int/jahia/Jahia/about-migration/key-migration-terms/lang/en#Push-pull-factors
5. Zhao, Y., and Liu, Q. (1997). A historical study of rural-to-urban migration in China: 1949–1985. *Chinese Journal of Population Science*, 9(3), 239–53.
6. Beijing Planning Office of Philosophy and Social Science. (2004). *Contemporary China's Floating Population* (Chinese). Retrieved from: http://www.bjpopss.gov.cn/bjpssweb/n10513c48.aspx
7. Ministry of Labour and Social Security. *On Widening Migrant Workers' Participation in Health Insurance Schemes*. Retrieved from: http://trs.molss.gov.cn/was40/mainframe.htm
8. Migrant population in China has reached 211 million. (2010). *People's Daily Newspaper*. Retrieved from: http://news.China.com.cn/rollnews/2010-06/26/content_2882643.htm
9. The Ministry of Public Security of the People's Republic of China. *Ministry Public Order No. 25*. Retrieved from: http://www.mps.gov.cn/n16/n1282/n3493/n3823/n443822/456893.html
10. Yue, Z., Li, S., Feldmen, M., and Du, H. (2010). Floating choices: a generational perspective on intentions of rural–urban migrants in China. *Environment and Planning*, 42, 545–62.
11. Hu, X., Cook, S., and Salazar, M. A. (2008). Internal migration and health in China. *Lancet*, 372(9651), 1717–19.
12. International Organization of Migration. *Migration & Gender*. Retrieved from: http://www.iom.int/jahia/Jahia/about-migration/developing-migration-policy/migration-gender
13. Chiang, Y. L., Hannum, E., and Kao, G. (2012, May). *Who Goes, Who Stays, and Who Studies? Gender, Migration, and Educational Decisions among Rural Youth in China*. University of Pennsylvania Department of Sociology Paper. Retrieved from: http://repository.upenn.edu/cgi/viewcontent.cgi?article=1030&context=gansu_papers
14. Gong, P., *et al.* (2012). Urbanisation and health in China. *Lancet*, 379(9818), 843–52.
15. Gao, Y., Li, L. P., Kim, J. H., Congdon, N., Lau, J., and Griffiths, S. (2010). The impact of parental migration on health status and health behaviours among left behind adolescent school children in China. *BMC Public Health*, 10, 56.
16. Liu, Z., Li, X., and Ge, X. (2009). Left too early: the effects of age at separation from parents on Chinese rural children's symptoms of anxiety and depression. *American Journal of Public Health*, 99(11), 2049–54.

17. State Council's Report. (2006). *Summary Report of Rural Migrant Workers in China.*
18. Fong, H. F. (2011). Policy implications of migration on the immunization of Chinese migrant children in Hong Kong and Shenzhen. Unpublished doctoral dissertation, The Chinese University of Hong Kong, Hong Kong, China.
19. McGivering, J. (2009, February 18). Aids takes deadly toll in China. *BBC News*. Retrieved from: http://news.bbc.co.uk/2/hi/asia-pacific/7896133.stm
20. Parish, W. L., Laumann, E. O., Cohen, M. S., *et al.* (2003). Population-based study of chlamydia infection in China. *JAMA*, 289, 1265–73.
21. Qian, Z. H., Vermund, S. H., and Wang, N. (2005). Risk of HIV/AIDS in China: subpopulations of special importance. *Sexually Transmitted Infections*, 81, 442–7.
22. Zheng, J., Zhou, Y., Wang, H., and Liang, X. (2010). The role of the China Experts Advisory Committee on Immunization Program. *Vaccine*, 28 Suppl 1, A84–7.
23. Mikolajczyk, R. T., Akmatov, M. K., Stich, H., Krämer, A., and Kretzschmar, M. (2008). Association between acculturation and childhood vaccination coverage in migrant populations: a population based study from a rural region in Bavaria, Germany. *International Journal of Public Health*, 53(4), 180–7.
24. Kim, S. S., Frimpong, J. A., Rivers, P. A., and Kronenfeld, J. J. (2007). Effects of maternal and provider characteristics on up-to-date immunization status of children aged 19 to 35 months. *American Journal of Public Health*, 97(2), 259–66.
25. World Health Organization. (2006). Joint Review on the Maternal and Child Survival Strategy in China. Retrieved from WHO WPRO publications online: http://www.wpro.who.int/NR/rdonlyres/E6 C29183-BC8E-4DEF-9A503606032E8CB4/0/MaternalandChildSurvivalStrategyinChinaENG.pdf
26. Cheng, Z., Ni, J., and Wang, S. (2007) Epidemiology characteristics of measles in the status of high coverage of MV and discussion on the necessity of immunization strategy adjustment. *Chinese Journal of Disease Control*, 11: 10–14.13.
27. Zheng, L. Q. Resurge of measles in China. *Health News* (Beijing), June 8, 2007. Retrieved from: http://www.chinacdc.net.cn/n272442/n272530/n272817/n272862/17878.html (accessed June 23, 2008).
28. Sun, M., Ma, R., Zeng, Y., Luo, F., Zhang, J., and Hou, W. (2010). Immunization status and risk factors of migrant children in densely populated areas of Beijing, China. *Vaccine*, 28(5), 1264–74.
29. Guo, W., Feng, Z., and Diao, L. (2000). Investigation of immunization status in children of floating population in Henan Province. *Zhonghua Yu Fang Yi Xue Za Zhi*, 34(5), 287–9.
30. Wang, Y. Y., Wang, Y., Zhang, J. X., Kang, C. Y., and Duan, P. (2007). Status of mother's KAP on child immunization in minority areas, Guizhou Province. *Beijing Da Xue Xue Bao*, 39(2), 136–9.
31. Global Forum for Health Research. Equitable Access: Research Challenges for Health in Developing Countries. Report on *Forum* 11, October 29–November 2, 2007, Beijing. Retrieved from: http://www.isn.ethz.ch/isn/Digital-Library/Publications/Detail/?ots591=0c54e3b3-1e9c-be1e-2c24- a6a8c7060233&lng=en&id=55106
32. Tobe, R. G., Xu, L., Song, P., and Huang, Y. (2001). The rural-to-urban migrant population in China: gloomy prospects for tuberculosis control. *Bioscience Trends*, 5(6), 226–30.
33. Jackson, S., Sleigh, A. C., Wang, G. J., and Liu, X. L. (2006). Poverty and the economic effects of TB in rural China. *International Journal of Tuberculosis and Lung Disease*, 10(10), 1104–10.
34. Wang, X., *et al.* (2011). Occupational health and safety challenges in China: focusing on township–village enterprises. *Archives of Environmental and Occupational Health*, 66(1), 3–11.
35. Zheng, Z., and Lian, P. (2005). Health vulnerability among temporary migrants in urban China. International Population Conference. Tours, France.
36. Occupational diseases haunt migrant workers. (2006, February 17). *China Daily*. Retrieved from: http://english.gov.cn/2006-02/17/content_202437.htm
37. China's State Council. (2006). *China Migrant Worker Investigation and Research Report.*
38. Government of People's Republic of China. (2011). United Nations Development Programme (UNDP) Project Document. Retrieved from: http://www.undp.org.cn/projectdocs/53962.pdf
39. Huo, X., *et al.* (2007, July). Elevated blood lead levels of children in Guiyu, an electronic waste recycling town in China. *Environmental Health Perspectives*, 115(7), 1113–17.
40. Tan, Y., and Guo, F. (2009, September). Environmentally induced migration in West China. Paper from the XXVI IUSSP International Population Conference. Morocco. Retrieved from: http://iussp2009.princeton.edu/download.aspx?submissionId=92044

41. Mou, J., Cheng, J., Dan, Z. D., Jiang, H., Lin, L., and Griffiths, S. M. (2009). Health care utilisation amongst Shenzhen migrant workers: does being insured make a difference? *BMC Health Services Research*, 9, 214.
42. Wagstaff, A., Yip, W., Lindelow, M., and Hsiao, W. C. (2009). China's health system and its reform: a review of recent studies. *Health Economics*, 18, S7–S23.
43. World Health Organization. (2009). Health care financing in rural China: new rural cooperative medical scheme. Retrieved from: http://www.who.int/health_financing/documents/pb_e_09_03-china_ nrcms.pdf
44. Guo, J., Liu, X., and Zhu, X. (2007). Migrant workers are not covered by NCMS (Chinese). *Outlook Weekly*, 47(2), S12.
45. China Ministry of Human Resources and Social Security, Ministry of Health, and Ministry of Finance. (2010). *Provisional Measures on the Transfer and Renewal of Medical Insurance of Migrant Workers.*
46. Zhang, D., Mou, J., Cheng, J. Q., and Griffiths, S. M. (2011). Public health services in Shenzhen: a case study. *Public Health*, 125(1), 15–19.
47. Shenzhen Government. Retrieved from: http://www.szsi.gov.cn/zxbs/wscx/ddyb/dg/201111/P020120706417068597872.xls
48. Li, Z., and Yang, J. M. (2009). Comparative study on the medical insurance models for the migrant populations in urban cities in China (Chinese). *Population Research*, 33(3). Retrieved from: http://www.youngmigrants.org/ew/uploadfile/20110324124653668.pdf
49. Liu, Q., Wang, B., Kong, Y., and Cheng, K. K. (2011). China's primary health-care reform. *Lancet*, 377(9783), 2064–6.
50. Li, X., *et al.* (2012). Predictors on delay of initial health-seeking in new pulmonary tuberculosis cases among migrant population in East China. *PLOSOne*, 7(2), e31995.
51. Meng, Q., and Tang, S. (2010). *Universal Coverage of Health Care in China: Challenges and opportunities.* WHO World Health Report: Health systems financing. Retrieved from: http://www.who.int/healthsystems/topics/financing/healthreport/7ChinaM_T.pdf
52. Tu, H., *et al.* (2012). Building clinical data groups for electronic medical records in China. *Journal of Medical Systems*, 36, 723–36.
53. Yang, T., *et al.* (2009). Smoking patterns among Chinese rural–urban migrant workers. *Public Health*, 123(11), 743–9.
54. Wan X., *et al.* (2011). Smoking among young rural to urban migrant women in China: a cross-sectional survey. *PLOSOne*, 6(8), e23028.
55. Mou, J., Fellmeth, G., Griffiths, S., Dawes, M., and Cheng, J. (2012). Tobacco smoking among migrant factory workers in Shenzhen, China. *Nicotine & Tobacco Research*. doi: 10.1093/ntr/nts085.
56. Lau, J. T., *et al.* (2012). Suicides in a mega-size factory in China: poor mental health among young migrant workers in China (Letter). *Occupational and Environmental Medicine*. Retrieved from: http://oem.bmj.com/content/early/2012/02/27/oemed-2011-100593.full
57. Phillips, M. R., Li, X., and Zhang, Y. (2002). Suicide rates in China, 1995–99. *Lancet*, 359, 835–40.
58. Blum, R., Sudhinaraset, M., and Emerson, M. R. (2012). Youth at risk: suicidal thoughts and attempts in Vietnam, China, and Taiwan. *Journal of Adolescent Health*, 50(3), S37–44.
59. Mou, J., Griffiths, S. M., Fong, H. F., Hu, Q., He, Y., Ma, H., and Cheng, J. (2010). Seroprevalence of rubella in female migrant factory workers in Shenzhen, China. *Vaccine*, 28(50), 7844–51.
60. Wang, W. *et al.* (2010). Prevalence and risks for sexually transmitted infections among a national sample of migrants versus non-migrants in China. *International Journal of STD & AIDS*, 21(6), 410–15.
61. Zhao, Q., Kulane, A., Gao, Y., and Xu, B. (2009). Knowledge and attitude on maternal health care among rural-to-urban migrant women in Shanghai, China. *BMC Women's Health*, 9, 5.
62. Lu, C., *et al.* (2012, January). Sexual and reproductive health status and related knowledge among female migrant workers in Guangzhou, China: a cross sectional survey. *European Journal of Obstetrics & Gynecology and Reproductive Biology*, 160(1), 60–5.
63. WHO Department of Reproductive Health and Research. (2002, May). Young female migrant workers in China in need of reproductive health information and services. *Social Science Research Policy Briefs*, 2(2). Retrieved from: www.who.int/reproductivehealth/publications/adolescence/policy_brief_china02.pdf

64. Li, X., Stanton, B., Fang, X., and Lin, D. (2006). Social stigma and mental health among rural-to-urban migrants in China: a conceptual framework and future research needs. *World Health & Population*, 8(3) 14–31.
65. Wang, D., Liu J., and Chin, D. (2007). Progress in tuberculosis control and the evolving public-health system in China. *Lancet*, 369, 691–6.
66. Zou, G., Wei, X., Walley, J. D., and Sun, Q. (2012). Factors influencing integration of TB services in general hospitals in two regions of China: a qualitative study. *BMC Health Services Research*, 12, 21. doi:10.1186/1472-6963-12-21
67. Wang, L., *et al.* (2008). Emergence and control of infectious diseases in China. *Lancet*, 372(9649), 1598–605.
68. Zhuo, J., *et al.* (2011). Impact of supplementary immunization activities in measles-endemic areas: a case study from Guangxi, China. *Journal of Infectious Diseases*, 204(suppl 1), S455–62.
69. Peng, Z. Q., *et al.* (2012). Evaluation of the mass measles vaccination campaign in Guangdong Province, China. *International Journal of Infectious Diseases*, 16(2), e99–103.
70. The Law of the People's Republic of China on Work Safety. (2002, June 29). Article 53.
71. Zhang, J., *et al.* (2010). Environmental health in China: progress towards clean air and safe water. *Lancet*, 375, 1110–19.
72. Changing migration patterns: Welcome home. (2012, February 25). *The Economist*. Retrieved from: http://www.economist.com/node/21548273
73. Qiu, P., Yang, Y., Zhang, J., and Ma, X. (2011). Rural-to-urban migration and its implication for new cooperative medical scheme coverage and utilization in China. *BMC Public Health*, 11, 520.
74. Shenzhen Government Online. (2008). Hospitalized and seriously ill children of Shenzhen: outpatient medical provisional measures on insurance. Retrieved from: http://www.szsi.gov.cn/sbjxxgk/zcfggfxwj/zctw/200810/t20081008_738.htm
75. XJRB Online. (2009). Shenzhen's Resident Card System has achieved full coverage in migrants (Chinese). Retrieved from: http://www.xjrb.net/news_view.asp?id=15404
76. Liu, Z., *et al.* (2011). Reproductive health knowledge and service utilization among unmarried rural-to-urban migrants in three migrant cities, China. *BMC Public Health*, 11, 74.
77. Jiang, Y., *et al.* (2009). Effectiveness evaluation of health warnings on cigarette packs in China (Chinese). *Chinese Journal of Health Education*, 25, 411–13.
78. Li, X., Stanton, B., Fang, X., and Lin, D. (2006). Social stigma and mental health among rural-to-urban migrants in China: a conceptual framework and future research needs. *World Health & Population*, 8(3), 14–31.
79. Griffiths, S., Jewell, T., and Donnelly, P. (2005). Public health in practice: the three domains of public health. *Public Health*, 119(10), 907–13.

# 4 The challenges of ageing in Japan

*Tomiko Hokama and Haley L. Cash*

## Introduction

Population ageing is a new and serious challenge for Japan, a country which has achieved the world's longest life expectancy. As Japan's life expectancy has increased over the past decades, its fertility rate has simultaneously decreased resulting in an increased elderly population. As of 2011, the population of Japan was 127.8 million of which 23.3 per cent (29.8 million) were elderly (over 65 years old) [1]. With this astounding figure, Japan currently has the world's highest elderly population.

In this chapter, we will present the challenges of ageing in Japan and the current strategies that are being utilized. We will describe the changes to Japan's population structure that have taken place since 1950 and discuss projected changes for the future. We will then present an overview of the challenges that Japan is currently facing, and will continue to face, due to its increasing elderly population and look at the major health reforms implemented by Japan to combat challenges of an ageing population.

## Japan's ageing population

Figure 4.1 demonstrates the dramatic changes to Japan's population pyramid. In 1950, Japan's age structure was pyramid-shaped with a large population of younger generations. Looking at the 2011 jar-shaped population pyramid, it shows a drastic shift in the age structure, with increased elderly and a substantial middle-aged population, including the two baby booms of 1947–49 and 1971–74. Following the second baby boom, the birth rate dropped considerably, from 19 (per 1,000 population) to 8.3 as of 2011. As this middle-aged generation continues to age while younger generations simultaneously get smaller, the highest proportion of the population will shift to older generations, as projected by the kite-shaped population pyramid of 2050 [1, 2].

By 2050, the elderly population (65 years and older) is projected to comprise 38.8 per cent of Japan's total population. With such rapid shifts in age structure, it is necessary for Japan to adapt its social security policies to suit this.

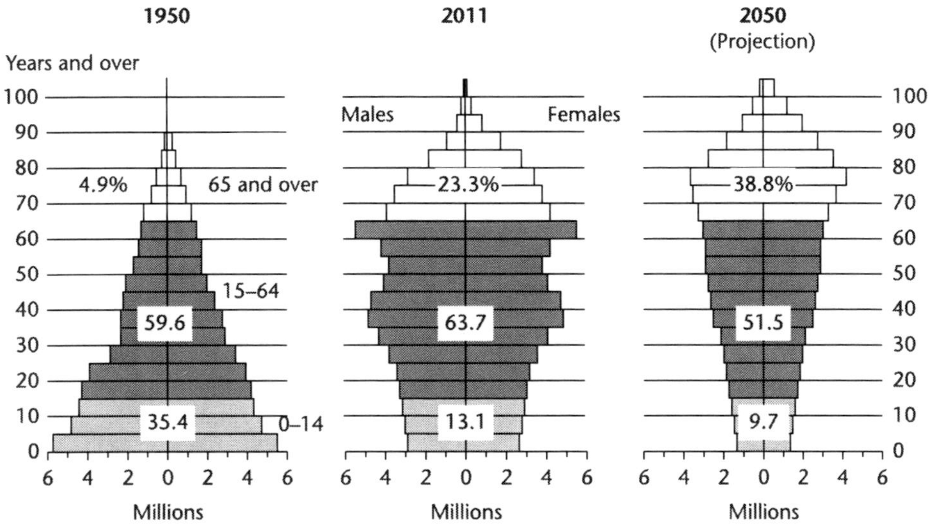


*Figure 4.1* Changes in the population pyramid, 1950–2050 [1]

## Challenges of ageing in Japan

### *Increasing social security expenditure*

In 1961, Japan introduced the 'universal coverage in public pension and health insurance' that provided all Japanese citizens with health insurance and a public pension from age 65 [3]. Income-based social insurance premiums are paid by all citizens based on their ability to pay and fund about 60 per cent of the total social security spending [3].

Due to a growing elderly population, social security expenditures are increasing annually as demonstrated in Figure 4.2. In 2009, expenditures were 99.9 trillion yen (29.4 per cent of Japan's total income) or 783,100 yen per person. Of this spending, pensions accounted for 51.8 per cent, medical care for 30.9 per cent and social welfare for 17.3 per cent [1]. Overall, social security benefits for elderly populations currently make up approximately 70 per cent of the total social security expenditures. This spending is projected to reach 141 trillion by 2025 [1].

Japan's healthcare system is globally praised for its universal coverage and exemplary health indicators, while having the lowest rate of healthcare spending to GDP of the developed nations [4]. Japan's high life expectancy is attributed to this universal healthcare system. This system relies on revenue from premiums in which working individuals support elderly populations. However, these dynamics are quickly changing with shifts in age structure. As of 1960, approximately 11.2 working-age individuals were supporting one elderly individual. This number is projected to fall to a 2:1 ratio by 2030 [5].

As the Japanese continue to live longer, there have been corresponding increases in age-associated disability including chronic disease, as well as physical and mental impairment. Therefore, medical care spending on the latter-stage elderly (75 years and older) has increased significantly since 1984. Japan's medical spending totalled 36.0 trillion yen in 2009 or 282,400 yen per person. Of this spending, latter-stage elderly medical costs totalled 12.0 trillion yen or 882,118 yen per person [1]. This spending increase in later life stages is due primarily to long-term care associated with elderly individuals [6].

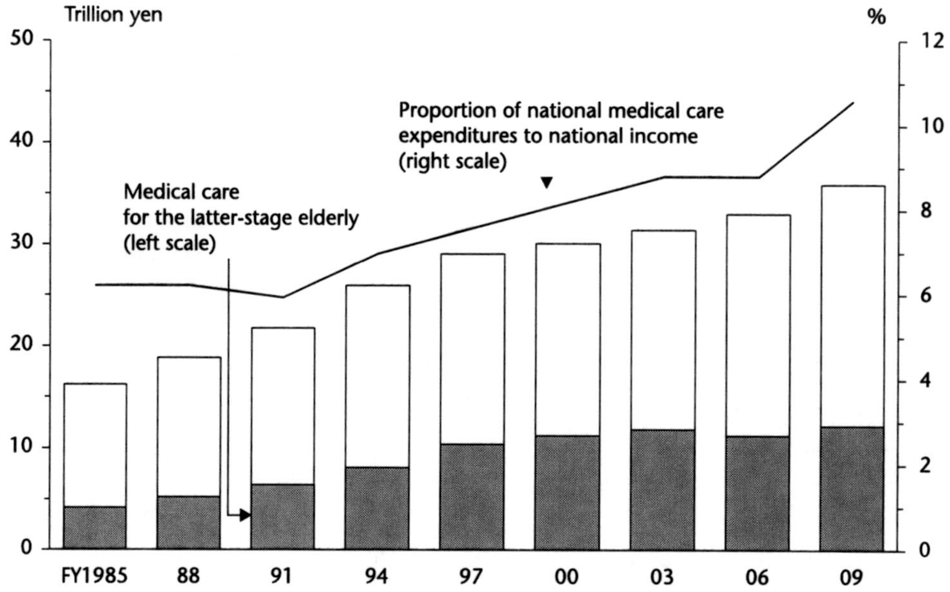


*Figure 4.2* Trends in medical care expenditures [1]

## *Increasing burden of elderly care*

In the past, elderly care was primarily a family responsibility, whereas the elderly are now increasingly living independently and relying on government support. For example, the percentage of elderly living with a child or relative has dropped from 87 per cent to 48 per cent between 1960 and 2006.

These changing family roles are due to various factors, including urbanization of youth to pursue education and work, as well an increasing acceptance of nuclear families [3, 5]. As job markets continue to get more competitive and the cost of living continues to increase, it is becoming essential that these youth work hard to compete for jobs and decent incomes. This generation must build their lives in the cities and they tend to create their own nuclear families in these areas while leaving their older relatives behind in rural areas to care for themselves.

Additionally, as Japanese women pursue higher education and professional careers, caring for elderly relatives becomes more burdensome. This is especially true for women who also have the responsibility of raising their own children. Many modern couples rely on dual incomes so women can no longer stay at home to care for elderly relatives.

Finally, as fertility rates continue to decrease, there are fewer children in families to provide physical and financial support to ageing parents. These factors combined result in an increasing reliance on government support among Japanese elderly.

## *Decreasing fertility rate*

In addition to increasing life expectancies, Japan is also experiencing a decreasing fertility rate. The fertility rate of Japan has decreased from 2.14 children per woman in 1973 [2] to 1.39 in 2011 [1].

A major contributing factor to this decrease in fertility rate is that of increased education and competition in the job market, specifically among women. As women strive for more education and professional careers, they are more likely to delay marriage and child bearing. The average ages for marriage and birth of first child for women have increased between 1984 and 2004 from 25.4 to 27.8 and from 26.6 to 28.9, respectively [7]. Additionally, divorce is becoming more commonplace in Japan and it is more socially acceptable to not marry at all. This detail is particularly important because only about 2 per cent of children are born out of wedlock in Japan compared to rates of about 40 per cent in most other developed nations [7]. Also, couples are finding it increasingly more expensive to raise children [5].

## Health reform policies and current strategies

### *National health promotion*

In order to promote healthy longevity in Japan, the Japanese Ministry of Health, Labour and Welfare issued a national plan in 2000 entitled the 'National Health Promotion Movement in the 21st Century', known as 'Healthy Japan 21' [8]. This was a ten-year plan that involved active participation at the local level. The main focus areas of this plan included: diet and nutrition, physical activity and exercise, leisure and mental health, smoking, alcohol, dental health, diabetes, cardiovascular disease and cancer. Specific goals were set for each of these focus areas and indicators were used to evaluate programme success.

In accordance with this national plan, each prefecture and municipality developed its own healthy programme that was tailored to its specific needs. Both national and local governments have provided citizens with educational information and healthier environments through collaboration with entities such as medical facilities, the media, the corporate sector, NGOs, as well as others.

The final evaluation of this programme indicated that 60 per cent of the initial target goals were met, including increased screenings for non-communicable diseases (NCDs), such as diabetes and cancer. These evaluation data were used to revise this programme into a second campaign with the same goal of promoting a healthier Japanese population. By reducing medical expenditures through primary prevention of NCDs, the Japanese government hopes to reduce overall healthcare spending even though it is promoting further longevity.

### *Long-term care insurance policy*

In order to effectively manage Japan's ageing population, the Japanese government has developed policies to combat the financial and social issues around elderly care. In 1989, Japan compiled an expert panel to develop a comprehensive community-based long-term care (LTC) system to promote senior independence and high-quality access to services. The LTC Insurance Act was enacted in 1997 and premium-based LTC social insurance was implemented in 2000 for Japanese citizens 65 years and over [9]. The vision of LTC was 'from care by family to care by society', in which seniors are provided in-home, community-based and institutional services [10]. Upon implementation, users skyrocketed, as did costs due to imperfections in the system design. This included an initial lack of eligibility screening, which resulted in many seniors opting for LTC housing due to the fact that it was less expensive than living on their own. Additionally, care management systems were initially weak, which would sometimes lead to care managers upping senior demands unnecessarily in order to increase profits.

A 2005 reform was developed to contain some of the costs. With this new system, seniors undergo an initial evaluation to determine an individualised care plan based on their needs. New preventive services were introduced to improve physical strength, nutritional status, oral function and mental health for those with lower needs in the hope that these seniors will maintain their independence. Additionally, income-adjusted room and board fees were introduced at all LTC nursing homes and institutions to make the cost of living in the LTC institutions more comparable to living on one's own.

From its inception in 2000, LTC users have increased from 1.5 million to 4.03 million as of April 2010. As Japan's population continues to age, it is projected that these numbers will continue to grow, likely provoking future adaptations to continue to cut costs while still providing exceptional elderly care that promotes healthy, independent lifestyles. This system is to undergo a re-evaluation every five years.

### *Policies to increase fertility and to support the next generation*

Due to a continually decreasing fertility rate, the Japanese government has made an effort to increase this rate by making it more convenient and affordable to have children. This movement began in 1990 with the creation of the committee Creating a Sound Environment for Bearing and Rearing Children to develop plans and policies to increase fertility.

In 1991, the Childcare Leave Act allowed either parent to take up to a one-year leave from their job. Child allowances which were originally designed to help low-income families with multiple children became pro-natalist in 1992 when they were extended to all parents [2]. Government-subsidized day care and after-school centres, babysitting services and fertility consultations were established through the 'Angel Plan' in 1994 and the 'New Angel Plan' in 1999. The 'New-new Angel Plan' of 2004 sought to promote marriage and children by focusing mainly on aiding younger generations to become independent through career services in order to achieve financial stability [11]. In 2009, publicly funded maternal health checks during pregnancy (14 check-ups in total throughout pregnancy) were added to this plan to promote sound maternal health and delivery.

Another plan developed in 2000, the 'Measures to Cope with a Fewer Number of Children Plus One' promoted a greater role for husbands in child rearing by requiring that they take at least a five-day leave upon the birth of their child. This plan also set a goal for 10 per cent of men taking childcare leave [2]. As of 2005, childcare leave was taken by 72.3 per cent of women and only 0.5 per cent of men [12]. Therefore, this ultimately led to the 2003 'Law for Measures to Support the Development of the Next Generation', in which all firms with 300+ employees are required to create a two-to-five year plan to raise fertility among employees, including targets and progress reports [2].

A State Minister for the Declining Birthrate and Gender Equality has been appointed since 2007 and is continuing to improve current policies in order to create an environment where parents feel secure about giving birth and raising children [13]. From 2007, the total fertility rate in Japan slightly increased from 1.34 to 1.39 in 2010, suggesting that these policies are in fact having a positive effect.

## Conclusion

The ageing population in Japan will continue to present economic and political challenges by straining Japan's economy through pensions and health care with a decreasing workforce to support them. To increase this workforce, Japan has attempted to increase its low fertility rate by making it easier for young adults to marry and raise children.

Although Japan is presently a highly homogenous country, with minimal immigration due to a difficult language that must be mastered for citizenship, an alternative solution involves immigration of foreign workers.

Finally, it is important to realize that Japan will have to support an enormous number of elderly citizens in the near future and it is critical that these elderly remain healthy and independent. In order for Japan to attain healthy and sustainable longevity, Japan must adapt to an ageing society through effective healthy longevity policies.

## References


1. Statistics Bureau, Japan. *The Statistical Handbook of Japan 2012.* [Online]. Available from: http://www.stat.go.jp/english/data/handbook/
2. Retherford, R. D. and Ogawa, N. *Japan's Baby Bust: Causes, Implications, and Policy Responses.* Population and Health Series, Honolulu: East–West Center, 2005.
3. Nishimura, N. *Social Security in Japan.* Tokyo: National Institute of Population and Social Security Research, 2011.
4. Idezuki, Y. Long Live the Health Care System in Japan. *Bioscience Trends* 2008; 2, 50–2.
5. Muramatsu, N. and Akiyama, H. Japan: Super-Ageing Society Preparing for the Future. *Gerontologist* 2011; 51, 425–32.
6. Hashimoto, H., Horiguchi, H. and Matsuda, S. Micro Data Analysis of Medical and Long-Term Care Utilization among the Elderly in Japan. *International Journal of Environmental Research and Public Health* 2010; 7, 3022–37.
7. Oshio, T. The Declining Birthrate in Japan. *Japan Economic Currents* 2008.
8. Sakurai, H. Healthy Japan 21. *Journal of the Japan Medical Association* 2003; 46, 47–49.
9. Tamiya, N., Noguchi, H., Nishi, A., Reich, M. R., Ikegami, N., Hashimoto, H., *et al.* Population Ageing and Wellbeing: Lessons from Japan's Long-Term Care Insurance Policy. *Lancet* 2001; 378, 1183–92.
10. Tsutsui, T. and Muramatsu, N. Japan's Universal Long-Term Care System Reform of 2005: Containing Costs and Realizing a Vision. *Journal of the American Geriatrics Society* 2007; 55, 1458–63.
11. Doteuchi, A. Focus on Policy Shifts from Boosting Fertility to Developing the Next Generation – The Socialization of Child-Raising. *Nli Research* 2005; 1–9.
12. Cabinet Office, Government of Japan, White Paper on Gender Equality, 2007.
13. Japan Ministry of Health, Labour and Welfare. Introduction to the Revised Child Care and Family Care Leave Law, 2009.

# 5

# Developing public health infrastructure in India

*K. Srinath Reddy and Manu Raj Mathur*

## Introduction

India combines the features of a historically ancient civilization, a mature and stable modern democracy and a demographically young nation where the largest fraction of the global population under 25 years of age resides. Over the last two decades, its economic growth has positioned it among the 'emerging economies', which are expected to play a major role in determining the direction and dimensions of global development in the twenty-first century.

Despite an impressive gain in life expectancy since independence from colonial rule (31 in 1947; 64 in 2010), India's health indicators have lagged behind other emerging economies and bear poor comparison to India's neighbours like China and Sri Lanka. While infectious diseases like tuberculosis, malaria and HIV/AIDS still remain major public health challenges, non-communicable diseases (NCDs) – cardiovascular disease, diabetes, cancers, chronic respiratory diseases – and mental illness are now the leading causes of death and disability [1]. While tobacco accounts for more than a million deaths per year [2], indoor air pollution has also been identified as a major contributor to death and disability [1].

At 44 per 1,000 live births, the infant mortality rate (IMR) in India is three times higher than in China, four times higher than in Sri Lanka and Thailand, and is even higher than that in Bangladesh and Nepal. The maternal mortality ratio (MMR) is 212 per 100,000 births. Immunization coverage in children is below par, ranging between 64 per cent and 72 per cent in the last decade. The spectre of undernutrition looms large, with 42 per cent of children under 5 years of age undernourished, while 70 per cent of children and 50 per cent of young women are anaemic [3]. At the same time, 14 per cent of urban adolescents (15 million) are reported to be overweight or obese [4].

The present health profile of India reflects the mixed effects of multiple transitions (demographic, nutrition and epidemiologic) superimposed on an uneven economic development, an under-resourced health system and inadequate multi-sectoral action on the determinants of health. There are wide-ranging disparities in health indicators across the different states in this large country of 1.21 billion people, with variations in the levels of development and nature of governance impacting upon the health status of different population groups.

## Architecture of the public health infrastructure

In the federal structure of the Indian polity, the constitutional mandate for delivering health services is mainly for the states. The central government designs and part funds national health programmes and also has the responsibility for international health agreements. The states and the centre contribute to health financing in a 2:1 ratio. Over time, primary health services have come to be substantially supported by central schemes, while the states have focused more on secondary and tertiary care.

The design for a three-tier healthcare system was developed for rural health care, extending from a sub-centre (for 5,000 persons) to the district hospital, with intermediate stations in the form of primary and community health centres. However, urban health care was not similarly designed, with primary health services delivered through an unplanned mix of providers, except in a very few municipalities. Due to long years of operational neglect, despite best policy intent, primary health care remains poor in many regions of the country [5].

India's mixed health system features a combination of public, private and voluntary service providers. Though the health system was originally designed to have most of the services delivered through the public sector, resource constraints progressively weakened its capacity to do so. The private sector grew in strength from the 1980s and has now become the major provider, by default, accounting for over 65 per cent of the services provided. However, it varies in composition ranging from the unqualified solo rural practitioner to the large urban corporate hospital. The weak regulatory systems do not ensure quality or cost control.

## Health system constraints

India's health system is burdened with multiple handicaps as it faces the concomitant challenges posed by the diseases of underdevelopment and the disorders of maladapted modernity. Public financing of health, at 1.04 per cent of GDP, is among the lowest in the world, especially when measured as per capita annual expenditure. As a result, out-of-pocket expenditure on health is over 70 per cent, again a mark of dubious distinction at the global level. About 60 million Indians are estimated to sink below the poverty line each year, due to unaffordable healthcare expenditure, while one out of five Indians does not even seek health care due to the deterrent effect of such costs [6, 7].

The health workforce is deficient in numbers and maldistributed, with an urban aggregation. There are shortages across the board of specialist and basic doctors, nurses, allied health professionals (technicians, paramedics, etc.) and community health workers [8]. At 0.9 hospital beds per 1,000 population, India is well below the global norm of 3 per 1,000 [9]. Public health expertise is not available for policy development or programme design, delivery and evaluation, since India neglected to establish Schools of Public Health until very recently. Managerial expertise is also sparse in the health sector.

The problem is compounded by the fact that the social determinants of health are in neglect. Clean drinking water is available only to 68.2 per cent of the people, while 53 per cent still practise open defecation in the absence of domestic toilets. Poverty, limited education and lack of women's empowerment are barriers to health, most visible in the northern and central Indian states which have the worst health indicators. The southern states of Kerala and Tamil Nadu stand out as models of public policy prioritizing population health, the former with its attention to social determinants and emphasis on equity and the latter with a robust public health system that boasts of the only formally constituted public health cadre in the country [10, 11].

India is among the countries described by the World Health Organization (WHO) as facing a 'health workforce crisis'. The number of medical colleges increased from 189 in 2000–1 to 335 in 2010–11. Similarly, the number of dental colleges has increased from 149 in 2001–2 to 291 in 2010–11. There are 2,028 colleges for nurses and midwives and 608 colleges for pharmacy [12]. However, there is maldistribution of health professional training institutions and the health workforce across states and urban–rural locales. The shortage of health workers is especially great in the central, northern and north-eastern states. Six 'high production states' (Andhra Pradesh, Karnataka, Kerala, Maharashtra, Puducherry and Tamil Nadu) represent 31 per cent of the population but have 58 per cent of the medical seats and 63 per cent of the nursing colleges. Eight 'low production states' account for 46 per cent of India's population but have only 21 per cent of the medical seats and 20 per cent of the nursing colleges [8].

Due to the inadequate amount of resources dedicated towards the development of the public health sector in India, public health has suffered as a teaching and practice discipline. Until 2006, India had very few institutions teaching public health as a discipline and a dedicated cadre in public health was missing from the majority of state health systems. However, positive trends have emerged since the launch of National Rural Health Mission (NRHM) in 2005, aiming to improve maternal and child health services to decrease IMR and MMR. To support the mission, the Central Ministry of Health and Family Welfare established a National Health Systems Resource Centre (NHSRC) to design training programmes for frontline health workers.

New institutions, with a mandate to develop public health as an educational stream and capacity building of existing health workforce in public health, have been created in many states in the past decade. The Public Health Foundation of India (PHFI) is a public–private initiative, launched in 2006, to establish a strong national network of public health and allied institutions, which would create a cadre of public health professionals and undertake policy and programme relevant research to advance prioritized public health goals. Presently, the PHFI runs several on-campus and distance learning courses through four institutions which have been established in different regions of the country to train new professionals in various disciplines of public health. Its postgraduate educational programme in public health management is linked to National Rural Health Mission (NRHM), and provides integrated training in public health and management to serving medical officers of the district health system. It provides short-term training in several theoretical and applied areas of public health to the existing health workforce of the country in order to build their capacity, while offering public health education to physicians as well as non-physicians through several application streams such as public health nutrition, health informatics, health promotion and health policy [13].

## National Health Mission: catalyst and vehicle for transforming public health

Since its implementation in 2007, the NRHM has provided the much-needed impetus to the development of public health infrastructure, workforce development and health systems strengthening in India. It initially focused only on maternal and child health, with incentives for institutional deliveries and immunization. It has positioned nearly a million women Accredited Social Health Activists (ASHA) in villages across the country, to act as social mobilizers for health and nutrition services.

It is now becoming a platform for progressive integration of other health programmes. With the initiation of the National Urban Health Mission (NUHM) in 2013, the flagship programme for public health will henceforth be called the National Health Mission (NHM), integrating both the NRHM and the NUHM.

## Towards Universal Health Care (UHC)

In October 2010, the Planning Commission of India set up a High Level Expert Group (HLEG) mandated to develop a framework for universal health coverage in India. The main objective was to create a system of health financing which would reduce the inordinately high out-of-pocket health expenditure and protect vulnerable segments of the population from the threat of impoverishment due to unaffordable costs of essential health care.

While adequate financing for health was the key objective, the framework proposed by the HLEG also included human resources for health; physical and financial norms for health services; strengthening of management systems; community participation; and access to drugs, vaccines and technologies. The HLEG emphasized that, without these, the entitlement envisaged by increased health financing cannot be delivered. The HLEG also included social determinants of health in the framework, recognizing that many of the determinants that lie outside of the conventional health sector have a profound influence on health and also need to be influenced for UHC to be realized [11].

The HLEG adopted a broad definition of UHC, which emphasizes access and affordability and assures quality of health care to all citizens. While encompassing promotive, preventive, therapeutic and rehabilitative services in the arena of UHC, it also brings other sectors relevant to public health (such as water, sanitation, nutrition and environment) into the ambit of action for UHC. The definition calls on the government to assume responsibility for guaranteeing the delivery of UHC, even though it may not be the sole provider of services [11].

## Developing public health infrastructure in India

The recommendations of the HLEG have been substantially incorporated into the twelfth Five Year Plan (2012–17), which provides the blueprint for national development. Public financing for health will rise to 1.87 per cent of GDP by 2017, with emphasis on primary health care and strengthening of district hospitals [14].

There is a proposal in the plan to open more medical, nursing and dental colleges in poorer, under-served and rural areas. These new colleges should be located in states with very few colleges and preferably in districts where no such colleges currently exist. Wherever feasible, they should be linked to district hospitals. There is also an urgent need to increase the number of functional beds in government hospitals and dispensaries.

The numbers of Auxiliary Nurse Midwife (ANM) schools too should be increased, especially in states where their numbers are very low. A large number of paramedical workers (allied health professionals) would also be required in many categories (ranging from laboratory technicians to radiographers and operation theatre assistants to mental health counsellors). Their production should be enabled by: the establishment of several new training institutions; improved training programmes with access to skill labs and simulation centres; and standardization of training and accreditation. To coordinate the training of several categories of health workers and to promote teamwork and inter-professional education, District Health Knowledge Institutes should be established with a link to the district hospital.

For strengthening primary health care in rural areas, the health workforce at the rural subcentre levels must be substantially augmented, while expanding the team of frontline health workers in each village. According to the recommendations of the HLEG on UHC, there should be two Accredited Social Health Activists (ASHAs) and two Anganwadi (government-sponsored childcare and mother-care centre) workers in every village to form an effective village-level team for maternal and child health, nutrition, sanitation, adolescent and reproductive health, and health promotion (including prevention of tobacco use, alcohol abuse and domestic violence). The health sub-centre (one for 5,000 population) should have two female ANMs, a male multi-purpose health worker (MPW), a mid-level health worker (community health officer) and a laboratory technician-cum-drug dispenser. The staff strength at both primary and continuing healthcare levels too should be augmented, especially with more nurses. Urban primary health care should be strengthened by establishing urban health sub-centres headed by a Nurse Practitioner and supported by Urban Social Health Activists (USHAs).

A well-designed and efficiently operated national disease surveillance programme, for both communicable as well as non-communicable diseases, is urgently needed [15]. The government of India launched the Integrated Disease Surveillance Programme (IDSP), with assistance from the World Bank, in 2004. The programme was mainly meant to track the outbreak of communicable diseases. The implementation of IDSP has been weak and has not extended across the district health system. With a rapid epidemiologic transition underway and clustering of risk behaviours like tobacco and alcohol use, there is a need to develop a robust surveillance system at the district level to track both communicable and non-communicable diseases as well as their risk factors, to rapidly detect and respond to disease outbreaks and also to effectively prevent them.

There is a need to develop a public health cadre at both central and state levels in India, with a defined career pathway. There is also a need to review existing cadre structures across a multilayered health workforce, create career tracks and professional advancement pathways, ensure incentives for health workers serving in difficult areas and strengthen human resource management in order to develop the functional infrastructure of public health. The twelfth Plan has incorporated the HLEG's recommendation for creation of public health and health management cadres at central and state levels. Even as schemes for implementing this recommendation are under development, medical colleges and universities have taken the cue to start new educational programmes in public health.

Coordination of health policies and programmes between the central and state governments must be improved, from design to delivery, with financing for impact evaluation. Public financing of health should rise to at least 3 per cent of the GDP, if UHC is to be meaningfully implemented. This requires greater contributions from both the centre and the states. Primary health care must be prioritized in both rural and urban settings, while the fragmented social insurance programmes operated by the centre and the states for hospitalized secondary and tertiary care must be unified under a UHC programme that provides comprehensive care through a predominantly tax-funded system.

## Conclusion

By taking these steps for capacity building, introducing Universal Health Care and implementing it through the National Health Mission, India would be on the path of developing a strong public health infrastructure. A comprehensive, coordinated and integrated approach between various components of India's health system would not only lead to a stronger and more responsive infrastructure but would also improve the health outcomes of the population. Prioritization of public health over mere clinical care and recognition of the health system as a necessary vehicle for delivering a wide range of health services are now features of, and are bringing greater attention to, public health after many years of neglect. There is hope that the health system will soon expand its outreach, improve the quality of health services and enhance health equity. This will assure the people of India that they will soon be provided the public health delivery system they desire, deserve and demand.

## References

1. Patel V, Chatterji S, Chisholm D, Ebrahim S, Gopalakrishna G, Mathers C, *et al.* Chronic diseases and injuries in India. *Lancet.* 2011; 377(9763): 413–28.
2. WHO. *WHO Report on the Global Tobacco Epidemic*, 2011; The MPOWER Package. Geneva; 2011.
3. International Institute of Population Sciences (IIPS) and Macro International. National Family Health Survey (NFHS–3), 2005–06: India, Volume 1. Key Indicators for India from NFHS–3. Mumbai; 2007. Accessible URL: http://www.rchiips.org/nfhs/volume_1.shtml (Accessed 12 June 2013).
4. Gupta N, Goel K, Shah P, Misra A. Childhood obesity in developing countries: epidemiology, determinants, and prevention. *Endocrine Reviews.* 2012; 33(1): 48–70.
5. Powell-Jackson T, Acharya A, Mills A. An assessment of the quality of primary health care in India. *Economic and Political Weekly.* 2013; 48(19).
6. Kumar AKS, Chen LC, Choudhury M, Ganju S, Mahajan V, Sinha A, *et al.* Financing health care for all: challenges and opportunities. *Lancet.* 2011; 377(9766): 668–79.
7. National Sample Survey Office (NSSO). Household consumer expenditure (NSS 61st Round: 2004–05). New Delhi; 2006.
8. Rao M, Rao KD, Kumar AKS, Chatterjee M, Sundararaman T. Human resources for health in India. *Lancet.* 2011; 377(9765): 587–98.
9. Central Bureau of Health Intelligence. National Health Profile of India 2010. New Delhi; 2011. Accesible URL: http://cbhidghs.nic.in/index2.asp?slid=1125&sublinkid=929 (Accessed 9 June 2013).
10. Dasgupta M, Rani M. India's public health system: how well does it function at the national level? Policy Research Working Paper 3447. 2004.
11. High Level Expert Group Report on Universal Health Coverage for India. New Delhi; 2011. Accesible URL: https://docs.google.com/viewer?url=http%253A%252F%252Fplanningcommission.nic.in%252F (Accessed 21 May 2013).
12. Central Bureau of Health Intelligence. National Health Profile of India 2011. New Delhi; 2011. Accesible URL: http://www.cbhidghs.nic.in/index2.asp?slid=1208&sublinkid=944 (Accessed 10 June 2013).
13. Sharma K, Zodpey S. Public health education in India: need and demand paradox. Indian Journal of Community Medicine: official publication of Indian Association of Preventive & Social Medicine. 2011; 36(3): 178–81.
14. Planning Commission of India. Twelfth Five Year Plan (2012–2017); Social Sectors. New Delhi; 2013. Accesible URL: http://planningcommission.gov.in/plans/planrel/12thplan/welcome.html (Accessed 4 June 2013).
15. Jacob John T, Muliyil J. Public health is infrastructure for human development. *Indian Journal of Medical Research.* 2009; 130(1): 9–11.

# 6

# Public health in the age of genomics, 'Big Data' and massively collaborative global science

*Vural Özdemir*

## Introduction

Until recently, public health and genomics have rarely come together although both have long aimed to improve population health. The emerging field of public health genomics represents this much-needed convergence. This new subspecialty of twenty-first-century public health is hybrid in its composition, made up of knowledge strands from public health and genomics sciences, and is defined as 'the responsible and effective translation of genome-based knowledge for the benefit of population health' [1]. This consensus definition was reached at an international meeting held in Bellagio, Italy, in 2005. Rather than viewing populations as a homogenous entity, public health genomics firmly recognizes the hitherto silent heterogeneity in population substructure as rooted in genomics and genome–environment interactions. Described in another way, public health genomics is an invitation to rethink the current efforts for stratified medicine in the broader context of populations.

This chapter introduces the reader to the basic concepts of public health genomics that rest on integration of inquiries from molecular and genomics sciences, population sciences, humanities and social sciences. Looking forward, this chapter underscores what we can anticipate from public health practice in the current age of genomics, 'Big Data' and massively collaborative global science [2].

## Twenty-first-century public health: the age of 'Big Data'

The twenty-first-century public health community has begun a new era since the completion of the Human Genome Project in 2001 [3, 4]. This is in part driven by the introduction of 'omics' technology applications in public health. Data-intensive omics technologies, such as genomics, have immensely increased our ability to generate data on an unprecedented scale. Public health sciences are now experiencing a 'data deluge' from these high-throughput biotechnologies. We are facing the challenges of exponential growth in data volume and variety, generated daily through massively parallel studies of biological pathways.

Omics science rests, first, on a 'systems approach' to human health and disease enabled by data-intensive technologies such as genomics. While the 1990s was named the 'decade of the brain', we are now in the 'decade of measurements' [5].

Second, omics data intensive research and development (R&D) starts with a 'commons' as the departure point for discovery science. The new science rests on an infrastructure science that includes, for example, international scientific consortia, cloud computing, educational and data standards, population biobanks and cyberinfrastructure that co-constitute the above digital commons, thus enabling and accelerating discovery science [6, 7, 8]. These two domains of twenty-first-century public health science – infrastructure science and discovery science – are inseparable and depend on each other (see Figure 6.1). As discussed later in this chapter, a new culture of collaboration and collective action between the digital commons created by various omics infrastructures and discovery science have become crucial for sustainable public health innovation in practice [7, 9].

These shifts in the architecture of twenty-first-century public health science have garnered international attention as seen in the recent release of policy reports about *Science as an Open Enterprise* by the Royal Society, London [10], and a *National Bioeconomy Blueprint* by the United States (USA) White House [11]. An important focus of these reports is a new form of scientific inquiry, data-intensive massively collaborative science and 'Big Data' R&D [3, 4, 12].

Big Data refers to a diverse array of unprecedentedly large datasets being created, for example, by genomics and proteomics, new biosensors, electronic health records, data simulation, social media and the Internet that are collectively shaping twenty-first-century public health sciences and practice. Edd Dumbill, the Editor-in-Chief of the journal *Big Data*,

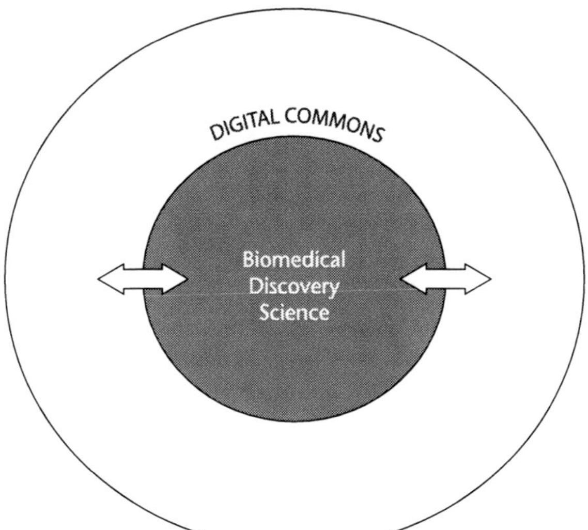


*Figure 6.1* Twenty-first-century public health is now embedded in, and draws from, the genomics commons

provided the following prescient definition: 'Big data is data that exceeds the processing capacity of conventional database systems. The data is too big, moves too fast, or doesn't fit the strictures of your database architectures. To gain value from this data, you must choose an alternative way to process it' [13].

Data-intensive collaborative science was also named the 'Fourth Paradigm of Science', preceded by the third (last few decades: *computational branch*, modelling and simulating complex phenomena); the second (last few hundred years: *theoretical branch*, using models leading to generalizations); and the first paradigm (a thousand years ago: *empirical description of natural phenomena*) [3].

The present convergence of public health and genomics is materializing against these broad and seismic shifts in the folklore of twenty-first-century science. Public health genomics is a multidisciplinary field that is concerned with the 'effective and responsible applications of genome-based knowledge and technologies to improve population health'. As mentioned above, this definition resulted from an international meeting held in Bellagio, Italy in 2005 [1]. As the name implies, the hybrid field is essentially rooted in principles of public health. It takes a population perspective to apply new genome-based technologies to improve health. It focuses on prevention; evidence-based multidisciplinary science; and ethical, legal and social implications, including addressing health disparities.

The availability of genomics applications has a significant impact on all areas of public health practice including infectious diseases, environmental and occupational health, and chronic diseases, in addition to the more traditional areas, such as prenatal diagnosis, newborn screening and genetic services delivery. In this sense, public health genomics is clearly cross-cutting and integrative.

## Defining the field of public health genomics

The early roots of convergence of knowledge strands from public health and genome-based science and technologies can be traced back to the 1990s with the establishment of public health genetics/genomics units in select locations in resource-rich countries. Enabled by support from the Rockefeller Foundation, interested individuals held the international multidisciplinary expert meeting in Bellagio, Italy, in 2005 to define the nascent field of 'public health genomics' (PHG). This inaugural Bellagio PHG meeting established several objectives for the field:

1 An international consensus definition of PHG was developed as described above;
2 'The Enterprise' was articulated as a conceptual model for knowledge generation, integration and application, describing the envisioned practice of PHG [1, 14];
3 The Genome-based Research and Population Health International Network (Graph-*Int*) was established as an international forum to promote the practice of PHG.

These have in turn enabled the scope and disciplinary diversity of PHG as a post-genomics 'field' of inquiry. An international PHG meeting was held at Ickworth House, Suffolk, United Kingdom (UK) 10–14 May 2010, and was attended by a multidisciplinary team of 27 experts from Argentina, Australia, Canada, France, Italy, the Netherlands, Switzerland, the UK and the USA [15].

## PHG applications ready for prime time

### *Antecedents: tracing the roots of PHG diagnostics*

Genomics science has a strong motive to characterize individual and population differences in biology. In this sense, the focus of PHG on 'variability questions' in population health is rooted in diagnostic medicine. In fact, understanding population heterogeneity and diagnosing individual differences in health and disease have been a preoccupation since ancient times, though not in the systematic and explicit manner of the PHG scholars in the twenty-first century. Early diagnosticians not only lacked the genomics tools such as microarrays that the modern-day PHG scientists now possess, but they were also limited in access to tissue specimens. In ancient times, patients could be observed and touched by physicians, but it was forbidden to practise invasive procedures. Access to diagnostic tissue specimens was essentially limited to those that were naturally passed from the body, such as urine. The Babylonians and Sumerians used urine to diagnose the health status of individuals as early as in 4,000 BCE, whereas Hippocrates (460–*ca.* 370 BCE, the Island of Cos, Greece) suggested the presence of bubbles in the urine to be an indication of chronic kidney disease [16]. Pythagoras in Croton (Calabria region), Italy, noted in 510 BCE that the ingestion of fava beans resulted in a potentially fatal reaction in some, but not all, individuals [5]. The scientific basis of this adverse reaction to food, that is, favism, was an inherited deficiency of glucose-6-phosphate dehydrogenase, one of the early documented accounts of metabolic genetic polymorphism.

### *Situating PHG in global science*

Before we discuss the current PHG applications ready for practice, and ways to evaluate those in transition from discovery, PHG innovations need to be situated within the context of global R&D. Such global perspectives are truly necessary to appreciate the present state of the field, while in parallel, developing foresight on future trajectories that will be built by the next generation of PHG scholars [17].

The annual investment in global R&D has doubled to US$1.1 trillion since 1996 [18]. Many countries, large and small, are embracing the concept of the knowledge society, whether because of hopeful expectations for a prosperous 'knowledge economy', tighter economic interdependence or decreasing cost of certain biotechnologies, such as genomics [17]. China, India, Korea, Singapore and Qatar are among the notable nations substantially investing in science and engineering research, education and workforce [19]. Consistent with this, a recent study on the globalization of science found, using quantitative indicators, that the current growth rate for state-level research funding in China greatly exceeds that in the USA and the European Union [20]. An analysis of the scientific publication data from the Web of Science over the past thirty years (1980–2009) showed that Asia's share of the world scientific output grew stupendously by 155 per cent, while the Middle East, as a region, displayed a growth of four times faster than at the world level [19].

In a recent federated effort to co-create merit standards for global science, the heads of major science and engineering research funding agencies from nearly 50 countries – primarily representing the G-20 and the Organization for Economic Co-operation and Development – have convened at the US National Science Foundation (NSF) in Virginia for the first Global Merit Review Summit [18]. This attests to the growing commitment of nations to ensure that global science and its practice function 'in a coherent and well-coordinated manner among developed and developing nations, maintain the public trust, and address each nation's unique needs for economic growth, national security and human capital development' [18].

The Asia-Pacific region is actively investing in a young generation of skilled professionals in response to global science. Based on the annual Open Doors report published by the Institute of International Education (IIE), the number of international students enrolled at colleges and universities in the USA was 690,923 during the 2009/10 academic year [21]. Of the top six-sending countries, five were from the Asia-Pacific region – mainland China and Taiwan, India, Japan and South Korea – representing more than half (52 per cent) of the total international student population.

Notably, PHG applications have broadened in the Asia-Pacific region over the past decade. These now include not only diagnostics for disease susceptibilities but also genomics tests for health outcomes related to drug therapy (pharmacogenomics), nutrition (nutrigenomics) and vaccines (vaccinomics) [22]. The bioinformatics community in the region has recently recognized the need to address the computational challenges of genomics/post-genomics high-throughput technologies, for example, at the annual conference of the Asia-Pacific Bioinformatics Network, held in September 2009 in Biopolis, Singapore [23]. In Sri Lanka, PHG practice includes, for example, hepatitis C diagnostics and clinical management by measurement of patients' baseline viral load and genotype [24]. Much of the fundamental research conducted within the Asia-Pacific leading research establishments – the Beijing Genomics Institute in China, the Eijkman Institute for Molecular Biology in Indonesia, the Institute of Molecular and Cell Biology in Singapore, the RIKEN Center for the Genomic Medicine in Japan, the Nutrigenomics New Zealand (the list is too extensive to do justice in this chapter) – now depend on genomics and other omics technologies, such as proteomics and metabolomics.

Within the Hong Kong Special Administrative Region (SAR), clinical genetics have provided public health service for nearly three decades led by Dr Stephen Lam, in addition to internationally recognized trailblazing academic research work, for example, by Professor Sir David Todd (haemoglobinopathies), Professor Lap-chee Tsui (cystic fibrosis), Professor Pak Sham (psychiatry) and Professor Dennis Lo (free foetal DNA). Notwithstanding these prominent bodies of work pertinent for PHG at the Chinese University of Hong Kong, Hong Kong University and the Genome Research Centre, there remains a serious need to establish a sound PHG strategy and attendant funding mechanisms in Hong Kong SAR and the Asia-Pacific region [25].

### *A three-tiered classification framework for 'PHG actionability'*

In the current post-genomics era, a growing number of candidate genomics applications are in transition from basic science to clinical and public health practice. Between 2009 and November 2012, more than 450 new genomic tests were identified from horizon scanning by the US Centers for Disease Control and Prevention [26]. In response to such rapid proliferation of genomics tests, some of which are being made available direct to the consumer, there is now a need for broadly framed evidentiary frameworks to evaluate genomics applications and their readiness for public health practice. Public health programmes have an important role in ensuring that any diagnostic, predictive or prognostic genomics tests used in health practice are properly evaluated in order to protect the public's health and assure validated health services.

A prevailing evaluation framework for genetic/genomics tests is the Analytical validity, Clinical validity, Clinical utility, and Ethical, legal and social implications (ACCE) evidentiary framework [27], using criteria originally proposed by the 1997 Task Force on Genetic Testing [28].

*Analytical validity*: The analytical validity is an assay's ability to measure accurately, in the case of a genomics test, the genotype or biomarker of interest. Analytical validity is the crucial first-level criterion that needs to be met for a candidate test to be considered. For most available PHG tests, analytical validity is usually available from the manufacturers, regulators or in the published literature.

*Clinical validity*: Clinical validity is the demonstration of robust statistical and epidemiological association between a genomics test result (e.g. the presence/absence of a genetic variant) and the disease or other phenotypes of interest (e.g. drug safety and efficacy). In addition, the clinical validity of a candidate test requires an understanding of the test performance such as sensitivity, specificity, positive and negative predictive values, likelihood ratios and the receiver operating characteristic (ROC) curve characteristics. It is important to bear in mind that a test can have a statistically significant association with the clinical phenotype and yet display a poor predictive value as a clinical diagnostic, thus having inadequate clinical validity.

*Clinical utility*: Clinical utility refers to the likelihood that a test will lead to an improved net health outcome. This outcome is measured in terms of the clinical course of the disease by way of reduced mortality or morbidity, or impact of the disease on the family. In cases of genomics tests that involve prediction of health intervention outcomes, such as drug toxicity, effectiveness of the clinical utility refers to these end points, and the net change therein in terms of risks and benefits. Other factors that influence utility include the availability of an effective intervention in case of a positive genomics test result, and the risks associated with any interventions and health economic assessment.

Among the above three evidence types, all face a contested future. Chief among them is the clinical utility of a test that varies markedly in terms of the associated stakeholder perceptions – the clinical utility is often in the eye of the beholder. It has been also underscored that the scope of ethics, considered as an integral part of the ACCE framework to evaluate candidate genomics applications, is presently expanding beyond classic issues such as informed consent and protection of research subjects to examine the issues related to genomics evidence: which evidence, generated or synthesized by whom, should be employed to adopt or reject genetic tests [29]?

Indeed, the task of evidence-based evaluation has become ever more challenging with the rapid growth in numbers and claims over candidate genomics applications. This has led to a need for a new taxonomy to classify genomics applications with a view to public health action. Notably, the previous binary (up or down) evidence-based recommendation for use of genomics tests frequently returns 'insufficient evidence' of clinical validity and utility for their use in clinical practice. Binary or insufficient evidence recommendations do not permit refined decision-making, especially for clinicians who need to provide advice in the face of insufficient evidence. In response to the need for criteria to determine an 'actionability gradient' for candidate genomics tests, Khoury *et al.* [30] have suggested a three-tier evidence-based classification of recommendations for use of genomic tests:

- *Tier 1*: 'use in practice' – These applications demonstrate analytic validity, clinical validity and clinical utility, and there are evidenced-based guidelines encouraging their use;
- *Tier 2*: 'promote informed decision-making' – These applications demonstrate analytic and clinical validity, display potential for clinical utility (e.g. well-designed trials with appropriately selected endpoints are known to be in progress), but there are no evidence-based guidelines recommending clinical use; and
- *Tier 3*: 'discourage use' – These applications have not yet demonstrated adequate analytic validity, clinical validity or clinical utility, or have demonstrated evidence of harms. The use of such applications is discouraged.

The intermediate category of promoting informed decision-making is particularly notable because it provides interim guidance for clinical and public health practice. The framework for assigning genomics applications to one of the above three tiers requires consideration, in the context of intended use, of the analytic validity, clinical validity and clinical utility of the test, and of the existence of an evidence-based recommendation.

As of 28 January 2013, the US Centers for Disease Control and Prevention (CDC) list a number of Tier 1 genomics applications, which can be seen in Table 6.1. Future updates by the US CDC to the Tier 1 to 3 PHG applications should be consulted to keep abreast of the emerging genomics tests, and to differentiate what is actionable, which tests are in the process of transition from discovery to practice and which tests are not ready or should not be used in practice.

## The road ahead

### *A strategic vision for the next generation of PHG innovation and scholarship*

These earlier efforts to develop PHG applications rested on a 'translation research' model that set out to show PHG implications for many different aspects of clinical and public health

*Table 6.1* Tier 1 genomic and family health history applications are recommended for clinical use by evidence-based panels based on a systematic review of analytic validity, clinical validity and utility for specific clinical scenarios

| *Test/application* | *Scenario* | *Evidence-based recommendation* |
|---|---|---|
| Newborn screening panel of 31 core conditions | Screening all newborns at birth through public health programs | Secretary's Advisory Committee on Heritable Diseases of Newborns and Children: Recommended Uniform Newborn Screening Panel (2011) |
| *BRCA* genetic counseling/*BRCA* genetic testing | Referral to genetic counseling of women with specific family history patterns of breast or ovarian cancer | US Preventive Services Task Force: Genetic Risk Assessment and BRCA Mutation Testing for Breast and Ovarian Cancer Susceptibility (2005)<br>*Additional information*:<br>NCCN Guideline: Genetic/Familial High-Risk Assessment: Breast and Ovarian Cancer (2012) |

| | | |
|---|---|---|
| Lynch syndrome testing | Screening newly diagnosed cases of colorectal cancer for Lynch syndrome and cascade testing of relatives of affected Lynch syndrome cases | Recommendations of the EGAPP Working Group: genetic testing strategies in newly diagnosed individuals with colorectal cancer aimed at reducing morbidity and mortality from Lynch syndrome in relatives (2009)<br>*Additional information*:<br>NCCN Task Force Report: Evaluating the Clinical Utility of Tumor Markers in Oncology (2011) |
| Familial hypercholesterolemia | Cascade cholesterol testing with/without DNA analysis among relatives of affected persons with familial hypercholesterolemia | NICE Guideline: identification and management of familial hypercholesterolemia (2008) |
| HLA testing for abacavir sensitivity | Testing HIV patients before starting abacavir to reduce adverse effects and inform drug choice | DHHS Advisory Committee on HIV treatment: Guidelines for the Use of Antiretroviral Agents in HIV-1-infected Adults and Adolescents (2012) |
| HER2 mutation testing in breast cancer | Routine testing for HER2 mutations in patients with invasive breast cancer to target therapy | NICE Guideline: early and locally advanced breast cancer: diagnosis and treatment (2009)<br>*Additional information*:<br>American Society of Clinical Oncology/College of American Pathologists guideline recommendations for human epidermal growth factor receptor 2 testing in breast cancer (2007) |
| EGFR mutation tumor analysis in non-small cell lung cancer | Predictive for therapy | NICE Guideline: erlotinib for the first-line treatment of locally advanced or metastatic EGFR-TK mutation-positive non-small cell lung cancer (2012)<br>*Additional Information*:<br>NCCN Clinical Practice Guidelines in Oncology: Non–Small Cell Lung Cancer. Version 3 (2012)<br>BCBSA Tec Evaluation – Epidermal Growth Factor Receptor Mutations and Tyrosine Kinase Inhibitor Therapy in Advanced Non-Small-Cell Lung Cancer (2011) |
| First-degree family history of breast cancer | To inform discussion of chemoprevention for breast cancer for women; consider age and other risk factors to identify high risk for breast cancer and low risk for adverse effects | US Preventive Services Task Force: Chemoprevention of Breast Cancer (2002) |

(*Continued overleaf*)

*Table 6.1* Continued

| *Test/application* | *Scenario* | *Evidence-based recommendation* |
|---|---|---|
| Family history of cardiovascular disease before 50 years of age in male relatives and 60 years of age in female relatives | To inform earlier start to screening for cholesterol abnormalities for men and women (starting at age 20); use to identify increased risk for lipid disorders | US Preventive Services Task Force: Screening for Lipid Disorders in Adults (2008) |
| Parental history of fracture | To inform (in combination with other risk factors) earlier start to screening for osteoporosis in women | US Preventive Services Task Force: Screening for Osteoporosis (2011) |
| Family history, especially siblings, with hereditary hemochromatosis | Counseling for genetic testing for hereditary hemochromatosis among asymptomatic people | US Preventive Services Task Force: Screening for Hemochromatosis (2006) |
| Family history of breast or ovarian cancer that includes a relative with a *known* deleterious *BRCA* mutation | Referral to counseling for BRCA genetic testing for women | US Preventive Services Task Force: Genetic Risk Assessment and BRCA Mutation Testing for Breast and Ovarian Cancer Susceptibility (2005) |

*Source*: Reproduced from [39].

practice. However, the changes in the practice and folklore of post-genomics science and technology noted above now demand a vision substantively broader than that earlier translation framework. In particular, general drivers of innovation, such as demography, technology, the environment, and the intersection of the global and local forces, the new 'GloCal' public health science, will necessitate a new approach to health in the twenty-first century [29, 31]. This new vision must:

- Encompass *all* the components of what has variously been called personalized, stratified or precision medicine across applications for disease and health interventions (e.g. drugs, nutrition, vaccines) [9];
- Have regard for the complexities of biological systems and the emerging set of post-genomic science including epigenetic science and the findings of systems biology;
- Take into account the novel post-genomics technologies (e.g. proteomics, metabolomics) developed as a consequence of our better understanding of genomic science and the issues around the development of various infrastructure science projects;
- Be cognizant of the changing epidemiology of disease, especially the rise in non-communicable diseases (NCDs) in emerging economies; and
- Chime with the changing social structures and dynamics of the twenty-first century.

The PHG work over the past decade has set the agenda and, by identifying a number of key issues, showed how an understanding of the scientific basis of modern biology and its ethical, social and legal implications would impact upon the practice of medicine and public health. As we move into the future, real-world implementation of this emerging knowledge and technologies will take on greater priority. Moving theory and evidence into practice will require capacity-building for PHG in the Asia-Pacific and other global regions to evaluate the impact and consequences of PHG for the practice of medicine and population health, while at the same time keeping a watch by real-time and dynamic horizon scanning for emerging post-genomic sciences, and their social and political science corollaries.

The end result of this next generation of PHG endeavour will produce real-life transformative changes across the entire healthcare system and a new understanding by both politicians and citizens of how these drivers must lead to a new way of organizing health care and practising medicine. This, we submit here, can be achieved by championing the creation of a global 'PHG innovation ecosystem' that will utilize the constituents of public health genomics as levers of change in the health and policy arena. We herein name this much-needed approach as the '*practice turn*' for PHG and data-intensive omics sciences [6, 31].

To be sure, creating healthy and sustainable modern societies in the twenty-first century – be it in 'developed' or 'developing' countries – requires *integrated knowledge ecosystems* (see Figure 6.2), with contributions from all sectors of science and society.

It is interesting to note that discussing the state of health at the beginning of the twenty-first century is not dissimilar to discussing the state of the environment. Both are in crisis and run counter to the notion of sustainable societies, both focus around inequities that have accrued over centuries in our societies and both indicate that transformative, if not radical, changes in our mindsets are required at the levels of both the '*science of whys*' and the '*science of hows*':

> Both our extensive knowledge about what creates health, as well as the exponentially rising rates of chronic disease, obesity and mental health problems, indicate that we need

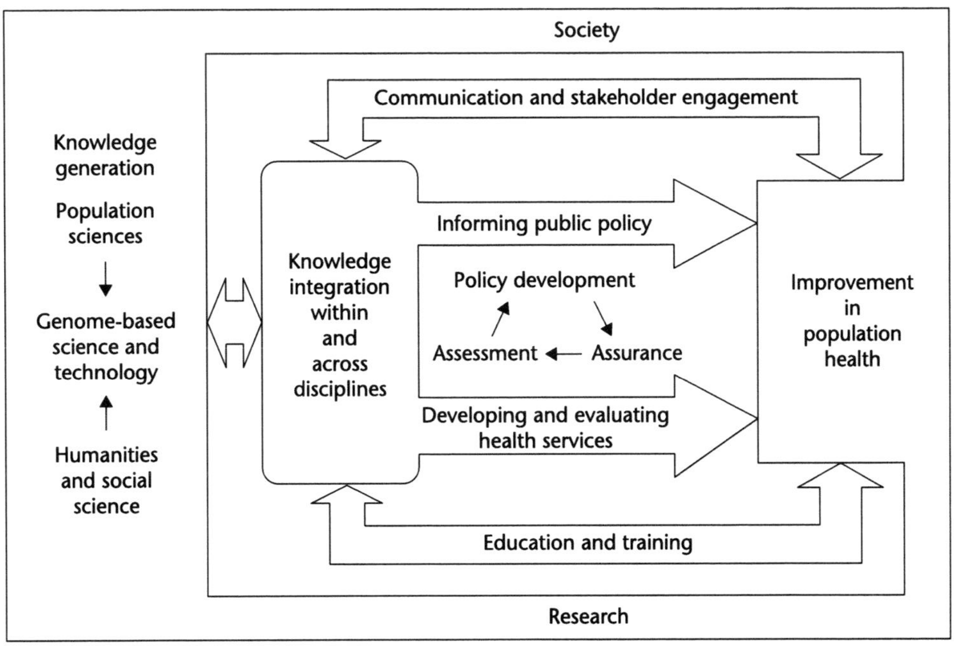


*Figure 6.2* Integrated knowledge ecosystems

> to shift course and apply a radically new mindset to health . . . Some warning voices state that the present generation of children – born at the turn of the century – might be the first to have a lower life expectancy than their parents. After the extraordinary gains in health and longevity over the last 100 years, such a development would indeed represent a phenomenal failure . . . Clearly if health is created by factors outside the remit of the traditional health sector then the creation of a healthy society needs commitment and action from all sectors of government, new partnerships for health, and citizens' participation [32].

The above analysis suggests ways forward for what is needed to transform the 'one-scientist-one-project paradigm' that has hitherto prevailed throughout nineteenth, as well as twentieth, century public health towards cross-disciplinary collaborative population health in the twenty-first century, including the need to work with, and include the view of, citizens for transdisciplinary knowledge co-production [7, 29]. Such *collective innovation* offers the promise of novel diagnostics for complex diseases and single gene disorders, as well as customized drug therapies, vaccines, cell-based therapies and nutrition.

This last point is important. The central tenet of PHG is recognizing and explaining population heterogeneity in host-environment interactions using genome-based science and technologies specifically, and the emerging tools of modern biology more broadly. Seen in this light, it becomes clearer that the field of PHG aims to bring modern science into public health science and practice; in particular to ensure that public health practitioners are mindful and responsive to individual differences in the population, for example, in the way we are differentially susceptible to illness and respond to health interventions, such as drugs, nutrition and vaccines. Seeing our societies as being comprised of both populations *and* individuals brings about a transformative perspective to centuries of public health practice that overlooked person-to-person real-life variations in health and sustainable well-being, and failed to define the dynamic relationships between the individual and the population.

Conversely, continuing to see human populations as a homogenous sea of identically constructed individuals only helps to create a 'straw man' whose foundations easily fall apart upon a real-life gaze into the public health practice – be they single gene disorders, birth defects or treatment-resistant tuberculosis that are increasingly devastating the resource-limited settings in the global North and South or the adverse drug reactions that rank as the fourth to sixth leading causes of death. More crucially, there are diagnostics – already in existence and accessible – that are not being used in public health practice. The question then becomes: how can we transform both the mindsets and the practice of twenty-first-century public health so that not only the concepts but also their day-to-day responsible applications can be realized now? Such bridging of theory and action is not, however, always tenable and may take years to decades to materialize.

To this end, it is noteworthy that the concept of 'global health' itself is presently undergoing transformative conceptual changes. While global health debates in the past have extensively focused on poverty in developing countries, this is only a partial incomplete account of the larger set of challenges that cuts across the traditional Westphalian model of independent sovereign nation states. That is, health inequities and poverty are vastly endemic throughout the globe and importantly impact health and well-being of individuals and communities in countries that are traditionally designated as 'developed' [33]. Hence, if we are to truly tackle global health, there is a need to focus on *resource-limited settings and communities per se*, and on the heterogeneity of human populations, regardless in which geographical location and nation-state they might be situated. Reorienting our population health focus on resource-limited contexts and on heterogeneity, both social and biological, rather than the artificial nation-state boundaries, is important for truly engaging in an inclusive 'global health' discourse.

Indeed, some of the major actors – previously defined as 'developing countries' – that are now shaping global policy have increasingly complex identities reflecting their rapid development. The need to think beyond the classic binaries of the 'developed' and 'developing' world has become markedly clear within the current global economic and health crisis. For example, at the global UN NCD Summit held in New York City in September 2011, India was among the low- and middle-income countries (LMICs) eligible to receive global aid to help curb the shared risk factors tied to Western-centric social and economic development. At the global Financial Summit in Washington in the same month, by contrast, India – along with fellow BRICS members China, Brazil, Russia and South Africa – debated how, and whether, their fast-growing economies and powerful emerging markets should help Europe contain its debt crisis.

The two very different realities embodied in a BRIC country like India are testament to how technological and economic progress is having a double-edged impact in a context of global health, reorienting its classic definitions. Recognizing that emerging powers such as India represent a *new hybrid* – in much the same way as the field of PHG or nations that are at once developing and affluent – is one important step toward strategically planning for how best to respond to the cross-cutting emerging needs in global health in the twenty-first century.

Adding to these game-changing complexities that define the need for a practice turn in PHG is the new challenge of Big Data. As noted earlier, data on the order of zettabytes are now sought as part of the solution, not the problem, in addressing the complex challenges we face in global health-related fields as diverse as pharmaceuticals and health care, watershed and ecosystem safety, global warming, climate change and oceanography. These collectively impact population health and sustainable well-being, serving as levers inside and outside the health sector that are ultimately inseparable and interconnected.

Public health scientists are not the only ones who are jumping on the Big Data bandwagon in global public health. We are increasingly witnessing global and distributed forms of knowledge production in the post-genomics era including, but well beyond, the ivory towers and academic experts. Direct-to-consumer (DTC) availability of products that rely on Big Data (e.g. whole genome sequencing for prediction of individual health risks) has brought consumers and scientists into closer proximity. Citizen-scientists now contribute to Big Data R&D, for example, in collection of high-granularity observations for ecosystem epidemiology where geographically distributed real-time science is crucial. Moreover, social media generates copious volumes of data that can reveal insights on consumer behaviours, computer hacker networking traffic or the spread of infectious diseases, to name a few.

Notably, population health science for too long rested on the individual-gain centred entrepreneurship model. The arrival of Big Data firmly challenges this long held (and often unexamined) assumption in translating science to innovative products [7, 34, 35]. New forms of collaboration ranging from open consortia, increased cross-disciplinary teaming, opening up to citizen-scientists for both data collection and analysis, as well as evolution of models of open data and open publication are transforming science rapidly. By virtue of its reliance on transdisciplinary expertise, not to mention consumers and citizen-scientists as explained above, a new kind of *hybrid* entrepreneurship model is emerging in the age of Big Data and PHG – one that recognizes and rewards both individuals' and groups' collective contributions

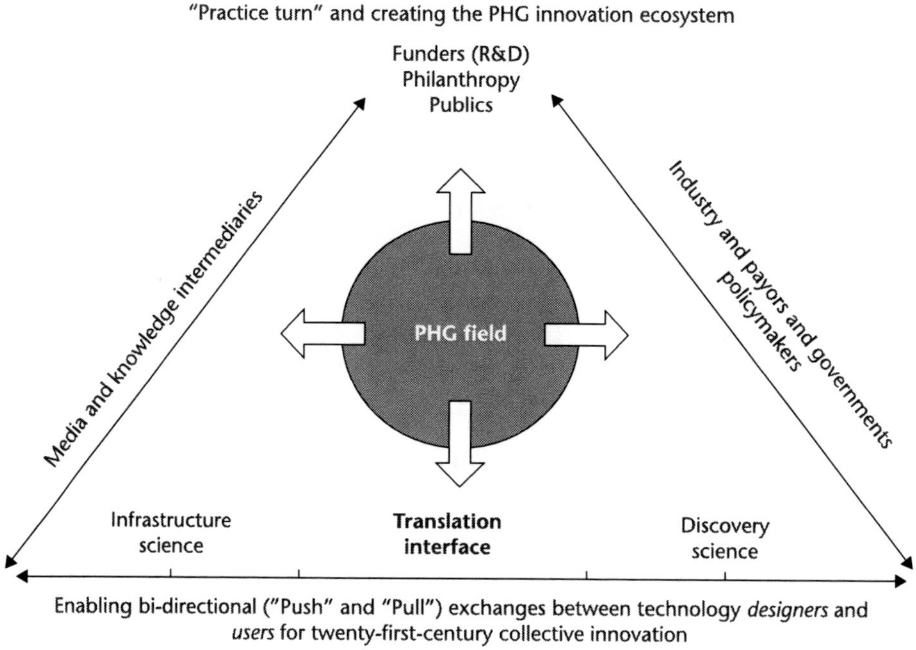


*Figure 6.3* Creating a PHG innovation ecosystem for global public health

so that large-scale datasets can be accessed, shared and analysed on the critical path to innovative products.

Big Data that underpins the modern twenty-first-century public health sciences calls for new modes of doing business in PHG and global health whereby the R&D actors, ranging from scientists, industry, regulators and policy makers, utilize the assistance of independent and standalone observatories – a type of 'innovation narrator' – that measure the performance of the Big Data innovation ecosystem with credible analytical distance from it while being firmly engaged with it at the same time.

Finally, there is much to be gained from a PHG 'practice' perspective to engage not only the 'push' factors (e.g. PHG scientists, academics, technology designers) but also the 'pull' factors (e.g. communities in resource-limited settings) within the framework of the proposed global PHG innovation ecosystem (see Figure 6.3).

## *Collaboration across PHG communities and epistemic cultures*

Introduction of genomics and Big Data to public health sciences and practice brings about new challenges. These challenges can be summed up in 'five Vs':

- Volume
- Velocity
- Variety
- Veracity and
- Valorization.

Together with the enormous increase in sheer amount (volume), speed (velocity) and type (variety) of data generated in biomedical sciences, the last two Vs refer to tensions posed by data validation (veracity) and lack of adequate understanding of knowledge co-production models that enable complex collaboration to move Big Data to value-added knowledge (valorization) [7, 34, 35].

The massively collaborative biomedical science that drives twenty-first-century discovery is put into action by consortia made up of thousands of scientists, distributed across different scales, geographical locales, disciplines and epistemologies. But rather than existing in a vacuum, the collective innovation practice (Big Data Science) coexists with the classic 'Edisonian discovery science' (single P-I, single lab, single project model) that promotes individual entrepreneurship and personal gain (e.g. withholding data for patents, first-authored publications, etc.). Never before in the long history of biomedical sciences have such conflicting values had to coexist in the same practice space and time. These promises and challenges of Big Data demand understanding the new and emergent forms of knowledge co-production, complex collaboration and organizing so as to link large-scale consortia science with discovery (small) science to ultimately harness the genome/omics commons. Table 6.2 provides a comparison of the discovery science and the collectivist consortia science.

It is interesting to note that we know very little about how individuals and the innovation actors are organizing themselves in the practice of data-enabled sciences, ways in which collaborations (e.g. cooperation, competition, pre-competitive collaboration and post-competitive collaboration) are developed, sustained or devolved, what human values guide and inform the knowledge ecologies emergent from collective innovation and, ultimately, how knowledge is created, transformed and transferred between innovators and users [36–38].

## Conclusion

Intersection of public health practice and genome-based knowledge and understanding how this new transdisciplinary knowledge co-production trajectory can be steered constructively to improve health and prevent disease or achieve rational therapeutics and health interventions through the principles of stratified medicine are among the salient grand challenges of twenty-first-century post-genomics biology. Ultimately, the field of PHG is an effort to

*Table 6.2* Comparison of discovery science and consortia science

| *Discovery (small-scale) science* | *Collective (consortia) science* |
|---|---|
| *Modus operandi* is 'single-scientist single-project' | *Modus operandi* is 'massively collaborative open science' |
| Primary objective is discovery of new knowledge using available lab and infrastructure science | Primary objective is 'infrastructure science', such as bioinformatics, cloud computing and biobanks, creating a 'digital commons' that can be creatively harvested by discovery science |
| Organization of practice centres on first-authored publications, grants, patents and individual entrepreneurship | Co-produced by both experts and non-professionals such as citizens, various publics and knowledge users; *individual* versus *group* level organization of practice and the tensions between them remain unexplored empirically |

bring modern biology and science to public health to address population heterogeneity in disease and health intervention outcomes. It is also a timely response to build global science and collaboration across epistemic cultures and diverse communities so as to respond in real time to the dynamic changes presently shaping population health with the availability of genomics sciences and technologies [9]. Identification of the *actionable diagnostics* to influence and shape twenty-first-century PHG practice will be an ongoing challenge and promises to move the field from its traditional epistemology and theory to evidence-based practice.

As we gaze into the future, building communities of practice to fulfil these promises and address gaps in traditional public health practice, particularly in hitherto unprecedented or neglected global locales [9], will help create innovative public spaces for, and by, the next generation of practitioners. The emerging sub-speciality of reflexive technology governance (RTG) within the PHG community offers further hope for sustainable applications of genomics in public health practice in developing countries [9]. As we move from a science where data collection was an essential locus of the scientific endeavour to one where data collection is automated or at least made easier and is available in digital form, we need to maintain an unassuming open mind to understand the new collaborative possibilities that emerge.

## Acknowledgements

The analysis, concepts and work reported herein were informed and supported by the following research grants to the author: Canadian Institutes of Health Research operating research grant, #84620, on pharmacogenomics policy, and a research grant from the Social Sciences and Humanities Research Council, 231644, on emerging biotechnology foresight research. The views expressed in this chapter are entirely the personal opinions of the author and do not necessarily represent the positions of their affiliated institutions or the funding agencies.

## References

1. Bellagio Statement. Genome-based Research and Population Health. Report of an expert workshop held at the Rockefeller Foundation Study and Conference Center, Bellagio, Italy, 14–20 April, 2005.
2. Özdemir V, Kolker E, Hotez PJ, Mohin S, Prainsack B, Wynne B, *et al.* Ready to put metadata on the post-2015 development agenda? Linking data publications to responsible innovation and science diplomacy. *OMICS: A Journal of Integrative Biology* 2014; 18(1): 1–9.
3. Hey T, Tansley S, Tolle K. *The Fourth Paradigm: Data-Intensive Scientific Discovery.* Redmond, WA: Microsoft Research, 2009.
4. Özdemir V, Smith C, Bongiovanni K, Cullen D, Knoppers BM, Lowe A, Peters M, Robbins R, Stewart E, Yee G, Yu YK, Kolker E. Policy and data-intensive scientific discovery in the beginning of the 21st century. *OMICS* 2011; 15(4): 221–225.
5. Özdemir V, Suarez-Kurtz G, Stenne R, Somogyi AA, Someya T, Kayaalp SO, Kolker E. Risk assessment and communication tools for genotype associations with multifactorial phenotypes: the concept of 'edge effect' and cultivating an ethical bridge between omics innovations and society. *OMICS* 2009; 13(1): 43–61.
6. Dove ES, Faraj SA, Kolker E, Özdemir V. Designing a post-genomics knowledge ecosystem to translate pharmacogenomics into public health action. *Genome Medicine* 2012; 4(11): 91.
7. Dereli T, Coskun Y, Kolker E, Guner O, Agirbasli M, Özdemir V. Big data and ethics review for health systems research in LMICs: understanding risk, uncertainty and ignorance – and catching the black swans? *American Journal of Bioethics* 2014 (in press).

8. Knoppers BM, Özdemir V. Biogenetics and the concept of humanity. In: *Research Project in Humanity*. Van Beers BB (Ed.) Cambridge: Cambridge University Press (forthcoming), 2013.
9. Dove ES, Özdemir V. All the postgenomic world is a stage: the actors and narrators required for translating pharmacogenomics into public health. *Personalized Medicine* 2013; 10(3): 213–16.
10. The Royal Society. *Science as an Open Enterprise*. London: The Royal Society, 2012.
11. The White House. *National Bioeconomy Blueprint*. 1550-9087. April, 2012.
12. Schofield PN, Eppig J, Huala E, de Angelis MH, Harvey M, Davidson D, *et al.* Research funding. Sustaining the data and bioresource commons. *Science* 2012; 330(6004): 592–3.
13. Dumbill E. Making sense of Big Data. *Big Data* January Preview Issue 2013, BD1–BD2. [Online]. Available from: http://www.liebertpub.com/mcontent/files/Big%20Data%20Preview%20Issue.pdf
14. Burke W, Khoury M, Stewart A, Zimmern R, Bellagio Group. The path from genome-based research to population health: development of an international public health genomics network. *Genetics in Medicine* 2006; 8(7): 451–8.
15. Burke W, Burton H, Hall AE, Karmali M, Khoury MJ, Knoppers B, Meslin EM, Stanley F, Wright CF, Zimmern RL; Ickworth Group. Extending the reach of public health genomics: what should be the agenda for public health in an era of genome-based and 'personalized' medicine? *Genetics in Medicine* 2010; 12(12): 785–91.
16. White WI. A new look at the role of urinalysis in the history of diagnostic medicine. *Clinical Chemistry* 1991; 37: 119–25.
17. Özdemir V, Knoppers BM. From government to anticipatory governance: responding to challenges set by emerging technologies and innovation. In: *Governance for Health in the 21st Century*. Kickbusch I (Ed.). New York: Springer (in press), 2013.
18. Suresh S. Moving toward global science. *Science* 2011; 333(6044): 802.
19. Science Metrix. 30 years in science. Secular movements in knowledge creation. 2010. [Online]. Available from: http://www.science-metrix.com/30years-Paper.pdf
20. Hather GJ, Haynes W, Higdon R, *et al.* The United States of America and scientific research. *PLoS One* 2010; 5(8): e12203.
21. Institute of International Education press release. Washington, DC: Nov. 15, 2010.
22. Bagnoli F, Baudner B, Mishra RP, Bartolini E, Fiaschi L, Mariotti P, Nardi-Dei V, Boucher P, Rappuoli R. Designing the next generation of vaccines for global public health. *OMICS* 2011; 15(9): 545–66.
23. Ranganathan S, Eisenhaber F, Tong JC, *et al.* Extending Asia Pacific bioinformatics into new realms in the '-omics' era. *BMC Genomics* 2009; 10(Suppl 3): S1.
24. Manamperi A, Huzair F. Capacity building in genomics medicine and molecular diagnostics: the case of Sri Lanka. *Current Pharmacogenomics and Personalized Medicine* 2012; 11(3): 185–94.
25. Zimmern RL. Genomic medicine: the future is now. Lessons for Hong Kong from the House of Lords Report on Genomic Medicine. *Hong Kong Medical Journal* 2009; 15(5): 324–5.
26. GAPP Finder. Genomic applications in practice and prevention (GAPP) Finder. Office of Public Health Genomics, Centers for Disease Control and Prevention (GAPP), Atlanta, 2012. [Online]. Available from: http://www.hugenavigator.net/GAPPKB/topicStartPage.do
27. Haddow J, Palomaki G. ACCE: A model process for evaluating data on emerging genetic tests. In: *Human Genome Epidemiology*. Khoury M, Little J, Burke W (Eds.), pp. 217–33. Oxford: Oxford University Press, 2004.
28. Holtzman NA, Watson MS (Eds.). Promoting safe and effective genetic testing in the United States. Final report of the Task Force on Genetic Testing. 1997. [Online]. Available from: http://www.genome.gov/10001733
29. Özdemir V, Joly Y, Kirby E, Avard D, Knoppers BM. Beyond ELSIs – Where to from here? From 'regulator' to anticipating and shaping the innovation trajectory in personalized medicine. In: *Pharmacogenomics: Challenges and Opportunities in Therapeutic Implementation*. Lam YWF, Cavallari L (Eds.). Amsterdam: Elsevier (in press), 2013.
30. Khoury MJ, Coates RJ, Evans JP. Evidence-based classification of recommendations on use of genomic tests in clinical practice: dealing with insufficient evidence. *Genetics in Medicine* 2010; 12(11): 680–3.
31. Özdemir V. OMICS 2.0: a practice turn for 21(st) century science and society. *OMICS* 2013; 17(1): 1–4.
32. Kickbusch I. Healthy societies: addressing 21st century health challenges. Adelaide: Department of the Premier and Cabinet, State of South Australia, 2008.

33. Hotez PJ, Bottazzi ME, Dumonteil E, Valenzuela JG, Kamhawi S, Ortega J, *et al.* Texas and Mexico: sharing a legacy of poverty and neglected tropical diseases. *PLoS Neglected Tropical Diseases* 2012; 6(3): e1497.
34. Özdemir V, Dove ES. Theranostics, the 21st century bioeconomy and 'one health'. Interview by Tikki Pang. *Expert Review of Molecular Diagnostics* 2012; 12(8): 807–9.
35. Özdemir V, Dove ES. Direct-to-consumer theranostics, 21st century collective innovation and entrepreneurship. Interview by Barbara Prainsack. *Expert Review of Molecular Diagnostics* 2012; 12(8): 803–5.
36. Petersen A. From bioethics to a sociology of bio-knowledge. *Social Science & Medicine* 2013; 98: 264–70.
37. Solbakk JH. Bioethics on the couch. *Cambridge Quarterly of Healthcare Ethics* 2013; 22(3): 319–27.
38. Ostrom E. *Governing the Commons: The Evolution of Institutions for Collective Action.* Cambridge: Cambridge University Press, 1990.
39. Office of Public Health Genomics, Centers for Disease Control and Prevention. Genomic Tests and Family History by Levels of Evidence. 2013. [Online]. Available from: http://www.cdc.gov/genomics/gtesting/tier.htm (Accessed 28 January 2013).

# 7

# Research challenges for public health in Asia

*Pascale Allotey, Daniel D. Reidpath and Julius Cheah*

## Introduction

Addressing public health in the current global environment encompasses a number of factors, including looking at improving health for whole populations and communities, the reduction of health inequalities within and between communities, and striving for sustained health environments [1]. In real terms, this means that public health practitioners need to understand the nature of *health* and disease, and the context in which health is experienced, enabled or hindered. Evidence is, therefore, the cornerstone of public health and it has traditionally been collected through various methods of surveillance, health information systems, administrative records and through research. Public health research is designed based upon either the systematic collection and analysis of primary data or on the analysis of existing secondary data sources.

However, the type of evidence that is sought, and how it is used, is often intensely political. Interventions for the purposes of making an impact on the health of populations, as opposed to individuals, involve a complex interplay of values, vested interests and political compromises that underpin the distribution of resources, public policy formulation and public health practice. Public health research in Asia therefore not only includes the challenges in undertaking the actual research on particular health-related issues, but also requires an understanding of the context in which that research evidence is gathered and used. Ultimately, for the end goal of improvements in the health of whole populations, the challenge for public health research is also to explore the approaches through which accountabilities can be monitored and analysed to ensure that the evidence generated is used to benefit the population and not for some other agenda.

In this chapter, we discuss the current research challenges in public health with a particular focus on the context of 'doing' public health in Asia. We present a brief overview of the notion of public health in Asia, which provides the context and parameters for current research, as well as identifying research gaps. We then discuss the challenges of extending public health research to a more comprehensive and inclusive agenda, and offer some suggestions as to how this might be achieved.

## Setting the scene: public health in Asia

Asia, defined here loosely to cover those countries within the Indian subcontinent and within the east and southeast of the continent, is home to about 60 per cent of the world's population, coming from a large number of different racial and ethnic groups. Asia has a rich and diverse cultural heritage and this diversity is also reflected in the political and colonial history, languages, systems of government, and religious and cultural practices. The heterogeneity which exists in the region has a significant impact on the range of issues affecting health, disease and the interaction of populations with the environment; the development of public health institutions; the nature of public health training, policy and practice; and, ultimately, the definition of public health research itself. Commonwealth countries, such as India and Malaysia, retain elements of a public health system defined by the British legacy, which places public health largely within the realm of medicine with a strong emphasis on regulation, administration, sanitation, food safety, vaccination and surveillance [2, 3]. Public health in the Philippines has its historical antecedents in the US public health system, which in turn is based on a 'public health as science' model, focusing heavily on disease control [4]. Various political changes have injected some social justice into public health care and the Philippines currently has very strong social science inputs into public health research and practice through professional lobby groups and technical expertise (often external to government). However, the general approach to public health at the national and professional levels remains largely clinical in focus and is disease driven. Countries such as Thailand, on the other hand, have consistently supported a notion of public health that acknowledges the need for social justice and access for the poor, and these issues remain within the purview of the Ministry of Public Health.

Asia has a rich history and culture in the area of promoting health and wellbeing. The importance of maintaining health is evident across the diversity of ethnic groups and is embedded in the cultural heritage, for instance, in the discourses of local food and drinks, social events and cultural practices, such as massage, herbal baths, and consumption of exotic plants and animals, all of which are believed to provide some protection from particular diseases or to improve health and vitality. Products for the self-management of health are one of the fastest-growing areas in economic development, including a large 'nutraceutical' industry providing products that are advertised for their health and medical benefits, particularly for protection against chronic disease. There is a thriving cosmetics industry that purports to enhance wellbeing, vitality and mental health, and products are available across markets, catering to all socio-economic groups. Prevention of disease and promotion of health are not difficult concepts to sell to the population – even if the products being sold are 'snake oil'.

The Alma Ata declaration on Primary Health Care, unanimously signed by all UN member states in 1978, has had an important influence on the development of health systems across most countries in Asia. The Declaration emphasized the responsibility of the state in ensuring health for all, and defined Primary Health Care as essential health care based on practical, scientifically sound and socially acceptable methods and technology, and made universally accessible to individuals and families through their full participation, and affordable for the individual, community and country. As signatories, governments were therefore committed to placing health systems within the realm of national politics and increasing the accountability of state bodies for equitable health care. Access to health care and public health interventions, such as immunization, were politicized through the People's Health Movement in countries such as India and Bangladesh. On the other hand, governments of Indonesia and

Malaysia were early proponents of universal access, particularly in poor rural communities. They therefore managed to significantly reduce maternal mortality from an estimated 141 per 100,000 live births in 1970 to less than 33 per 100,000 births to date and infant mortality from 41 per 1,000 live births to 6.3 per 1,000 live births over the same period. This has been achieved through a range of public health strategies that include the provision of basic primary healthcare services, emergency obstetric care and close monitoring of outcomes at the community level. More recent influences on developments in health systems come from various models of health sector reforms, the rapid growth of a regional and global private health sector, medical tourism and various others models that run in addition – and sometimes in opposition – to the persistent drivers for universal health coverage, equity and social justice.

The Millennium Development Goals (MDGs), particularly those relating to health, have been a significant driver for countries to begin to undertake, or support, research in non-disease areas of public health. Currently, many countries in Asia report on non-disease indicators such as poverty, gender parity, hunger and environmental sustainability. These have provided some impetus for generating research and data across sectors that have not been traditionally under the health portfolio. Public health research is also largely driven by agencies and researchers external to Asia, often from Europe, the USA and Australia. Less than half of the publications on public health research from low- and middle-income countries in Asia are first authored by researchers affiliated with institutions in the region [5].

Major pandemics over recent decades have been a big influence on the need for public health research. The rapid spread of HIV in countries such as Thailand was a catalyst for research to explore the risk factors and develop interventions that could be appropriately targeted. Similarly, the spread of the viruses causing SARS, H5N1 and H1N1 influenza over the last decade have resulted in joint efforts by national governments, international health agencies and global health funding bodies to increase research and monitor efforts for prevention and control of these diseases. Other catalysts for research have included a series of environmental disasters, and political and civil conflicts that forced movements of populations displaced by these events.

Evidence required and generated for the purposes of public health policy formulation often comes out of government agencies that focus and place a greater emphasis on data about disease distribution and evaluation of intervention outcomes. Although some evidence might be generated on non-disease challenges and outcomes, it often does not come from health agencies and, therefore, requires a dissemination and advocacy strategy to support its translation into policy and practice.

## Public health research capacity

Research, specifically the generation of primary data, is still predominantly undertaken by higher education institutions and research institutes. A recent review commissioned by the International Association of Epidemiology showed that countries such as China supported epidemiological research through academic institutions and agencies, such as the Chinese Academy of Medical Sciences, public health agencies and international organizations. Governments of other countries tend to be reactive and commission research in response to a crisis. Malaysia has the National Institutes of Health, a dedicated arm of the Ministry of Health that undertakes or commissions research projects to support disease control programmes.

Public health practice necessarily defines the training of public health researchers and practitioners in order to ensure that the workforce retains the competencies that are at the core of the values embodied by a particular approach to public health. An example of this can be seen in the fact that tertiary public health training is mostly undertaken by the departments of the schools of medicine. Until about ten years ago, public health as a professional qualification was, in most parts of Asia, open only to physicians as an area of specialization. Schools of public health within higher education institutions are beginning to open up to encourage greater multidisciplinary engagement. Capacity in the low- and middle-income countries is a particular challenge and for several countries this is addressed through 'sandwich' programmes, which support research being conducted in the home country of the student, while taking advantage of the formal educational structures and economic support in higher-income regions, particularly in Australia and in European countries. Other related professional areas of public health are offered as technical qualifications, including environmental health officers and food hygiene inspectors. Research generated under these models focuses largely on surveillance. Non-award programmes and short courses have provided alternative training methods for public health and public health researchers largely through the non-government sector.

The Blakely and Dhillon reviews on the status of epidemiology and capacity in the region report on the heterogeneity of training [5, 6]. The majority of publications (in English-language peer-reviewed journals) on public health research are generated from institutions and researchers in China, India, Thailand, Singapore and Bangladesh. Publication rates out of China are currently low but growing exponentially. In 2005, over 19,000 papers were submitted for publication from China alone. This number grew to over 113,000 by 2010 [7]. The lowest numbers of submissions for publications are reported from Korea, Vietnam and the Philippines [5, 6] (approximately 20,000 with an acceptance rate of 0.3 per cent) [7]. It is important to note that the focus of these publications is largely on epidemiology. Publications on topics relating to applied social sciences in public health are generated predominantly by researchers from India, the Philippines and Thailand.

An important aspect of research capacity relates to the funding available. Although several countries across the region have made commitments to support health research, very few have the formal infrastructure, such as national research councils, to promote or support local investigator-driven research [8]. Domestic funding for health research is negligible. This means that outside of the directly government-funded research and surveillance data generated through the Ministry of Health and related bodies, public health research is mostly driven by external institutions. The result of this is poor ownership by relevant national stakeholders of the results generated by the research.

## Public health research priorities: disease burden and risk factors

In most countries, health research priorities are generally driven by disease control, which provides the need for ongoing epidemiological research to reflect current and emerging diseases. The variation in the disease burden reflects the state of development across high-income countries, such as Singapore and Brunei; middle-income countries, such as Thailand, Malaysia and India; and low-income countries, such as Cambodia, Laos and Vietnam. Based on the World Health Statistics 2012 [9], the mean life expectancy across the region is 70 years; the lowest being 62 years in Cambodia and Lao People's Democratic Republic and the highest being 83 years in Japan. Most countries in the region are experiencing the epidemic of chronic non-communicable diseases (NCDs), such as heart disease, stroke, cancer and chronic obstructive pulmonary disease, which account for 60 per cent of deaths in the region [10]. Death rates from NCDs were highest in the lower-income countries, namely Myanmar, Cambodia, Laos and Vietnam, with a third of these deaths occurring in the 15 to 59 age group, accounting for 51 per cent of deaths in that age group [10]. However, adjusted for age, proportions of deaths due to chronic NCDs were greatest in higher-income countries, such as Singapore, Malaysia and Brunei. The incidence of cancers is also unacceptably high in the region with liver cancers in both men and women recorded as the second highest in the world. Prevalence rates of other cancers reflect trends in other parts of the world [11].

Risk factors for chronic NCDs include alcohol and tobacco use, high blood pressure, occupational risk, high blood glucose, indoor air pollution, being overweight or obese, unsafe water, sanitation and hygiene, and low fruit and vegetable intake. This pattern suggests a transition to environmentally conditioned behavioural risk factors [5]. This also suggests that these risk factors are modifiable with effective public health interventions.

The work of global initiatives, such as the UN Summit on Non-Communicable Diseases, encourages governments to focus attention on the prevention and management of chronic conditions, and also to improve research and surveillance systems for monitoring and evaluating interventions. The evidence collected is an important mechanism for ensuring accountability. Furthermore, monitoring the status of these conditions needs to remain a significant part of the public health research agenda, not only to map how the trends change with increasing levels of development, but also to be able to continue exploring the evolution of risks. There is evidence to suggest that there is a range of biomarkers for several chronic diseases, but the precise effects of biological risk, and how these interact with environmental factors, are not well understood. There is also significant evidence that needs to be collected on appropriate interventions that take into account the cultural, ethnic and religious diversity, gender and socio-economic circumstances, health systems effects, availability of treatment and other contextual factors, and the mechanisms for ensuring that these interventions are effectively implemented [12].

The disease burden from many of the more traditional causes of morbidity and mortality in lower-income countries in Asia remains unacceptably high, again highlighting the extent of disparities in the region. The under-5 mortality per 1,000 is 68 for Lao PDR and 60 for Cambodia, as compared to 3 per 1,000 in countries such as Singapore and Japan. While, in general, the region has made some progress in reducing maternal mortality, countries such as Timor Leste still record a ratio of 420 per 100,000 live births, as compared to Malaysia with 30 per 100,000 [13]. Infectious diseases of poverty remain a problem, with rates of tuberculosis, diarrhoeal diseases and lower respiratory infections accounting for more than one-fifth of the world's mortality burden [14]. Access to safe drinking water and sanitation is not guaranteed, particularly for rural populations, and children continue to die from malnutrition and vaccine-preventable diseases. Based on a coverage index measured across family planning, maternal health, infant immunization and treatment of sick children, low-income countries in the region such as Cambodia and the Philippines still have a coverage gap of over 25 per cent of the expected coverage to achieve the health-related MDGs [5].

Limited resources often mean that compromises have to be made in order to focus on the priorities, although the criteria for prioritization are not always transparent. Small-scale studies by specific interest groups and by universities in various countries across Asia highlight a plethora of other health research challenges that require further investigation. Adolescent health poses persistent questions relating to risk taking in sexual practices, including teenage pregnancies and sexually transmissible diseases, drug and alcohol use, injuries related to road traffic accidents and violence, mental health and mood-related disorders, high suicide rates and general poor sexual health, often relating to confusion of sexual identity and sexual orientation. Non-fulfilment of sexual and reproductive health and rights presents challenges in low-, middle- and high-income countries in Asia across the lifespan. These problems relate to fertility and infertility, sexual identity, choice of partner and forms of domestic violence, and reproductive choices. The gap in these areas of research is particularly problematic because of the strong emotions engendered by sexuality and sexual practices in a region where religious, social and moral values, while complex and diverse, are also often conservative.

Occupational health, within an increasingly stressed and often unstable employment environment, also presents important challenges that do not attract the level of interest or funding given their global significance. Within the older population groups in the region, there is a dearth of public health evidence on rates and management of dementia, sequelae of stroke and cardiovascular conditions, other common age-related conditions and contextual factors, such as social isolation and social support, financial management of health-related expenditure and so on.

Also requiring public health research attention are special populations, such as migrant groups (see Chapter 3) and sex workers. Asia has the most mobile population in the world with many countries largely reliant on remittances from their temporary emigrant workforce (e.g. the Philippines), while others rely on an unskilled, temporary migrant workforce (e.g. Malaysia). The region is also an important hub for human trafficking. The vulnerabilities of these populations present clear public health challenges. Very few countries in Asia have provisions in health (and immigration) policy and practice that are inclusive of migrant groups within health-related programmes. There is a level of discrimination against migrants because they undertake the lower paid jobs that citizens are unwilling to do and are perceived to be competing for resources. In addition, migrants raise the subject of the traditional public health regulatory problem of the transmission of infectious diseases across borders. Available research across these health issues and sub-populations tends to cover basic areas, such as documenting communicable diseases in migrants, or HIV and risk factors in sex workers.

Essentially, areas of public health, such as epidemiology, continue to dominate public health research. A commissioned review by the International Epidemiological Association on the state of epidemiology across the WHO regions provides a detailed analysis of epidemiological research in the South-East Asia (SEARO) and Western Pacific (WPRO) regions [5, 6]. Methodologies for disease surveillance are well established and, for the most part, would be considered standard in public health research and practice. These areas of research continue to be important in public health and still provide challenges in disease surveillance in many Asian countries. Cause of death statistics are notoriously inaccurate and improving the situation is hampered not only by a lack of infrastructure and capacity, but also by cultural and religious edicts in countries that preclude post-mortems and require burial within 24 hours of death. This notwithstanding, epidemiological surveillance, and the provision of basic health statistics, probably constitutes the 'low-hanging fruit' within a much larger public health agenda.

There are several other areas of public health research where there are significant gaps. Research on environmental influences on health and disease, and on the effects of climate and climate change, are fast-growing areas of public health expertise. Social epidemiology has generated evidence that has opened up a major global health agenda on the social determinants of health. It has now been clearly demonstrated, for instance, that poverty and socio-economic status, geography, migration, gender and human rights violations all have a significant effect on health and outcomes of disease [15]. Understanding the associations of these factors with disease and health is critical to public health. Any associations also have to be understood in the context in which they occur, and herein lies another major challenge for the region. Available data for analyses on the social determinants of health support are epidemiologically based on a measure of socio-economic status. Therefore most of our current knowledge on the broader determinants of health is based on data from high-income countries and it cannot be assumed that the associations would be universal.

The systems for delivering primary, secondary and tertiary care are the core, but often forgotten, aspect of public health and public health research. The structure of a health system is a significant determinant of health. The implementation of the comprehensive primary health care model in Malaysia three decades ago was an important determinant in improving maternal and child health outcomes in the country, although these have stagnated in recent times. Structural choices about universal coverage (what that means and who is covered), the public–private mix and healthcare workforce training will all have an impact on the health of a population. The immediate effect will be seen by those seeking health care, but the more wide-reaching effect will be on these individuals' family and the community. This is a critical area of research just beginning in the region, particularly given the rising epidemic of chronic NCDs, as well as the multiple burdens faced by the disadvantaged communities [16, 17, 18]. There is still, however, relatively little research actually conducted within the region that traces the impact of health system choices and public health.

The growing burden of chronic diseases has supported the endurance of strong traditional, complementary and alternative health systems and healthcare practices [19]. While there is an established and growing body of evidence on complementary and alternative medicines in the region, much of the current practice is embedded within the cultures of the various ethnic groups. Religion also has a strong influence on attitudes towards health, and practices that promote health and prevent disease. Given the role they play in the lives of the population, these traditional practices need to be part of the broader public health research agenda.

Evidence-based, or at least well-evaluated, health policy is rare. Governments do not generally want to know whether a policy works – they want to know that the policy choice *they made* worked. The search is for evidence of success. The capacity in the region to engage with the health policy process independent of government is heavily constrained by political needs. This is not peculiar to the region but some governments are more sensitive and fail to distinguish between critique and criticism. There is also a capacity gap within the region. Because public health is so strongly associated with quantitative analysis and surveillance, less effort has been put into developing a cadre of health policy analysts.

## Envisioning public health

To conclude, it is worth speculating where the future of public health research is headed in Asia. This vision is probably not so different from the vision for public health research for the rest of the world, except that the emphasis on context would mean that distinctly Asian factors would arise.

The current trend of public health research is important and is likely to continue. There are two areas of public health research that are likely to be significant in the future: implementation research and developing an understanding of the values basis for public health interventions.

## Implementation research

Globally, public health knowledge has been focused on knowing the facts, such as the cause of a disease and the treatment for a health issue. The problem with a fact-based approach to public health is that it assumes that, once armed with the knowledge, the solution is self-evident. Just deliver the drug, stop the harmful behaviour or undertake the health-promoting behaviour. The 'just' attitude, however, is an issue of implementation. How does one deliver the drug or promote a new behaviour? Currently, there is hardly any research on this.

Research reveals facts and technocrats implement. Once pointed in the right direction, the Ministry of (Public) Health slowly grinds out the solution. For some issues, this can work extremely well as seen by the many ministries in Asia that have successfully rolled out a new vaccine. But this may fail when the target group is marginalized and/or resistant. When well-tried approaches do not work, when the 'just' attitude fails, there is no strong basis for public health research into implementation. Knowing that something is true and knowing how to intervene are distinct kinds of public health knowledge, requiring distinct kinds of research. Unfortunately, current research is concerned with knowing 'what', rather than knowing 'how'.

Future public health research will need to develop a much stronger evidence base for implementation. Acknowledging the diversity of cultural groups across South, East and Southeast Asia, and the variation in health-promoting/diminishing practices this implies, the research approaches that are required need to support the implementation of public health interventions. These may result in 'one-size-fits-all' solutions or may require additional research to investigate specific interventions for specific (sub-)groups.

A decade ago, there was a disease outbreak in South Asia that was otherwise well controlled by vaccination. The ministries of health mobilized to re-vaccinate the populations. The epidemiological evidence quickly showed the outbreak occurred mainly within the children of a marginalized sub-group. A subsequent investigation revealed little commitment to the vaccination by the community when other more pressing needs relating to housing remained unaddressed. This is exactly the kind of situation when knowing that a particular vaccine is protective, and knowing how to maintain routine vaccination, are far from being the same kind of knowledge.

The way implementation research has been described leads to a definition of it always being a forensic investigation of the cultural practices of one group or another, and the beliefs that impede the application of an intervention, and this is certainly part of it. But, there is another aspect of implementation, which relates to broader systems issues. For example, it is well known that smoking affects an individual's health and significant work has been done on factors that affect the success of smoking interventions. Some of the research has looked at individual factors, family factors and cultural practices within groups, but these seem to get us only so far in reducing smoking rates at the population level. Research has also been conducted on the larger systems issue of the relationship between ministries within government (health, finance, agriculture); between government and industry; and between government, industry, researchers and non-government organizations – some of which support the tobacco industry and some of which do not. The 'just' kind of solution is 'just ban smoking' or 'just raise excise on tobacco'. However, in the absence of a contextually specific understanding of the systems issues, and ways of successfully engaging with the system politically, implementing these kinds of interventions is likely to fail. The research base for systems engagement is scant and regarded as being more of an art than a science. This perception may be correct or it may be a combination of both.

### *The values basis of public health*

Whenever resources are limited, decisions need to be made about their allocation and this is also true when dealing with health, as it is in other areas such as agriculture and education. Rationally, one should seek as much gain as possible for the resource inputs available (i.e. one should seek efficiency in the achievement of goals). Knowing that efficiency makes sense, however, does not provide any insight into the domains over which efficiency should be achieved. Given the limited resources available to support health, and the certainty that the health desires of a community will usually exceed the available resources, the question of where these resources should be directed needs to be asked.

There have been rigorous technocratic attempts to define universal, objective measures of population health. If these measures are correct, then resources should be directed with the goal of achieving these improvements most efficiently. Although debate around the universal and objective nature of this has generally been resisted, it is clear that the way in which a population's health is defined is historically and culturally varied. This variation has an impact on the emphasis that is placed on resource allocation and this is a significant value issue for public health.

The manner in which health is valued in a population raises questions about whose health is most important: Does every child count? Does every child count more than every person over the age of 70? Do women in their reproductive years count more than men? One could add as many nuances to the descriptors around health conditions and life expectancies, years lived and potential years lost of community members, but the reality is that the answer will often not be definitive and change according to the situation. Furthermore, the answers from one group will be in discord with answers from another group. Populations with different health and demographic profiles will have different needs. It is almost impossible to disentangle this from broader social, economic and demographic views about the nature of a good society. Some will want to emphasize population growth, others will want to emphasize population reduction. Some will want to emphasize rights and equity, others will (possibly silently) disengage from that agenda seeking to emphasize some other notion of a healthy population.

These ideas should be open to debate – vigorous, sometimes inharmonious, debate. However, unless the values that are being promoted explicitly in policies and speeches, and implicitly in the kinds of measures being used, are congruent with the actual allocation of resources, then inefficiencies will most certainly occur.

## Conclusion

The Asian region is, economically, one of the fastest growing in the world. With this growth comes a range of public health challenges as highlighted in this chapter. There is an extensive potential for the production of rich health research that not only could have a significant impact on the populations in the region, but could also contribute to evidence for health in poorer and aspiring middle-income countries in other regions. To realize this potential, there needs to be a clear definition of the public health research priorities, and significant strengthening of research funding, governance and ownership.

## References

1. McMichael, AJ, Beaglehole, R. The scope of public health. In Robert Beaglehole and R. Bonita, eds. *Global Public Health: A New Era*. Oxford: Oxford University Press; 2009.

2. Fee, E, Bu, L. Models of public health education: choices for the future? *Bulletin of the World Health Organization* 2007; 85(12): 977–9.
3. Porter, D. *Health, Civilization and the State: A History of Public Health from Ancient to Modern Times* 1st ed. London: Routledge; 1999.
4. Fee, E, Bu, L. Models of public health education: choices for the future? *Bulletin of the World Health Organization* 2007; 85(12): 977–9.
5. Blakely, T, *et al.* Health status and epidemiological capacity and prospects: WHO Western Pacific Region. *International Journal of Epidemiology* 2011; 40(4): 1109–21.
6. Dhillon, PK, *et al.* Status of epidemiology in the WHO South-East Asia region: burden of disease, determinants of health and epidemiological research, workforce and training capacity. *International Journal of Epidemiology* 2012; 41(3): 847–60.
7. Thomas Reuters. Global Publishing: changes in submission trends and impact on scholarly publishers 2012 [online]. Available at: http://scholarone.com/about/industry_insights/ SSR 1203 037 [Accessed 1 September 2012].
8. Rani, M. Future directions for 'research for health' in the Western Pacific Region [online]. Available at: http://www.nus.edu.sg/globalasiainstitute/events/forums/downloads/NIHA_PPT_ManjuRani.pdf [Accessed 11 December 2012].
9. World Health Organization. *World Health Statistics 2012* [online]. Available at: http://www.who.int/healthinfo/EN_WHS2012_Full.pdf [Accessed 24 October 2012].
10. Dans, A, *et al.* The rise of chronic non-communicable diseases in Southeast Asia: time for action. *The Lancet* 2011; 377(9766): 680–9.
11. Ferlay, J, *et al.* Estimates of worldwide burden of cancer in 2008: GLOBOCAN 2008. *International Journal of Cancer* 2010; 127(12): 2893–917.
12. Allotey, P, *et al.* Efficacious, effective, and embedded interventions: implementation research in infectious disease control. *BMC Public Health* 2008; 8(1): 343.
13. World Health Organization. Country Cooperation Strategy at a glance – Malaysia [online]. Available at: http://www.who.int/countryfocus/cooperation_strategy/ccsbrief_mys_en.pdf [Accessed 22 October 2012].
14. World Health Organization. Global Health Risks 2009. Mortality and burden of disease attributable to selected major risks [online]. Available at: http://www.who.int/healthinfo/global_burden_disease/GlobalHealthRisks_report_full.pdf [Accessed 5 November 2012].
15. Marmot, M, *et al.* Closing the gap in a generation: health equity through action on the social determinants of health. *The Lancet* 2008; 372(9650): 1661–9.
16. Allotey, P, *et al.* Rethinking health-care systems: a focus on chronicity. *The Lancet* 2011; 377(9764): 450–1.
17. Reidpath, DD, *et al.* The fallacy of the equity-efficiency trade off: rethinking the efficient health system. *BMC Public Health* 2012; 12(Suppl 1): S3.
18. Yasin, S, *et al.* Contextualizing chronicity: a perspective from Malaysia. *Globalization and Health* 2012; 8: 4.
19. Moissinac, K, *et al.* Treatment by practitioners of traditional healing in Malaysia. *Tropical Doctor* 2004; 34(3): 191.

# 8

# Developing the public health workforce in Asia

*Tim Evans and Syed Masud Ahmed*

## Introduction

The health workforce represents one of the most important determinants of population health since 'in health systems, workers function as gatekeepers and navigators for the effective or wasteful application of all other resources such as drugs, vaccines and supplies' [1]. Under the changing health scenario in Asia, developing an appropriate health workforce, including a public health workforce, has become of utmost priority for the governments and health systems across Asian countries. In this chapter, we provide an overview of the current state of the public health workforce in Asia followed by an analysis of the current state of public health education instruction and institutions.

## The public health workforce in Asia: current state of development and what lies ahead

### *Current state of development*

Generalizations related to the current state of development of the public health workforce in Asia are difficult to make due to the immense diversity of the region. From small island states to continental giants and from low-, middle-, to high-income economies, there is an enormous mix of contexts that underlie and inform the specific challenges countries are facing across this vast region. However, the challenges countries are facing have much more in common than one might think. Across the region – and indeed across the world – public health workforce development suffers from a general neglect in terms of policy attention and robust or comprehensive frameworks for its development. This deficit in policy and programmatic efforts is reflected in the widespread crisis that characterizes the public health workforce in most countries: (1) a massive shortage of public health workers required to perform core public health functions; (2) inequitable concentrations of workers in well-off urban areas leaving remote, rural and disadvantaged populations perilously underserved; (3) skews in skill-mix with yawning gaps in new competency areas required to deal with new types of problems; and (4) a crisis-to-crisis, band-aid approach to addressing problems that systematically fails to invest in the career paths and institutional arrangements for a ready and responsive public health workforce.

## *The public health context of the twenty-first century*

Public health needs of twenty-first century Asia are reflected by rapid transitions both within and beyond the health sector. Beyond the health sector, demographic change (e.g. urbanization, ageing, international migration), economic forces of global markets, the connected world facilitated by Information and Communication Technologies (ICT) and transport, and concerns related to food, fuel and climate security are reflected in the Asian region's remarkable economic resurgence, striking inequalities and growing interdependencies in virtually all realms of social and economic activity. Nested within this complex global and regional context, the health sector is both surging forward with improvements and exponential expansion of healthcare systems, while struggling with its own set of problems related to massive shifts in disease burden from, primarily, infectious diseases to non-communicable diseases (NCDs), and challenges related to the provision of safe, appropriate, accessible and affordable services according to need. The public–private mix in health services, a constant flow of new health technologies, and irrepressible expectations of the population with respect to their health rights and entitlements are among the myriad of factors that characterize the complex and dynamic health landscape in the countries across the region.

## *Development of the public health workforce in the twenty-first century*

It is the context of this brave new world that is defining the 'needs' that one must consider the development of the public health workforce in Asia. Health workers are central to the health system insofar as they constitute the glue that holds the various building blocks of the health systems together, define the values in practice that characterize the system as responsive and compassionate and, ultimately, are the ones that can lead important changes on a day-to-day basis in terms of improvements, as well as leading more fundamental reforms of the system.

Distinguishing the public health workforce from the clinical workforce is not always precise. Many clinical health workers (dealing with individual patients) can, do and should play an important role in public health. Similarly, there is an increasing number of professionals who would not characterize themselves as health professionals but for whom public health competencies are of growing importance (e.g. people involved in urban policy related to recreation or green spaces, water and sanitation, transport and housing). As such, any approach to the development of the public health workforce must embrace the diverse professional cadres and disciplines that are critical to addressing public health problems and not limit itself to just full-time public health professionals and workers. Furthermore, it is essential not to limit workforce development to 'professionals' but embrace the broader spectrum of the public health workforce from professional through to para-professionals to the public (see Box 8.1).

According to the World Health Organization (WHO) health workforce framework, 'development' of the health workforce refers to the 'formation' of the health workforce through a deliberate 'professional' training or education [1]. It is thus associated with the preparation/education of the health workforce as opposed to the deployment or employment of health workers. Beside the needs of the health sector (as expressed in a demand for health workers), development of the public health workforce is also contingent on the state of the

## Box 8.1 Who constitutes the public health workforce?

The public health workforce comprises a broad swathe of health and non-health workers who work full-time and part-time, and may be either formally or informally employed. Clarity with regards to these diverse target groups is critical in terms of establishing the appropriate range of opportunities for public health workforce development.

### *Professionals for public health*

At the apex of the public health workforce are professionals who are university trained with depth skills and competencies spanning the key knowledge domains of public health. These include professionals who work in the policy and practice of public health, e.g. departments of public health, NGOs or CSOs; or those who work as public health academics or researchers, e.g. epidemiologists, demographers and policy analysts. The professional workforce also includes many in the healthcare workforce whose clinical practice requires or benefits from public health competencies.

### *Para-professionals for public health*

In many settings, 'professionals' are too few and too expensive to deal with the totality of public health needs especially in settings of severe resource constraints as found in many countries in the Asian region. In this regard, there exists a diverse set of para-public health professionals that includes but is not limited to medical assistants, community nutritionists, laboratory technicians, pharmacists, supply-chain managers/logisticians, community outreach workers, surveillance officers, enumerators and emergency relief workers. In addition to providing critical public health functions, there is a growing experience of task shifting whereby well-defined tasks are shifted from higher-level professionals to these para-professionals with appropriate supervision thereby extending the coverage of critical public health functions [2].

### *People as public health agents*

While not formally part of the public health workforce, people are increasingly being called upon to take individual, household and community responsibility for public health. This group's development has lacked any systemic approach; rather efforts have been characterized by very specific issue-based campaigns and interventions related to health behaviours such as smoking cessation. However, in the twenty-first century – with the ubiquitous availability of knowledge – the role of the people in public health represents an important opportunity that can no longer be ignored. Comprehensive training efforts for public health – linked to primary/secondary schools and continuing adult education – will help to empower the public with respect to their rights, responsibilities and diverse roles as promoters of health in the home and community.

education sector in terms of the supply and effective functioning of the education institutions. It is the intersection of these health and education systems that defines, in many respects, the performance of the health workforce in terms of having the right workers with the right skills in the right place at the right time.

On the supply side, the production of health workers depends on both instructional and institutional reforms [3]. Instructionally, one considers the content and shape of curricula that constitute diplomas, degrees and continuing education, the range and quality of pedagogic modalities, as well as the mechanisms of evaluating the acquisition of critical competencies. Institutionally, the number, type, location, financing, staffing, infrastructure, governance and regulation/accreditation of education institutions are critical, but too often overlooked.

## Instructional reforms

The instructional reforms of public health education refer to the different types of curricula, their content, the pedagogic process, including faculty development, and the measures of education achievement and performance.

### *Curricular spectrum in public health*

At the university level, there are a wide range of degrees and qualifications that define public health professionals. Following in the American tradition of the Welch–Rose Report of 1915, there are many schools of public health in Asia that provide graduate degrees in public health at the Master's (MPH, MSc, MPhil) and Doctoral (DPH, DPhil, DMed) levels. In many countries following the British tradition, specialization in public health takes place primarily through medical schools, most often referred to as fellowship qualification in 'community medicine'. There is a growing trend for universities in the region, and elsewhere, to provide undergraduate degrees in public health.

In addition to specifically denominated degrees in public health, there are a wide number of other types of degrees and programmes from where the public health workforce draws its qualifications. These include undergraduate and graduate degrees in subjects such as public administration, business administration, political science, urban planning, economics, sociology, law, anthropology, informatics, statistics, nutrition, food sciences, pharmacology and many others.

Alongside full-time public health teaching, there is growth in part-time learning opportunities that allow professionals to continue to work full-time and acquire a degree qualification or a specific skills-set over a longer period of time. While this represents a demand for 'continuing education', unlike medical education, public health tuition has not developed an explicit practice of 'continuing education' partly due to a general absence of clear standards of practice that must be met by public health professionals.

### *Core curricula responsive to changing public health needs*

The intrinsic interdisciplinary nature of public health coupled with the rapidly changing public health landscape pose a major challenge in the identification of a 'core' set of competencies around which to base the curriculum. Existing curricula for public health professionals suffer from a growing mismatch between the rapid emergence of complex 'twenty-first-century' global health challenges and a static, discipline-defined curricular legacy that is resistant to change. While there are a number of efforts to (re-)define the 'core' of public health education [4] (see Figure 8.1), the model of public health education is struggling to accommodate the diverse set of competencies required for the new public health landscape.

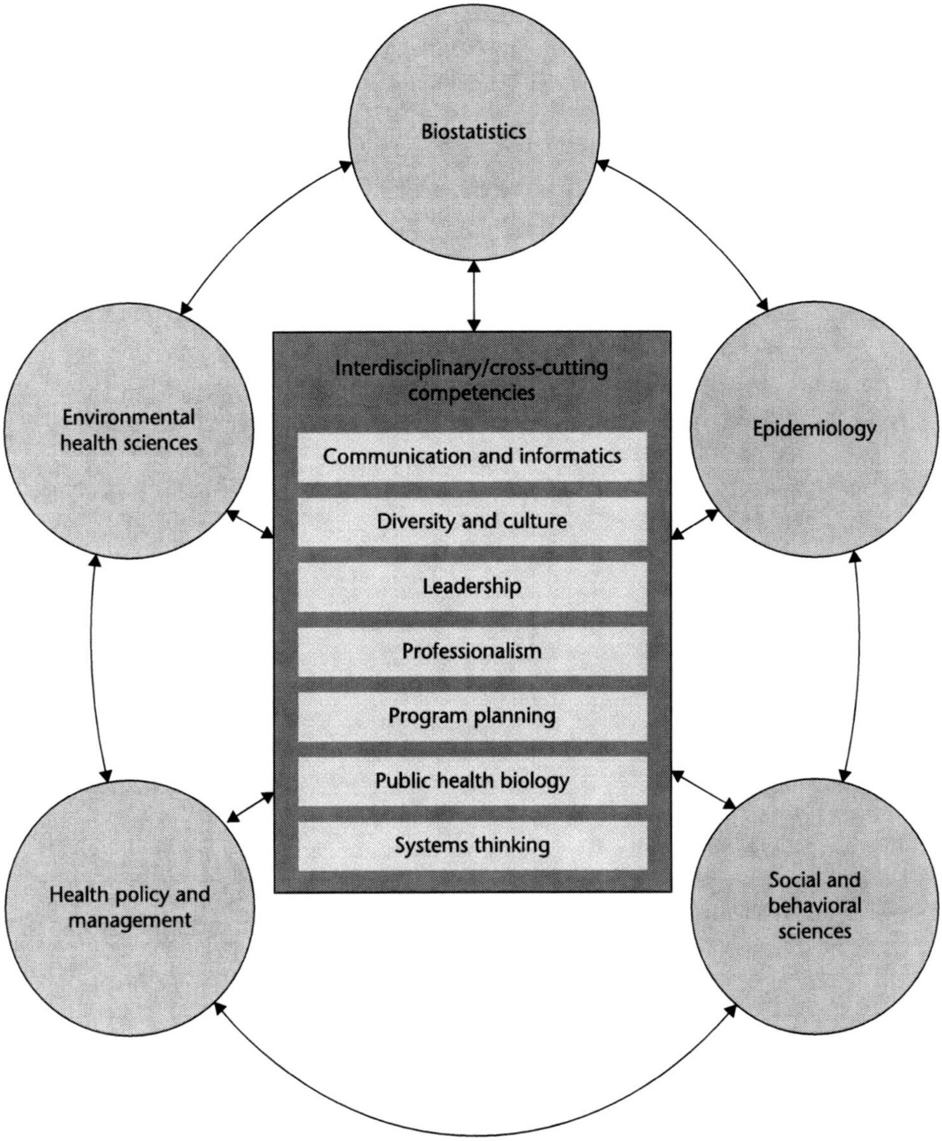


*Figure 8.1* Master in Public Health core competencies [4]

In many respects, this is the same challenge medical education faced in the 1960s when McMaster University introduced the revolutionary problem-based approach to medical education, marking a definitive departure from the discipline and disease-based curriculum advocated by the Flexner Report of 1913. Public health education is ripe for a similar change and a new 'praxis model' is currently being elaborated as part of a larger reform agenda of public health education (see Box 8.2).

Critical to education reform in public health is the ability to use public health problems as the basis for informing the pursuit and acquisition of knowledge required to address these problems. Four core domains of public health knowledge in relation to any given problem

**Box 8.2 The Savar Statement – a seven-point agenda for reform of public health education in the twenty-first century**

Reflecting renewed and growing interest in health professional education, a group of public health educators from diverse regions in the world met in Savar, Bangladesh, in June 2012, to flesh out key components of an agenda to transform professionals' education in public health.

1. The development and articulation of a *unifying theory of knowledge and action*, or praxis, for public health as a common conceptual foundation for public health education.
2. The development of *core content for public health education* that builds on the theory of knowledge and encompasses three types of learning: informative, formative and transformative.
3. The development of an online library of 'illustrative' and 'representative' *teaching cases or problems* that illuminate the spectrum of knowledge necessary to address public health issues.
4. The identification of a common, or *core, set of competencies*, linked to the foundational framework, that can be used to guide the formulation of curricula and to facilitate standardized evaluation of students and accreditation of programmes both within and across countries and across levels of education – undergraduate through graduate, generalist to sub-specialist.
5. The development of an open-source, *shared resource on innovative approaches to public health education* that describes in a succinct and common manner the specific efforts of institutions around the world to reform their programmes.
6. The creation of a *network for pedagogic excellence and innovation in public health education* that would develop an inventory of, and criteria for evaluating, the array of pedagogic approaches for public health education, including instructor-led, self-directed, student-to-student, team-based, field-based, exchange and ICT-facilitated.
7. A concerted effort to look at how public health education as articulated in the six points above can inform *reforms in the training of 'clinical' health professionals* recognizing the growing demand for public health education among these diverse cadres.

referred to as the 4Ds – description, development, delivery and Did it work? – structure a comprehensive big picture that helps students from getting lost in a myriad of facts and details (see Figure 8.2).

To complement these domains are three levels of learning: (1) informative; (2) formative; and (3) transformative (see Figure 8.3). The resulting matrix of domains and levels of learning can be used to guide knowledge and learning around the diverse spectrum of public health problems as they are found in diverse contexts.

The move to a more problem-centred curriculum permits greater flexibility to adapt and tailor learning to new issues and specific contexts. Some of the more common topics that are on the 'waiting list' for inclusion in public health curricula include the health system's building blocks, management of public–private enterprises and emerging public health challenges, such as the rise of NCDs and injuries, emergency response in disasters including conflict/post-conflict situations and the health impact of climate change. Rather than try to accommodate these in new 'add-on' courses – often referred to as the 'laundry list'

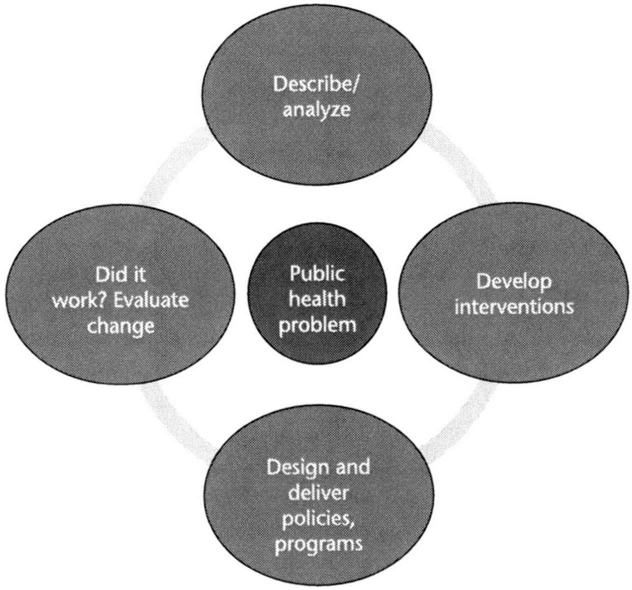


*Figure 8.2* Four core knowledge domains for problem-based public health education [10]

| Level | Objectives | Outcome |
|---|---|---|
| Informative | • Information<br>• Skills | Experts |
| Formative | • Socialization<br>• Values | Professionals |
| Transformative | • Leadership attributes | Change agents |

*Figure 8.3* Three levels of learning [3]

approach – problems can be developed to reflect the nature of these issues and act as a stimulus for the four domains of knowledge and the three levels of learning described above.

## *Pedagogic and faculty development*

In contrast to medical education where pedagogic innovation has been an active field of study for many years through departments of medical education, there is a near absence of academic reflection on the pedagogic approach in public health [3]. While there is general recognition of the limitations of the predominant teacher-centred, lecture-based, didactic approach, there is very little systematic effort to look at the different types of pedagogic approaches that are required to effectively acquire public health competencies. Many curricula include 'field-based' learning; however, there are very few guidelines related to the optimal amount of time that should be spent in the field, and the ways in which learning in the field can be optimized in terms of both competency acquisition and efficiency. There is growing recognition of the importance of peer-to-peer or student-to-student learning insofar as public health programmes draw students from different cultural, geographic and professional backgrounds; however, there is no formalization of this as a pedagogic tool. Similarly, group-work, team-based learning, mentoring, internships and even international exchange are growing dimensions of public health programmes that require greater attention to their pedagogic value-added and assessment of what constitutes good (or not-so-good) practice. New ICTs are facilitating greater access to distance courses, especially through the Massive Open Online Courses (MOOC), and leading to major changes in the teaching timetable with, for example, courses and lectures being viewed independently by students in the evening or at home, and the class time being used for more interactive discussions.

With public health education on the cusp of a major change in pedagogic methods, the role of faculty cannot be overemphasized. Faculty development is thus a critical but missing part of the public health education development agenda. In many respects, it is faculty who are pushing the modernization of pedagogic approaches. However, in too many public health schools, faculty are limited in numbers and without formal pedagogic training, and thus a major constraint to change. Given these challenges as well as the rapid growth of new types of public health problems, old models of having a 'full stable' of qualified faculty housed within a single teaching institution are being replaced with innovative ways of sourcing faculty. These include part-time or visiting appointments, recruitment of 'greying' professionals who have more time (and interest) in teaching, as well as accessing pedagogic resources online. Beyond instruction and qualification in pedagogic methods, the faculty development challenge links to broader structural and institutional issues in education, such as career paths, financing of salaries (often on soft monies that are research or project based), and in these complex contexts the extent to which faculty time for education is valued financially, as well as in terms of performance, and being related to career progression.

### *Monitoring and evaluation of education effectiveness*

Most training of public health professionals is evaluated through the norms and standards that govern degrees and diplomas in universities. Credits are accumulated based on successful completion of courses and put towards the minimum required for the degree. Likewise, the forms of student evaluation within courses – multiple choice questions, short answer, essays, papers and theses, as well as participation – are widespread and in no way specific to public health. As a profession, however, public health, unlike medicine, has yet to adopt across-institution national 'licensure' examinations. Nor has public health innovated new forms of evaluation as in medicine like the observed, standardized, clinical evaluation (OSCE). However, like many other areas of clinical training, there has been a move in recent years towards identifying 'competencies' defined as knowledge that relates to undertaking specific tasks as a standard currency of evaluation. Agreement on core competencies may help give more clarity and inter-institutional comparability on whether a Master's of Public Health (MPH) degree from one institution is similar to or different from an MPH granted by another institution. Similarly, a map or inventory of core competencies may allow students to understand better where they have particular strengths or weaknesses and thereby (re-)direct their learning efforts.

In addition to evaluation of students, most schools have some form of evaluation of faculty as teachers. This evaluation comes most commonly as feedback from students at the end of a course. Other forms of faculty evaluation, such as peer assessment and performance in the different forms/media of pedagogic instruction, are much less common.

Beyond individual evaluation of students and faculty, there is neither a framework nor a standardized practice of measurement that assesses the performance of public health education institutions. As such, the relative performance of one school of public health compared to another is a purely subjective assessment. The whole area of institutional performance assessment is beginning to get more attention – both from an inter-institutional comparison (i.e. student measures such as diversity, drop-out, strength of graduates, employment, etc.), as well as for the public health education system as a whole (i.e. Are there sufficient institutions? Are the right students getting access to the right type of training? Are education institutions responsive to shifting demands amongst employers?) [5].

## Institutional reforms

The institutional landscape of education institutions responsible for the training of public health workers in the Asian region, like in many other parts of the world, reflects the absence of clear policies and strategies for development of the public health workforce. China, for example, had 72 schools of public health in 2000, while India had just 4 [6, 7]. This skew is in part a reflection of the dominance of medical education institutions and the absence of systematic strategies to develop public health training. In many countries, especially in South Asia and Austral-Asia, the predominant forms of public health professional training reflect the colonially inherited British system of providing doctors postgraduate training in community medicine or family medicine. While the limitations of defining public health training opportunities to doctors is clear, the institutional landscape for medical professionals also suffers from widespread neglect with nearly half of all countries globally having either one or no medical school [8]. In other countries, such as China, a soviet-style model of 'hygiene' has driven the development of public health infrastructure and institutions [7].

In recent years, however, there appears to be more widespread recognition of the need and demand for stand-alone public health institutions. India now has 20 schools of public health, and Bangladesh had one school of public health in 2000 and, by 2010, had 18. This growth reflects market forces with private sector institutions leading the way but is accompanied by a growing array of regional initiatives that aim to strengthen the development of public health institutional capacity across the Asian region (see Box 8.3).

### *Institution location and education infrastructure*

Despite the encouraging growth in the number of public health institutions in the Asian region, there are still many countries with a vastly inadequate institutional infrastructure relative to need. In low-income countries such as Laos, Cambodia, Papua New Guinea and many small island states, there is only one or no schools of public health. Furthermore, in countries with one or more schools of public health, these are often concentrated in prosperous urban areas delinked from the harsh realities of remote and disadvantaged high public health needs populations and drawing a skew of students from the top tiers of the socio-economic ladder who are able to afford private tuition fees. In Bangladesh, for example,

## Box 8.3 Initiatives to develop institutional capacity for public health in the Asia region

In response to the widespread sense of a crisis in the quantity and quality of the public health workforce, in the last ten years, a significant number of initiatives in the region that are attempting to bring more systematic attention to public health workforce development have emerged. The South-East Asian Public Health Education Institutes Network (SEA PHEIN) was formed in 2004 by the South East Asia Regional Office of WHO to encourage technical cooperation for capacity building of the public health institutes and improve public health education. The Asia-Pacific Academic Consortium for Public Health (APACPH) with 81 member institutes in 23 countries is dedicated to improve professional education for public health. To address the unmet need for greater public health expertise in India, the Public Health Foundation of India (PHFI) was formed as a public–private partnership involving academia at home and abroad, government institutions at state and central level, bilateral and multilateral agencies and civil society organizations. It aims to 'initiate and catalyse action for better health outcomes' through building the capacity of the public health institutions and public health workforce, and set a benchmark of quality standards for public health education.

of 14 private sector schools of public health, all are located in the capital city of Dhaka. This raises legitimate concerns that public health schools may be less-than-optimally connected to the communities they are supposed to serve.

Beyond the numbers and location of public health institutions, there are a myriad of important issues related to education infrastructure. Increasingly, the public health classroom is one without walls. One manifestation of this is the extent to which core-learning materials can be accessed online through, for example, Massive Open Online Courses (MOOCs), and learning at distance is now facilitated through technology. Less frequently, but perhaps more importantly, are the set of learning infrastructures outside the classroom in terms of access to populations and institutions – governmental, private, NGO, research – that constitute the 'field-based' or 'problem-based' realities to complement 'desk-based or class-room-based' learning.

### *Accreditation*

The recent growth in private sector public health institutions raises many unresolved questions with regards to the accreditation of education. Concerns about market-driven provision of degrees with little or no guarantee of quality are raising important issues with regards to both the standards and the institutional mechanism for accreditation. The accreditation mechanism for public health in the Asian region (or for any region in the world) is not well established: in some countries it is linked to the medical education regulatory authority and in others it is part of a university education regulatory authority. The outstanding need for greater definition of minimum or common standards, as well as the development of appropriate institutional mechanisms for public health education regulation, is receiving concerted attention through the Asia-Pacific Academic Consortium for Public Health [APACPH] [9].

### *Admissions and placement*

A critical institutional function of schools of public health relates to the entry and exit of students. Selection or admissions criteria of students are opportunities to bring the requisite numbers and qualities of students that are deemed critical to be represented in the public health workforce. Merit criteria are the most commonly used in identifying eligible candidates – this includes past academic performance, as well as performance on standardized tests for quantitative, logic/reasoning, written and linguistic skills. Less often included but perhaps as, or more, important are criteria related to diversity including gender, professional/disciplinary background (beyond clinical medicine), socio-economic status, geographical status/residence and ethnic/religious background.

These diverse criteria for admissions are not simply important to maximize the richness of the learning environment, but are also important in supplying the workforce with the appropriate skills and background that will respond appropriately to needs. This relates to the important function of 'placement' or facilitating employment opportunities for graduates and tracking career trajectories. In the absence of registries of public health professionals, education institution alumni tracking of careers can provide important labour market information related to the types of jobs and employers graduates are able to get, as well as important issues such as migration out of the public health workforce or even migration to work in other countries (i.e. brain-drain). The placement function also relates to developing opportunities for prospective employers to influence the supply side of public health education through providing feedback on the performance of public health graduates and developing applied/ experiential learning opportunities for students or recent graduates through internships or fellowships.

## Conclusion

Asia, like many other regions in the world, is facing severe shortages, skews in skill-mix and an inequitable distribution of health workers, be they clinical or public health professionals. Public health education has for too long been considered a sub-specialization of clinical medicine as opposed to a field in and of itself that requires full-time professionals in its own right, as well as making a critical contribution to the training of clinical health professionals. With rapid and complex transitions in health affecting all countries in Asia, such as population ageing and the emergence of NCDs, urbanization, health effects of climate change, disasters and injuries, there is an urgency to take forward more systematic reforms in public health education such that the public health workforce is an asset rather than an anchor in managing these transitions. Adequate investment in such reforms can lead to vibrant institutions with cutting-edge instruction that can educate more and better public health professionals capable of mobilizing knowledge and other resources necessary to achieve equitable 'patient and population-centred' health systems in the twenty-first century.

## References

1. World Health Organization. *World Health Report 2006. Working Together for Health.* Geneva: WHO, 2006.
2. World Health Organization. *Task shifting to tackle health workers shortage.* Geneva: WHO, 2007.
3. Frenk J, Chen L, *et al.* Health professionals for a new century: transforming education to strengthen health systems in an interdependent world. *Lancet* 2010; 376: 1923–58.

4. Calhoun JG, Kalpana R, Weistet EM, *et al.* Development of a core competency model for the Master of Public Health Degree. *American Journal of Public Health* 2008; 98(9): 1598–607.
5. Workshop on 'Cross-country Health Professional Education Situation Assessment'; Hanoi, April, 2011.
6. Gupta MD. Public Health in India: an overview. World Bank Policy Research Working Paper No. 3787, 2005.
7. Lee L. The current state of public health in China. *Annual Review of Public Health* 2004; 25: 327–39.
8. Bhutta ZA, Chen L, Cohen J, Crisp N, Evans T, Fineberg H, *et al.* Education of health professionals of the 21st century: a global independent Commission. *Lancet* 2010; 375(9721): 1137–8.
9. Patrick WK and Charupoonphal P, *et al.* Accreditation policy on public health education in Asia Pacific region and preliminary steps. [Online]. Available from: www.apacph.org/wp/wp-content/. . ./Compiled-Agenda-Papers-Seoul.pdf
10. Evans TG, Afifi R, Adams AM, Rashid S, and Newman S. Towards a theory of knowledge to guide public health education reform in the 21st century. Joint working paper of the James P Grant School of Public Health, BRAC University Bangladesh and the School of Public Health, American University of Beirut, 2013.

# Part II

# Epidemiology as research methodology and its applications

# Introduction to Part II: epidemiology as research methodology and its applications

*Jin Ling Tang*

## Epidemiology: research methods in public health

As described in other chapters, public health has evolved from integrating sanitation and hygiene, to including social medicine, community medicine and preventive medicine. If public health is regarded as a discipline that views and tackles issues of disease, and health and health care at the population or societal level, with the aim of finding ways of continually improving the health of the population, epidemiology provides the theories and methods for conducting scientific research in human populations in public health.

Epidemiology originated from investigating the causes of outbreaks and epidemics of communicable diseases to identify measures for prevention and control. Epidemiology may still be known to many as a discipline about communicable diseases, and/or as research findings on causes, risk factors, prevalence, incidence and mortality of diseases as shown in many clinical textbooks. Modern epidemiology [1, 2], which began in the middle of the twentieth century and came of age in the 1980s, has become the methodology of studying quantitatively general issues in disease, and health and health care in human populations. Its major methods include cohort studies, case-control studies, cross-sectional studies, randomized controlled trials and systematic reviews.

Epidemiology along with biostatistics is a foundation of public health, but also widely used in clinical medicine in the name of clinical epidemiology. For example, epidemiology provides methods for studying causes and risk factors of diseases, the prognosis of diseases, assessing the accuracy of diagnostic methods, and evaluating the efficacy and harms of interventions.

As demonstrated in Chapter 9 by Chung and Kim, epidemiology has played an important role in identifying the causes of outbreaks and epidemics of communicable diseases. The classic example is John Snow's comparison of geographical distribution of deaths from cholera in Broad Street, London. He found that the number of deaths near some water pumps was much higher than that around other pumps and postulated that contaminated drinking water was responsible for the spread of cholera in the 1854 epidemic in London. Importantly, this preposition of contaminated water as the cause of the cholera outbreaks was made a few decades before bacterium *Vibrio cholerae* was discovered.

Since the middle of the twentieth century, cohort studies were invented and conducted to investigate the causes of non-communicable chronic diseases. Notably, the British doctors study [3] discovered that smoking was the cause of lung cancer and the Framingham Heart Study [4] revealed that elevated blood cholesterol among other risk factors was associated with higher risk of cardiovascular diseases. Randomized controlled trials are widely used to evaluate the efficacy of interventions, while cohort and case-control studies are used to investigate rare chronic harms of drugs and other medical interventions, after they have been used in practice.

By the end of the twentieth century, many epidemiological studies, in particular randomized controlled trials, have been conducted and cumulated. Their findings provided scientific evidence that should be used to inform clinical practice as well as decision making in health care.

In 1992, the concept of evidence-based medicine was proposed, which urges all healthcare decisions to be consistent with current best evidence [5]. Epidemiology encompasses the research methods for studying practical issues in health care in human populations. Results from epidemiological studies provide requisite evidence for making healthcare decisions. Evidence-based medicine is about how to make use of such evidence in clinical medicine, and evidence-based health care is about how to make evidence-based decisions for populations.

In Chapter 10, Chung and Tang review the relationship between epidemiology and evidence-based medicine, and describe the early models for practising evidence-based medicine. The chapter goes on to describe what constitutes evidence and how existing evidence can be most effectively summarized, disseminated and used, and concludes with a comparison of evidence-based decision making in clinical medicine and public health [6, 7].

In addition, epidemiology has also been used to detect potential genes that may be related to a certain disease. Typically, gene–disease association studies compare the genes of individuals with a certain disease with individuals free of the disease in question. Genes that are related to the disease would show a difference between those with and those without the disease. In terms of study design, a typical case-control study in epidemiology is used, in which the exposure of interest is genes – the cases are those with the disease and the control group of those free of the disease. Similar to case-control studies of traditional risk factors of disease such as age and smoking, control of biases and confounding must be considered [8].

As described in Part I in Chapter 6 by Özdemir, with the availability of Big Data on the Internet or collected in routine practices, such as electronic patient records in primary care or hospitals, retrospective cohort studies on causes of disease, harms of treatments and prognosis of patients can be conducted much more easily [9–11]. Large data indeed help to reduce costs and improve precision of results. But precision cannot replace validity. Cohort studies based on large routine data would have more difficulties in controlling biases and confounding as compared to traditional cohort studies. The major problems are not computing difficulties but missing data and varying accuracy in measuring exposure and outcomes amongst different patients.

Finally in Chapter 11, Shen uses cancer as an example and demonstrates the use of epidemiology in investigating the burden and causes of cancer in China, which is followed by a brief summary of the strategies for prevention of cancer including the topical issue of cancer screening.

## References

1. Rothman KJ. *Modern Epidemiology.* Boston, MA: Little, Brown, 1986.

2. Feinstein AR. *Clinical Epidemiology*. Philadelphia, PA: WB Saunders, 1985.
3. Doll R, Peto R, Boreham J, Sutherland I. Mortality in relation to smoking: 50 years' observations on male British doctors. *BMJ* 2004; 328: 1519–28.
4. Castelli WP. Cholesterol and lipids in the risk of coronary artery disease – the Framingham Heart Study. *Canadian Journal of Cardiology* 1988; 4(Suppl A): 5A–10A.
5. Guyatt G, Cairns J, Churchill D, Cook D, Haynes B, Hirsh J, *et al*. Evidence-based medicine: a new approach to teaching the practice of medicine. *AMA* 1992; 268(17): 2420–5.
6. Gray M, Tang JL. *Evidence-Based Decision Making in Health Care* [Chinese]. Beijing: Peking University Medical Press, 2004.
7. Tang JL, Griffiths S. Review paper: epidemiology, evidence-based medicine, and public health. *Asia-Pacific Journal of Public Health* 2009; 21(3): 244–51.
8. Tang JL. Selection bias in meta-analyses of gene–disease associations [perspective]. *PLoS Medicine* 2(12): e409.
9. Matok I, Gorodischer R, Koren G, Sheiner, E, Wiznitzer A, Levy A. The safety of metoclopramide use in the first trimester of pregnancy. *New England Journal of Medicine* 2009; 360: 2528–35.
10. Goldberger ZD, Chan PS, Berg RA, *et al*. Duration of resuscitation efforts and survival after in-hospital cardiac arrest: an observational study. *The Lancet* 2012; 380(9852): 1473–81.
11. Bhaskaran K, Douglas I, Evans S, van Staa T, Smeeth L. Angiotensin receptor blockers and risk of cancer: cohort study among people receiving antihypertensive drugs in UK General Practice Research Database. *BMJ* 2012; 344: e2697.

# 9

# Epidemiology

## From observation to public health action

*Roger Y. Chung and Jean H. Kim*

The superior physician helps before the early budding of the disease.

*(Huang Ti)*

## Introduction

This chapter aims to describe epidemiology and its role in public health. The chapter begins with a brief history of epidemiology, and then goes on to discuss how disease occurrence is measured and how the burden of disease is quantified. We then look at the common sources of data for public health research, provide an overview of epidemiological study designs and conclude with an example of research being translated into public health action by looking at a case study of alcohol harm reduction in Hong Kong.

## A brief history of epidemiology and its role in public health

Epidemiology is the academic field that constitutes one of the core areas of public health. It is the discipline that examines 'the distribution and determinants of health-related conditions in human populations in order to control or prevent health problems' [1]. Although epidemiology did not exist as a formally recognized discipline until the twentieth century, the rudiments of epidemiological thought can be traced back to ancient times. The Greek physician, Hippocrates (460–377 BC), the father of Western medicine, noted the strong relationship that exists between disease occurrence and environmental influences [2]. In the Eastern Hemisphere, observational study methods were used in Traditional Chinese Medicine (TCM) that date back to the eleventh to fourteenth centuries BC during the Shang dynasty in China [3]. Moreover, the concept of disease prevention had been emphasized as the job of a 'superior physician' in the *Yellow Emperor's Inner Canon* [4], the oldest and most fundamental work of Chinese medical theory compiled around the first century BC.

Despite its long coexistence with medicine, the birth of modern epidemiology is widely considered to have occurred in the nineteenth century. In 1854, Dr John Snow undertook an investigation of the cholera epidemic of London by spatially mapping the outbreak on a street map. He noted that residents obtaining water from the Southwark and Vauxhall Company had an eight-fold higher risk of cholera mortality than those that obtained their water elsewhere. The ensuing removal of the water source stopped the outbreak that had killed over 5,000 residents and provided strong evidence that cholera was not an airborne disease, as previously believed. Technological developments since then have allowed more sophisticated methods to be used for such investigations, including geographic information systems, high-speed computing, advanced laboratory techniques and complex mathematical models. Despite these scientific advances, the role of epidemiology in public health remains fundamentally unchanged since the time of John Snow.

Together with biostatistics, epidemiology is needed to conduct most quantitative public health studies. The term *study* encompasses both *surveillance* and *research*. *Surveillance* refers to the monitoring of disease occurrence and distribution for the purpose of effective control [5], whereas *research* refers to the expansion of the general knowledge that consists of theories, principles and relationships [1]. Epidemiological research seeks to examine disease risk factors or uncover mechanisms of disease causation that may, in turn, alter clinical guidelines, health services or governmental policies towards preventive actions. For instance, a recent epidemic of urinary tract stones among children in China prompted the Chinese government to institute a free screening program on urinary tract stones that was targeted at children [6]. This was then followed by an epidemiological study that confirmed an association between the exposure to melamine-contaminated formula milk powder and urinary stones among infants. Similar to John Snow's discovery of the association between contaminated water sources and cholera, consumption of various food products were noted to be significant risk factors for illnesses. These findings led to public health actions, such as the seizure and recall of food products and more stringent cross-border food safety legislation [8].

Similarly, in 2003, epidemiological surveillance of infectious diseases investigated a clustering of acute respiratory illnesses in Hong Kong that led to the discovery of a novel SARS coronavirus and resulted in the release of guidelines for personal hygiene in public spaces [9]. By identifying risk factors for adverse health conditions in the population, epidemiology provides an evidence base for preventive action, as well as for clinical practice. Epidemiological studies allow public health scientists to make scientific observations and develop rational programmes to protect the health of the public. In addition to guiding preventive actions, epidemiology is also used to assess the effectiveness of these actions and existing programmes.

As a result of the enormous public health burden historically associated with infectious diseases, such as influenza, polio and tuberculosis, topics such as outbreak investigations and infectious disease surveillance have long been the primary focus of modern epidemiology. However, as non-communicable diseases (NCDs) gradually came to the forefront of the global disease burden in the second half of the twentieth century, the scope of epidemiology has broadened to include NCDs (such as cancer and cardiovascular diseases) and lifestyle behaviours (such as cigarette smoking, alcohol consumption and Internet addiction). With the advent of sophisticated statistical models and modern computing, epidemiological methods are now employed to forecast disease trends, project healthcare needs and conduct studies comparing treatment modalities. In contemporary society, modern epidemiologists often collaborate with an interdisciplinary team of researchers from such diverse fields as natural sciences, clinical medicine, biostatistics, engineering and social sciences for a better understanding of the health issues they are investigating. Specifically, the primary aims of epidemiology are to:

- Study the prognosis of different diseases;
- Estimate the burden of different diseases on a population;

- Identify risk/protective factors for health conditions;
- Apply evidence to inform health policy and measures regarding disease prevention and health promotion; and
- Evaluate existing healthcare measures and interventions.

## Measuring disease occurrence

In order to examine the prognosis of the disease and the burden of the disease on a population, it is necessary to quantify the illness in said population. In measuring the occurrence of disease morbidity, there are two basic concepts that require elaboration: *prevalence* and *incidence.*

### *Prevalence*

In epidemiology, prevalence is the *proportion* of people affected by a disease in a specified population (e.g. a country; a city; a sub-population, such as an ethnic group) at a particular instant in time. In addition to clinically recognized diseases, prevalence can be also used to describe the proportion of the population having an attribute (e.g. blood type) or a condition (e.g. nearsightedness, drug addiction). It is defined as the number of persons who have the disease divided by the total number of individuals in the specified population at that particular time (or midway through the time period). Prevalence is often calculated using the formula shown in Figure 9.1.

For instance, the prevalence of HIV in Vietnam in 2011 among 15–49-year-olds is estimated to be 0.45 per cent while the prevalence among injection drug users and female sex workers in Vietnam was estimated to be 13.4 per cent and 3 per cent, respectively [10]. These statistics give a snapshot of the distribution of HIV in Vietnam and help to identify population subgroups for targeting HIV interventions. Prevalence data can be used to track health trends over time. For instance, a study of displaced Thai children living in camps after the 2004 Indian Ocean tsunami showed that the prevalence of post-traumatic stress disorder was 13 per cent at eight weeks post-disaster. The prevalence at nine months had only decreased to 10 per cent, demonstrating the persistence of this mental health condition among displaced children and the continued need for psychological treatment [11].

Nonetheless, it must be noted that prevalence reflects both the number of new cases, as well as the duration that people have the condition. It is not difficult to imagine that the more new cases there are for a disease, the greater the prevalence of that disease will be in the population. However, even with small numbers of new cases, the prevalence of disease can be very high in a population if the condition is long-lasting (incurable and/or not rapidly fatal) due to the accrual of individuals with that condition. In high-income countries, illnesses such as diabetes, hypertension and even HIV have higher than expected prevalence despite low numbers of new cases. This is due to the duration of survival time from improvements in clinical management. For example, the availability of highly active antiretroviral therapies in developed countries has greatly extended the survival of HIV patients,

$$\frac{\text{(Number of persons who have the disease in the population at a specified time)}}{\text{(Number of persons in the population at that specified time)}}$$

*Figure 9.1* Formula to calculate the prevalence of disease

resulting in a higher prevalence of HIV in the population. Due to these limitations, prevalence is primarily useful for descriptive purposes, such as examining trends and measuring the health burden of a disease in a population, rather than for assessing a person's *risk* of getting that disease.

## Incidence

In epidemiology, *incidence* of a disease refers to the occurrence of *new disease cases* rather than existing cases. In contrast to prevalence, which measures the probability *of having the disease*, incidence quantifies the *risk of developing a disease*. Incidence is defined as the number of new cases of the disease that occur in a population *at risk of developing such a disease* during a defined period. In calculating incidence, it is important to only include the people who are potentially *at risk* of developing the disease of interest in the denominator. For example, if the objective of the study is to estimate the incidence rate of cervical cancer, it would not be meaningful to include women who have had a hysterectomy or men. These individuals would be excluded from the denominator since they are not at risk of developing cervical cancer. Moreover, the time period of observation must also be clearly defined in calculating incidence (e.g. a neighbourhood homicide rate of 1/1,000 individuals *per decade* is clearly very different to a homicide rate of 1/1,000 *per week*).

Incidence is commonly calculated as cumulative incidence for large epidemiological studies (or as an incidence rate for greater precision in etiological studies). Cumulative incidence is defined as the probability of the occurrence of a disease during a defined period and is calculated using the formula shown in Figure 9.2.

Figure 9.3 is of a world map that shows the estimated cumulative incidence rate of tuberculosis in all countries in 2011. This is a common presentation that allows easy comparison of the incidence of the disease of interest internationally.

For greater precision or in studies where there is a significant dropout or admissions on an ongoing basis, researchers may opt to use the incidence rate rather than cumulative incidence. As with cumulative incidence, the numerator is the number of new cases of a disease. The denominator for the incidence rate, however, uses person-time (e.g. person-years or person-months) as a unit of comparison. Person-time is calculated as the sum of each individual's period of observation that he/she was free of the disease. For instance, if all people at risk in the population are observed throughout the defined study period, the denominator is simply the number of persons at risk of developing such a disease during that defined period and cumulative incidence will be calculated. On the other hand, if not all people are observed for the full study period, the incidence rate is the preferred measure using total person-time in the denominator.

## Mortality

Death from an illness thereby represents just the tip of the iceberg of the total health burden of that disease. Nevertheless, death is of great interest since mortality allows us to compare

$$\frac{\text{(Number of new disease cases in a defined period)}}{\text{(Number of individuals at risk at the beginning of the time period)}}$$

*Figure 9.2* Formula to calculate the cumulative incidence of disease

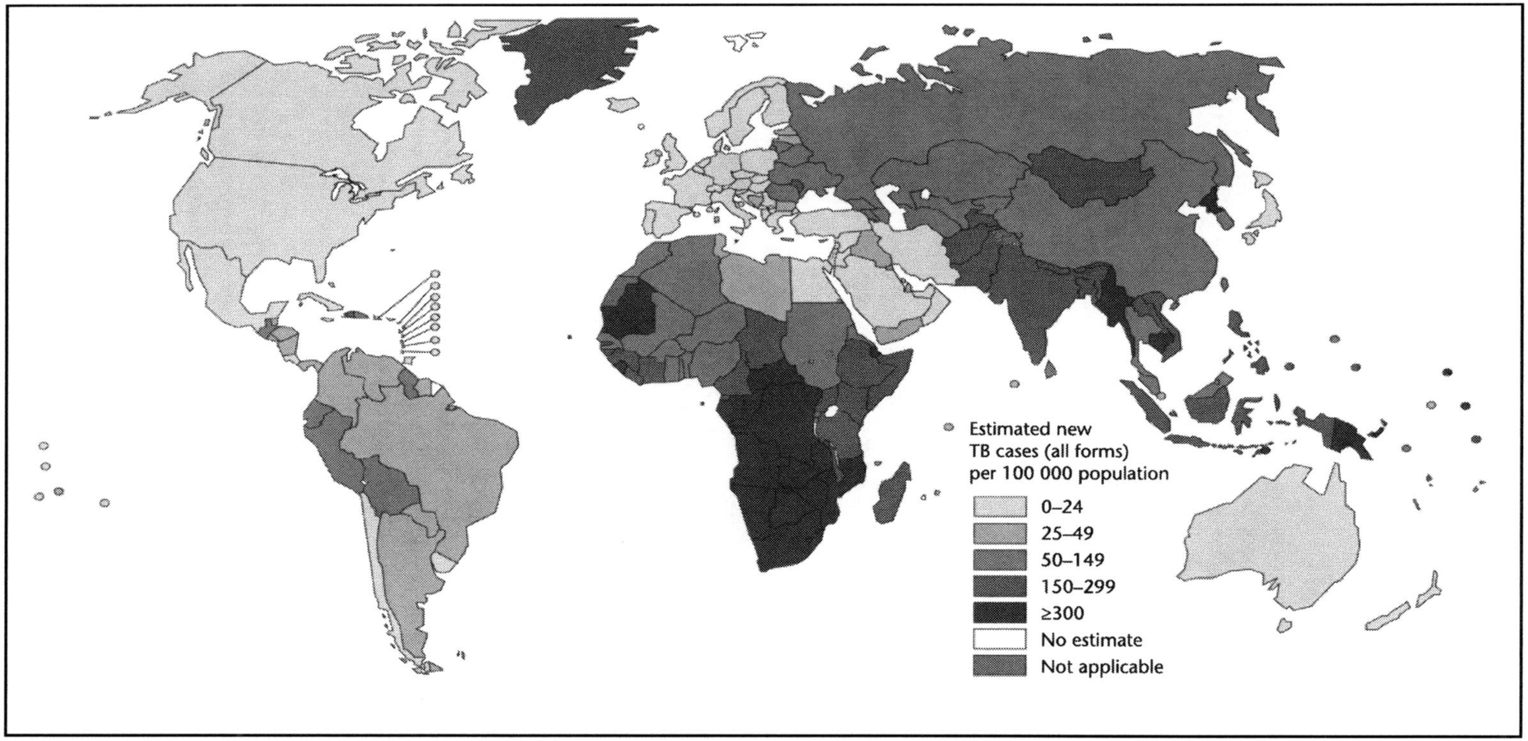


The boundaries and names shown and the designations used on this map do not imply the expression of any opinion whatsoever on the part of the World Health Organization concerning the legal status of any country, territory, city or area or of its authorities, or concerning the delimitation of its frontiers or boundaries. Dotted and dashed lines on maps represent approximate border lines for which there may not yet be full agreement.

Source: *Global Tuberculosis Report 2012*.WHO,2012.

World Health Organization

*Figure 9.3* World map of estimated tuberculosis incidence rates, 2011 [39]

the risk of death across different diseases, across different populations and across time for the same disease. For example, it is interesting to observe that despite relatively rapid socio-economic development, Hong Kong's mortality rate for ischemic heart disease has not reached the level of other developed countries, such as the USA, Japan and Singapore, and has been decreasing over the past thirty years, albeit to a lesser extent compared to other disease outcomes [12]. Mortality also allows us to measure the disease severity and determine whether treatments of the disease have improved over time. Lastly, mortality also serves as a proxy of incidence when the disease of interest is a very lethal one.

Mortality rate is the most commonly used measure to quantify death in a population. Essentially, mortality rate is an incidence rate where the event being measured is death itself. The numerator is the number of persons dying during a defined period, while the denominator is the number of people at risk of dying during that period, as shown in Figure 9.4.

If the annual mortality rate from all causes of death is to be calculated, the population at risk is the entire population of interest because it is assumed that every person in the population is at risk of dying from any cause. In addition to *all-cause* mortality, *cause-specific* (or *disease-specific*) mortality rates may also be calculated for different causes of death such as ischemic heart disease. Similarly, we can also place restrictions on age, giving *age-specific* mortality rates or on sex, giving *sex-specific* mortality rates. Time must also be specified in any mortality rate – it can be calculated over one year, giving an annual mortality rate or over five years, giving a five-year mortality rate, so on and so forth. For example, the infant mortality rate of a country (estimating the number of deaths of children younger than 1 year old per 1,000 live births) is often calculated to compare the level of general health with other countries, since it is believed that the level of general health of a population can be reflected by the health condition of their babies. According to the United Nations [13], the world average infant mortality rate is approximately 45.6 per 1,000 live births during 2005–2010, whereas it is 2.0 per 1,000 live births for Hong Kong, reflecting an exceedingly better level of general health in Hong Kong in comparison with the rest of the world.

## Common sources of epidemiologic data

In order to conduct public health research and inform public health policies, reliable and accurate sources of information must first be obtained. Each of these data sources has their advantages and limitations.

Routinely collected government data, such as vital statistics, census data and disease surveillance data are commonly employed in epidemiological research as a starting point for examining health issues. The majority of the industrialized countries in the world maintain up-to-date birth and death records that include demographic characteristics of the individual (e.g. sex, race, marital status, address) as well as cause(s) of death for death records and other information, such as mother's age and birth abnormalities, for birth certificates. Even in less developed countries, vital statistics are commonly accessible and may represent the most

$$\frac{\text{(Number of deaths occured during a defined period)}}{\text{(Number of person X time at risk of dying during that defined period)}}$$

*Figure 9.4* Formula to calculate the mortality rate in a population

complete source of population data available. In addition to vital statistics, population census also provides population-wide statistics, which can be used to analyse the prevalence of the disease of interest and to project future trends.

Other sources of routine morbidity data include hospital records and infectious disease surveillance data from the government. The World Health Organization (WHO) requires all its member states to report certain infectious diseases deemed notifiable. In addition to notifiable infectious diseases, many countries also maintain cancer registries that document the clinical details of cancer cases of its citizens similar to the Surveillance, Epidemiology and End Results (SEER) database maintained by the US Cancer Institute. As well as that, the WHO regularly publishes international statistics collated from its member states on specific health topics. In addition to the data described above, many countries also periodically conduct national household surveys, which often include questions on various health issues. For example, the Hong Kong government regularly conducts the Thematic Household Survey to collect data on different topics, including health outcomes, ageing, healthcare utilization, lifestyle, as well as others. In addition to routinely collected government data, other important sources of routine morbidity data include school health reports, sickness benefit forms, health insurance claims, military records, accident statistics, and records of vaccinations and immunizations.

The advantages of routine data are that they are relatively cheap and easily accessible, and even authoritative in nature when official records are being used (e.g. government or census official data). The main limitation of using these types of data is that they are typically conducted for purposes other than the research question at hand and are thereby unlikely to yield enough detail or adequate information for investigating the research question. Instead, the primary uses of these data are for generating hypotheses and examining general health trends rather than looking for disease risk factors or uncovering disease etiologies.

In cases where routine data may not provide sufficient information for examining risk factors for health conditions, surveys can be conducted to obtain such data. Questionnaires, clinical examinations and biological testing are common surveying methods. Epidemiological studies may examine a wide variety of exposures that may include population-level macro-environment exposures (e.g. regional socio-economic development, national income inequality levels), physical environment exposures (e.g. air pollution, ambient noise levels) and individual level exposures (e.g. personal health behaviours, educational attainment, medical history). For instance, surveys can be conducted to query alcohol-drinking habits of the population in question and these self-reported data can be supplemented with more objective physical measurements, such as the blood alcohol levels of the subjects.

## Overview of the types of epidemiological studies

As described earlier in this chapter, epidemiology is a scientific discipline which studies the distribution and determinants of health-related phenomena in human populations. The ultimate objective of epidemiological research is to use data to control or reduce the harms of disease. In this section, we will describe several major epidemiologic study designs commonly used to achieve this goal, and their common applications.

### *Preliminary descriptive epidemiological studies*

In epidemiological and clinical research, many initial clues of disease causation or disease therapies are derived from case reports. Case reports, which represent the first interface between clinical medicine and epidemiology, are simply a detailed clinical description of unusual cases of patients from clinicians. Such reports may provide information about newly emerging diseases, such as HIV in the 1980s [14] or SARS in 2003 [9], or may provide early warnings of previously unknown harms, such as toxicity or drug interactions from patients showing previously unreported adverse events. Lastly, case reports may also provide an early clue for newfound therapies from noteworthy beneficial effects seen in a patient. The main limitation of case reports is that they typically study only a handful of patients who may not be representative of the general population. Hence, case reports are taken as a preliminary study that may generate a hypothesis for more rigorous study designs.

The second type of descriptive study that is commonly used to provide initial clues for disease etiology is correlational studies, also known as ecological studies. Correlational studies examine groups of people or populations, such as countries (rather than individuals), as the units of analysis in order to search for high- and low-risk populations for a disease of interest. For instance, a correlational study may begin by comparing heart disease rates across countries to search for high- and low-risk countries. Once these countries are identified, further correlational studies can be conducted to compare the diseases, such as cardiovascular diseases, with a hypothesized risk factor, such as average red meat consumption levels or a hypothesized protective factor, such as average fish consumption levels. Another well-known example of an ecological study is the Atherosclerosis Risk in Communities Study conducted by Diez Roux and colleagues that studied the relationship between neighbourhood characteristics and incidence of coronary heart disease, of which the unit of analysis is neighbourhood [15]. They found that coronary heart disease was more likely to develop in people living in the most disadvantaged neighbourhoods than in those living in the most advantaged ones. However, since the units of analysis of correlational studies are groups of people rather than individuals, caution must be exercised in extrapolating findings to individuals. Ecological fallacy describes such misinterpretation when a causal relationship that exists at a group or population level is interpreted to also exist at an individual level. While ecological study design has lost a great deal of its creditability due to ecological fallacy, it has recently become apparent that such a study design is especially useful for developing further hypotheses to test the relationship between risk factors and the disease of interest at an individual level, and to test whether valid ecological risk factors actually exist for a health outcome that individual-level studies may not be able to capture. Moreover, ecological studies are important in public health for their cost-effectiveness. Since correlational studies typically use existing data sources, such as government or trade data, these studies can be conducted very quickly.

### *Observational study designs*

From initial hypotheses that may be generated from case reports, correlational studies or simply from existing knowledge of disease mechanisms, observational studies are usually conducted to examine the association between presumed exposures and health outcomes with more scientific rigour. In observational studies, the investigators observe health and disease-related records without any intervention and conduct statistical analyses on these observed data. Even though observational studies are conducted under less controlled circumstances than experimental studies, such as clinical trials, observational studies represent a valuable source of health information. Observational studies are the only manner in which researchers can study exposures that are known to be harmful to humans under accepted standards of ethical scientific research. By contemporary standards of research ethics, it is not an acceptable practice to expose humans to high doses of ionizing radiation or to have subjects ingest harmful substances. In fact, the deleterious effects of such hazards as cigarette smoke have been primarily uncovered by the famed British doctors study, which is observational in nature. In October 1951, the research team, headed by the renowned epidemiologists Richard Doll and Austin Bradford Hill, wrote to all registered doctors in the United Kingdom and obtained responses from 40,701 about their smoking history and habits. Subjects were subsequently followed up, and in 1956 [16], the findings were published and provided the first official link of tobacco smoking to serious illnesses using observational methods. In this section, we will describe three types of observational studies that are commonly used to test hypotheses: cross-sectional, cohort and case-control studies.

## Cross-sectional studies

A cross-sectional study, also known as a disease frequency or a prevalence survey, simultaneously obtains information about each individual's level of the presumed risk factor (e.g. smoking status, blood type, mental stress) and whether the individual has the health outcome of interest (e.g. bronchitis, metabolic conditions, anxiety disorders) at a particular point in time. A cross-sectional study is analogous to taking a 'snapshot' of the disease and exposure status of people in a particular instant, without follow-up; thus, it is descriptive in nature. Due to the lack of a follow-up, a major limitation of cross-sectional studies is that the temporal sequence of the presumed exposure and health outcome is often obscured unless the exposure is an unchanging attribute, such as genetic traits (e.g. blood type). That is, since the presumed exposure and presumed outcome are assessed simultaneously, there often is a 'chicken and egg' issue whereby it is uncertain which variable preceded the other. Although cross-sectional studies may not be able to provide conclusive evidence of disease etiology, the main reason for their popularity is that studies can be conducted in a time-efficient manner and at low cost. Also, similar to political opinion polls, serial cross-sectional studies can be done on the population to quickly examine changes in health behaviours. This can be useful for assessing health interventions (i.e. a pre- and post-intervention study) and also for tracking changes in a population over time. For example, serial cross-sectional studies were conducted to assess changes in personal hygiene behaviours after SARS among the general public [17] and among medical staff [18]. These studies showed that there was a greater uptake of positive health behaviours such as improved hand hygiene resulting from a large-scale infectious disease epidemic. Such studies are useful for quickly ascertaining the pervasiveness of behavioural risk factors and preventive behaviours in the population so that risk communication messages can be quickly tailored to the most up-to-date information.

## Cohort studies

A cohort study, also known as a longitudinal study, is designed to examine putative associations between risk factors and outcomes by taking the study sample and dividing it by the exposure levels of the individuals who do not have the health condition of interest at the beginning. The participants are followed longitudinally from the beginning of the study to anywhere from a few days to several decades to determine whether the incidence of disease differs between exposure groups. Despite the attractiveness of a clear temporal sequence and detailed exposure levels, the main drawback of cohort studies is the potentially high dropout rate of subjects, also known as a loss to follow-up. For this reason, this study design is logistically unsuited for itinerant or hard-to-locate populations, such as homeless people. The other main limitation of this study design is that it is inefficient for rare health outcomes since an extremely large study sample must be initially assembled in order to obtain sufficient numbers of cases to conduct statistical analysis. The high cost of cohort studies is another consideration that limits their use. Nonetheless, large-scale cohort studies spanning decades, such as the famous Framingham Heart study [19] and Harvard University's Nurses' Health Studies [20], have contributed enormously to the knowledge we have about chronic illnesses, such as cardiovascular disease and cancer. Specifically, the Framingham Heart study began in 1948 and recruited 5,209 men and women aged 30–62 years old who were free of cardiovascular disease at the beginning of the study. They were then examined every two years for new cardiovascular events and by daily surveillance of hospitalizations at the only hospital in Framingham. It was the first study to identify various epidemiological determinants of cardiovascular disease. Similarly, the Harvard Nurses' Health Study (established in 1976) and the Nurses' Health Study II (established in 1989) have followed 121,700 and 116,000 female registered nurses, respectively, and are the definitive prospective observational studies on women's health to date.

### Case-control studies

For studying rare health outcomes or when resources are limited, case-control studies offer a cost-effective option for examining associations between diseases and their presumed risk factors. In a case-control study, subjects who have the disease or outcome – the *cases* – and subjects who do not have the disease – the *controls* – are first identified. While cohort studies follow study participants based on their exposure levels to see whether they develop the disease, case-control studies go backwards from disease onset to the postulated risk factors. The proportion of the cases that report the exposure of interest is statistically compared with the proportion of the non-diseased controls that have had the exposure. For example, this study design was used to identify the factors associated with the breakthrough transmission of the SARS virus among hospital workers infected in hospital settings during the SARS outbreak in Hong Kong in 2003 [21]. However, a main concern of this study design is that of recall by subjects, including both limitations in recall, as well as bias in recall when the subjects try harder to identify their exposures due to them contracting the disease of interest.

Figure 9.5 shows a schematic comparison of the study designs among cross-sectional, cohort and case-control studies.

## *Experimental study designs*

Historically speaking, experimental studies in epidemiology refer to those that tested epidemics among experimental animals. In more recent literature, they refer to studies in which the investigator actively assigns the exposure status of the study participants.

### Randomized controlled trials

Randomized controlled trials (RCTs) are the most common type of epidemiological experiment, and widely regarded as the most scientifically rigorous method of hypothesis testing available in epidemiology and medicine [1]. In an RCT, subjects in a population are randomized or randomly allocated, into either the *study* (or experimental) group or *control* (or *placebo*) group to

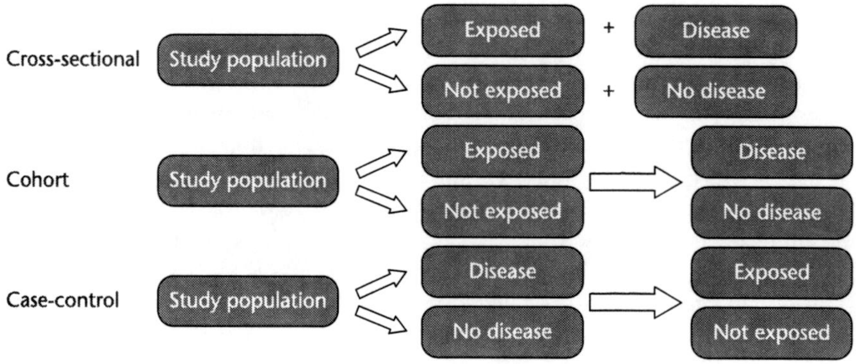


*Figure 9.5* Designs of cross-sectional, cohort and case-control studies

receive or not receive an exposure, which is usually an experimental preventive or therapeutic procedure, manoeuvre or intervention [1]. The usual purpose is to test the effectiveness and efficacy of such exposure. Differences in disease rates, recovery, death and other relevant outcomes will be tested between the *study* and the *control* groups. Testing efficacy of a pharmaceutical drug (e.g. Viagra), new preventive vaccines (e.g. HPV vaccines) or a new intervention strategy (e.g. web-based mental health interventions) are all examples of common RCTs.

## Community trials

Community trials, or community-based clinical trials, are another type of epidemiologic experiment in which the unit of allocation to receive a preventive or therapeutic procedure, manoeuvre or intervention is an entire community or political subdivision. For example, this study design was used to test the feasibility and effectiveness of an intervention to increase condom use rates and increase HIV/AIDS knowledge among female sex workers in China, in which 30 establishments in Chengjiang were randomized [22].

Figure 9.6 shows an illustration of the design of a randomized controlled trial. The study population is the individual subjects in an RCT, whilst the study population is an entire community or political subdivision in a community trial.

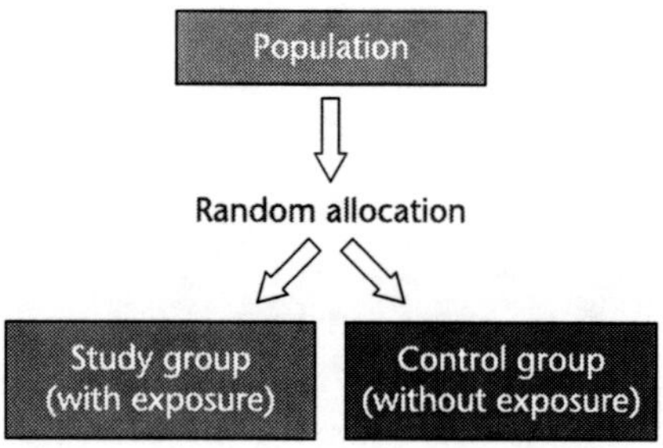


*Figure 9.6* Design of a randomized controlled trial

## Translation of research into public health action: a brief case study of alcohol harm reduction in Hong Kong

As mentioned above, the findings of epidemiological research aim to alter clinical guidelines, health services or governmental policies towards preventive actions. In this section, we present an example of the application of epidemiological research to public health action for alcohol harm reduction in Hong Kong.

After the 1997 handover, Hong Kong has retained its laissez-faire capitalist economy under China's 'one country, two systems' policy and the Westernizing effects of global commerce have continued to influence the lifestyle habits of its 7.1 million residents. Hong Kong is historically considered to be a low-alcohol consumption region and has been slow to implement alcohol policies. Unlike countries such as the USA, Hong Kong has no restrictions on alcohol advertising and there is very little enforcement against underage drinking.

Alcohol-related deaths currently comprise approximately 3.2 per cent of all global mortality [23], but great variations exist internationally of the harms associated with alcohol consumption in accordance with socio-cultural drinking norms and alcohol policies. Research to guide public health policy on alcohol, however, was lacking in Hong Kong. Alcohol consumption data were mainly limited to routinely collected government data from the Hong Kong Behavioural Risk Factor Surveillance surveys, which obtained basic information on a wide range of health behaviours and sporadically conducted surveys on students. Despite the lack of detailed information at that time, the data were nevertheless able to show that less than half of adult males and about one-sixth of adult females drank in the past month [24] and that drinking levels in young people were much lower than in American students [25–27].

In order to provide evidence for alcohol policies, special population-based surveys on alcohol-related attitudes and drinking behaviours were conducted by the Chinese University of Hong Kong to provide serial data for changes in drinking patterns. In 2006, a cross-sectional study of nearly 10,000 adults, interviewed by telephone, showed that Hong Kong has lower population rates of ever drinking (66.6 per cent), past-year drinking (47.3 per cent), past-month binge drinking (9.0 per cent), past-year alcohol abuse (3.3 per cent) and alcohol dependence (1.5 per cent) [28] than the prevalence reported in the USA and most of Western Europe [29–30]. Only 60.7 per cent of males and 39.3 per cent of females had consumed alcohol in the past year in stark contrast to countries such as France, Germany and the United Kingdom (> 85 per cent of both sexes) [30]. The cross-sectional data nonetheless showed high levels of lifetime 'ever drinking' in younger age groups, giving strong evidence of the secular trends of the increasing alcohol intake in Hong Kong. This study also showed that the past-year prevalence of drink driving was relatively low with only 5.2 per cent of males and 0.8 per cent of females driving within two hours of consuming alcohol [31].

Since the 2006 baseline study, however, the Hong Kong government has embarked on an active campaign to promote Hong Kong as a regional wine hub as part of an economic stimulus plan to counter the effects of the 2007 global financial crisis. The 80 per cent excise taxes on wine and 40 per cent taxes on beer were eliminated in February 2008 and the government began to foster alcohol-related training programmes to support the hospitality industry. These actions led to a rapidly burgeoning wine culture, as evidenced by year-on-year wine import growths of 80 per cent, 45 per cent and 73 per cent for 2008–9, 2009–10 and 2010–11, respectively [32]. Since greater accessibility of alcoholic beverages has been correlated with higher levels of alcohol-related traffic accidents in international literature

[33–36], the Hong Kong government began to implement evidence-based international best practices to combat alcohol-related traffic accidents. Based on the research from other countries, the government implemented random blood alcohol testing on roadways, introduced stiffer penalties (higher fines, longer imprisonment and longer minimum driving disqualification period), and commenced a media campaign that included giving voluntary breath tests to bar patrons, making TV commercials and distributing informational pamphlets.

A subsequent cross-sectional study conducted in 2011 indeed showed that the reduction in alcohol prices had resulted in the prevalence of those ever drinking alcohol to have significantly increased from the 2006 baseline level of 66.6 per cent to 81.7 per cent in 2011 [37]. The 2011 study also demonstrated that Hong Kong's combined strategy of random breath testing, awareness-raising campaigns and increasing penalties appears to be effective in reducing the harms of alcohol use. After the implementation of random breath testing in 2009, there was a decline of alcohol-related traffic accidents, indicating that some of the hazards of alcohol consumption can be effectively mitigated by appropriate legal controls even in an environment of heavy alcohol promotion and increasing drinking levels. Nonetheless, binge drinkers in Hong Kong remained a high-risk group for drink driving, indicating that these heavy drinkers may require clinical management or additional deterrents. Based on previous studies showing a high co-morbidity of alcohol abuse and dependence among binge drinkers, cohort studies of binge drinkers should be conducted to examine the risk of developing alcohol abuse and/or alcohol dependence in Hong Kong.

In 2011, the Hong Kong government officially launched an ongoing 'Action Plan to Reduce the Alcohol-related Harm in Hong Kong' after reviewing the international and local research on alcohol harms and consulting community stakeholders. The action plan outlines the collaborative work to be undertaken to reduce the harms of alcohol in Hong Kong in the coming years [38]. Currently, ongoing alcohol research is examining ways to improve the clinical management of patients at-risk for alcohol misuse and studies are being conducted to provide culturally relevant drinking advice to the general public.

## Conclusion

For readers unfamiliar with public health research methods, this chapter introduces basic epidemiological concepts and provides a brief overview of common study designs that will be mentioned in later chapters of this book. As an applied science, this discipline helps students of public health critically evaluate public health literature and medical studies. In the larger picture, epidemiology's ultimate objective is to provide a strong evidence base for informing clinical practice, disease prevention measures and health policy. We have presented a case study of real life applications of epidemiology for alcohol policy in Hong Kong. In doing so, we have tried to illustrate how public health improvement is a continual process that requires well-designed and properly conducted studies. We hope to convey to readers that the complexities of contemporary health problems increasingly require a dialogue between researchers and a diverse group of stakeholders that may include not only clinicians and policy makers, but also law enforcement agencies, trade organizations as well as the public.

## References

1. Porta M. *A Dictionary of Epidemiology*. Oxford: Oxford University Press; 2008: 10–11.
2. Hippocrates. Airs, waters, places. In: Buck C (ed.) *The Challenge of Epidemiology: Issues and Selected Readings*. Washington, DC: Pan American Health Organization; 1988: 18–19.

3. Unschuld PU. *Medicine in China: A History of Ideas*. Berkeley: University of California Press; 1985.
4. Huang Ti Nei Ching Su Wen. In: Veith I (ed.) *The Yellow Emperor's Classic of Internal Medicine*. Berkeley: University of California Press; 1970.
5. Benenson AS. *Control of Communicable Diseases in Man*. 15th ed. Washington, DC: American Public Health Association; 1990.
6. Chinese Ministry of Health. Report from the Ministry of Health of the People's Republic of China on Sanlu infant milk powder incident and medical treatment situation [in Chinese]. 2008 [Online]. Available from: http://www.moh.gov.cn/sofpro/cms/previewjspfile/mohbgt/cms_0000000000000000144_tpl.jsp?requestCode=38386&CategoryID=4800 [Accessed 21 October 2009].
7. Guan N, Fan Q, Ding J, Zhao Y, Lu J, Ai Y, *et al*. Melamine-contaminated powdered formula and urolithiasis in young children. *New England Journal of Medicine* 2009; 360: 1067–74.
8. Hong Kong Food and Health Bureau. Third Report of the Expert Group on Melamine Incident. 2009 [Online]. Available from: http://www.fhb.gov.hk/download/press_and_publications/otherinfo/081020_melamine/e_report20090415.pdf [Accessed 14 February 2013].
9. Chan-Yeung M, Yu WC. Outbreak of severe acute respiratory syndrome in Hong Kong Special Administrative Region: case report. *BMJ* 2003; 326: 850–2.
10. National Committee for AIDS, Drugs, and Prostitution Prevention and Control. Viet Nam AIDS Response Progress Report 2012. Hanoi, March 2012. [Online]. Available from: http://www.unaids.org/en/dataanalysis/knowyourresponse/countryprogressreports/2012countries/ce_VN_Narrative_Report.pdf [Accessed 30 January 2013].
11. Thienkrua W, Cardozo BL, Chakkraband ML, Guadamuz TE, Pengjuntr W, Tantipiwatanaskul P, *et al*. Symptoms of posttraumatic stress disorder and depression among children in tsunami-affected areas in southern Thailand. *JAMA* 2006; 296(5): 549–59.
12. Chung RY, Schooling CM, Cowling BJ, Leung GM. How does socioeconomic development affect risk of mortality? An age–period–cohort analysis from a recently transitioned population in China. *American Journal of Epidemiology* 2010; 171(3): 345–56.
13. United Nations. World population prospects: the 2010 revision. 2011. New York: Population Division of the Department of Economic and Social Affairs of the United Nations Secretariat [Online]. Available from: http://esa.un.org/unpd/wpp/Excel-Data/mortality.htm [Accessed 4 March 2013].
14. Centers for Disease Control and Prevention. Pneumocystis pneumonia. Los Angeles. *Morbidity and Mortality Weekly Report* 1981; 30: 250–2. [Online]. Available from: http://www.cdc.gov/mmwr/pdf/wk/mm5021.pdf [Accessed 30 January 2013].
15. Diez Roux AV, Nieto FJ, Muntaner C, Tyroler HA, Comstock GW, Shahar E, *et al*. Neighborhood environments and coronary heart disease: a multilevel analysis. *American Journal of Epidemiology* 1997; 146(1): 48–63.
16. Doll R, Hill AB. Lung cancer and other causes of death in relation to smoking; a second report on the mortality of British doctors. *BMJ* 1956; 2(5001): 1071–81.
17. Lau JT, Yang X, Tsui HY, Kim JH. Impacts of SARS on health-seeking behaviors in general population in Hong Kong. *Preventive Medicine* 2005; 41(2): 454–62.
18. Wong TW, Tam WW. Handwashing practice and the use of personal protective equipment among medical students after the SARS epidemic in Hong Kong. *American Journal of Infection Control* 2005; 33(10): 580–6.
19. Kannel WB. CHD risk factors: a Framingham Study update. *Hospital Practice* 1990; 25(7): 93–104.
20. The Nurses' Health Study [Online]. Available from: http://www.channing.harvard.edu/nhs/ [Accessed 6 March 2013].
21. Lau JT, Fung KS, Wong TW, Kim JH, Wong E, Chung S, *et al*. SARS transmission among hospital workers in Hong Kong. *Emerging Infectious Diseases* 2004; 10(2): 280–6.
22. Wu Z, Rou K, Jia M, Duan S, Sullivan SG. The first community-based sexually transmitted disease/HIV intervention trial for female sex workers in China. *AIDS* 2007; 21(Suppl 8): S89–94.
23. World Health Organization. Management of substance abuse: Alcohol. 2007. [Online]. Available from: http://www.who.int/substance_abuse/facts/global_burden/en/index.html [Accessed 3 January 2013].
24. Centre for Health Protection. Statistics on behavioural risk factors. Department of Health, Hong Kong. 2006. [Online]. Available from: http://www.chp.gov.hk [Accessed 1 August 2007].

25. Abdullah AS, Fielding R, Hedley, AJ. Patterns of cigarette smoking, alcohol use and other substance use among Chinese university students in Hong Kong. *American Journal on Addictions* 2002; 11: 235–46.
26. Griffiths S, Lau JTF, Chow JKW, Lee SS, Kan PYMY, Lee S. Alcohol use among entrants to a Hong Kong University. *Alcohol & Alcoholism* 2006; 41: 560–5.
27. Youth Research Center. A study on the alcohol drinking habits among youth in Hong Kong. Hong Kong SAR: Hong Kong Federation of Youth Groups; 2000.
28. Kim JH, Lee S, Chow J, Lau J, Tsang A, Choi J, Griffiths S. Prevalence and factors associated with binge drinking, alcohol abuse and alcohol dependence: a population-based study of Chinese adults in Hong Kong. *Alcohol & Alcoholism* 2008; 43(3): 360–70.
29. Dawson, D. Gender differences in the risk of alcohol dependence: United States, 1992. *Addiction* 1996; 91: 1831–42.
30. World Health Organization. Department of Mental Health and Substance Abuse. *Global Status Report on Alcohol 2004*. Geneva: WHO; 2004.
31. Kim JH, Lee S, Chan KC, Lau JT, Tsang A, Griffiths SG. A population-based study on the prevalence and correlates of drinking and driving in Hong Kong. *Accident Analysis & Prevention* 2010; 42(4): 994–1002.
32. Chan KC. LCQ15: Impact of the abolition of estate duty and duty on alcoholic beverages. Information Services Department, Hong Kong. 15 December 2010. [Online]. Available from: http://www.ird.gov.hk/eng/ppr/archives/10121503.htm [Accessed 30 January 2013].
33. Wagenaar AC, Tobler AL, Komro KA. Effects of tax and price policies on mobility and mortality: a systematic review. *American Journal of Public Health* 2010; 100(11): 2270–8.
34. Anderson P, Chisholm D, Fuhr DC. Effectiveness and cost-effectiveness of policies and programmes to reduce the harm caused by alcohol. *Lancet* 2009; 373(9682): 2234–46.
35. Gruenewald PJ, Johnson FW, Treno AJ. Outlets, drinking and driving: a multilevel analysis of availability. *Journal of Studies on Alcohol* 2002; 63: 460–8.
36. Treno AJ, Grube JW, Martin SE. Alcohol availability as a predictor of youth drinking and driving: a hierarchical analysis of survey and archival data. *Alcohol Clinical and Experimental Research* 2003; 27: 835–40.
37. Kim JH, Wong A, Goggins WB, Lau J, Griffiths SM. Drink driving in Hong Kong: the competing effects of random breath testing and alcohol tax reductions. *Addiction* 2013; 108(7): 1217–28.
38. Hong Kong Department of Health. Action Plan to Reduce Alcohol-related Harm in Hong Kong. 2011. [Online]. Available from: http://www.dh.gov.hk/english/pub_rec/pub_rec_ar/pub_rec_ncd_ap2.html [Accessed 30 January 2013].
39. World Health Organization. *Global Tuberculosis Report 2012*. Geneva. [Online]. Available from: http://www.who.int/tb/publications/global_report/en/ [Accessed 3 January 2013].

# 10

# Evidence-based decision making in health care

*Vincent C. H. Chung and Jin Ling Tang*

## Epidemiology, public health and evidence-based medicine

Epidemiology as a discipline originated in the search for causes of outbreaks and epidemics of communicable diseases with the aim of finding effective ways of preventing and controlling them [1]. A disease can be effectively prevented only after its causes or risk factors are known. Epidemiological research is thus the prerequisite for prevention, and epidemiology forms a core discipline of public health, a modern and broader version of preventive medicine. However, public health deals with health issues at the population or societal level as opposed to clinical medicine that works at the individual level. Epidemiology that is used to study and understand health issues in populations thus forms the foundation for public health, and has long been known as a discipline relevant only to public health.

Since the middle of the twentieth century, chronic non-communicable diseases (NCDs) have become the major cause of suffering and death in most human populations. Epidemiological concepts and methods were used to study the cause of chronic diseases, and new study methods such as randomized controlled trials were invented for evaluating the efficacy of medical interventions. Since then epidemiology has rapidly evolved. Modern epidemiology, including clinical epidemiology as a subdiscipline, is a discipline of research methodology for studying, quantitatively and in human populations, general issues of disease, health and health care, such as etiology of disease, epidemics of disease, disease burdens and health needs; accuracy of diagnostic methods; prognosis of diseases; and efficacy of interventions including treatments, screening and management and policies [2].

From the 1980s when medical research involving various epidemiological studies started to gain maturity, research evidence, particularly from randomized control trials on the effectiveness of medical interventions, continued to cumulate. Systematic reviews and meta-analyses of epidemiological research evidence, in the early 1990s, showed that some routinely used medical interventions were ineffective or of marginal value. The importance of epidemiological evidence began to be more widely recognized, and evidence-based medicine (EBM) that urges clinical practice and decisions to be made consistent with current best evidence was proposed in 1992. Evidence here is primarily referred to as the findings from

*Table 10.1* Definitions of epidemiology, evidence-based medicine and evidence-based health care

| | |
|---|---|
| *Epidemiology* | The science and art of studying, quantitatively and in human populations, general laws and issues about disease, health and health care. Findings of epidemiological research are directly relevant to medical and public health practice and thus provide the essential evidence for making decisions in medicine and public health. |
| *Evidence-based medicine* | The science and art of making patient care decisions which are consistent with current best evidence. Evidence-based decisions should also consider available resources and values of the individual patient in addition to evidence. |
| *Evidence-based health care* | The science and art of making healthcare decisions for populations or communities which are consistent with current best evidence. Evidence-based decisions in health care should also consider available resources and values of people in addition to evidence. The major difference between evidence-based medicine and evidence-based health care is that the former is about individuals and the latter is about populations. |

*Sources*: [6, 7].

epidemiological research such as randomized controlled trials, cohort studies, case-control studies, surveys, and systematic reviews and meta-analyses.

In EBM, ineffective interventions should be discarded, interventions with marginal or uncertain effectiveness should be recommended with caution and powerful interventions should be used in any suitable circumstances whenever appropriate [3]. Increasing the use of effective interventions in health care can greatly improve the quality of clinical and health-care services provided [4].

Many concepts, theories and methods in EBM are rooted in, or related to, epidemiology or clinical epidemiology [5]. However, evidence-based medicine and epidemiology are different. The latter is research methods that help generate reliable and robust scientific evidence about issues in healthcare practice, whereas the former is the science and art of making use of this evidence to inform healthcare practice. The two disciplines work closely together to reach the common goal of improving the health of the popualtion. Evidence-based medicine was proposed originally for clinical practice. Decision making in public health is more complicated and differs from clinical care. Special issues in applying EBM to public health must be highlighted (see Table 10.1) [6, 7]. In this chapter, we will discuss EBM in further detail and then move on to describe the recent attempts in translating EBM principles into public health practice.

## Evolution of evidence-based medicine (EBM)

The early approach of teaching EBM to physicians was focused on critical appraisal skills by using the following five steps [8]:

1 Forming an answerable practice-related question;
2 Locating the current best evidence which may answer the question;
3 Evaluating the validity, results and applicability of that evidence using critical appraisal;
4 Incorporating the evidence with clinical expertise, patients' needs and values to make the decision or recommendation; and

5 Studying and forming ways to increase the efficiency and effectiveness of the previous steps.

The fourth step is the core concept of the practice of EBM. Steps before it are about making the fourth step possible and can be achieved through the efforts of individuals or by society collectively. Great efforts internationally have been made in the past twenty years in identifying, appraising, summarizing and disseminating research evidence for decision makers. The Cochrane Collaboration (www.cochrane.org) is a good example: it carries out the aforementioned tasks in preparing evidence, and helps save time for busy medical workers and decision makers in using evidence for making decisions. It was founded in 1993 with a vision that 'healthcare decision making throughout the world will be informed by high quality, timely research evidence', and it has now become a large international organization. The Cochrane Database of Systematic Review (CDSR, http://www.thecochranelibrary.com/view/0/index.html) is the most important sources of systematic reviews and meta-analyses of medical interventions and plays a pivotal role in the production and dissemination of evidence across all areas of health care. Currently, more than 5,000 full-text Cochrane systematic reviews are available on the CDSR database.

In recent years, there have been two major shifts of focus in the practice of EBM: first, the practice of EBM has evolved from building critical appraisal skills to mastering the timely use of pre-appraised evidence, and second, EBM has extended its scope from evidence-based clinical practice for individuals to evidence-based health care for populations.

## Validity of evidence

What constitutes evidence? Generally speaking, evidence is the 'available body of facts and information indicating whether a belief or proposition is true or valid' [9]. Any piece of information may be considered evidence, yet each piece differs in how relevant, valid and trustworthy it is for patient care [10]. Evidence of high validity is needed as it allows reliable decisions to be made. In the era of information explosion, decision makers need to be competent in identifying the best available evidence applicable to the questions at hand amongst a vast volume of published information.

An example can be made by showing the varying validity of different sources of evidence on efficacy of intervention. Evidence may come from animal and *in vitro* laboratory studies, pathophysiological reasoning, clinical experience, observational studies, randomized controlled trials and systematic reviews [10]. According to how valid, generalizable and relevant the evidence is to patient care, there is a hierarchy of evidence with the validity decreasing from systematic reviews to randomized controlled trials, to observational studies, to clinical experience, and finally to animal and *in vitro* studies. When all sorts of evidence exist, systematic reviews and large randomized clinical trials have the highest relevance and quality, and should always be used in decision making. Evidence of lower quality can be considered and used only when higher quality evidence is absent. Decisions should be made based on the best evidence currently available.

The Levels of Evidence document produced by the Oxford Centre for Evidence-based Medicine in 2011 can be used as a quick guide for assessing the validity of evidence for various questions relating to day-to-day clinical practice [11]. It can be used as a heuristic so that clinicians, policy makers and patients can answer clinical questions quickly without performing their own critical appraisals. It can also be used as a guide to search for literature which should always start from the best possible evidence and continue until the evidence is found. In Table 10.2, each column represents the evidence of various degrees of validity,

*Table 10.2* Oxford Centre for EBM Levels of Evidence 2011

| *Question* | *Step 1 (Level 1*)* | *Step 2 (Level 2*)* | *Step 3 (Level 3*)* | *Step 4 (Level 4*)* | *Step 5 (Level 5)* |
|---|---|---|---|---|---|
| **How common is the problem?** | Local and current random sample surveys (or censuses) | Systematic review of surveys that allow matching to local circumstances** | Local non-random sample** | Case-series** | n/a |
| **Is this diagnostic or monitoring test accurate?** (Diagnosis) | Systematic review of cross sectional studies with consistently applied reference standard and blinding | Individual cross-sectional studies with consistently applied reference standard and blinding | Non-consecutive studies, or studies without consistently applied reference standards** | Case-control studies, or poor or non-independent reference standard** | Mechanism-based reasoning |
| **What will happen if we do not intervene with a therapy?** (Natural prognosis) | Systematic review of inception cohort studies | Inception cohort studies | Cohort study or control arm of randomized trial* | Case-series or case-control studies, or poor quality prognostic cohort study** | n/a |
| **Does this intervention help?** (Treatment benefits) | Systematic review of randomized trials | Randomized trial or observational study with dramatic effect | Non-randomized controlled cohort/follow-up study** | Case-series, case-control studies or historically controlled studies** | Mechanism-based reasoning |
| **What are the COMMON harms?** (Treatment harms) | Systematic review of randomized trials, systematic review of nested case-control studies, *n*-of-1 trial with the patient you are raising the question about, or observational study with dramatic effect | Individual randomized trial or (exceptionally) observational study with dramatic effect | Non-randomized controlled cohort/follow-up study (post-marketing surveillance) provided there are sufficient numbers to rule out a common harm. (For long-term harms the duration of follow-up must be sufficient.)** | Case-series, case-control or historically controlled studies** | Mechanism-based reasoning |

| | | | | | |
|---|---|---|---|---|---|
| **What are the RARE harms?** (Treatment harms) | Systematic review of randomized trials | Randomized trial or (exceptionally) observational study with dramatic effect | | | |
| **Is this (early detection) test worthwhile?** (Screening) | Systematic review of randomized trials | Randomized trial | Non-randomized controlled cohort/follow-up study** | Case-series, case-control or historically controlled studies** | Mechanism-based reasoning |

*Source*: [12].

*Notes*: * Level may be graded down on the basis of study quality, imprecision, indirectness (study PICO does not match questions PICO), because of inconsistency between studies, or because the absolute effect size is very small; level may be graded up if there is a large or very large effect size.

** As always, a systematic review is generally better than an individual study.

starting from the strongest at the top (Level 1) to the weakest at the bottom (Level 5). The first column presents the type of questions clinicians would ask in the order they encounter them in normal practice. For a single condition, clinicians and public health practitioners would need to know its prevalence in the community, the diagnostic accuracy of the test for confirming the presence of the condition, the prognosis of the condition, therapeutic effects of available treatments, the harms of the chosen treatment and, finally, the usefulness of screening for the condition (see Table 10.2) [12].

## Providing evidence for practice

The central idea of EBM is to make healthcare decisions based on the best evidence available. Although great efforts have been made to educate individual clinicians in conducting critical appraisals of original research articles and systematic reviews, the process of refining research findings to usable information is time consuming and does not fit in the busy clinicians' daily work routine. After many years of efforts, critical appraisal skills are still lacking in many clinicians throughout the world. In view of this, collective efforts from information experts have been made for creating databases that contain concise pre-appraised information. Clinicians can use the pre-appraised information in their practice without going through the process of searching, appraising and summarizing the evidence themselves [13, 14]. These databases are particularly important in areas for which updated clinical guidelines are not available.

The '6S' model for the evolution of evidence summarizes the international effort for preparing evidence for decision making in health care in the past twenty years [15]. The result of these efforts can be summarized in Figure 10.1, which we call the Evidence Pyramid. Common sources of information in each 'S' are listed in Table 10.3. Under this model, decision makers should begin their search at the *system* level, which entails the use of computerized decision support systems. In these systems, the best available evidence is automatically linked to electronic health records and clinicians would be provided with key evidence-based instructions on management strategies for each patient. If this system is unavailable, clinicians should explore *summaries*, which provide overviews on the best available evidence in the forms of clinical pathways, textbook summaries or practice guidelines.

When existing summaries do not cover the condition in question, systematic reviews (*syntheses*) and their synopses (*synopses of syntheses*) should be sought. Since many busy clinicians and policy makers do not have the skills and time to appraise and extract useful information from systematic reviews, synopses of syntheses are highly useful as they aim to provide succinct information that is essential for decision making. Moreover, they are often supplemented with commentaries on clinical applicability, as well as the original systematic reviews' methodological quality.

If there are no systems, summaries, synopses of syntheses or syntheses related to the clinical problem, the next stop is *synopses of single studies*. Similar to synopses of syntheses, they provide a brief overview of high-quality clinical studies that inform practice, often accompanied by expert commentaries that contextualize the findings in day-to-day clinical settings. The difference between synopsis and summary is that the latter generally covers a wider scope of relevant evidence for patient care. The last resort would be primary *studies*, which are often available in traditional databases without pre-appraisal.

Although the use of pre-appraised evidence would bring knowledge closer to the point of care, the '6S' model is not without limitations. The transformation of studies into higher 'S' levels takes time and this causes a time lag between availability and usability of evidence, which sometimes could be long. Also, high-quality evidence may not be available for certain

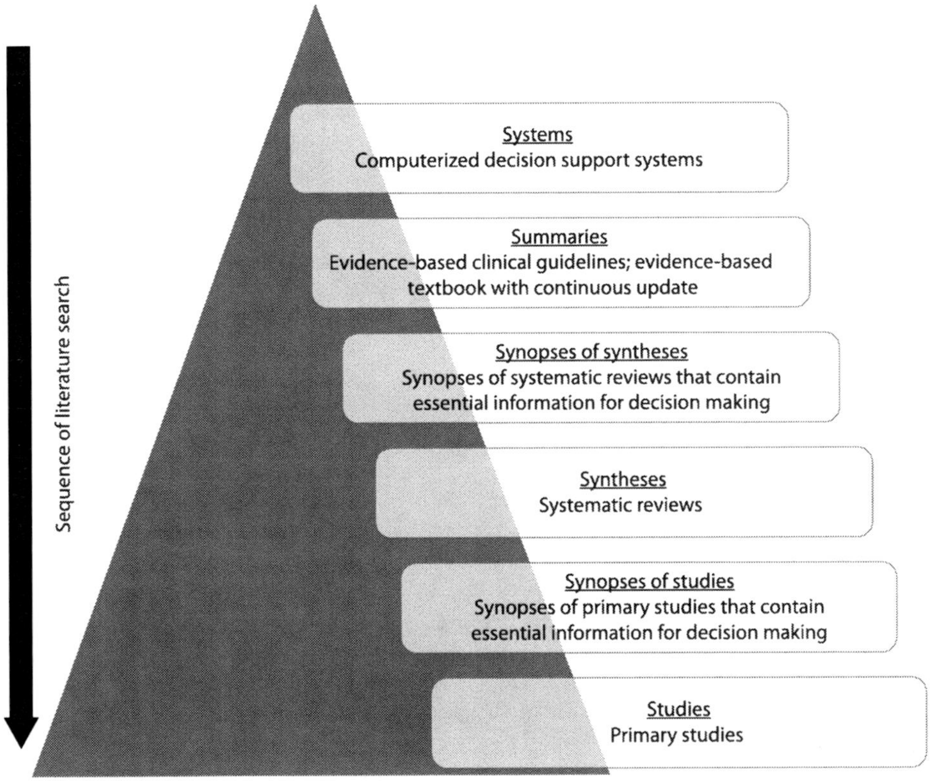


*Figure 10.1* The evidence pyramid and the '6S' evolution of healthcare

clinical questions and, at times, evidence from other health systems may not be applicable to the patient population which the clinicians or policy makers are taking care of. End users remain responsible for making sound choices based on the available evidence. Finally, regardless of the form of evidence a clinician has in hand, he or she should always consider the following questions before making the final decision [11]:

- Do your patients closely resemble those in the studies that you are reading?
- Does the treatment that you are about to use carry clinically meaningful benefit without posing significant harm to the patient?
- Are there any alternatives? How do they compare to the current choice?
- Does the proposed treatment fit with the patient's values and circumstances?

## Making evidence-based decisions

The ultimate goal of EBM is not merely to make evidence more accessible but the application of such evidence in practice for making good decisions. *Clinical Evidence* has reviewed evidence and provided summaries of more than 2,500 medical interventions for over 300 common clinical problems, such as diabetes mellitus and hypertension (www.clinicalevidence.com). It has shown that 36 per cent of the available interventions were effective or likely to be effective, 10 per cent were unlikely to be beneficial or likely to be ineffective or harmful and 46

*Table 10.3* Common sources of pre-appraised evidence

| *Level of pre-appraised evidence* | *Resources for clinical medicine: examples* | *Resources for public health: examples* |
|---|---|---|
| **System** | Zynxhealth (www.zynxhealth.com/)<br>Map of Medicine (www.mapofmedicine.com/) | *To be developed* |
| **Summaries** | Clinical Evidence (www.clinicalevidence.com)<br>Dynamed (www.ebscohost.com/dynamed/default.php) | National Guidelines Clearinghouse (NGC) (http://guideline.gov)<br>National Institute for Health and Clinical Excellence Public Health Guidance (http://guidance.nice.org.uk/PHG?textonly=false) |
| **Synopses of syntheses** | *ACP Journal Club* (www.acpjc.org)<br>Database of Abstracts of Reviews of Effects (www.crd.york.ac.uk/crdweb/Home.aspx?DB=DARE) | Health Evidence (www.health-evidence.ca)<br>CDC Guide to Community Preventative Services (www.thecommunityguide.org) |
| **Syntheses** | Evidence Updates (http://plus.mcmaster.ca/evidenceupdates)<br>The *Cochrane Library* (www.thecochranelibrary.com/) | McMaster Health Knowledge Refinery – Public Health+ (www.nccmt.ca/tools/public_health_plus-eng.html)<br>The *Cochrane Library* (www.thecochranelibrary.com/)<br>The Campbell Collaboration (www.campbellcollaboration.org/) |
| **Synopses of studies** | *ACP Journal Club* (www.acpjc.org)<br>*Evidence-Based Medicine* (ebm.bmj.com) | Trip Database (filter by evidence-based synopses) (www.tripdatabase.com)<br>Evidence Updates (http://plus.mcmaster.ca/EvidenceUpdates/) |
| **Studies** | MEDLINE<br>EMBASE | |

per cent were of unknown effectiveness. Such information is of vital importance in making healthcare decisions: interventions that are ineffective or unlikely to be beneficial should be prevented or discarded from use in practice and those that are of uncertain effectiveness should be used with caution. These two recommendations affect the use of more than 50 per cent of common interventions. Elimination of ineffective interventions and reduction in use of interventions with uncertain efficacy can easily spare 10–20 per cent of current healthcare resources for interventions that are proved to be effective.

On the other hand, interventions found to be effective or likely to be effective should not necessarily be recommended in all circumstances. Sometimes, available resources will dominate the decision. For example, an intervention as expensive as a liver transplant is likely to be unaffordable to a patient in rural China without medical insurance to cover it. Even when effective interventions are made affordable, people with different values may make different choices in accepting them. For example, a professional basketball player may consult the doctor for a minor elbow pain, while a housewife may not. Generally, people who have more resources tend to buy intervention of moderate or small values as compared to those with fewer resources.

In making evidence-based decisions, evidence, resources and values should all be considered [16]. Evidence provides us with information on what the benefit (or harm) is, how large it could be and how valid the claim may be. Further consideration on resources available and people's values will determine whether we will eventually use a certain intervention or not. The more we emphasize the role of values in making healthcare decisions, the greater the value for money will be achieved for the population.

## Evidence-based decision making in public health

Public health has long embraced the central idea of making decisions based on evidence [17], yet there is considerable room for improvement in public health in terms of adopting a systematic approach in classifying and grading evidence, in searching and evaluating evidence, in identifying contextual determinants of effectiveness and appraising the generalizability of evidence, and in studying the theories and methods of making evidence-based decisions. Better evidence-based decision making in the fields of clinical medicine and public health will benefit from mutual learning and cross-fertilization of ideas. For instance, the '6S' hierarchy of pre-processed evidence has recently extended to include sources relevant to public health practitioners [18]. Nevertheless, there is a striking difference between evidence-based public health and evidence-based care of individual patients. Unlike treatment for individual patients, public health takes collective measures and makes decisions for the entire population whether the interventions be preventive or therapeutic. In addition, it is usually difficult to evaluate public health interventions in a randomized controlled trial due to political and organizational difficulties [19]. Public health programmes are typically multifaceted and their

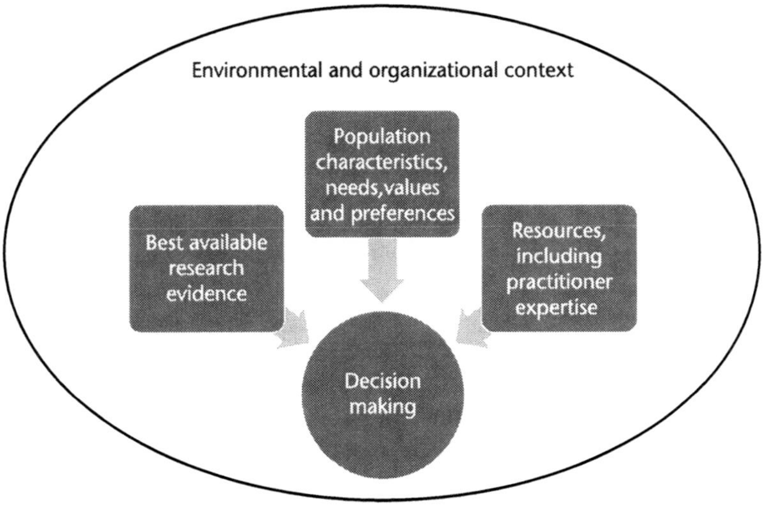


*Figure 10.2* Domains that influence evidence-based decision making [20]

success hinges not on any single but on multiple factors (see Figure 10.2) [20]. With such limitations, even if a randomized controlled trial could be conducted, the results of such a trial may not be easily generalized to other settings. Given such complexities, normally, a wide array of evidence is needed in making public health decisions (see Table 10.4) [21].

Evidence for public health decision making is most often derived from observational studies, but etiological evidence alone is not enough to make sound public health decisions. For example, the public health benefits of air pollution control are grounded on observations. However, such evidence only provides public health practitioners with information on the direction and size of the effect – it does not provide guidance on how an effective intervention should be implemented (e.g. how to resolve political challenges of encouraging the use of cleaner energy). Answers to this type of question would usually come from rigorous research and case studies, but the direct applicability of such findings would usually be confined to health systems with similar infrastructures. Decision makers from other health systems should develop knowledge translation strategies that will facilitate implementation [22]. For instance, successful emission reduction measures in developed countries may not be applicable in developing countries where values and priorities are substantially different.

Furthermore, in terms of consequences or outcomes, public health programmes and policies outnumber clinical treatments of individual patients [23, 24]. For instance, an anti-hypertension drug may lower blood pressure and the risk of cardiovascular events while causing some side effects. The number of outcomes that could happen to the patient is relatively small and often known. Therefore, in consideration of whether to take the drug or not, one may consider the gains and losses, the willingness to pay, the opportunity cost and possibly even the allocation of resources (i.e. money) among one's family. It is relatively straightforward for views to be expressed and equity issues to be settled for an individual patient. On the other hand, decisions made in public health affect not one, but many. It is hard to balance the values that are held by different stakeholders as they may vary. Hence, the equity issue in public health settings is more prominent than in clinical settings. In general, public health practitioners should answer the following four questions before making a decision [25]:

1 What is the size of the public health problem?
2 Are there effective interventions for addressing the problem?
3 What information about the local context and this particular problem is helpful in deciding its potential use in the situation at hand?
4 Is a particular programme or policy worth doing? And will it provide a satisfactory return on investment?

These questions demonstrate that making decisions in public health is much more complex than in clinical settings: decision makers must consider 'what works for whom in what circumstances' [26]. To demonstrate this, let's take the decision on drug treatment of hypertension as an example. Results from cohort studies show that blood pressure is almost linearly related to the future risk of cardiovascular events. This implies that no ideal cut-off values can be set to define hypertension, and who will and will not benefit from anti-hypertensive treatment [27, 28]. This also implies that it will be arbitrary no matter where the cut-off is drawn. If the cut-off value is set to be high, then fewer people will be considered as hypertensive and require treatment, whereas a lower cut-off value would mean more people would be considered as hypertensive and requiring treatment. As long as the blood pressure is not particularly low, potentially everyone can benefit from using an anti-hypertensive treatment and the

*Table 10.4* Typology of evidence in evidence-based public health decision making

| *Research question* | *Qualitative research* | *Survey* | *Case-control studies* | *Cohort studies* | *RCTs* | *Quasi-experimental studies* | *Non-experimental evaluations* | *Systematic reviews* |
|---|---|---|---|---|---|---|---|---|
| ***Effectiveness*** | | | | | | | | |
| Does this work? Is doing this better than doing nothing? | | | | + | ++ | + | | +++ |
| ***Process of service delivery*** | | | | | | | | |
| How does it work? | ++ | + | | | | | + | +++ |
| ***Salience*** | | | | | | | | |
| Does it matter? | ++ | ++ | | | | | | +++ |
| ***Safety*** | | | | | | | | |
| Will it do more good than harm? | + | | + | + | ++ | + | + | +++ |
| ***Acceptability*** | | | | | | | | |
| Will the users be willing to or want to take up the service offered? | ++ | + | | | + | + | + | +++ |
| ***Cost effectiveness*** | | | | | | | | |
| Is it worth buying this service? | | | | | ++ | | | +++ |
| ***Appropriateness*** | | | | | | | | |
| Is this the right service for this population? | ++ | ++ | | | | | | ++ |
| ***Satisfaction with the service*** | | | | | | | | |
| Are users, providers and other stakeholders satisfied with the service? | ++ | ++ | + | + | | | | + |

*Source*: [21].

*Key*: A larger number of '+' denotes greater appropriateness of evidence.

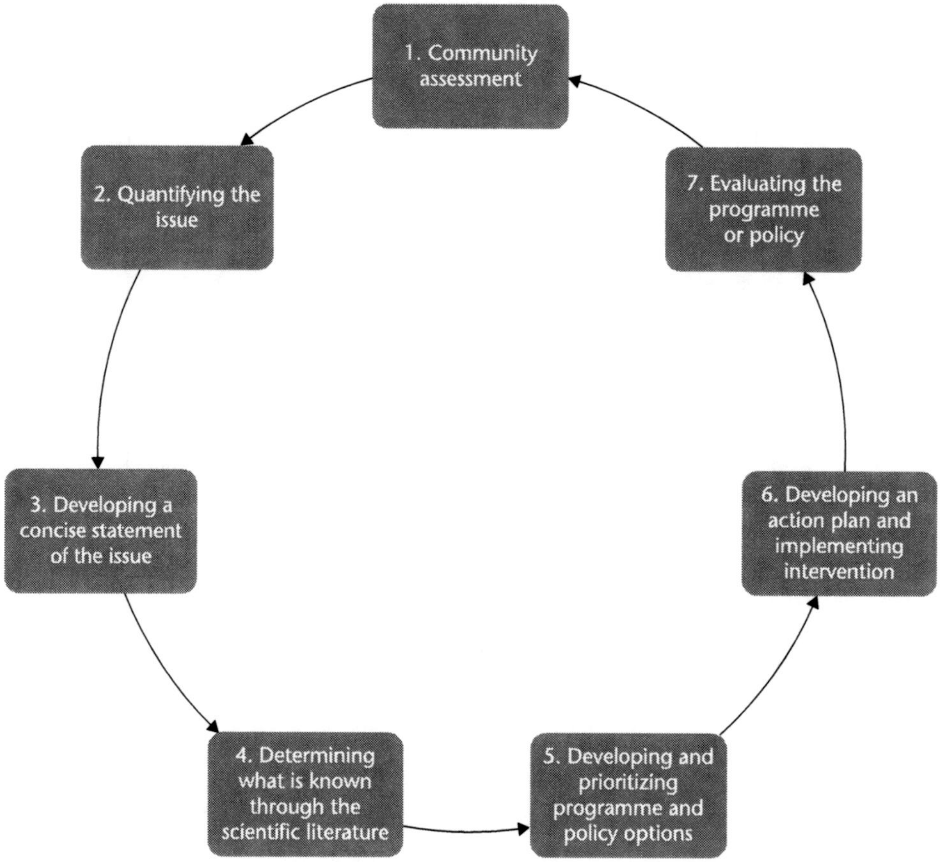


*Figure 10.3* **Steps in practising evidence-based public health [25]**

difference lies in the varying magnitude of benefits amongst individuals [28]. In order to solve the cut-off issue, one attempt is to reflect on the amount of resources available in the community. Further, the actual amount invested on hypertension in each society depends on the level of importance that cardiovascular diseases are given, relative to all other health problems that the society faces. When resources are limited, a high blood pressure cut-off point which gives rise to a low cost–benefit ratio for the whole community should be adopted, and vice versa. Any values above that should not be recommended [29, 30]. Whichever cut-off point is chosen, an evaluation of the programme should be conducted. The whole process can be conceptualized as a cycle, as demonstrated in Figure 10.3 [31]. In this process, an evidence-based practitioner should make the decision on the basis of the best available, peer-reviewed evidence, using data and information systems systematically, applying programme planning frameworks, engaging the community in decision making, conducting sound evaluation and disseminating what is learned [25].

## Conclusion

Epidemiology is the research methodology for investigating, quantitatively and by using a human individual as the basic study unit, the general issues about disease, health and health care. Unlike basic biomedical research, findings of epidemiological research are directly applicable to clinical and healthcare decisions. Remarkable efforts have been made internationally to identify, distil, integrate and disseminate evidence for decision makers' easy access, often in electronic forms. Clinicians and policy makers must take advantage of this and utilize this distilled evidence in their practice. In making evidence-based decisions, multiple factors are considered, including evidence, resources and values [32]. As we step into the future, continued effort has to be made to develop a systematic approach to promote the use of evidence in decision making [33].

The great potential of evidence-based health care will not be realized until medical and public health practices are brought in line with current best evidence. Implementation of clinical and public health practice guidelines produced by organizations, such as the UK National Institute for Health and Clinical Excellence (http://www.nice.org.uk/) are important ways of translating evidence into practice. It must be re-emphasized that collecting evidence does not immediately equate with making decisions. Many factors are at play in decision making, including cost-effectiveness, acceptability by patients in communities, experience of practitioners and clinicians, and political concerns. For example, there is insufficient evidence supporting the screening of prostate cancer using prostate-specific antigen. However, the UK government has made this test available on request because of strong public demand. Decision making in both medicine and public health would require careful consideration on values amongst patients and communities [34].

Evidence, available resources and values all affect what will be done in health care. For decision makers in Asia, two important points are worth noting. First, as most of the major research is conducted in Caucasians, decision makers in Asia must consider the applicability of the evidence to their own populations [35, 36]. This lack of local evidence also calls for more research in Asian populations to address important local health issues. Second, as views on the importance of a disease and benefit of treatment differ from individual to individual and from population to population, no single recommendation can be suitable for all individuals or populations, and recommendations and guidelines made for other populations should be adapted before they are recommended in local populations.

Even with locally relevant guidelines, experience suggests that successful implementation require involvement of stakeholders in research management, setting realistic goals, nurturing long-term relationships between researchers and policy makers, and empowering end users in driving change [37].

Finally, education on evidence-based practice, including a wide dissemination of locally relevant guidelines, is needed for promoting evidence-based decision making in Asia [38].

## References

(1) Morabia A. (ed.) *A history of epidemiologic methods and concepts.* Basel: Birkhäuser; 2004.

(2) Feinstein AR. *Clinical epidemiology: the architecture of clinical research.* Philadelphia, PA: W.B. Saunders; 1985.

(3) Cochrane A. *Effectiveness and efficiency: random reflections on health services.* London: Nuffield Provincial Hospitals Trust; 1972.

(4) Sackett DL, Rosenberg W, Gray J, Haynes RB, Richardson WS. Evidence-based medicine: what it is and what it isn't. *BMJ* 1996; 312(7023): 71–2.

(5) Evidence-Based Medicine Working Group. Evidence-based medicine. A new approach to teaching the practice of medicine. *JAMA* 1992; 268(17): 2420–5.

(6) Last JM. *A dictionary of public health.* Oxford: Oxford University Press; 2007.

(7) Rychetnik L, Hawe P, Waters E, Barratt A, Frommer M. A glossary for evidence-based public health. *Journal of Epidemiology and Community Health* 2004; 58(7): 538–45.
(8) Straus SE, Richardson WS, Glasziou P, Haynes RB. *Evidence-based medicine: how to practice and teach EBM.* 4th ed. Edinburgh: Churchill Livingstone; 2011.
(9) Jewell EJ, Abate F. (eds) *The new Oxford American dictionary.* New York: Oxford University Press; 2001.
(10) GRADE Working Group. Grading quality of evidence and strength of recommendations. *BMJ* 2004; 328: 1490–7.
(11) Howick J, Chalmers I, Glasziou P, Greenhalgh T, Heneghan C, Liberati A, *et al.* The 2011 Oxford CEBM Levels of Evidence (introductory document). Oxford: Oxford Centre for Evidence-based Medicine. http://www.cebm.net/index.aspx?o=5653
(12) OCEBM Levels of Evidence Working Group. The Oxford 2011 Levels of Evidence. Oxford: Oxford Centre for Evidence-based Medicine. http://www.cebm.net/index.aspx?o=5653
(13) Guyatt GH, Meade MO, Jaeschke RZ, Cook DJ, Haynes RB. Practitioners of evidence-based care: not all clinicians need to appraise evidence from scratch but all need some skills. *BMJ* 2000; 320(7240): 954–5.
(14) Tang JL, Wang S. Guest editorial: defining and providing essential evidence for practice. *Clinical Evidence* November 17, 2008. http://clinicalevidence.bmj.com/downloads/17-11-2008.pdf (Accessed April 9, 2009).
(15) DiCenso A, Bayley L, Haynes RB. Accessing pre-appraised evidence: fine-tuning the 5S model into a 6S model. *Evidence-Based Nursing* 2009; 12(4): 99–101.
(16) Haynes RB, Devereaux P, Guyatt GH. Physicians' and patients' choices in evidence-based practice: evidence does not make decisions, people do. *BMJ* 2002; 324(7350): 1350.
(17) Rosen G. *A history of public health.* Baltimore, MD: Johns Hopkins University Press; 1993.
(18) Paula R, Maureen D, Kara DC, Daiva T. Facilitating access to pre-processed research evidence in public health. *BMC Public Health* 2010; 10: 95.
(19) Victora CG, Habicht JP, Bryce J. Evidence-based public health: moving beyond randomized trials. *American Journal of Public Health* 2004; 94(3): 400–5.
(20) Satterfield JM, Spring B, Brownson RC, Mullen EJ, Newhouse RP, Walker BB, *et al.* Toward a transdisciplinary model of evidence-based practice. *Milbank Quarterly* 2009; 87(2): 368–90.
(21) Petticrew M, Roberts H. Evidence, hierarchies, and typologies: horses for courses. *Journal of Epidemiology and Community Health* 2003; 57(7): 527–9.
(22) Rychetnik L, Bauman A, Laws R, King L, Rissel C, Nutbeam D, *et al.* Translating research for evidence-based public health: key concepts and future directions. *Journal of Epidemiology and Community Health* 2012. doi:10.1136/jech-2011-200038.
(23) Brownson RC, Baker EA, Leet TL, Gillespie KN. *Evidence-based public health.* Oxford: Oxford University Press; 2003.
(24) Davies H, Nutley SM, Smith PC. (eds) *What works?: Evidence-based policy and practice in public services.* Bristol: Policy Press; 2000.
(25) Brownson RC, Fielding JE, Maylahn CM. Evidence-based public health: a fundamental concept for public health practice. *Annual Review of Public Health* 2009; 30: 175–201.
(26) Russo F. Public health policy, evidence, and causation: lessons from the studies on obesity. *Medicine Health Care and Philosophy* 2012; 15(2): 141–51.
(27) Lawes CM, Rodgers A, Bennett DA, *et al.* Asia Pacific Cohort Studies Collaboration. Blood pressure and cardiovascular disease in the Asia Pacific region. *Journal of Hypertension* 2003; 21(4): 707–16.
(28) Tang JL, Hu YH. Drugs for preventing cardiovascular disease in China [editorial]. *BMJ* 2005; 330(7492): 610–11.
(29) Gray JAM. *How to get better value healthcare.* Oxford: Offox Press; 2007.
(30) Donabedian A, Bashshur R. *An introduction to quality assurance in health care.* Oxford: Oxford University Press; 2003.
(31) Brownson RC, Diem G, Grabauskas V, Legetic B, Potemkina R, Shatchkute A, *et al.* Training practitioners in evidence-based chronic disease prevention for global health. *Promotion and Education* 2007; 14(3): 159–63.
(32) Tang JL, Glasziou P. (eds) *Essentials in evidence-based medicine.* Beijing: Peking University Medical Press; 2010.
(33) Muir Gray, Tang JL. *Evidence-based decision making in healthcare.* Beijing: Peking University Medical Press; 2004.

(34) Hill A, Griffiths S, Gillam S. *Public health and primary care: partners in population health*. Oxford: Oxford University Press; 2007. Chapter 4, The essential public health toolkit.
(35) Zhao D, Hu D. Barriers to translating EU and US CVD guidelines into practice in China. *Nature Reviews Cardiology* 2012; 9(7): 425–9.
(36) Sgaier SK, Claeson M, Gilks C, *et al*. Knowing your HIV/AIDS epidemic and tailoring an effective response: how did India do it? *Sexually Transmitted Infections* 2012; 88(4): 240–9.
(37) Hawkes S, Zaheer HA, Tawil O, *et al*. Managing research evidence to inform action: influencing HIV policy to protect marginalised populations in Pakistan. *Global Public Health* 2012; 7(5): 482–94.
(38) Short J, McDonald S, Turner T, *et al*. Improving capacity for evidence-based practice in South East Asia: evaluating the role of research fellowships in the SEA-ORCHID Project. *BMC Medical Education* 2010; 10: 37.

# 11
# The challenges of cancer in China

*Hongbing Shen*

## Introduction

Over the past few decades, there has been a dramatic increase of cancer incidence and mortality all over the world. According to the estimation from the International Agency for Research on Cancer (IARC), there were nearly 12.7 million new cancer cases and 7.6 million cancer deaths in 2008 worldwide [1]. With the growing ageing population and increasing adoption of cancer-causing behaviours, such as tobacco smoking, physical inactivity and obesity [2], the IARC also indicated that the incidence of cancer worldwide would grow by 75 per cent by the year 2030 and nearly double in some developing countries [3]. Although North America had the highest cancer incidence rate in the world, Eastern Asia had the largest amount of new cases (3.7 million in 2008) [3, 4]. The burden of cancer continues to increase in this region, and in this century, cancer becomes the major cause of death in many Asian countries [5].

China, accounting for approximately one-third of the Asian population, is facing a big challenge from cancer due to the high incidence and mortality rates. Among all the countries in Eastern Asia, China had the most new cases (more than 2.8 million) and deaths (more than 1.9 million), accounting for nearly 75.7 per cent and 80.2 per cent of new cases and deaths from cancer in Eastern Asia in 2008, respectively. Moreover, China can expect nearly 4.9 million new cases in 2030. According to the Third National Retrospective Sampling Death Survey, cancer has been the second cause of death after cerebrovascular disease in China [6]. As a key chronic disease, cancer is much more expensive in diagnosis, treatment and care than acute infectious diseases. The increase of cancer incidence will put a much larger burden on the developing healthcare system in China. Therefore, cancer prevention and control becomes one of the most important issues for the Chinese government to address.

In this chapter, we reviewed the prevalence and the underlying risk factors of cancer in China, with the aim to promote better strategies in cancer prevention and control.

## The cancer burden in China

Reliable assessment of the impact of cancer on the general population is predicated upon the availability of measurements related to cancer incidence and mortality. Given the lack of national cancer registration in China, we have estimated the cancer incidence and mortality in the country based on the latest available data from the GLOBOCAN 2008 database compiled by the IARC, covering 36 cancer registries in China [3, 4]. In addition, data from Chinese cancer registry annual report in 2008 were also selected for regional data estimation of cancer incidence and mortality, and for comparisons of the rates in rural and urban China [7]. Because of the lack of long-time surveillance data of cancer incidence, data from three national death cause surveys in China [6, 8, 9] were used for trend analysis of cancer in China over the last few decades. An age-standardized rate (ASR) based on world standard population proposed by Segi and modified by Doll [10, 11] was adapted for the description and comparison with other countries.

## *Number of new cancer cases and deaths in China*

According to the GLOBOCAN 2008 data, more than 2.8 million cancer cases and 1.9 million cancer deaths were estimated to have occurred in China in 2008, accounting for 22.2 per cent of the cases and 25.9 per cent of the deaths worldwide. For such a large population, China nearly had the most new cases and deaths of cancer among all of the countries in Eastern Asia and even worldwide (see Table 11.1).

Table 11.2 shows the estimated cancer incidence, mortality and five-year prevalence rates for both males and females in China. As shown in Table 11.2, lung cancer was the most frequently diagnosed cancer both in males and females accounting for 21.7 per cent and 14.3 per cent of the total new cancer cases in China, respectively. This differed from economically developed regions where prostate cancer and breast cancer were most common among males and females, respectively. In addition to lung cancer, cancers of the digestive system were also common in Chinese males, such as stomach cancer, liver cancer, oesophageal cancer and colorectal cancer, while in Chinese females, cancers of breast, stomach, liver and colorectum were most frequently diagnosed.

Parallel to the incidence of cancer, except for lung cancer which was the leading cause of cancer deaths, accounting for 25.9 per cent and 20.2 per cent of the total deaths in Chinese males and females, respectively, cancers of the digestive system, including liver cancer, stomach cancer, oesophageal cancer and colorectal cancer were also the main causes of cancer deaths in China. However, although breast cancer is now the most frequently diagnosed cancer in females in China, the number of deaths was ranked sixth among all site specific cancers in Chinese females.

According to the estimates of the IARC, the number of new cancers and deaths in both males and females will keep growing in the next twenty years. Compared to those in 2008, the numbers of incidence and mortality of cancer are expected to grow by 72.7 per cent and 84.0 per cent by the year 2030, respectively.

## *Incidence and mortality rates for all cancers in China*

In 2008, crude incidence and mortality rates for cancer were 209.5/100,000 and 145.6/100,000 in China, respectively. Also estimated by the IARC, after standardization by age, the adjusted incidence and mortality rates were 181.0/100,000 and 124.6/100,000, respectively. Although China had the most new cases of cancer among all the countries in Eastern/South-Eastern Asia, the age-standardized incidence rate was relatively lower than that in Japan, Korea and Singapore, and ranked fourth among all the countries in Eastern/South-Eastern Asia. However, age-standardized mortality rates for Chinese males and females ranked third among

*Table 11.1* Estimated incidence and mortality of cancer for males and females by region

| *Region* | *Male* | | | | | | *Female* | | | | | |
|---|---|---|---|---|---|---|---|---|---|---|---|---|
| | *Incidence*[1] | | | *Mortality*[1] | | | *Incidence*[1] | | | *Mortality*[1] | | |
| | *Numbers* | *Crude rate*[2] | *ASR (W)*[2] | *Numbers* | *Crude rate*[2] | *ASR (W)*[2] | *Numbers* | *Crude rate*[2] | *ASR (W)*[2] | *Numbers* | *Crude rate*[2] | *ASR (W)*[2] |
| World | 6617844 | 193.8 | 202.8 | 4219626 | 123.6 | 127.9 | 6044710 | 180.0 | 164.4 | 3345176 | 99.6 | 87.2 |
| More developed regions | 2964206 | 496.2 | 299.2 | 1522368 | 254.9 | 143.1 | 2591075 | 409.5 | 226.3 | 1222472 | 193.2 | 87.2 |
| Less developed regions | 3653638 | 129.7 | 159.1 | 2697258 | 95.7 | 118.4 | 3453635 | 126.7 | 137.2 | 2122704 | 77.9 | 84.9 |
| Africa | 324958 | 66.0 | 114.1 | 267014 | 54.3 | 95.7 | 390613 | 78.9 | 118.1 | 274765 | 55.5 | 86.5 |
| Europe | 1700526 | 482.4 | 292.9 | 956284 | 271.3 | 155.3 | 1508356 | 397.0 | 217.2 | 758956 | 199.8 | 89.8 |
| South America | 318031 | 167.1 | 186.7 | 200625 | 105.4 | 116.6 | 332066 | 170.6 | 162.8 | 185256 | 95.2 | 88.2 |
| Northern America | 831767 | 488.6 | 334.0 | 332455 | 195.3 | 122.4 | 772103 | 441.7 | 274.4 | 305873 | 175.0 | 91.5 |
| Asia | 3241249 | 154.5 | 170.6 | 2353611 | 112.2 | 124.2 | 2851110 | 142.6 | 139.6 | 1718721 | 85.9 | 83.2 |
| Eastern Asia | 2135271 | 264.2 | 222.1 | 1511750 | 187.0 | 155.5 | 1585387 | 208.1 | 158.1 | 928601 | 121.9 | 87.3 |
| South-Eastern Asia | 336689 | 117.6 | 143.9 | 258582 | 90.3 | 112.3 | 388757 | 134.4 | 141.6 | 242464 | 83.8 | 89.4 |
| China | 1622502 | 232.6 | 211.0 | 1222199 | 175.2 | 158.6 | 1194708 | 184.5 | 152.4 | 736148 | 113.7 | 91.5 |
| Japan | 361600 | 582.9 | 247.3 | 206002 | 332.1 | 129.4 | 253907 | 389.1 | 167.6 | 136212 | 208.7 | 68.0 |
| Korea | 89463 | 375.3 | 309.4 | 43514 | 182.5 | 149.9 | 79065 | 325.2 | 234.4 | 25238 | 103.8 | 64.0 |
| Singapore | 6434 | 277.3 | 208.2 | 3446 | 148.5 | 110.0 | 6482 | 282.4 | 188.4 | 2660 | 115.9 | 73.3 |
| Mongolia | 2225 | 170.3 | 281.5 | 1767 | 135.2 | 230.3 | 2082 | 156.0 | 210.8 | 1364 | 102.2 | 147.2 |
| Thailand | 50407 | 152.0 | 146.0 | 35484 | 107.0 | 102.6 | 62259 | 181.9 | 156.1 | 34850 | 101.8 | 85.9 |
| Vietnam | 55045 | 128.1 | 154.4 | 43688 | 101.7 | 122.6 | 56536 | 128.1 | 127.7 | 38318 | 86.8 | 85.0 |

*Source*: Data from [3].

*Notes*: [1] Incidence and mortality data for all ages.
[2] Crude and age-standardized rates (ASR) per 100,000.

*Table 11.2* Estimated incidence, mortality and five-year prevalence for males and females in China

| Rank | Cancer | *Incidence*[1] | | | *Mortality*[1] | | | *5-year prevelance*[2] | | |
|---|---|---|---|---|---|---|---|---|---|---|
| | | *Number* | *%* | *ASR(W)*[3] | *Number* | *%* | *ASR(W)*[3] | *Number* | *%* | *Proportions*[3] |
| **Male** | | | | | | | | | | |
| 1 | Lung | 351713 | 21.7 | 45.9 | 304020 | 24.9 | 39.6 | 329891 | 15.1 | 60.3 |
| 2 | Stomach | 315843 | 19.5 | 41.3 | 231193 | 18.9 | 30.1 | 466415 | 21.3 | 85.3 |
| 3 | Liver | 292966 | 18.1 | 37.4 | 266830 | 21.8 | 34.1 | 219844 | 10.1 | 40.2 |
| 4 | Oesophagus | 175863 | 10.8 | 22.9 | 143718 | 11.8 | 18.7 | 177114 | 8.1 | 32.4 |
| 5 | Colorectum | 125461 | 7.7 | 16.3 | 61908 | 5.1 | 8.0 | 289330 | 13.2 | 52.9 |
| 6 | Bladder | 42686 | 2.6 | 5.5 | 15935 | 1.3 | 2.0 | 110657 | 5.1 | 20.2 |
| 7 | Leukemia | 38635 | 2.4 | 5.3 | 30243 | 2.5 | 4.2 | 42986 | 2.0 | 7.9 |
| 8 | Prostate | 33802 | 2.1 | 4.3 | 14297 | 1.2 | 1.8 | 75535 | 3.5 | 13.8 |
| 9 | Brain, nervous system | 33244 | 2.0 | 4.3 | 25253 | 2.1 | 3.3 | 45962 | 2.1 | 8.4 |
| 10 | Pancreas | 24841 | 1.5 | 3.2 | 22173 | 1.8 | 2.9 | 17186 | 0.8 | 3.1 |
| **Female** | | | | | | | | | | |
| 1 | Breast | 169452 | 14.2 | 21.6 | 44908 | 6.1 | 5.7 | 631171 | 26.1 | 120.8 |
| 2 | Lung | 170337 | 14.3 | 21.3 | 148793 | 20.2 | 18.3 | 157924 | 6.5 | 30.2 |
| 3 | Stomach | 148596 | 12.4 | 18.5 | 121122 | 16.5 | 14.6 | 214409 | 8.9 | 41.0 |
| 4 | Liver | 109242 | 9.1 | 13.7 | 105249 | 14.3 | 13.1 | 76238 | 3.2 | 14.6 |
| 5 | Colorectum | 95852 | 8.0 | 12.2 | 48578 | 6.6 | 5.9 | 219810 | 9.1 | 42.1 |
| 6 | Corpus uteri | 86066 | 7.2 | 11.1 | 19126 | 2.6 | 2.4 | 324484 | 13.4 | 62.1 |
| 7 | Oesophagus | 83372 | 7.0 | 10.5 | 67366 | 9.2 | 8.2 | 80238 | 3.3 | 15.4 |
| 8 | Cervix uteri | 75434 | 6.3 | 9.6 | 33914 | 4.6 | 4.3 | 232465 | 9.6 | 44.5 |
| 9 | Leukemia | 32191 | 2.7 | 4.7 | 24363 | 3.3 | 3.5 | 36412 | 1.5 | 7.0 |
| 10 | Brain, nervous system | 33210 | 2.8 | 4.5 | 20320 | 2.8 | 2.7 | 45487 | 1.9 | 8.7 |

*Source*: data from [3].

*Notes*: [1] Incidence and mortality data for all ages.
[2] Five-year prevalence for adult population only.
[3] ASR(W) and proportions per 100,000.

all the countries in Eastern/South-Eastern Asia (see Table 11.1). The ratio of mortality to incidence was 0.75 and 0.60 in Chinese males and females, respectively, which was higher than that in Japan (0.52 in males and 0.41 in females), Korea (0.48 in males and 0.27 in females) and Singapore (0.53 in males and 0.39 in females). The higher ratio of mortality to incidence, to some extent, suggested that early detection and treatment for cancer still needs to be much improved in China.

## *Incidence and mortality rates for all cancers in China by region*

Because of the large population and imbalance of economic development and health resource settings, cancer burdens varied by regions in China. Data from the Chinese Cancer Registry Annual Report showed that by the year of 2008, cancer incidence was 332.2/100,000 and 281.5/100,000 in urban males and females, respectively, while it was 322.6/100,000 and 215.2/100,000 in rural males and females respectively. Crude incidence in Chinese urban males and females was 3.0 per cent and 30.8 per cent higher than that in rural males and females, respectively. However, after age standardization, the incidence of cancer in urban males was 218.0/100,000, which was 13.6 per cent lower than that in rural males (247.6/100,000). Meanwhile, age-standardized incidence of cancer in urban females was 175.2/100,000, which was 15.0 per cent higher than that in rural females (152.3/100,000).

Mortality rates were 332.2/100,000 and 281.52/100,000 among males and females in urban China, while it was 322.6/100,000 and 215.2/100,000 in males and females in rural China, respectively. After age standardization, the mortality rate of cancer in males in urban areas was 13.6 per cent lower than that in males in rural areas, while age-standardized mortality rates for cancer in urban females was 15.0 per cent higher than that in rural females.

Lung cancer and breast cancer were the most frequently diagnosed cancers in urban males and females, respectively, followed by colorectal cancer. However, cancers of the upper digestive tract, including stomach cancer and oesophageal cancer, were still the most common cancers in rural males and females (see Table 11.3). The difference of the cancer incidence of the digestive tract between urban and rural Chinese populations might be due to the different regional diet styles. Strategies for cancer prevention and control should therefore be more individualized according to the regional exposures.

## *Incidence and mortality rates for all cancers in China by gender*

According to the 2008 pooled data from the IARC, the crude incidence rate of cancer was 232.6/100,000 in males, while it was 184.5/100,000 in females. Mortality rates for cancer were 175.2/100,000 in males which was higher than in females (113.7/100,000). After age standardization, both the adjusted incidence (211.0/100,000) and mortality rate (152.4/100,000) in Chinese males were higher than those in females (158.6/100,000 for adjusted incidence rate and 91.5/100,000 for adjusted mortality rate) (see Table 11.1).

Moreover, the incidence and mortality of site specific cancers also varied by gender. In males, lung cancer was the most common cancer with the highest age-standardized incidence and mortality rate, followed by cancers of stomach, liver, oesophagus and colorectum. Yet in females, breast cancer and lung cancer were the most common cancers, followed by stomach, liver and colorectal. It is worth noting that although the age-standardized incidence rate of breast cancer was highest among all site specific cancers, the age-standardized mortality rate

*Table 11.3* Estimated incidence and mortality of major cancers for males and females among urban and rural China, 2008

| *Rank* | *Urban* | | | | | *Rural* | | | | |
|---|---|---|---|---|---|---|---|---|---|---|
| | *Cancer* | *Incidence*[1, 2] | *ASR(W)*[2] | *Mortality*[1, 2] | *ASR(W)*[2] | *Cancer* | *Incidence*[1, 2] | *ASR(W)*[2] | *Mortality*[1, 2] | *ASR(W)*[2] |
| **Male** | | | | | | | | | | |
| 1 | Lung | 76.7 | 48.7 | 65.6 | 40.4 | Stomach | 77.0 | 59.4 | 55.4 | 42.2 |
| 2 | Stomach | 44.8 | 29.1 | 30.5 | 19.0 | Oesophagus | 61.2 | 47.3 | 47.8 | 36.4 |
| 3 | Colorectum | 38.6 | 24.7 | 17.5 | 10.7 | Lung | 60.0 | 45.5 | 50.8 | 38.5 |
| 4 | Liver | 37.8 | 25.0 | 34.4 | 22.4 | Liver | 52.8 | 39.9 | 48.5 | 36.4 |
| 5 | Oesophagus | 19.9 | 13.0 | 15.6 | 9.9 | Colorectum | 16.7 | 12.6 | 8.8 | 6.6 |
| **Female** | | | | | | | | | | |
| 1 | Breast | 54.7 | 35.6 | 11.5 | 6.9 | Oesophagus | 35.7 | 25.0 | 27.2 | 17.9 |
| 2 | Lung | 39.0 | 22.2 | 31.7 | 17.0 | Stomach | 33.8 | 23.4 | 26.8 | 17.8 |
| 3 | Colorectum | 32.5 | 18.7 | 15.4 | 8.1 | Lung | 25.2 | 17.1 | 20.9 | 13.9 |
| 4 | Stomach | 21.3 | 12.4 | 14.7 | 8.0 | Breast | 21.2 | 15.5 | 6.4 | 4.6 |
| 5 | Liver | 13.7 | 8.0 | 13.1 | 7.3 | Liver | 20.5 | 14.4 | 17.9 | 12.3 |

*Source*: Data from [7].

*Notes*: [1] Incidence and mortality data for all ages.
[2] Incidence, mortality and ASR(W) per 100,000.

of lung cancer was highest in females, followed by stomach cancer, liver cancer, colorectal cancer and oesophageal cancer (see Table 11.2).

## Incidence and mortality rates for all cancers in China by age

Both in males and females, incidence and mortality of cancer increase with age. However, although the overall incidence of cancer in males was higher than that in females, the age-specific curve of cancer incidence showed that the incidence rate in females was higher than in males younger than 40 years of age and conversely afterwards. The mortality rate of cancer in males was always higher than that in females in each age group. Moreover, mortality rates in males far outpaced mortality rates in females, especially for those older than 40 years of age (see Figure 11.1).

## Incidence and mortality rates for all cancers in China by calendar period

Although there are no national data on cancer incidence, the three national death cause surveys conducted in the 1970s, 1990s and 2004–05 provided us with a grave picture of the variation of cancer burden in China over the last few decades [6, 8, 9]. In general, the cancer mortality rate has been increasing rapidly and continuously over the past three decades, from 74.2/100,000 in the 1970s to 108.3/100,000 in the 1990s and to 135.9/100 000 in 2004–05 (see Figure 11.2).

However, after age standardization, a different trend of cancer mortality was shown. Age-standardized cancer mortality rates increased between the 1970s and 1990s, but declined a little afterwards until 2004–05 (see Figure 11.3). This trend revealed that the ageing population played a more important role in the pattern of disease in China since the 1990s, which corresponds with the fact that China became an ageing society around the year 2000.

Different changing trends of mortality rate were shown by site specific cancer. Unlike the decreasing lung cancer death rate of lung cancer in males in most Western countries, including

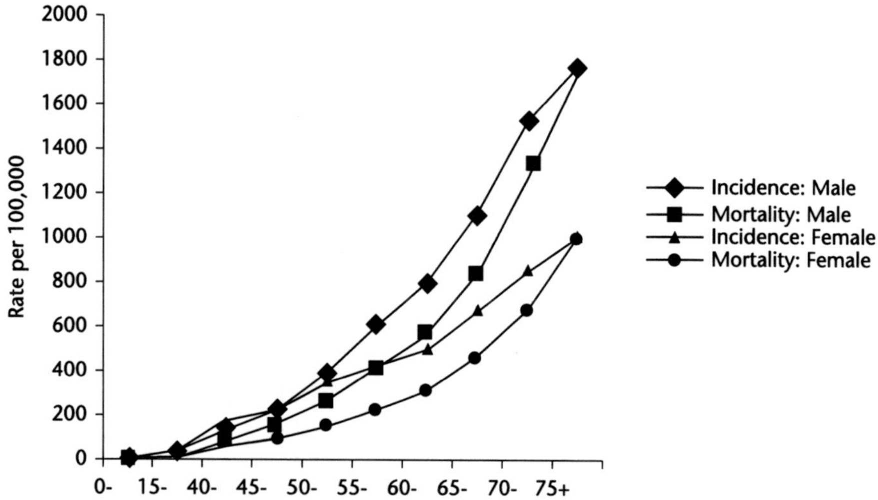


*Figure 11.1* Age-specific incidence and mortality of cancer in China, 2008 [3]

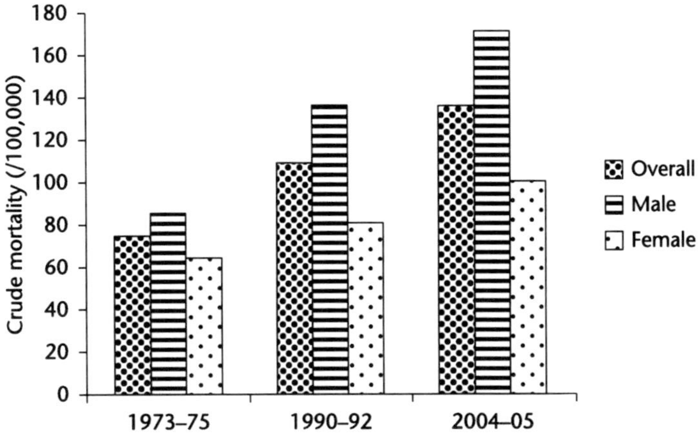


*Figure 11.2* Crude cancer mortality in China, 1970s, 1990s and 2004–05
*Note*: The population from census of China in 1982 was used as standard population.

many European countries, North America and Australia, the mortality rate of lung cancer increased by 465 per cent in China over the past thirty years [12] (see Figures 11.4 and 11.5). Why this is the case is difficult to stipulate until a national investigation on risk factors of lung cancer and a further analysis on age–period–cohort trends of the past thirty years is conducted. This increase may be partially attributed to increased diagnosis and reporting, but we cannot exclude the possibility that may be due to smoke exposure, air pollution and other factors, which are on the increase in China. According to data from the China National Cancer Registration, there was an obvious increase in the incidence rate of lung cancer from 2004 to 2008 (see Figures 11.6 and 11.7). If this trend continues, the World Health Organization (WHO) estimates that by 2025, more than 800,000 Chinese will be diagnosed with lung cancer.

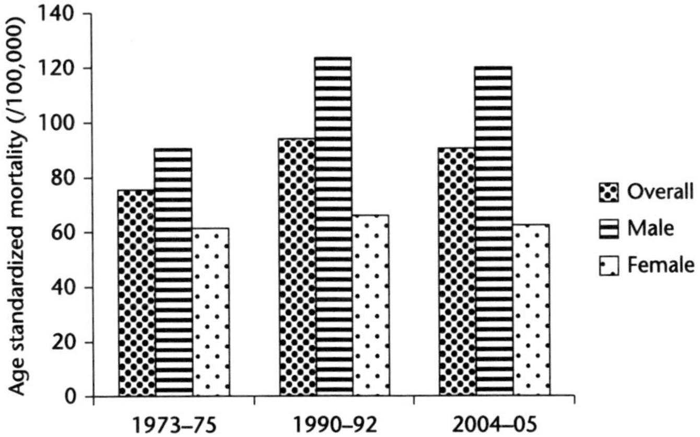


*Figure 11.3* Age-standardized cancer mortality in China, 1970s, 1990s and 2004–05
*Note*: The population from census of China in 1982 was used as standard population.

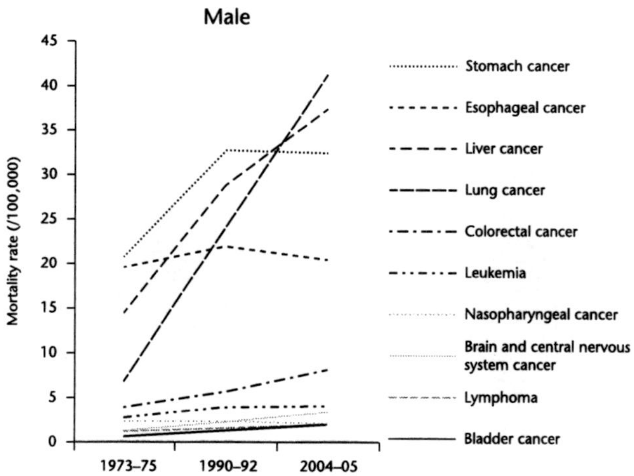


*Figure 11.4* Cancer mortality rate (ASW) of 10 most common cancers in males, 1970s, 1990s and 2004–05

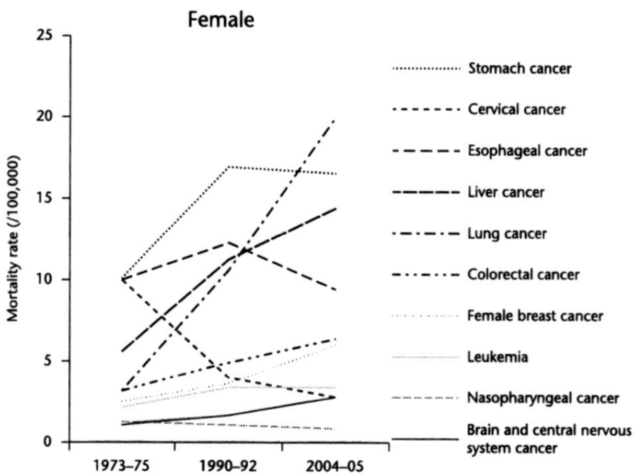


*Figure 11.5* Cancer mortality rate (ASW) of 10 most common cancers in females, 1970s, 1990s and 2004–05

In addition to lung cancer, liver cancer and colorectal cancer also showed a marked increase of mortality in both Chinese males and females over the last thirty years (see Figures 11.4 and 11.5). In particular, liver cancer cases are increasing with an estimate of 402,208 Chinese cases of primary liver cancer reported in the GLOBOCAN 2008 data, and accounts for more than half of the world's liver cancer cases. The mortality of female breast cancer has also increased in the last thirty years, suggesting the potential increase of incidence of female breast cancer in China. However, the decreased mortality of upper digestive tract cancers, such as stomach and oesophageal cancer, was observed in both Chinese males and females from 1990 to 2005 (see Figures 11.4 and 11.5). The recent data on cancer incidence from 2004 to 2008 also shows the increase in lung cancer, colorectal cancer and female breast cancer, but the decrease in oesophageal cancer (see Figures 11.6 and 11.7).

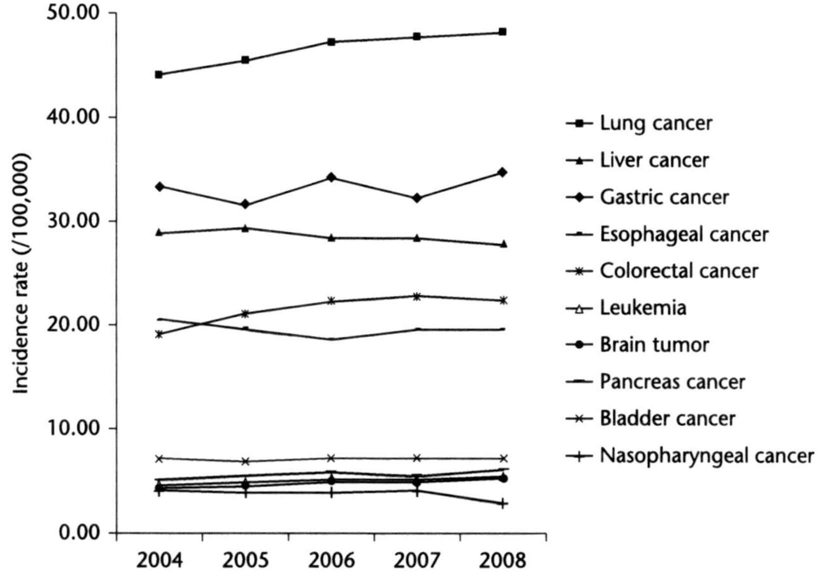


*Figure 11.6* Incidence (ASW) of 10 most common cancers in males in China, 2004–08

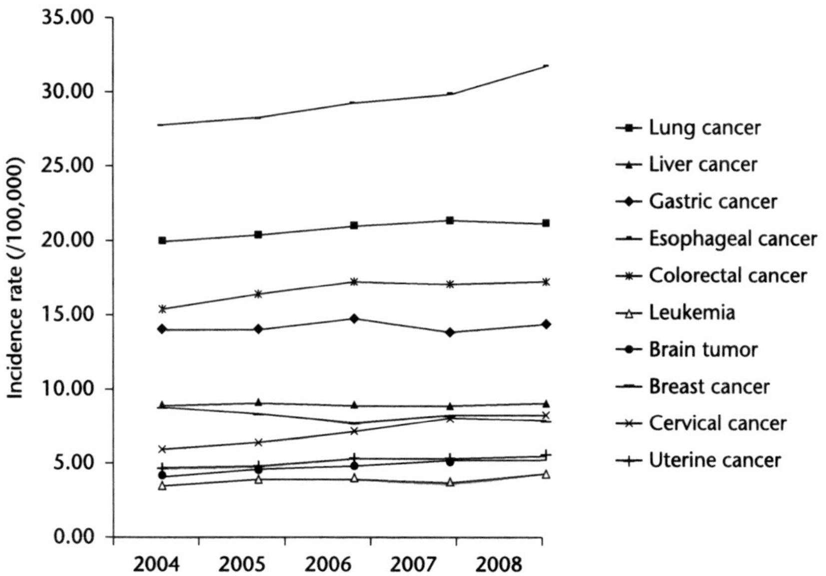


*Figure 11.7* Incidence (ASW) of 10 most common cancers in females in China, 2004–08

## The causes of cancer

Certain subgroups are at an elevated risk for various cancers and there has been accumulative evidence relating lifestyle and other environmental factors to cancer onsets [13]. By the early 1980s, epidemiologists had identified many important risk factors of cancer and a 'multi-stage' model of carcinogenesis had also been proposed [14]. However, causal interpretation becomes problematic when the epidemiological association is fairly convincing but the biological rationale is uncertain. Over the past two decades, the remarkable advances in cell and molecular biology have transformed the scope and methods of cancer epidemiology, and modern epidemiological studies depending on genetic, biochemical or viral assays have clarified the mechanism of many specific causes of cancer and precisely estimated many long-suspected minor risks. Many important causes of cancer are now known, including smoking, obesity and various oncogenic viruses. It is also observed that the risk factors for cancer, such as an ageing population, deterioration of the environment and Western lifestyles, are increasing in many Asian countries, including China, which result in the increasing incidence of cancers, such as breast cancer and colorectum cancer [12].

## *Tobacco*

The carcinogenicity of tobacco and tobacco smoke to humans has been supported by extensive mechanistic evidence [15]. Although nicotine is probably not a classic tumour initiator, it may function as a promoter or co-carcinogen, and many carcinogens and promoters are formed during the smoking of tobacco, including polycyclic aromatic hydrocarbon (e.g. benzo(a)pyrene), aromatic amines (e.g. naphthylamine), aldehydes (e.g. formaldehyde), other phenolic compounds (e.g. phenol, catechol), a variety of free radicals and tobacco-specific nitrosamines [16]. Carcinogens and procarcinogens from tobacco smoke reach most tissues in the body through either direct exposure to tobacco leaf and/or smoke, or indirect exposure to substances dissolved in saliva and swallowed, absorbed, circulated systemically in the bloodstream, or accumulated and excreted in urine or stool [17].

The cancer risks of tobacco use, especially cigarette smoking, have been extensively investigated. Based predominantly on epidemiologic evidence, active cigarette smoking is considered causally related to multiple cancers [17]. In addition to the obvious link between tobacco consumption and cancer of the lung and oral cavity, there is increasing evidence that carcinogens in smoke also have an impact on cancers of many other organs [18]. An intensive review on the smoking-related research in Asian-Pacific countries suggested that smoking increased the risk of cancers in the respiratory, gastrointestinal and genitourinary tracts [19]. As well as that, smoking was also reported as a possible risk factor for breast cancer in the Asian population [20].

As smoking is known to be a strong risk factor for lung cancer, second-hand smoke was also reported to moderately increase the risk of lung cancer incidence and mortality. Based on data from the Shanghai women's health study, a population-based cohort study of approximately 75,000 Chinese women who were recruited between 1997 and 2000, a high proportion of study participants (83.1 per cent) were exposed to second-hand smoke from their husbands, at work and/or from family members in early life [21]. After following up until 2004, non-smoking women who were exposed to second-hand smoke showed a 1.79-fold higher risk of lung cancer mortality than those unexposed [21].

It is noteworthy that China is the world's largest tobacco production and consumption country [22]. Despite China having endorsed the Framework Convention on Tobacco Control (WHO FCTC) on 9 January 2006, sales of tobacco have been increasing in the country. Based on data from the 2010 WHO global adult tobacco survey, 53 per cent of Chinese men and 2 per cent of Chinese women were current tobacco smokers, with a total number being more than 300 million. As well as that, 7 in 10 non-smoking adults are exposed to second-hand smoke. Of note, 15 million regular smokers and 40 million casual smokers were aged between 13 and 18 years, and the average age to start smoking is decreasing (age 22 in 1984, age 19 in 1996 and age 18 in 2002). In addition, the number of female smokers is increasing rapidly by 10 per cent annually, particularly among young women [22].

## *Infections*

*Helicobacter pylori* (*H. pylori*), hepatitis B virus (HBV), hepatitis C virus (HCV), human papilloma virus (HPV) and Epstein–Barr virus (EBV) have been considered as important risk factors for the development of cancers of the stomach, liver, uterine cervix and nasopharynx in Asia [18]. A high percentage of the cancer burden in China is attributable to these infections [12].

The role of *H. pylori* in causing stomach cancer has been well documented. The IARC classified *H. pylori* as a group 1 human carcinogen for stomach cancer in 1994. The infection rates of *H. pylori* in Asian countries are considerably higher than in the world population [23]. In the high-risk area of stomach cancer, Linqu County (Shandong Province, China), a 68 per cent positive rate of *H. pylori* infection was reported among adults aged 35 to 64 years [24].

Chronic infection with HBV and/or HCV is a well-known risk factor for hepatocellular carcinoma, with a twenty-fold and a twenty-five-fold higher risk among carriers than non-carriers, respectively [25]. It was reported that China had about 120 million HBV carriers [26] and the overall prevalence of HBsAg carriers was 9.75 per cent according to data from a 1992 nationwide cross-sectional seroepidemiologic study of hepatitis virus infections. However, only a small population of HBV carriers would develop hepatocellular carcinoma. Factors attributing to the inter-individual variation include aflatoxin exposures and lifestyle factors, such as alcohol consumption and cigarette smoking [27].

Persistent infection with high risk 'oncogenic' types of HPV has been a well-established necessary cause for cervical cancer, which is the second most frequently diagnosed female cancer worldwide, especially in developed countries [18]. There is a high prevalence of HPV in Asia, especially in India and China [28, 29]. Based on the data from multi-central HPV prevalence in China performed from 2003 to 2006, HPV positivity was about 15 per cent in both rural and urban areas. Although there has been a dramatic decrease of mortality from cervical cancer, the incidence of cervical cancer was still high before the HPV vaccine or national screening programme was implemented all over the country.

The role of EBV in causing nasopharyngeal carcinoma, one of the carcinomas common in Southeast China, has been also well documented. Serological screening for EBV could significantly increase the rate of early detection of nasopharyngeal cancer [30].

In addition, chronic parasitic infections have long been thought to be human carcinogenics. Infection with three species of liver flukes has been associated with cholangiocarcinoma of the liver: *Opisthorchis viverrini*, *Opisthorchis felineus* and *Clonorchis sinensis*. In China, *Clonorchis sinensis* can be found at highly endemic levels and is known as a predisposing factor for liver cancer [31].

## *Occupational and environmental carcinogens*

With rapid industrialization and economic development, China is facing great environmental health challenges and many places in China are famously known as 'cancer villages' due to pollution of the environment [32]. Well-established human carcinogens, such as polycyclic aromatic hydrocarbons (PAHs), have been detected in high levels in major cities in Asia, and air pollution has been associated with increased cancer risk, mortality and other health problems in China [1]. Both outdoor and indoor air pollution can elevate the risk of lung cancer. An increased risk of lung cancer was related to coal used for heating and cooking in rural areas [33–36]. Radon and asbestos are other known environmental factors to elevate the risk of lung cancer. Miners were intensively studied to show a significant association between inhalation of high levels of radioactive radon gas and an increased risk of lung cancer. Residential radon exposure also appears to be able to increase the risk of lung cancer in China [37, 38].

Arsenic exposure in drinking water has also been associated with cancer. High mortality rates from bladder and lung cancer were observed in highly arsenic-exposed villages in Taiwan, with a significant dose–response relationship. Liver cancer mortality also appeared to be associated with arsenic exposure [39]. In China, a three-fold increased risk of lung cancer was reported in smelter workers who were exposed to inorganic arsenic [34].

## *Diet, physical activity and overweight*

The proportion of people who are overweight or obese is increasing rapidly in China, especially in the urban areas [12]. This is probably due to an increasingly Westernized lifestyle, which includes greater consumption of animal meat products and a lack of physical activity. The 2009 China Health and Nutrition Survey reported 17.1 per cent of Chinese men and 4.4 per cent of Chinese women were overweight (body mass index, BMI: 25–27.49 $kg/m^2$) and an additional 11.4 per cent of men and 10.1 per cent of women had general obesity (body mass index, BMI ≥ 27.5 $kg/m^2$). Besides this, the prevalence of abdominal obesity (waist circumference ≥ 90cm for men and ≥ 80cm for women) was 27.8 per cent among men and 45.9 per cent among women [40].

Reports have also shown the association between food or nutrients and cancer risk [18]. High total caloric and fat consumption was found to increase the risk of breast and colorectal cancers. A study in China reported a 2.9-fold increased risk of breast cancer from red meat and animal fat consumption [41]. High red meat and animal fat intake have also been associated with the risk of colorectal cancer in the Chinese population [42, 43]. Low consumption of fruits and vegetables is associated with an increased cancer risk in Asian countries [44–47], although there are some inconsistent findings. On the other hand, some Asian diet staples, such as soy and green tea, are suspected to play a protective role in cancer risk with growing epidemiologic evidence suggesting this [48–51]. As well as that, *in vivo* and animal studies on a number of compounds in green tea, such as polyphenols, have reported its chemopreventive properties against cancer. However, soy intake was also suspected to be a marker of other factors associated with a degree of Westernization that is causally associated with cancer risk and further evaluation is needed [52, 53].

Low physical activity has also been associated with a significantly increased risk of breast and colorectal cancer in numerous studies [54]. Regular and frequent physical activity over a long time period was reported to decrease the risk of colon cancer in the Chinese population [55].

## *Reproductive and hormonal factors*

Late age at first child birth, early menarche, late menopause, oral contraceptive intake and shorter duration of lifetime lactation are known to increase the risk of breast cancer by the effects of hormones [18]. Several Chinese studies have demonstrated that menstrual and reproductive factors, oral contraceptive use and hormone replacement therapy are associated with breast cancer risk in China [56, 57]. The Western diet and obesity can impact on the influence of reproductive factors and increase endogenous oestrogen production, which hence increases breast cancer risk [41, 58]. Hormone replacement therapy also increases the chances of developing ovarian cancer [59], however, an increased number of parities is a protective factor [60]. In contrast to breast cancer, early age at first child birth increased the risk of cervical cancer [61]. Women with multiple parities also had an increased risk of cervical cancer than nulliparous women [61]. The reproductive factors in relation to other cancers are inconclusive.

### *Inherited susceptibility*

Accumulated evidence suggests that inherited susceptibility is an important attributer to most types of cancer. The occurrence of many cancers tends to run in families. Mutations in *BRCA1* or *BRCA2* was found in most multiple-case families of breast cancer [62]. However, only a few percent of cases are attributable to the high penetrance genes discovered to date. More recently, genome-wide association studies have been widely conducted to identify the low penetrance genes, so too in China. Several novel genetic susceptibility loci have successfully been identified for multiple types of cancers in the Chinese population, including lung [63], stomach [64], oesophageal [65, 66], liver [67], nasopharyngeal [68] and pancreatic [69]. However, taking all the identified genes together only accounts for a small proportion of predisposition to cancer [70]. Further studies are required to determine the precise genetic determinants and their interactions with environmental exposures and host factors in the carcinogenic process.

## Cancer prevention and control

Cancer is currently one of the most important public health problems in many Asian countries, including China. Active strategies for cancer control have been developed in Asia, focusing on prevention, screening, early diagnosis and treatment. The prevention programme includes national cancer registries, cancer screening programmes, education programmes for public awareness, anti-smoking campaigns, changes in dietary habits, eradication of *H. pylori*, and vaccination against HBV and HPV. Specifically for China, with the hope to accelerate cancer prevention and control efforts, the Ministry launched a new National Cancer Control Plan together with the Hepatitis B Prevention and Control Plan in 1992, aiming to reduce the incidence and mortality rates of cancer, and to improve the survival and quality of life of cancer patients [71]. Tobacco control, vaccination against HBV and screening for breast and cervix cancers are outlined. In addition, public education and promotion campaigns for healthy lifestyles are also essential and have been actively carried out all over China. National healthy lifestyle action was initiated in 2007. In addition, demonstration plots of chronic diseases, including cancer prevention and treatment in communities, had been established in more than 30 provinces by the end of 2012.

### *Primary prevention*

By the 1960s, cancer epidemiologists had concluded that most of the cancers are, in principle, preventable and many could be avoided by a suitable choice of lifestyle and environment [13]. Smoking is a primary lifestyle-related risk factor for cancer and lung cancer is largely avoidable by smoking cessation. Anti-smoking programmes are therefore the most important element in cancer prevention. As recommended by the FCTC to which China is a signatory, an effort to reduce smoking prevalence should include raising cigarette prices, putting warning labels on cigarette packets, banning tobacco smoking in public places and running smoking cessation clinics [18]. The inverse dose–response relationship between the duration of smoking cessation and lung cancer risk should be taught to smokers. Also, the risk of former smokers may never reach as low as that of non-smokers. Thus, in addition to making an effort to promote smoking cessation, educating adolescents not to start smoking is of equal importance [18]. In China, an anti-smoking campaign was initiated a couple of years ago and several programmes are ongoing. In 1999, the Law of the People's Republic of China on the Protection of Minors (younger than 18 years of age) prohibited the sale of cigarettes to minors. In 2005 and 2006, the Chinese government provided a special fund of more than 10 million RMB for tobacco control by building the national tobacco control network, creating smoke-free places, establishing surveillance systems on tobacco smoking among high-risk populations and providing services for quitting smoking [12]. In 2007, a special fund from the Bloomberg School of Public Health of the Johns Hopkins University initiated a programme to prevent passive smoking in China.

Chronic HBV infection (see Chapter 17) is a well-known risk factor for hepatocellular carcinoma. However, the infection of HBV is approximately 80–90 per cent preventable with the hepatitis B vaccination and it is generally accepted that vaccination with HBV will prevent the disease [5]. Initiated in 1992, national vaccination of infants against HBV has been implemented in China [12]. In 2005, the overall coverage of the hepatitis B vaccine in infants reached more than 95 per cent in urban and 97.0 per cent in rural areas. Although no obvious decline has been observed for liver cancer, the nationwide mass HBV vaccination has reduced chronic HBV infections by more than 30 million, with the chronic HBV carrier rate decreasing from 10 per cent to 7.8 per cent in the general population, and decreasing from 10 per cent to 1–2 per cent in children younger than 10 years of age [26]. In June 2009, China launched a programme giving booster shots of the hepatitis B vaccine to those under the age of 15. An effective HPV vaccination programme for pre-adolescent girls may also reduce mortality from cervical cancer; however, the high cost of vaccine, poor awareness of the linkage between HPV infection and cervical cancer, and social stigmatizing for a sexually transmitted disease are barriers that still need to be overcome [72].

Health education is also of great importance for cancer control in today's China, where Westernized lifestyle-related cancers are rapidly increasing. Lifestyle is an avoidable risk factor of cancer, thus more efforts should be paid to promote a healthy lifestyle, such as a balanced diet that includes high consumption of fruits and vegetables, and lower consumption of salty foods, red meat and alcohol; more physical activity; and not taking up smoking or ceasing smoking. Breast self-examination should be recommended for women and risky sexual behaviour should be warned against.

### *Cancer screening*

As secondary prevention of cancer, early detection for cancer cases through screening programmes is important, providing an alternative approach to cancer control. Many studies in Asia have shown the effectiveness of cancer screening in reducing cancer mortality rates. However, breast cancer is usually presented and diagnosed at a later stage of development in Asian women possibly due to a lack of population-based breast cancer screening programmes in the majority of Asia [5]. In 2004, a special fund from the China Ministry of Health initiated screening programmes for breast cancer and cervical cancer, with 530,000 and 113,000 female participants, respectively. The population coverage of these screening programmes is now expanding and screening for cervical cancer and breast cancer is now covered by medical insurance in urban areas, and supported by a programme initiated in 2009. Screening for these two cancers is now free for all women in 200 counties in rural areas (more than 1,500 counties in total in China). Moreover, a programme to screen digestive tract cancers including gastric, liver and oesophageal cancer is ongoing with the provision of a special fund in some high-risk areas in the Huaihe region. Also funded by the China Ministry of Health, programmes for cancer early detection and treatment for specific-site cancers was performed in rural China in 2004, such as liver cancer screening in Qidong, Jiangsu Province, and Fusui, Guangxi Province; colorectal cancer screening in Haining and Jiashan, Jejiang Province; and stomach cancer screening in Zhuanghe, Liaoning Province. More importantly, considering the discrepancy of the cancer burden between rural and urban China, the China Ministry of Health has funded a new programme for early detection and treatment of cancer in urban China in 2012. Unlike screening for site specific cancer in certain rural high-risk areas, the six most common cancers in urban areas, including lung, liver, oesophageal, stomach, colorectal and female breast cancer, are screened free of charge, simultaneously for urban inhabitants. By the end of 2012, nine cities in seven provinces were covered by the programme and by the end of 2013, five more cities will be included in this ongoing programme.

## Conclusion

China is facing a big challenge from cancer due to the higher incidence and mortality rates of cancer and the more complicated cancer spectrum. Although some programmes for cancer prevention and control are being carried out, there is still a long way to go. The recent medical reforms aiming at building the basic medical network will accelerate the process of cancer prevention and control in China. The progress in cancer prevention and control in China will be helpful for the decline of the cancer burden in Asia, as well as globally.

## References

1. A. Jemal, F. Bray, M.M. Center, J. Ferlay, E. Ward, D. Forman, Global cancer statistics, *CA: A Cancer Journal for Clinicians*, 61 (2011) 69–90.
2. H.R. Shin, E. Masuyer, J. Ferlay, M.P. Curado, Cancer in Asia – Incidence rates based on data in cancer incidence in five continents IX (1998–2002), *Asian Pacific Journal of Cancer Prevention*, 11 Suppl 2 (2010) 11–16.
3. J. Ferlay, H.R. Shin, D. Forman, C. Mathers, D.M. Parkin, GLOBOCAN 2008 v2.0, Cancer Incidence and Mortality Worldwide: IARC CancerBase No. 10 [Internet]. Lyon, France: International Agency for Research on Cancer, 2010. Available from: http://globocan.iarc.fr [Accessed 25 December 2012].
4. F. Bray, J.S. Ren, E. Masuyer, J. Ferlay, Global estimates of cancer prevalence for 27 sites in the adult population in 2008, *International Journal of Cancer*, 132 (2013) 1133–45.
5. K.Y. Yoo, Cancer prevention in the Asia Pacific region, *Asian Pacific Journal of Cancer Prevention*, 11 (2010) 839–44.
6. Ministry of Health, People's Republic of China, *Report on the Third National Sampling Survey of Causes of Death*, Beijing: People's Health Publishing House, 2008.
7. Z.P. He, J. W. Chen, *et al.*, *Chinese Cancer Registry Annual Report*, Beijing: Military Medical Science Press, 2011.
8. L. Li, F. Lu, S. Zhang, Analysis of cancer modality and distribution in China from year 1990 through 1992 – an epidemiologic study, *Zhonghua Zhong Liu Za Zhi*, 18 (1996) 403–7.
9. National Cancer Prevention Research Office, Ministry of China, *Investigate for Malignant Tumor Mortality in China*, Beijing: People's Health Publishing House, 1979.

10. M. Segi, S. Fujisaku, M. Kurihara, Y. Narai, K. Sasajima, The age-adjusted death rates for malignant neoplasms in some selected sites in 23 countries in 1954–1955 and their geographical correlation, *Tohoku Journal of Experimental Medicine*, 72 (1960) 91–103.
11. R. Doll, P. Payne, J. Waterhouse, International Union against Cancer. Cancer incidence in five continents: a technical report, New York: International Union Against Cancer/Springer Verlag, 1966.
12. P. Zhao, M. Dai, W. Chen, N. Li, Cancer trends in China, *Japanese Journal of Clinical Oncology*, 40 (2010) 281–5.
13. R. Doll, R. Peto, The causes of cancer: quantitative estimates of avoidable risks of cancer in the United States today, *Journal of the National Cancer Institute*, 66 (1981) 1191–308.
14. J. Peto, Cancer epidemiology in the last century and the next decade, *Nature*, 411 (2001) 390–5.
15. S.S. Hecht, Cigarette smoking and lung cancer: chemical mechanisms and approaches to prevention, *Lancet Oncology*, 3 (2002) 461–9.
16. D. Hoffmann, I. Hoffmann, K. El-Bayoumy, The less harmful cigarette: a controversial issue. a tribute to Ernst L. Wynder, *Chemical Research in Toxicology*, 14 (2001) 767–90.
17. D. Schottenfeld, F.F. Joseph, *Cancer Epidemiology and Prevention*, New York: Oxford University Press, 2006.
18. S. Park, J. Bae, B.H. Nam, K.Y. Yoo, Aetiology of cancer in Asia, *Asian Pacific Journal of Cancer Prevention*, 9 (2008) 371–80.
19. M.A. Moore, H. Tsuda, Smoking-related research in the Asian-Pacific countries, *Asian Pacific Journal of Cancer Prevention*, 3 (2002) 291–304.
20. C. Nagata, T. Mizoue, K. Tanaka, I. Tsuji, K. Wakai, M. Inoue, S. Tsugane, Tobacco smoking and breast cancer risk: an evaluation based on a systematic review of epidemiological evidence among the Japanese population, *Japanese Journal of Clinical Oncology*, 36 (2006) 387–94.
21. W. Wen, X.O. Shu, Y.T. Gao, G. Yang, Q. Li, H. Li, W. Zheng, Environmental tobacco smoke and mortality in Chinese women who have never smoked: prospective cohort study, *BMJ*, 333 (2006) 376.
22. J. Zhang, J.X. Ou, C.X. Bai, Tobacco smoking in China: prevalence, disease burden, challenges and future strategies, *Respirology*, 16 (2011) 1165–72.
23. C. Prinz, S. Schwendy, P. Voland, *H. pylori* and gastric cancer: shifting the global burden, *World Journal of Gastroenterology*, 12 (2006) 5458–64.
24. J.L. Ma, W.C. You, M.H. Gail, L. Zhang, W.J. Blot, Y.S. Chang, *et al.*, *Helicobacter pylori* infection and mode of transmission in a population at high risk of stomach cancer, *International Journal of Epidemiology*, 27 (1998) 570–3.
25. H. Tsukuma, H. Tanaka, W. Ajiki, A. Oshima, Liver cancer and its prevention, *Asian Pacific Journal of Cancer Prevention*, 6 (2005) 244–50.
26. Y.H. Zhou, C. Wu, H. Zhuang, Vaccination against hepatitis B: the Chinese experience, *Chinese Medical Journal* (English Edition), 122 (2009) 98–102.
27. P. Srivatanakul, H. Sriplung, S. Deerasamee, Epidemiology of liver cancer: an overview, *Asian Pacific Journal of Cancer Prevention*, 5 (2004) 118–25.
28. S. Franceschi, R. Herrero, G.M. Clifford, P.J. Snijders, A. Arslan, P.T. Anh, *et al.*, Variations in the age-specific curves of human papillomavirus prevalence in women worldwide, *International Journal of Cancer*, 119 (2006) 2677–84.
29. M.A. Moore, K. Tajima, Cervical cancer in the Asian Pacific: epidemiology, screening and treatment, *Asian Pacific Journal of Cancer Prevention*, 5 (2004) 349–61.
30. C. Desgranges, G.W. Bornkamm, Y. Zeng, P.C. Wang, J.S. Zhu, M. Shang, G. De-The, Detection of Epstein-Barr viral DNA internal repeats in the nasopharyngeal mucosa of Chinese with IgA/EBV-specific antibodies, *International Journal of Cancer*, 29 (1982) 87–91.
31. Y.I. Kim, Liver carcinoma and liver fluke infection, *Arzneimittelforschung*, 34 (1984) 1121–6.
32. J. Watts, China's environmental health challenges, *Lancet*, 372 (2008) 1451–2.
33. Y. Zhao, S. Wang, K. Aunan, H.M. Seip, J. Hao, Air pollution and lung cancer risks in China: a meta-analysis, *Science of the Total Environment*, 366 (2006) 500–13.
34. A.H. Wu-Williams, X.D. Dai, W. Blot, Z.Y. Xu, X.W. Sun, H.P. Xiao, *et al.*, Lung cancer among women in north-east China, *British Journal of Cancer*, 62 (1990) 982–7.
35. Z.Y. Xu, W.J. Blot, H.P. Xiao, A. Wu, Y.P. Feng, B.J. Stone, *et al.*, Smoking, air pollution, and the high rates of lung cancer in Shenyang, *China, Journal of the National Cancer Institute*, 81 (1989) 1800–6.

36. R.A. Kleinerman, Z. Wang, L. Wang, C. Metayer, S. Zhang, A.V. Brenner, *et al.*, Lung cancer and indoor exposure to coal and biomass in rural China, *Journal of Occupational and Environmental Medicine*, 44 (2002) 338–44.
37. J.H. Lubin, Z.Y. Wang, J.D. Boice, Jr., Z.Y. Xu, W.J. Blot, L. De Wang, R.A. Kleinerman, Risk of lung cancer and residential radon in China: pooled results of two studies, *International Journal of Cancer*, 109 (2004) 132–7.
38. Z. Wang, J.H. Lubin, L. Wang, S. Zhang, J.D. Boice, Jr., H. Cui, *et al.*, Residential radon and lung cancer risk in a high-exposure area of Gansu Province, China, *American Journal of Epidemiology*, 155 (2002) 554–64.
39. K.H. Morales, L. Ryan, T.L. Kuo, M.M. Wu, C.J. Chen, Risk of internal cancers from arsenic in drinking water, *Environmental Health Perspectives*, 108 (2000) 655–61.
40. B. Xi, Y. Liang, T. He, K.H. Reilly, Y. Hu, Q. Wang, Y. Yan, J. Mi, Secular trends in the prevalence of general and abdominal obesity among Chinese adults, 1993–2009, *Obesity Reviews*, 13 (2012) 287–96.
41. J.M. Yuan, Q.S. Wang, R.K. Ross, B.E. Henderson, M.C. Yu, Diet and breast cancer in Shanghai and Tianjin, China, *British Journal of Cancer*, 71 (1995) 1353–8.
42. B.C. Chiu, B.T. Ji, Q. Dai, G. Gridley, J.K. McLaughlin, Y.T. Gao, J.F. Fraumeni, Jr., W.H. Chow, Dietary factors and risk of colon cancer in Shanghai, China, *Cancer Epidemiology, Biomarkers & Prevention*, 12 (2003) 201–8.
43. A. Seow, S.R. Quah, D. Nyam, P.T. Straughan, T. Chua, T.C. Aw, Food groups and the risk of colorectal carcinoma in an Asian population, *Cancer*, 95 (2002) 2390–6.
44. C. Sauvaget, J. Nagano, M. Hayashi, E. Spencer, Y. Shimizu, N. Allen, Vegetables and fruit intake and cancer mortality in the Hiroshima/Nagasaki Life Span Study, *British Journal of Cancer*, 88 (2003) 689–94.
45. M.R. Forman, S.X. Yao, B.I. Graubard, Y.L. Qiao, M. McAdams, B.L. Mao, P.R. Taylor, The effect of dietary intake of fruits and vegetables on the odds ratio of lung cancer among Yunnan tin miners, *International Journal of Epidemiology*, 21 (1992) 437–41.
46. K. Hirose, T. Takezaki, N. Hamajima, S. Miura, K. Tajima, Dietary factors protective against breast cancer in Japanese premenopausal and postmenopausal women, *International Journal of Cancer*, 107 (2003) 276–82.
47. A.S. Malin, D. Qi, X.O. Shu, Y.T. Gao, J.M. Friedmann, F. Jin, W. Zheng, Intake of fruits, vegetables and selected micronutrients in relation to the risk of breast cancer, *International Journal of Cancer*, 105 (2003) 413–18.
48. M. Zhang, C.D. Holman, J.P. Huang, X. Xie, Green tea and the prevention of breast cancer: a case-control study in Southeast China, *Carcinogenesis*, 28 (2007) 1074–8.
49. A.H. Wu, M.C. Yu, C.C. Tseng, J. Hankin, M.C. Pike, Green tea and risk of breast cancer in Asian Americans, *International Journal of Cancer*, 106 (2003) 574–9.
50. K. Hirose, N. Imaeda, Y. Tokudome, C. Goto, K. Wakai, K. Matsuo, *et al.*, Soybean products and reduction of breast cancer risk: a case-control study in Japan, *British Journal of Cancer*, 93 (2005) 15–22.
51. S. Yamamoto, T. Sobue, M. Kobayashi, S. Sasaki, S. Tsugane, Soy, isoflavones, and breast cancer risk in Japan, *Journal of the National Cancer Institute*, 95 (2003) 906–13.
52. A.H. Wu, D. Yang, M.C. Pike, A meta-analysis of soyfoods and risk of stomach cancer: the problem of potential confounders, *Cancer Epidemiology, Biomarkers & Prevention*, 9 (2000) 1051–8.
53. A.H. Wu, R.G. Ziegler, A.M. Nomura, D.W. West, L.N. Kolonel, *et al.*, Soy intake and risk of breast cancer in Asians and Asian Americans, *American Journal of Clinical Nutrition*, 68 (1998) 1437S–43S.
54. K. Hirose, N. Hamajima, T. Takezaki, S. Miura, K. Tajima, Physical exercise reduces risk of breast cancer in Japanese women, *Cancer Science*, 94 (2003) 193–9.
55. L. Hou, B.T. Ji, A. Blair, Q. Dai, Y.T. Gao, W.H. Chow, Commuting physical activity and risk of colon cancer in Shanghai, China, *American Journal of Epidemiology*, 160 (2004) 860–7.
56. Y.L. Xu, Q. Sun, G.L. Shan, J. Zhang, H.B. Liao, S.Y. Li, *et al.*, A case-control study on risk factors of breast cancer in China, *Archives of Medical Science*, 8 (2012) 303–9.
57. L. Li, J. Ji, J.B. Wang, M. Niyazi, Y.L. Qiao, P. Boffetta, Attributable causes of breast cancer and ovarian cancer in China: reproductive factors, oral contraceptives and hormone replacement therapy, *Chinese Journal of Cancer Research*, 24 (2012) 9–17.
58. K.Y. Yoo, H. Kim, H.R. Shin, D. Kang, M. Ha, S.K. Park, *et al.*, Female sex hormones and body mass in adolescent and postmenopausal Korean women, *Journal of Korean Medical Science*, 13 (1998) 241–6.

59. B. Zhou, Q. Sun, R. Cong, H. Gu, N. Tang, L. Yang, B. Wang, Hormone replacement therapy and ovarian cancer risk: a meta-analysis, *Gynecologic Oncology*, 108 (2008) 641–51.
60. J.T. Casagrande, E.W. Louie, M.C. Pike, S. Roy, R.K. Ross, B.E. Henderson, 'Incessant ovulation' and ovarian cancer, *Lancet*, 2 (1979) 170–3.
61. W.D. Guo, A.W. Hsing, J.Y. Li, J.S. Chen, W.H. Chow, W.J. Blot, Correlation of cervical cancer mortality with reproductive and dietary factors, and serum markers in China, *International Journal of Epidemiology*, 23 (1994) 1127–32.
62. J. Peto, T.M. Mack, High constant incidence in twins and other relatives of women with breast cancer, *Nature Genetics*, 26 (2000) 411–14.
63. Z. Hu, C. Wu, Y. Shi, H. Guo, X. Zhao, Z. Yin, *et al.*, A genome-wide association study identifies two new lung cancer susceptibility loci at 13q12.12 and 22q12.2 in Han Chinese, *Nature Genetics*, 43 (2011) 792–6.
64. Y. Shi, Z. Hu, C. Wu, J. Dai, H. Li, J. Dong, *et al.*, A genome-wide association study identifies new susceptibility loci for non-cardia gastric cancer at 3q13.31 and 5p13.1, *Nature Genetics*, 43 (2011) 1215–18.
65. C. Wu, Z. Hu, Z. He, W. Jia, F. Wang, Y. Zhou, *et al.*, Genome-wide association study identifies three new susceptibility loci for esophageal squamous-cell carcinoma in Chinese populations, *Nature Genetics*, 43 (2011) 679–84.
66. L.D. Wang, F.Y. Zhou, X.M. Li, L.D. Sun, X. Song, Y. Jin, *et al.*, Genome-wide association study of esophageal squamous cell carcinoma in Chinese subjects identifies susceptibility loci at PLCE1 and C20orf54, *Nature Genetics*, 42 (2010) 759–63.
67. H. Zhang, Y. Zhai, Z. Hu, C. Wu, J. Qian, W. Jia, *et al.*, Genome-wide association study identifies 1p36.22 as a new susceptibility locus for hepatocellular carcinoma in chronic hepatitis B virus carriers, *Nature Genetics*, 42 (2010) 755–8.
68. J.X. Bei, Y. Li, W.H. Jia, B.J. Feng, G. Zhou, L.Z. Chen, *et al.*, A genome-wide association study of nasopharyngeal carcinoma identifies three new susceptibility loci, *Nature Genetics*, 42 (2010) 599–603.
69. C. Wu, X. Miao, L. Huang, X. Che, G. Jiang, D. Yu, *et al.*, Genome-wide association study identifies five loci associated with susceptibility to pancreatic cancer in Chinese populations, *Nature Genetics*, 44 (2012) 62–6.
70. J. Peto, R.S. Houlston, Genetics and the common cancers, *European Journal of Cancer*, 37 Suppl 8 (2001) S88–96.
71. X. Liang, S. Bi, W. Yang, L. Wang, G. Cui, F. Cui, *et al.*, Evaluation of the impact of hepatitis B vaccination among children born during 1992–2005 in China, *Journal of Infectious Diseases*, 200 (2009) 39–47.
72. P.W. Lee, T.T. Kwan, K.F. Tam, K.K. Chan, P.M. Young, S.S. Lo, *et al.*, Beliefs about cervical cancer and human papillomavirus (HPV) and acceptability of HPV vaccination among Chinese women in Hong Kong, *Preventive Medicine*, 45 (2007) 130–4.

# Part III

# Infectious diseases

# Introduction to Part III: infectious diseases

*Siân M. Griffiths*

In this part, we describe the challenges of infectious diseases, and the need for robust organizations to carry out effective surveillance and control. The examples of the Shanghai Centre for Disease Control (CDC) and the Centre for Health Protection (CHP) in Hong Kong provide insights into the work underpinning health protection in two large Chinese cities. As well as looking at some specific and important diseases – HIV/AIDS, hepatitis, TB and malaria – authors also examine the future threats of emerging diseases.

Just as understanding epidemiology is an essential skill for public health practice so too is an understanding of infectious diseases. Epidemiological skills are needed for identification of the source and spread of an infectious disease, as well as for tracking the course of an epidemic. Early public health heroes Pasteur, Jenner and Koch are those who developed germ theory, immunization and antibiotics. And it was the sanitary reformers of nineteenth-century England, such as Chadwick, who understood that the workforce producing the country's wealth would be more productive if the workers were healthier, and living and working in better conditions with sufficient income for better diets and able to withstand the ravages of infection. The interrelationship between poverty and disease, and the need to break the vicious cycle that exists between them, remains a cornerstone of public health. In their chapter on the neglected diseases of poverty, Utzinger and colleagues discuss the complexity of the links that exist between poverty and the diseases not commonly perceived as direct threats to industrialized countries despite hundreds of millions of people being affected. Comparatively few deaths are attributable to these neglected tropical diseases, common in low-income countries in Asia, and this low stature makes it difficult to seek international attention and funds. Whilst non-communicable diseases (NCDs) are often now the leading public health concern, neglected chronic infectious diseases are still widespread, particularly among people who live in poor or marginalized communities. The remaining, ever widening, inequalities are reflected by statistics, such as that more than one out of two people in Cambodia, Indonesia and Lao PDR currently live on less than US$2 per day. Lack of access to clean water, poor sanitation and inadequate hygiene behaviour contribute to the sustained transmission of disease and favour the proliferation of vectors and intermediate hosts. Uneven access to health services, low literacy levels and inadequate nutrition (both qualitatively and quantitatively) result in increased vulnerability to infection, and future threats such as climate change may well impact on these diseases in the future. It is also amongst some of these poorer communities in Asia that new infections, such as H5N1, H7N9 and SARS, have arisen. The lack of attention to the need for robust systems for surveillance and response to new and emerging infectious diseases was amply demonstrated in the 2003 SARS epidemic in Hong Kong. The emergence of the new coronavirus was unexpected and reviews of the systems in place at the time highlighted their inadequacies. The next two chapters describe perspectives from institutions whose role is reflective of the lessons from SARS in 2003, and of the need for vigilant systems, resilience in response and good communication. In Chapter 13 Tsang writes from experience as Director of the Centre for Health Protection (CHP), established in Hong Kong post-SARS. In his view, governments are a vital source of health information and are key players in health education and promotion activities. In partnership with community groups, government agencies contribute to disease control in many different domains including health research and development, training and capacity building, and monitoring and evaluation of health services. At a supranational level, government agencies form versatile networks to share information, tackle global issues and provide mutual support in disease control. Over the years, the CHP's role in disease control has undergone a gradual evolution. First, following global trends, more emphasis is being put on intersectoral collaboration and community engagement, whether in the setting of health priorities or in planning or execution of programmes and activities. The CHP is moving away from the role of a dominant, autonomous player to that of a facilitator, coordinator and funder. Risk communication plays a core role in disease control and the credibility of a government agency can be damaged irrevocably by mishandling a single aspect of a disease outbreak, no matter how good its track record.

Whilst Hong Kong's population is around 7 million, Shanghai's is now over 23 million, of which 14 million are registered residents and 9 million are migrants. Over 24 per cent of the total population is aged over 60 years. Using the Shanghai Municipal Centre for Disease Control and Prevention (SCDC) as a case study to discuss how Centres for Disease Control (CDC) operate in China, in Chapter 14 Fan Wu describes the structure, function and future challenges facing the CDC. The most important part of this system is the vertical interaction between the SCDC, district CDCs and community health service centres (CHSC). The SCDC fulfils the municipal government's public health function and its essential tasks include: implementation of disease control and prevention programmes, surveillance on health-related risk factors, responding to public health emergency events, conducting research on applied preventive medicine, and promoting international cooperation and exchange. The CDC is responsible for vital statistics in Shanghai and has a relatively complete database for death and birth registry. It also conducts surveillance and intervention programmes on health-related risk factors in occupational health, environmental health, food safety, nutritional health, school health and radiation protection. In order to provide early warning and detection of outbreaks of infectious diseases, a real-time online reporting system based on individual cases, as well as an online student absentee reporting system, have been developed. In 2010, the SCDC, in cooperation with the district and county CDCs, was successfully responsible for public health security for the Shanghai Expo, monitoring surveillance data in real time, ready to respond if needed at the Expo sites.

Understanding the patterns of acute and chronic infections is reliant on the countrywide CDC system in China where, despite the increase in NCDs, infectious diseases still remain a burden. The case studies of three common and potentially chronic diseases highlight different aspects of the challenges of their control. Lau *et al.* in Chapter 15 examine the new emergent approaches to HIV/AIDS amongst a high-risk and often stigmatized group – men who have sex with men (MSM) – and the potential gains to be achieved from social marketing. They describe the emergence and implications of the use of electronic social media, the key and underdeveloped roles of NGOs and the importance of translating research findings into policy and practice. In Chapter 16 Walley and Wei focus on local control of tuberculosis (TB). Over 60 per cent of all new TB cases in the world occur in Asia. The top three countries with the highest burdens of TB are all in Asia, namely India, China and Indonesia. The infection is more likely to become a disease in people with reduced immunity due to undernutrition, diabetes or HIV infection. In general, about one in ten people infected with TB later develop the disease. However, for those who are already infected with TB and HIV, around half will get active TB. In countries or provinces with high rates of HIV, an increased incidence of TB disease occurs. The most significant cause of drug resistant TB is inappropriate treatment of normal TB cases, for example, if TB drugs are not taken correctly or not taken for the full six months (treatment default). The global average prevalence for multidrug resistant (MDR) strains in newly diagnosed TB cases (not previously treated for TB) is 3.4 per cent, while it is 6 per cent in China, 4 per cent in the Philippines and 2 per cent in India. Around half of the people with both HIV and TB infections will develop active TB disease and they are also more susceptible to new infections or re-infection. Tuberculosis is also a major cause of death in people with HIV/AIDS. Conversely, TB patients are more likely to rapidly progress to full-blown AIDS when infected with the HIV virus. The TB/HIV situation is more serious in countries such as Myanmar, Cambodia and Thailand where HIV prevalence rates are generally higher.

The burden of disease from hepatitis in Asia, described by Li in Chapter 17, is another serious and interrelated public health issue. Whilst vaccination, safe blood supply, safe injections, and safe food and water can all reduce the transmission of viral hepatitis infections – and all WHO member states of the region have included the hepatitis B vaccine in their routine NIPs (National Immunization Programs) – it is estimated that there are 100 million people with chronic hepatitis B infection and 30 million people with chronic hepatitis C infection living in the region. Injecting drug use is also widespread in most countries in Southeast Asia. Bangladesh, India, Indonesia, Myanmar, Nepal and Thailand also have a high prevalence of double infection – with HIV and hepatitis C virus (HCV) – and 50–100 per cent of HIV-positive injecting drug users (IDUs) are co-infected with HCV. Over 50 per cent of global hepatitis E deaths occur in Asia and since hepatitis E is a waterborne disease, poor sanitation (especially in the form of contaminated water or food supplies) has been a factor in major outbreaks, such as those involving refugees residing in overcrowded temporary camps after natural disasters.

The close juxtaposition of animals and humans in many parts of Asia has stimulated debate about the One Health concept, a worldwide strategy for expanding interdisciplinary collaborations and communications in all aspects of health care for humans, animals and the environment. This is not least, as argued by Horby in Chapter 18, because Asia is considered a hotspot for emerging infectious diseases (EIDs) due to increasing population density, population growth, latitude, rainfall and richness of its wildlife host species. Emerging infectious diseases are defined as diseases that are increasing in their incidence, geographic or host species range or their impact (due to, for instance, the acquisition of resistance to antimicrobial drugs or vaccines, or the acquisition of new virulence factors). This encompasses both newly recognized pathogens, such as SARS, and known pathogens that are 're-emerging' including multi-resistant TB. Horby describes the paradox of the macroeconomic success of Asia – industrialization and urbanization have resulted in better socio-economic gains, but also create large demand for natural resources such as hard wood, fire wood, pulp, agricultural and grazing land, living space, roads and minerals. These demands have led to deforestation and alterations in habitat, which change species composition and the interaction between wild animals, domestic animals, insect vectors and humans, thereby providing new opportunities for disease emergence. Horby reminds us that reduced access to clean water for low-income families increases the risk of water-washed diseases such as trachoma and scabies, and water-borne diseases such as typhoid, cholera, and hepatitis A and E. Additional unquantified risks also arise, for example, from the use of pesticides and fertilizers in the intensification of agriculture, as well as changes in agricultural practice. On the one hand, China and India have together taken 125 million people out of slum conditions between 2000 and 2010, and urbanization and urban infrastructures have played an important role in Asia's success in improving access to safe water and sanitation, with almost half of the world's population (living in China and India) gaining access to improved sources of drinking water between 1990 and 2008. However, the rate of increase in access to improved drinking water sources is barely keeping up with the rate of urban population growth and in 2010 an estimated 500 million people were living in slums in Asia, de facto in poor sanitary conditions.

The recognition of the linkage between anthropogenic changes and disease emergence has resulted in repeated calls for a more holistic and interdisciplinary approach to the study of infectious diseases. The theme of climate change and its impact on disease is illustrated further in the case study in Chapter 19 by Guo-Jing Yang and Xiao-Nong Zhou which stresses the urgent need to explore whether climate change will have an effect on the transmission of major infectious diseases in Southeast Asia, in particular on malaria, and how to increase understanding of the impact on distribution and transmission patterns for malaria. Climate change alters the transmission of vector-borne diseases by

- changing the survival and reproduction rate of the vector,
- changing the development behaviour of the pathogen inside the vector,
- changing vector activities of contacting human beings.

The authors describe their work to identify key environmental risk factors that govern malaria transmission and pinpoint high transmission regions, thus providing guidance for malaria control. Mitigation and adaptation strategies to reduce the potential impacts of climate change on vector-borne diseases are recommended.

# 12

# Chronic neglected diseases of poverty in Asia

## Challenges and opportunities ahead

*Jürg Utzinger, Peiling Yap, Shan Lv, Guo-Jing Yang, Xiao-Nong Zhou, Peter Steinmann and David Molyneux*

### Introduction

The past two decades have seen considerable achievements in population health. Indeed, as revealed by the Global Burden of Disease Study 2010 (GBD 2010) [1], life expectancy for men and women has increased, whilst the public health impact of many communicable diseases, including HIV/AIDS and malaria, has declined. Consequently, compared to the situation in 1990, non-communicable diseases (NCDs) are now the predominant public health issue in most regions of the world and a higher proportion of deaths occur in people aged 70 years and above. Infant and child mortality, on the other hand, has declined [1, 2]. It must be noted, however, that these global estimates hide local and national idiosyncrasies and trends. Hence, there is a need to deepen our understanding of rates and trends of diseases, injuries and risk factors at local, national and regional levels. In turn, such an understanding will shape current and future national health priorities, and should thus set the terms for social and health policy and planning. Another issue that must be recognized is health inequalities, particularly the gap between the rich and the poor, which continues to widen in many parts of the industrialized and developing world [3–5]. Finally, diseases, disabling conditions and risks that primarily affect the 'bottom-billion' warrant special attention and concerted action. Neglecting these issues will hamper progress towards achieving the Millennium Development Goals (MDGs) [6–8] and jeopardize the post-2015 era of sustainable development [9].

This chapter focuses on chronic neglected diseases of poverty with a particular emphasis on East and Southeast Asia. Although malaria, tuberculosis (TB) and HIV/AIDS are considered perhaps the three most important diseases of poverty [10, 11], we will exclude reference to TB (see Chapter 16) and HIV/AIDS (see Chapter 15), as these diseases are covered elsewhere in this book [12, 13]. Malaria, on the other hand, will be discussed from a specific perspective, thus complementing the malaria case study that is part of the climate change chapters (Chapters 19 and 20) [14]. Inclusion of malaria is further justified by its grouping together with neglected tropical diseases in the recent GBD 2010 [1, 2]. Of note, the majority of malaria encountered in Asia is due to *Plasmodium vivax*, which is considered a neglected malaria parasite [15–18].

This chapter is structured as follows: first, we summarize the major changes that have occurred in population health since 1990. We describe trends at the global level and then focus on ten countries in East and Southeast Asia. Second, we highlight the multi-causal and extremely complex nature of poverty and emphasize that poverty is a key driver of poor health. We review recent data and national statistics and highlight the proportion of people living on less than US$ 2 per day and below the national poverty lines in our selection of Asian countries. Third, the centrepiece of our chapter is the section pertaining to chronic neglected diseases of poverty, summarizing their epidemiology, and current tools and strategies for their control and eventual elimination. Fourth, we review major drivers of global change and discuss how these might influence the frequency and transmission dynamics of chronic neglected diseases of poverty. Finally, we discuss the remaining challenges and new potential threats, and discuss opportunities to reduce chronic neglected diseases of poverty and underlying inequalities to improve people's health and wellbeing.

## Current state of population health

### *The global situation*

The GBD 2010 is a landmark publication, as it represents the most comprehensive systematic effort undertaken thus far to describe the global distribution of a wide array of diseases, injuries and risk factors [19]. Over a five-year period, some 500 scientists investigated a total of 291 diseases and 67 risk factors. Using sophisticated modelling, specific mortality and burden estimates were calculated and stratified for 21 regions of the world [2]. Mortality estimates were derived for 235 causes of death for 20 different age groups [1]. Moreover, in early 2013, the Institute for Health Metrics and Evaluation (IHME) at the University of Washington in Seattle released national-level estimates for 192 countries, including an innovative web-based interactive visualization interface (http://www.healthmetricsand evaluation.org/gbd).

What are the key findings of the GBD 2010? At the global level, men and women now can expect to live longer than they could 20 years ago, but this gain in life expectancy has come at the price of spending additional years of life with more illnesses and morbid sequelae – in other words, in poorer health. Particularly striking is a 60 per cent drop in under-5 mortality. Infectious diseases, maternal and child illnesses, and malnutrition cause fewer deaths and less illness than they did in the 1990s. Chronic diseases are replacing premature mortality as leading causes of death everywhere, except in Africa. Physical inactivity and inappropriate diet (e.g. low fruit intake and excess consumption of salt) are new leading risk factors for poor health, already accounting for 10 per cent of the disability-adjusted life years (DALYs). For the first time in human history, overweight has replaced under-nutrition as a major health risk factor. These global trends underscore the remarkable achievements made in population health. However, global averages hide important information at local, national and regional levels and they fail to shed light on health inequalities within populations. High-quality data at smaller scales and for different socio-economic strata are required to define current and future health priorities, particularly for disadvantaged population groups and communities, and to shape evidence-based action, social and health policy and planning.

## *Health trends in East and Southeast Asia*

In our chapter, we focus on ten countries in East and Southeast Asia, namely Cambodia, Indonesia, Lao People's Democratic Republic (Lao PDR), Malaysia, Mongolia, Myanmar, the People's Republic of China (P.R. China), the Philippines, Thailand and Vietnam. Using readily available country-specific data from the IHME, Table 12.1 summarizes changes that occurred between 1990 and 2010 in two key health indicators, namely the age-standardized death rate and life expectancy at birth. In each of the ten countries investigated, age-standardized death rates decreased, with particularly encouraging changes observed in P.R. China and Vietnam, where age-standardized death rates in 2010 were approximately 600 per 100,000, a reduction of more than 30 per cent over the past 20 years. The smallest changes were observed in the Philippines and Mongolia with relatively modest reductions of 4.5 per cent and 5.1 per cent, respectively. In Mongolia, Myanmar and Lao PDR the age-standardized death rate in 2010 was still above 1,000 per 100,000. With regard to life expectancy at birth, Lao PDR made the greatest gain as people in 2010, on average, lived up to 8.5 years longer when taking 1990 as the reference benchmark. Among the countries considered here, P.R. China and Vietnam currently have the highest average life expectancy at above 75 years (see Table 12.1).

Table 12.2 summarizes the 25 leading causes of DALYs in 2010, stratified by (i) communicable, maternal, neonatal and nutritional causes; (ii) NCDs; and (iii) injuries. The data underscore that NCDs are the main drivers of the total burden – in the ten selected countries, they make up a minimum of 10 (Lao PDR) and a maximum of 19 (P.R. China) positions out of the 25 listed here. With regard to communicable, maternal, neonatal and nutritional causes of DALYs, lower respiratory infections are the most important issue, currently ranked first in four countries (Cambodia, Lao PDR, Myanmar and the Philippines). Although not considered in any greater detail in this chapter, it is noteworthy that TB and HIV/AIDS figure among the top 25 causes of DALYs in nine and five of the ten investigated

*Table 12.1* Changes in two selected health indicators between 1990 and 2010 in ten selected countries of East and Southeast Asia

| *Region* / *Country* | *Age-standardized death rate (per 100,000)* | | | *Life expectancy at birth (in years)* | | |
|---|---|---|---|---|---|---|
| | *1990* | *2010* | *Difference (%)* | *1990* | *2010* | *Difference (%)* |
| ***East Asia*** | | | | | | |
| Mongolia | 1,283 | 1,218 | −65 (5.1) | 60.5 | 64.6 | +4.1 (6.8) |
| P.R. China | 896 | 607 | −289 (32.3) | 69.3 | 75.7 | +6.4 (9.2) |
| ***Southeast Asia*** | | | | | | |
| Cambodia | 1,355 | 957 | −398 (29.4) | 50.1 | 58.0 | +7.9 (15.8) |
| Indonesia | 1,033 | 867 | −166 (16.1) | 65.0 | 69.7 | +4.7 (7.2) |
| Lao PDR | 1,532 | 1,094 | −438 (28.6) | 56.2 | 64.7 | +8.5 (15.1) |
| Malaysia | 825 | 726 | −99 (12.0) | 71.6 | 73.7 | +2.1 (2.9) |
| Myanmar | 1,640 | 1,185 | −455 (27.7) | 56.5 | 63.9 | +7.4 (13.1) |
| Philippines | 909 | 868 | −41 (4.5) | 67.8 | 70.1 | +2.3 (3.4) |
| Thailand | 712 | 663 | −49 (6.9) | 72.4 | 74.1 | +1.7 (2.3) |
| Vietnam | 876 | 595 | −281 (32.1) | 68.9 | 75.6 | +6.7 (9.7) |

*Source*: [134].

*Table 12.2* Top 25 causes of disability-adjusted life years (DALYs) in 2010 in selected countries of East and Southeast Asia

| ***Region*** *Country* | *No. of leading causes of DALYs (among top 25)* | | | *Most important communicable disease (rank)* |
|---|---|---|---|---|
| | *Communicable, maternal, neonatal and nutritional* | *Non-communicable* | *Injuries* | |
| ***East Asia*** | | | | |
| Mongolia | 5 | 15 | 5 | Lower respiratory infection (2) |
| P.R. China | 2 | 19 | 4 | Lower respiratory infection (15) |
| ***Southeast Asia*** | | | | |
| Cambodia | 9 | 13 | 3 | Lower respiratory infection (1) |
| Indonesia | 8 | 15 | 2 | Tuberculosis (2) |
| Lao PDR | 10 | 10 | 5 | Lower respiratory infection (1) |
| Malaysia | 6 | 16 | 3 | Lower respiratory infection (4) |
| Myanmar | 9 | 12 | 4 | Lower respiratory infection (1) |
| Philippines | 7 | 15 | 3 | Lower respiratory infection (1) |
| Thailand | 5 | 15 | 5 | HIV/AIDS (1) |
| Vietnam | 5 | 17 | 3 | HIV/AIDS (6) |

*Source*: [134].

countries, respectively. The only country where TB is not listed among the top 25 causes of DALYs is P.R. China despite hosting the second-largest population of TB patients in the world. Malaria was among the top 25 causes of DALYs in three of the ten Asian countries considered here: Myanmar (rank: 6), Cambodia (rank: 14) and Lao PDR (rank: 20).

## Poverty and health

### *The intimate connection between poverty and health*

Although the links and mutual reinforcement between poverty and health have been recognized for centuries [20], we often still do not fully understand whether a specific disease (e.g. malaria) is a cause or a consequence of people's low socio-economic status. This might be explained by the extremely complex and multi-causal nature of poverty. Indeed, poor health is only one of myriad factors that drive poverty. With the publication of the World Development Report in 1993 by the World Bank, a sea change has occurred. The report, entitled *Investing in health*, made a compelling case that investment to improve public health spurs economic development. Prioritization of health interventions was – for the first time – based on the DALY metric, which was a novel concept from the early 1990s, and combinined the loss of life from premature deaths with the loss of healthy life due to disability [21]. Put simply, the underlying rationale was to get the 'biggest bang for the buck' in health dollars invested.

Subsequent work by the Commission on Macroeconomics and Health, chaired by the economist Jeffrey D. Sachs, reinforced the World Bank's prior position, as can be seen by the following quote:

> Although health is widely understood to be both a central goal and an important outcome of development, the importance of investing in health to promote economic development and poverty reduction has been much less appreciated. We have found that extending the coverage of crucial health services, including a relatively small number of specific interventions, to the world's poor could save millions of lives each year, reduce poverty, spur economic development, and promote global security [10].

At the height of the HIV/AIDS pandemic, it is not surprising that the Commission placed so much emphasis on it [10]. The catastrophic impact at the individual and household level, and the growing awareness of its public health significance, particularly in Africa, are key features that might explain why HIV/AIDS – along with malaria – was explicitly mentioned in MDG 6: *Combat HIV/AIDS, malaria and other diseases.* It is clear that the specific naming of HIV/AIDS and malaria raised the profile of these diseases, whilst other communicable and non-communicable diseases were sidelined, even though the 'other diseases' also perpetuate the cycle of poverty in the developing world to perhaps a far greater extent given the absolute numbers of individuals infected or at risk. Perhaps the most important outcome of putting the spotlight on specific diseases was a reconfiguration of development aid for health. Indeed, a number of high-level, multi-billion US dollar global health initiatives were launched, including the Global Fund to Fight AIDS, Tuberculosis and Malaria (the 'Global Fund'), the President's Emergency Plan for AIDS Relief (PEPFAR) and the President's Malaria Initiative (PMI). While these initiatives averted hundreds of thousands of deaths and millions of DALYs [22, 23], they marshalled an unprecedented number and scale of vertical programmes, and diverted both funds and human resources away from existing health programmes, and might have also undermined already fragile health and social systems in developing countries [24].

The neglected tropical diseases represent some of the 'other diseases' in MDG 6 and it has been argued that their successful control is critical for achieving progress on multiple MDGs [6, 8, 25, 26]. In May 2013, during the 66$^{th}$ World Health Assembly (WHA), resolution EB132.R7 was passed on neglected tropical diseases, and hence all 17 neglected tropical diseases listed by the World Health Organization (WHO) are now specifically included alongside HIV/AIDS, TB and malaria in the recently published high-level panel report by Eminent Persons to the Secretary-General of the United Nations in connection with the post-2015 development agenda. Goal 4e reads: '*Reduce the burden of disease from HIV/AIDS, tuberculosis, malaria, neglected tropical diseases and priority non-communicable diseases*' [27].

Recognizing the central role of research, in 2008, the Special Programme for Research and Training in Tropical Diseases (TDR) set up a global 'think tank' to develop the research agenda on infectious diseases of poverty. More than 130 experts were convened into six disease-specific and four thematic reference groups. Along with extensive stakeholder consultation to ensure input from disease-endemic countries, the expert groups reviewed and synthesized the literature, and put forward top research priorities. Key findings were published in the peer-reviewed literature [28–31] and in stand-alone technical report series publications [32, 33]. Importantly, the expert groups' analyses and identification of priorities and research-related actions fed into the *Global report for research on infectious diseases of poverty*, published by WHO in 2012 [20]. In order to further promote research and to provide an open-access forum for addressing essential public health issues related to infectious diseases of poverty, in October 2012, BioMed Central launched a specialized journal – *Infectious Diseases of Poverty* (www.idpjournal.com). This journal provides a unique platform to discuss and disseminate trans-disciplinary and multi-sectoral research, including health systems, eco-health and innovative technology towards a better understanding of the epidemiology, control and elimination of infectious diseases of poverty.

## *How much poverty is there in the target countries discussed here?*

Using a diversity of recent national statistics, Table 12.3 shows the proportion of the population living on less than US$ 2 per day and the percentage of the population living below the national poverty line in the ten selected countries of East and Southeast Asia. Strikingly, more than one out of two people in Cambodia, Indonesia and Lao PDR currently live on less than US$ 2 per day. In rural parts of the P.R. China, the respective percentage is almost 50 per cent. At the other end of the spectrum are Malaysia, Thailand and urban areas of P.R. China, where 5 per cent or less of the population are currently living on less than US$ 2 per day.

Regarding the percentage of the population living below the national poverty line, the available data suggest that it currently ranges between 2.8 per cent in P.R. China and 39.2 per cent in Mongolia. No data are currently available for Myanmar. The striking differences between the internationally recognized cut-off of US$ 2 per day and the national definitions of poverty highlight important differences in national concepts of poverty and political considerations (see Table 12.3).

*Table 12.3* List of low- and middle-income countries[a] in the East Asia and Southeast Asia regions, including their respective poverty indicators

| ***Region*** *Country* | *Percentage of population living below US$ 2 per day (%)* | *Percentage of population living below the national poverty line (%)* | *Year* |
|---|---|---|---|
| ***East Asia*** | | | |
| Mongolia | n.d. | 39.2 | –/2010 |
| P.R. China | 29.9 | 2.8 | 2008/2004 |
| Rural | 48.9 | n.d. | 2008/– |
| Urban | 4.8 | n.d. | 2008/– |
| ***Southeast Asia*** | | | |
| Cambodia | 53.5 | 30.1 | 2008/2007 |
| Indonesia | 54.6 | 12.5 | 2008/2011 |
| Lao PDR | 66.2 | 27.6 | 2008/2008 |
| Malaysia | 2.0 | 3.8 | 2008/2009 |
| Myanmar | n.d. | n.d. | – |
| Philippines | 42.4 | 26.5 | 2008/2009 |
| Thailand | 5.0 | 7.8 | 2008/2010 |
| Vietnam | 43.6 | 14.2 | 2008/2010 |

*Notes:* [a] South Korea, Japan, Brunei and Singapore belong to these regions but are considered as high-income countries by the World Bank.
n.d., not determined.

## Chronic neglected diseases of poverty

### *Malaria*

Malaria is a typical disease of poverty (see also Chapter 19). Once the parasite causing malaria and its mode of transmission were discovered more than a century ago, efforts were soon made to quantify the economic impact of malaria. However, in view of the complexity of both poverty and the epidemiology of malaria, the evidence base for describing the nature, determinants and direction of the causal relationship between malaria and poverty remains weak [34, 35]. A 25-year cross-country regression analysis (1965–1990) concluded that the annual growth rate in countries characterized by intense malaria transmission was 1.3 per cent lower than that in less malaria-prone countries [36], particularly in sub-Saharan Africa, possibly because of the virulence of the dominant species in Africa, *Plasmodium falciparum*, together with the efficiency of the principal vector, *Anopheles gambiae*. These estimates at the macroeconomic level were at the root of launching the aforementioned Global Fund and the PMI, and provided strong leverage to massively scale-up malaria control interventions and renewed efforts for elimination, as laid out in the 2008 Global Malaria Action Plan [37]. A recent systematic review and meta-analysis provides new evidence of the negative association between malaria and poverty. Indeed, a total of 15 studies met the investigators' inclusion criteria and the meta-analysis revealed that the odds of parasitologically confirmed or clinical malaria among the poorest children was approximately twice that in economically better-off children (adjusted odds ratio 2.1, 95 per cent confidence interval 1.4–3.0) [38].

### *Neglected tropical diseases*

The neglected tropical diseases, often abbreviated as NTDs, are now a well-established and widely used brand identity [39, 40]. The origin can be traced to two three-day workshops held in Berlin, the first one in December 2003 and the second in April 2005. Co-hosted by WHO, the German Technical Cooperation (GTZ), the German Ministry for Development and Technical Cooperation, 'Kreditanstalt für Wiederaufbau' (KfW), the German Ministry for Health and Social Security and TDR, the workshops brought together researchers and a broad range of experts from public health, economics, human rights, non-governmental organizations (NGOs) and industry. Discussions and deliberations pertained to neglected diseases (note: without the term 'tropical'), including key challenges to intensify and scale-up efforts to tackle them [41]. The pressing need to control neglected diseases was emphasized and justified on moral, human rights and economic grounds, and from global public goods and societal perspectives. It was acknowledged that, although the neglected diseases are biologically and medically diverse, they share many common features, which are intimately tied to conditions of poverty. For example, lack of access to clean water, no or unimproved sanitation and unhygienic behaviour sustain the transmission of many diseases and favour the proliferation of vectors and intermediate hosts. Additionally, uneven access to health services, low literacy levels and inadequate nutrition (both qualitatively and quantitatively) result in increased vulnerability to infection. Initially, a set of 13 diseases were grouped together and collectively phrased neglected tropical diseases [42]. The WHO currently lists 17 neglected tropical diseases [26, 43]. However, it must be noted that many more diseases fit the criteria of general neglect. It is thus not surprising that a recent comprehensive review came up with an extensive list of over 40 neglected tropical diseases. The causative agents can be grouped into helminths, bacteria, protozoa, viruses, fungi and ectoparasites [40].

The issue of neglect occurs at different levels. First, at the individual and community level, as many of the neglected diseases are associated with fear and suffering (e.g. human African trypanosomiasis), disfigurement (e.g. Buruli ulcer and lymphatic filariasis) and stigma (e.g. leprosy) [40, 44, 45]. Second, the neglected tropical diseases are underappreciated at the national level, because they mainly affect poor and marginalized groups and communities with little political voice. Hence, the neglected tropical diseases are given no or only very low priority by the ministries of health and finance. Third, the neglected tropical diseases lack visibility at the international level. The diseases are not commonly perceived as direct threats to industrialized countries and, although hundreds of millions of people are affected, the conditions are mostly chronic and comparatively few deaths are attributable to them. Nevertheless, it has been argued that, directly or indirectly, the annual mortality due to neglected tropical diseases is at least as high as that attributed to maternal mortality [42], excluding the numbers of death attributable to snake bite, which is a major neglected and unrecognized problem in many developing countries [46]. This low stature and the neglect at all levels make it difficult to seek international attention and adequate funding for research and control [40, 41, 47].

Importantly though, papers published in high-impact factor journals made a compelling case for their low-cost community-based control by highlighting the considerable global burden due to neglected tropical diseases, and the availability of safe, highly efficacious and inexpensive drugs (at present usually donated by pharmaceutical companies) [42, 48–50]. These messages were reinforced at scientific meetings and symposia held at annual conferences of tropical medicine and hygiene societies. The launch of *PLoS Neglected Tropical Diseases* in October 2007 was also a milestone towards further raising the profile of the neglected tropical diseases (http://www.plosntds.org/). *PLoS Neglected Tropical Diseases* publishes original research on all aspects of the neglected tropical diseases, including epidemiology, diagnosis, pathogenesis, clinical features, pharmacology and treatment, vector biology, vaccinology and prevention. Cultural, demographic, ecological, economic and social determinants, public health, and policy aspects of the diseases are also considered. As of 10 June 2013, more than 2,000 papers had been published in *PLoS Neglected Tropical Diseases* and the journal has become the leader in tropical medicine [51].

As shown in Table 12.4, we discuss a total of 15 neglected tropical diseases which are endemic in East and Southeast Asia. The majority of these neglected tropical diseases are caused by helminths (schistosomiasis, soil-transmitted helminthiasis, food-borne trematodiasis, angiostrongyliasis, echinococcosis, cysticercosis and lymphatic filariasis). We include three viral infections (dengue, rabies and Japanese encephalitis), two bacterial infections (trachoma and leprosy) and one protozoal infection (leishmaniasis). Finally, we include malaria, which is caused by protozoa and not usually grouped with the neglected tropical diseases (see Table 12.4).

## Schistosomiasis

Schistosomiasis is a parasitic worm infection caused by blood flukes of the genus *Schistosoma*. Transmission occurs via skin penetration by the infective stage of the parasite (i.e. cercariae), usually during freshwater contact. Two species occur in Asia: *S. japonicum* affecting approximately one million people in P.R. China and the Philippines [52, 53] and a few thousand people in Indonesia [54], and *S. mekongi*, parasitizing an estimated 40,000 people in Cambodia and Lao PDR [55].

Experiences and lessons from the national schistosomiasis control programme in P.R. China are worth highlighting [56]. Indeed, efforts to control the 'plague of God' in this

*Table 12.4* List of neglected tropical diseases and malaria with their disease burden in 2010 and recent trends, stratified by region

| Disease | Southeast Asia | | | East Asia | | | Reference(s) |
|---|---|---|---|---|---|---|---|
| | No. of deaths | Burden (x 1000 DALYs) | Trend[a] | No. of deaths | Burden (x 1000 DALYs) | Trend[a] | |
| ***Helminth infection*** | | | | | | | |
| Schistosomiasis | 777 | 29 | ⇑ | 8,520 | 252 | ⇓ | (1, 2) |
| Soil-transmitted helminthiosis | 354 | | | 369 | | | |
| Ascariasis | n.d. | 303 | ⇓ | | 97 | ⇓ | (1, 2) |
| Trichuriasis | n.d. | 326 | ⇓ | | 14 | ⇓ | (1, 2) |
| Hookworm disease | n.d. | 573 | ⇓ | | 977 | ⇓ | (1, 2) |
| Strongyloidiasis | n.d. | n.d. | n.d. | n.d. | n.d. | n.d. | (40) |
| Food-borne trematodiasis | 1,808 | 164 | ⇑ | 4,925 | 1,599 | ⇑ | (1, 2) |
| Angiostrongyliasis | n.d. | n.d. | n.d. | n.d. | n.d. | n.d. | (77) |
| Echinococcosis | n.d. | n.d. | n.d. | 254 | 45 | ⇑ | (1, 2, 132) |
| Cysticercosis | 0 | 22 | ⇓ | 38 | 68 | ⇓ | (1, 2) |
| Lymphatic filariasis | 0 | 196 | ⇓ | n.d. | n.d. | n.d. | (1, 2) |
| ***Viral infection*** | | | | | | | |
| Dengue | 6,630 | 421 | ⇑ | 1,103 | 52 | ⇓ | (1, 2) |
| Rabies | 3,306 | 167 | ⇓ | 1,197 | 46 | ⇓ | (1, 2) |
| Japanese encephalitis | n.d. | 71 | n.d. | 158[b] | 20[b] | n.d. | (97, 133) |
| ***Bacterial infection*** | | | | | | | |
| Trachoma | 0 | <0.5 | n.a. | 0 | 40 | ⇑ | (1, 2) |
| Leprosy | n.d.[b] | <0.5 | n.a. | n.d. | <0.5 | n.a. | (1, 2, 32) |
| ***Protozoal infection*** | | | | | | | |
| Leishmaniasis | 304 | 18 | ⇓ | 1,845 | 111 | ⇓ | (1, 2) |
| Malaria | 45,118 | 2,311 | ⇓ | 58 | 12 | ⇓ | (1, 2) |

*Sources*: [1, 2].

*Notes*: DALYs, disability-adjusted life years; n.a., not applicable; n.d. not determined.

[a] Trend, in terms of DALYs, from 1990 to 2010.

[b] Estimates of deaths and DALYs for P.R. China only.

country have a history of more than sixty years. The political will and resources allocated for a multi-faceted, dynamic national control programme are unprecedented [57]. Thus far, *S. japonicum* has been eliminated in 7 of the 12 provinces where the disease was endemic, and the individual suffering and public health burden have been greatly reduced. Yet, schistosomiasis shows important temporal fluctuations, partially explained by changing patterns of coverage and intensity of interventions, coupled with climatic factors and environmental changes, such as floods and alteration in land-use patterns. Recent evidence suggests that an integrated control package consisting of chemotherapy, improved water supply and sanitation at the unit of the household, mechanization of agriculture, fencing of water buffaloes and health education can reduce the prevalence of infection in humans to below 1 per cent [58]. These experiences were made in the lake and marshland regions of central P.R. China and have encouraged the central government to adopt this approach as its national control strategy. Hence, the current goal is to achieve transmission control by 2015 (prevalence < 1 per cent), a goal that might be attained [59].

Given the clear geographical restriction of *S. japonicum* in Indonesia and the small endemic area, elimination could be feasible and hence should be tackled without delay. However, control of *S. japonicum* in the Philippines is a greater challenge because of the existence of a wider spectrum of reservoir hosts, particularly water buffaloes [60], but also rats, cats, pigs and dogs [61]. In a recent high-level meeting held in Lao PDR, researchers, disease control experts, and representatives of national and international organizations (e.g. WHO and Asian Development Bank) discussed prospects for the elimination of *S. mekongi* in Cambodia and Lao PDR.

## Soil-transmitted helminthiasis

Arguably, the three most prevalent parasitic worm infections in tropical and subtropical areas are the soil-transmitted helminths, roundworm (*Ascaris lumbricoides*), whipworm (*Trichuris trichiura*) and hookworm (*Ancylostoma duodenale* and *Necator americanus*). Simultaneous infections with two or more soil-transmitted helminths are commonly observed among people who live in poor or marginalized communities [62, 63]. More than one billion people are infected and the global burden is estimated at 5.2 million DALYs [2, 64]. In Asia, a comparison of data from 1994 and 2003 reveals that the prevalence and absolute numbers of soil-transmitted helminth infections have declined considerably. This is mainly attributed to control activities and general socio-economic development [65]. Using P.R. China as an example, the second national survey pertaining to parasitic diseases, in 2001–2004, revealed national prevalences of *A. lumbricoides*, hookworm and *T. trichiura* of 12.7 per cent, 6.1 per cent and 4.6 per cent, respectively. Compared to the first nationwide survey conducted in the late 1980s/early 1990s, the observed prevalences declined by more than 60 per cent for each of the three soil-transmitted helminth species [66].

Morbidity due to soil-transmitted helminth infections is often sub-clinical and ranges from abdominal pain, dysentery and physiological abnormalities in the intestinal tract to pruritus, skin eruptions, and impaired physical and cognitive development and performance. To control morbidity due to chronic soil-transmitted helminth infections, the WHO recommends the periodic administration of the deworming drugs albendazole or mebendazole to at-risk populations, most importantly school-aged children. This strategy has been termed 'preventive chemotherapy' in consideration of its potential to prevent chronic morbidity and other negative outcomes mentioned above [67]. However, preventive chemotherapy is unable to prevent re-infections, and hence, it is essential to combine deworming with interventions targeting the transmission of infections, e.g. health education focusing on proper personal and food hygiene, supply of safe water and improved sanitation [68, 69]. These interventions are subsumed under the acronym WASH (i.e. water, sanitation and hygiene). These non-chemotherapeutic interventions should be combined with sustained efforts to address under-nutrition, further cognitive development, and address other deficits resulting from – and possibly also promoting – soil-transmitted helminth infections [70].

## Food-borne trematodiasis

Food-borne trematodiasis is a cluster of zoonotic infections caused by liver flukes (e.g. *Clonorchis sinensis*, *Fasciola* spp. and *Opisthorchis* spp.), lung flukes (e.g. *Paragonimus* spp.) and intestinal flukes (e.g. *Echinostoma* spp.). Transmission occurs via the ingestion of raw or undercooked aquatic foodstuff (e.g. freshwater fish, crabs and water plants). More than one billion people are estimated to be at risk of infection and 56 million people were infected in 2005, mainly in Asia and Latin America [71]. The global burden due to food-borne trematodiasis has been estimated at between 0.7 and 1.9 million DALYs [2, 72]. Food-borne trematodiasis is associated with a variety of signs, symptoms and pathologies which depend on the fluke species and the intensity of infection. The most severe clinical outcome of a chronic infection with the liver flukes *Opisthorchis viverrini* (in Lao PDR and Thailand) and *C. sinensis* (in P.R. China) is cholangiocarcinoma, cancer of the bile duct [73].

Food-borne trematodiasis is an emerging public health issue, partially explained by the exponential growth of freshwater aquaculture [74]. In P.R. China, for example, the number of infections with *C. sinensis* has tripled in recent years [75]. A recent outbreak of fascioliasis (due to infection with *Fasciola gigantica*) has been documented in Yunnan province in south-western P.R. China [76]. The habit of raw food consumption is culturally deeply rooted in many parts of Asia, which is a key driver in maintaining the transmission of food-borne trematodiasis. Hence, concerted action is required to control food-borne trematodiasis, including setting-specific information, education and communication (IEC) strategies [71, 73].

## Angiostrongyliasis

Angiostrongyliasis, caused by an infection with the rat lung worm, *Angiostrongylus cantonensis*, is characterized by eosinophilic meningitis. The nematode worm is transmitted between rats and molluscs. Humans occasionally acquire an infection through consumption of raw snails harbouring third stage larvae ($L_3$) of *A. cantonensis*. Southeast Asia is considered the original home range of angiostrongyliasis. Although infections have first been described in the mid-1940s, the bio-invasion of the snails *Pomacea* spp. and *Achatina fulica* drove the emergence of angiostrongyliasis in the region [77]. For example, more than three-quarters of human cases are definitively attributed to these invasive snails in P.R. China [78]. Since 1997, nine outbreaks due to the consumption of snails have been documented in P.R. China. A total of 336 human cases were involved in these outbreaks.

Angiostrongyliasis is truly neglected and a key reason is the lack of sensitive diagnostic tools [77]. Conventional parasitological diagnosis rests on the discovery of the young worms from cerebrospinal fluid, but this diagnosis is rarely performed. In view of the global distribution of definitive hosts (*Rattus rattus* and *R. norvegicus*), the key intermediate host of *A. cantonensis* (i.e. *Pomacea* spp. and *A. fulica*) may play an increasingly important role in the transmission of angiostrongyliasis. Indeed, recent modelling studies suggest that the expanded range of the snails, along with wider distances food is being transported, will place many more people at risk. Climate change is an important determinant that governs the distribution of such invasive snails and predictions for P.R. China show considerable expansion of climate suitability areas for the snails in twenty years from now [79].

## Echinococcosis

Echinococcosis (hydatid disease) is caused by the larval stages of cestodes (tapeworms) of which the definitive hosts are wild and domestic canids (foxes and dogs). The two major species that infect humans are *Echinococcus granulosus* and *E. multilocularis*, which manifest themselves as cystic echinococcosis (CE) and alveolar echinococcosis (AE). Herbivores and rodents are the usual hosts of the cystic stages. Once the larval stage emerges from an ingested egg, a hydatid cyst develops and enlarges over time. Cysts are mainly located in the liver and lungs and the severity of the disease in humans is dependent on the location, size and type of the cyst, as well as their number. Death can ensue if the disease is not managed properly [80].

In P.R. China, *E. granulosus* is endemic in at least 21 of the 31 provinces and autonomous regions. The highest prevalences are found in Xinjiang, Qinghai, Gansu, Ningxia, Inner Mongolia, Tibet and parts of Sichuan and Yunnan. Limited information is available for Mongolia even though CE is suspected to be a public health problem in this country. On the other hand, only sporadic CE cases have been recorded in Lao PDR, Thailand, Vietnam, Malaysia, Indonesia and the Philippines. Likewise, the distribution of AE is restricted to Xinjiang, Qinghai, Gansu, Ningxia, Inner Mongolia, Sichuan and Tibet [81].

In terms of interventions for their control, screening and subsequent treatment of human populations, treatment of dogs four to five times a year with praziquantel, and health education to increase awareness for the disease, are important strategies. In P.R. China, these interventions resulted in the number of seropositives dropping from 2.4 per cent in 2008 to 0.3 per cent in 2010 in Sichuan province. A long-term national prevention and control programme has been further extended to the north-western parts of the country in 2010 [82]. Control efforts are especially important in poor and marginalized populations, as a recent study showed the true socio-economic impact of echinococcosis in poor underdeveloped rural communities [83]. AE has also been linked to changing land-use patterns as a result of agricultural change on the rodent populations (which host the cysts) and wild canid hosts. Transmission and resultant human disease was more effectively predicted from landscape features that supported increases of small mammal host species that were prone to population outbreaks, rather than host species richness. It has therefore been suggested that landscape management and climate can be utilized to predict disease risk to control this disease [84, 85].

## Cysticercosis

Cysticercosis occurs if humans take the place of pigs in the natural life cycle of the pork tapeworm *Taenia solium*, which depends on humans for its reproductive stage and on pigs for the larval stage. Poor hygiene and sanitation, and the use of 'night soil' in agriculture, can result in the ingestion of *T. solium* eggs by humans in whom the cysticerci then develop, most often in muscles but also in other organs including the brain and eyes.

Neurocysticercosis (i.e. the development of cysticerci in the central nervous system) can cause epilepsy and is the most serious form of the disease. Thailand, Vietnam, Lao PDR, the

Philippines, Cambodia, P.R. China, and parts of Malaysia and Indonesia – essentially everywhere where pork is consumed – are known to be endemic for cysticercosis. No data are available for Myanmar [86].

Control strategies mainly aim at the prevention of human infections through improved hygiene behaviour and a reduction of the environmental contamination with human faeces, which contain the eggs of *T. solium* or at least access of pigs to human faeces. This is achieved through improved farm management that prevents the consumption of contaminated feed or water by the animals. Taeniasis control, for example, through meat inspection to identify and impound infected pig carcasses according to the Joint Food and Agriculture Organization (FAO) and the WHO Food Standards Programme also reduces the number of eggs in the environment.

## Lymphatic filariasis

Lymphatic filariasis is caused by three parasites transmitted by several genera of mosquitoes. The predominant parasite in East and Southeast Asia is *Wuchereria bancrofti*, but *Brugia malayi* and *B. timori* also cause disabling and debilitating disease. Lymphatic filariasis is the subject of a global elimination campaign spearheaded by the strategy of preventive chemotherapy. This disease is one of the most disabling of all infectious conditions and has been suggested as an indicator of poverty as it occurs in both urban and rural settings [87, 88].

Currently in Asia, several countries have active programmes using annual treatment with albendazole and diethylcarbamazine (DEC) to reduce the microfilaria loads in order to reduce transmission. The annual treatment is given over a five- to seven-year period. The latest WHO report shows the number of treatments targeting lymphatic filariasis in endemic countries for 2011 and the status of the programmes [89]. Vietnam and Cambodia have stopped mass drug distribution following several years of treatment, whilst preventive chemotherapy is continuing in Malaysia, Lao PDR and the Philippines where 19.4 million people were treated in 2011. However, the biggest success in the region was the historic programme carried out in P.R. China over a period of 40 years starting in 1949 culminating in the certification by the WHO of the absence of active transmission in a population of some 350 million people. These efforts are summarized in a 230-page seminal piece published by the WHO Western Pacific Regional Office in 2003 [90]. However, the initial strategy used in P.R. China was based on treatment of microfilaraemic individuals with DEC as well as integrated vector control. The strategy of the use of DEC medicated salt was introduced in the 1970s to reduce the febrile reactions produced by DEC, an approach facilitated by the existence of a commercial network for salt distribution. DEC medicated salt was found to produce no fever or other adverse events. These efforts on a large scale resulted in cessation of transmission over wide areas as supported and validated by extensive monitoring and surveillance. This success provided a platform for later global efforts, initiated by WHA resolution 50.29 and put forth in May 1997, to aim for the elimination of lymphatic filariasis as a public health problem by 2020. Later on, this resolution was followed by a decision of GlaxoSmithKline (GSK) to donate albendazole for a global programme, while, in Africa ivermectin, donated by Merck & Co. Inc. At present over 500 million annual treatments are given globally for lymphatic filariasis in more than 50 countries. However, a major problem remains, as many at-risk in Indonesia are still to be treated, although the programme is expanding in Myanmar with a high coverage of those treated to date [91].

## Viral infection: dengue, rabies and Japanese encephalitis

Mosquito-borne viral infections provide amongst the most important examples of emerging diseases of global significance. Of particular note are dengue and Japanese encephalitis – indeed, dengue is the most rapidly spreading mosquito-borne viral disease in the world. Over the past 50 years, the incidence has increased thirty-fold with increasing geographic expansion to new countries and, most recently, from urban to rural settings. An estimated 50 million dengue infections occur annually and approximately 2.5 billion people live in dengue-endemic countries. Some 1.8 billion (more than 70 per cent) of the population at risk for dengue worldwide live in member states of the WHO Southeast Asian Region and the Western Pacific Region, which bear nearly 75 per cent of the current global disease burden due to dengue [92]. The spread of *Aedes aegypti* is the leading cause for the epidemic of dengue in the world. Initially, this mosquito species was spread around the world via sailing ships at the time of shipping industry and commerce. World War II dramatically changed the global epidemiology and transmission dynamics of dengue. Vector control programmes can significantly influence the transmission of dengue. For example, dengue was absent from the Americas before the 1970s, when there was intensive vector control against yellow fever. However, mosquitoes invaded many countries from the 1970s onwards, coinciding with control programmes being abandoned, and hence, dengue started to occur and spread accompanied by the urbanization in the Asian region and the associated expansion of breeding sites (artificial containers) [93]. Climate change is an important determinant that might explain the expanding range of mosquitoes carrying the dengue virus [94]. The exponential growth in international travel of people and goods (e.g. used tyres) contributes to the epidemiological pattern of dengue [95].

Japanese encephalitis was first reported in Japan in the 1920s before it expanded to Korea and eastern P.R. China in the 1950s. In the meantime, Japanese encephalitis has become endemic in large parts of Asia and the Pacific and is transmitted by the mosquito *Culex tritaeniorhynchus*, and there are signs of further geographical spread into new territories. More than 3 billion people are at risk of Japanese encephalitis, the disease affects over 50,000 people and might result in 15,000 deaths per year [96]. Due to the availability of an effective vaccine, improved living standards and mechanized agriculture, Japanese encephalitis has declined considerably in Japan and South Korea. However, transmission is likely to increase in other parts of East and Southeast Asia because of population growth, expanded agriculture and lack of vaccination programmes [97], whilst control is constrained by the presence of animal reservoirs (e.g. pigs) and birds (especially herons).

Rabies caused by the bite of an infected dog occurs in more than 150 countries and territories. Although the prevalence has declined in the recent past, there are more than 4,000 deaths due to rabies in East and Southeast Asia every year (see Table 12.4). There is an active rabies control programme in the Philippines. It is facilitated thanks to more than 300 treatment centres providing increased access to free post-exposure prophylaxis immunization, complemented with a multi-sectoral approach based on dog vaccinations, vaccinating high-risk groups (i.e. school-aged children) in endemic areas, improving health education and promoting responsible pet ownership. The establishment of rabies-free zones is part of such a process as the country seeks to become rabies free by 2020 [98].

## Bacterial infection: trachoma and leprosy

Trachoma is caused by ocular infections with *Chlamydia trachomatis* that might result in chronic inflammation of the eye lids, which is the leading cause of infectious blindness worldwide, particularly in children aged 1 to 5 years and women. Trachoma is most prevalent where extreme poverty persists, characterized by limited access to healthcare services and clean water. Trachoma is considered to be endemic in 57 countries. In the Southeast Asia region discussed here, Myanmar and Vietnam are reported to have achieved trachoma elimination targets and are undertaking surveillance, but Cambodia has yet to define its strategy, whilst Lao PDR is evaluating progress to date of its control and elimination programme. P.R. China plans to launch its programme with the objective of eliminating trachoma by 2020 [99, 100]. The SAFE strategy (i.e. surgery, antibiotics, facial cleanliness and environmental improvement) has been endorsed by the WHO for the elimination of blinding trachoma. The antibiotic azithromycin ('Zithromax') as an oral dose given annually has been the important driver of the expansion of global trachoma programmes and is donated by Pfizer. Importantly, the SAFE strategy has ancillary benefits on other neglected tropical diseases, most importantly soil-transmitted helminthiasis and intestinal protozoa infections.

Leprosy, also known as Hansen's disease, is a chronic infection caused by *Mycobacterium leprae* and *M. lepromatosis*. This disease remains endemic in Africa, Latin America and Asia. According to a report by the WHO, there are still 200,000–400,000 newly detected cases annually [101]. Eighteen countries are currently considered to have incidence rates of more than 1,000 new cases per year, of which eight are in Asia, including P.R. China, Indonesia, Myanmar and the Philippines.

## Leishmaniasis

Leishmaniasis is caused by protozoan parasites of the genus *Leishmania* that are transmitted through the bites of phlebotomine sandflies (*Phlebotomus*). The four major clinical presentations are: (i) the cutaneous form, most frequently observed in infected patients and presenting as a skin ulcer at the bite site. These lesions usually heal with time, leaving a disfiguring permanent scar, but might also progress to any of the following three forms: (ii) the diffuse cutaneous form, which is difficult to treat as it is characterized by disseminated and chronic skin lesions, resembling leprosy; (iii) the mucocutaneous form damaging the mucous membranes, often in the mouth, nose and throat cavities; and (iv) the visceral form (kala azar) which is the most serious manifestation and presents as high fever, weight loss, swelling of the spleen and liver and anaemia. Death might result if proper treatment is not given [102]. The disease has a complex epidemiology and ecology, and incidence data are difficult to obtain although WHO estimates suggest a global incidence of cutaneous disease at 1.2 million new cases per year. Recent estimates put the annual number of reported visceral leishmaniasis cases in P.R. China and Thailand at 378 and 2, respectively. Importantly, outbreaks result in major fluctuations in case numbers between years. For example, a total of 268 visceral leishmaniasis cases were recorded in Jiashi county, Xinjiang Uyghur autonomous region between January 2008 and May 2009 alone [103]. No cutaneous leishmaniasis cases have been reported in the other East and Southeast Asian countries covered by our chapter [104].

Active surveillance, treatment of infected individuals and the use of insecticide-treated nets reduce the number of human reservoir hosts and transmission. Likewise, the number of canine reservoir hosts should be limited by the screening and treatment or culling of seropositive dogs. Indeed, historically, P.R. China used culling of dogs to control visceral disease. Finally, vector control with insecticides or through environmental management, but ideally integrated approaches targeting different vector-borne diseases simultaneously, reduce transmission through the suppression of sandfly populations, and when malaria control has been initiated, sandfly vectors have also been controlled [105]. Leishmaniasis is less of a public health problem in the region under discussion. It should be noted, however, that control, where it occurs, is difficult as there is limited awareness of the disease. Indeed, leishmaniasis often occurs in the visceral form, which is particularly difficult to diagnose.

### Malaria

Malaria is an infectious disease caused by protozoan parasites (i.e. *Plasmodium*), which are transmitted by female *Anopheles* mosquitoes. Among the five *Plasmodium* species parasitizing man, *P. falciparum* is the most virulent and is responsible for most of the malaria-related deaths, particularly in children up to 5 years of age in sub-Saharan Africa. *P. vivax* and *P. ovale* are less virulent but the ability of these parasites to remain dormant in the liver makes them difficult to be resolved in the host [106]. According to the *World malaria report 2011*, malaria transmission occurs in all the countries in East and Southeast Asia discussed here, with the exception of Mongolia [107]. Interestingly, some hundred years ago, the bulk of the global malaria burden was concentrated in Asia [108]. Nowadays, *P. vivax* in Southeast Asia is responsible for up to 50 per cent of clinical malaria cases due to this species [16]. The public health importance of *P. vivax* has been exacerbated by the spread of resistance to widely used antimalarial drugs (e.g. chloroquine and sulfadoxine/pyrimethamine) over large parts of Southeast Asia. New research has shown that *P. knowlesi* is a zoonotic infection of humans occasionally acquired from monkeys in Malaysia [109].

Historically, there is a long list of chemotherapeutic agents used for the treatment of malaria. At present, artemisinin-based combination therapy (ACT), a combination of artemisinin derivatives with other active antimalarial medication, is the most effective form of treatment as studies have shown that using two or more drugs in combination has the potential to delay the development of resistance [110]. On the Thailand–Myanmar border, there is a well-known hotspot of multi-drug resistant *P. falciparum* [111], and hence, the artemisinins remain the only effective antimalarial drugs there. The recent emergence of artemisinin resistance in the border areas of Thailand with Myanmar and Cambodia is thus of utmost public health concern [112].

While high malaria incidence rates have been reported from 24 out of the 31 provinces of P.R. China several decades ago, in 2010, the country embarked on a programme to eliminate malaria. The goal is to interrupt malaria transmission by 2015 with the exception of the border areas of Yunnan province due to the challenge of cross-border transmission. There, malaria elimination is scheduled for 2020. Importantly, large-scale control activities facilitated through primary healthcare networks and strong community participation already achieved elimination of *P. falciparum* malaria in P.R. China, except in the provinces of Yunnan and Hainan. *P. vivax* has therefore become the predominant species. A key strategy of the national elimination programme is the establishment of effective surveillance–response systems that are tailored to the local transmission patterns [14, 113].

## Major drivers of global change

### *General considerations*

The growth of the human population and increases in per capita levels of consumption, coupled with the interconnectedness of contemporary human activities, are the principal drivers of global change [114–116]. Such human domination of the biosphere resulting from agricultural intensification, land clearance, habitat degradation and fragmentation, urban expansion and industrialization is historically unprecedented, and has far-reaching consequences for global atmospheric and hydrological systems, as well as chemical flows and balances. Together, the changes have started to disrupt many of the ecosystems and the services they provide [33]. Such changes are complex, have a myriad of consequences as they adversely impact ecological systems and therefore threaten the foundations of human health and livelihood, such as food yields, water availability, quality of the air, soil and water, constraints on infectious disease outbreaks, and buffers against extreme weather and environmental events [33]. However, the implications of these drivers of global change on the frequency and transmission dynamics of chronic neglected diseases of poverty and other issues of health and livelihood are exceedingly hard to predict and quantify.

### *Population growth, urbanization and industrialization*

Towards the end of 2011, the world's human population exceeded 7 billion [117]. Population growth continues at a rapid pace and predictions for the year 2050 suggest that the population will have grown to 9 billion. Most of the recent, current and future population growth is concentrated in developing countries, particularly in the urban areas. Indeed, in 2009, for the first time in human history, more people were estimated to live in urban rather than rural settings. Table 12.5 shows the development over the past twenty years in terms of total population growth and the proportion of people living in urban settings in the ten selected countries of East and Southeast Asia. Particularly high population growth over the past twenty years has occurred in Malaysia, the Philippines, Cambodia and Lao PDR as the total population of these countries grew between 48 per cent and 56 per cent. The lowest rate of growth was observed in P.R. China (+ 17.1 per cent), but given the high population in this country,

*Table 12.5* Changes in total population and percentage of population residing in urban areas between 1990 and 2010 in ten selected countries of East and Southeast Asia

| *Region* / *Country* | *Total population (thousands)* | | | *Population residing in urban areas (%)* | | |
|---|---|---|---|---|---|---|
| | *1990* | *2010* | *Difference (%)* | *1990* | *2010* | *Difference (%)* |
| ***East Asia*** | | | | | | |
| Mongolia | 2,193 | 2,756 | +25.7 | 57.0 | 67.6 | +18.4 |
| P.R. China | 1,145,195 | 1,341,335 | +17.1 | 26.4 | 49.2 | +86.2 |
| ***Southeast Asia*** | | | | | | |
| Cambodia | 9,532 | 14,138 | +48.3 | 15.5 | 19.8 | +27.5 |
| Indonesia | 184,346 | 239,871 | +30.1 | 30.6 | 49.9 | +63.2 |
| Lao PDR | 4,192 | 6,201 | +47.9 | 15.4 | 33.1 | +114.6 |
| Malaysia | 18,209 | 28,401 | +56.0 | 49.8 | 72.0 | +44.6 |
| Myanmar | 39,268 | 47,963 | +22.1 | 24.6 | 32.1 | +30.4 |
| Philippines | 61,629 | 93,261 | +51.3 | 48.6 | 48.6 | +0.1 |
| Thailand | 57,072 | 69,122 | +21.1 | 29.4 | 33.7 | +14.6 |
| Vietnam | 67,102 | 87,848 | +30.9 | 20.3 | 30.4 | +50.1 |

*Source*: [135].

in absolute numbers, this represents the largest absolute increase in the number of people in all countries considered here. With regard to the proportion of people residing in urban areas, many of the focus countries have approached the 50 per cent level in 2010 (Indonesia, 49.9 per cent; P.R. China, 49.2 per cent; and the Philippines, 48.6 per cent). The lowest proportion of urban dwellers is currently registered in Cambodia (19.8 per cent), followed by Vietnam (30.4 per cent) (see Table 12.5).

Figure 12.1, a picture from Shanghai in 2008, illustrates the transformation of a traditional Asian city of relatively limited size into a modern megacity. Its population grew exponentially from approximately 1 million in 1900 to over 23 million in 2010. Figure 12.2 shows the construction site of the power station, the tailrace channel and the regulating pond of the Nam Theun 2 hydroelectric project in rural central Lao PDR in the midst of construction activities in 2008. Rapid industrialization and urbanization has resulted in massive demographic, environmental and social transformations, and it is evident that these changes have major ramifications on public health, with NCDs rapidly replacing infectious diseases as the main issues of burden of disease, a process often driven by changes in lifestyle choices, nutrition and, not least, air, soil and water pollution that is concentrated in urban and peri-urban environments [118–120]. The release of chemical toxins into the urban environment, dumping of industrial waste without prior consent and traffic-related accidents are additional issues that worsen the quality of the urban environment and represent major public health threats for urban dwellers [118–120].

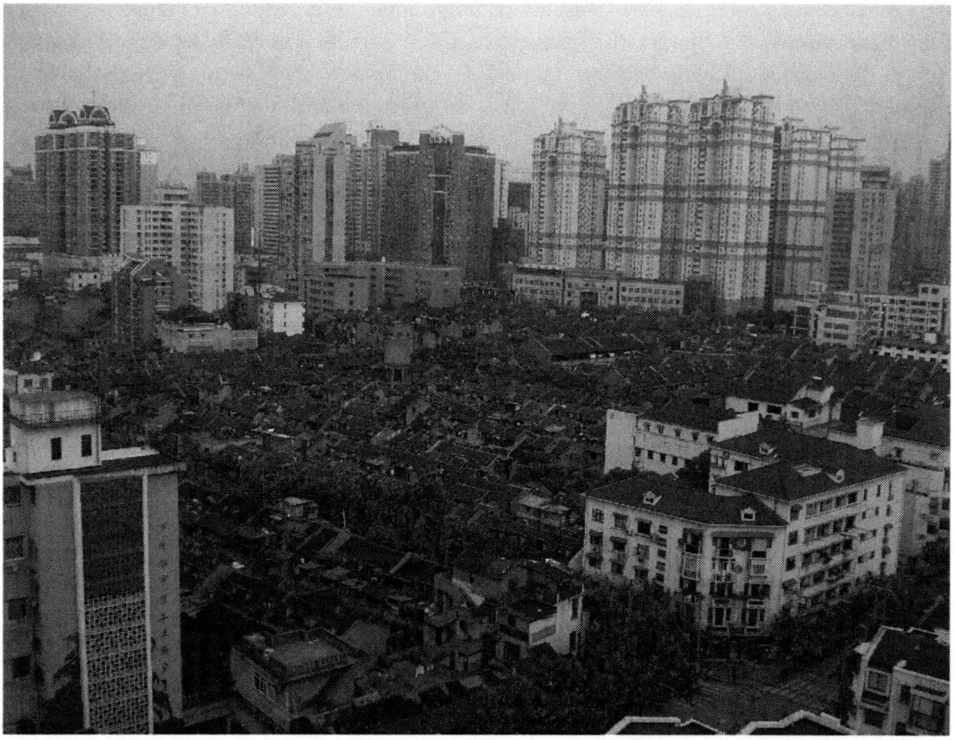

*Figure 12.1* Snapshot picture of Shanghai, P.R. China in 2008. Photo: P. Steinmann

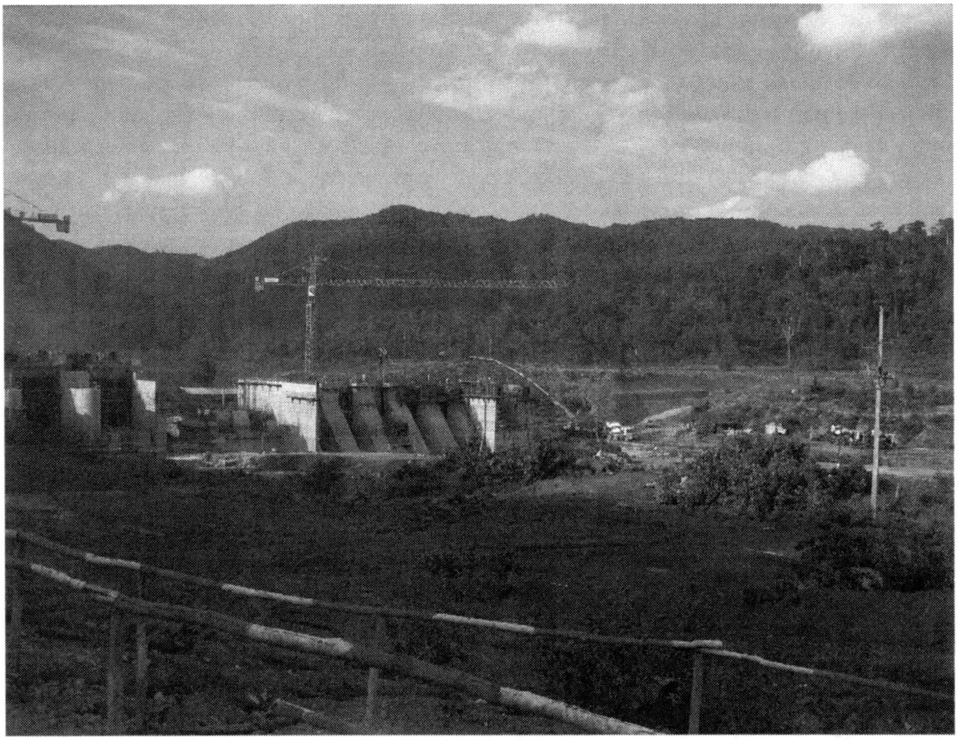

*Figure 12.2* Construction work at the power station, tailrace channel and regulating pond of the Nam Theun 2 hydroelectric project in rural central Lao PDR in 2008. Photo: J. Utzinger

### *Climate change*

There is growing evidence that suggests that climate change already adversely affects crop yields and nutrient content, and hence local economies, food availability and security, and global food prices [121, 122] (see also Chapter 20). Climate change is therefore likely to exacerbate poverty, and thus jeopardize progress towards reaching the MDGs and the post-2015 era of sustainable development. Indeed, since poverty and under-nutrition are inextricably linked with many infectious and non-infectious diseases that in turn lead to poor nutrition, this development further 'locks in' poverty [33]. Potential impacts of climate change and land use on the epidemiology of chronic neglected diseases of poverty, including case studies pertaining to schistosomiasis, angiostrongyliasis, AE and malaria in P.R. China, have been discussed elsewhere [14, 79, 85, 123, 124].

## Challenges ahead

There are two major challenges regarding the control and elimination of the diseases we discussed in this chapter. First, the recognition of the conditions themselves as drivers of poverty by national authorities, particularly as disabling conditions which disproportionately affect the poorest of the poor. Second, the drain such avoidable and preventable conditions have had not only on the health systems, but also on the individual, the household and the community in terms of workforce and economic loss, and thus the loss of ability of individuals to realize their full potential. Additionally, families are often confronted by medical expenses, which push them into the poverty trap as urgent medical care drives families into debt and irreversible poverty. The stress on health systems will also increase as climate change creates more severe and unpredictable weather events at increased frequency, often with catastrophic consequences as seen in recent flood and typhoon disasters in the region. The long-term impact on the epidemiology of infectious diseases, including chronic neglected diseases of poverty that such events have, has yet to be investigated, whilst the impact of explosive urban growth and rapid industrialization is generating widespread pollution with consequences for chronic NCDs at a scale and over a time period which remains to be projected [120]. In addition, changes of diet and lifestyle choices associated with urban living will also have long-term health consequences, in particular obesity and diabetes [121]. Particularly in the built-up urban environment, there is a growing overlap of traditional, modern and emerging environmental dilemmas, and a deeper understanding of their interactions is needed to implement setting-specific actions [118].

The transmission and epidemiology of the chronic neglected diseases discussed here are well recognized in East and Southeast Asia, and the strategies for their control are well established. The region also offers remarkable examples of how these diseases can be addressed when there is sustained political will and adequate resources are deployed – schistosomiasis in P.R. China and Cambodia, lymphatic filariasis in P.R. China and Vietnam, rabies in the Philippines and trachoma in Myanmar – are compelling examples [53, 55, 57, 125–128]. The progress towards the elimination of some of these infections has been impressive, but there remains the challenge of sustained resourcing, of raising the level of prioritization of the conditions to increase the commitment of national governments to implement appropriate policies and the need for increased human capacity to allow the implementation of programmes within decentralized health systems. Allied to this are requirements for targeted research as outlined in the recent WHO/TDR reports on infectious diseases of poverty, which will allow further improvement of the existing interventions [20, 32, 33]. These challenges, together with rapid population growth and industrialization, must be overcome while acknowledging that resources for health are constrained by the rapidly increasing need for ever more costly interventions to address the emerging non-communicable conditions driven by lifestyle changes and the threat of the emergence of pandemic viruses, such as severe acute respiratory syndrome (SARS), H5N1, Nipah, among others, which often originate from this region and require urgent attention as soon as they are recognized [129–131]. Both of these pressures on the health systems – one chronic, the other acute – challenge the capacity of the healthcare system to embark on elimination initiatives targeting neglected chronic diseases despite the availability of cheap tools, often via donated drugs. However, the non-technical approaches of high-quality health education and particularly safe water supply and improved sanitation, often not motivated by public health considerations but rather convenience and modernization, remain fundamental to improve population health.

## Conclusion

Our chapter provides some insights into chronic neglected diseases in East and Southeast Asia and their intimate connection with poverty. Most importantly, we hope that our chapter will inform students, public health experts, policy makers and disease control managers about recent progress made towards control and local elimination of certain chronic neglected diseases, important challenges that remain and new threats that might emerge as a result of major global drivers of change. Infectious agents and their vectors and intermediate hosts display a recognized ability to evolve rapidly in the face of environmental pressures; the rate of change and the implications of which are not predictable. The current capacity of health services to respond to that change is limited. The need will remain for awareness that in the decades to come flexible deployment of both existing and new tools for the control or elimination of neglected diseases of poverty is necessary. Such interventions are feasible, but strategies need to be adaptable to the many variables that will increase the complexity of the social, political and economic environment upon which the drivers of global change will impinge.

## References


1. Lozano R, Naghavi M, Foreman K, Lim S, Shibuya K, Aboyans V, *et al.* Global and regional mortality from 235 causes of death for 20 age groups in 1990 and 2010: a systematic analysis for the Global Burden of Disease Study 2010. *Lancet* 2012; 380(9859): 2095–128.
2. Murray CJL, Vos T, Lozano R, Naghavi M, Flaxman AD, Michaud C, *et al.* Disability-adjusted life years (DALYs) for 291 diseases and injuries in 21 regions, 1990–2010: a systematic analysis for the Global Burden of Disease Study 2010. *Lancet* 2012; 380(9859): 2197–223.
3. Barros AJD, Ronsmans C, Axelson H, Loaiza E, Bertoldi AD, Franca GVA, *et al.* Equity in maternal, newborn, and child health interventions in Countdown to 2015: a retrospective review of survey data from 54 countries. *Lancet* 2012; 379(9822): 1225–33.
4. Bleich SN, Jarlenski MP, Bell CN, LaVeist TA. Health inequalities: trends, progress, and policy. *Annu Rev Public Health* 2012; 33: 7–40.
5. Di Cesare M, Khang YH, Asaria P, Blakely T, Cowan MJ, Farzadfar F, *et al.* Inequalities in non-communicable diseases and effective responses. *Lancet* 2013; 381(9866): 585–97.
6. Molyneux DH. Combating the 'other diseases' of MDG 6: changing the paradigm to achieve equity and poverty reduction? *Trans R Soc Trop Med Hyg* 2008; 102(6): 509–19.
7. Hotez PJ, Fenwick A, Savioli L, Molyneux DH. Rescuing the bottom billion through control of neglected tropical diseases. *Lancet* 2009; 373(9674): 1570–5.
8. Molyneux DH, Malecela MN. Neglected tropical diseases and the millennium development goals: why the 'other diseases' matter: reality versus rhetoric. *Parasit Vectors* 2011; 4: 234.
9. Horton R. GBD 2010: understanding disease, injury, and risk. *Lancet* 2012; 380(9859): 2053–4.
10. WHO. *Macroeconomics and health: investing in health for economic development.* Geneva: World Health Organization; 2001.
11. Vitoria M, Granich R, Gilks CF, Gunneberg C, Hosseini M, Were W, *et al.* The global fight against HIV/AIDS, tuberculosis, and malaria: current status and future perspectives. *Am J Clin Pathol* 2009; 131(6): 844–8.
12. Lau J, *et al.*, Reflections on public health challenges for the HIV epidemic among men who have sex with men in China. *Routledge Handbook of Global Public Health in Asia.* Abingdon, UK; 2014, 212–29.
13. Walley J, Wei, X. Tuberculosis control in Asia: the case of China. *Routledge Handbook of Global Public Health in Asia.* Abingdon, UK; 2014, 230–9.
14. Yang G-J, Zhou X-N. Climate change and its impact on the patterns of disease: malaria in the People's Republic of China as a case study. *Routledge Handbook of Global Public Health in Asia.* Abingdon, UK; 2014, 265–74
15. Mendis K, Sina BJ, Marchesini P, Carter R. The neglected burden of *Plasmodium vivax* malaria. *Am J Trop Med Hyg* 2001; 64(1–2 Suppl): 97–106.
16. Price RN, Tjitra E, Guerra CA, Yeung S, White NJ, Anstey NM. Vivax malaria: neglected and not benign. *Am J Trop Med Hyg* 2007; 77(6 Suppl): 79–87.
17. Mueller I, Galinski MR, Baird JK, Carlton JM, Kochar DK, Alonso PL, *et al.* Key gaps in the knowledge of *Plasmodium vivax*, a neglected human malaria parasite. *Lancet Infect Dis* 2009; 9(9): 555–66.
18. Guerra CA, Howes RE, Patil AP, Gething PW, Van Boeckel TP, Temperley WH, *et al.* The international limits and population at risk of *Plasmodium vivax* transmission in 2009. *PLoS Negl Trop Dis* 2010; 4(8): e774.

19. Murray CJL, Ezzati M, Flaxman AD, Lim S, Lozano R, Michaud C, *et al.* GBD 2010: design, definitions, and metrics. *Lancet* 2012; 380(9859): 2063–6.
20. WHO. *Global report for research on infectious diseases of poverty.* Geneva: World Health Organization on behalf of the Special Programme for Research and Training in Tropical Diseases; 2012.
21. World Bank. *World Development Report 1993: investing in health.* New York: Oxford University Press; 1993.
22. Bendavid E, Bhattacharya J. The President's Emergency Plan for AIDS Relief in Africa: an evaluation of outcomes. *Ann Intern Med* 2009; 150(10): 688–95.
23. Global Fund. *The Global Fund 2010: innovation and impact.* Geneva: The Global Fund to Fight AIDS, Tuberculosis and Malaria; 2010.
24. Shiffman J. Has donor prioritization of HIV/AIDS displaced aid for other health issues? *Health Policy Plan* 2008; 23(2): 95–100.
25. Fenwick A, Molyneux D, Nantulya V. Achieving the Millennium Development Goals. *Lancet* 2005; 365(9464): 1029–30.
26. WHO. *Neglected tropical diseases: hidden successes, emerging opportunities.* Geneva: World Health Organization; 2006.
27. United Nations. *A new global partnership: eradicate poverty and transform economies through sustainable development.* New York: United Nations; 2013.
28. Molyneux D, Hallaj Z, Keusch GT, McManus DP, Ngowi H, Cleaveland S, *et al.* Zoonoses and marginalised infectious diseases of poverty: where do we stand? *Parasit Vectors* 2011; 4: 106.
29. Butler CD. Infectious disease emergence and global change: thinking systemically in a shrinking world. *Infect Dis Poverty* 2012; 1: 5.
30. Lustigman S, Prichard RK, Gazzinelli A, Grant WN, Boatin BA, McCarthy JS, *et al.* A research agenda for helminth diseases of humans: the problem of helminthiases. *PLoS Negl Trop Dis* 2012; 6(4): e1582.
31. Utzinger J. A research and development agenda for the control and elimination of human helminthiases. *PLoS Negl Trop Dis* 2012; 6(4): e1646.
32. WHO. Research priorities for zoonoses and marginalized infections: technical report of the TDR Disease Reference Group on Zoonoses and Marginalized Infectious Diseases of Poverty. *WHO Tech Rep Ser* 2012; 971: 1–119.
33. WHO. Research priorities for the environment, agriculture and infectious diseases of poverty: technical report of the TDR Thematic Reference Group on Environment, Agriculture and Infectious Diseases of Poverty. *WHO Tech Rep Ser* 2013; 976: 1–125.
34. Worrall E, Basu S, Hanson K. Is malaria a disease of poverty? A review of the literature. *Trop Med Int Health* 2005; 10(10): 1047–59.
35. Castro MC, Fisher MG. Is malaria illness among young children a cause or a consequence of low socioeconomic status? Evidence from the United Republic of Tanzania. *Malar J* 2012; 11: 161.
36. Gallup JL, Sachs JD. The economic burden of malaria. *Am J Trop Med Hyg* 2001; 64 (1–2 Suppl): 85–96.
37. Roll Back Malaria Partnership. *The global malaria action plan: for a malaria free world.* Geneva: Roll Back Malaria Partnership; 2008.
38. Tusting LS, Willey B, Lucas H, Thompson J, Kafy HT, Smith R, *et al.* Socioeconomic development as an intervention against malaria: a systematic review and meta-analysis. *Lancet* 2013; 382(9896): 963–72.
39. Molyneux DH. The 'Neglected Tropical Diseases': now a brand identity; responsibilities, context and promise. *Parasit Vectors* 2012; 5: 23.
40. Utzinger J, Becker SL, Knopp S, Blum J, Neumayr AL, Keiser J, *et al.* Neglected tropical diseases: diagnosis, clinical management, treatment and control. *Swiss Med Wkly* 2012; 142: w13727.
41. WHO. Intensified control of neglected diseases: report of an international workshop, Berlin, 10–12 December 2003. Geneva: World Health Organization; 2004.
42. Hotez PJ, Molyneux DH, Fenwick A, Ottesen E, Ehrlich Sachs S, Sachs JD. Incorporating a rapid-impact package for neglected tropical diseases with programs for HIV/AIDS, tuberculosis, and malaria. *PLoS Med* 2006; 3(5): e102.
43. WHO. *Working to overcome the global impact of neglected tropical diseases.* First WHO report on neglected tropical diseases. Geneva: World Health Organization; 2010.
44. Hotez PJ. Stigma: the stealth weapon of the NTD. *PLoS Negl Trop Dis* 2008; 2(4): e230.

45. Weiss MG. Stigma and the social burden of neglected tropical diseases. *PLoS Negl Trop Dis* 2008; 2(5): e237.
46. Williams D, Gutierrez JM, Harrison R, Warrell DA, White J, Winkel KD, *et al.* The Global Snake Bite Initiative: an antidote for snake bite. *Lancet* 2010; 375(9708): 89–91.
47. Hotez PJ, Molyneux DH, Fenwick A, Savioli L, Takeuchi T. A Global Fund to Fight Neglected Tropical Diseases: is the G8 Hokkaido Toyako 2008 Summit ready? *PLoS Negl Trop Dis* 2008; 2(3): e220.
48. Molyneux DH. 'Neglected' diseases but unrecognised successes: challenges and opportunities for infectious disease control. *Lancet* 2004; 364(9431): 380–3.
49. Molyneux DH, Hotez PJ, Fenwick A. 'Rapid-impact interventions': how a policy of integrated control for Africa's neglected tropical diseases could benefit the poor. *PLoS Med* 2005; 2(11): e336.
50. Hotez PJ, Molyneux DH, Fenwick A, Kumaresan J, Ehrlich Sachs S, Sachs JD, *et al.* Control of neglected tropical diseases. *N Engl J Med* 2007; 357(10): 1018–27.
51. Hotez PJ, Aksoy S. Now we are six. *PLoS Negl Trop Dis* 2012; 6(10): e1862.
52. Steinmann P, Keiser J, Bos R, Tanner M, Utzinger J. Schistosomiasis and water resources development: systematic review, meta-analysis, and estimates of people at risk. *Lancet Infect Dis* 2006; 6(7): 411–25.
53. Zhou XN, Bergquist R, Leonardo L, Yang GJ, Yang K, Sudomo M, *et al.* Schistosomiasis japonica: control and research needs. *Adv Parasitol* 2010; 72: 145–78.
54. Garjito TA, Sudomo M, Abdullah, Dahlan M, Nurwidayati A. Schistosomiasis in Indonesia: past and present. *Parasitol Int* 2008; 57(3): 277–80.
55. Muth S, Sayasone S, Odermatt-Biays S, Phompida S, Duong S, Odermatt P. *Schistosoma mekongi* in Cambodia and Lao People's Democratic Republic. *Adv Parasitol* 2010; 72: 179–203.
56. Wang L, Utzinger J, Zhou XN. Schistosomiasis control: experiences and lessons from China. *Lancet* 2008; 372(9652): 1793–5.
57. Utzinger J, Zhou XN, Chen MG, Bergquist R. Conquering schistosomiasis in China: the long march. *Acta Trop* 2005; 96(2–3): 69–96.
58. Wang LD, Chen HG, Guo JG, Zeng XJ, Hong XL, Xiong JJ, *et al.* A strategy to control transmission of *Schistosoma japonicum* in China. *N Engl J Med* 2009; 360(2): 121–8.
59. McManus DP, Gray DJ, Li Y, Feng Z, Williams GM, Stewart D, *et al.* Schistosomiasis in the People's Republic of China: the era of the Three Gorges Dam. *Clin Microbiol Rev* 2010; 23(2): 442–66.
60. Wu HW, Qin YF, Chu K, Meng R, Liu Y, McGarvey ST, *et al.* High prevalence of *Schistosoma japonicum* infection in water buffaloes in the Philippines assessed by real-time polymerase chain reaction. *Am J Trop Med Hyg* 2010; 82(4): 646–52.
61. Carabin H, Balolong E, Joseph L, McGarvey ST, Johansen MV, Fernandez T, *et al.* Estimating sensitivity and specificity of a faecal examination method for *Schistosoma japonicum* infection in cats, dogs, water buffaloes, pigs, and rats in Western Samar and Sorsogon provinces, The Philippines. *Int J Parasitol* 2005; 35(14): 1517–24.
62. Bethony J, Brooker S, Albonico M, Geiger SM, Loukas A, Diemert D, *et al.* Soil-transmitted helminth infections: ascariasis, trichuriasis, and hookworm. *Lancet* 2006; 367(9521): 1521–32.
63. Steinmann P, Utzinger J, Du ZW, Zhou XN. Multiparasitism a neglected reality on global, regional and local scale. *Adv Parasitol* 2010; 73: 21–50.
64. Pullan RL, Brooker SJ. The global limits and population at risk of soil-transmitted helminth infections in 2010. *Parasit Vectors* 2012; 5: 81.
65. de Silva NR, Brooker S, Hotez PJ, Montresor A, Engels D, Savioli L. Soil-transmitted helminth infections: updating the global picture. *Trends Parasitol* 2003; 19(12): 547–51.
66. Li T, He S, Zhao H, Zhao G, Zhu XQ. Major trends in human parasitic diseases in China. *Trends Parasitol* 2010; 26(5): 264–70.
67. WHO. *Preventive chemotherapy in human helminthiasis: coordinated use of anthelminthic drugs in control interventions: a manual for health professionals and programme managers.* Geneva: World Health Organization; 2006.
68. Ziegelbauer K, Speich B, Mäusezahl D, Bos R, Keiser J, Utzinger J. Effect of sanitation on soil-transmitted helminth infection: systematic review and meta-analysis. *PLoS Med* 2012; 9(1): e1001162.
69. Bieri FA, Gray DJ, Williams GM, Raso G, Li YS, Yuan L, *et al.* Health-education package to prevent worm infections in Chinese schoolchildren. *N Engl J Med* 2013; 368(17): 1603–12.

70. Hall A. Micronutrient supplements for children after deworming. *Lancet Infect Dis* 2007; 7(4): 297–302.
71. Fürst T, Sayasone S, Odermatt P, Keiser J, Utzinger J. Manifestation, diagnosis, and management of foodborne trematodiasis. *BMJ* 2012; 344: e4093.
72. Fürst T, Keiser J, Utzinger J. Global burden of human food-borne trematodiasis: a systematic review and meta-analysis. *Lancet Infect Dis* 2012; 12(3): 210–21.
73. Sripa B, Kaewkes S, Intapan PM, Maleewong W, Brindley PJ. Food-borne trematodiases in Southeast Asia: epidemiology, pathology, clinical manifestation and control. *Adv Parasitol* 2010; 72: 305–50.
74. Keiser J, Utzinger J. Food-borne trematodiases. *Clin Microbiol Rev* 2009; 22(3): 466–83.
75. Lun ZR, Gasser RB, Lai DH, Li AX, Zhu XQ, Yu XB, *et al.* Clonorchiasis: a key foodborne zoonosis in China. *Lancet Infect Dis* 2005; 5(1): 31–41.
76. Gu W, Su HY, Zou J, Li QC, Chen BY, Lin CS, *et al.* [Clinical diagnosis and treatment in an outbreak of *Fasciola gigantica* infection in Yunnan province]. Chin J Parasitol Parasit Dis 2012;30(6):455–9 (in Chinese).
77. Lv S, Zhang Y, Steinmann P, Zhou XN, Utzinger J. Helminth infections of the central nervous system occurring in Southeast Asia and the Far East. *Adv Parasitol* 2010; 72: 351–408.
78. Lv S, Zhang Y, Steinmann P, Zhou XN. Emerging angiostrongyliasis in Mainland China. *Emerg Infect Dis* 2008; 14(1): 161–4.
79. Lv S, Zhang Y, Steinmann P, Yang GJ, Yang K, Zhou XN, *et al.* The emergence of angiostrongyliasis in the People's Republic of China: the interplay between invasive snails, climate change and transmission dynamics. *Freshw Biol* 2011; 56: 717–34.
80. McManus DP, Gray DJ, Zhang W, Yang Y. Diagnosis, treatment, and management of echinococcosis. *BMJ* 2012; 344: e3866.
81. WHO/OIE. *WHO/OIE manual on echinococcosis in humans and animals: a public health problem of global concern.* Eds. J, Eckert, MA, Gemmell, F-X, Meslin, ZS, Pawlowski. Paris; 2001.
82. WHO. *Report of the WHO informal working group on cystic and alveolar echinococcosis surveillance, prevention and control, with the participation of the Food and Agriculture Organization of the United Nations and the World Organization for Animal Health.* Geneva; 2011.
83. Yang YR, Williams GM, Craig PS, McManus DP. Impact of increased economic burden due to human echinococcosis in an underdeveloped rural community of the People's Republic of China. *PLoS Negl Trop Dis* 2010; 4(9): e801.
84. Giraudoux P, Raoul F, Afonso E, Ziadinov I, Yang Y, Li L, *et al.* Transmission ecosystems of *Echinococcus multilocularis* in China and Central Asia. *Parasitology* 2013; 140(13): 1655–66.
85. Giraudoux P, Raoul F, Pleydell D, Li T, Han X, Qiu J, *et al.* Drivers of *Echinococcus multilocularis* transmission in China: small mammal diversity, landscape or climate? *PLoS Negl Trop Dis* 2013; 7(3): e2045.
86. WHO. *Report of the WHO expert consultation on foodborne trematode infections and taeniasis/cysticercosis.* Vientiane; 2011.
87. Galvez Tan JZ. The elimination of lymphatic filariasis: a strategy for poverty alleviation and sustainable development – perspectives from the Philippines. *Filaria J* 2003; 2(1): 12.
88. Durrheim DN, Wynd S, Liese B, Gyapong JO. Lymphatic filariasis endemicity: an indicator of poverty? *Trop Med Int Health* 2004; 9(8): 843–5.
89. WHO. Global programme to eliminate lymphatic filariasis: progress report, 2011. *Wkly Epidemiol Rec* 2012; 87(37): 346–56.
90. WHO. *Control of lymphatic filariasis in China: the editorial board of control of lymphatic filariasis in China.* Manila; 2003.
91. WHO. Integrated preventive chemotherapy for neglected tropical diseases: estimation of the number of interventions required and delivered, 2009–2010. *Wkly Epidemiol Rec* 2012; 87(2): 17–27.
92. WHO. *Dengue: guidelines for diagnosis, treatment, prevention and control.* Geneva; 2009.
93. Gubler DJ. Epidemic dengue/dengue hemorrhagic fever as a public health, social and economic problem in the 21st century. *Trends Microbiol* 2002; 10(2): 100–3.
94. Hales S, de Wet N, Maindonald J, Woodward A. Potential effect of population and climate changes on global distribution of dengue fever: an empirical model. *Lancet* 2002; 360(9336): 830–4.
95. Wilder-Smith A, Schwartz E. Dengue in travelers. *N Engl J Med* 2005; 353(9): 924–32.
96. Misra UK, Kalita J. Overview: Japanese encephalitis. *Prog Neurobiol* 2010; 91(2): 108–20.

97. Erlanger TE, Weiss S, Keiser J, Utzinger J, Wiedenmayer K. Past, present, and future of Japanese encephalitis. *Emerg Infect Dis* 2009; 15(1): 1–7.
98. WHO. *The control of neglected zoonotic diseases: community-based interventions for prevention and control.* Geneva; 2011.
99. WHO. Global WHO Alliance for the Elimination of Blinding Trachoma by 2020. *Wkly Epidemiol Rec* 2012; 87(17): 161–8.
100. Mariotti SP, Pascolini D, Rose-Nussbaumer J. Trachoma: global magnitude of a preventable cause of blindness. *Br J Ophthalmol* 2009; 93(5): 563–8.
101. WHO. Global leprosy situation, 2012. *Wkly Epidemiol Rec* 2012; 87(34): 317–28.
102. Desjeux P. Human leishmaniases: epidemiology and public health aspects. *World Health Stat Q* 1992; 45(2–3): 267–75.
103. Wang JY, Gao CH, Yang YT, Chen HT, Zhu XH, Lv S, *et al.* An outbreak of the desert sub-type of zoonotic visceral leishmaniasis in Jiashi, Xinjiang Uygur autonomous region, People's Republic of China. *Parasitol Int* 2010; 59(3): 331–7.
104. Alvar J, Velez ID, Bern C, Herrero M, Desjeux P, Cano J, *et al.* Leishmaniasis worldwide and global estimates of its incidence. *PLoS One* 2012; 7(5): e35671.
105. WHO. Control of the leishmaniases. Report of a WHO expert committee. *World Health Organ Tech Rep Ser* 1990; 793: 1–158.
106. Greenwood BM, Fidock DA, Kyle DE, Kappe SH, Alonso PL, Collins FH, *et al.* Malaria: progress, perils, and prospects for eradication. *J Clin Invest* 2008; 118(4): 1266–76.
107. WHO. *World malaria report 2011.* Geneva; 2011, 248.
108. Carter R, Mendis KN. Evolutionary and historical aspects of the burden of malaria. *Clin Microbiol Rev* 2002; 15(4): 564–94.
109. Lee KS, Divis PC, Zakaria SK, Matusop A, Julin RA, Conway DJ, *et al. Plasmodium knowlesi*: reservoir hosts and tracking the emergence in humans and macaques. *PLoS Pathog* 2011; 7(4): e1002015.
110. White NJ. Antimalarial drug resistance. *J Clin Invest* 2004; 113(8): 1084–92.
111. Newton PN, Hampton CY, Alter-Hall K, Teerwarakulpana T, Prakongpan S, Ruangveerayuth R, *et al.* Characterization of 'Yaa Chud' medicine on the Thailand–Myanmar border: selecting for drug-resistant malaria and threatening public health. *Am J Trop Med Hyg* 2008; 79(5): 662–9.
112. Na-Bangchang K, Karbwang J. Emerging artemisinin resistance in the border areas of Thailand. *Expert Rev Clin Pharmacol* 2013; 6(3): 307–22.
113. Yang GJ, Tanner M, Utzinger J, Malone JB, Bergquist R, Chan EY, *et al.* Malaria surveillance–response strategies in different transmission zones of the People's Republic of China: preparing for climate change. *Malar J* 2012; 11: 426.
114. McMichael AJ. Globalization, climate change, and human health. *N Engl J Med* 2013; 368(14): 1335–43.
115. Rabinowitz P, Conti L. Links among human health, animal health, and ecosystem health. *Annu Rev Public Health* 2013; 34: 189–204.
116. Winkler MS, Krieger GR, Divall MJ, Cissé G, Wielga M, Singer BH, *et al.* Untapped potential of health impact assessment. *Bull World Health Organ* 2013; 91(4): 298–305.
117. *Lancet* Editorial. A world of 7 billion people. *Lancet* 2011; 378(9802): 1527.
118. Zhang J, Mauzerall DL, Zhu T, Liang S, Ezzati M, Remais JV. Environmental health in China: progress towards clean air and safe water. *Lancet* 2010; 375(9720): 1110–19.
119. Gong P, Liang S, Carlton EJ, Jiang Q, Wu J, Wang L, *et al.* Urbanisation and health in China. *Lancet* 2012; 379(9818): 843–52.
120. Yang G, Wang Y, Zeng Y, Gao GF, Liang X, Zhou M, *et al.* Rapid health transition in China, 1990–2010: findings from the Global Burden of Disease Study 2010. *Lancet* 2013; 381(9882): 1987–2015.
121. Gregory PJ, Ingram JS, Brklacich M. Climate change and food security. *Philos Trans R Soc Lond B Biol Sci* 2005; 360(1463): 2139–48.
122. Cordell D, Drangert J-O, White S. The story of phosphorus: global food security and food for thought. *Global Environmental Change* 2009; 19: 292–305.
123. Zhou XN, Yang GJ, Yang K, Wang XH, Hong QB, Sun LP, *et al.* Potential impact of climate change on schistosomiasis transmission in China. *Am J Trop Med Hyg* 2008; 78: 188–94.
124. Yang GJ, Utzinger J, Lv S, Qian YJ, Li SZ, Qiang W, *et al.* Regional network for Asian

schistosomiasis and other helminth zoonoses (RNAS+): target diseases in face of climate change. *Adv Parasitol* 2010; 73: 101–35.
125. Wilde H, Khawplod P, Khamoltham T, Hemachudha T, Tepsumethanon V, Lumlerdacha B, *et al.* Rabies control in South and Southeast Asia. *Vaccine* 2005; 23(17–18): 2284–9.
126. Durkin SR, Casson RJ, Newland HS, Aung TH, Shein WK, Muecke JS, *et al.* Prevalence of trachoma-related trichiasis and corneal opacity in rural Myanmar: the Meiktila Eye Study. *Ophthalmology* 2007; 114(5): e7–11.
127. Sinuon M, Tsuyuoka R, Socheat D, Odermatt P, Ohmae H, Matsuda H, *et al.* Control of *Schistosoma mekongi* in Cambodia: results of eight years of control activities in the two endemic provinces. *Trans R Soc Trop Med Hyg* 2007; 101(1): 34–9.
128. Sudomo M, Chayabejara S, Duong S, Hernandez L, Wu WP, Bergquist R. Elimination of lymphatic filariasis in Southeast Asia. *Adv Parasitol* 2010; 72: 205–33.
129. Weiss RA, McMichael AJ. Social and environmental risk factors in the emergence of infectious diseases. *Nat Med* 2004; 10(12 Suppl): S70–6.
130. Jones KE, Patel NG, Levy MA, Storeygard A, Balk D, Gittleman JL, *et al.* Global trends in emerging infectious diseases. *Nature* 2008; 451(7181): 990–3.
131. Snowden FM. Emerging and reemerging diseases: a historical perspective. *Immunol Rev* 2008; 225: 9–26.
132. McManus DP. Echinococcosis with particular reference to Southeast Asia. *Adv Parasitol* 2010; 72: 267–303.
133. Carlton EJ, Liang S, McDowell JZ, Li H, Luo W, Remais JV. Regional disparities in the burden of disease attributable to unsafe water and poor sanitation in China. *Bull World Health Organ* 2012; 90(8): 578–87.
134. Institute for Health Metrics and Evaluation (IHME). University of Washington in Seattle. Global Burden of Disease Country Profiles. [Online]. Available from: http://www.healthmetricsandevaluation.org/gbd/country-profiles. [Accessed 10 June 2013].
135. United Nations. World Urbanization Prospects, the 2011 Revision. United Nations Department of Economic and Social Affairs, Population Division, Population Estimates and Projection Section. [Online]. Available from: http://esa.un.org/unup/. [Accessed 10 June 2013].

# 13

# Role of government agencies in controlling disease

## Hong Kong's Centre for Health Protection as a case study

*Thomas Tsang Ho-Fai*

## Introduction

Health is a common goal shared by virtually all societies and their governments. Across the globe, countries show interesting similarities and differences in the way their government agencies interact with societies in fostering citizens' health. Such interactions have become increasingly dynamic in the contemporary era of globalization, information technology revolution and shifting social, political and economic landscapes. In this chapter, we examine, in broad terms, the government's role in controlling diseases and follow with a case study from the Centre for Health Protection (CHP), which is the corresponding government agency for health control in Hong Kong, China.

## Role of government agencies in controlling diseases [1–5]

Government agencies enjoy certain privileged roles when it comes to the subject of controlling diseases. Some government agencies can even achieve monopoly, one example being the enactment and enforcement of certain legislations (e.g. smoking bans). When a national health crisis strikes, whether it is due to a natural disaster or acute epidemic, government agencies have the unequalled capacity to mobilize vast amounts of health manpower and resources at short notice. Thanks to their public health mandate and neutrality, governments are also in a prime position to set public health goals and priorities, formulate national strategies, publish standards and best practices, and build consensus among diverse community stakeholders. Similarly, governments have the advantages of guiding and coordinating the work of different community groups and organizations, especially if said group's work is supported by public funds or government staff.

Nearly all governments provide some form of health services in controlling diseases, but they vary greatly in how much healthcare financing they provide and in which delivery systems they operate. Governments are a vital source of health information and are key players in health education and promotion activities. In partnership with community groups, government agencies contribute to disease control in many different domains including health research and development, training and capacity building, monitoring and evaluation of health services, as well as others. At a supranational level, government agencies form versatile networks to share information, tackle global issues and provide mutual support in disease control.

While the pivotal role of government agencies in disease control can hardly be questioned, one can argue there are soft spots and gaps. By necessity, governments are oriented to controlling diseases from the general population perspective. Certain marginal populations and hard-to-reach groups (e.g. ethnic minorities, religious groups, sex workers) are often served better by non-government organizations (NGOs) that provide tailor-made services to these groups. Compared with government bureaucracy, NGOs and the private sector tend to be more responsive to changing health needs and more ready to adopt technological innovations in controlling diseases. The academic sector and NGOs are less bound than government agencies in deploying unconventional approaches in health advocacy (e.g. launching petitions, lobbying legislators). As it is often the case, government agencies and their non-government counterparts can work complementarily each playing to their own strengths.

In the past two decades, there has been a movement for governments across the world to assume greater roles and responsibilities in controlling communicable diseases (CDs) and non-communicable diseases (NCDs). In the wake of the SARS pandemic in 2003, health legislation and infrastructure in relation to CDs were considerably strengthened, at both the national and international levels. Under the International Health Regulations (2005), governments are required to have more power and capacity to deal with large-scale public health crises of international concern.

In the realm of NCDs, the past two decades have seen governments introducing more stringent laws and tax hikes in various areas of disease control: smoking ban, alcohol tax and sales restriction of unhealthy food (e.g. forbidding sale of soft drinks in schools and government premises). Part of this momentum comes from international treatises, as exemplified by the Framework Convention on Tobacco Control (FCTC). In an unprecedented move, NCDs were elevated to the agenda of the United Nations Summit in September 2011. There is an increasing recognition of social and environmental determinants for health, and whole-government approaches in controlling NCDs are being studied and tried in some places.

Interestingly, many social, political, economic and technological factors account for the government taking a more escalating role in disease control. Recent global economic crises may have resulted in a larger number of people who lost their jobs and financial security to become more reliant on the government providing health services. In the information age, mass media put severe demands on governments to respond almost instantaneously to all kinds of disease outbreaks and incidents of media interest. As far as disease control is concerned, public sentiment in general demands governments respond quickly and do more.

## The CHP's role in disease control

The CHP is a government agency serving the Hong Kong special administrative region, which is a metropolitan city of 7 million people in southern China. The CHP was established in June 2004 in the aftermath of the SARS epidemic, which claimed the lives of 300 people. Its mission is to achieve effective prevention and control of diseases in Hong Kong in collaboration with local and international stakeholders. Staffed with some 1,500 employees, the CHP's jurisdiction falls under the Department of Health and is headed by a civil servant, known as the Controller, and served by a Board of Scientific Advisers. Its legal mandate is provided by the Prevention and Control of Disease Ordinance (Cap. 599).

The CHP's functions are broadly similar to those of Centres for Diseases Control in many countries. It is organized in six branches, which are Surveillance and Epidemiology, Emergency Response and Information, Infection Control, Public Health Laboratory Services, Public Health Services, and Program Management and Professional Development. The CHP draws upon external professional expertise via six Scientific Committees comprised of esteemed experts.

At the strategy level, the CHP supports priority setting and formulation of disease control strategies through research and analysis. It brings together major stakeholders to build consensus and coordinate actions. Representative examples include the NCD Prevention and Control Framework (2008) [6] and the Strategy on HIV/AIDS (2012–16) [7]. From these, action plans targeted on diet, physical activity, alcohol abuse, injuries and HIV are produced and put into practice. In a similar vein, the CHP publishes a substantial body of scientific recommendations on the prevention and control of miscellaneous CDs/NCDs, ranging from immunization schedules to cancer prevention and screening guidelines.

At the programme level, the CHP conducts a wide range of health protection programmes against major CDs/NCDs affecting Hong Kong. Examples include immunization programmes, the cervical cancer screening programme, healthy eating programmes at schools and restaurants, organ donation campaigns, as well as others. Health promotion programmes aimed at empowering the community in disease control feature prominently in the CHP's portfolio.

At the operations level, the CHP plays a dominant and statutory role in the surveillance, investigation and control of CDs and NCDs, the latter also encompassing environmental health risk assessment and toxicovigilance. The CHP's Public Health Laboratory provides comprehensive laboratory diagnostic services and acts as a Reference Laboratory and training centre for laboratory personnel. From the experience of the SARS outbreak, the CHP devotes much effort to emergency preparedness and crises management, such as developing contingency plans, and coordinating exercises and drills on major disease outbreaks. The CHP also takes a leading role in nosocomial outbreaks, infection control guidelines and training of healthcare staff.

At the service level, the CHP provides clinical specialist treatment services for patients with tuberculosis, HIV/AIDS and sexually transmitted infections (STI) through 24 outpatient clinics. The CHP is the major service provider for treating these diseases: up to 80 per cent of tuberculosis cases, 75 per cent of HIV/AIDS and 40 per cent of STI in Hong Kong are observed in these clinics.

## Lessons from the CHP

An interesting question is: should a publicly funded disease control agency be put under government (as in the case of the CHP) or better set apart from government (as per the model in the UK or Canada)? The chief theoretical advantage of the latter model is a superior image of scientific independence. However, in a city like Hong Kong, the amount of surge capacity and depth of professional expertise may not compare with those of large countries. As a government agency, the CHP can readily draw upon government resources in the face of major outbreaks and health crises. Furthermore, some key statutory disease control functions (e.g. port health, tobacco control) reside outside the CHP's realm. By staying under the same roof, the CHP can work closely with other government agencies involved in disease control.

Due to the special historical circumstances (i.e. SARS epidemic) leading to its birth, the CHP's role was focused almost exclusively on CDs during its initial years. More resources and attention were gradually shifted to NCDs after CD control became well established. Despite the clear public health fact that NCDs account for far greater disease burden than CDs, public attention and expectations of the CHP's role are still fixated on the latter. Apart from factors like fear perception and newsworthiness, CD control is widely regarded as an exclusive government obligation while NCD control is everybody's business. This has proved extremely difficult to change and poses a major obstacle to better NCD control. More innovative techniques in social marketing and risk communication are being explored by the CHP to reduce this risk perception parallax. A recent example is the idea to pictorially depict central obesity as a bomb-in-the-waist to underline its seriousness and urgency, just as if it was a CD.

Over the years, the CHP's role in disease control has undergone gradual evolution. First, following global trends, more emphasis is being put on intersectoral collaboration and community engagement, whether in the setting of health priorities, planning or execution of programmes and activities. The CHP is moving away from the role of a dominant, autonomous player to that of a facilitator, coordinator and funder. Hong Kong is particularly suited to this model because of its rich and diversified community organizations and services. The AIDS Trust Fund managed by the CHP, for example, allocates HK$300 million for HIV/AIDS related projects for NGOs. As well as that, there is other government funding for disease control and health research. Second, the CHP is playing a greater role in creating more health conducive environments rather than simply providing health education as research has shown that knowledge often does not translate into practice especially in the absence of an enabling environment. In two healthy eating programs (eatsmart@school and eatsmart@restaurant), lots of healthy recipes are created and promoted through schools and restaurants so that students and customers have easy access to nutritious food. Some of Hong Kong's tobacco control legislation, such as the smoking ban in public parks and bus terminals, is considered to be one of the world's most progressive legislations in creating a smoke-free environment.

The mass media in Hong Kong is well known for its news efficiency and ability to sway public opinion and sentiment. Disease outbreaks inevitably generate media interest and the CHP handles press enquiries on a daily basis. Hence at the CHP, risk communication takes on a core role in disease control, and the CHP is expected to provide timely health alerts and health advice at all times. To the public, the credibility of a government agency can be damaged irrevocably by mishandling a single aspect of a disease outbreak, no matter how good its track record has been. The CHP produces a risk communication document under the auspices of the Risk Communication Advisory Group with contributions from different walks of society. Besides conventional communication channels like television, radio, press releases and advertisements in public places, the CHP is embracing novel platforms like social media and apps. Where possible, the CHP adopts a proactive, pre-emptive approach in risk communication, alerting people and telling them what the agency is going to do before an outbreak turns serious. These have worked sometimes but not always. During the vaccination campaign for human swine influenza (pandemic H1N1) in 2009, people stopped requesting vaccinations after widespread media reports of serious adverse effects following the vaccination (such as Guillain–Barré Syndrome and intra-uterine deaths), and despite all efforts in risk communication, vaccination rates never recovered.

Hong Kong's status as a foremost international travel hub poses special challenges to CD control. Epidemiologically, the Pearl River Delta (including Hong Kong, Guangdong and Macau) may be viewed as one entity particularly with regards to some respiratory and enteric infections. Every day, some 500,000 passengers traverse the Hong Kong/Guangdong borders. Successful disease control requires the government's role to be extended beyond its normal jurisdiction and for it to work closely with its neighbours. After SARS, direct regular and emergency channels of communication were established between senior officials of the CHP and their Guangdong/mainland China counterparts. These rapid, direct channels prove exceedingly useful and important in exchanging outbreak intelligence and clarifying rumours. Other collaboration includes annual expert meetings, conjoint research projects and professional staff attachments.

## Conclusion

Disease control at the present time, and probably in the next decade, will face daunting challenges from several megatrends, including globalization, urbanization, population ageing, emerging infections, an escalating burden of NCDs, information and biotechnology revolution, and socio-economic upheaval. Many governments are met with a rising public expectation to play a greater role in disease control and not leave it up to the individual to take care of. To fulfil their responsibilities, government agencies need to develop extensive networks, invest in technology and expertise, adopt multisectoral approaches, review regulatory functions and, above all, communicate with the public effectively and earn their trust.

## References

1. The role of the government in public health: a national perspective. Adshead F, Thorpe A. *Public Health* 2007; 121(11): 835–9.
2. Nanny or steward? The role of government in public health. Jochelson K. *Public Health* 2006; 120(12): 1149–55.
3. Health and well-being: the role of government. Hunt P. *Public Health* 2012; 126 Suppl 1: S19–23.
4. The roles of government in improving health care quality and safety. Tang N, Eisenberg JM, Meyer GS. *Jt Comm J Qual Saf* 2004; 30(1): 47–55.
5. The role of government in health care: a societal issue. DeBakey ME. *Am J Surg* 2006; 191(2): 145–57.
6. Promoting Health in Hong Kong: A Strategic Framework for Prevention and Control of Non-communicable Diseases. Department of Health, Hong Kong Special Administration Region Government. [Online]. Available from: http://www.chp.gov.hk/en/epidemiology/29/134/504/505.html.
7. Recommended HIV/AIDS Strategies for Hong Kong 2012–16. Hong Kong Advisory Council on AIDS. [Online]. Available from: http://www.aca.gov.hk/publication/g253.pdf.

# 14

# The role of Centres for Disease Control in China

## Shanghai as a case study

*Fan Wu*

### Introduction

This chapter uses the Shanghai Municipal Centre for Disease Control and Prevention (SCDC) as a case study to discuss how Centres for Disease Control (CDC) operate in China. A brief summary of Shanghai and the health status of its residents is presented first, followed by a detailed study of how the CDC system works and its partnership in Shanghai. The chapter goes on to describe control and response plans for various infectious diseases, as well as the role of the CDC in non-communicable diseases (NCDs). Then, a discussion of the involvement of the SCDC and CDCs in public health security in the city is presented, and the chapter concludes with an overview of the public health challenges and opportunities Shanghai faces in the wake of globalization.

### Health status of Shanghai residents and its disease control and prevention system

Located on the west coast of the Pacific Ocean, Shanghai lies at the mouth of the Yangtze River Delta and is the midpoint of China's east coast. Shanghai's excellent geographic location has contributed to its development as a modern metropolis. Relying on the vast hinterland of China and ease of accessibility, the city has become a domestic and international hub for human and material resources. Shanghai has a land area of 6340.5 square kilometres, which is divided into 16 districts and one county. Currently, Shanghai has a population of 23 million, of which 14 million are registered residents and 9 million are migrants. Over 24 per cent of the total population is aged over 60 years [1].

Currently, the health indictors of Shanghai residents have already reached a level comparable to those of developed countries. According to the statistics provided by the SCDC, the average life expectancy for Shanghai residents, in 2011, was 82.51 years of age, the infant mortality rate was 5.7/100,000 and the maternal mortality rate was 7.36/100,000.

The great achievements that Shanghai has made in disease control and prevention are owed not only to the local government's long-term commitment to public health, but also to a comprehensive disease control and prevention system. The most important part of this system is the vertical interaction between the SCDC, district CDCs and community health service centres (CHSC). Receiving technical guidance from the Chinese Centres for Disease Control and Prevention, and under direct leadership of the Shanghai Municipal Health Bureau, the SCDC manages and coordinates disease control and prevention citywide. The SCDC also provides technical guidance to district CDCs and oversees their performance.

District CDCs share similar functions and responsibilities with the SCDC at the district level. They organize disease control and public health work in their jurisdictions and guide CHSCs to perform their public health functions through tangible public health programmes. As the grassroots players in this system, CHSCs are responsible for public health and infectious disease control, which includes the management of patients in their respective communities. As an important supplement to the disease control and prevention network, clinical agencies of all types at all levels play a major role in the detection, registration, reporting, treatment and clinical prevention of infectious diseases and chronic diseases. In addition, the SCDC has fostered extensive collaboration with related medical schools, research institutes, hospitals, NGOs and professional committees, such as the Fudan University Medical School and the Shanghai Jiaotong University Medical School.

SCDC is the key professional agency which fulfils the municipal government's public health function and its essential tasks include: implementation of disease control and prevention programmes, surveillance on health-related risk factors, responding to public health emergency events, conducting research on applied preventive medicine and promoting international cooperation and exchange.

Since 1949, when the People's Republic of China was founded, infectious diseases in Shanghai have been effectively controlled. In the past two decades, the incidence of infectious diseases has maintained a consistent downward trend. The reported incidence of notifiable infectious diseases (including Class I and Class II as categorized by the law) among the local Shanghai population has been reduced by over 90 per cent when compared with the statistics from the early 1950s, and by 56.48 per cent since the establishment of the SCDC in 1998. When analysing cause of death statistics, the ranking of infectious diseases has dropped from the number one cause of death as it was in the early 1950s (accounting for 36.98 per cent of deaths), to the seventh spot in 2011 (accounting for 1.19 per cent of deaths).

In the area of chronic disease control and prevention, Shanghai was one of the first cities in China to start chronic diseases prevention and control planning, and has achieved substantial progress in this area. The Shanghai Cause-of-Death Registry was set up as early as 1954 and the Shanghai Birth Registry was established in 2004. Shanghai CDC is responsible for vital statistics in Shanghai and has a relatively complete database for death and birth registry. Starting in 1963, the Shanghai Cancer Registry at Shanghai CDC has developed into a population-based system covering all the Shanghai residents in 2001 and it is the earliest cancer registry in China, as well as being the largest in the world. Shanghai CDC also guides district CDCs and CHSCs to build electronic health record systems, which lay the foundation for monitoring risk factors of chronic diseases and conducting health promotion programmes. So far, 1.60 million hypertension patients and 425,000 diabetes patients are managed at the community level across Shanghai. Besides, a hospital-based injury surveillance network has been preliminarily established and specific programmes are conducted at the community level according to the population characteristics.

The SCDC also conducts surveillance and intervention programmes on health-related risk factors in occupational health, environmental health, food safety, nutritional health, school health and radiation protection. In recent years, the SCDC has also gone ahead with the application of information technology in disease control and prevention by setting up and improving the public health information database in order to strengthen capacity for evidence-based decision making and practice.

## Shanghai disease control and prevention practice

### *Surveillance programmes on infectious diseases*

Shanghai started infectious disease surveillance at a comparatively early time in China. In order to meet the ever-changing need for infectious disease control, Shanghai has continuously refined what has now become a well-functioning surveillance system. So far, Shanghai has conducted surveillance programmes on 39 notifiable diseases [2]. Furthermore, a surveillance programme for certain non-notifiable infectious diseases, such as chickenpox and fever with thrombocytopenia syndrome, was also established. The city monitors the density and positive rates of infectious agents among vectors, such as mice, cockroaches, mosquitoes and flies. It also monitors the work of disinfection and infection control groups. As well as that, 5,708 surveillance sites for 15 categories of infectious diseases have been set up across Shanghai.

The development of infectious disease surveillance systems in Shanghai has gone through three stages. The earliest surveillance was passive surveillance, focusing on case reports for notifiable diseases. Using infectious disease report cards, hospitals would report cases to anti-epidemic stations at district level, which served the function of the district CDC at the time.

In the 1990s, China saw a major development in the field of public health. Scientists became more knowledgeable about infectious diseases and their epidemic patterns, while both laboratory testing techniques and information technology developed rapidly. This advancement in the field allowed for the evolution of surveillance systems to reach the next stage where passive surveillance was combined with active surveillance using laboratory testing and information technology. In accordance with the unified plan of the Ministry of Health in China [3], Shanghai developed a real-time online reporting system based on individual cases. In association with the city's education departments, the SCDC also set up an online student absentee reporting system, which covered 1,708 kindergartens, and 1,596 middle, primary and intermediate vocational schools. This reporting system has moved forward the possibility for early warning and detection of outbreaks of infectious diseases. In addition, a case registry has been established and a pathogenic search targeting high-risk populations has been introduced in Shanghai. Etiological tests for bacillary dysentery are conducted for staff from key occupations such as kindergarten workers, primary and middle school workers, and catering service staff. Monitoring is also carried out on targeted populations such as sex workers, drug addicts, and MSM and STD patients.

Moreover, the city has also been monitoring the levels of antibodies among healthy populations, as well as pathogenic drug resistance. Pathogenic monitoring of common modes of transmission for infectious disease transmission, such as food, water sources, breeding water, soils, and faeces of poultry and domestic animals, has also been initiated.

The past few years have seen a rise in the number of surveillance systems catering to individual infectious diseases in Shanghai. In order to consolidate existing surveillance resources and link similar or related surveillance programmes more effectively, the development of an integrated surveillance system combining intestinal infectious disease surveillance and food-borne disease surveillance is being explored in Shanghai. These two surveillance systems have significant overlap in the populations they monitor, as well as in their methodology, their surveillance content and their surveillance sites. Recognizing these similarities, the SCDC began redesigning the surveillance plan and formed an integrated system in which unified monitoring sites were set up to carry out surveillance for diarrhoea cases, syndromes, pathogens and drug resistance. Going forward, the SCDC plans to use this model to establish more integrated surveillance systems for other diseases such as respiratory infections.

### *Response to infectious disease outbreaks*

In accordance with Shanghai's public health contingency plans for emergency response, and infectious disease, once an infectious disease outbreak happens, investigation and response will be conducted according to a grading system of the outbreak's severity. District CDCs will conduct an investigation and draw up a response plan for outbreaks in their jurisdiction or will assist the SCDC to deal with any major outbreaks.

Hospitals follow a system in which the first doctor who consults on the case is accountable for handling and reporting the disease. Once the infectious disease case is detected in hospitals, the doctor will immediately log on to the China Disease Control and Prevention Information System to report the case online, especially if it is a whole group of cases. In the meantime, hospitals will quarantine, diagnose, collect, record samples and treat patients. Hospitals also initiate iatrogenic infection control protocols under the guidance of the CDC staff. Professional disinfection protection and self-protection by doctors and nurses are conducted in hospitals to prevent secondary contamination.

After receiving the reports of a suspected infectious disease outbreak, district CDCs will enact a wide range of preventive and control measures, which include case investigation, contact tracing of close contacts, sample collection, pathogenic testing, disinfection of epidemic points and vector control. For ordinary to severe outbreaks, the SCDC will provide technical assistance to district CDCs and retest the positive samples. For major outbreaks, the SCDC staff will go to the field site and mobilize district CDCs, and they will collaboratively carry out the investigation and implement a response plan.

Furthermore, being the grassroots level of a three-tier network, the CHSCs play a vital role in the process of outbreak control by providing an ongoing response. Implicated CHSCs are responsible for the quarantine of patients, medical observation of close contacts, health education and vector control in their communities.

### *Chronic infectious disease control and prevention*

China and Shanghai place great importance on the control and prevention of chronic infectious diseases, such as HIV and tuberculosis (TB). China has successively issued a number of policies such as the Regulation on the Prevention and Treatment of HIV/AIDS [4], China's 'Twelfth Five-Year' action plan for Containment and Control of HIV/AIDS [5], the National Tuberculosis Control Program (2011–2015) [6], the 'Four Frees and One Care' policy for HIV/AIDS, the cost-reduction/free treatment policy for tuberculosis patients, as well as others. These policies provide a favourable environment for chronic infectious disease control and prevention.

In line with China's 'Twelfth Five-Year' action plan to control and treat HIV/AIDS, the goal is to reduce newly infected cases of HIV and the fatality rate of HIV/AIDS, and decrease discrimination against the HIV-infected population so as to improve the survival of HIV-infected persons and patients. By the end of 2015, the rapid rise of the HIV epidemic in key areas and populations will be controlled. The number of newly infected AIDS patients will decrease by 25 per cent and the fatality rate by 30 per cent, as compared with 2010. The number of people living with HIV infection and HIV patients will be controlled to 1.2 million. According to China's 'Twelfth Five-Year' action plan TB control program, the aim is to further decrease infection, prevalence and death of TB; lessen the disease burden of TB; improve the health level of people; and promote the development of the national economy, and stability and harmony of society.

Shanghai has set up a megalopolis integrated prevention and control model for TB, which is coordinated by the CDCs, hospitals and the CHSCs, and an efficient model for chronic infectious disease control and prevention has been evolving [7]. The CDC is responsible for TB control, prevention and disease management, which includes formulating the plan, coordinating management, providing technical guidance and training, quality control and outcome evaluation. General hospitals are responsible for screening patients with suspicious symptoms, referring patients with probable and confirmed diseases, reporting infectious diseases and educating affected patients. According to the guidelines for implementing the National Tuberculosis Control Program in China [8], the designated TB hospitals offer normalized diagnoses, standardized treatment, health education and reporting of TB cases. CHSCs are responsible for full-course supervision chemotherapy management for confirmed cases, follow-up and management of close contacts with smear-positive cases, as well as for providing health education. According to a report from World Health Organization (WHO) experts who visited Shanghai, its TB control model is regarded as the future direction for TB control in large and medium-sized cities in China.

Regarding HIV/AIDS control and prevention, Shanghai has built a laboratory testing network, a case report network and an integrated intervention network. The laboratory testing network uses clinical agencies, maternal and child health agencies, and blood centres as screening laboratories. The district CDCs are used as confirmatory laboratories while the SCDC is the only confirmed central laboratory and is also responsible for quality accreditation and oversight of all other HIV laboratories in Shanghai. The case report network covers all the health organizations in Shanghai. Organized by the SCDC and dependent on CHSCs, hospitals and maternal and child health agencies, an active sentinel surveillance for HIV/AIDS, covering 18,000 people across nine categories, has also been set up. The primary feature of the HIV/AIDS control and prevention initiative is the integrated intervention programme for high-risk populations conducted mainly by CHSCs. The CHSCs provide integrated interventions, such as free condom dissemination, in high-risk areas (recreation centres and places where mobile populations gather) and provide health education. The CDC offers technical support, supervision and evaluation for these integrated inventions.

### *Immunization programmes and vaccine-preventable diseases control and prevention*

According to the National Vaccine Circulation and Vaccination Management regulations, two categories of vaccines are currently offered in Shanghai [9]. Vaccines in Category I are provided by the national or local government and are free of charge for citizens. Vaccines in Category II are those that citizens can obtain at their own expense. Currently, Shanghai has 11 types of Category I vaccines and 15 types of Category II vaccines. Introduction to Category II and Category I vaccines will be available on the English website of SCDC very soon.

According to the principle of graded management, the SCDC takes responsibility for formulating and implementing the technical planning of immunization programmes in Shanghai. District CDCs provide technique training and guidance for clinics that are responsible for administering vaccines. Vaccination clinics offer vaccination services and undertake Adverse Effect Following Immunization (AEFI) through monitoring systems.

Currently, the immunization coverage rate of the Shanghai registered population for vaccines in Category I remains above 99 per cent. The immunization coverage rate of the migrant population has increased from 60 per cent in 2000 to over 99 per cent in 2011. The incidence of every vaccine-preventable disease currently remains at a record low. The SCDC also recently established the Shanghai Immunization Program Information System to facilitate vaccination services provided to the public. Citizens can now access services in any vaccination clinic at their convenience by using their personal Vaccination Record Card and can also receive an up-to-date short message service alerting them to important vaccination information.

## *Shanghai public health security*

In order to protect public health security of the city and efficiently respond to public health emergencies, the SCDC has established an Office of Public Health Emergency Response and Preparedness Department, and set up professional response teams. This has gradually perfected the public health emergency response mechanism by combining routine management and emergency response with coordination between sectorial authorities and local governments to form 29 emergency response contingency plans and technique proposals in eight categories. These include plans for overall emergency response contingency, infectious diseases, poisoning incidents, environmental incidents, mass diseases of unknown origin, vaccination and prophylaxis, anti-terrorism and other events. The SCDC guides district and county-level CDCs to establish and improve similar professional teams in order to build functional and integrated emergency response teams that permeate all levels of society.

Due to these complete disease prevention and control systems, Shanghai has been able to effectively respond to infectious diseases such as SARS, highly pathogenic avian influenza and novel H1N1 influenza. The city has also safely and successfully held mass gatherings such as the APEC conference, some events as part of the Beijing Olympic Games and the 2010 Shanghai Expo, which is discussed in more detail below.

In 2010, the SCDC, in cooperation with the district and county CDCs, fully guaranteed public health security for the Shanghai Expo. It was the first time in China that dynamic public health risk assessment approaches were applied to a large-scale event, where the priority areas and periodic key points in the Expo's public health security were scientifically determined. The Attendance Abnormalities Monitoring System, developed by the SCDC, utilized real-time collection, synchronized analyses and promptly alarmed any attendance abnormalities at the Expo sites. The system included integrated response plans thereby forming a complete public health surveillance system, allowing for immediate responses.

Understanding that laboratory testing capacity building is at the core of public health, the SCDC recently increased the range of pathogens being screened by 28.7 per cent in order to decisively respond to uncommon diseases and high-risk events. Now the SCDC has substantially gained the capability to handle any public health emergency events in a quick and effective way. The SCDC compiled and distributed 100,000 pamphlets containing travel health information to all the three-star hotels and above, as well as to other Expo-related areas. This methodology generated a new intervention model of how to approach mass gathering events in China from a public health perspective. In addition, the SCDC has locally cooperated with the CDCs of Zhejiang and Jiangsu to launch the synchronic defence and control system of the Yangtze River Delta. The SCDC has also engaged nationally to set up an information communication and interaction control system with the Chinese CDC. The SCDC has even extended their reach internationally by establishing regular risk communication mechanisms and global technical support networks with organizations such as the WHO, European Centre for Disease Prevention and Control (ECDC) and Centers for Disease Control and Prevention of the United States (USCDC). During the 2010 Expo, infectious diseases incidence remained at historically low levels and no serious infectious diseases emergence happened at an Expo site or in Shanghai in general.

## Conclusion: challenges and opportunities

In the twenty-first century, emerging infectious diseases are continuously threatening human health. As globalization accelerates, infectious diseases are more likely to break through geographical barriers, to cause quick transmission or even to turn into epidemics or pandemics. The goal related to infectious disease control and prevention increasingly relies on development of technical and human resources which are not conventional. As Shanghai becomes a megalopolis, it faces increasing challenges with floating population health management, which includes infectious disease control and prevention.

Urbanization and population ageing make the health threats from chronic diseases more prominent. Apart from this, SCDC faces daunting challenges from other factors such as public health emergencies, threat from nuclear–biological–chemical terrorism and global warming.

The CDCs in Shanghai will strengthen urban disease control and prevention to meet the ever-increasing challenges facing this industrious city. The CDCs seek to expand cooperation with hospitals to fully develop their role in clinical prevention of diseases, which will be done by improving their early detection systems, diagnosis and reporting, and by standardizing the treatment of these diseases. The CDCs will help to solidify the CHSCs, which are the foundation of the public health network, and strengthen their functions in order to be able to fulfil basic public health needs. It is the municipal and district CDCs that guide hospitals, medical care, prevention agencies and CHSCs to substantially carry out public health service programmes, and elevate the equity and accessibility of these basic health services to the public. Public health services will be accordingly adjusted and developed based on residents' health demands and socio-economic statuses. Shanghai will not only cooperate with other provinces and cities to control diseases, but will also further enhance collaborations with international organizations.

## Acknowledgements

The author would like to acknowledge staff from the Shanghai Municipal Centre for Disease Control and Prevention, in particular, Xiaogang Feng, Yuan Dong, Yi He and Xiaojing Yu, for their contributions to this chapter.

## References

1. *Shanghai Statistical Yearbook*. Shanghai Statistics Bureau, China Statistics Press, 2011.
2. Law of the People's Republic of China on the Prevention and Treatment of Infectious Diseases. Standing Committee of the National People's Congress, 2004.
3. Regulation on report management of public health emergency and infectious diseases epidemic. Ministry of Health, 2003.
4. Regulation on the Prevention and Treatment of HIV/AIDS. The State Council, 2006.

5. China's 'Twelfth Five-Year' action plan for Containment and Control of HIV/AIDS. The State Council, 2012.
6. National Tuberculosis Control Program (2011–2015). The State Council, 2011.
7. Zhang, S., Yuan, Z. A. and Mei, J. The effectiveness of the new TB control network in Shanghai. *Journal of the Chinese Antituberculosis Association*, 2007, 29, 74–7.
8. Guidelines for implementing the national tuberculosis control program in China, Ministry of Health, 2009.
9. Regulation on the Administration of Circulation and Vaccination of Vaccines. The State Council, 2005.*

* Refer to the footnote at Chapter 40.

# 15

# Reflections on public health challenges of the HIV epidemic among men who have sex with men in China

*Joseph T. F. Lau, Eric P. F. Chow, Jing Hua Li and Lei Zhang*

## Introduction

The HIV epidemic among men who have sex with men (MSM) is a global one. The HIV prevalence among MSM in Western countries rebounded after the initial decline observed during the 1980s and early 1990s [1–4]. In various Asian countries, a sharp increase in HIV prevalence has been observed. For instance, the HIV prevalence among MSM increased rapidly from 17 per cent in 2003 to 28 per cent in 2009 in Bangkok, Thailand [5] and from 5.2 per cent in 2007 to 8.5 per cent in 2011 in Indonesia [6, 7]. Concentrated prevention efforts have shown to be effective in controlling HIV epidemics in some heterosexual populations, such as the well-known 100 per cent condom campaign conducted in Thailand [8, 9] and the effective HIV prevention campaign conducted in Cambodia [10].

In China, where there are about 0.78 million HIV cases [11] within a large population of 1.35 billion [12] and an estimated prevalence of about 2–5 per cent of MSM among the sexually mature and active male population [13], the HIV epidemic among MSM would dominate the future number of HIV cases in the country. As it will be demonstrated in this chapter, it is evident that the HIV epidemic among MSM is not under control despite a lot of attention being paid to it and intensive efforts being made. In-depth reflections on some of the major problems involved are necessary and may draw useful insights not only for HIV prevention in China, but also for other countries where the epidemic trends share similar patterns.

## The HIV epidemic among MSM in China

The national HIV epidemic among MSM has increased rapidly in the last decade and is now spreading at an alarming rate across the country, from 1.4 per cent in 2001 to 6.3 per cent in 2011 [11, 14], while Southwest China has the highest HIV prevalence (11.4 per cent; 95 per cent CI: 9.6–13.5 per cent) [14]. Consistently, growing trends of HIV epidemic among MSM have been observed in many Chinese provinces and municipalities, such as Beijing

(1.5 per cent in 2004 to 7.9 per cent in 2011) [15, 16], Chongqing (from 0.0 per cent in 2004 to 19.0 per cent in 2009) [17, 18], Guangdong (1.7 per cent in 2003 to 5.8 per cent in 2010) [19, 20], Henan (from 0.9 per cent in 2003 to 12.5 per cent in 2011) [16], Heilongjiang (from 1.2 per cent in 2003 to 10.3 per cent in 2011) [16], Liaoning (from 1.9 per cent in 2006 to 8.1 per cent in 2009) [21, 22], Shanghai (from 1.5 per cent in 2005 to 5.0 per cent in 2009) [21, 23], Sichuan (from 0.6 per cent in 2003 to 16.3 per cent in 2011) [16, 24] and Yunnan (from 2.4 per cent in 2004 to 11.6 per cent in 2010) [25, 26]. In 2011, the HIV prevalence among MSM in Chongqing, Chengdu and some other cities exceeded 20 per cent (personal correspondence with provincial CDC). Alarmingly high HIV incidence rates have been observed in different parts of China, such as Beijing city (from 2.9 to 8.1 per 100 person-years during 2005–2009) [27, 28], Chongqing (from 7.3 to 9.4 per 100 person-years during 2006–2008) [29–31], Nanjing city of Jiangsu province (from 3.4 to 4.2 per 100 person-years during 2008–2010) [32, 33] and Shenyang city of Liaoning province (from 4.7 to 10.2 per 100 person-years during 2007–2009). Such extremely high incidence rates imply that HIV prevalence would increase sharply in the absence of new effective interventions. As expected, the proportion of all reported diagnosed HIV/AIDS cases in China that are attributed to male homosexual exposure is rising sharply, from 7.3 per cent in 2005 [34] to 12.2 per cent in 2007 [35] to 32.5 per cent in 2009 [36]. In Kunming city of Southwest China, the proportion has increased from 2.2 per cent in 2000 to 42.2 per cent in 2007 [37].

## HIV-related risk behaviours among MSM in China

The high HIV prevalence is not surprising when its behavioural context is revealed. In 2006, a large study conducted in nine major cities estimated that 85 per cent of the MSM in China engage in anal sex [38, 39], each of them has had an average of 6.6 ± 15.6 anal sex partners in the past six months [39] and 18.6 per cent of them have involved in group sex [39]. In addition, the majority of Chinese MSM reported to have multiple male sex partners. The national statistics showed that the proportion of Chinese MSM who had multiple male sex partners in the past six months increased from 68.0 per cent in 2008 to 85.4 per cent in 2011 [16]. Of the MSM in China, 4.2 to 13.7 per cent have paid a male partner for sex in the past six months in 2010 [40–43]. The prevalence of unprotected anal sex is also high. The low condom use rate is mainly due to the preference of better sexual sensation and the fear of making partners feeling untrusted [39]. A recent meta-analysis summarized that MSM with regular male partners had the lowest consistent condom use rate over the past six months (19.9 per cent) during 2003–2007, as compared with non-commercial casual (30.4 per cent) during 2003–2007 and commercial partnerships (58.0 per cent) during 2006–2008 [44]. It was estimated that 6.0 to 26.4 per cent of the MSM in China in 2010 were male sex workers, usually known as money boys (MBs) [43, 45–53]. Furthermore, use of psychoactive substances may become a new trend among MSM in China. Although previous data showed low prevalence (3–4 per cent) of substance use among MSM in China [54], drug use is more common among MBs than among non-MB MSM [55], and our unpublished data show that about half of the MSM in Beijing use a new substance called RUSH before having anal sex with men and the use was associated with unprotected anal sex. This substance is illegal in several Western countries (e.g. the USA and France), but is still legal in China. It remains a challenge to promote public health interventions to this population [56].

Despite a significant increasing trend of HIV annual testing among MSM in China (from 11.0 per cent in 2003 to 50.4 per cent in 2011) [16, 57], about 87.0 per cent of all HIV-infected MSM in China remained undiagnosed in 2007 [37]. A recent report revealed that 26 per cent of Chinese medical staff exhibited discriminatory attitudes toward people living with HIV (PLWH) in 2009 [58]. In addition, a high proportion of MSM in China are not aware of the locations of any HIV testing sites in their neighbourhood [39, 59, 60], likely due to the lack of outreach of HIV/AIDS intervention programmes for MSM in China. Furthermore, double social stigma against gay men and PLWH in China hinders MSM to disclose their sexual orientation and/or HIV positive status to others, including their male sex partners [39, 59, 60].

Several studies have shown that active bisexual behaviours are common among MSM in China. Approximately one-third of the MSM in China are currently married to a woman [39, 61–63] and over 70 per cent have married or would marry a woman during their lifetime, mostly due to social and family pressures [53, 64]. To fulfil parental expectation, it is common for MSM to marry women and to have unprotected sex with their wives. A study showed that 63.8 per cent of married MSM felt guilty for not disclosing their sexual orientation to their wives and 27.2 per cent regretted getting married [64]. Recent studies reported that consistent condom use between MSM and female couples in the past six months decreased from 32.6 per cent in 2005 to 16.5 per cent in 2008 [50]. Another recent study estimated that the HIV incidence among female partners of bisexual MSM has significantly increased by 5.3 fold, from 0.18 per 1,000 person-years in 2002 to 0.88 per 1,000 person-years in 2010 in China [65]. Bisexual behaviours of MSM pose potential threats to bridging HIV transmission from the population of MSM to their female partners, spreading the epidemic into the general female population [65–67]. Only 11 per cent of married MSM in China have disclosed their homosexuality to their wives [64]. There are almost no HIV-related interventions for female sex partners of MSM in China. Disclosure of HIV status to female sex partners among HIV-infected MSM is also rare (25.8 per cent) [68].

To summarize, we are witnessing very complex behavioural patterns that would actively contribute to the serious HIV epidemic among MSM in China: high prevalence of unprotected anal sex, multiple sex partners, high-risk sex work, substance use, unprotected bisexual sex and low disclosure rates together with low prevalence of regular HIV testing. Each of these problems is extremely difficult to deal with, and they also intertwine, and previous studies have shown that various risk behaviours tend to cluster together [69–71]. Furthermore, we have hinted at the complex roles of socio-cultural and contextual obstacles hindering effective interventions, such as stigma [72], cultural factors [24, 70, 73] and internal migration [74, 75]. HIV prevention for MSM in China is an uphill battle.

## The importance of interdisciplinary partnerships

Governmental leadership is absolutely essential in controlling HIV. The political context for HIV prevention among MSM in China has been improved only within the last 15 years, as homosexuality was decriminalized in 1997 and subsequently removed from the list of psychiatric disorders by the Chinese National Psychiatric Association in 2001 [76]. There was only one surveillance site for HIV epidemic among MSM in the entire country from 2002 to 2005 [77]; HIV-related interventions for MSM in China only largely started in 2005 after a number of national consultative meetings involving the government and gay community leaders took place. Since then, the Chinese government has placed a very high priority for HIV prevention targeting MSM and related research also flourished. However, it takes a long time for healthcare workers in China to develop effective HIV prevention programmes and the epidemic, which has been growing at a much faster pace, will not wait. There is a global consensus that HIV prevention services need to be backed up by quality care services. In China, free antiretroviral treatment is available but there are restrictions for those who are not local residents due to the currently in-place residence registration (*hukou*) system [74, 75]. As many HIV-infected MSM are internal migrants from small towns or rural areas, many of them experience difficulties accessing general health care and HIV-related medical treatment [74, 75].

Furthermore, it is known that the prevalence of syphilis among MSM in China is higher than that of HIV. For instance, it exceeds 20 per cent among MBs in many Chinese cities, such as Beijing [51] and Tianjin [78]. A systematic review suggested that the national prevalence of syphilis among MSM was 13.5 per cent (95 per cent CI: 11.8–15.3 per cent) in 2009 [79]. Syphilis and other STDs, such as herpes simplex virus, increase the risk of HIV transmission by two- to three-fold [50, 80]. Co-infection of HIV and syphilis hence aggravates the already rampant epidemic of HIV [79]. It makes sense to seek a more comprehensive integration of HIV and STD prevention programmes, which have largely been managed by two separate systems in China. The CDC is responsible for HIV prevention and care, whilst the National Centre for STD Control is responsible for STD prevention and care. Treatment and prevention of STDs are essential for HIV prevention, both because of the co-infection effects and having condom use as the same key preventive method in common. The two systems need to show better integration and collaboration [81–83]. Partnerships and coordination across governmental departments need to be improved. High-level inter-departmental coordination committees have been formed at the national and provincial levels. It is, however, much less clear if active, organized and systematic coordination is in existence at local levels.

Partnerships with gay communities and non-governmental organizations (NGOs) are definitely essential in controlling HIV/AIDS [84–86]. They should have different but complementary roles and duties. It is important for HIV prevention programmes for MSM to be sensitive to the subcultures, needs and values of MSM. Peer educators and peer workers play an important role in provision of various services, such as outreach to MSM in the community for peer education, voluntary counselling and testing (VCT) and follow-up of HIV-infected MSM. NGOs for MSM in China serve as trustworthy mediators between the government and MSM communities, without which the government may have difficulties accessing this special population to conduct effective epidemic surveillance and other interventions [87–89]. Development of NGOs in China is, however, very primitive as compared to those of developed countries. The political environment in China tends to tightly restrict the establishment of NGOs [90]. As a result, almost all the NGOs for HIV prevention in China can only be registered as commercial firms rather than civil organizations [84, 90]. The majority of these NGOs are very small in size, underfunded, and have little experience in project development, management and strategic planning [91]. Recently, we have contacted about 70 such NGOs in about 20 cities in China, discovering that about 39 per cent (28/72) of them had no employed staff and 40 per cent (29/72) had two or fewer employed staff (unpublished data). Therefore, whilst many NGOs have been collaborating with the local Centres of Disease Control and Prevention (CDCs), most of those collaborations may be of the nature of implementing specific tasks, such as condom distribution and surveys, which are routine responsibilities of the CDCs. It is uncertain whether there is enough technical and resource support obtained from the government for long-term development and capacity building for such NGOs. It is important that NGOs become very strong partners of CDCs in China in order to formulate feasible and effective strategic plans and interventions. In this regard, a huge gap exists.

Partnerships with interdisciplinary trainers and researchers are also needed. The CDCs at different levels are responsible for HIV prevention services, which have mainly been provided by clinicians. The teams implementing HIV-related services need to include many more nurses, social workers, psychologists and interdisciplinary researchers. Capacity building is essential for HIV prevention. For instance, VCT is one of the very few evidence-based means of HIV prevention [92, 93] that has been used widely in HIV prevention services targeting MSM in China. It has shown to be a means of case detection and can reduce risky behaviours [92, 93]. However, the counselling component of VCT may be quite weak in China [94–96]. Behavioural health theories, such as stages of change theories [97], and counselling methods, such as motivational interviewing [98], have shown to be useful in increasing effectiveness of VCT [99–102]. However, very few of the VCT service providers in China have been trained accordingly. Partnership between trainers and researchers hence needs to be strengthened.

In the past decade, academicians have been collaborating with the CDCs of different provinces and levels, and have generated many journal papers. However, not much of this collaborative research seems to have been translated into regular and effective services. The reasons are complex but attention is needed. The development of behavioural health in China may be lagging behind as compared to that of Western countries. According to our investigation, the majority of the schools of public health in Chinese universities do not have faculty members trained with doctorate degrees in psychology or other behavioural health disciplines. Stable and long-term partnership with international and local academic institutions may need to go beyond implementation of ad hoc research projects, but be extended to include the generation of research agenda, problem identification and problem solving through systematic operation research and strategic planning. Improvements are warranted.

## Pros and cons of the expanding social networking among MSM in China

A decade ago, MSM were almost invisible in China. This is understandable as the Chinese culture does not find same-sex behaviours among men acceptable and strong stigma exists. When HIV prevention campaigns in China first started targeting MSM, this was considered a very hard-to-reach population. The picture has changed completely over the last few years. Unlike female sex workers and injecting drug users, MSM have not been harassed by police as same-sex activity is not illegal in China. Gay activities and operations of gay venues, such as gay bars and saunas, have become much more open and flourish in most of the major cities in China as long as they do not involve commercial sex. This is also part of the globalization trend as gay movements spread from Western countries to Asian countries. Celebrities come out and disclose their homosexual and bisexual orientations. MSM have become not only visible, at least within the sight of healthcare workers, but they also concentrate in major cities where there are more gay venues, having a relatively open culture for same-sex activities, and easy access to friends and partners who are MSM. As a result, the majority of the MSM in many cities, such as Shenzhen (88.2 per cent) [103], Shanghai (78 per cent) [23], Chengdu (52.6 per cent) [104] and Beijing (75.6 per cent) [104] are internal migrants – many of them coming from smaller towns to find a new, more enjoyable life as an MSM in a big city. The internal migrant status contributes to high prevalence of risk factors of HIV-related behaviours, such as stress and poor mental health, lack of social support and unstable relationships, as well as financial burden that may result in sex work [105, 106]. Availability of medical treatments for MSM who move away from their hometowns is another potential problem [74, 75].

The rapid socio-economic development in China further speeds up the process of building up MSM communities across the country. High proportions of MSM in urban China are relatively well educated. Previous studies have shown that 47.7 per cent to 79.6 per cent had attended colleges or universities in 2010 [20, 46, 107]. The concentration of critical masses of educated MSM who are relatively stable in their financial situation in Chinese cities allows for creation of NGOs for self-help and advocacy among MSM in China. Though small in size, most of these NGOs have been operated by peer workers and peer volunteers, serving MSM in the community not only on HIV prevention, but also on social functions. MSM may see these NGOs as a home away from home where they can share their emotional feelings with others. Therefore, the ability for these NGOs to attract and build up MSM communities is disproportionate to their size and should not be underestimated. For instance, one of the NGOs in Chengdu which has 12 paid staff, was able to create a gay-friendly social media platform which has enrolled over 10,000 MSM members within a year (personal communication), and the NGO is currently actively serving about 1,400 or about 80 per cent of all the HIV-infected MSM that have been identified in the city.

The rapid development of electronic social media completes the process of community building for MSM in China. Gay-friendly websites have been created for MSM in most cities. Smart phones and the Internet have become widely available and are very affordable in China (as low as 100 RMB or 16 USD per month). In Chengdu, it is estimated that over 80 per cent of the MSM are using one of the social media platforms, QQ, which is the most widely used Chinese instant messaging and social networking tool and has multiple functions including one-to-one and group chat, sharing photos, videos, notes and links, blogs and other functions. New social networking platforms and applications (e.g. Sina micro-blog, Jack'd, Pengpeng and M2 date) make it even more convenient to find male sex partners over the Internet and using smart phones. About 51.7–79.6 per cent of the MSM in China sourced male sex partners through the Internet in 2009 [108–115], compared with only 27.2–38.8 per cent in 2004 [15, 116–118]. Previous studies have, however, suggested that sex partnership involving partners recruited via the Internet may also be associated with risk behaviours, such as unprotected anal sex [119].

It is apparently good news for HIV prevention workers to know that a large number of MSM are networking intensively with each other. The China CDCs greatly need such platforms to conduct HIV-related surveillance and to recruit MSM for testing and hence case detection, often in collaboration with the local NGOs. The financial support provided by the CDCs for collaborative work may be small but it is essential and critical for sustaining these NGOs. Fundraising for NGOs is rare in China and the income obtained from CDCs may hence be the major source of support for these NGOs. Besides financial support, collaborations with CDCs justify the existence of such NGOs, making them more socially and politically acceptable. Therefore, collaboration with CDCs is one of the several factors contributing to the rapid building up of MSM communities in China.

The potential extension of social networking, either through NGOs or electronic media, provides a potential platform for HIV prevention. Peer education and online HIV prevention services have been delivered to MSM in different cities in China, such as Chengdu and Shenzhen. Some of such interventions have been conducted with success in Western countries [120–122]. This should, however, be approached with caution, as such intensive social networks could also mean concentrations of large numbers of individuals practising high risk behaviours, as multiple partnership and unprotected anal sex are very prevalent among MSM in China [44, 54, 84, 123]. Our study showed that peer influences among MSM could be negative [124] rather than positive. Those with higher proportions of friends who are involved in various high risk behaviours and related attitudes were more likely to practise similar risk behaviours [124]. Such findings corroborate with those of the literature that the characteristics of a social network can potentially increase risk behaviours of its members [125–127], and this also applies to MSM [125, 126].

Unfortunately, very few effective theory-based and evidence-based intervention programmes for HIV prevention targeting MSM in China have been documented in the literature, possibly due to the short history of HIV prevention for MSM in China and the lack of interdisciplinary support, as mentioned previously. Therefore, in the absence of effective interventions, the gathering of numerous high-risk MSM in the calling of NGOs is potentially a mixed blessing and a curse. It might have become much easier to access a larger number of male sex partners since the establishment of these new organizations and networks than it has been in the past. There are very few studies investigating the impact of expanded social networking and the prevention versus the spread of HIV among MSM in China via these networks. Such studies are warranted. Research is greatly needed to document changes in levels of risk before and after MSM move to cities and join the local MSM community through NGO activities and electronic networking. It is hence potentially important to understand and to shape up social norms for HIV testing and safer sex through these physical and electronic networks. However, review of the literature and discussion with NGO members at different places suggest that such opportunities have not been fully explored.

## The unfavourable social environment

Social scientists have placed high importance on social norms in understanding various types of behaviours [128–130]. We have seen that concurrent sexual partnerships are popular among MSM in China [23, 131]. Monogamy is the norm for Chinese heterosexual couples [132], but it is less clear whether that is the case for MSM in the country. Homosexual marriage has been controversial. It is legally recognized nationwide in some countries [133], such as Canada [134], Denmark [135] and Spain [136], but not in China. There are contentions that social rejection of MSM leads them to engage in unstable relationships [137], amongst other reasons. This reasoning may only be partial as multiple partnerships might be normative to a large number of MSM. Unlike heterosexual relationships, the social control for monogamy among MSM might be relatively weak or even absent. Our literature review finds no discussion on this topic. It is potentially important to strengthen norms on monogamy among MSM engaging in regular partnerships, which make up 56.7 to 70.1 per cent of partnership networks of the population [104]. Despite multiple sex partnerships, romantic love exists among MSM. Norm building is possible and successful interventions have been reported [122].

Discussion about the HIV epidemic among MSM would be incomplete without mentioning stigma. Stigma toward MSM originates not only from the general public [138, 139], but also from employers, friends, service providers and even family members [140]. The one-child policy and emphasis on continuation of the family line as an important criterion of filial conduct [73, 141] compound the feeling of shame and guilt with stigma in family settings. Layered stigma has been described in the literature [133] – MSM who are sex workers and/or who are HIV-infected and/or are transgender would have double or more sources of stigma. MSM in China tend to face many stressors and hence have prevalent psychological problems, such as depression [142]. One study showed that 57.5 per cent of the sampled MSM were depressed; other studies reported high prevalence of attempted suicide of 6.9 to 36.0 per cent [143–145]. Stigma has shown not only to be one of the strongest determinants of mental health problems and quality of life among MSM [72, 146, 147] in China, but it has also shown to be associated with risk behaviours, such as unprotected sex, less utilization of HIV-prevention services and poor adherence to HIV-related medical treatments [59]. Stigma toward MSM is hence very consequential.

Besides being stigmatized, MSM may stigmatize themselves. Self-stigma is prevalent among Chinese MSM [137, 148] and has been associated with problems that are similar to those associated with social stigma. Self-stigma can be reduced through interventions and such interventions need to be developed. It may be difficult to reduce social stigma overnight, but it is possible to enhance resilience and coping of MSM to deal with stigma and its associated stress among MSM in China. Positive psychology is a rapidly developing discipline and evidence-based interventions have been developed [149–152]. It has been applied to many populations that face severe stress [153] and such interventions should also be applied to MSM in China.

Stigma inevitably limits the social space of MSM in China. Gay venues, such as gay bars and gay saunas, become important meeting places and, often, places for action. Previous studies have shown that about 8.3–25.5 per cent and 5.3–31.4 per cent of the MSM in China recruit their male sex partners mainly through gay bars and gay saunas respectively [39, 104]. Our cohort study showed that sourcing male sex partners mainly from gay saunas is a strong factor predicting HIV sero-conversion among MSM in China [32]. Our meta-analysis of ten surveys also showed that the behaviour was associated with a higher risk of HIV transmission among MSM in China [154]. Other studies conducted in China have also pointed out that gay saunas are high-risk venues for sexual transmission of HIV [61, 155, 156]. Condom availability is still a problem at these venues [154, 157]. Interventions do exist in some gay saunas in China, which largely involve condom distribution and peer education. Consistent structural interventions at gay saunas are required, including convenient and continual supply of condoms, arrangement of physical space to reduce risk behaviours, availability of regular HIV testing and counselling, dissemination of risk information about unprotected sex taking place at saunas and establishment of social norms for sexual behaviours taking place at the saunas. Such structural interventions have been reported [158], but have not been common in China.

## Importance of segmentation

One potential problem of HIV interventions in China is inadequate segmentation of the MSM population. Segmentation is an important strategy of social marketing which has proven to be able to increase effectiveness of health promotion campaigns [159] by providing tailored interventions to subgroups that have homogeneous values and needs [160, 161]. Current HIV-related intervention programmes targeting MSM in China do not seem to have differentiated enough across different subgroups of MSM. Transgender MSM in China have seldom been mentioned in research reports and there are very few services targeting this group. Interventions may not have been adequately tailored to promote condom use involving different types of male sex partners. Condom usage rate varies across different types of sexual partnerships [44]. Previous studies have shown that MSM had an average number of 0.96 regular and 5.36 non-regular sex partners over a six-month period [162]. Our recent cohort study further showed that unprotected sex with male regular sex partners is a predictor of HIV sero-conversion among MSM in China [155]. MBs form another very important segment in HIV prevention. Most of the MBs are highly mobile [38, 105, 163], facilitating HIV transmissions across geographical locations. A recent review showed that MBs among MSM was associated with high risk of HIV infection (OR = 1.29; 95 per cent CI: 1.09–1.54) [105]. Additionally, 43 per cent of the MBs have had a heterosexual partnership but only 36 per cent used condoms consistently with their female partners in the past six months in 2007 [164]. They are also more likely than other MSM to have unprotected sex with multiple male clients [105, 163–165]. HIV-infected MSM are another very important segment for HIV interventions. It is shown that 67.5 to 82.5 per cent of these MSM still engaged in unprotected anal sex during 2005–2009 [166]. Interventions targeting MSM who are college students may require different strategies as compared to other types of MSM, such as those who are migrant workers, and may require better use of the settings approaches [167]. Underage and older MSM may also have different needs. HIV interventions for MSM in China may hence need to consider more about segmentation. The top-down approach may have made decisions on the preventive strategies at the national level and may hinder effective segmentation at the local levels.

## Conclusion: knowing the problems but not knowing what to do

Our impression, after discussions with various health workers and NGO members working on HIV prevention for MSM in China, can be summarized by the following quotation: 'We are aware of the problems but we don't know what to do.' It seems that the plans for HIV prevention have largely been top-down. In the consultancy work performed by one of this chapter's authors, Joseph Lau, for the completion of the China–UK HIV prevention project in 2011, we found out that workers at the local level in some provinces in China are seldom involved in any service planning. Instead, they only implement programmes assigned to them from the provincial office. Capacity building for service planning at all levels is warranted. Participation in planning ensures contextual appropriateness and avoids alienation from the planned and assigned HIV prevention services. As China is a big country with diverse geographic differences in terms of economic development and service development, strategic planning needs to involve genuine horizontal partnerships with NGOs, researchers, STD doctors and gay communities, and vertical partnerships with policy makers and local workers. NGOs have a unique important role to play not only because they can access MSM, but also because they understand the culture and norms of the community and the changes. More importantly, NGOs can provide extremely useful feedback about HIV-related policies and services provided by CDCs, allowing for adjustments and improvement. Their role in policy formation definitely needs to be enhanced. Coordinating bodies should be set up at various levels. An example can be found in Hong Kong, where the Hong Kong Advisory Council of AIDS represents the government and holds regular forum meetings with the HIV-related NGOs and other stakeholders, and involves them fully in preparing its strategic plans. The published strategic plans were drafted by groups involving the government and stakeholders and were led by members of the NGOs [168]. Advocacy is warranted.

Capacity building and policy support to stakeholders are also essential. Service providers may need to become more interdisciplinary in the areas of counselling and provision of psycho-social support, and NGO workers may benefit from training in organization management and programme planning. It is important to provide long-term support for the development of NGOs for HIV prevention in China, both financially and technically.

Without effective interventions, grouping of high-risk individuals together might do harm instead of social good. Health workers should pay attention to potential side effects of expanded social networking. Intensive efforts need to be paid to develop online prevention programmes through social networking. In the literature, some of those programmes have shown to be effective [120–122]. Effective programmes should be developed systematically and should be both theory-based and evidence-based, instead of the current state of seemingly piecemeal interventions and detachment between research and practice. Specific research funding for development of operation research on HIV prevention for MSM, carefully monitored by both interdisciplinary academic researchers and practitioners, may generate pilot studies which can potentially be translated into regular services. Intervention research that does not involve NGOs or CDCs, or other local health workers serving MSM in China, should be discouraged. Planning of intervention research should consider fully scalability, sustainability and dissemination of results. Norm building on monogamy, mental health promotion, disclosure to male and female sex partners, improvement of regular testing rates, structural HIV prevention at gay saunas, prevention of substance use, prevention through electronic social networking, STD check-up and treatments (e.g. syphilis) and communication on condom use between regular male sex partners are all very important topics discussed in this chapter that should receive high priorities in funding support.

Lastly, social marketing is a promising approach that can be used to tackle the complex and challenging problems in developing effective interventions. It has been shown to be an effective approach that has been used successfully in many areas of health promotion, including HIV prevention [169–172]. Its benchmark criteria [173, 174], such as customer orientation (i.e. importance of understanding the target population), segmentation, exchange (cost and benefits of engaging in risk and safer behaviours), theory base and marketing mix (considering product, place, price, promotion) are all highly relevant to HIV prevention for MSM in China. The use of a well-recognized approach would facilitate systematic training and accumulation of meaningful experiences. Social marketing is a potentially useful approach for planning HIV prevention programmes for MSM in China as it emphasizes that programmes aiming at behavioural changes should not be overly top-down but should instead consider fully the 'needs and wants' of the clients and 'create services to satisfy such needs and wants' by involving the stakeholders [175].

The ultimate message for researchers, practitioners and stakeholders of HIV prevention for MSM in China is that they need to form regular, trustful and genuine partnerships to answer the question: 'What to do?' There seems to be no other alternative.

## References


1. Beyrer C, Baral SD, van Griensven F, Goodreau SM, Chariyalertsak S, Wirtz AL, *et al.* Global epidemiology of HIV infection in men who have sex with men. *Lancet* 2012, 380: 367–377.
2. Stall R, Duran L, Wisniewski SR, Friedman MS, Marshal MP, McFarland W, *et al.* Running in place: implications of HIV incidence estimates among urban men who have sex with men in the United States and other industrialized countries. *AIDS Behav* 2009, 13: 615–629.
3. Sullivan PS, Hamouda O, Delpech V, Geduld JE, Prejean J, Semaille C, *et al.* Reemergence of the HIV epidemic among men who have sex with men in North America, Western Europe, and Australia, 1996–2005. *Ann Epidemiol* 2009, 19: 423–431.
4. Van Griensven F, de Lind van Wijngaarden JW, Baral S, Grulich A. The global epidemic of HIV infection among men who have sex with men. *Curr Opin HIV AIDS* 2009, 4: 300–307.
5. National AIDS Prevention and Alleviation Committee. UNGASS Country Progress Report Thailand; 2010.
6. Indonesian National AIDS Commission. Republic of Indonesia Country Report on the Follow up to the Declaration of Commitment on HIV/AIDS (UNGASS) Reporting Period 2010–2011, 2012.
7. Indonesian National AIDS Commission. Country report on the Follow up to the Declaration of Commitment on HIV/AIDS (UNGASS) Reporting Period 2006–2007, 2008.
8. Mastro T, Limpakarnjanarat K. Condom use in Thailand: how much is it slowing the HIV/AIDS epidemic? *AIDS* 1995, 9: 523–525.
9. Rojanapithayakorn W, Hanenberg R. The 100% condom program in Thailand. *AIDS* 1996, 10: 1–7.
10. Rojanapithayakorn W. The 100% condom use programme in Asia. *Reprod Health Matters* 2006, 14: 41–52.

11. Ministry of Health of the People's Republic of China. *2012 China AIDS Response Progress Report*, 2012: 70.
12. National Bureau of Statistics of China. *2012 China Statistical Yearbook*. Beijing, China: China Statistics Press; 2012.
13. Zhang B, Li X, Shi T, Yang L, Zhang J. Primary estimation on population size and HIV prevalence of gay men and bisexual men in China. *Journal for China AIDS/STD* 2002, 8: 197–199.
14. Chow EPF, Wilson DP, Zhang J, Jing J, Zhang L. Human immunodeficiency virus prevalence is increasing among men who have sex with men in China: findings from a review and meta-analysis. *Sex Transm Dis* 2011, 38: 845–857.
15. Ma X, Zhang Q, He X, Sun W, Yue H, Chen S, *et al.* Trends in prevalence of HIV, syphilis, hepatitis C, hepatitis B, and sexual risk behavior among men who have sex with men. Results of 3 consecutive respondent-driven sampling surveys in Beijing, 2004 through 2006. *J Acquir Immune Defic Syndr* 2007, 45: 581–587.
16. Wang L, Norris JL, Li DM, Guo W, Ding ZW, Wang N. HIV prevalence and influencing factors analysis of sentinel surveillance among men who have sex with men in China, 2003–2011. *Chin Med J (Engl)* 2012, 125: 1857–1861.
17. Wei SL, Zhou SJ, Zhang BC, Zeng Y, Xu H, Chen L. Analysis on the high risk behaviors and other STI/AIDS factors in men who have sex with men in a southwestern city of China. *Journal of Chongqing Medical University* 2005, 30: 679–682.
18. Ding X, Feng L, Lu R, Xu J, Guo X, Xu S, *et al.* Analysis on sexual behavior, prevalence of HIV and syphilis among male homosexuals from 2006 to 2009 in Chongqing. *Journal of Tropical Medicine* 2011, 11: 689–692.
19. He Q, Wang Y, Lin P, Zhang Z-b, Zhao X-x, Xu H-f. KAP study on AIDS among men who have sex with men in Guangzhou, Guangdong province. *Chinese Journal of Disease Control & Prevention* 2005, 9: 106–108.
20. Jiang Y, Dai L. Analysis of HIV infection and its associated factors among 1454 men who have sex with men. *Chinese Community Doctors* 2011, 13: 331–332.
21. Key Laboratory of Immunology of AIDS – The First Hospital of China Medical University. Analysis in the characteristics and trends of HIV/AIDS epidemics among men who have sex with men in seven cities of China in 2010; 2010.
22. Xiao Y, Sun J, Li C, Lu F, Allen KL, Vermund SH, *et al.* Prevalence and correlates of HIV and syphilis infections among men who have sex with men in seven provinces in China with historically low HIV prevalence. *J Acquir Immune Defic Syndr* 2010, 53 Suppl 1: S66–73.
23. Choi KH, Ning Z, Gregorich SE, Pan QC. The influence of social and sexual networks in the spread of HIV and syphilis among men who have sex with men in Shanghai, China. *J Acquir Immune Defic Syndr* 2007, 45: 77–84.
24. Feng Y, Wu Z, Detels R, Qin G, Liu L, Wang X, *et al.* HIV/STD prevalence among men who have sex with men in Chengdu, China and associated risk factors for HIV infection. *J Acquir Immune Defic Syndr* 2010, 53 Suppl 1: S74–80.
25. Ma AB, An XJ, Yu HF, Zhang Y, Yang ZM, Zhang RD, *et al.* HIV seropositivity in 78 MSM from Yunnan Provence in 2005. *Chinese Journal of AIDS & STD* 2007, 13: 60–61.
26. Chen H, Luo W, Li Y, Lo Z. Analysis on HIV and syphilis infection among 831 men who have sex with men. *Journal of Dermatology and Venereology* 2011, 33: 236–237.
27. Li SW, Zhang XY, Li XX, Wang MJ, Li DL, Ruan YH, *et al.* Detection of recent HIV-1 infections among men who have sex with men in Beijing during 2005–2006. *Chin Med J (Engl)* 2008, 121: 1105–1108.
28. Li D, Li S, Liu Y, Gao Y, Yu M, Yang X, *et al.* HIV incidence among men who have sex with men in Beijing: a prospective cohort study. *BMJ Open* 2012, 2.
29. Feng TJ, Liu XL, Cai YM, Pan P, Hong FC, Jiang WN, *et al.* Prevalence of syphilis and human immunodeficiency virus infections among men who have sex with men in Shenzhen, China: 2005 to 2007. *Sex Transm Dis* 2008, 35: 1022–1024.
30. Han M, Feng LG, Jiang Y, Shen S, Ling H, Ding XB, *et al.* Surveillance on HIV-1 incidence among men who have sex with men in Chongqing, China, 2006–2008. *Zhonghua Liu Xing Bing Xue Za Zhi* 2009, 30: 878–881.
31. Wang MJ. Research on BED-CEIA in detecting recent infections and on drug resistance in recent HIV-l infections in Dehong prefecture and Chongqing Municipal: Chinese CDC; 2007.

32. Hao C, Yan H, Yang H, Huan X, Guan W, Xu X, *et al.* The incidence of syphilis, HIV and HCV and associated factors in a cohort of men who have sex with men in Nanjing, China. *Sex Transm Infect* 2011, 87: 199–201.
33. Yan H, Yang H, Zhao J, Wei C, Li J, Huan X, *et al.* Long-chain peer referral of men who have sex with men: a novel approach to establish and maintain a cohort to measure HIV incidence, Nanjing, China. *J Acquir Immune Defic Syndr* 2012, 59: 177–184.
34. Ministry of Health of the People's Republic of China, UNAIDS, WHO. 2005 Update on the HIV/AIDS Epidemic and Response in China. Beijing, China: Ministry of Health; 2006.
35. State Council AIDS Working Committee Office, UN Theme Group on HIV/AIDS in China. A Joint Assessment of HIV/AIDS Prevention, Treatment and Care in China. Beijing, China: China Ministry of Health; 2007.
36. Ministry of Health of the People's Republic of China. China 2010 UNGASS Country Progress Report. Beijing, China: Ministry of Health; 2010.
37. Chow EPF, Wilson DP, Zhang L. The next era of HIV in China: rapidly spreading epidemics among men who have sex with men. *J Acquir Immune Defic Syndr* 2010, 55: 32–34.
38. Zeng G, Xiao Y, Xu P, Feng N, Jin CR, Lu F. Evaluation of effect of community-based HIV/AIDS interventions among men who have sex with men in eighteen cities, China. *Zhonghua Yu Fang Yi Xue Za Zhi* 2009, 43: 977–980.
39. Zhang B, Li X, Chu Q, Wang N, Wang Z, Zhou S, *et al.* A survey of HIV/AIDS related behaviors among 2250 MSM in nine major cities of China. *Chinese Journal of AIDS & STD* 2008, 14: 541–547.
40. Qu L, Gao Y, Liu J, Yao J, Yang Y, Tao B. Prevalence of HIV infection and its associated factors among 805 MSM in Inner Mongolia. *Practical Preventive Medicine* 2011, 18: 2081–2083.
41. Hu JF, Wang YN, Li J. Study on HIV, syphilis and HCV infection and high risk behaviors among men who have sex with men in Donghu, Jiangxi Province. *World Health Digest* 2011, 8: 68–69.
42. Gao LM, Chen L, Ma Y, Lu JB, Li LX, Zhang YL. HIV/STD infection and KABP status among men who have sex with men in Yuxi city, Yunnan province, 2009–2010. *Soft Science of Health* 2010, 24: 547–549, 553.
43. Mao FY. Survey on HIV/STI high risk behaviors among 211 men who have sex with men in Yichang city, Huebi province. *World Health Digest* 2010, 7: 246–247.
44. Chow EP, Wilson DP, Zhang L. Patterns of condom use among men who have sex with men in China: a systematic review and meta-analysis. *AIDS and Behavior* 2012, 16: 653–663.
45. Chen XX, Yu JP, Li M, Su QX. Survey on infection of HPV and HIV among men who have sex with men in Beijing. *International Journal of Virology* 2011, 18: 101–105.
46. Chen XX, Yu JP, Li M, Su QX. A survey on HIV and syphilis infection among men who have sex with men in Beijing. *Capital Journal of Public Health* 2011, 5: 153–156.
47. Xi S. Study on AIDS prevention knowledge, behavioral characteristics, HIV infection and its influencing factors among men who have sex with men (MSM) in Hangzhou City [Master Thesis]: Zhejiang University; 2011: 65.
48. Choi KH, Gibson DR, Han L, Guo Y. High levels of unprotected sex with men and women among men who have sex with men: a potential bridge of HIV transmission in Beijing, China. *AIDS Educ Prev* 2004, 16: 19–30.
49. Zhang D, Bi P, Lv F, Zhang J, Hiller JE. Changes in HIV prevalence and sexual behavior among men who have sex with men in a northern Chinese city: 2002–2006. *Journal of Infection* 2007, 55: 456–463.
50. Ruan Y, Li D, Li X, Qian HZ, Shi W, Zhang X, *et al.* Relationship between syphilis and HIV infections among men who have sex with men in Beijing, China. *Sex Transm Dis* 2007, 34: 592–597.
51. Li Q, Wu H, Sun L, Huang X, Liu Y. Infections of STDs/HIV and assessment of risk factors in male sex workers. *Journal of Capital University of Medical Sciences* 2006, 27: 754–757.
52. Choi KH, Liu H, Guo Y, Han L, Mandel JS, Rutherford GW. Emerging HIV-1 epidemic in China in men who have sex with men. *Lancet* 2003, 361: 2125–2126.
53. Zhang B, Liu D, Li X, Hu T. A survey of men who have sex with men: mainland China. *Am J Public Health* 2000, 90: 1949–1950.
54. He Q, Xia Y, Raymond HF, Peng R, Yang F, Ling L. HIV trends and related risk factors among men having sex with men in mainland China: findings from a systematic literature review. *Southeast Asian J Trop Med Public Health* 2011, 42: 616–633.

55. Guo Y, Li X, Stanton B. HIV-related behavioral studies of men who have sex with men in China: a systematic review and recommendations for future research. *AIDS Behav* 2011, 15: 521–534.
56. Bull SS, Piper P, Rietmeijer C. Men who have sex with men and also inject drugs: profiles of risk related to the synergy of sex and drug injection behaviors. *Journal of Homosexuality* 2002, 42: 31–51.
57. Chow EPF, Wilson D, Zhang L. The rate of HIV testing is increasing among men who have sex with men in China. *HIV Medicine* 2012, 13: 255–263.
58. UNAIDS. *The China Stigma Index Report*, 2009.
59. Song Y, Li X, Zhang L, Fang X, Lin X, Liu Y, *et al.* HIV-testing behavior among young migrant men who have sex with men (MSM) in Beijing, China. *AIDS Care* 2011, 23: 179–186.
60. Choi KH, Lui H, Guo Y, Han L, Mandel JS. Lack of HIV testing and awareness of HIV infection among men who have sex with men, Beijing, China. *AIDS Educ Prev* 2006, 18: 33–43.
61. Feng L, Ding X, Lu R, Liu J, Sy A, Ouyang L, *et al.* High HIV prevalence detected in 2006 and 2007 among men who have sex with men in China's largest municipality: an alarming epidemic in Chongqing, China. *J Acquir Immune Defic Syndr* 2009, 52: 79–85.
62. Qu SQ, Zhang DP, Wu YH, Zhu H, Zheng XW. Seroprevalence of HIV and risk behaviors among men who have sex with men in a northeast city of China. *Chinese Journal of STD & AIDS Prevention and Control* 2002, 8: 145–147, 161.
63. Xiao Y, Ding X, Li C, Liu J, Sun J, Jia Y. Prevalence and correlates of HIV and syphilis infections among men who have sex with men in Chongqing Municipality, China. *Sex Transm Dis* 2009, 36: 647–656.
64. Zhang B, Li X, Chu Q, Wang N, Wang Z, Zhou S, *et al.* Correlation between AIDS and homosexuals: a study of 2046 male homosexuals in nine major cities of China. *Chinese Journal of Human Sexuality* 2008, 17: 6–10.
65. Chow EPF, Wilson D, Zhang L. Estimating HIV incidence among female partners of bisexual men in China. *International Journal of Infectious Diseases* 2012, 16: e312–320.
66. He Q, Wang Y, Lin P, Liu Y, Yang F, Fu X, *et al.* Potential bridges for HIV infection to men who have sex with men in Guangzhou, China. *AIDS and Behavior* 2006, 10: S17–23.
67. Chow EPF, Wilson DP, Zhang L. What is the potential for bisexual men in China to act as a bridge of HIV transmission to the female population? Behavioural evidence from a systematic review and meta-analysis. *BMC Infect Dis* 2011, 11: 242.
68. Mi G, Zeng Y, Huang W, Zhang L, Li T, Wang X, *et al.* A survey on the utilization of AIDS/STD related health services in HIV carriers of MSM, Chengdu city. *Chin Prev Med* 2010, 11: 328–331.
69. Taleski SJ, Myers T, Remis RS, Husbands W, *et al.* Unprotected anal intercourse (UAI) with casual sex partners clusters with other risk behaviours among men who have sex with men (MSM): results from the Lambda Study. *Can J Infect Dis Med Microbiol* 2009, 20: SB (Abstract P214).
70. Lau JT, Wang M, Wong HN, Tsui HY, Jia M, Cheng F, *et al.* Prevalence of bisexual behaviors among men who have sex with men (MSM) in China and associations between condom use in MSM and heterosexual behaviors. *Sex Transm Dis* 2008, 35: 406–413.
71. Lau JT, Cheng F, Tsui HY, Zhang Y, Zhang J, Wang N, *et al.* Clustering of syringe sharing and unprotected sex risk behaviors in male injecting drug users in China. *Sex Transm Dis* 2007, 34: 574–582.
72. Feng Y, Wu Z, Detels R. Evolution of men who have sex with men community and experienced stigma among men who have sex with men in Chengdu, China. *J Acquir Immune Defic Syndr* 2010, 53 Suppl 1: S98–103.
73. Cai Y, Liu H, Pan P, Hong F, Feng T. Social psychological stress and sex dysfunction among 458 men who have sex with men in Shenzhen. *South China Journal of Preventive Medicine* 2008, 34: 23–25.
74. Todrys KW, Amon JJ. Within but without: human rights and access to HIV prevention and treatment for internal migrants. *Global Health* 2009, 5: 17.
75. Vail J. Managing infectious diseases among China's migrant populations. In: *China's Capacity to Manage Infectious Diseases*. Edited by Freeman CW, Lu X. Washington, DC: Center for Strategic and International Studies; 2009: 17–25.
76. Psychiatric department of Chinese Medical Association. Diagnostic criteria of mental disorders (CCMD-3). Jinan: Scientific and Technological Publishing House of Shandong; 2001.
77. Sun X, Wang N, Li D, Zheng X, Qu S, Wang L, *et al.* The development of HIV/AIDS surveillance in China. *AIDS* 2007, 21 Suppl 8: S33–38.

78. Liu Z, Zhu X, Xu P. The prevalence of HIV and syphilis infection among money boys in Tianjin. *Chinese Journal of AIDS & STD* 2009, 15: 279–281.
79. Chow EP, Wilson DP, Zhang L. HIV and syphilis co-infection increasing among men who have sex with men in China: a systematic review and meta-analysis. *PLoS One* 2011, 6: e22768.
80. Buchacz K, Patel P, Taylor M, Kerndt PR, Byers RH, Holmberg SD, *et al.* Syphilis increases HIV viral load and decreases CD4 cell counts in HIV-infected patients with new syphilis infections. *AIDS* 2004, 18: 2075–2079.
81. Chen XS, Peeling RW, Yin YP, Mabey DC. The epidemic of sexually transmitted infections in China: implications for control and future perspectives. *BMC Med* 2011, 9: 111.
82. Liu H, Yang H, Li X, Wang N, Wang B, Zhang L, *et al.* Men who have sex with men and human immunodeficiency virus/sexually transmitted disease control in China. *Sex Transm Dis* 2006, 33: 68–76.
83. Choi K, Diehl E, Guo Y, Qu S, Mandel J. High HIV risk but inadequate prevention services for men in China who have sex with men: an ethnographic study. *AIDS and Behavior* 2002, 6: 255–266.
84. Lau JT, Lin C, Hao C, Wu X, Gu J. Public health challenges of the emerging HIV epidemic among men who have sex with men in China. *Public Health* 2011, 125: 260–265.
85. Chen Z, Hu J, Peng Y. Status quo and problems of NGO's participation in HIV/AIDS control and prevention in Henan. *Chinese Journal of AIDS & STD* 2010, 16.
86. Su Q, Zhou F, Tian X, Zhang K, Wu Z. Capacity of nongovernmental organizations for men who have sex with men at grassroots involving in HIV/AIDS prevention and control. *Chin J Dis Control Prev* 2010, 14: 296–299.
87. Huang SQ, Luo M. Discussion on the HIV/AIDS prevention programs and grassroots organization. *Chinese Journal of AIDS & STD* 2007, 13: 363–365.
88. Zhang XH. Utilitarianism and absence of trust: the reflection on utilitarianism guide in the movement of preventing and curing AIDS. *Medicine & Philosophy: Humanistic & Social Medicine Edition* 2008, 29: 43–45.
89. Duan Y. Sustainable development of NGOs' HIV/AIDS prevention and control in transition period. *Soft Science of Health* 2010, 24: 209–212.
90. Yu F. *Challenges for NGOs in China*, 2009.
91. Niu CX. A survey of grassroots NGOs involved in China's HIV/AIDS prevention and control. *Chinese Journal of Human Sexuality* 2005, 14: 8–17.
92. Cleary PD, Van Devanter N, Rogers TF, Singer E, Shipton-Levy R, Steilen M, *et al.* Behavior changes after notification of HIV infection. *Am J Public Health* 1991, 81: 1586–1590.
93. Higgins DL, Galavotti C, O'Reilly KR, Schnell DJ, Moore M, Rugg DL, *et al.* Evidence for the effects of HIV antibody counseling and testing on risk behaviors. *JAMA* 1991, 266: 2419–2429.
94. Hesketh T, Duo L, Li H, Tomkins AM. Attitudes to HIV and HIV testing in high prevalence areas of China: informing the introduction of voluntary counselling and testing programmes. *Sex Transm Infect* 2005, 81: 108–112.
95. Koralage N. China to offer free HIV testing and treatment. *BMJ* 2004, 328: 975.
96. Wu Z, Sun X, Sullivan SG, Detels R. Public health. HIV testing in China. *Science* 2006, 312: 1475–1476.
97. Prochaska JO, Velicer WF, Rossi JS, Goldstein MG, Marcus BH, Rakowski W, *et al.* Stages of change and decisional balance for 12 problem behaviors. *Health Psychol* 1994, 13: 39–46.
98. Miller WR, Rollnick SR. *Motivational interviewing, preparing people for change*. 2nd ed. New York: Guilford Press; 2002.
99. Weinhardt LS, Carey MP, Johnson BT, Bickham NL. Effects of HIV counseling and testing on sexual risk behavior: a meta-analytic review of published research, 1985–1997. *Am J Public Health* 1999, 89: 1397–1405.
100. Choi KH, Yep GA, Kumekawa E. HIV prevention among Asian and Pacific Islander American men who have sex with men: a critical review of theoretical models and directions for future research. *AIDS Educ Prev* 1998, 10: 19–30.
101. Gullette DL, Turner JG. Stages of change and condom use among an Internet sample of gay and bisexual men. *J Assoc Nurses AIDS Care* 2004, 15: 27–37.
102. Hao C, Huan X, Yan H, Yang H, Guan W, Xu X, *et al.* A randomized controlled trial to evaluate the relative efficacy of enhanced versus standard voluntary counseling and testing on promoting condom use among men who have sex with men in China. *AIDS Behav* 2012, 16: 1138–1147.

103. Lai Y, Cai Y, Zheng X, Liu H. STD/HIV high risk behavior survey among men who have sex with men in Shenzhen. *Southern China Journal of Dermato-Venereology* 2006, 13: 146–149.
104. Xu J, Han DL, Liu Z, Ma XY, Wang LL, Xu J, *et al.* The prevalence of HIV infection and risk factors among MSM in 4 cities, China. *Chin J Prev Med* 2010, 44: 975–980.
105. Chow EP, Iu KI, Fu X, Wilson DP, Zhang L. HIV and sexually transmissible infections among money boys in China: A data synthesis and meta-analysis. *PLoS One* 2012, 7: e48025.
106. Wong FY, Huang ZJ, He N, Smith BD, Ding Y, Fu C, *et al.* HIV risks among gay- and non-gay-identified migrant money boys in Shanghai, China. *AIDS Care* 2008, 20: 170–180.
107. She Y, Zhong XN, Zhang Y, Peng B, Liang J, Zou YF, *et al.* Knowledge and behaviors related to HIV/AIDS among men who have sex with men in western China. *Journal of Chongqing Medical University* 2010, 35: 1902–1905.
108. Zhang DD, Zhang Y, Li HL, Wang JX, Zhang S, Zhou WY, *et al.* Investigation of HIV, syphilis and HCV infection situation and sexual behavioral characteristics among MSM in Ningbo City, Zhejiang. *Preventive Medicine* 2010, 22: 1–3.
109. Gong CT, Zhang QH. Results of AIDS monitoring of 252 MSM in Quanzhou City. *China Tropical Medicine* 2010, 10: 1496–1497.
110. Liu YY, Tian B, Song WW. Study on the prevalence of HIV, HCV and syphilis and demographic characteristics among 507 men who have sex with men. *Practical Preventive Medicine* 2010, 17: 788–790.
111. Huang W, Xiao Y, Yang X, Li Y, He FN, Tang YL, *et al.* Survey on HIV/STD infection and the related knowledge and behavior among 260 MSM in Jiujiang City. *Practical Preventive Medicine* 2011, 18: 2275–2277.
112. Xu JJ, Reilly KH, Lu CM, Ma N, Zhang M, Chu ZX, *et al.* A cross-sectional study of HIV and syphilis infections among male students who have sex with men (MSM) in northeast China: implications for implementing HIV screening and intervention programs. *BMC Public Health* 2011, 11: 287.
113. Mu L, Huang A, Peng H, Feng Y, Feng J, Yang F, *et al.* AIDS-related knowledge, attitudes and behaviors: a prevalence survey among 309 homosexual men in a Chinese city. *Zhonghua Nan Ke Xue Za Zhi* 2011, 17: 401–405.
114. Wang WW, Yu SL, Chen K, Lan P. Effect of AIDS comprehensive intervention with core peer education on men having sex with men population. *Journal of Preventive Medicine Information* 2011, 27: 590–593.
115. Wang Y, Xu J, Li ZJ, Zhang GG, Li LL, Fan J. The relationship within awareness of AIDS prevention among MSM, social Internet and preventive service. *Journal of Preventive Medicine Information* 2011, 27: 852–856.
116. He Q, Wang Y, Lin P, Liu Y, Yang F, Fu X, *et al.* Potential bridges for HIV infection to men who have sex with men in Guangzhou, China. *AIDS Behav* 2006, 10: S17–23.
117. Cai WD, Fen TJ, Tan JQ, Chen L, Shi XD, Chen PL, *et al.* A survery of the characteristics and STD/HIV infection of homosexuality in Shenzhen. *Modern Preventive Medicine* 2005, 32: 328–330.
118. Yang HT, Ding JP, Chen GH, Li XF, Zhang BC, Guan WH. Behavioral features of men who have sex with men in Jiangsu. *Jiangsu Prev Med* 2006, 17: 1–4.
119. Mustanski BS. Are sexual partners met online associated with HIV/STI risk behaviours? Retrospective and daily diary data in conflict. *AIDS Care* 2007, 19: 822–827.
120. Amirkhanian YA, Kelly JA, Kabakchieva E, Kirsanova AV, Vassileva S, Takacs J, *et al.* A randomized social network HIV prevention trial with young men who have sex with men in Russia and Bulgaria. *AIDS* 2005, 19: 1897–1905.
121. Amirkhanian YA, Kelly JA, Kabakchieva E, McAuliffe TL, Vassileva S. Evaluation of a social network HIV prevention intervention program for young men who have sex with men in Russia and Bulgaria. *AIDS Educ Prev* 2003, 15: 205–220.
122. Hays RB, Rebchook GM, Kegeles SM. The Mpowerment Project: community-building with young gay and bisexual men to prevent HIV1. *Am J Community Psychol* 2003, 31: 301–312.
123. She M, Zhang HB, Wang J, Xu J, Duan YW, Song DD, *et al.* Investigation of HIV and syphilis infection status and risk sexual behavior among men who have sex with men in four cities of China. *Zhonghua Yu Fang Yi Xue Za Zhi* 2012, 46: 324–328.
124. Hao C, Lau JT, Zhao X, Yang H, Huan X, Yan H. Associations between characteristics of the peer social network of significant others and risk of HIV transmission among men who have sex with men in China. *AIDS and Behavior* 2013, 5 May.

125. Amirkhanian YA, Kelly JA, Kukharsky AA, Borodkina OI, Granskaya JV, Dyatlov RV, *et al.* Predictors of HIV risk behavior among Russian men who have sex with men: an emerging epidemic. *AIDS* 2001, 15: 407–412.
126. Kegeles SM, Hays RB, Coates TJ. The Mpowerment Project: a community-level HIV prevention intervention for young gay men. *Am J Public Health* 1996, 86: 1129–1136.
127. Latkin CA, Hua W, Forman VL. The relationship between social network characteristics and exchanging sex for drugs or money among drug users in Baltimore, MD, USA. *Int J STD AIDS* 2003, 14: 770–775.
128. Scott J, Marshall G. *A Dictionary of Sociology*, Oxford: Oxford University Press; 2009.
129. Ajzen I. From intention to actions: a theory of planned behaviour. In: *Action Control: from Cognition to Behavior.* Edited by Julius K, Beckmann J. New York: Springer-Verlag; 1985: 10–39.
130. Ajzen I. The theory of planned behaviour. *Organizational Behavior and Human Decision Processes* 1991, 50: 179–211.
131. Ha TH, Liu H, Cai Y, Feng T. Concurrent sexual partnerships among men who have sex with men in Shenzhen, China. *Sex Transm Dis* 2010, 37: 506–511.
132. Hare-Mustin RT. China's Marriage Law: a model for family responsibilities and relationships. *Fam Process* 1982, 21: 477–481.
133. Altman D, Aggleton P, Williams M, Kong T, Reddy V, Harrad D, *et al.* Men who have sex with men: stigma and discrimination. *Lancet* 2012, 380: 439–445.
134. An Act respecting certain aspects of legal capacity for marriage for civil purposes. Civil Marriage Act. S.C. 2005, Government of Canada.
135. Sanners P. Gay marriage legalised. *Copenhagen Post*; 7 June 2012.
136. Spain approves liberal gay marriage law. *St. Petersburg Times*; 1 June 2005.
137. Neilands TB, Steward WT, Choi KH. Assessment of stigma towards homosexuality in China: a study of men who have sex with men. *Arch Sex Behav* 2008, 37: 838–844.
138. Cloete A, Simbayi LC, Kalichman SC, Strebel A, Henda N. Stigma and discrimination experiences of HIV-positive men who have sex with men in Cape Town, South Africa. *AIDS Care* 2008, 20: 1105–1110.
139. Dowshen N, Binns HJ, Garofalo R. Experiences of HIV-related stigma among young men who have sex with men. *AIDS Patient Care STDS* 2009, 23: 371–376.
140. Gill B. China's HIV/AIDS crisis: implications for human rights, the rule of law and U.S.–China relations. Testimony before the Congressional-Executive Commission on China, Roundtable on HIV/AIDS; 9 September 2002.
141. Liu JX, Choi K. Experiences of social discrimination among men who have sex with men in Shanghai, China. *AIDS Behav* 2006, 10: S25–33.
142. Zheng Y, Xu J, Zhang H. Anxiety, depression and high-risk behaviors among men who have sex with men. *Chinese Mental Health Journal* 2005, 19: 699–701.
143. Wu H, Sun Y, Zhang X, Zhang Z, Cao H. Study on the social psychology influencing factors of suicidal ideation in people living with AIDS. *Chin J Dis Control Prev* 2007, 11: 342–345.
144. Jin H, Hampton Atkinson J, Yu X, Heaton RK, Shi C, Marcotte TP, *et al.* Depression and suicidality in HIV/AIDS in China. *J Affect Disord* 2006, 94: 269–275.
145. Lau JT, Yu XN, Mak WW, Cheng YM, Lv YH, Zhang JX. Suicidal ideation among HIV+ former blood and/or plasma donors in rural China. *AIDS Care* 2010, 22: 946–954.
146. Wong WC, Zhang J, Wu SC, Kong TS, Ling DC. The HIV related risks among men having sex with men in rural Yunnan, China: a qualitative study. *Sex Transm Infect* 2006, 82: 127–130.
147. Chen G, Li Y, Zhang B, Yu Z, Li X, Wang L. Psychological characteristics in high-risk MSM in China. *BMC Public Health* 2012, 12: 58.
148. Lau JT, Kim JH, Lau M, Tsui HY. HIV related behaviours and attitudes among Chinese men who have sex with men in Hong Kong: a population based study. *Sex Transm Infect* 2004, 80: 459–465.
149. Emmons RA, McCullough ME. Counting blessings versus burdens: an experimental investigation of gratitude and subjective well-being in daily life. *Journal of Personality and Social Psychology* 2003, 84: 377–389.
150. Lyubomirsky S, Tkach C, Sheldon KM. Pursuing sustained happiness through random acts of kindness and counting one's blessing: tests of two 6-week interventions. Unpublished manuscript, Department of Psychology, University of California, Riverside; 2005.

151. Seligman MEP, Steen TA, Park N, Peterson C. Positive psychology progress: empirical validation of interventions. *American Psychologist* 2005, 60: 410–421.
152. Sheldon KM, Lyubomirsky S. How to increase and sustain positive emotion: the effects of expressing gratitude and visualizing best possible selves. *Journal of Positive Psychology* 2006, 1: 73–82.
153. Sin NL, Lyubomirsky S. Enhancing well-being and alleviating depressive symptoms with positive psychology interventions: a practice-friendly meta-analysis. *Journal of Clinical Psychology* 2009, 65: 467–487.
154. Lau JT, Zhao J, Wu X, Gu J, Hao C. Gay saunas and the risk of HIV and syphilis transmissions in China: results from a meta-analysis. *Journal of Sexual Medicine* 2012, 10, 3: 642–652.
155. Yang H, Hao C, Huan X, Yan H, Guan W, Xu X, *et al.* HIV incidence and associated factors in a cohort of men who have sex with men in Nanjing, China. *Sex Transm Dis* 2010, 37: 208–213.
156. Hong FC, Zhou H, Cai YM, Pan P, Feng TJ, Liu XL, *et al.* Prevalence of syphilis and HIV infections among men who have sex with men from different settings in Shenzhen, China: implications for HIV/STD surveillance. *Sex Transm Infect* 2009, 85: 42–44.
157. Lau JT, Cai W, Tsui HY, Chen L, Cheng J, Lin C, *et al.* Unprotected anal intercourse behavior and intention among male sex workers in Shenzhen serving cross-boundary male clients coming from Hong Kong, China – prevalence and associated factors. *AIDS Care* 2012, 24: 59–70.
158. Reisner SL, Mimiaga MJ, Skeer M, Vanderwarker R, Gaucher MJ, O'Connor CA, *et al.* Differential HIV risk behavior among men who have sex with men seeking health-related mobile van services at diverse gay-specific venues. *AIDS Behav* 2009, 13: 822–831.
159. Rimal RN, Brown J, Mkandawire G, Folda L, Bose K, Creel AH. Audience segmentation as a social-marketing tool in health promotion: use of the risk perception attitude framework in HIV prevention in Malawi. *Am J Public Health* 2009, 99: 2224–2229.
160. Forthofer MS, Bryant CA. Using audience-segmentation techniques to tailor health behavior change strategies. *Am J Health Behav* 2000, 24: 36–43.
161. Slater MD, Flora JA. Health lifestyles: audience segmentation analysis for public health interventions. *Health Educ Q* 1991, 18: 221–233.
162. Zhang L, Chow EP, Wilson DP. Distributions and trends in sexual behaviors and HIV incidence among men who have sex with men in China. *BMC Public Health* 2012, 12: 546.
163. He N, Wong FY, Huang ZJ, Ding YY, Fu CW, Smith BD, *et al.* HIV risks among two types of male migrants in Shanghai, China: money boys vs. general male migrants. *AIDS* 2007, 21: S73–79.
164. Liu H, Cai Y, Rhodes AG, Hong F. Money boys, HIV risks, and the associations between norms and safer sex: a respondent-driven sampling study in Shenzhen, China. *AIDS and Behavior* 2009, 13: 652–662.
165. Xi SJ, He YF, Zhou XH. Analysis of influencing factors of risk behaviors associated with AIDS among money boys in Hangzhou, Zhejiang. *Disease Surveillance* 2009, 24: 839–842.
166. He Q, Peng WJ, Zhang JQ, Wang BX, Wang J. Prevalence of unprotected anal intercourse and unprotected vaginal intercourse among HIV-positive men who have sex with men in China: a meta-analysis. *Sex Transm Infect* 2012, 88: 229–233.
167. Green LW, Poland B, Rootman I. The setting approach to health promotion. In: *Setting for Health Promotion; Linking Theory and Practice.* Edited by Poland B, Green LW, Rootman I. Thousand Oaks, CA: Sage; 2000.
168. Hong Kong Advisory Council on AIDS. Recommended HIV/AIDS strategies for Hong Kong 2012–2016. Hong Kong: Hong Kong Advisory Council on AIDS (Secretariat); 2012.
169. Giordano TP, Rodriguez S, Zhang H, Kallen MA, Jibaja-Weiss M, Buscher AL, *et al.* Effect of a clinic-wide social marketing campaign to improve adherence to antiretroviral therapy for HIV infection. *AIDS Behav* 2012.
170. Harris AO, Jubwe S, Kennedy SB, Taylor CH, Martin RB, Bee EM, *et al.* Condom social marketing program to prevent HIV/AIDS in post-conflict Liberia. *Afr Health Sci* 2011, 11 Suppl 1: S77–81.
171. Pedrana A, Hellard M, Guy R, El-Hayek C, Gouillou M, Asselin J, *et al.* Stop the drama Downunder: a social marketing campaign increases HIV/sexually transmitted infection knowledge and testing in Australian gay men. *Sex Transm Dis* 2012, 39: 651–658.
172. Wei C, Herrick A, Raymond HF, Anglemyer A, Gerbase A, Noar SM. Social marketing interventions to increase HIV/STI testing uptake among men who have sex with men and male-to-female transgender women. *Cochrane Database Syst Rev* 2011: CD009337.

173. Andreasen A. Marketing social marketing in the social change marketplace. *Journal of Public Policy & Marketing* 2002, 21: 3–13.
174. French J, Blair-Stevens C. *Social Marketing Pocket Guide* (1st Edition). National Social Marketing Centre for Excellence; 2005.
175. Kotler P, Zaltman G. Social marketing: an approach to planned social change. *J Mark* 1971, 35: 3–12.

# 16
# Tuberculosis control in Asia
## The case of China

*John Walley and Xiaolin Wei*

## Introduction

Tuberculosis (TB) is an air-borne communicable disease caused by bacteria mostly affecting the lungs. People with TB transmit the disease through coughing and sneezing. TB has been widely spread across the world. In 2011, there were 8.7 million new cases and 990,000 deaths of TB, including 430,000 deaths among HIV positive patients [1]. Over 90 per cent of people with HIV eventually died from TB because TB is more likely to infect people with immune deficiency.

Asia holds over 60 per cent of all new TB cases in the world. The top three countries with the highest burdens of TB are all in Asia, namely India, China and Indonesia. However, TB prevalence rates in Asian countries are much lower than in the Sub-Saharan African countries due to the relatively low HIV prevalence in Asia. TB is curable and preventable and under the World Health Organization's TB Programme, over 85 per cent of TB cases can be cured with six months of treatment.

## What is tuberculosis?

Tuberculosis (TB) infection is one of the biggest causes of death in Asia, particularly in adults. It is caused by bacteria called *Mycobacterium tuberculosis*. Around one in three people in the world have live TB bacteria in their chest, but might not experience symptoms as their immune system is keeping it under control. This is known as latent TB. People with latent TB do not fall ill with the disease and cannot transmit TB. A person with active TB transmits the infection to an average of ten other people. The transmission of infection is at its highest in crowded places or in places with poor ventilation. It is therefore important to promote improved housing with better ventilation systems.

The infection is more likely to become a disease in people with reduced immunity due to under-nutrition, diabetes or HIV infection. In general, about one in ten people infected with TB later develop the actual TB disease. However, for those who are already infected with TB and HIV, around half will get active TB. In countries or provinces with high rates of HIV, an increased incidence of TB disease has occurred.

TB can be treated and cured with a six-month multi-drug treatment. The WHO Stop TB strategy for effective control includes identification, treatment, adherence support and monitoring. This strategy is commonly called DOTS, because originally the emphasis was on the Directly Observed Treatment part of the TB Short course treatment (DOTS). In most Asian countries with functional TB programmes – where TB is effectively identified and cured – the rates of TB are decreasing. More than 85 per cent of new TB cases should be cured if treated by this programme.

All health professionals have to be alert to the possibility of TB in any patient who exhibits a chronic cough. TB symptoms include a productive cough, weight loss, fever or coughing up blood. Patients with a cough that has lasted for more than two weeks should be screened for TB, which is done by sending two or three sputum smears for microscopy. If any smear is positive, then treatment for TB must commence. If all smears are negative, then treatment should be for the most likely infection. The doctor may diagnose sputum negative TB if there are persistent clinical symptoms and an X-ray result which is suggestive of TB.

When a new case is diagnosed, patients and accompanying relatives are asked whether there are any other family members coughing. Close contacts of the patient are people who live or work in the same house or office as them. If they have a cough, they should also have sputum smears examined for TB. Child contacts should be given a vaccine called Bacille Calmette Guerin (BCG). Chemoprophylaxis is given to any child under 6 years of age and/or any contact who is positive for HIV.

## TB prevalence in China and other Asian countries

Asia has the largest number of new TB cases, accounting for 60 per cent of new cases globally, although Africa has higher incidence rates [1]. The burden of TB (numbers of cases and deaths) is highest in India, followed by China, Indonesia, Afghanistan, Bangladesh, Cambodia, Myanmar, Pakistan, the Philippines, Thailand and Vietnam.

In 2011, China had an estimated 1.4 million TB cases, in which one million were new TB cases, accounting for 11 per cent of the new TB cases globally [1]. China's TB prevalence rate was relatively lower compared with other countries with high TB burdens in Asia. Table 16.1 shows estimates of cases and prevalence rates for all types of TB in Asian countries with high TB burdens in 2011 [1].

*Table 16.1* WHO estimates of TB cases and prevalence rates for all cases* in Asian countries with high TB burdens in 2011

| *Country* | *Cases (in thousands)* | *Prevalence rate per 100,000* |
|---|---|---|
| India | 3,100 | 249 |
| China | 1,400 | 104 |
| Pakistan | 620 | 350 |
| Philippines | 460 | 484 |
| Vietnam | 290 | 323 |
| Indonesia | 281 | 281 |
| Myanmar | 240 | 506 |
| Cambodia | 99 | 817 |

* All TB cases include positive and negative pulmonary cases and extra-pulmonary cases.

*Source*: [1].

These figures, however, may be underestimated, as surveys in a number of Asian countries have shown higher actual prevalence rates. Vietnam, for example, reported a prevalence rate of 145 per 100,000 for confirmed smear positive cases in 2006, much higher than the WHO estimate for Vietnam (89 per 100,000) for that same year [2]. One reason for this is that rates from prevalence surveys are based on community surveys (active case finding) whereas the WHO estimates are based on numbers of cases notified from those (passively) identified at health facilities, such as clinics. As a result, there may be an international overestimation of the decline in TB prevalence [3].

## TB control

The main TB control strategies include BCG vaccination of newborns, as well as identification and treatment of all TB cases. Treating all cases effectively depends on the engagement of all health providers, including hospitals and private partners. Also important is active case finding and contact tracing. These can be better achieved by strengthening and monitoring the performance of laboratories and TB drug supplies. The service will be delivered though general health workers and facilities with technical inputs by the national TB programme.

### *BCG vaccination*

Vaccination by BCG induces cell-mediated immunity (that is alerting the body's blood cell defences, rather than producing immunity from specific antibodies as with most other vaccines). In low- and middle-income (and some developed) countries, BCG is given at birth or as soon as possible as part of the Expanded Programme of Immunization (EPI). After a BCG vaccination, a primary infection will still take place, but a dissemination of severe infection is less likely. For this reason BCG protects against the worst kinds of childhood TB, which are disseminated to the chest and the lining of the brain (TB meningitis). However, BCG has less of an effect on adults with TB disease who commonly cough and transmit the infection to others.

### *Identification and treatment of TB*

The main focus of TB programmes is to ensure early identification, diagnosis and treatment. All patients with a cough that has lasted for more than two weeks need to be screened for TB using sputum microscopy.

Sputum smear microscopy is a simple technique for screening patients. All contacts of a confirmed case should have two or three sputum smears taken. Quality assurance means an overarching laboratory has to re-check the slides and give a report on the percentage of slides with which it agrees or disagrees. If there is a significant percentage of slides that doesn't agree with the results of the original laboratory, then supervision and in-service training is given to that laboratory.

The treatment of TB cases reduces onward transmission and therefore reduces morbidity and mortality. The earlier the TB treatment starts, the better it can reduce the number and period of infectious cases. Good TB programmes help prevent the emergence of resistant strains. Unfortunately, due to poor implementation of TB care, a significant percentage of cases in many countries are multi-drug resistant (MDR) and need to be on MDR regimens, as the TB strains are likely to develop resistance when treatment is incomplete and/or disrupted (see section below on multi-drug resistance). It is therefore very important to implement TB care systematically and with standardized procedures (called the StopTB strategy or 'DOTS'). A similar public health approach can be applied to other chronic diseases, such as HIV or diabetes.

Until 2006, WHO Stop TB recommended that all TB cases should have directly observed treatment to ensure compliance. However, trial evidence has shown that direct observation of each dose of tablets, especially at health facilities, does not improve cure rates [4, 5, 6]. Watching patients swallow tablets makes patients passive [7]. The opportunity costs, such as time, distance and cost of attending facilities daily for some months, make it difficult for patients and can lead to defaults from treatment [8, 9]. Anyway, studies have found that only a small proportion of TB patients were actually having direct observation during their treatment [5, 11, 12, 13, 14]. As a consequence, WHO now recommends directly observed treatment only for certain cases such as prisoners, mentally ill people and people being re-treated for TB [15].

However, it is still very important to ensure treatment support and other adherence measures. Treatment supervision is done at the monthly follow-up in health centres. As well as that, the treatment supporter is chosen by the patient after a discussion with a healthcare worker. The treatment supporter should be someone who is accessible, concerned and reliable, such as a family member or a community health worker. The treatment supporter encourages the patient when they are feeling unmotivated, encourages them to attend follow-up appointments and encourages them to take the right tablets for the full course of treatment. If the patient is late attending, or has defaulted from treatment, they should be contacted. This may be by mobile phone.

A newly diagnosed case of TB should begin to be treated with a four-drug regimen for two months. Preferably these should be in fixed-dose combination tablets, as this helps with adherence. The WHO approved regimen consists of isoniazid, rifampicin, pyrazinamide and ethambutol. This is followed by isoniazid and rifampicin taken daily for a further four months. Recent trials have shown that replacing ethambutol with moxifloxin is more effective and will allow the total period of treatment to be reduced to four months. In re-treatment cases, the initial four-drug treatment is extended by a third month and for the first two months, streptomycin injections are given daily.

The TB programme includes a thorough system of follow-up of all diagnosed cases. It requires the health worker and clinic to:

- Record details on the patient's TB treatment card;
- Register the case in the unit TB register on diagnosis;
- Ensure the patient receives regular follow-up treatment or go and find them if they default; and
- Record the treatment outcome (e.g. cured or treatment) in the register when the patient is discharged.

The TB coordinator (in China, this is a doctor at the TB dispensary) should check the TB record cards, update the district TB register, as well as supervise the quality of care. Reminders and double-checks can be built into the system, for example, the central registry conducting quarterly checks on each patient. Treatment adherence can be improved through new technologies such as reminders and recall using mobile phones. As well as that, tablets can be put in drug boxes with a memory chipped cap recording when it is opened. These methods have been employed to improve follow-up of TB patients in Asia and Africa.

China's national TB programme has been expanding since the 1990s. It is a semi-vertical system of TB control consisting mostly of TB dispensaries from the national to local levels.

The county/district TB dispensary is responsible for clinical tasks, such as TB diagnosis and treatment, and public health tasks, such as data reporting, supply of first-line anti-TB drugs, and training and coordination with hospitals. The higher levels are mainly responsible for the quality control of dispensaries at lower levels.

## Major challenges of TB control

### *Multi-drug resistance*

Drug resistance by the TB bacteria is an increasing problem. When a patient has bacteria that are resistant to two or more anti-TB drugs, this is called multi-drug resistance (MDR). Diagnosing and treating MDR cases is more complicated and much more expensive than diagnosing normal TB cases. Drug sensitivity analysis has to be used to diagnose MDR and other TB drugs have to be used to treat MDR. These 'second-line' drugs are not as readily available, more expensive and have more side effects. Treating an MDR case takes at least 24 months and costs up to US$5,000, compared to six months and an average of US$20 in treating a normal TB case [16]. When TB bacteria are resistant to even these drugs, this is called extensively drug-resistant TB (XDR-TB).

The most significant cause of drug-resistant TB is inappropriate treatment of normal TB cases, for example, if TB drugs are not taken correctly or not taken for the full six months (treatment default). The global average prevalence for MDR strains in newly diagnosed TB cases (not previously treated for TB) is 3.4 per cent, while it is 6 per cent in China, 4 per cent in the Philippines and 2 per cent in India [16, 17]. China's 2007 MDR survey found that most MDR cases in China were from newly diagnosed cases [17]. Of MDR TB patients who have received TB treatment before, most of the MDR strains were infected when the patients first caught TB [18, 19, 20]. This indicates that primary transmission of MDR strains is the major cause of MDR spread in China. Treatment of these patients is even more problematic when there is resistance to the 'second-line' drugs, including drugs from the 'floxacin' group. One reason for this is that 'floxacins' are often given unnecessarily for less serious infections where other drugs could be used. They are even given to patients with viral upper respiratory infections such as influenza. Unnecessary antibiotic use is costly for patients and the health system.

### *HIV/AIDS*

Around half of the people with both HIV and TB infections will develop active TB disease. They are also more susceptible to new infections or re-infection. TB is also a major cause of death in people with HIV/AIDS. Conversely, TB patients are more likely to rapidly progress to full-blown AIDS when infected with the HIV virus. All HIV positive cases should therefore be examined for TB and all TB cases should be tested for HIV. All people infected with HIV should receive long-term cotrimoxazole preventive treatment, including those that also have TB.

Preventive treatment (prophylaxis) consisting of daily isoniazid for a duration of six months is given for contacts of smear positive TB cases and for patients found to have both HIV and TB infections, thereby clearing the TB bacilli and preventing progression to TB disease with the treatment. However, it is important to note that patients may become re-infected, especially if they have HIV. Prophylaxis with isoniazid can be given to close contacts under 35 years of age and to babies (five mg/kg) born to mothers who develop TB shortly before or after delivery.

Most TB/HIV incident cases in Asia were found in India (110,000), Myanmar (37,000), Indonesia (18,000) and China (18,000). The TB/HIV situation is more serious in countries such as Myanmar, Cambodia and Thailand where HIV prevalence rates are generally higher. In China, the highest HIV rates are in Yunnan where transmission is high amongst intravenous drug addicts and their sexual partners.

## Programme monitoring

Evaluation of the TB control programmes occurs by measuring the proportion of new smear positive cases that are cured or are certified to have completed treatment. The WHO target is 85 per cent. The other main target is to achieve at least a 70 per cent case finding, that is diagnosing and registering at least 70 per cent of the estimated incidence of new smear positive TB cases. Commonly, the rate is lower than this because health workers often do not request sputum smears for people with coughs lasting more than two weeks or with other symptoms related to TB. In addition, many patients attend private practitioners who do not consider TB as being the infection the patient has or do not register the patient.

The registration of cases in the TB register is very important. The register is usually held at the TB dispensary or a TB unit in a hospital, or by the district TB coordinator. Every three months, the TB coordinator reports the case finding rate (percent), which is the quarterly 'cohort' of patients entering the register during these months. For the quarter ending the year before, the TB coordinator calculates the treatment outcomes. The outcomes are the numbers of patients who are cured (were sputum positive and are now sputum negative), completed their treatment (smear positive but no final sputum smear or originally sputum negative), defaulted, failed their treatment (still sputum positive) or died due to the disease. TB programmes use these treatment outcomes to monitor whether the programme in that district, province or country is improving or not.

China's case detection rates were substantially lower than the WHO target in 2005 [21, 22] and this was largely due to the lack of referrals from public hospitals to TB dispensaries. The hospital TB collaboration has improved since then due to the implementation of an online communicable disease reporting system developed after the outbreak of severe acute respiratory syndrome (SARS), which required all public hospitals to report TB suspects and cases online within 24 hours [23]. In addition, the Ministry of Health published guidelines to improve the collaboration between hospitals and TB dispensaries [24]. Efforts above, as well as government commitment and a strengthened public health system as a result of SARS, have eventuated in a substantial improvement of case detection in China and not only achieved but trumped the 70 per cent WHO target by 2005 [25].

## Engaging all providers in TB services in China

Engaging all providers in TB control is an essential component of WHO's new Stop TB strategy. TB symptoms such as cough and fever are not specific so the majority of TB patients commonly seek care from general healthcare providers, such as hospitals, and public and private clinics. It is vital for the national TB programmes to include other health providers, such as parastatal and private hospitals, and private doctors in the treatment programme, and ensure they follow the international standards of TB care.

Public–private partnership (PPM) for TB care has been successfully implemented in many countries to improve case findings and treatment. This has been seen in India with their revised national TB control programme [26], Kenya [27] and Pakistan [28]. Social franchising in Myanmar [29] and Vietnam [30] was used to contact private physicians and pharmacists to promote TB care. Evidence has shown that involving private providers was cost effective as compared with treatment provided by the national TB programme only [31, 32]. Though owned by the government, hospitals in China are focused on revenue generation and so this public–private (CDC/TB programme–hospital) partnership approach determines whether the TB programme can achieve its targets for case detection and treatment success.

There are three models of public–private partnership for hospital TB collaboration in China. These illustrate the options that may be relevant to other Asian countries regarding how to integrate big hospitals into TB control, because treatment in hospitals out of the TB programme tends to be more expensive, longer and not following the WHO DOTS regimens [33, 34]. The three hospital TB models in China are:

*The Dispensary Model* – This is currently the most prevalent model of TB practice in China. The TB dispensary is usually a department of the Centre for Disease Control (CDC). General hospitals take a passive role in this model, as they are supposed to refer those with suspected TB to dispensaries for diagnosis and treatment. Hospitals should only treat complicated TB cases. TB dispensaries have the responsibility to trace cases referred to them by hospitals if they have not shown up within three days. Free treatment is provided to TB patients treated in TB dispensaries. The free treatment policy covers the costs of TB drugs, TB sputum smears and cultures, and X-ray examinations for the first and last months. The policy does not cover hospitalization costs, 'second-line' anti-TB drugs and any other drugs or medical examinations in TB treatment.

*The Specialist Model* – This model is similar to the dispensary model except that a specialist TB hospital is located in the same area, usually a district in the urban area. The specialist hospital should only treat severe TB cases, while uncomplicated cases should be treated in the district TB dispensary. Treatment cost in the specialist hospitals is not covered by the free treatment policy. This model is practised in northern China such as the Shandong, Henan, Liaoning and Helongjiang provinces.

*The Integrated Model* – This model is a new development. A clinic providing TB care under the free treatment policy is established in a general hospital. A general hospital is designated the TB hospital. Patients are diagnosed and treated in the designated hospital without being referred to the TB dispensary. The TB dispensary provides public health services, such as training, mass education, case supervision and reporting, and ensures that other hospitals refer suspected TB cases to the designated hospital. The model has been running since 2002 in eastern China, in places such as Shanghai, Zhejiang, Jiangsu and Guangxi.

Current policy debates focus on the best TB control model for the future. The rise of MDR TB and other complicated cases challenges the clinical capacity of TB dispensaries. Furthermore, the dispensary model is to be phased out after the tightening of the Law for Licensing Medical Practitioners in 2002, which called for restricting medical practice in public health organizations such as the TB dispensaries in CDCs [35].

The policy debates are whether the integrated model or the specialist model should be the option for the future. One argument put forward is that treating TB should be the main responsibility of specialist hospitals because they may have better clinical capacity to deal with TB. Another argument favours the integrated model, as patients can be treated under one hospital without referral because patients normally seek care from the general hospital designated. However, phasing out the TB dispensary model will take time due to the organizational changes required in both CDCs and hospitals.

At the community level in China, health workers in the township hospitals or Community Health Centres provide treatment supervision and follow-up with patients during the TB treatment period at the guidance of the TB dispensary. TB patients normally receive a visit from the health workers or phone calls on a monthly basis to check their adherence to drug treatments. Village 'doctors' (mostly private upgraded community health workers) are required to conduct the direct observation of treatment with patients by the DOTS policy. However this observation usually does not happen because patients with TB are afraid of being stigmatized. These health workers are often poorly motivated and the contribution from village doctors to TB care has been low in China, as reflected by several studies [10, 36, 37, 38]. Because of this, and the lack of evidence for directly observed treatment, other approaches to treatment support and supervision are required.

## Active case finding and contact tracing

Passive case finding is the current normal practice in all countries where patients with TB symptoms present themselves to healthcare providers. Only those suspected of having TB are investigated for TB diagnosis. Passive case finding does not require intensive resources, but it may miss TB patients not seeking health care or those who sought health care but were not referred to the TB programme.

Active case finding strategies should be encouraged, where resources are available, in a range of population groups that have a higher risk of TB. Effective active case-finding strategy aims to facilitate easy access and early diagnosis and treatment for TB patients among high-risk groups [39]. Examples include the intensified TB case finding among people living with HIV, diabetic patients and close contacts of TB patients. Close contacts of TB cases have a higher chance of being infected with TB. Active case finding among TB contacts has provided a significant yield within acceptable additional costs [40, 41, 42]. A systematic review of contact screening in China revealed that the majority of studies achieved yield rates of active TB of around 1 per cent [43]. Congregate settings such as schools and workshop dormitories may have a higher yield than family members [44].

## Conclusion

TB is one of the major communicable diseases in Asia but it can be controlled. New diagnostic tests, vaccines and drugs are much needed and will become available in the coming years. All hospital and other practitioners need to be engaged in TB identification and referral for care. TB treatment should include adherence support and supervision. Implementing effective MDR TB services will be expensive and complex, but is essential given the major problem it poses for TB treatment. TB programmes have to be designed with the population in mind and all health providers in the country have to be engaged to collaboratively provide more effective TB care.

## Acknowledgements

We would like to acknowledge Charlotte Woodhead for her help in preparing this chapter.

## References


1. WHO. *Global Tuberculosis Report 2012*. Geneva: World Health Organization, 2012.
2. Hoa NB, Sy DN, Nhung NV, Tiemersma EW, Borgdorff MW and Cobelens FG. National survey of tuberculosis prevalence in Viet Nam. *Bull World Health Organ* 2011; 88: 273–280.
3. Lancet. Global funding for infectious diseases: TB or not TB? *Lancet* 2011; 378: 1439.
4. Newell JN, Baral SC, Pande SB, Bam DS and Malla P. Family-member DOTS and community DOTS for tuberculosis control in Nepal: cluster-randomised controlled trial. *Lancet* 2006; 367: 903–909.
5. Volmink J and Garner P. Directly observed therapy for treating tuberculosis. *Cochrane Database of Systematic Reviews* 2006; 2.
6. Walley J, Newell J and Khan A. Directly observed therapy and treatment adherence. *Lancet* 2000; 356: 1031–1032.
7. Leinhardt C and Ogden J. Tuberculosis control in resource poor countries: have we reached the limits of our universal paradigm? *Tropical Medicine and International Health*, 2004; 9: 833–841.
8. Khan MA, Walley JD, Witter SN, Imran A and Safdar N. Costs and cost effectiveness of different DOT strategies for the treatment of tuberculosis in Pakistan. *Health Policy and Planning* 2002; 17: 178–186.
9. Khan MA, Walley JD, Witter SN, Shah SK and Javeed S. Tuberculosis patient adherence to direct observation: results of a social study in Pakistan. *Health Policy and Planning* 2005; 20: 354–365.
10. Sun Q, Meng QY, Yip W, Yin X and Li H. DOT in rural China: experience from a case study in Shandong Province, China. *International Journal of Tuberculosis and Lung Disease* 2008; 12: 625–630.
11. Wei X, Chen J, Chen P, Newell JN, Li H, Sun C, Mei J and Walley JD. Barriers to TB care for rural-to-urban migrant TB patients in Shanghai: a qualitative study. *Trop Med Int Health* 2009; 14: 754–760.
12. Wei X, Liang X, Walley J, Liu F and Dong B. Analysis of care-seeking pathways of tuberculosis patients in Guangxi, China, with and without decentralised tuberculosis services. *International Journal of Tuberculosis and Lung Disease* 2009; 13: 514–520.
13. Wei X, Walley J, Zhao J, Yao H, Liu J and Newell J. Why financial incentives did not reach the poor tuberculosis patients? A qualitative study of a Fidelis funded project in Shanxi China. *Health Policy* 2009; 90: 206–213.
14. Xu B, Dong HJ, Zhao Q and Bogg L. DOTS in China – removing barriers or moving barriers? *Health Policy and Planning* 2006; 21: 365–372.
15. WHO. *The STOP TB Strategy: Building on and enhancing DOTS to meet the TB related Millennium Development Goals*. Geneva: World Health Organization, 2006, 15.
16. WHO. *Global Tuberculosis Control: WHO Report 2011*. Geneva: World Health Organization, 2011.
17. Zhao Y, Xu S, Wang L, Chin DP, Wang S, Jiang G, Xia H, Zhou Y, Li Q, Ou X, Pang Y, Song Y, Zhao B, Zhang H, He G, Guo J and Wang Y. National survey of drug-resistant tuberculosis in China. *N Engl J Med* 2012; 366: 2161–2170.
18. Li X, Zhang Y, Shen X, Shen G, Gui X, Sun B, Mei J, Deriemer K, Small PM and Gao Q. Transmission of drug-resistant tuberculosis among treated patients in Shanghai, China. *Journal of Infectious Diseases* 2007; 195: 864–869.
19. Zhao M, Li X, Xu P, Shen X, Gui XH, Wang LL, DeRiemer K, Mei J and Gao Q. Transmission of MDR and XDR tuberculosis in Shanghai, China. *PLoS One* 2009; 4: e4370.
20. Shen G, Xue Z, Shen X, Sun B, Gui X, Shen M, Mei J and Gao Q. The study recurrent tuberculosis and exogenous reinfection, Shanghai, China. *Emerging Infectious Diseases* 2006; 12: 1776–1778.
21. WHO. *Global Tuberculosis Control: Surveillance, Planning and Financing*. Geneva: World Health Organization, 2005, 75–78.
22. WHO. Tackling poverty in tuberculosis control. *Lancet* 2005; 366: 2063.
23. Ministry of Health. Notice about Further Strengthening of TB Report and Patient Management. Beijing: Disease Control Department, 2004.
24. Wang L, Cheng S, Xu M, Huang F, Xu W, Li R and Chin DP. Model collaboration between hospitals and public health system to improve tuberculosis control in China. *International Journal of Tuberculosis and Lung Disease* 2009; 13: 1486–1492.
25. Wang L, Liu J and Chin D. Progress in tuberculosis control and the evolving public-health system in China. *Lancet* 2007; 369: 691–696.

26. Kelkar-Khambete A, Kielmann K, Pawar S, Porter J, Inamdar V, Datye A and Rangan S. India's Revised National Tuberculosis Control Programme: looking beyond detection and cure. *International Journal of Tuberculosis and Lung Disease* 2008; 12: 87–92.
27. Chakaya JM, Meme H, Kwamanga D, Githui WA, Onyango-Ouma WO, Gicheha C, Karimi F, Mansoer J and Kutwa A. Planning for PPM-DOTS implementation in urban slums in Kenya: knowledge, attitude and practices of private health care providers in Kibera slum, Nairobi. *International Journal of Tuberculosis and Lung Disease* 2005; 9: 403–408.
28. Ahmed J, Ahmed M, Laghar A, Lohana W, Ali S and Fatmi Z. Public private mix model in enhancing tuberculosis case detection in District Thatta, Sindh, Pakistan. *Journal of Pakistan Medical Association* 2009; 59: 82–86.
29. Lonnroth K, Aung T, Maung W, Kluge H and Uplekar M. Social franchising of TB care through private GPs in Myanmar: an assessment of treatment results, access, equity and financial protection. *Health Policy and Planning* 2007; 22: 156–166.
30. Lönnroth K, Karlsson M, Lan NTN, Buu TN and Dieu TTN. Referring TB suspects from private pharmacies to the National Tuberculosis Programme: experiences from two districts in Ho Chi Minh City, Vietnam. *International Journal of Tuberculosis and Lung Disease* 2003; 7: 1147–1153.
31. Ferroussier O, Kumar MK, Dewan PK, Nair PK, Sahu S, Wares DF, Laserson K, Wells C, Granich R and Chauhan LS. Cost and cost-effectiveness of a public–private mix project in Kannur District, Kerala, India, 2001–2002. *International Union Against Tuberculosis and Lung Disease* 2007; 11: 755–761.
32. Floyd K, Arora VK, Murthy KJ, Lonnroth K, Singla N, Akbar Y, Zignol M and Uplekar M. Cost and cost-effectiveness of PPM-DOTS for tuberculosis control: evidence from India. *Bulletin of the World Health Organization* 2006; 84: 437–445.
33. Chiang C, Trébucq A and Billo N. A survey of TB services in hospitals in seven large cities in Asia and North Africa. *International Journal of Tuberculosis and Lung Disease* 2007; 11: 739–746.
34. Singh AA, Frieden TR, Khatri GR and Garg R. A survey of tuberculosis hospitals in India. *International Journal of Tuberculosis and Lung Disease* 2004; 8: 1255–1259.
35. Zou G, Wei X, Walley J, Yin J and Sun Q. Factors influencing integration of TB services in general hospitals in two regions of China: a qualitative study. *BMC Health Services Research* 2012; 12: 21.
36. Hu D, Liu X, Cheng J, Wang Y, Wang T, Zeng W, Smith H and Garner P. Direct observation and adherence to tuberculosis treatment in Chongqing, China: a descriptive study. *Health Policy and Planning* 2008; 23: 43–55.
37. Hu S, Tang S, Liu Y, Zhao Y, Escobar ML and de Ferranti D. Reform of how health care is paid for in China: challenges and opportunities. *Lancet* 2008; 372: 1846–1853.
38. Yao H, Wei X, Liu J, Zhao J, Hu D and Walley J. Evaluating the effects of providing financial incentives to tuberculosis patients and health providers in China. *International Journal of Tuberculosis and Lung Disease* 2008; 12: 1166–1172.
39. WHO. *Regional Strategy to Stop Tuberculosis in the Western Pacific 2011–2015*. Manila: WPRO, World Health Organization, 2011.
40. Golub J, Mohan C and Comstock G. Active case finding of tuberculosis: historical perspective and future prospects. *International Journal of Tuberculosis and Lung Disease* 2007; 9: 1183–1203.
41. Kilicaslan Z, Kiyan E, Kucuk C, *et al.* Risk of active tuberculosis in adult household contacts of smear positive pulmonary tuberculosis cases. *International Journal of Tuberculosis and Lung Disease* 2009; 13: 93–98.
42. Sprinson JE, Flood J, Fan CS, Shaw TA, Pascopella L, Young JA and Royce SE. Evaluation of tuberculosis contact investigations in California. *International Journal of Tuberculosis and Lung Disease* 2003; 7: S363–368.
43. Liu E, Cheng S and Xuejing W. A systematic review of the investigation and management of close contacts of tuberculosis in China. *Journal of Public Health* 2010; 32: 461–466.
44. Zhang X, Wei X, Zou G, Walley J, Zhang H, Guo X, Zhu L and Liu Z. Evaluation of active tuberculosis case finding through symptom screening and sputum microscopy of close contacts in Shandong, China. *Tropical Medicine and International Health* 2011; 16: 1511–1517.

# 17

# Viral hepatitis in Southeast Asia

*Lanjuan Li*

## Introduction

Viral hepatitis is an infectious disease caused by several different kinds of hepatovirus. Mostly it causes prolonged inflammation and necrotic lesions in the liver. It is highly contagious with a high incidence in Southeast Asia and is widely transmitted via complex routes. To date, five types of hepatitis have been discovered: hepatitis A to E. Among these, hepatitis A and E generally cause acute hepatitis, while hepatitis B, C and D may be related to acute or chronic hepatitis, and most likely lead to cirrhosis and hepatocellular carcinoma (HCC).

Viral hepatitis shows degeneration, necrosis and an inflammatory response of the hepatocyte as pathological characteristics. It causes nausea, vomiting, oil detestation, fatigue, appetite loss, hepatomegaly and other clinically abnormal liver functions. Some patients may also develop jaundice, an asymptomatic infection or a self-limited latent infection. Some symptoms can evolve into chronic hepatitis or liver failure.

There are different transmission routes for the different types of viral hepatitis. For example, hepatitis A and E are mainly transmitted through the digestive tract (fecal–oral transmission). The virus can cause large-scale epidemics through contaminated food and/or water. In China, an outbreak of hepatitis A occurred in Shanghai due to contaminated clam ingestion in 1988. A hepatitis E epidemic that lasted from September 1986 to April 1988 in southern Xinjiang was caused by unclean water sources. Hepatitis B, C and D are transmitted through blood, body fluids and pregnancy. Due to the hepatitis B immunization programmes promoted in Asia, the mother-to-child transmission rate has decreased considerably [1]. The spread caused by intravenous drug use has aroused much attention in recent years [2]. Hepatitis D can only flourish in a person already infected with hepatitis B.

According to scientific journals and World Health Organization (WHO) documents and publications, the estimated status for the regional burden in Asia is shown in Table 17.1.

The deaths directly or indirectly caused by viral hepatitis and its complications in Asia outnumber the total from malaria, dengue and HIV/AIDS combined. More than 500,000 people died and millions of people suffer from hepatitis every year. Moreover, with long-term hospitalization and costly medicine, viral hepatitis also leads to a heavy financial burden for the patients, their families and health systems.

*Table 17.1* The estimated status for the regional burden of hepatitis in Asia

| *Disease* | *New cases annually* | *Deaths annually* |
|---|---|---|
| Hepatitis A | 400,000 | 800 |
| Hepatitis B* | 1,380,000 | 300,000 |
| Hepatitis C* | 500,000 | 120,000 |
| Hepatitis E | 6,500,000 | 160,000 |
| Acute hepatitis of unknown etiology | 200,000 | 5,000 |
| ***Total*** | 8,980,000 | 585,800 |

* Includes cirrhosis and liver cancer.

*Source*: [3].

## Types of hepatitis

### *Hepatitis A*

Hepatitis A is a liver infection caused by the hepatitis A virus (HAV). The virus is transmitted by fecal–oral transmission, which means uninfected or unvaccinated individuals can be infected when in contact with something contaminated by the stool of an HAV-infected person. Hepatitis A can cause fatigue, appetite loss, hepatomegaly, other clinically abnormal liver functions and jaundice. In most cases, a hepatitis A infection causes acute hepatitis and often develops asymptomatically. People can be infected at any age, but particularly in infancy and adolescence. Clinical symptoms in adults are usually more serious than those in children. The peak incidence of hepatitis A is often seen in the winter and the spring. For hepatitis A, the infection is self-limiting, as it does not develop into chronic liver disease. Hepatitis A has been controlled effectively with the help of an inactivated vaccine throughout the world.

In Asia, the endemicity for the hepatitis A virus infection is different from region to region. Some countries or regions have low prevalence, such as Japan, Taiwan, Singapore and Hong Kong. In Indonesia, Thailand, Sri Lanka and Malaysia, the burden is moderate, and in India, China, Nepal, Bangladesh, Pakistan, Myanmar and the Philippines, the burden is high [4].

It is known that an epidemic of hepatitis A relies on living standards and the socio-economic environment. With living standards improving, the peak age of exposure to the virus has changed from childhood to adolescence/early adulthood. Korea has experienced a very typical cycle in that among those individuals aged 10 to 14 years, almost all of the population (96 per cent) had antibodies to HAV (anti-HAV) in 1980. However, by 1990, only 60 per cent of the same age group had been exposed to HAV and by 1995 an even smaller percentage (13 per cent) was exposed [5, 6, 7]. A similar cycle has occurred in Malaysia, where in 1985, 100 per cent of individuals under the age of 30 were positive for anti-HAV, but only 45 per cent of the same age group were positive by 1992 [8].

Currently, vaccination of high-risk groups in developed countries with a low endemicity is recommended by WHO. The groups of people who are likely to be exposed to the infection are people who travel to high-risk areas, use drugs, men who have sex with men and those who participate in certain ethnic or religious practices. Nevertheless, it is worth noting that vaccination programmes aimed at high-risk groups may not have universal influence on the general situation of the national incidence of the disease.

In Southeast Asia, the majority of people gain immunity to hepatitis A due to early childhood infection with HAV when infections are usually asymptomatic. Therefore at present, countries are not advised to adopt universal hepatitis A immunization programmes.

## *Hepatitis B and C*

As a major global health problem, hepatitis B is a potentially life-threatening liver infection caused by the hepatitis B virus (HBV). This virus is a hepadnavirus, which mainly exists in the liver, leading to cell damage and putting people at high risk of death from inflammation, necrosis and fibrosis of liver cells. Hepatitis B can result in an acute disease accompanied by several months of sustained symptoms, including jaundice, dark urine, exhaustion, feeling sick, vomiting and abdominal pain. It takes from several months to a year to recover from the symptoms. HBV can also cause a chronic liver infection, which may develop into cirrhosis or HCC. About 90 per cent of infants infected before 1 year of age, and 30 per cent to 50 per cent of children infected between 1 to 4 years of age, will develop chronic infections. About 90 per cent of healthy adults infected with HBV will recover and the virus will be completely gone within six months.

Whilst acute hepatitis B is a self-limiting disease that will resolve, chronic hepatitis B infections can be divided into three groups: chronic hepatitis B carrier status, chronic active hepatitis B and hepatitis B cirrhosis. Globally, about 2 billion people are infected with HBV and more than 240 million have chronic liver infections [9].

In developing countries, the common modes of transmission are: maternal–neonatal transmission (from mother to child at birth), early childhood infections (apparent infections through close contact with infected households), unsafe injection practices, blood transfusion and sexual contact [10].

Countries in Asia can be broadly classified into regions of high (> 8 per cent), intermediate (2–8 per cent) and low HBV endemicity (< 2 per cent). East and Southeast Asia are highly infected areas, with the following prevalence rates: Taiwan (15–20 per cent), the Philippines (5–16 per cent) and Vietnam (10–20 per cent). Korea (2.8 per cent), the Indian continent (3.34 per cent), Thailand (3–6 per cent), Malaysia (5.24 per cent), Singapore (4 per cent) and China (7.18 per cent) are considered intermediate infection areas. Japan (0.2–1.9 per cent) is classified as a low prevalence country [11]. There are approximately 100 million hepatitis B carriers in Southeast Asia, with more than 5.6 per cent of the population living in this region. Because of the chronic consequences of hepatitis B, especially cirrhosis and HCC, over 300,000 people may die each year in this region.

Hepatitis C infection is a viral infection caused by the hepatitis C virus (HCV) and is mainly transmitted via blood transfusions, acupuncture and drug injection. The virus attacks liver cells and can cause a number of complications over a long period of time. Up to 30 per cent of HCV sufferers recover completely, but the remaining individuals become chronic carriers, whether they have symptoms or not [12]. Among these individuals, 20 per cent will suffer cirrhosis of the liver [13] and 11 to 19 per cent of this group will develop HCC [14]. According to estimates from WHO, over 150 million people have been chronically infected with HCV. The global prevalence is 3 per cent and about 350,000 infections are emerging each year [15]. It is predicted that in the next 20 years, the mortality associated with HCV infection (death caused by liver failure and hepatocellular carcinoma) will continue to increase, and HCV will become a serious social and public health issue.

HCV is no longer a concern in industrialized countries. In Asia, the estimated prevalence of HCV infection is 1–1.9 per cent, which is comprised of more than 48 countries with more than 3.6 billion people. Each year, more than 120,000 people in Southeast Asia are estimated to die due to cirrhosis or liver cancer associated with hepatitis C.

Since 1992, the prevalence of HCV was reported to be in the range of 0.29–9.6 per cent in Southeast Asia [16, 17, 18]. However, there are no systematic estimates available. In 2003, an investigation involving 13,620 volunteer blood donors in China reported a prevalence rate of 0.49 per cent, which increased up to 0.86 per cent in the 40 to 49 age group, which was the highest percentage [16] of all age groups.

In Southeast Asia, chronic hepatitis B and C infections are the leading causes of preventable deaths. It is estimated that 100 million people with chronic hepatitis B infection and 30 million people with chronic hepatitis C infection live in this region. However, hepatitis B and C are asymptomatic in the early stages of infection. About 60 per cent of infected people are not aware of their condition until they suffer from complications, such as cirrhosis or HCC. Cirrhosis and HCC are irreversible, and usually lead to death.

Due to the low level of knowledge of these infections among health professionals, hepatitis B and C infections are often not diagnosed early enough. Many care providers do not conform to the WHO and national guidelines or recommendations for hepatitis B and C prevention, screening, treatment and follow-up services. To date, there is an effective vaccine available for HBV, but there is still a lack of a vaccine or an effective cure for HCV.

Currently, all member states of the region have included the hepatitis B vaccine in their routine NIPs (National Immunization Programs). The birth rate of India is higher than any other country, but India has complete hepatitis B vaccine coverage. It is well accepted by the community and health workers. All countries where the hepatitis B vaccine has been introduced have reached a coverage rate of 71.5 per cent. However, there is a lack of accurate prevalence data for viral hepatitis, which has led to limited access to testing in the region – more than half of those infected are not able to receive the limited free testing. Furthermore, some countries have not implemented mandatory hepatitis B surface antigen (HBsAg) screening of blood, blood products and blood transfusion. So far, no government will provide free treatment to chronic hepatitis B patients. Apart from establishing effective access to testing, improving diagnosis requires that those exposed to the hepatitis B virus are more aware of the risk factors and transmission routes. This is also important for prevention of the disease. Recently, a community-based investigation of 761,544 residents in China from 12 counties reported that there was a dramatic reduction in the HBV prevalence rate among individuals born after 1992, when a national neonatal HBV vaccination programme was implemented. Prior to 1992, the HBsAg carrier rate was as high as 8 per cent [19] (see Figure 17.1).

However, government-funded campaigns are not common, and more awareness and resources are needed to combat this disease. In addition to government efforts, civil society and non-governmental organizations have to be involved in promoting HBV vaccination, and better coordination with the national health authorities is needed. Hepatitis B is also regarded as a developing public health problem in the Southeast Asia region. Many blood banks in the region screen blood for HIV and hepatitis B, but not for HCV.

Injecting drug use is also widespread in most countries in Southeast Asia. Bangladesh, India, Indonesia, Myanmar, Nepal and Thailand also have a high prevalence of HIV and HCV infection and 50–100 per cent of HIV-positive injecting drug users (IDUs) are co-infected with HCV. All countries with HCV in this area have common challenges. The low degree of awareness about the seriousness of the problem among the general population

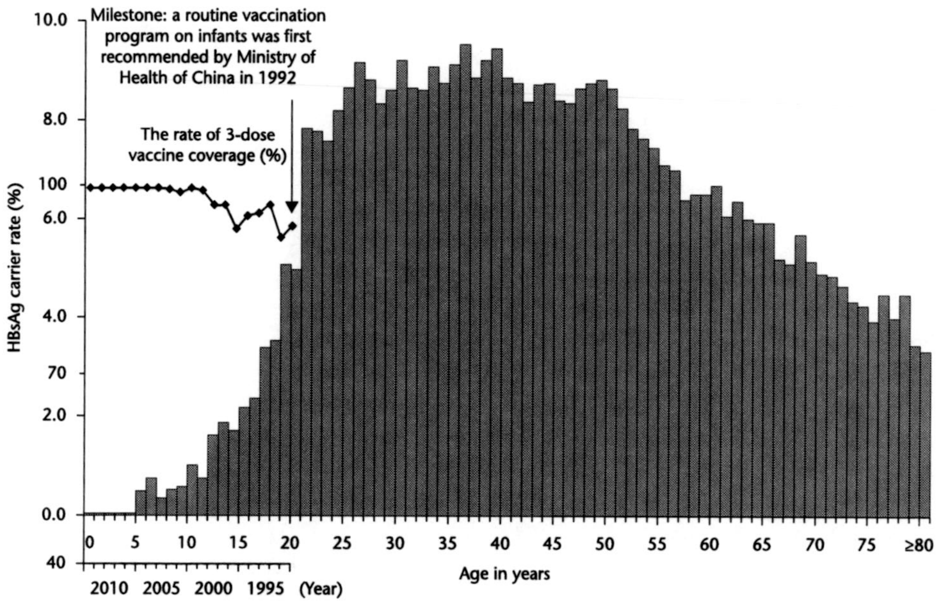


*Figure 17.1* Distribution of the HBsAg carrier rate by age in China [19]

and public health workers is one of the most important factors. In addition, current clinical knowledge of HCV is also insufficient.

## *Hepatitis D*

Hepatitis D is caused by a defective RNA virus, the hepatitis D virus (HDV). The replication of the virus requires the assistance of a hepadnavirus, such as HBV. Hepatitis D invariably occurs in the form of co-infection or super-infection with HBV [20]. HDV has three genotypes, identified by the analysis of the HDV genomes worldwide. In Asia, genotypes I and II are the most epidemic – genotype I is mostly found in the Middle East [21] and genotype II is predominantly found in the Far East [22].

HDV is transmitted percutaneously or sexually via direct contact with infected blood or blood products, and it is present worldwide and in all age groups. Due to the approach of HDV replication, chronic HBV carriers are more inclined to become infected with HDV. Individuals who are not infected with HBV, or who have no immunity against HBV, are also at risk of becoming infected with HBV simultaneous or subsequent infection with HDV [23]. Further, intravenous drug abuse, contaminated needles of therapeutic injections and maternal–fetal transmission are all risk factors.

Since HDV requires the assistance of a hepadnavirus for its multiplication, its distribution parallels that of HBV infection, although with different prevalence rates. In some HBV-prevalent countries in Asia such as China, HDV infection is disproportionately low [23]. According to a recent report about the epidemiology of HDV in the Asia-Pacific region, it is apparent that prevalence rates in different parts of Asia are variable. The rate is 3–8 per cent in Saudi Arabia and 3–10 per cent in India. In the Middle East, the prevalence is higher:

2–20 per cent in Iran and 18 per cent in Afghanistan. In China, the prevalence ranges from 1–13 per cent [24].

### *Hepatitis E*

Hepatitis E is caused by the hepatitis E virus (HEV), which is transmitted through the fecal–oral route, principally through contaminated water and food supplies, similar to HAV. Hepatitis E has four major genotypes. In Asia, epidemics have been found in the majority of Central Asia and Southeast Asia. Genotype I has been found in countries such as Burma and India, and in North and Central Asia (for example, Pakistan and Kyrgyzstan). Genotype IV is found mostly in Taiwan and also in mainland China [25].

As an acute disease, hepatitis E presents a global epidemic. According to a report from the regional office for Southeast Asia of the World Trade Organization (WTO), symptomatic cases of hepatitis E are estimated at 6.5 million every year, including 160,000 deaths and 2,700 stillborns. Therefore, over 50 per cent of global hepatitis E deaths occur in Asia.

Symptomatic HEV infection is rare in children and most common in 15 to 40 year olds, often with males outnumbering females. Overall infection rates during the epidemics of HEV have ranged from 1–15 per cent and the mortality varies from 0.5–4 per cent of the overall population of patients. Pregnant women with HEV are more likely to develop fulminant hepatitis (15–22 per cent) or to have a fatal consequence (20 per cent within the third trimester) [25].

Since hepatitis E is a waterborne disease, poor sanitation (especially in the form of contaminated water or food supplies) has been a factor in major outbreaks, such as those involving refugees residing in overcrowded temporary camps after natural disasters. Additionally, individuals who have chronic liver disease are at a higher risk of contracting the disease. Since zoonotic spread of the virus has been proven in primates and several other animal species, working with non-human primates, pigs, cows, sheep, goats and rodents are also risk factors [26].

## Prevention and control

In Southeast Asia, hepatitis is a serious public health issue and the four main viral types (A, B, C and E) are a particular problem. All these types may lead to epidemic spread and even outbreaks, while B and C result in a chronic infection in a large segment of the population. Multiple practices, such as vaccination, safe blood supply, safe injections, and safe food and water, can reduce the transmission of viral hepatitis infections [27].

### *Primary prevention*

To reduce transmission, advocacy and raising awareness of viral hepatitis should be top priority. A safe and effective vaccination programme is also widely recommended. Most countries in Southeast Asia have passed legislation to implement these measures and some regional organizations, including the Coalition for the Eradication of Viral Hepatitis in Asia Pacific (CEVHAP), enhance the cooperation between countries in Southeast Asia.

In the last two decades, according to Centre for Disease Control (CDC) in China and WHO, the incidence of new cases of viral hepatitis has decreased due to use of safe injection and safe sex practices that have helped prevent hepatitis B and C, and the availability of vaccines for hepatitis A and hepatitis B. In 2011, an HEV vaccine was registered in China and this may also lead to improved HEV prevention.

Health education is as important for the public as it is for policy makers and health professionals in order to be able to strengthen preventive measures and remove discrimination against infected patients. Currently in Southeast Asia, there have been mass media campaigns, whilst individuals have been engaged in making proposals for safe sex, harm reduction and occupational safety measures, resulting in increased visibility of the issues arising from viral hepatitis and the available solutions for the disease. Policy makers can also obtain accurate data concerning hepatitis from the CDC in their country or from the WHO, and then prepare evidence-based and cost-effective policies. By 2011, China had built an online monitoring platform for contagious diseases, with a coverage of 1,700 million people in three provinces. This network will expand to cover the whole country over the next few years.

Vaccination is an important prevention of transmission. As well as safe food and water, the HAV vaccine has been identified as providing efficient protection. To date, most countries in Southeast Asia have included the HBV vaccine in their infant immunization programmes. Although there are regional differences, which we can see from the Statistical Yearbook of the Ministry of Health of P. R. China, there has been a sharp decline in the carrier rate of HBsAg in newborns. In China, the HBV vaccine has been included in infant immunization programmes since 2002, with a coverage rate of 85–99 per cent, depending on the province. This has resulted in the carrier rate of HBsAg in newborns significantly declining from 10.19 per cent to 0.2–3.2 per cent [28].

Moreover, guidance and technical support from the CDC, the WHO and other organizations have assisted countries in improving the safety of injections and blood transfusions, with a view to prevent the transmission of hepatitis, especially HBV and HCV.

## *Secondary prevention and tertiary prevention*

Early diagnosis allows the infected person to promptly receive effective medical support. It also allows people to take precautions regarding additional harm of the liver and further spread of the disease. In conjunction with a patient's history and a physical examination, diagnosis can be made by dipping various hepatitis biochemical markers in serum (see Table 17.2).

Table 17.3 shows recommendations for screening for different types of hepatitis, which will be implemented in different ways across Southeast Asia. Since HDV can only propagate in the presence of the hepatitis B virus, it is considered to be a subviral satellite [30], and the risk factor for HDV screening is the same as for HBV infection. There are huge differences between regions in Southeast Asia, and more still needs to be done to ensure access to, and availability of, reliable and low-cost diagnostics [27].

For people with hepatitis, tertiary prevention, which refers to efficient and specific medical care, reduces mortality and accelerates recovery. In recent years, multiple new methods have emerged in both etiological and symptomatic therapeutics.

*Etiological therapeutics* – Antiviral agents against HBV and HCV, including oral drugs and immune system modulators for injection, are being used as effective treatments. As of 2012, there are five types of oral antiviral drugs licensed for HBV in China: lamivudine, adefovir, tenofovir, telbivudine and entecavir. The two immune system modulators, interferon alpha-2a and alpha-2b, were licensed in the mid-1980s. Similar to the HBV therapy, technical progress and intense research have led to the development of many

*Table 17.2* Biochemical markers used in the diagnosis of hepatitis

| *Classification* | *Marker* | *Significance* |
|---|---|---|
| Viral Hepatitis A | HAV-IgM | Acute infection |
| | HAV-IgG | Previous exposure |
| | HBV-DNA | Active infection |
| | HBsAg | HBV infections status |
| | Anti-HBs | Previous exposure |
| Viral Hepatitis B | HBeAg | Active replicating |
| | Anti-HBe | To monitor the infection and treatment |
| | Anti-HBc | HBV infections status |
| Viral Hepatitis C | HCV RNA | Viral load |
| | Anti-HCV | Exposure to HCV |
| | HDV-RNA | Viral load |
| Viral Hepatitis D | HDAg | Acute infection |
| | HDV-IgM | Recent infection |
| | HDV-IgG | Chronic infection |
| Viral Hepatitis E | HEV-IgM | Acute infection |
| | HEV-IgG | Previous exposure |

*Source*: [29].

*Table 17.3* Recommendations for hepatitis screening

| *Factors* | *Hepatitis group* | | | |
|---|---|---|---|---|
| | *HAV* | *HBV* | *HCV* | *HEV* |
| Individuals who have abnormal liver symptoms, signs or liver tests result | + | + | + | + |
| Individuals who are willing to be vaccinated | + | + | – | – |
| Injecting drug users | + | + | + | + |
| Individuals with poor sanitation or lack of safe water, especially those who are affected by natural disasters | + | – | – | + |
| Individuals who have close contact with an infected person, especially sexual partners | + | + | + | + |
| Individuals travelling to highly endemic areas without being immunized | + | – | – | + |
| Individuals who had received blood, blood products or organs before screening for hepatitis virus was implemented | – | + | + | – |
| Health-care workers | – | + | + | – |
| HIV carriers | – | + | + | – |
| Infants born to infected mothers | – | + | + | – |
| Immunosuppressed or immunocompromised people | – | + | + | + |

*Key*: + = recommended for screening test; – = not necessary for screening test.

new therapies for HCV infection. However, due to the high prices of these two antiviral drugs, access to etiological therapeutics remains an issue in many countries in Southeast Asia.

*Symptomatic therapeutics* – In patients with liver failure caused by a single or multiple pathogen, a sudden and severe impairment or loss of hepatocyte function may lead to death or, in less serious cases, end-stage liver disease, which would require a liver transplant. Considering the scarcity of donors and the self-regenerating specialty of the liver, a temporary hepatic support device, termed 'Artificial Liver', should also be considered. 'Artificial Liver' is essentially based on a blood purification device and, with or without the addition of physiological active substances, can partially carry out the functions of the liver, including detoxification, substance synthesis and metabolic functions [31].

The following are therapeutic principles associated with different hepatitis infections.

*Viral hepatitis A and E* – Hepatitis A and E are typically caused by ingestion of contaminated food or water. They are usually self-limiting and have no specific treatment. Recovery from the infection of these two viruses may be slow and take several weeks or months, but the patient won't necessarily be hospitalized. However, pregnancy or fulminant manifestation requires hospitalization and intensive care. Therapy is focused on adequate nutrition, acid–base balance and body fluid equilibrium. In principle, patients with viral hepatitis A or E are advised to rest, avoid fatty foods and alcohol (these may be poorly tolerated for some additional months during the recovery phase and cause minor relapses), eat a well-balanced diet, and stay hydrated [32].

*Viral hepatitis B* – Most adults do not need medications for acute HBV infection, as it can be cleared spontaneously [33]. But in chronic HBV infection, antiviral treatment, including oral drugs and interferon injections, is necessary to reduce the risk of cirrhosis or carcinoma. Oral antiviral drugs are the most frequently used medication due to their effectiveness, safety and ability to provide sustained viral suppression. The most important reasons for selecting interferon therapy were effectiveness, fixed duration of treatment and the lack of drug resistance [34]. In patients without a specific genotype, interferon should be used for at least one year. Patients with persistently normal alanine aminotransferase (ALT) values should not be treated with interferon outside of clinical trials because treatment might actually induce liver enzyme abnormalities.

*Viral hepatitis C* – HCV-positive patients should be evaluated for the presence and severity of chronic liver disease [35]. A chronic asymptomatic HCV carrier does not need immediate treatment. However, some patients may have severe histological changes, which may lead to cirrhosis gradually, and the diagnosis should be made carefully. Combination therapy with interferon and ribavirin is recommended for the patient with a definite diagnosis [36].

For patients suffering from alcohol addiction or drug abuse, treatment should be delayed until these behaviours have been discontinued for more than six months. Currently, the best indicator of effective treatment is an sustained virological response (SVR), defined by the absence of detectable HCV RNA in the serum as shown by a qualitative HCV RNA assay with a limit of detection lower than 50 IU/mL at 24 weeks after the end of treatment.

*Viral hepatitis D* – Hepatitis D infection only occurs as a co-infection or a super-infection in individuals infected with HBV. Co-infection with HBV and HDV often leads to more severe forms of acute hepatitis. There is no specific effective treatment for HDV, but the antiviral therapy of HBV may have benefits for HDV recovery. That is to say, treatment with interferon for six months or more may improve the patient's condition. However, relapse is common when treatment is stopped. Since no effective therapy is currently available for treatment of HDV, liver transplantation may be considered for cases of fulminant acute and end-stage chronic hepatitis D. To date, the best approach to HDV co-infection is the treatment and control of hepatitis B itself.

## Conclusion

The most common cause of hepatitis at present is by viral transmission. By raising awareness of these diseases, as well as by an implementation of a vaccination policy, the incidence of these diseases would be kept under control at the country level. With the help of the developing techniques for early diagnosis, infected persons would take precautions regarding additional harm or further transmission. Even for the sufferers, there would be new efficient therapies in the foreseeable future. Because medicine is constantly advancing, it is believed that viral hepatitis will become another eliminated disease in the near future, as was the case of smallpox in the 1980s.

## Acknowledgements

This work was financially supported by the Technology Group Project for Infectious Disease Control of Zhejiang Province (No.: 2009R50041).

## References

1. André F. Hepatitis B epidemiology in Asia, the Middle East and Africa. *Vaccine* 2000, 18(Suppl 1): S20–2.
2. Merican I, Guan R, Amarapuka D. Chronic hepatitis B virus infection in Asian countries, *J Gastroenterol Hepatol* 2000, 15(12): 1356–61.
3. WHO. Viral Hepatitis in the WHO South-East Asia Region, 2011. Available at: http://www.who.int/topics/hepatitis/en/ [Accessed 16 October 2012].
4. Gust ID. Epidemiological patterns of hepatitis A in different parts of the world. *Vaccine* 1992, 10(Suppl): S5–58.
5. Hong WS, Kim JR. The epidemiologic study of seroprevalence of hepatitis A and B antibodies in Seoul. *Kor J Intern Med* 1992, 25: 19.
6. Byun KS, Kweon SY, Shin SW, *et al.* Epidemiology of hepatitis A in Kyungin area. *Kor J Intern Med* 1991, 20.
7. Jung KM, Teon JE, Park YT, *et al.* Epidemiology of HAV infection in Seoul. *J Kor Gastroenterol* 1995, 27(Suppl): S117.
8. Malik YA, Baharin R. Changing prevalence of hepatitis A in Malaysia. In: *Proceedings of the 4th Western Pacific Congress on Chemotherapy and Infectious Diseases*, Ab, 1994, OP 63.
9. WHO. *Hepatitis B.* 2012. Available at: http://www.who.int/mediacentre/factsheets/fs204/en/ [Accessed 15 October 2012].
10. Elisabetta F, Barbara B, Laura Z. Hepatitis B: epidemiology and prevention in developing countries. *World Journal of Hepatology* 2012, 4(3): 74–80.
11. Yun FL. Antiviral therapy of chronic hepatitis B: opportunities and challenges in Asia. *Journal of Hepatology* 2009, 51(2).
12. Klenerman P, Gupta PK. Hepatitis C virus: current concepts and future challenges. *QJM* 2012, 105(1): 29–32.
13. John G, Bruce R. Chronic hepatitis C: an age wave of disease burden. *American Journal of Managed Care* 2005, 11(10): S286–95.

14. Leonard B. Natural history of hepatitis C. *Hepatology* 1997(Suppl 1), 26(3): 21–8.
15. WHO. *Hepatitis C.* 2012. Available at: http://www.who.int/mediacentre/factsheets/fs164/en/ [Accessed 15 October 2012].
16. Zhao SM, Jiang TL, Li RQ. HCV infection in voluntary donors and its influence on recruitment of donors in Chongqing area. *Zhongguo Shi Yan Xue Ye Xue Za Zhi* 2008, 16: 676–80.
17. Liu F, Chen K, He Z. Hepatitis C seroprevalence and associated risk factors, Anyang, China. *Emerg Infect Dis* 2009, 15: 1819–22.
18. Zhang YY, Guo LS, Hao LJ. Antibodies to hepatitis C virus and hepatitis C virus RNA in Chinese blood donors determined by ELISA, recombinant immunoblot assay and polymerase chain reaction. *Chin Med J* 1993, 106: 171–4.
19. Yang SG, Wang B, Li LJ. Effectiveness of HBV vaccination in infants and prediction of HBV prevalence trend under new vaccination plan: findings of a large-scale investigation. *PLoS ONE* 2012, 7(10): e47808.
20. Mehwish R, Muhamad I, Hifza K. An overview of triple infection with hepatitis B, C and D viruses. *Virology Journal* 2011, 8: 368.
21. Farci P. Delta hepatitis: an update. *J Hepatol* 2003, 39(Suppl 1): S212–19.
22. Moatter T, Abbas Z, Shabir S, Jafri W. Clinical presentation and genotype of hepatitis delta in Karachi. *World J Gastroenterol* 2007, 13: 2604–7.
23. WHO. *Hepatitis D.* 2012. Available at: http://www.who.int/csr/disease/hepatitis/whocdscsrncs20011/en/index1.html#what/ [Accessed 16 October 2012].
24. Abbas Z, Jafri W, Raza S. Hepatitis D: scenario in the Asia-Pacific region. *World J Gastroenterol* 2010, 16(5): 554–62.
25. WHO. *Hepatitis E.* 2001. Available at: http://www.who.int/csr/disease/hepatitis/whocdscsredc200112/en/ [Accessed 16 October 2012].
26. Harrison TJ. Hepatitis E virus – an update. *Liver* 1999, 19(3): 171–6.
27. WHO. *Prevention and Control of Viral Hepatitis Infection: Framework for Global Action.* 2012.
28. Shizhu C. Immunological status of hepatitis B in newborn, child. *World Chinese Journal of Digestology* 2006, 14(27): 2708–12.
29. AACC. *Hepatitis.* 2012. Available at: http://labtestsonline.org/understanding/conditions/hep/ [Accessed 2 October 2012].
30. Makino S, Chang MF, Shieh CK, Kamahora T, Vannier DM, Govindarajan S, Lai MM. Molecular cloning and sequencing of a human hepatitis delta (delta) virus RNA. *Nature* 1987, 329: 343–6.
31. Li, L. *Artificial Liver.* Hangzhou: Zhejiang University Press. 2012.
32. Hepatitis A. 2011, 2012. Available at: PubMed Health http://www.ncbi.nlm.nih.gov/pubmedhealth/PMH0001323/
33. Hollinger FB, Lau DT. Hepatitis B: the pathway to recovery through treatment. *Gastroenterol Clin North Am* 2006, 35: 895–931.
34. Asselah T, *et al.* Interferon therapy for chronic hepatitis B. *Clin Liver Dis* 2007, 11(4): 839–49, viii.
35. NIH. National Institutes of Health Consensus Development Conference Statement: Management of hepatitis C. *Hepatology* 2002, 36: S3–20.
36. Farrell, GC. New hepatitis C guidelines for the Asia-Pacific region: APASL consensus statements on the diagnosis, management and treatment of hepatitis C virus infection. *J Gastroenterol Hepatol* 2007, 22: 607–10.

# 18

# Emerging infectious diseases in Asia

*Peter Horby*

## Introduction

The former US Surgeon General William H. Stewart is often quoted as having said, in the 1960s, 'It is time to close the book on infectious diseases and declare the war against pestilence won.' Although it seems he was misquoted and never actually said this, it is true that the 1960s was a period of optimism for the health sector, when the power of sanitation, antibiotics, vaccination and vector control seemed to herald an end to infectious diseases [1, 2]. This optimism, however, was dashed when HIV emerged and the term 'emerging infectious disease' (EID) rose in popularity throughout the 1980s. The use of the term reached a high in 1992 following the publication of the US Institute of Medicine report, 'Emerging Infections: Microbial Threats to Health in the United States'. The journal *Emerging Infectious Diseases* was subsequently launched in 1995 and the National Library of Medicine added the medical sub-heading 'Communicable Diseases, Emerging' to PubMed in 2001.

Emerging infectious diseases are often thought of as 'novel' (newly recognized) pathogens of humans, but are actually defined as diseases that are increasing in their incidence, geographic or host species range or their impact (due, for instance, to the acquisition of resistance to antimicrobial drugs or vaccines or the acquisition of new virulence factors). The definition therefore encompasses both newly recognized pathogens and known pathogens that are 're-emerging'. The development and introduction over time of new, more sensitive technologies for identifying microbial diversity, such as molecular methods to identify elements of the microbial genome, coupled with geographical heterogeneities in the availability of these technologies, make it difficult to accurately assess where and when new infectious diseases first emerge. The difficulty is further compounded by changes over time in the ease of publishing articles in bio-medical literature. Attempts have nevertheless been made and 335 emerging infectious disease events were identified between 1940 and 2004, an average of five per year, with a peak in the 1980s relating to the emergence of HIV/AIDs and its associated opportunistic infections [3].

## Asia as a 'hotspot' for emerging infectious diseases

One analysis has identified Asia as a 'hotspot' for EIDs and indeed some of the most high profile EIDs in the last decade, such as SARS and highly pathogenic avian influenza H5N1, arose in Asia. Conversely, however, equally notorious EIDs such as HIV, bovine spongiform encephalopathy (BSE or mad-cow disease) and pandemic influenza H1N1 (swine flu) arose outside Asia. The premise that Asia is a hotspot for EIDs is based on the distribution of 335 EIDs after correcting for spatial differences in disease reporting and the distribution of some putative 'drivers' of EID events (population density, population growth, latitude, rainfall and richness of wildlife host species) [3]. This assessment of Asia as a hotspot for EIDs must be balanced against the fact that only 17 per cent (56/335) of EID events identified were detected in Asia.

Table 18.1 shows 59 EID events that were first identified in Asia from 1940 to 2011 (56 were identified by Jones *et al.* and three additional ones are more recent events). This table shows that the emergence of a previously unrecognized human pathogen that results in a significant number of human infections is rare. Since their identification, SARS and H5N1 have together resulted in fewer than 1,400 deaths globally, 1,000 times fewer than the estimated 1.4 million childhood deaths from pneumonia every year [4]. The potential for SARS and H5N1 to evolve into devastating epidemics does however necessitate that they are taken seriously and the fear of this 'potential' has resulted in economic consequences that far outweigh the actual, realized health impacts. The economic consequences of SARS, for example, have been estimated at US$3–10 million per case [5].

*Table 18.1* Emerging infectious diseases (EID) identified in Asia, 1940–2011

| *Pathogen* | *Year* | *Pathogen type* | *Driver* | *Location* |
|---|---|---|---|---|
| Acinetobacter baumannii multi-drug-resistant | 1998 | Bacteria | Antimicrobial agent use | Taiwan |
| Angiostrongylus cantonensis | 1945 | Protozoa | International travel and commerce | Taiwan |
| Banna | 1985 | Virus | Medical industry changes | China |
| Burkholderia pseudomallei | 1965 | Bacteria | War and famine | Vietnam |
| Chlamydia pneumonaie TWAR strain | 1965 | Bacteria | Unspecified | Taiwan |
| Dengue | 1954 | Virus | War and famine | Philippines |
| Ehrlicia sennetsu | 1953 | Rickettsia | International travel and commerce | Japan |
| Escherichia coli O118:H2 | 1996 | Bacteria | Food industry changes | Japan |
| Escherichia coli O145:H5 | 1990 | Bacteria | Food industry changes | Japan |
| Far Eastern tick borne encephalitis | 1993 | Virus | Land use changes | Japan |
| Haemophilus influenzae amp/cm/tmp-smz-res | 1979 | Bacteria | Antimicrobial agent use | Thailand |
| Haemophilus influenzae chlor/amp-res | 1979 | Bacteria | Antimicrobial agent use | Thailand |
| Hantaan | 1941 | Virus | Land use changes | China |

| | | | | |
|---|---|---|---|---|
| Hepatitis E | 1955 | Virus | Unspecified | India |
| Human T-lymphotropic virus 1 | 1974 | Virus | Human susceptibility to infection | Japan |
| Influenza A (H5N1) | 1997 | Virus | Agricultural industry changes | China (Hong Kong) |
| Klebsiella pneumoniae | 1981 | Bacteria | Human susceptibility to infection | Taiwan |
| Kyasanur forest disease virus | 1957 | Virus | Land use changes | India |
| Leptospira interrogans | 1950 | Bacteria | War and famine | Malaysia |
| Leptospira weilii | 2000 | Bacteria | Land use changes | Malaysia |
| Mycobacterium shimoidei | 1975 | Bacteria | Human susceptibility to infection | Japan |
| Mycobacterium tuberculosis isoniazid-res | 1981 | Bacteria | War and famine | North Korea, South Korea |
| Neisseria gonorrhoeae pen/tet/cipr-res | 1996 | Bacteria | Antimicrobial agent use | Japan |
| Neisseria meningitidis serogroup A termed subgroup III | 1966 | Bacteria | International travel and commerce | China |
| New Delhi metallo-beta-lactamase1 (NDM-1) | 2009 | Bacteria | Antimicrobial agent use | India |
| Nipah virus | 1998 | Virus | Agricultural industry changes | Malaysia |
| Nosema connori | 1973 | Protozoa | Human susceptibility to infection | Japan |
| Plasmodium falciparum artemisinin-res | 2009 | Protozoa | Antimicrobial agent use | Cambodia |
| Plasmodium falciparum mefloquine-res | 1982 | Protozoa | Antimicrobial agent use | Thailand |
| Plasmodium falciparum multiple drug-res | 1991 | Protozoa | Land use changes | Thailand |
| Plasmodium falciparum proguanil-res | 1948 | Protozoa | Antimicrobial agent use | Malaysia |
| Plasmodium falciparum quinine-res | 1960 | Protozoa | Antimicrobial agent use | Thailand |
| Plasmodium falciparum sulfadoxine-primethamine-res | 1981 | Protozoa | Antimicrobial agent use | Thailand |
| Plasmodium vivax | 1964 | Protozoa | Breakdown of public health measures | India |
| Plasmodium vivax proguanil-res | 1948 | Protozoa | Antimicrobial agent use | Malaysia |
| Poliovirus type 2 | 2003 | Virus | Human demographics and behaviour | India |
| Pseudomonas aeruginosa imipenem-res | 1988 | Bacteria | Antimicrobial agent use | Japan |
| Rickettsia honei | 1990 | Rickettsia | International travel and commerce | Thailand |
| Rickettsia japonica | 1984 | Rickettsia | Unspecified | Japan |

*(Continued overleaf)*

*Table 18.1* Continued

| *Pathogen* | *Year* | *Pathogen type* | *Driver* | *Location* |
|---|---|---|---|---|
| Salmonella enterica serovar typhi 3rd generation cephalosporin-res | 1999 | Bacteria | Agricultural industry changes | Bangladesh |
| Salmonella enterica serovar typhi cipro-res | 1991 | Bacteria | Antimicrobial agent use | Nepal |
| Salmonella enterica serovar typhi CT-18 | 1993 | Bacteria | Antimicrobial agent use | Vietnam |
| Salmonella enterica serovar typhi multi drug-res | 1990 | Bacteria | Antimicrobial agent use | Pakistan |
| Salmonella paratyphi multidrug-res | 1997 | Bacteria | Antimicrobial agent use | Pakistan |
| SARS coronavirus | 2002 | Virus | Bushmeat | China |
| Schistosoma japonicum | 1950 | Helminth | War and famine | China |
| Serratia marcescens fluoroquinolone-res | 1986 | Bacteria | Antimicrobial agent use | Taiwan |
| Shigella dysenteriae | 1998 | Bacteria | Breakdown of public health measures | Indonesia |
| Shigella dysenteriae multidrug-res | 1955 | Bacteria | Antimicrobial agent use | China |
| Shigella dysenteriae sulfa-res | 1949 | Bacteria | Antimicrobial agent use | Japan |
| Shigella dysenteriae tet-res | 1953 | Bacteria | Antimicrobial agent use | Japan |
| Staphylococcus haemolyticus multidrug-res | 1997 | Bacteria | Antimicrobial agent use | India |
| Streptococcus suis serotype 2 | 2005 | Bacteria | Agricultural industry changes | China |
| Strongyloides stercoralis | 1949 | Helminth | War and famine | Vietnam |
| Vibrio cholera O1 El Tor | 1961 | Bacteria | Breakdown of public health measures | Indonesia |
| Vibrio cholera O139 | 1992 | Bacteria | International travel and commerce | India |
| Vibrio fluvialis | 1965 | Bacteria | Climate and weather | Bangladesh |
| Vibrio parahaemolyticus | 1950 | Bacteria | Climate and weather | Japan |
| Zika virus | 1977 | Virus | Climate and weather | Indonesia |

Over 60 per cent of the world's population lives in Asia and the region is home to some of the fastest developing economies in the world. Yet despite tremendous advances, infectious diseases still remain a major burden in Asia. Of the estimated 2.1 million deaths in children aged less than 5 years in Southeast Asia in 2010, 47 per cent were attributed to infectious causes [4]. As such, Asia is both vulnerable to imported EIDs and is a powerhouse of social and environmental change that may facilitate the emergence of new pathogens. However, it would be simplistic and disingenuous to present the extensive changes in Asia as inevitably increasing the risk of EIDs. Many of the socio-economic changes, such as urbanization; industrialization and commercialization of agriculture and food production; increased international connectivity; and globalization of information and trade, may reduce the risk of disease emergence.

## Causes of emergence: conditions and events

The world is laden with microbes. They are the second most abundant life form on earth (after plants) and they are essential to our survival: fixing nitrogen, degrading organic materials, and ensuring the functioning and integrity of the gut, genital tract, and immune system of animals [6]. Each of us hosts many more microbial cells than we have cells of our own (99 per cent of all cells in a human body are microbial) but this symbiotic relationship hides a 'universal struggle for life', with each species trying to blindly optimize its own survival [7]. Our relationship with microbes is therefore interdependent and whilst most of them are beneficial or harmless, occasionally they are harmful and are responsible for causing diseases.

Ecological factors (specifically the environmental living conditions) rather than genetic or geographic constraints seem to critically define pathogen niches, and whilst the conditions or events that result in the emergence of new human pathogens are not well understood, they are often precipitated by changes to ecological or biological systems that result in pathogen dispersal or pathogen adaptation (through natural selection). The most successful EIDs are characterized by a process of both dispersal and adaptation [8]. The events leading to dispersal or adaptation can take many forms and occur on many scales, such as altered patterns of domestic and wild animal contact (e.g. Nipah virus) or human and animal contact (e.g. HIV, SARS), drug pressure (e.g. artemisinin resistant malaria) and changes in species diversity (e.g. Lyme disease).

Species diversity, including the diversity of pathogenic microbes, increases closer to the equator [9] and a correlation between the emergence of zoonotic pathogens and the diversity of mammalian wildlife species has been reported [3]. Indeed, around 60 per cent of emerging infections identified since 1940 have arisen from animals and primarily from wild animals [3, 10]. Whilst wild animal and pathogen species diversity may be associated with an increased burden of infectious diseases and a consequent risk of disease emergence, a reduction of species diversity may, perhaps counterintuitively, be associated with increased disease transmission. Species diversity loss directly disrupts the functioning and stability of ecosystems, producing effects that can extend well beyond the particular species lost [11]. As such, a variety of mechanisms may favour pathogen dispersal, including reduced predation and competition resulting in increased abundance of competent hosts, and the loss of 'buffering species' leading to increased contact between amplifying host species and pathogens [12]. Tropical regions with a rich pool of existing and potential pathogens that are increasingly connected, but that are also experiencing high rates of ecosystem disruption and biodiversity loss, may therefore be at a particularly high risk of disease emergence.

Even though new human pathogens occasionally emerge as a result of dynamics that apparently do not involve humans, for example the emergence of *Vibrio cholera* O139 and *Cryptococcus gattii*, most ecological disturbances resulting in an EID seem to originate in the actions of humans. A wide range of factors have been linked to infectious disease emergence, including changes in land use, travel, trade, demographics and climate, but nearly all of these associations are speculative, with little hard data [13]. This is because ecological and biological systems are highly complex and multilayered, and predicting the impact of particular conditions or events on the functioning of a system is difficult, with further inference of the impact of any changes on the risk of pathogen emergence posing a formidable challenge. There are a handful of well-researched case studies where the ecosystem disruption that has resulted in increased disease risk to humans has been identified, for example, the emergence of Lyme disease in the United States and the Nipah virus in Malaysia, but general principles or rules are hard to identify from these specific examples.

## *Economic development and altered ecosystems*

Over the past two decades, Asia has been home to many of the top performing world economies and this macroeconomic success has resulted in large increases in demand for natural resources. The demand for hardwood, firewood, pulp, agricultural and grazing land, living space, roads, minerals and power has had an enormous impact on the landscapes of Asia. Deforestation occurred throughout the 1990s and the area of primary forest in Asia has continued to decline, with net forest loss continuing in Myanmar, Cambodia, Indonesia and Papua New Guinea. However, the last decade has seen net increases in the overall forested areas of Asia due to active afforestation (which includes commercial plantations) in China, India, the Philippines and Vietnam [14]. Deforestation, forest fragmentation and afforestation are all, however, alterations in habitat, which changes species composition and the interaction between wild animals, domestic animals, insect vectors and humans, thereby providing new opportunities for disease emergence. There are well-documented examples of deforestation and forest encroachment resulting in increases in infectious diseases, such as the Oropouche virus, Chagas disease and Hantaan virus [15]. Across much of Asia, however, there are already very high pressures on productive land and the peak in land-use change in Asia has probably passed, with much of the continent now in an era of increasing intensification of land productivity. This intensification is driven largely by demographic pressures, which are predicted to result in a 70 per cent increase in food production by 2050, with decreased consumption of grains and increased demand for meats, fruits and vegetables [16].

The increased demand for food (and meat in particular), when combined with demands for natural resources from industry and domestic consumers and river damming for hydroelectric power, is increasing the stress on water resources [16]. The consequences of intensified agricultural production include the depletion and degradation of river and groundwater, reduced soil quality and biodiversity loss. A direct and predictable effect of reduced access to clean water for low-income families is an increased risk of water-washed diseases such as trachoma and scabies, and water-borne diseases such as typhoid, cholera, and hepatitis A and E. However, unquantified risks arising from the intensification of agriculture include fresh water pollution with pesticides and fertilizers, loss of biodiversity and land abandonment by small-scale farmers. The potential consequences of these changes on the risk of infectious disease emergence have not yet been assessed.

## *Livestock production*

Demand for livestock products in Asia has risen dramatically over the last 50 years, with the per capita consumption of meat in developing countries more than tripling since the early 1960s and egg consumption increasing five-fold [17]. The increased demand for animal products has been met by more intensive and geographically concentrated production of livestock, especially pigs and poultry. Much of this has been through expansion of small-scale production units but industrial-style commercial premises are also increasing. High-density monoculture of domestic animals is a form of low biodiversity that poses a particular threat to the spread of infectious diseases from wild animal reservoirs to humans. Genetic diversity within an individual host species is important since genetic diversity limits the potential for devastating epidemics [18]. The Nipah virus outbreak in Malaysia and Singapore in 1998–1999 is a good example. Once the Nipah virus crossed from wild bats to domesticated pigs, an explosive outbreak in high-density pig farms resulted in widespread exposure of humans and over 250 human cases of encephalitis [19]. Highly pathogenic avian influenza H5N1 is another example, where crossover from wild aquatic birds (the normal reservoirs of influenza A viruses) to humans arose via massive amplification in domestic poultry. However, the intensification of livestock farming often entails improvements in the separation of domestic and wild animals, improved veterinary supervision and input, reduced movement and species mixing.

Reducing contact between domestic and wild animals, whether the wild animals are wild or captive in markets, is a key tactic of the Food and Agriculture Organization (FAO) to decrease the risk to human health and is part of the wider FAO strategy of 'biosecurity'. The reduction of risk in live animal markets (wet-markets) involves the separation of species, not allowing animals to remain in the market for more than 24 hours, not allowing live animals to exit the market, improved cleaning and disinfection, and weekly rest-days, when all animals are removed and the market is thoroughly cleaned. Improving biosecurity in farms is a major challenge since a large proportion of farming in Asia is small-scale backyard production, and there is often a mix of commercial and backyard farming in any one location.

Achieving improvements in biosecurity without adversely affecting the livelihoods of small-scale farmers requires an approach to risk management that is 'As Low As Reasonably Achievable'. The longer-term vision is to restructure the livestock production sector towards a more commercialized and controlled system, which benefits animal health, human health and commercial profitability. Increasing intensification of animal husbandry in Asia may be a trade-off between a lower risk of emergence events, as animals are 'healthier' and better isolated, but should an EID even occur, there may be a greater risk of massive amplification in large, naive monocultures. Perhaps the greatest risk arises when there is a mixed economy with substantial backyard farming with little or no biosecurity, linked through extensive and poorly regulated market chains to large international commercial organizations. This is the situation throughout much of Asia and, as such, the risk of the dispersal and adaptation of zoonotic infections via domestic animals remains substantial.

Wild animal products are popular in Asia and are used in traditional medicines, tonics and delicacies, or appear as symbols of wealth. Although all ten countries in the Association of Southeast Asian Nations (ASEAN) are signatories to the Convention on International Trade in Endangered Species of Wild Fauna and Flora (CITES), Asia continues to host the largest illegal wildlife trade in the world [20]. The capture and use of wild animals for food (bushmeat) has been implicated in the emergence of HIV and SARS, although the animal species that transmitted SARS to humans, the civet cat, is not the reservoir species for SAR-coronavirus (the reservoir is bats) [21]. Growing wealth has increased the demand for wild animal products, and whilst the development and enforcement of regulations on the capture and trading of wild animals has improved, regulation is a weak tool in the face of intense consumer demand.

Many large cities in Asia have begun to ban, or more tightly regulate, live animal markets in the wake of SARS and H5N1, but complex and poorly regulated food manufacturing and distribution chains still offer ample opportunities for disease outbreaks. A critical challenge in the control of foodborne outbreaks is the traceability of foodstuffs, particularly fresh meat and vegetables. Food safety is, however, high on the agenda of many Asian countries following a number of high-profile food contamination scandals, such as the adulteration of formula milk with melamine in China.

Rudolf Virchow was one of the earliest proponents of a concept that is now known as 'One Health', which states that 'between animal and human medicine there are no dividing lines – nor should there be'. 'One Health' has gained popularity recently as a concept to stimulate cross-sectoral solutions to animal and human health problems. Whilst this has had some success at higher levels of decision-making, the real difficulty remains at the local, implementing level, where the day-to-day activities of animal health workers and human health workers rarely intersect.

Antibiotics are used extensively in the livestock and aquaculture sector in Asia to treat or prevent infections, or as growth promoters. Non-therapeutic use of antibiotics as growth promoters involves the prolonged administration of sub-therapeutic doses. This practice has a demonstrable effect on the emergence and prevalence of resistant microorganisms in food, animals and their environment, as well as resulting in the excretion of antibiotics into the environment where environmental bacteria may be subject to antibiotic selection pressures [22]. While there remains some debate about the overall impact of these factors on human health, it is clear that the continued use of non-therapeutic antibiotics in an agriculture industry that is rapidly increasing in scale and intensity, poses a very real threat.

### *Travel and trade*

Cities are mixing vessels and hubs of connectivity, and can play a central role in the amplification and dissemination of EIDs. SARS is a classic example of the role of contemporary cities in the emergence of an EID. The initial international dissemination of SARS was via a hotel in Hong Kong where international travellers crossed paths, and it was then further amplified and dispersed through large urban hospitals. Global connectivity continues to increase, with only 10 per cent of the world now classified as remote (more than 48 hours travel time to a big city) and 95 per cent of the world's population living on just 10 per cent of the land. The development of a regional road transport network within East and Southeast Asia may be especially important since, compared to air travel, roads offer a more egalitarian form of connectivity that includes animals and goods as well as humans. Whilst this provides opportunities for pathogens to disperse beyond their traditional niche [23], it may also benefit mankind by ensuring that no populations are completely unexposed to a pathogen species, thereby avoiding the devastating epidemics that often followed the first contact with isolated populations in the past [24].

### *Human demographics and behaviour*

Between 2011 and 2050, the world's population is expected to increase by 2.3 billion (a 32 per cent increase) and over the same period, the global urban population is expected to rise from 3.6 billion to 6.3 billion (a 72 per cent increase). Therefore, all of the population increase in the next 40 years will be concentrated in cities [25]. Most of this growth will occur in developing countries, particularly Asia, which will experience an increase in its urban population of 1.4 billion people. Whilst mega-cities (cities with a population of at least 10 million) receive a lot of attention, most urban dwellers live in small cities, with half of the global urban population in 2011 living in cities of less than 500,000 people.

In many ways, this is a good thing and the popularity of cities is a testament to the fact that cities generally offer better economic opportunities, better education opportunities, better living conditions, better nutrition, better sanitation and, therefore, better health, than underdeveloped rural areas. However, given the scale of urbanization, urban humanitarian crises, including epidemic diseases, are a particular concern for the future [26].

Cities are important in the epidemiology of many infectious diseases as they may act as 'pacemakers' of local epidemiology (e.g. dengue), become hubs for national and global spread (e.g. SARS and HIV) or act as a bridge between human and animal ecosystems (e.g. H5N1). Increasing travel and medical tourism in Asia adds a new dimension, with the potential for the generation and dissemination of healthcare associated infections, such as the bacterial enzyme New Delhi metallo-beta-lactamase-1 (NDM-1) that confers resistance to a range of potent antibiotics, the carbapenems.

Urbanization and urban infrastructures have played an important role in Asia's success in improving access to safe water and sanitation, with almost half of the world's population, living in China and India, gaining access to improved sources of drinking water between 1990 and 2008. However, the rate of increase in access to improved drinking water sources is barely keeping up with the rate of urban population growth. With large growths anticipated in urban populations in Asia and water scarcity predicted by the United Nations (UN) to be a major challenge of the twenty-first century, there is a risk that the pace of urban population growth will outstrip the delivery of a healthy infrastructure. Although better on average, cities are also home to great inequalities and the health of the urban poor can be as bad as, or even worse than, that of the rural poor. Whilst China and India have together taken 125 million people out of slum conditions between 2000 and 2010, urban slums remain a concern, with an estimated 500 million people living in slums in Asia in 2010 [27]. In China, at the end of 2008, the number of rural migrant workers was estimated at around 140 million [28]. Circular and temporary migration between rural and urban settings may allow the introduction of pathogens from wild or rural ecosystems and amplification in settings with high concentrations of migrant workers.

The tropical urban environment suits certain vector species, particularly *Aedes aeypti* and *Aedes albopictus* mosquitoes, which breed in water containers of urban households. Increasing urbanization is one factor that has contributed to the inexorable spread of dengue in the last 50 years and of chikungunya since 2000, such that these are now major public health problems in large parts of tropical and subtropical Asia [29]. Vector control in tropical urban settings is a major challenge, as demonstrated by the experience of one of the richest and most developed cities in Asia, Singapore, which spends an estimated US$4,500 per Disability Adjusted Life-Year averted and yet has failed to eliminate dengue transmission [30]. Whilst vector control is not currently a cost-effective solution for most countries in Asia, the development of genetically modified sterile male mosquitoes, and of mosquitoes infected with the intracellular bacterium *Wolbachia* (which limits the susceptibility of the mosquito to dengue), perhaps offer new hopes for vector control.

In addition to changes in the physical living environment, urbanization is accompanied by many different lifestyles changes. Urbanization often results in an expansion of social and sexual behaviours, which may offer new opportunities for diseases transmitted by social or sexual contact. The apparent emergence of enterovirus 71 (one of the viruses causing hand, foot and mouth disease) in Asia over the past decade may be in part attributable to changes in childcare practices and the increasing concentration of young children in pre-school environments.

## Health systems

Almost 40 per cent (23/59) of EIDs identified in Asia since 1940 represent the emergence of a new pattern of antimicrobial resistance (see Table 18.1). The most important driver of antimicrobial resistance is drug pressure. The sequential development of resistance by malaria parasites in Asia to chloroquine, sulphadoxine-pyrimethamine, mefloquine and, now, artemisinin is a measure of both the adaptive capacity of the parasite and the failure of health systems to implement effective drug combination and cycling strategies to avoid resistance. Bacteria in Asia show alarmingly high rates of resistance to anti-bacterial agents, including multi-drug resistant *Acinetobacter baumanii*, *Salmonella enterica*, *Enterobacteriaceae* and tuberculosis. The recent emergence of the NDM-1 resistance gene in Asia and its rapid dissemination to other regions highlights the serious threat of antimicrobial resistance. The growth of multi-drug resistant (MDR) and extensively drug-resistant (XDR) tuberculosis in Asia is also alarming, with China's rates of MDR TB in 2007 being twice the global average. Although drug resistance initially develops as a consequence of inadequate treatment, the majority of detected MDR and XDR TB cases in China are now the result of primary acquisition of resistant strains, without prior treatment [31].

Whilst malaria remains a serious problem in Asia (with an estimated 658 million people in Central, South and East Asia living in areas with stable *Plasmodium falciparum* transmission and 876 million people living in areas with stable *P. vivax* transmission in 2010), improved living conditions, vector control, rapid case identification and treatment, and insecticide impregnated bed nets have resulted in a substantial decline in the burden of malaria in Asia and a contraction of the areas where malaria transmission is stable [32, 33]. However the threat of artemisinin resistance, now detected in western Cambodia and western Thailand, is substantial and, together with insecticide resistance, threatens to reverse some of these health gains.

A high level of antimicrobial resistance is a marker of a failure of health systems to control access to antibiotics and to influence prescribing behaviours. Antibiotics are easily available over the counter from pharmacists and drug-sellers without a prescription throughout much of Asia, including in Pakistan, India, Bangladesh, China, Vietnam, Thailand and Indonesia, even though antibiotics are officially prescription-only medicines in most of these countries. A vast number of people are therefore receiving unnecessary or inappropriate antibiotics, creating a massive pressure for the development of resistance. There is also unnecessary and inappropriate prescription of antibiotics within the primary and secondary healthcare systems, which is a particular issue for tuberculosis and healthcare associated infections. Self-medication with antibiotics in the community is driven by easy access, convenience, cost savings (no doctors' fees) and the unregulated profit motive of pharmacy owners. Within the public healthcare sector, under-funded providers seek to balance hospital finances by over-prescribing, whilst poorly paid healthcare workers seek to augment meagre salaries. Meanwhile, weak monitoring and regulation of the public and private healthcare sectors further complicate the situation.

Unchecked, these supply and demand side incentives have led to a region awash with antibiotics and an incipient public health disaster. This disaster is comprised not only of untreatable infections, which are already happening, but also the unmeasured economic and social burden of the need for hospitalization and treatment with expensive second and third lines when the cheap first-line therapies fail.

Weak enforcement of regulations on the sale of antimicrobials and a lack of adherence to best practice in prescribing antimicrobials need to be urgently addressed. World Health

Day in 2011 was 'Antimicrobial resistance: no action today, no cure tomorrow', and there is increasing global and regional advocacy for action against antimicrobial resistance. Such initiatives need to bring together all sectors including the public (whose expectations need to be adjusted), medical professionals (whose duty of care to future, as well as current, patients must be reinforced), and the drug sellers, pharmacists and pharmaceutical companies (who need to take their corporate social responsibilities seriously).

The prevention and control of healthcare associated infections is an essential function of all healthcare systems, yet infection control teams throughout the world struggle to encourage hand hygiene and 'standard precautions'. In poorly resourced hospitals in low- and middle-income countries of Asia, where more than one patient may share a bed, infection control is usually a low priority. Although financial resources play a role, infection control is more about attitudes, working practices and governance structures. Within the constraints of affordable infrastructure and materials, health managers need to establish and monitor infection control standards, which should be publicly available core indicators of the quality of care for all healthcare institutions.

## The internal human ecology

An exciting new area of exploration is the effect of disturbances of our own microbial ecology (the collection of microbes living on and inside us, known as our microbiome) on the emergence of both infectious and non-communicable diseases (NCDs). It is becoming increasingly clear that our internal microbial ecology plays a critical role in our health, influencing our susceptibility to both infectious diseases and NCDs, such as obesity, asthma and diabetes [34]. The Human Microbiome Project is part of the ongoing effort to explore this ecology. As knowledge accumulates, new insights will emerge of how changes in lifestyles and living conditions influence the emergence of new pathogens and new diseases – some of which may not yet be recognized as infectious in nature [35].

## Disease surveillance and response

The International Health Regulations 2005 (IHR) place a requirement on member states to ensure that 'core capacities' in disease surveillance and response are 'present and functioning throughout their territories by June 2012' and to report 'Public Health Emergencies of International Concern' (PHEIC) to the WHO. Importantly, the IHR allows the WHO to unilaterally announce a PHEIC in the event of the WHO becoming aware of a public health emergency of international concern, if the implicated member state refuses to acknowledge the event or collaborate with the WHO.

A number of events and trends have converged to improve the reporting of EIDs in Asia. These include the revised IHR, the SARS and H5N1 epidemics, and advances in information technology. Whilst the Internet and social media have rendered it almost impossible to completely suppress information on emerging health crises, reporting first requires detection and the ability to detect EIDs at an early stage is still largely dependent on astute clinicians with close personal links to public health professionals. These human networks are crucial to successful surveillance and must not be neglected in the race to embrace new technologies.

Epidemic preparedness in the region has substantially improved as a result of SARS, H5N1 and pandemic influenza H1N1. The SARS outbreak is the most striking modern example of the aggressive and successful application of traditional public health interventions to contain an epidemic. The interventions included 'source control' (case-finding and isolation, quarantine of contacts), increasing social distance (such as by closing schools and cancelling mass gatherings), limiting spread of infection by domestic and international travellers (travel alerts, screening and restrictions), and infection control and hygiene measures (hand and cough hygiene, wearing masks or respirators). This success coloured the approaches taken to pandemic H1N1, with an unrealistic expectation by some that the pandemic could be contained. Informed by the eventful previous decade of EIDs the region is nevertheless much better placed to implement epidemic control interventions in a measured, thoughtful way. However, privatization, deregulation and provider diversification of the health sector is a regional trend that, without robust protection of public health interests, may have an adverse impact on disease surveillance systems.

## Conclusion

A major shift is underway in the global centre of gravity, from West to East. Asia is becoming the dominant force of economic, social and environmental change, and whilst rapid development has brought many benefits, it has also resulted in widening health inequalities, increased social stratification, environmental degradation, increased migration and urbanization, and a concentration of people, food production and economic activity. These changes pose new risks to the populations' health.

Amongst these health risks, infectious diseases remain critically important. Whilst inroads have been made, infectious diseases are dynamic and resilient, and continue to challenge local, national and global public health systems [36]. The recognition of the linkage between anthropogenic changes and disease emergence has resulted in repeated calls for a more holistic and interdisciplinary approach to the study of infectious diseases. The task ahead is to better understand how social and environmental changes occurring in Asia are altering the landscape of infectious disease risks and how future risks may be mitigated [37].

## Acknowledgements

The author wishes to thank Dirk Pfeiffer for helpful discussions on livestock production systems in Asia.

## References

1. Spellberg, B. Dr William H. Stewart: Mistaken or Maligned? *Clin Infect Dis*, 2008; 47, 294.
2. Snowden, F. M. Emerging and Reemerging Diseases: A Historical Perspective. *Immunol Rev* 2008; 225, 9–26.
3. Jones, K. E, Patel, N. G, Levy, M. A, Storeygard, A, Balk, D, Gittleman, J. L, Daszak, P. Global Trends in Emerging Infectious Diseases. *Nature* 2008; 451, 990–3.
4. Liu, L, Johnson, H. L, Cousens, S, Perin, J, Scott, S, Lawn, J. E, *et al*. Global, Regional, and National Causes of Child Mortality: An Updated Systematic Analysis for 2010 with Time Trends since 2000. *Lancet* 2012; 379, 2151–61.
5. Smith, R. D. Responding to Global Infectious Disease Outbreaks: Lessons from SARS on the Role of Risk Perception, Communication and Management. *Social Science & Medicine* 2006; 63, 3113–312.
6. Whitman, W. B, Coleman, D. C, Wiebe, W. J. Prokaryotes: The Unseen Majority. *Proc Natl Acad Sci USA* 1998; 95, 6578–83.

7. Costello, E. K, Stagaman, K, Dethlefsen, L, Bohannan, B. J, Relman, D. A. The Application of Ecological Theory toward an Understanding of the Human Microbiome. *Science* 2012; 336, 1255–62.
8. Wolfe, N. D, Dunavan, C. P, Diamond, J. Origins of Major Human Infectious Diseases. *Nature* 2007; 447, 279–83.
9. Guernier, V, Hochberg, M. E, Guegan, J. F. Ecology Drives the Worldwide Distribution of Human Diseases. *PLoS Biol* 2004; 2, E141.
10. Taylor, L. H, Latham, S. M, Woolhouse, M. E. Risk Factors for Human Disease Emergence. *Philos Trans R Soc Lond B Biol Sci* 2001; 356, 983–9.
11. Hooper, D. U, Adair, E. C, Cardinale, B. J, Byrnes, J. E, Hungate, B. A, Matulich, K. L, *et al.* A Global Synthesis Reveals Biodiversity Loss as a Major Driver of Ecosystem Change. *Nature* 2012; 486, 105–8.
12. Keesing, F, Belden, L. K, Daszak, P, Dobson, A, Harvell, C. D, Holt, R. D, *et al.* Impacts of Biodiversity on the Emergence and Transmission of Infectious Diseases. *Nature* 2010; 468, 647–52.
13. Woolhouse, M. How to Make Predictions about Future Infectious Disease Risks. *Philos Trans R Soc Lond B Biol Sci* 2011; 366, 2045–54.
14. FAO. *State of the World's Forests*, Rome; 2011.
15. WHO. *Globalization and Infectious Diseases: A Review of the Linkages*, Geneva; 2004.
16. FAO. *The State of the World's Land and Water Resources for Food and Agriculture*, Rome; 2011.
17. FAO. *The State of Food and Agriculture 2010–2011*, Rome; 2011.
18. King, K. C, Lively, C. M. Does Genetic Diversity Limit Disease Spread in Natural Host Populations? *Heredity* 2012 (Edinb).
19. Pulliam, J. R, Epstein, J. H, Dushoff, J, Rahman, S. A, Bunning, M, Jamaluddin, A. A, *et al.* Agricultural Intensification, Priming for Persistence and the Emergence of Nipah Virus: A Lethal Bat-Borne Zoonosis. *J R Soc Interface* 2012; 9, 89–101.
20. Rosen, G. E, Smith, K. F. Summarizing the Evidence on the International Trade in Illegal Wildlife. *Ecohealth* 2012; 7, 24–32.
21. Li, W, Shi, Z, Yu, M, Ren, W, Smith, C, Epstein, J. H, *et al.* Bats Are Natural Reservoirs of SARS-Like Coronaviruses. *Science* 2005; 310, 676–9.
22. Marshall, B. M, Levy, S. B. Food Animals and Antimicrobials: Impacts on Human Health. *Clin Microbiol Rev* 2011; 24, 718–33.
23. Eisenberg, J. N, Cevallos, W, Ponce, K, Levy, K, Bates, S. J, Scott, J. C, *et al.* Environmental Change and Infectious Disease: How New Roads Affect the Transmission of Diarrheal Pathogens in Rural Ecuador. *Proc Natl Acad Sci USA* 2006; 103, 19460–5.
24. Shanks, G. D, Brundage, J. F. Pacific Islands which Escaped the 1918–1919 Influenza Pandemic and their Subsequent Mortality Experiences. *Epidemiol Infect* 2012; 1–4.
25. UN-DESA. *World Urbanization Prospects: The 2011 Revision*; 2012.
26. Patel, R. B, Burke, T. F. Urbanization – An Emerging Humanitarian Disaster. *N Engl J Med* 2009; 361, 741–3.
27. UN-Habitat. *State of the World's Cities: 2010/2011 – Cities for All: Bridging the Urban Divide*; 2010.
28. UN-DESA. *Population Distribution, Urbanization, Internal Migration and Development: An International Perspective*, Geneva; 2011.
29. Burt, F. J, Rolph, M. S, Rulli, N. E, Mahalingam, S, Heise, M. T. Chikungunya: A Re-Emerging Virus. *Lancet* 2012; 379, 662–71.
30. Carrasco, L. R, Lee, L. K, Lee, V. J, Ooi, E. E, Shepard, D. S, Thein, T. L, *et al.* Economic Impact of Dengue Illness and the Cost-Effectiveness of Future Vaccination Programs in Singapore. *PLoS Negl Trop Dis* 2011; 5, e1426.
31. Zhao, Y, Xu, S, Wang, L, Chin, D. P, Wang, S, Jiang, G, *et al.* National Survey of Drug-Resistant Tuberculosis in China. *N Engl J Med* 2012; 366, 2161–70.
32. Gething, P. W, Elyazar, I. R, Moyes, C. M, Smith, D. L, Battle, K. E, Guerra, C. A, *et al.* A Long Neglected World Malaria Map: Plasmodium Vivax Endemicity in 2010. *PLoS Negl Trop Dis* 2012; 6, e1814.
33. Gething, P. W, Patil, A. P, Smith, D. L, Guerra, C. A, Elyazar, I. R, Johnston, G. L, *et al.* A New World Malaria Map: Plasmodium Falciparum Endemicity in 2010. *Malar J* 2011; 10, 378.
34. Cho I, Blaser M. J. The Human Microbiome: At the Interface of Health and Disease. *Nat Rev Genet* 2012; 13(4): 260–70.

35. Hanski, I, Von Hertzen, L, Fyhrquist, N, Koskinen, K, Torppa, K, Laatikainen, T, *et al.* Environmental Biodiversity, Human Microbiota, and Allergy Are Interrelated. *Proc Natl Acad Sci USA* 2012; 109, 8334–9.
36. Fauci, A. S, Morens, D. M. The Perpetual Challenge of Infectious Diseases. *N Engl J Med* 2012; 366, 454–61.
37. Woolhouse, M. How to Make Predictions about Future Infectious Disease Risks. *Philos Trans R Soc Lond B Biol Sci* 2011; 366, 2045–54.

# 19

# Climate change and its impact on the patterns of disease

## Malaria in the People's Republic of China as a case study

*Guo-Jing Yang and Xiao-Nong Zhou*

### Introduction

The impact of climate change on the transmission of infectious diseases has been given much attention since the start of the new millennium. The topic was hotly debated by the board of the World Summit on Sustainable Development held in Johannesburg, South Africa, in 2002 [1]. The World Health Organization (WHO) further called on its member states to 'Protect health from climate change' as the theme of the World Health Day in 2008 [2]. Scientists and policymakers took these actions because research has supported the fact that climate change had impacted on human health and increased the burden of diseases, whether directly or indirectly. For instance, some reports showed that global climate change might already be responsible for over 150,000 deaths annually, including the loss of about 5 million disability-adjusted life years (DALYs) globally [3]. The direct impact is that human beings are exposed directly under the scenario of warmer temperatures, more extreme climate events and so on. The indirect impacts are that climate change also causes changes in water, air, food quality/quantity, ecosystems, agriculture, livelihoods and infrastructure, which are also huge impacts on human health [4]. These facts support the conclusion that climate change will not only affect public health (see Box 19.1), but also conservation biology, agriculture, aquaculture, fishery and livestock production [5–11].

This chapter will mainly focus on the impact of climate change on the transmission of infectious diseases since changes in the temperature provide more opportunities for transmission of infectious diseases, particularly vector-transmitted diseases, to develop or expand [12, 13]. For instance, malaria will climb into higher altitude places which were previously non-transmission areas, but may not be the same as the highland malaria in East Africa [14]. Exploring impacts of climate change on the transmission of major infectious diseases in Southeast Asia, with a particular focus on malaria, is not sufficient but urgent [15]. In this chapter, we are only able to provide one example from the rapidly growing body of literature with respect to the impact of climate change on malaria transmission [2, 12, 16–23].

### Box 19.1 Factors affecting the health status of people

The health status of millions of people is affected through:

- increases in malnutrition;
- increased deaths, diseases and injury due to extreme weather events;
- increased burden of diarrhoeal diseases;
- increased diseases due to higher concentrations of ground-level ozone related to climate change; and
- the altered spatial distribution of some infectious diseases.

*Source*: [1].

## The interplay between climate change and infectious diseases

Climate change denotes a long-term process, characterized by spatial changes of weather distribution and significant temporal fluctuations ranging from short-term periods to millions of years. The drivers of climate change include both natural variability and anthropogenic activities with the latter growing in importance since the last century [24, 25]. There is a growing consensus that the combustion of fossil fuels is the key driver of the recent global warming due to anthropogenic activities [26]. The fourth assessment of the Intergovernmental Panel on Climate Change (IPCC) predicted that the average temperature will rise by 0.2°C per decade over the next 20 years according to the increased patterns of global atmospheric concentrations of $CH_4$ and $N_2O$ between the pre-industrial era and 2005. The first report of the IPCC in 1990 projected global average temperature increases between about 0.15°C and 0.3°C per decade from 1990 to 2005, which was proved by comparing it with observed values of about 0.2°C per decade. It further strengthened confidence in near-term projections [26, 27]. Besides rises in surface air temperature, climate change also alters free atmospheric temperature, sea level pressure, the height of the tropopause (the boundary of the Earth's atmosphere between the troposphere and the stratosphere), ocean heat content, and precipitation at local, regional and global levels [7, 28–31].

Climate change is likely to cause changes in ecological systems that will alter the risk of infectious diseases globally [15, 32]. These risks affect seasonal activity of local vectors and invasion patterns of tropical and semi-tropical species in areas where they previously could not be distributed due to the restrictions of temperature and environmental conditions. In other words, the potential impact of climate change will result in shifts in the spatio-temporal distribution of disease vectors, causing changes in transmission dynamics of vector-borne diseases [33–35]. Sensitive infectious diseases affected by climate change include ancient diseases, such as malaria, lymphatic filariasis, schistosomiasis, etc., and invasive diseases, such as dengue fever, chikungunya fever and angiostrongyliasis. Table 19.1 summarizes the key findings obtained from studies focusing on climate change and vector-borne diseases, including diseases other than malaria, i.e. lymphatic filariasis, schistosomiasis, leishmaniasis, onchocerciasis, human African trypanosomiasis and arboviral diseases (e.g. dengue, yellow fever and Japanese encephalitis) [1, 36–38].

*Table 19.1* Impacts of climate change on the sensitive vector-borne diseases with the likely change in their distribution

| *Disease* | *At-risk population (million)* | *Present distribution* | *Likelihood of change of disease distribution due to climate change*[a] |
|---|---|---|---|
| ***Parasitic diseases*** | | | |
| Malaria | 2,211[b] | Tropics and subtropics | +++ |
| Lymphatic filariasis | >1,000[b] | Tropics and subtropics | + |
| Schistosomiasis | 779[b] | Tropics and subtropics | ++ |
| Leishmaniasis | 350[b] | Asia, Africa, South America and South Europe | n.k. |
| Onchocerciasis | 120[b] | Africa and Latin America | + |
| Human African trypanosomiasis | >60[b] | Africa | + |
| ***Arboviral diseases*** | | | |
| Dengue | n.k. | Tropics and subtropics | ++ |
| Yellow fever | n.k. | Africa and Latin America | + |
| Japanese encephalitis | n.k. | East Asia and Southeast Asia | + |

*Notes*: [a] Likelihood of change stratified as follows: 0, unlikely; +, likely; ++, very likely; +++, almost certain; n.k., not known.
[b] *Source*: [2].

The potential impact of climate change on vector-borne diseases can be explained by the mechanism that vectors survive and reproduce within certain temperature ranges along with the optimal ecosystems. Climate change, therefore, alters the transmission of vector-borne diseases in the following three ways [2, 3, 18, 34, 39]:

- by changing the survival and the reproduction rate of the vector;
- by changing the development behaviour of the pathogen inside the vector; and
- by changing vector activities of contacting human beings.

The following three main lines of investigation have been undertaken in the last decade [40]:

1 the relationship between climactic parameters and the transmission of vector-borne diseases, and an assessment of whether transmission is likely to change in a future warmer world;
2 the application of methodologies in statistical models to simulate the potential increase in transmission intensity and geographic distribution; and
3 the use of biology-based models, in which key biological parameters are derived from experimental studies and field observations, and inference is derived from extrapolations.

## Case study on malaria in the People's Republic of China (P.R. China)

Malaria kills about 1 million people each year, and most of them are children below the age of 5 [39, 41]. Currently, over 80 per cent of all malaria-related deaths, and the global burden due to malaria, are concentrated in sub-Saharan Africa [39, 42–44]. In recent years, biology-driven and statistical models have been developed and used in the field of the impact of climate change on the transmission scale and intensity of malaria. For example, Craig *et al.* developed a fuzzy-logic, climate-based distribution model and suggested that such a model can be used to study the impact of climate change on malaria transmission [29]. When integrated with multi-source data including population, morbidity and mortality datasets, this model can be applied to assess the burden of disease and provide solid information in formulating a malaria control strategy. In fact, both the regression approach and the statistical model have been used in predicting the potential effects of climate change on highland malaria transmission intensity and distribution [45–46].

Yang and her team have applied both biology-driven and statistical models supported by information-theoretical methods [47–48] and GIS techniques in predicting the transmission patterns and risk factors for *Plasmodium vivax* malaria epidemics in P.R. China [23]. Their specific objectives were to:

1 identify the key environmental risk factors related to malaria transmission;
2 predict the transmission intensity and potential risk areas of *P. vivax* malaria in P.R. China;
3 highlight the high-transmission regions' hotspots; and
4 provide a practical guide for malaria control in the field.

Similar results of impact factors on malaria transmission were illustrated by both Delphi analysis and multinomial statistic analysis. First, through two rounds of Delphi analysis with 23 questionnaires, it was revealed that three environmental factors – temperature, precipitation and relative humidity (RH) – had a particular influence on malaria transmission in P.R. China. Second, based on multinomial statistical analysis, results showed that the greatest support was for the fully saturated model, which also included the factors of temperature, rainfall and RH. The percentage deviance (%-DE) suggested that the parameters used in this model had a good level of prediction [23]. Both results are in agreement with the biological requirements of the parasite's life cycle, which illustrated that once the basic knowledge of the ecology of vectors is clear enough, and the weak points in the life cycle are identified, a strategy can be formulated [49–51].

Utilizing previous findings, temporal variations of malaria transmission in P.R. China were further explored. First, monthly temperature and yearly relative humidity (YRH), for the period 1961–2000, were investigated based on the environmental data obtained from 676 locations across P.R. China. Second, the smoothed surface maps of the monthly mean temperature and YRH revealed the number of months suitable for parasite survival. Finally, the malaria prediction map of each decade was overlaid by two mask maps, namely a map showing the number of months suitable for parasite survival and a map showing when YRH was in excess of 60 per cent [31]. The final malaria prediction map (see Figure 19.1) derived from classified environmental factors predicted that *P. vivax* malaria has been mainly distributed in the south-eastern part of P.R. China, with the potential risk increasing steadily from north to south [31]. This prediction map was very much in agreement with the ground truth data of malaria transmission patterns. Three vulnerable zones were identified as high-risk malaria transmission areas due to climate change. This study gave another sample that multiple environmental factors with seasonality analysis were essential to determine the transmission risk or vulnerable zones.

The risk maps indicating the transmission intensity of malaria in various localities provided smarter guidance for malaria control, and hence facilitated surveillance and intervention.

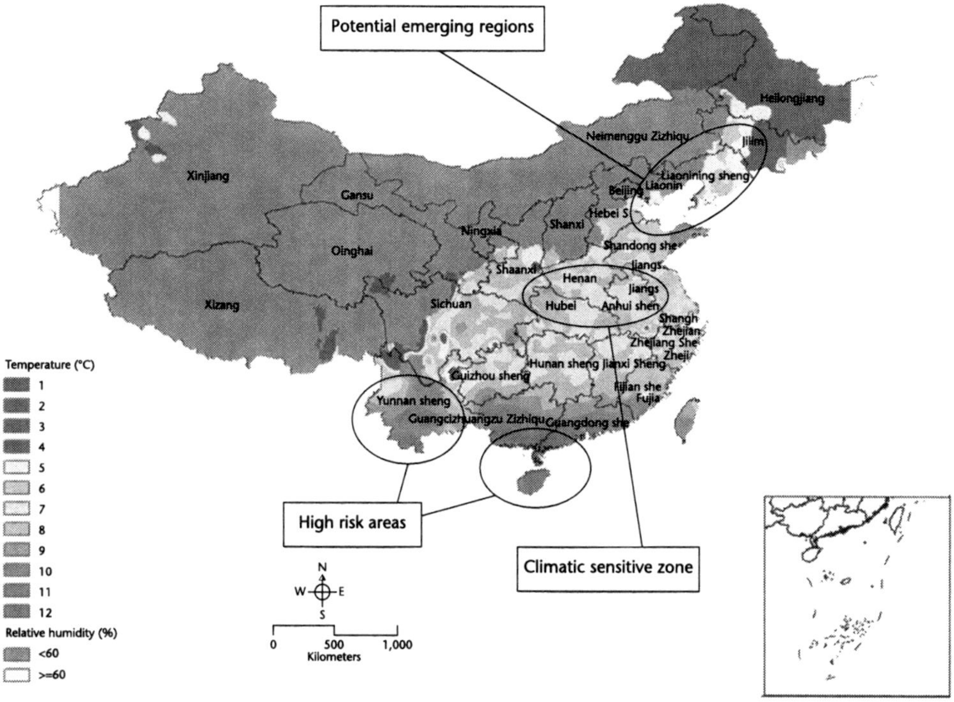


*Figure 19.1* The prediction of malaria transmission in P.R. China by integrated modelling, along with three vulnerable zones identified based on the potential risk of malaria transmission under a warmer world posed by climate change in P.R. China

*Note*: Prediction maps, based on data derived from 1991–2000, created by combining two factors which are (i) the number of months in which temperature is suitable for malaria transmission, and (ii) relative humidity (%). Grey colour screens the regions where relative humidity is less than 60 per cent. The dark colour catalogued as 1–4 under the temperature legend indicates the regions where number of months suitable for malaria transmission is less than four successive months, which is located in the most northeast and sporadically distributed area of the western region of the country.

This will be useful information for the National Malaria Control Programme, particularly the national malaria elimination project launched in 2010, which aims to eliminate malaria in most regions of P.R. China by 2015, and in the whole country by 2020 [52–53]. Based on the transmission intensity map, it was recommended that interventions, including vector control and swift case management within a surveillance strategy, should be focused on the high-intensity transmission areas such as Hainan, Yunnan and Guangxi provinces. On the other hand, the surveillance to detect and treat all imported cases needs to be strengthened in low-risk regions which are highly sensitive to climate change, such as Shandong, Henan, Shaanxi and Gansu provinces (see Figure 19.1) [31]. Clearly, the National Malaria Elimination Programme needs to shift its focus from extensive monitoring and evaluation towards surveillance and response strategies to reach the expected elimination targets [54].

## Research priorities

The impact of climate change is related to a myriad of issues, including environmental factors, economic performance, social behaviour, infrastructure and other aspects of human existence

*Table 19.2* Gap analysis and identified research priorities with regard to climate change, including adaptation and mitigation measures of snail-borne diseases

| *Disease* | *Biological variables for threshold determinants* | *Assessment* | *Adaptation* | *Mitigation* |
|---|---|---|---|---|
| Schistosomiasis | Lowest and highest developing temperature of *Schistosoma japonicum* and *Oncomelania hupensis*; GDD of *S. japonicum* and *O. hupensis* | Only in P.R. China | Only in P.R. China | Only in P.R. China |
| Clonorchiasis | N.a. | None | None | None |
| Opisthorchiasis | N.a. | None | None | None |
| Fascioliasis | GDD of *Fasciola hepatica* and *Fasciola gigantica* | None | None | None |
| Angiostrongyliasis | GDD of *Angiostrongylus cantonensis* and *Pomacea canaliculat* | Only in P.R. China | None | None |

*Source*: Adapted from [63].

*Notes*: N.a., not available. GDD, growing degree delays.

[55]. It is therefore important to predict the changes sooner rather than later. It is also noted that very few studies have been carried out on the issues of adaptation and mitigation strategies related to vector-borne diseases in the face of climate change (for a notable exception, see [56]).

We have highlighted some approaches to study the potential impacts of climate change on vector-borne infectious diseases, particularly in Asia [32, 57]. The research gaps on the impact of climate change on the transmission of vector-borne infectious diseases have been identified (see Table 19.2), and five areas for research priorities, including adaptation and mitigation measures and strategies, have been discussed through series workshops and seminars in the last decade (see Box 19.2 for the research priorities) [1, 40].

In spite of there being a long way to go to systematically examine these complex questions, progress is able to be made if more interdisciplinary research groups work together on innovative methodologies and approaches rather than compete with one another [55, 58–59]. It is important for the region to highlight its own priorities at the local level, under the platform of sustainably maintaining the long-term meteorological and ground epidemiological datasets, in order to achieve the 'ground-truth' data and validate predictions so as to improve the surveillance and early-warning systems [60]. The concept on the health co-benefits will create a different paradigm or a 'win–win' model for all of people living on the planet [57].

## Conclusion

The impact of climate change on infectious diseases has been investigated for several decades, showing the most negative effect on the transmission of vector-borne diseases. However, research on the impact of climate change on vector-borne diseases is still limited in Asia. Climate change may asymmetrically affect transmission of vector-borne diseases due to special transmission features of each disease which call for different considerations in selection of model parameters. Mitigation and adaptation strategies to reduce the potential impacts of

**Box 19.2 Research priorities to mitigate and adapt climate changes in the field of vector-borne diseases**

- The transmission risks in the vector-borne diseases posed by climate change, importantly, an understanding of the relative significance of those risks, in order to provide wide education for the public.
- Assessment on the potential impact of the distribution and transmission patterns of the vector-borne diseases in Asia and neighbourhood countries, particularly on the integrated impacts of climate change and other demographic, ecological and social transformations.
- The impact determinants of climate change on vector-borne diseases, including variability at the regional level, along with the consequences of responses to these determinants in terms of the environment and human communities.
- The smarter strategy of mitigation and adaptation in the face of climate change to effectively reduce the impacts on increasing transmission risks and burden of vector-borne diseases supported by disease surveillance and early-warning systems.
- Evaluation approaches on the cost-effectiveness and cost–benefit analysis of adaptation strategies, essentially on the feasibility analysis to scale up those approaches in the future.

climate change on vector-borne diseases are recommended in five areas, which could be listed on the agendas of high-level discussion. Therefore, the platforms of 'ground-truth' and validated predictions, surveillance and early-warning systems, and smarter adaptation strategies, need to be strengthened or initiated as soon as possible in the region [61].

## References


1. WHO. *Global Report for Research on Infectious Diseases of Poverty*. Geneva: World Health Organization; 2012.
2. Yang GJ, Utzinger J, Lv S, Qian YJ, Li SZ, Wang Q, *et al.* The Regional Network for Asian Schistosomiasis and Other Helminth Zoonoses (RNAS(+)) target diseases in face of climate change. *Advances in Parasitology*. 2010; 73: 101–35.
3. Ebi KL, Hartman J, Chan N, McConnell KJ, Schlesinger M, Weyant J. Climate suitability for stable malaria transmission in Zimbabwe under different climate change scenarios. *Climatic Change*. 2005; 73: 375–93.
4. McMichael AJ, Powles JW, Butler CD, Uauy R. Food, livestock production, energy, climate change, and health. *Lancet*. 2007; 370(9594): 1253–63.
5. Harvell CD, Mitchell CE, Ward JR, Altizer S, Dobson AP, Ostfeld RS, *et al.* Climate warming and disease risks for terrestrial and marine biota. *Science*. 2002; 296(5576): 2158–62.
6. Solomon S, Qin D, Manning M, Chen Z, Marquis M, Averyt KB, *et al. Climate Change 2007: The Physical Science Basis*. Cambridge: Cambridge University Press; 2007.
7. Forman S, Hungerford N, Yamakawa M, Yanase T, Tsai HJ, Joo YS, *et al.* Climate change impacts and risks for animal health in Asia. *Rev Sci Tech*. 2008; 27(2): 581–97.
8. Crabbe MJ. Climate change and tropical marine agriculture. *J Exp Bot*. 2009; 60(10): 2839–44.
9. Lafferty KD. The ecology of climate change and infectious diseases. *Ecology*. 2009; 90(4): 888–900.

10. Mas-Coma S, Valero MA, Bargues MD. Climate change effects on trematodiases, with emphasis on zoonotic fascioliasis and schistosomiasis. *Vet Parasitol*. 2009; 163(4): 264–80.
11. Miraglia M, Marvin HJ, Kleter GA, Battilani P, Brera C, Coni E, *et al*. Climate change and food safety: an emerging issue with special focus on Europe. *Food Chem Toxicol*. 2009; 47(5): 1009–21.
12. Butler CD. Infectious disease emergence and global change: thinking systemically in a shrinking world. *Infectious Diseases of Poverty*. 2012; 1(1): 5.
13. Easterling DR, Meehl GA, Parmesan C, Changnon SA, Karl TR, Mearns LO. Climate extremes: observations, modeling, and impacts. *Science*. 2000; 289: 2068–74.
14. Chaves LF, Koenraadt CJ. Climate change and highland malaria: fresh air for a hot debate. *Q Rev Biol*. 2010; 85(1): 27–55.
15. Bergquist R, Whittaker M. Control of neglected tropical diseases in Asia Pacific: implications for health information priorities. *Inf Dis Poverty*. 2012; 1(1): 3.
16. Epstein PR. Climate change and emerging infectious diseases. *Microbes and Infection*. 2001; 3(9): 747–54.
17. Knowlton K, Rosenthal JE, Hogrefe C, Lynn B, Gaffin S, Goldberg R, *et al*. Assessing ozone-related health impacts under a changing climate. *Environmental Health Perspectives*. 2004; 112(15): 1557–63.
18. Patz JA, Graczyk TK, Geller N, Vittor AY. Effects of environmental change on emerging parasitic diseases. *International Journal for Parasitology*. 2000; 30: 1395–405.
19. Haines A, Patz JA. Health effects of climate change. *Journal of the American Medical Association*. 2004; 291: 99–103.
20. Beggs PJ. Impacts of climate change on aeroallergens: past and future. *Clinical and Experimental Allergy*. 2004; 34: 1507–13.
21. Diza JH. The public health impact of global climate change. *Family and Community Health*. 2004; 27(3): 218–29.
22. Lv S, Zhang Y, Steinmann P, Yang GJ, Yang K, Zhou XN, *et al*. The emergence of angiostrongyliasis in the People's Republic of China: the interplay between invasive snails, climate change and transmission dynamics. *Freshwater Biology*. 2011; 56: 717–34.
23. Yang GJ, Gao Q, Zhou SS, Malone JB, McCarroll JC, Tanner M, *et al*. Mapping and predicting malaria transmission in the People's Republic of China, using integrated biology-driven and statistical models. *Geospatial Health*. 2010; 5(1): 11–22.
24. Crowley TJ. Causes of climate change over the past 1000 years. *Science*. 2000; 289(5477): 270–7.
25. Huang SP, Rollack HN, Shen PY. Temperature trends over the past five centuries reconstructed from borehole temperatures. *Nature*. 2000; 403: 756–8.
26. IPCC. *Climate Change 2007: Synthesis Report*. Cambridge: Cambridge University Press; 2007.
27. IPCC. *Climate Change 2001: Impacts, Adaptation and Vulnerability*. Cambridge: Cambridge University Press; 2001.
28. Ye Y, Hoshen M, Kyobutungi C, Louis VR, Sauerborn R. Local scale prediction of Plasmodium falciparum malaria transmission in an endemic region using temperature and rainfall. *Glob Health Action*. 2009; 2.
29. Craig MH, Snow RW, le Sueur D. A climate-based distribution model of malaria transmission in sub-Saharan Africa. *Parasitol Today*. 1999; 15(3): 105–11.
30. Amano T, Smithers RJ, Sparks TH, Sutherland WJ. A 250-year index of first flowering dates and its response to temperature changes. *Proc Biol Sci*. 2010; 277(1693): 2451–7.
31. Yang GJ, Tanner M, Utzinger J, Malone JB, Bergquist R, Chan EY, *et al*. Malaria surveillance–response strategies in different transmission zones of the People's Republic of China: preparing for climate change. *Malaria Journal*. 2012; 11: 426.
32. Zhou XN, Olveda R, Sripa B, Yang GJ, Leonardo L, Bergquist R. From gap analysis to solution and action: The RNAS model. *Acta Tropica*. 2013.
33. Reiter P. Climate change and mosquito-borne disease. *Environmental Health Perspectives*. 2001; 109 Suppl. 1: 141–61.
34. Hunter PR. Climate change and waterborne and vector-borne disease. *Journal of Applied Microbiology*. 2003; 94 Suppl: 37S–46S.
35. Sutherst RW. Global change and human vulnerability to vector-borne diseases. *Clinical Microbiology Reviews*. 2004; 17(1): 136–73.

36. WHO. Sustaining the drive to overcome the global impact of neglected tropical diseases – Second WHO report on neglected tropical diseases. 2013. Available: wwwwhoint/iris/bitstream/10665/77950//9789241564540_engpdf (Accessed March 1, 2013).
37. Zhou XN, Yang GJ, Yang K, Wang XH, Hong QB, Sun LP, *et al.* Potential impact of climate change on schistosomiasis transmission in China. *Am J Trop Med Hyg.* 2008; 78(2): 188–94.
38. Zhou XN, Lv S, Yang GJ, Kristensen TK, Bergquist R, Utzinger J, *et al.* Spatial epidemiology in zoonotic parasitic diseases: insights gained at the 1(st) International Symposium on Geospatial Health in Lijiang, China, 2007. *Parasit Vectors.* 2009; 2.
39. Hay SI, Guerra CA, Tatem AJ, Noor AM, Snow RW. The global distribution and population at risk of malaria: past, present, and future. *Lancet Infect Dis.* 2004; 4(6): 327–36.
40. WHO. Research priorities for the environment, agriculture and infectious diseases of poverty. World Health Organization technical report series. 2013; 976: i–xiii, 1–125.
41. Brooker S, Clarke S, Snow RW, Bundy DA. Malaria in African school children: options for control. *Trans R Soc Trop Med Hyg.* 2008; 102(4): 304–5.
42. Brooker S. Estimating the global distribution and disease burden of intestinal nematode infections: adding up the numbers: a review. *Int J Parasitol.* 2010; 40(10): 1137–44.
43. Hay SI, Omumbo JA, Craig MH, Snow RW. Earth observation, geographic information systems and Plasmodium falciparum malaria in sub-Saharan Africa. *Advances in Parasitology.* 2000; 47: 173–215.
44. WHO. *World Malaria Report 2009.* Geneva: World Health Organization; 2009.
45. Hay SI, Cox J, Rogers DJ, Randolph SE, Stern DI, Shanks GD, *et al.* Climate change and the resurgence of malaria in the East African highlands. *Nature.* 2002; 415(6874): 905–9.
46. Rogers DJ, Randolph SE. The global spread of malaria in a future, warmer world. *Science.* 2000; 289: 1763–6.
47. McCarthy MA. *Bayesian Methods for Ecology.* Cambridge: Cambridge University Press; 2007.
48. Burnham KP, Anderson DR. Multimodel inference – understanding AIC and BIC in model selection. *Sociological Methods & Research.* 2004; 33(2): 261–304.
49. Yang GJ, Brook BW, Whelan PI, Cleland S, Bradshaw CJA. Endogenous and exogenous factors controlling temporal abundance patterns of tropical mosquitos. *Ecological Applications.* 2008; 18(8): 2028–40.
50. Juliano SA, Lounibos LP. Ecology of invasive mosquitoes: effects on resident species and on human health. *Ecol Lett.* 2005; 8(5): 558–74.
51. Whelan PI, Jacups SP, Melville L, Broom A, Currie BJ, Krause VL, *et al.* Rainfall and vector mosquito numbers as risk indicators for mosquito-borne disease in central Australia. *Communicable Diseases Intelligence.* 2003; 27(1): 110–16.
52. Wang DQ, Xia ZG, Zhou SS, Zhou XN, Wang RB, Zhang QF. A potential threat to malaria elimination: extensive deltamethrin and DDT resistance to Anopheles sinensis from the malaria-endemic areas in China. *Malaria Journal.* 2013; 12: 164.
53. Yin JH, Wang RB, Xia ZG, Zhou SS, Zhou XN, Zhang QF, *et al.* Students' awareness of malaria at the beginning of national malaria elimination programme in China. *Malaria Journal.* 2013; 12: 237.
54. Zhou XN, Bergquist R, Tanner M. Elimination of tropical disease through surveillance and response. *Infectious Diseases of Poverty.* 2013; 2(1): 1.
55. Zhou XN. Prioritizing research for 'One health–One world'. *Inf Dis Poverty.* 2012; 1(1): 1.
56. Beebe NW, Cooper RD, Mottram P, Sweeney AW. Australia's dengue risk driven by human adaptation to climate change. *PLoS Negl Trop Dis.* 2009; 3(5): e429.
57. Chen JH, Wang H, Chen JX, Bergquist R, Tanner M, Utzinger J, *et al.* Frontiers of parasitology research in the People's Republic of China: infection, diagnosis, protection and surveillance. *Parasit Vectors.* 2012; 5: 221.
58. Haines A, McMichael AJ, Smith KR, Roberts I, Woodcock J, Markandya A, *et al.* Public health benefits of strategies to reduce greenhouse-gas emissions: overview and implications for policy makers. *Lancet.* 2009; 374(9707): 2104–14.
59. Tanser FC, Sharp B, le Sueur D. Potential effect of climate change on malaria transmission in Africa. *Lancet.* 2003; 362(9398): 1792–8.
60. Ostrom E. A general framework for analyzing sustainability of social–ecological systems. *Science.* 2009; 325: 419–22.

61. Brooker S, Utzinger J. Integrated disease mapping in a polyparasitic world. *Geospatial Health*. 2007; 1(2): 141–6.

# Part IV

# Environment and sustainability

# Introduction to Part IV: environment and sustainability

*Siân M. Griffiths*

Early public health practice was predominantly concerned with the environmental factors contributing to ill-health. While doctors, civil servants and legislators all played a role, architects and engineers also made key contributions. For example, Joseph Bazalgette built the London sewer system following the 'Big Stink' of 1858 when the Houses of Parliament became so smelly that the members demanded action. In response to politicians' concerns, his sewer network diverted raw sewage downstream, a masterpiece of engineering which is still admired. The need to provide clean water, clean air and safe food is linked to further discussions of the challenges of climate change/global warming, sustainability and resilience in response to disasters.

In their chapter, Samet and Zhang describe the health implications of climate change as occurring through both direct and indirect pathways. They highlight the particular risk for Asia and the increasing pressure on natural resources and the environment – such as deforestation, floods, droughts and disrupted ecosystems – as the population grows. Climate change will alter the distributions of some causal factors affecting morbidity and mortality, disproportionately adversely affecting poorer and vulnerable communities. The impact of climate change is complex, involving the multilevel social, economic, health and governmental systems that determine the health of individuals and populations. Morbidity and mortality associated with high temperatures, increased risks of allergy, changing patterns of infectious diseases, as well as the health risks of both ozone and airborne particles are all potential risks. Climate change can also threaten food security, lead to desertification and threaten water supplies, and have a negative effect on agricultural productivity as a result. In Asia, a sea-level rise would cause large-scale inundation along the vast Asian coastline and cause recession of flat sandy beaches, forcing migration from coastal areas, leading to crowding and potentially to cross-border migration. The ecological stability of mangroves and coral reefs around Asia would be put at risk. Mitigation and adaptation strategies are needed at individual and population level, particularly in Asia where, as the authors point out, compared to the 'global average', several of the pathways through which climate change affects human health may be amplified within areas already experiencing a scarcity of resources, environmental degradation, high rates of infectious diseases, as well as weak infrastructure and overpopulation. The poor are highly vulnerable to climate change because of their limited access to stable livelihood opportunities, and limited access to areas that are fit for safe and healthy habitation. Consequently, those who are impoverished are more likely to be at increased risk from floods, droughts, and contaminated water and food.

The need for advocacy to mitigate the impact of climate change is demonstrated in the case study from Atkinson *et al.* in Chapter 21. They describe the work of the Climate and Health Council (CHC), which is based in the UK and brings together doctors, nurses and other health professionals who recognize the urgent need to address climate change. The council's work focuses on the already apparent and predicted health effects of climate change. The CHC is an advocacy group which is dedicated to raising awareness of the adverse health effects of climate change and promoting the health co-benefits of tackling these issues. The model it uses could be adapted by most Asian countries.

Additional threats to Asia's future livelihood come from the rapid urbanization and economic transition that has improved socio-economic conditions but has resulted in high levels of air pollution and an increasing burden of associated disease. A major public health threat, pollution in many Asian cities has climbed to unacceptable levels. According to the WHO, roughly 1.3 million deaths worldwide are caused by urban outdoor air pollution every year. Tze Wai and Andromeda Wong use Hong Kong as a case study in Chapter 22 to exemplify the contributors to air pollution, the harm it poses to health, the possibilities for control, and the need for political will, new legislation and public advocacy to address this issue. Drawing on the history, research base and examples from cities such as London and Los Angeles, the authors track the relocation of manufacturing industries and factories from Hong Kong across the border to mainland China. This gradual but relentless removal of Hong Kong's manufacturing base resulted in a reduction in air pollutant emissions from local factories, and at the same time in the rapid development of the neighbouring Pearl River Delta as the 'factory of the world', which soon posed a regional air pollution problem to Hong Kong. At the same time, the problem of pollution from local sources remained – predominantly – from increasing numbers of motor vehicles as well as shipping traffic in the harbour. Local research has shown that children living in the more polluted districts had poorer lung functions than those living in districts with cleaner air and children living closer to a pollution source had three times the prevalence of respiratory illnesses compared with children living in a district farther away from the source. Other studies in primary care indicated that high air pollution levels affect not only those with serious illnesses requiring hospitalization, but also the much larger population at risk for minor respiratory illnesses. Although some steps have been taken to reduce pollution levels, the emissions reduction targets have been based on what can practically be done rather than on what needs to be done, and the authors emphasize the need for political will and public engagement to improve the air in Hong Kong and the region.

In addition to clean air, clean water is also a prerequisite of good health. Lack of safe water is a major contributor to poverty and the Millennium Development Goal (MDG) to ensure environmental sustainability includes halving the proportion of people without sustainable access to safe drinking water and basic sanitation by 2015. According to the World Water Council report, around 1.1 billion people (approximately one in every six people) worldwide do not have access to safe drinking water and around 2.6 billion people do not have improved sanitation facilities. Only 46 per cent of people in Africa have access to safe drinking water. Thousands of students, especially girls, drop out of school each year because of water insecurity or because they have to help fetch water for their families. Achieving the MDG would prevent 470,000 diarrhoeal deaths and this would result in an extra 320 million productive working days per year. In economic terms, each dollar invested in water and sanitation would bring back US$3–34.

Drawing on examples from Asia and beyond, in Chapter 23 Mitra highlights the problems of water scarcity, water pollution and water security, linking with themes already described in other chapters, such as climate change, changing patterns of vectors and increased risks of infectious diseases. Urbanization, industrialization and demand from the influx of a large number of people from rural to urban areas have increased the need for available water. At the same time, more rivers in China become contaminated by industrial waste and heavy metals and the potential impact of climate change on availability of water becomes a reality.

Food safety and food security are also important environmental health safeguards and are increasingly becoming global issues. Providing safe food is another key environmental challenge, particularly in large urban areas. The role of the Centre for Food Safety in Hong Kong, described by Ho and Chan in Chapter 24, provides a case study for implementing public health policy. Hong Kong depends almost entirely on imported food, in particular, fresh food from mainland China, and China meets some 50 per cent of Hong Kong's food demand. Due to the globalization of the food trade, food from every corner of the world is also available in Hong Kong. With rising expectations of the community on food safety, food safety management is increasingly difficult and challenging. This chapter describes risk analysis, the food safety regulatory framework adopted in Hong Kong and how its three components work together. It also uses the incident caused by melamine abuse in milk as a case study to describe how food safety can have a long-standing impact on a country's supply of a certain product (in this case, on China's milk supply).

Safe environments, response to climate change, safe water and safe food are all important considerations for protecting the population from the impact of disasters. The Asia-Pacific region includes some of the most disaster-prone areas thus disaster preparedness and disaster response are important elements in public health practice since they affect large segments of the population and can play a role in mitigating the adverse impacts of disasters. Like many other public health programmes, responses to disasters need to be addressed as long-term sustainable efforts.

In Chapter 25 Chan describes the need for disaster response strategies particularly in low-income territories where effective response is often hindered by lack of development. She outlines approaches to be taken to mitigate the health impacts of disasters. Two case studies for public health response also illustrate these principles in practice. In Chapter 26 Southgate describes the Japanese earthquake of 2011 and how it and the tsunami it started together precipitated the third event of the '3/11 triple disaster' – three reactors at the Fukushima Daiichi Nuclear Power Plant lost all power and went into meltdown with fires, explosions and radiation that contaminated the land, groundwater and the atmosphere. In Chapter 27 Charupoonphol, like Southgate, details the public health response and lessons from natural disaster in his case study of the public health challenges of the floods in Thailand in 2011. Floodwaters swamped more than two-thirds of the country, submerging rice fields and shutting down hundreds of factories. Severe flooding started at the end of July and spread through the provinces of northern, north-eastern and central Thailand along the Mekong and Chao Phraya river basins. In October, floodwaters inundated parts of Bangkok. Flooding persisted in some areas until mid-January 2012, and resulted in a total of 815 deaths and 13.6 million people affected.

Another impact of the transition from rural to urban economies has been the change in working conditions and practices. Protecting the health of the population – particularly the more vulnerable – places massive strains on government agencies, local employers and communities. Occupational health aims to promote and maintain the highest degree of physical, mental and social wellbeing of workers in all occupations, preventing harm from working conditions and protecting workers in employment from risks. An estimated 2 million people or more worldwide die annually of occupational injuries and work-related diseases, 160 million people suffer from work-related diseases and 270 million people suffer fatal and non-fatal work-related accidents per year. The WHO's *World Health Report 2002* indicates that 1.5 per cent of the global burden in terms of disability-adjusted life years (DALYs) results from only a selected subset of occupational risks. In developing countries, the risks are estimated to be 10 to 20 times higher than in established market economies. At present, rapid changes in working life are affecting both the health of workers and the environment. For example, in the African region the introduction of new technologies, new chemical substances and materials have led to new occupational and work-related diseases and injuries, while traditional hazards, such as high dust or noise levels in workplaces, have not yet been dealt with adequately.

The basic tasks of occupational health are the recognition, evaluation, prevention and control of harmful occupational working conditions and they involve the production process, the labour process and securing the working environment. In Chapter 28, Chen and Wu describe the approaches taken to occupational health and safety, highlighting some of the distinct characteristics of occupational hazards in developing countries in Asia, including the traditional occupational hazards and health injuries, such as pneumoconiosis, acute and chronic poisoning, injuries and hearing loss as well as new types of occupational injuries caused by new technologies and materials, such as nano dust, new occupational hazards including adverse ergonomic design, forced posture and psychological stress related to work and pesticide poisoning and agricultural occupational health. In addition they highlight the need to protect the occupational health of migrant floating populations.

Occupational accidents and occupational diseases also have an impact not only on the lives of individual workers, but also on the productivity and profitability of their enterprises and, ultimately, on the welfare of the whole society. How to intervene effectively to reduce the risk of workplace hazards is receiving increased attention in low-income countries where reforms include establishing information systems; training health personnel, labour inspectors and other relevant actors; and developing policies and guidelines.

# 20
# Climate change and health

*Jonathan M. Samet and Junfeng (Jim) Zhang*

## Introduction: climate change – the need for regional assessments

While uncertainty persists about the pace of climate change, there is scientific consensus that the build-up of greenhouse gases has resulted in global warming and climate change. The Intergovernmental Panel on Climate Change (IPCC), an effort of a global collective of scientists, projects that the Earth's temperature could rise by as much as 4°C by the year 2100 depending on future trends of greenhouse gas emissions [1, 2]. The magnitude of the health consequences resulting from climate change will reflect the actual increase in temperature. The consequences of greenhouse gas emissions for climate are not simply a warming uniformly across the globe, but rather the warming is anticipated to be variable by place and over time, and extremes of weather will be enhanced. The direct weather consequences of climate change include warmer temperatures and more extreme conditions, and an associated sea-level rise, whereas the indirect consequences are broad with implications for human health (see Table 20.1). Beyond the adverse consequences listed in Table 20.1, some regions may benefit from warming through expanded agriculture and less need for heating.

The health implications of climate change reflect both direct and indirect pathways (see Figure 20.1). Climate change will not lead to new causes of morbidity and mortality, but will change the distributions of some causal factors that affect the occurrence of morbidity and mortality. For vector-borne infectious diseases (e.g. malaria), changes in the geographic distributions of vectors may lead to the emergence of diseases in places that have been previously free from the particular diseases. There is concern, for example, about the potential for malaria to re-enter places where it has long been eliminated if the range of its vector, the *Anopheles* mosquito, expands. Changes in flora may bring new allergens and crop yields may drop. Air pollution may worsen from fossil fuel combustion for power generation to meet increasing cooling needs due to warming and other energy demands to adapt to climate change. Rising sea levels and weather changes with consequences for agriculture and availability of water may displace people and lead to social and economic disruption with diverse potential implications for health.

The consequences of climate change for human health will be manifested differentially across broad regions of the world. The extent of change is projected to be variable, at least on

*Table 20.1* Potential threats and health consequences of climate change

| *Threat* | *Consequence* |
|---|---|
| Increased frequency and intensity of heatwaves | Increased mortality from heatwaves, particularly in elderly |
| Altered distributions of aeroallergens | Increased frequency and severity of allergic diseases and symptoms |
| Altered distributions of vectors of infectious diseases | Spread of infectious diseases and increased frequency |
| Increased air pollution | Increased morbidity and premature mortality |
| Changing agricultural yields | More undernourished people in low-income countries |
| Social and economic disruptions, displacement | Various, with acute and chronic consequences |

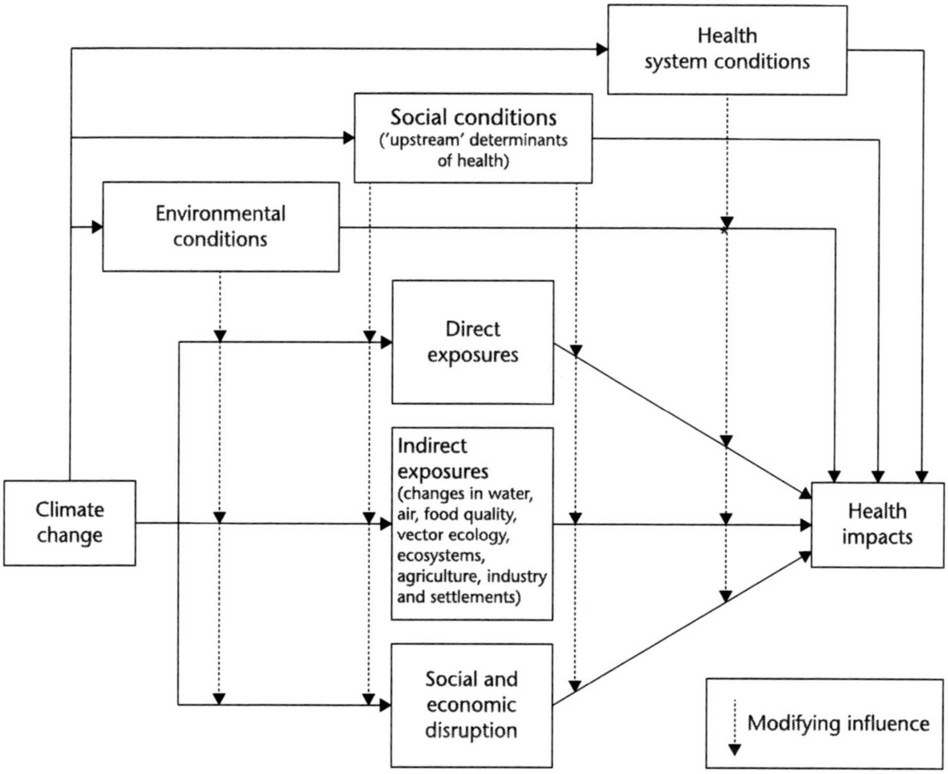


*Figure 20.1* Schematic diagram of pathways by which climate change affects health, and concurrent direct-acting and modifying (conditioning) influences of environmental, social and health-system factors [2]

the regional scale – populations vary in their vulnerability and resilience, and adaptive capacity and resources also differ. Consequently, the IPCC provides regional assessments giving specific insights into anticipated impacts of climate change, including effects on human health. In its Fourth Assessment Report, the IPCC includes a chapter on Asia that offers findings used in this chapter [1, 2]. Additionally, in 2012, the World Health Organization (WHO) and the World Meteorological Organization (WMO) collaborated in the publication of the *Atlas of Health and Climate*, which provides useful maps that highlight the geographic diversity of the health consequences of climate change [3].

This chapter begins with an overview of the health consequences of climate change, covering effects that result through both direct and indirect paths. It considers not only the health consequences, but also the specific measures that might be taken to reduce impact. We then turn to the health consequences of climate change that are projected for South/East Asia. Of necessity, our coverage of this wide-ranging set of topics is brief. For further information, we recommend the reports of the IPCC, as well as the series in *Lancet* on climate change and health [4, 5].

## Mechanisms by which climate change affects health

Climate change has been labelled as 'the biggest global health threat of the 21st century'. In so labelling it, the *Lancet* and the University College London Institute for Global Health Commission cited the far reach of climate change and its diverse threats to human health [6]. Estimates of the potential burden of premature mortality and additional morbidity from climate change, while subject to great uncertainty, indicate a looming, substantial impact. For the year 2000, climate change was estimated to have caused the premature loss of about 150,000 lives and about 5.5 million disability-adjusted life-years (DALYs), representing 0.3 per cent of total deaths and 0.4 per cent of all DALYs, respectively [7].

Climate change affects health within the complex, multilevel system that determines the health of individuals and populations, including social, economic and health systems and governmental determinants (see Figure 20.1). The time domains of the stressor and adaptive and mitigative responses are also relevant. The acute stress of a catastrophic and large-scale weather event may overwhelm countering responses and mitigating mechanisms – the devastation caused by Hurricane Sandy to the East Coast of the United States (US) in 2012 is exemplary. The health status of the population affected is also a key consideration, as is the adequacy of its health system. Responses to the stressors associated with climate change may vary with the age structure of the population, the prevalence of chronic diseases and the capacity of the health system to provide care for the burden of disease that might arise from a climate-change driven event. There is concern that climate change could cause large-scale social and economic disruption through drought, famine and sea-level rise, and migration could lead to instability and conflict. For such consequences, the geopolitics of the world at the time will be critical [8].

There is the additional conceptual complexity of determining that health consequences are attributable to climate change. The assignment of causation is based on the concept of comparing actual events to scenarios of what might have happened absent climate change – the so-called counterfactual. For weather events, for example, a comparison is between the number of extreme events with health consequences, compared with the number generated by climate models in the absence of human-forced climate change. Such comparisons are conceptually challenging and not readily communicated to decision-makers and the public.

## Heat stress and heatwaves

Temperature has long been associated with adverse effects on health and mortality. At extreme temperatures, the well-known clinical entities of hypothermia and hyperthermia are documented causes of death [9]. For climate change, exposure to heat and hyperthermia are of particular concern, given the resulting warming and increased frequency of extreme events with dangerously high temperatures. Hyperthermia occurs when temperatures are high among persons carrying out physical activities that lead to thermal stress, as well as among people who are susceptible to heat because of limited adaptive capacity, such as infants, the elderly and persons taking medications that impair responses to thermal stress (e.g. medications widely used for hypertension and heart disease). Even in developed countries, excess deaths from heat and heatwaves remain common and dramatic heatwaves with large numbers of deaths continue to occur. For example, in recent decades, the dramatic and well-documented epidemics of death associated with heatwaves in Chicago in 1995 (about 750 excess deaths [10]) and in Europe in 2003 (about 35,000 or more excess deaths [11, 12]), have alerted the public to the dangers of heatwaves and led to protective actions by governments and public health agencies.

Warmer temperatures are associated with mortality even in times when heatwaves are not in progress [9, 12]. The relationship between temperature and mortality has been characterized as 'J-shaped', such that mortality increases with both colder and warmer temperatures from an optimum temperature at which it is the lowest [13, 14]. Figure 20.2 provides

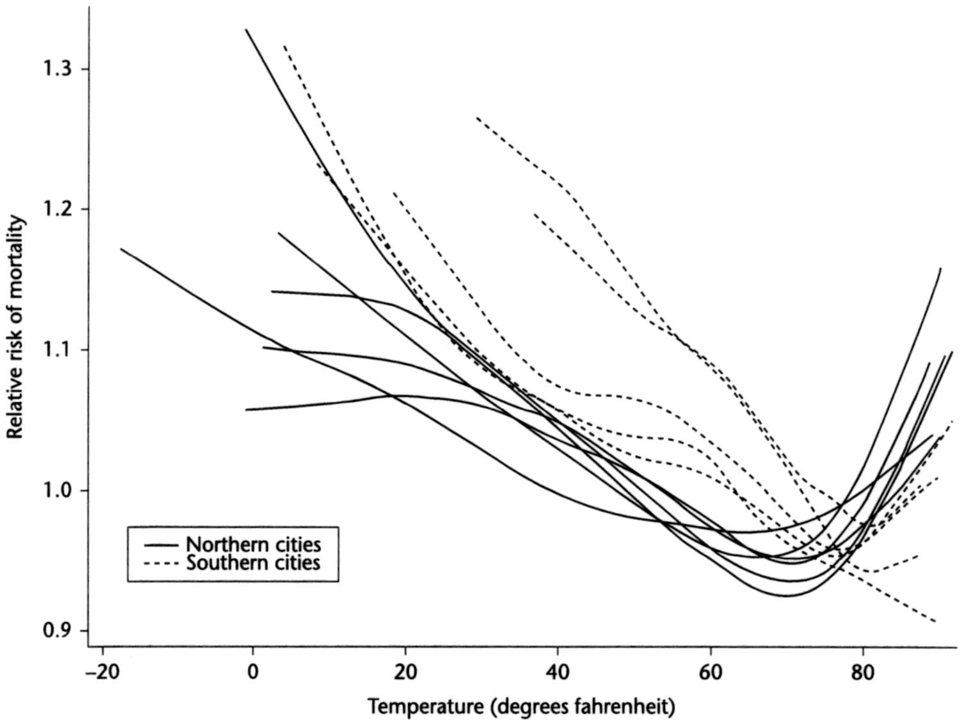


*Figure 20.2* Temperature–mortality relative risk functions for 11 US cities, 1973–1994 [13]
*Note*: °C = 5/9 x (°F – 32).

illustrative analyses from 11 US cities. In almost all cities, the temperature with the lowest risk for mortality is evident and the upturn with higher temperature is more prominent in northern cities. The optimum temperature varies inversely with average temperature, and hence latitude, as well as the extent to which adaptive measures, such as air conditioning, are in place for buffering warmer or colder temperatures [12, 13, 15]. This J-shaped relationship has implications for the potential overall effect of global warming consequent to climate change on heat-associated mortality. Warming would reduce the cold-associated mortality while increasing heat-associated mortality, minus the new adaptive measures [13]. However, beyond the rise in average temperature, climate change is also projected to increase the variability of temperature and the frequency of heatwaves [1, 2]. There is an effect of heatwaves per se and the temperature profile of heatwaves seems to be a critical determinant of excess mortality [16].

Evidence suggests that the risk of heat-related excess mortality has declined on longer time frames. Carson and colleagues [17] examined weekly mortality in London during the twentieth century and assessed temperature-associated mortality over a period during which a major shift occurred in the underlying causes of death, the population became progressively older and the proportion affected by chronic diseases increased. They found declines in susceptibility to dying from both cold and heat. Carson *et al.* attributed this finding to factors related to social and environmental conditions, behaviour and health care. Davis *et al.* [18] examined heat-related mortality over the period between 1964 and 1998 in the US and also found declining heat mortality, which they attributed to various adaptations, including the increased availability of air conditioning. Barnett [19] found that the association of warm temperature with cardiovascular mortality during the summer declined substantially over the period between 1987 and 2004.

Population characteristics also affect the impact of heatwaves. The elderly and persons with underlying chronic diseases, such as coronary heart disease and congestive heart failure, are particularly at risk. Additionally, individuals taking diuretics, or taking some drugs used for blood pressure control and/or other drugs may have impaired cardiovascular responses to thermal stress, as may those who are obese. In the ageing populations of the more developed countries, these at-risk groups are increasing. Epidemiological analyses have identified additional risk factors for mortality during heatwaves, including a lack of social support, socio-economic status and housing characteristics. In urban areas, the 'urban heat island' phenomenon tends to increase the risk of mortality associated with heatwaves [20]. Determinants of risk in less developed countries have received little research attention. In such countries, there is a very low prevalence of air conditioning.

Because the elderly and people with underlying chronic diseases are particularly susceptible, the hypothesis has been advanced that the excess mortality associated with heatwaves comes from a brief advancement of the time of dying, a phenomenon sometimes referred to as 'mortality displacement' or 'harvesting'. If such mortality displacement is occurring, a reduction in mortality would be anticipated following the excess associated with the heatwave and, indeed, analytical approaches have been developed for assessing mortality displacement [21, 22]. Regarding the 2003 heatwave in France, the extent of mortality displacement was found to be modest [23]. Parallel analyses of heat-related deaths in Delhi, São Paulo and London, using distributed lag models, found some mortality displacement in London and a lesser indication of this phenomenon in Delhi [24], with the pattern being intermediate for São Paulo. These results, as well as descriptive observations on the ages of individuals dying during heatwaves, suggest that heatwaves do not affect only the most vulnerable.

Where there is little evidence on temperature-associated mortality in developing countries, greater excess mortality might be anticipated because of limited penetration of air conditioning, the density of megacities and limited attention to the problem by public health authorities. The ISOTHURM project examined the temperature–mortality relationship in 12 urban areas, including several in low- and middle-income countries [14]. The data from most of the cities showed the typical J-shaped relationship with temperature. In Delhi and Salvador, mortality did not increase at colder temperatures, nor did an increase occur at hotter temperatures in Chiang Mai and Cape Town.

## Aeroallergens and allergic diseases

Aeroallergens – biological agents associated with allergic responses – are ubiquitous in indoor and outdoor environments. The two principal and most prevalent diseases associated with aeroallergens are allergic rhinitis, also referred to as hay fever and asthma [25]. Aeroallergens are known to exacerbate asthma and trigger attacks of allergic rhinitis.

For persons with allergic rhinitis and asthma, climate change might increase the risk of exacerbation through altered local and regional pollen production. Warming has already caused an earlier onset of the spring pollen season in the Northern Hemisphere [1, 2]. It may also lengthen the pollen season, change the spatial distribution of vegetation and possibly alter pollen production [1, 2, 26, 27]. Evidence suggests that climate change has changed exposures of populations to aeroallergens [1, 2, 28]. Vegetation patterns have changed and pollination is occurring earlier for some species in some places. New species could potentially become successful in additional areas, leading to exposures of populations to new antigens. More prolonged and intense exposure to aeroallergens could result in more severe disease and greater morbidity, and even increased mortality from asthma. Beggs and Bambrick [27] have proposed that climate change could be contributing to the global rise in asthma as a consequence of greater pollen exposure.

## Changes in endemic and epidemic infectious diseases

Worldwide, in both developed and developing countries, infectious agents remain a leading cause of disease and death [29]. Warming from climate change has the potential to affect the transmission of infectious diseases across the globe. The transmission of these diseases is conceptually described by the 'epidemiological triangle' (see Figure 20.3), which captures the interplay between its components: the agent, the environment and the vector. Environmental conditions that promote or extend the geographic range of the vector increase the potential for infection. In addition to potentially affecting vector-borne diseases, climate change may also extend or change the geographic regions in which an infectious agent is present. Climate change may affect both endemic disease (i.e. disease generally occurring in a population) and epidemic disease (i.e. disease occurring in excess of normal expectancy). The time frames over which climate change could affect infectious diseases extend from relatively short, as even the temperature rise to date has had apparent impact, to relatively long, as continued temperature increases would be predicted to continue to alter vector distributions and densities.

Mathematical models of infectious disease transmission provide quantitative insight into the potential for climate change to increase rates of vector-borne diseases. The potential for transmission of infectious diseases is characterized by the basic reproductive rate ($R_0$) which describes the number of new cases of infection arising from one case in a population of

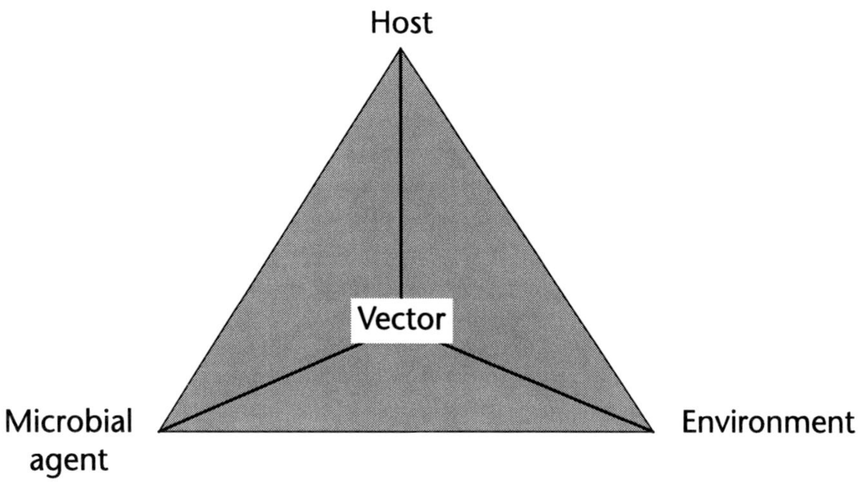


*Figure 20.3* The epidemiological triangle of epidemics

susceptible persons [30]. Values above unity imply the possibility of epidemic disease – a value of unity means that endemic disease will be maintained and a value below unity means that the disease will decline. Warming can increase $R_0$ through its effect on vector numbers, transmission probabilities and biting rates for insect vectors [30]. The geographic spread of vectors may also be affected by the extension of their ranges resulting from warmer conditions. Several vector-borne diseases are considered to be potentially sensitive to climate change [31] (see Table 20.2).

Waterborne and airborne diseases may also be affected by climate change. For diseases transmitted by water, warming may enlarge the geographic area in which conditions are suitable for survival of disease-causing organisms and for propagation of infection [32, 33]. The occurrence of waterborne infections has also been linked to extreme weather events [34]. Increased air conditioning and more time spent indoors, because of warming, might affect patterns for diseases that are transmitted in indoor environments by droplets or by contact, such as influenza and the common cold.

*Table 20.2* Examples of vector-borne diseases likely to be sensitive to climate change

| *Vector* | *Major diseases* |
|---|---|
| Mosquitoes | Malaria, filariasis, dengue fever, yellow fever, West Nile fever |
| Sandflies | Leishmaniasis |
| Triatomines | Chagas disease |
| Ixodes ticks | Lyme disease, tick-borne encephalitis |
| Tsetse flies | African trypanosomiasis |
| Blackflies | Onchocerciasis |
| Snails (intermediate host) | Schistosomiasis |

*Source*: [31].

Cholera illustrates the complexity of understanding how climate change can alter the occurrence of infectious diseases [32, 33]. The disease-causing organism, *Vibrio cholera*, is endemic and widely found in water. Multiple global cholera pandemics have been documented – the seventh, which began in 1961, is still ongoing. The present epidemic began with the emergence of a new biotype, the El Tor biotype of *V. cholerae* 01, in Indonesia. In 1991, the pandemic moved to South America, with outbreaks along the Pacific coast. The epidemic's occurrence was linked to a plankton bloom that was driven by the El Niño Southern Oscillation (ENSO). The planktonic copepod organism harbours the *V. cholera* organisms on its surface. Consequently, a higher concentration of plankton increases the dose of the infectious agent received from drinking contaminated water. A time-series analysis of cholera in Bangladesh found a link with the ENSO phenomenon [35]. Lipp and colleagues [33] propose that climate change could affect each step in their model for cholera transmission. Checkley and colleagues [36] carried out a time-series analysis of temperature changes associated with the ENSO and all hospital admissions for diarrhoea in children in Peru. Over the period between 1993 and 1998, they found that the numbers of admissions were positively associated with temperature and also with the ENSO, which had an effect on the admissions rate beyond that expected from the temperature increase alone.

Changes in the epidemiological characteristics of other infectious diseases have been examined in relation to climate change. Dengue transmission was addressed in the IPCC report [1, 2] and in specific studies [37]. In Western Australia, Woodruff *et al.* [38] found that climate data predicted epidemics of the Ross River virus disease (which is spread by mosquitoes) reasonably well, particularly if data on mosquitoes were incorporated into the model. Studies have also addressed tick-borne disease [39, 40] and food-borne disease [41]. The potential for malaria to increase as a consequence of climate change has been controversial and malaria is receding globally in spite of some predictions that it would intensify as the world warms [42] (see chapters 18 and 19).

Many factors determine susceptibility to infection and the severity of the resulting illness, including mortality risk. In developed countries, key factors include age, immunocompetence, presence of comorbid chronic diseases (e.g. coronary heart disease, chronic obstructive pulmonary disease and diabetes), access to vaccines and to medical care, and the quality of the medical care available. In developing countries, additional determinants of severity include general nutritional status and specific micronutrient deficiencies. The level of sanitation, the availability and use of preventive measures (such as bed nets and vector control), and the availability of vaccinations determine transmission probabilities. In both developed and developing countries large populations are at risk for more severe infections and mortality.

## Ambient air pollution

Climate change may worsen air pollution, either directly (through increased tropospheric – ground-level – ozone production) or indirectly (through greater power plant emissions as power generation increases to meet the demand for air conditioning capacity). Ozone is a secondary pollutant formed via sunlight-driven photochemical reactions involving precursor hydrocarbons and oxides of nitrogen. Together with ozone, other secondary products are generated, forming the complex mixture of photochemical smog. Ozone pollution is projected to increase because warmer temperatures increase ozone production [1, 2]. Warmer temperatures enhance the chemical reactions that generate ozone. Under various scenarios, increases of several parts per billion are projected over the next two decades [43] and up to a range of 10 to 30 parts per billion by the end of this century [44]. Fossil fuel combustion contaminates the atmosphere with the primary particles generated by combustion and with the secondary particles formed from gaseous components of power plant emissions through complex chemical and physical processes. Increased fossil fuel burning could also worsen particulate air pollution, beyond predictions from climate change scenarios [1, 2, 45].

The health risks of both ozone and airborne particles have been characterized in numerous epidemiological studies, with supporting evidence coming from in vivo and in vitro toxicological research [46, 47, 48]. Both ozone and particulate matter (PM) air pollution have been associated with an increased risk of mortality in time-series studies of daily mortality [49, 50, 51] and airborne particles have also been associated with an increased risk of death on longer time frames [47, 51, 52]. Both types of pollution are also associated with morbidity, including an increased risk for hospitalization [51, 53] and other adverse outcomes [48]. A quickly expanding body of evidence links particulate air pollution to adverse cardiovascular effects [52]. As for temperature and infection, a substantial proportion of the population is at increased risk because of older age and comorbidity, particularly respiratory and cardiac diseases.

Analyses that link climate change model outputs to ozone concentrations have been carried out for cities in the US. Knowlton *et al.* [54] projected future increases in ozone concentration for 31 counties of the New York metropolitan region. Considering the impact of climate change alone on ozone concentration, they estimated a median 4.5 per cent increase in summertime ozone-related, acute, all-cause mortality for all the counties. Bell *et al.* [55] performed a similar modelling for 50 cities in eastern US. They estimated the average increase in daily one-hour maximum concentration as 4.8 parts per billion. Depending on the concentration–response relationship used, the increase in ozone concentration corresponded to an increase in daily, all-cause mortality of 0.11 to 0.27 per cent.

Analyses have also addressed particulate air pollution, considering potential risks of increased fossil fuel combustion and benefits for health of reducing air pollution through greenhouse gas mitigation [45, 56]. In one assessment, enhanced energy consumption based on fossil fuel combustion was projected as leading to substantial increase in premature mortality [45]. In a scenario of business as usual that results in increased exposure to PM air pollution, an additional 700,000 premature deaths were forecast. Similarly, in an analysis of four of the world's major cities (Mexico City, New York City, Santiago and São Paulo), Cifuentes *et al.* [56] predicted that reductions of ozone and particles from mitigation would substantially reduce premature mortality.

In addition, air pollution and thermal stress may act synergistically: both affect the same susceptible populations and mean that hot temperatures will increase ozone production. A few studies have addressed such synergism. In Athens, the short-term effect of sulphur dioxide on daily mortality was independent of temperature over the period between 1975 and 1982 [57]. An analysis of mortality in Athens during a 1987 heatwave suggested synergism of air pollution with higher temperatures [58]. Filleul and colleagues [59] examined the contributions of ozone and temperature to the excess mortality observed in nine French cities during the 2003 heatwave. They estimated that both ozone and heat contributed to the excess and found that the relative contributions varied from city to city. Fischer *et al.* [60] published similar findings for the Netherlands during the 2003 heatwave. Neither analysis tested for synergism between ozone and temperature. Synergistic effects of aeroallergens and urban air pollutants (such as ozone and particulate matter) on asthma and allergenicity have been examined in epidemiological and toxicological studies [61, 62]. A recent study showed that ragweed pollen collected along high-traffic roads induced higher allergenicity than ragweed pollen sampled in vegetated areas, suggesting that traffic-related pollution enhances pollen allergenicity [63].

## Climate change and social and economic disruption

The possibility of social and economic disruption from climate change looms large for much of the world, including Asia. Climate change can threaten food security, lead to desertification and threaten water supplies [5]. Agricultural productivity is likely to suffer as a result. Sea-level rise may force migration from coastal areas, leading to crowding and potentially to cross-border migration. In Asia, sea-level rise would cause large-scale inundation along the vast Asian coastline and recession of flat sandy beaches. The ecological stability of mangroves and coral reefs around Asia would be put at risk. The potential implications for health of the social and economic impacts of these broad consequences of climate change are enormous, including inadequate food and water supplies, breakdown of governmental services and failure of health systems. There is also potential for conflict over resources, possibly water access and agricultural land.

## Specific health outcomes and adaptation measures

The inevitable consequences of climate change, as described above, require responsible actions to mitigate the problem. Central to the mitigation debate is the reduction of $CO_2$ emissions by using renewable energy sources, cleaner fossil fuels and improving energy efficiencies. Given that $CO_2$ has a long-term half-life in the atmosphere, proposals to mitigate short-lived warming pollutants such as methane and black carbon have gained support in recent years, especially under the notion of 'co-benefits'. In addition to having a larger warming potential than $CO_2$ on a per-molecule basis, methane is a precursor of troposphere ozone and black carbon (BC) is considered to be a more toxic component of airborne fine particulate matter. In a recent assessment of 14 specific emission control measures targeting BC and methane to reduce the rate of climate change over the next 20–40 years, Anenberg *et al.* [64] found that in addition to climate benefits, the methane and BC emission control measures would have substantial co-benefits for air quality and public health worldwide, potentially reversing trends of increasing air pollution concentrations and mortality in Africa, and South, West and Central Asia. The projected benefits are independent of $CO_2$ mitigation measures.

Perhaps more urgent than mitigating greenhouse pollutants is developing adaptation strategies. We consider a number of adaptation measures, at both societal and individual levels, that are specific to pathways through which climate change affects health outcomes. Across all pathways, assessment of the impact of climate change is the first step for exploring adaptation strategies. In general, disease surveillance systems are essential for acquiring data needed for impact assessment. Specifically, monitoring of diseases, along with related meteorological data and ecological factors, is needed to track the impact of weather factors by each pathway, as shown in Table 20.3. Disease monitoring is also necessary for assessing the effectiveness and efficiency of adaptation measures [65]. For example, heat watch and warning systems implemented in the US have proven effective in helping to minimize the impact of heatwaves [66]. A similar system has been recently initiated in Shanghai, China [67].

Other adaptation strategies include improvements in assuring safe water and food distribution, disaster preparedness and management, and improvements in public infrastructure, such as healthcare facilities and emergency shelters [68]. Improving socio-economic status through sustainable and equitable socio-economic development can substantially enhance social capital and reduce the vulnerability of developing countries of Asia to climate change. Adaptations to deal with sea-level rise, potentially more intense cyclones and threats to

*Table 20.3* Examples of climate change-related health outcomes and possible adaptation measures

| *Pathways* | *Health outcome* | *Adaptation measures* |
|---|---|---|
| Direct effects of heat | Mortality, dehydration, hypothermia, hyperthermia | Using air conditioners, heat warning systems and shelters for the public |
| Effects of urban air pollution | Cardio-respiratory mortality and morbidity, adverse birth outcome | Staying indoors, adding filters to building ventilation systems |
| Effects of aeroallergens | Asthma, allergic rhinitis, sinusitis, allergies | Staying indoors, using filters, medical therapies |
| Water-borne/food-borne diseases | Diarrhoeal diseases, bacillary dysentery | Enhancing monitoring of water and food quality, enhancing personal hygiene practices |
| Vector-borne diseases | Malaria, dengue, Japanese encephalitis, West Nile virus | Enhancing mosquito controls, enhancing disease surveillance and infectious disease controls |
| Disasters (drought, floods, forest fires, etc.) | Drowning, injury, mental health problems, increased susceptibility to infections | Improving public infrastructures (e.g. forecast and evacuation capacities) in response to natural disasters |
| Malnutrition | Underweight, increased susceptibility to disease and infections | Advancing technologies to improve crop yields, especially in poor agriculture communities; implementing policies and other means to reduce poverty |

ecosystems and biodiversity are recommended as high-priority actions in coastal areas of temperate and tropical countries [1, 2].

## Climate change in South/East Asia

In the following sections, we focus on several sub-regions of Asia: South Asia and Southeast Asia based on the definition in the IPCC report [1, 2]. We use the term 'South/East Asia' when referring non-specifically to South Asia and Southeast Asia.

Asia is the most populous continent, covering 30 per cent of the Earth's land surface, but home to over 4 billion people in 2010 or about 60 per cent of the world's total. During the twentieth century, Asia's population nearly quadrupled. The majority of the region's population growth is projected to come from South Asia, which is anticipated to add 570 million people in India, 200 million in Pakistan and 130 million in Bangladesh over the next 50 years [69]. The projected population growth, especially in regions with high baseline population densities, implies increased pressure on the natural resources and the environment (e.g. deforestation, floods, droughts and disrupted ecosystems) [70]. For example, in the developing regions of Asia, the remaining natural flood plains are disappearing at an accelerating rate, due primarily to changes in land use and hydrological cycle. The most threatened flood plains may be those in South and Southeast Asia [71], and this loss of flood plains makes the region more vulnerable to climate change.

Southeast Asia is characterized by tropical rainforests, monsoon climates with high and constant rainfall, and heavily leached soils. The coastlines in monsoon Asia are cyclone-prone with approximately 40 per cent of the world's total tropical cyclones occurring in this region [72]. This region has reportedly undergone a 0.1°C to 0.3°C increase per decade from 1951 to 2000 [73]. Furthermore, extreme weather events associated with El Niño were reported to be more frequent and intense in the past 20 years [74, 75]. For example, increased occurrence of extreme rains caused flash floods in Vietnam, landslides and floods in 1990 and 2004 in the Philippines and floods in Cambodia in 2000 [76, 77]. Since 1970, the frequency and intensity of tropical cyclones originating in the Pacific have increased [78], while cyclones originating from the Bay of Bengal and Arabian Sea have decreased in frequency but increased in intensity [79]. In both cases, the damage caused by intense cyclones has risen significantly in the affected countries, particularly India, the Philippines, Vietnam and Cambodia, as well as Japan and China [1, 2].

Temperature projections for the twenty-first century, based on the Fourth Assessment Report of IPCC [1, 2], suggest a significant acceleration of warming over that observed in the twentieth century [80, 81]. Given that South/East Asia has vast coastlines and consists of many islands, sea-level rise due to warming is a practical and serious concern. Fundamental thermodynamics and climate models suggest that dry regions will become drier and wet regions will become wetter in response to global warming [82]. These model results suggest that the absence of climate mitigation will further increase the intensity and frequency of typhoons, tropical storms, floods and landslides in South/East Asia.

## Health impacts of climate change in South/East Asia

Compared to the 'global average', several of the pathways through which climate change affects human health may be amplified in South/East Asia, with some areas already experiencing a scarcity of resources, environmental degradation and high rates of infectious disease, in the context of weak infrastructure and overpopulation [83, 84]. In particular, tropical regions of South/East Asia will experience significant changes in human–pathogen relationships due to climate change [85, 86]. Changing temperatures and precipitation patterns linked to climate change will further affect health by changing the ecology of various vector-borne diseases, such as malaria, dengue, chikungunya, Japanese encephalitis, kala-azar and filariasis [87, 88]. The numbers within the vulnerable groups are large [89, 90].

## Impact on urban populations and population migration

Major cities, including Bangkok, Jakarta, Manila and Ho Chi Minh City, are at risk as the sea rises [91]. In general, cities are vulnerable to the health impacts of climate change, partly because of urban heat island effects and urban air pollution. Long heatwaves and urban smog are indeed a potent and injurious combination to which urban areas in South/East Asia are vulnerable [83, 91].

Additionally, populations in cities throughout South/East Asia are growing rapidly. Rapid population growth and urbanization force poor people to move to fragile and high-risk areas prone to natural hazards. Moreover, the rapid growth of industries in urban areas drives people to migrate from rural areas to urban/industrialized areas. Such population migration brings substantial challenges for implementing many of the adaptation measures described earlier in this chapter because it is difficult to expand the infrastructure at a pace matching the speed of population growth. A further complication to this socio-economic-driven migration is the expected population movement following extreme weather events. Such unplanned migration has significant public health implications at its origins, along the migration routes and in the receptor areas [92]. The countries/areas that can be potentially affected by climate-induced population migration (often accompanied by pathogen migration) need to develop preparedness and adaptation strategies to minimize the potential for resulting catastrophic damage [93].

## Impact on vector-borne and infectious diseases

Mortality and morbidity from diarrhoeal diseases and malnutrition attributable to climate change were already the largest in South/East Asian countries including Bangladesh, Bhutan, India, Maldives, Myanmar and Nepal in 2000 [94]. In this region, endemic morbidity and mortality due to diarrhoeal disease have been linked to poverty and hygiene behaviour, accelerated by the effect of high temperatures on bacterial proliferation [36]. Incidence rates and frequency of outbreaks of diarrhoeal and other infectious diseases (e.g. cholera, hepatitis, malaria, dengue fever) have also been linked to climate-related factors, such as floods, droughts, rising sea-surface temperatures and rainfall. Other relevant factors include the scope of the susceptible population, e.g. children, the elderly and the impoverished; lack of access to safe drinking water; and inadequate sewer systems [1, 2, 95]. Increases in sea-surface temperature due to climate change will increase the growth of phytoplankton along the coastlines of South/East Asia. Phytoplankton blooms are excellent habitats for survival and spread of bacteria responsible for infectious diseases such as cholera [96]. Increases in the frequency and intensity of floods from increased precipitation and sea-level rise in the future, absent of adequate mitigation/adaptation measures, will lead to drinking water contamination and consequently increased water-borne infectious diseases. Based on the trends in temperature and rainfall, it is projected that the frequency of vector-borne and water-borne infectious diseases in Southeast Asia will remain the highest in the world in 2030 [94].

The distribution of vector-borne diseases such as malaria and dengue fever is influenced by the spread of vectors (e.g. mosquitoes) and the climate dependence of the infectious pathogens. A warmer and more humid climate is favourable for propagation and invasiveness of infectious insect vectors. For example, evidence shows that dengue incidence in metropolitan Manila varies with changing rainfall patterns [97]. As Singapore experienced higher weekly mean temperatures and cumulative precipitation in the years 2004–2007, a significant increase in intensity and number of dengue fever cases could be attributed to climate factors [98]. As the increasing trends in surface temperature and rainfalls are likely to continue in South/East Asia, intensified surveillance and control of mosquitoes during periods with high rainfalls are recommended [97].

## Poverty and vulnerability

A significant portion of the Asian population is living below social and economic poverty thresholds [99]. Most of the world's poor reside in South Asia and, within the region, the majority resides in rural areas [100], although rural-to-urban migration continues to increase. The poor are highly vulnerable to climate change because of their limited access to stable livelihood opportunities and limited access to areas that are fit for safe and healthy habitation. Consequently, those who are impoverished are more likely to be at increased risks from floods, droughts, and contaminated water and foods [101]. Without appropriate measures, climate change will likely exacerbate the poverty situation and increase social inequity [102], as those who live in poverty contribute far less greenhouse gases on a per capita basis than wealthier persons. Consequently, there needs to be equity in assuring that those living in poverty advance economically in order to have enhanced capacity for adaptation. Crucial infrastructure should be designed and constructed to withstand extreme events for all who will be potentially affected. Health care and education should be strengthened, inequality addressed, and resources directed to communication and surveillance systems/technologies. Intensive development in very low-lying areas should be avoided, although large numbers of people are living at sea level in South/East Asia [91].

## Conclusion

South/East Asia, with vast coastal areas and a vector-prone climate, is one of the most vulnerable regions, facing a range of adverse health outcomes of climate change. It has many impoverished inhabitants and its coastal cities and megacities are at risk from the direct and indirect stressors associated with climate change. For the short term, adaptive strategies are needed for heatwaves and other extreme weather events. For the longer term, the success of global mitigation strategies will be critical, particularly if sea-level rise is to be slowed, and the threat to agriculture and water security minimized.

## Acknowledgements

The authors thank Athena Foong, Department of Preventive Medicine, Keck School of Medicine, and Institute for Global Health, University of Southern California, USA, for editorial assistance and research support in preparing this chapter.

## References

1. Intergovernmental Panel on Climate Change (IPCC). *Contribution of Working Group I to the Fourth Assessment Report of the Intergovernmental Panel on Climate Change, 2007: The Physical Science Basis.* S. Solomon, D. Qin, M. Manning *et al.* Cambridge, Cambridge University Press; 2007.
2. Intergovernmental Panel on Climate Change (IPCC). *Contribution of Working Group II to the Fourth Assessment Report of the Intergovernmental Panel on Climate Change, 2007: Impacts, Adaptation and Vulnerability.* M. L. Parry, O. F. Canziani, J. P. Palutikof, P. J. van der Linden and C. E. Hanson. Cambridge, Cambridge University Press; 2007.
3. World Health Organization and World Meteorological Organization. *Atlas of Health and Climate.* Geneva, WHO Press; 2012.
4. Intergovernmental Panel on Climate Change (IPCC). Intergovernmental Panel on Climate Change Assessment Reports. Available at: http://www.ipcc.ch/publications_and_data/publications_and_data_reports.shtml [accessed 26 November 2012].
5. The Lancet. The Lancet Series on Health and Climate Change. Available at: http://www.thelancet.com/series/health-and-climate-change [accessed 26 November 2012].
6. Costello, A., M. Abbas, *et al.* Managing the health effects of climate change: Lancet and University College London Institute for Global Health Commission. *Lancet* 2009; 373(9676): 1693–1733.
7. Ezzati, M., A. D. Lopez, *et al.* Selected major risk factors and global and regional burden of disease. *Lancet* 2002; 360(9343): 1347–1360.
8. Parenti, M. *The Face of Imperialism.* Boulder, CO, Paradigm Publishers; 2011.
9. Basu, R. and J. M. Samet. Relation between elevated ambient temperature and mortality: a review of the epidemiologic evidence. *Epidemiol Rev* 2002; 24(2): 190–202.
10. Semenza, J. C., C. H. Rubin, *et al.* Heat-related deaths during the July 1995 heatwave in Chicago. *New England Journal of Medicine* 1996; 335(2): 84–90.
11. Vandentorren, S., F. Suzan, *et al.* Mortality in 13 French cities during the August 2003 heat wave. *Am J Public Health* 2004; 94(9): 1518–1520.
12. Kovats, R. S., G. Jendritzky, *et al.* Heatwaves and human health. *Climate Change and Adaptation Strategies for Human Health.* Darmstadt, Germany, Steinkopff-Verlag; 2006; 63–97.
13. Curriero, F. C., K. S. Heiner, *et al.* Temperature and mortality in eleven cities of the eastern United States. *American Journal of Epidemiology* 2002; 155(1): 80–87.

14. McMichael, A. J., P. Wilkinson, *et al.* International study of temperature, heat and urban mortality: the 'ISOTHURM' project. *Int J Epidemiol* 2008; 37(5): 1121–1131.
15. The Eurowinter Group. Cold exposure and winter mortality from ischaemic heart disease, cerebrovascular disease, respiratory disease, and all causes in warm and cold regions of Europe. *Lancet* 1997; 349(9062): 1341–1346.
16. Gasparrini, A. and B. Armstrong. The impact of heat waves on mortality. *Epidemiology* 2011; 22(1): 68–73.
17. Carson, C., S. Hajat, *et al.* Declining vulnerability to temperature-related mortality in London over the 20th century. *American Journal of Epidemiology* 2006; 164(1): 77–84.
18. Davis, R. E., P. C. Knappenberger, *et al.* Changing heat-related mortality in the United States. *Environmental Health Perspectives* 2003; 111(14): 1712–1718.
19. Barnett, A. G. Temperature and cardiovascular deaths in the US elderly: changes over time. *Epidemiology* 2007; 18(3): 369–372.
20. Buechley, R. W., B. J. Van, *et al.* Heat island equals death island? *Environ Res* 1972; 5(1): 85–92.
21. Zanobetti, A., J. Schwartz, *et al.* The temporal pattern of mortality responses to air pollution: a multicity assessment of mortality displacement. *Epidemiology* 2002; 13(1): 87–93.
22. Zeger, S. L., F. Dominici, *et al.* Harvesting-resistant estimates of air pollution effects on mortality. *Epidemiology* 1999; 10(2): 171–175.
23. Toulemon, L. and M. Barbieri. The mortality impact of the August 2003 heat wave in France: investigating the 'harvesting' effect and other long-term consequences. *Popul Stud (Camb.)* 2008; 62(1): 39–53.
24. Hajat, S., B. G. Armstrong, *et al.* Mortality displacement of heat-related deaths: a comparison of Delhi, São Paulo, and London. *Epidemiology* 2005; 16(5): 613–620.
25. Avila-Tang, E., E. Matsui, *et al.* Epidemiology of asthma and allergic diseases. *Allergy: Principles and Practices*, 7th edn. N. F. Adkinson, W. W. Busse, B. S. Bochner, *et al.* Edinburgh, Mosby-Elsevier; 2008.
26. Beggs, P. J. Impacts of climate change on aeroallergens: past and future. *Clin Exp Allergy* 2004; 34(10): 1507–1513.
27. Beggs, P. J. and H. J. Bambrick. Is the global rise of asthma an early impact of anthropogenic climate change? *Environmental Health Perspectives* 2005; 113(8): 915–919.
28. Shea, K. M., R. T. Truckner, *et al.* Climate change and allergic disease. *J Allergy Clin Immunol* 2008; 122(3): 443–453.
29. Nelson, K. E., C. F. Masters Williams, *et al.* *Infectious Disease Epidemiology: Theory and Practice.* Sudbury, MA, Jones and Bartlett; 2007.
30. Rogers, D. J. and S. E. Randolph. Climate change and vector-borne diseases. *Adv Parasitol* 2006; 62: 345–381.
31. Haines, A., R. S. Kovats, *et al.* Climate change and human health: impacts, vulnerability, and mitigation. *Lancet* 2006; 367(9528): 2101–2109.
32. Colwell, R. R. Global climate and infectious disease: the cholera paradigm. *Science* 1996; 274(5295): 2025–2031.
33. Lipp, E. K., A. Huq, *et al.* Effects of global climate on infectious disease: the cholera model. *Clin Microbiol Rev* 2002; 15(4): 757–770.
34. Charron, D., M. Thomas, *et al.* Vulnerability of waterborne diseases to climate change in Canada: a review. *J Toxicol Environ Health* 2004; A 67(20–22): 1667–1677.
35. Rodo, X., M. Pascual, *et al.* ENSO and cholera: a nonstationary link related to climate change? *Proc Natl Acad Sci USA* 2002; 99(20): 12901–12906.
36. Checkley, W., L. D. Epstein, *et al.* Effect of El Niño and ambient temperature on hospital admissions for diarrhoeal diseases in Peruvian children. *Lancet* 2000; 355(9202): 442–450.
37. Cazelles, B., M. Chavez, *et al.* Nonstationary influence of El Niño on the synchronous dengue epidemics in Thailand. *PLoS Med* 2005; 2(4): e106.
38. Woodruff, R. E., C. S. Guest, *et al.* Early warning of Ross River virus epidemics: combining surveillance data on climate and mosquitoes. *Epidemiology* 2006; 17(5): 569–575.
39. Lindgren, E. and R. Gustafson. Tick-borne encephalitis in Sweden and climate change. *Lancet* 2001; 358(9275): 16–18.
40. Ogden, N. H., L. St-Onge, *et al.* Risk maps for range expansion of the Lyme disease vector, Ixodes scapularis, in Canada now and with climate change. *International Journal of Health Geographics* 2008; 7(24).

41. D'Souza, R. M., G. Hall, *et al.* Climatic factors associated with hospitalizations for rotavirus diarrhoea in children under 5 years of age. *Epidemiol Infect* 2008; 136(1): 56–64.
42. Gething, P. W., D. L. Smith, *et al.* Climate change and the global malaria recession. *Nature* 2010; 465(7296): 342–345.
43. Dentener, F., D. Stevenson, *et al.* The global atmospheric environment for the next generation. *Environ Sci Technol* 2006; 40(11): 3586–3594.
44. Wilson, S. R., K. R. Solomon, *et al.* Changes in tropospheric composition and air quality due to stratospheric ozone depletion and climate change. *Photochem Photobiol Sci* 2007; 6(3): 301–310.
45. Davis, D. L. and Working Group on Public Health and Fossil-Fuel Combustion. Short-term improvements in public health from global-climate policies on fossil-fuel combustion: an interim report. *Lancet* 1997; 350(9088): 1341–1349.
46. US Environmental Protection Agency. Integrated Science Assessment of Ozone and Related Photochemical Oxidants (Third External Review Draft). Washington, DC, US Environmental Protection Agency; 2012.
47. US Environmental Protection Agency. Integrated Science Assessment for Particulate Matter (final report). Washington, DC, US Environmental Protection Agency; 2009.
48. World Health Organization. Air Quality Guidelines: Global Update 2005–Particulate Matter, Ozone, Nitrogen Dioxide and Sulfur Dioxide. Copenhagen, World Health Organization; 2006.
49. Samet, J. M., F. Dominici, *et al.* Fine particulate air pollution and mortality in 20 U.S. cities, 1987–1994. *N Engl J Med* 2000; 343(24): 1742–1749.
50. Bell, M. L., A. McDermott, *et al.* Ozone and short-term mortality in 95 US urban communities, 1987–2000. *Journal of the American Medical Association* 2004; 292(19): 2372–2378.
51. Pope, C. A., III and D. W. Dockery. Health effects of fine particulate air pollution: lines that connect. *J Air Waste Manag Assoc* 2006; 56(6): 709–742.
52. Brook, R. D., S. Rajagopalan, *et al.* Particulate matter air pollution and cardiovascular disease: an update to the scientific statement from the American Heart Association. *Circulation* 2010; 121(21): 2331–2378.
53. Dominici, F., R. D. Peng, *et al.* Fine particulate air pollution and hospital admission for cardiovascular and respiratory diseases. *Journal of the American Medical Association* 2006; 295(10): 1127–1134.
54. Knowlton, K., J. E. Rosenthal, *et al.* Assessing ozone-related health impacts under a changing climate. *Environmental Health Perspectives* 2004; 112(15): 1557–1563.
55. Bell, M. L., F. Dominici, *et al.* Spatial and temporal variation in PM(2.5) chemical composition in the United States for health effects studies. *Environmental Health Perspectives* 2007; 115(7): 989–995.
56. Cifuentes, L., V. H. Borja-Aburto, *et al.* Assessing the health benefits of urban air pollution reductions associated with climate change mitigation (2000–2020): Santiago, São Paulo, Mexico City, and New York City. *Environmental Health Perspectives* 2001; 109(Suppl 3): 419–425.
57. Hatzakis, A., K. Katsouyanni, *et al.* Short-term effects of air pollution on mortality in Athens. *Int J Epidemiol* 1986; 15(1): 73–81.
58. Katsouyanni, K., A. Pantazopoulou, *et al.* Evidence for interaction between air pollution and high temperature in the causation of excess mortality. *Archives of Environmental Health* 1993; 48(4): 235–242.
59. Filleul, L., S. Cassadou, *et al.* The relation between temperature, ozone, and mortality in nine French cities during the heat wave of 2003. *Environmental Health Perspectives* 2006; 114(9): 1344–1347.
60. Fischer, P. H., B. Brunekreef, *et al.* Air pollution related deaths during the 2003 heat wave in the Netherlands. *Atmospheric Environment* 2004; 38(8): 1083–1085.
61. Knox, R. B., C. Suphioglu, *et al.* Major grass pollen allergen Lol p 1 binds to diesel exhaust particles: implications for asthma and air pollution. *Clin Exp Allergy* 1997; 27: 246–251.
62. Wyler, C., C. Braun-Fahrlander, *et al.* Exposure to motor vehicle traffic and allergic sensitization. The Swiss Study on Air Pollution and Lung Diseases in Adults (SAPALDIA) Team. *Epidemiology* 2000; 11(4): 450–456.
63. Ghiani, A., R. Aina, *et al.* Ragweed pollen collected along high-traffic roads shows a higher allergenicity than pollen sampled in vegetated areas. *Allergy* 2012; 67(7): 887–894.
64. Anenberg, S. C., J. Schwartz, *et al.* Global air quality and health co-benefits of mitigating near-term climate change through methane and black carbon emission controls. *Environmental Health Perspectives* 2012; 120(6): 831–839.

65. Wilkinson, P., D. H. Campbell-Lendrum, *et al.* Monitoring the health effects of climate change. *Climate Change and Human Health: Risks and Responses.* A. J. McMichael, D. H. Campbell-Lendrum, C. F. Corvalan, *et al.* Geneva, World Health Organization; 2003: 204–219.
66. Ebi, K. L., T. J. Teisberg, *et al.* Heat watch/warning systems save lives – estimated costs and benefits for Philadelphia 1995–98. *Bulletin of the American Meteorological Society* 2004; 85(8): 1067–1073.
67. Tan, J. G., L. S. Kalkstein, *et al.* An operational heat/health warning system in Shanghai. *International Journal of Biometeorology* 2004; 48(3): 157–162.
68. Beggs, P. J. and C. M. Bennett. Climate change, aeroallergens, natural particulates, and human health in Australia: state of the science and policy. *Asia Pac J Public Health* 2011; 23(2 Suppl): 46S–53.
69. UN-DESA-PD. *World Population Prospects, 2002.* New York, United Nations Department of Economic and Social Affairs – Population Division; 2002.
70. Zeqiang, F., C. Yunlong, *et al.* Research on the relationship of cultivated land change and food security in China. *Journal of Natural Resources* 2001; 16: 313–319.
71. Pulhin, J. M., U. Chokkalingam, *et al.* Historical overview of forest rehabilitation in the Philippines. *One Century of Forest Rehabilitation in the Philippines: Approaches, Outcomes and Lessons.* U. Chokkalingam, A. P. Carandang, J. M. Pulhin, R. D. Lasco and R. J. J. Peras. Bogor, CIFOR-CFNR UPLB-FMB DENR; 2006: 6–41.
72. Ali, A. Climate change impacts and adaptation assessment in Bangladesh. *Climate Research* 1999; 12(2–3): 109–116.
73. Manton, M. J., P. M. Della-Marta, *et al.* Trends in extreme daily rainfall and temperature in Southeast Asia and the South Pacific: 1961–1998. *International Journal of Climatology* 2001; 21(3): 269–284.
74. Aldhous, P. Land remediation: Borneo is burning. *Nature* 2004; 432(7014): 144–146.
75. Trenberth, K. E. and T. J. Hoar. El Niño and climate change. *Geophysical Research Letters* 1997; 24(23): 3057–3060.
76. Cruz, R. V. O., R. D. Lasco, *et al.* Climate change impact on water resources in Pantabangan Watershed, Philippines. Assessments of Impacts and Adaptations to Climate Change (AIACC), Project No. AS 21; 2006: 9–107.
77. Tran, V. L., D. C. Hoang, *et al.* Building of climate change scenario for Red River catchments for sustainable development and environmental protection. Preprints, Science Workshop on Hydrometeorological Change in Vietnam and Sustainable Development. Hanoi, Ministry of Natural Resource and Environment; 2005: 70–82.
78. Fan, D. D. and C. X. Li. Complexities of Chinese coast in response to climate change. *Advances in Research on Climate Change* 2005; 1: 111–114.
79. Lal, M. Tropical cyclones in a warmer world. *Current Science* 2001; 80(9): 1103–1104.
80. Christensen, J. L., B. Hewitson, *et al.* Regional climate projections. Climate Change 2007: The Scientific Basis. Contribution of Working Group I to the Fourth Assessment Report of the Intergovernmental Panel on Climate Change. S. Solomon, D. Qin, M. Manning, *et al.* Cambridge, Cambridge University Press; 2007: 847–940.
81. Ruosteenoja, K., T. R. Carter, *et al.* Future climate in world regions: an intercomparison of model-based projections for the new IPCC emissions scenarios. Helsinki, Finnish Environment Institute; 2003.
82. Durack, P. J., S. E. Wijffels, *et al.* Ocean salinities reveal strong global water cycle intensification during 1950 to 2000. *Science* 2012; 336(6080): 455–458.
83. Patz, J. A., D. Campbell-Lendrum, *et al.* Impact of regional climate change on human health. *Nature* 2005; 438(7066): 310–317.
84. Wiley, L. F. and L. O. Gostin. The international response to climate change: an agenda for global health. *JAMA* 2009; 302(11): 1218–1220.
85. Bush, K. F., G. Luber, *et al.* Impacts of climate change on public health in India: future research directions. *Environmental Health Perspectives* 2011; 119(6): 765–770.
86. Sattenspiel, L. Tropical environments, human activities, and the transmission of infectious diseases. *Am J Phys Anthropol Suppl* 2000; 31: 3–31.
87. Bhattacharya, S., C. Sharma, *et al.* Climate change and malaria in India. *Current Science* 2006; 90(3): 369–375.
88. Dhiman, R. C., S. Pahwa, *et al.* Climate change and malaria in India: interplay between temperature and mosquitoes. *Regional Health Forum* 2008; 12: 27–31.

89. Ebi, K. L. and J. A. Paulson. Climate change and child health in the United States. *Curr Probl Pediatr Adolesc Health Care* 2010; 40(1): 2–18.
90. O'Neill, M. S. and K. L. Ebi. Temperature extremes and health: impacts of climate variability and change in the United States. *J Occup Environ Med* 2009; 51(1): 13–25.
91. Butler, C. D. A stormy future for population health in Southeast Asia? *Lancet* 2011; 377(9769): 885–886.
92. Munslow, B. and T. O'Dempsey. Globalisation and climate change in Asia: the urban health impact. *Third World Q* 2010; 31(8): 1339–1356.
93. Pelling, M. *The Vulnerability of Cities: Natural Disasters and Social Resilience*. Sterling, VA, Earthscan Publications; 2003.
94. McMichael, A. J., D. Campbell-Lendrum, *et al. Global Climate Change. Comparative Quantification of Health Risks*, Vol. 2. Geneva, World Health Organization; 2004: 1543–1649.
95. Chou, W. C., J. L. Wu, *et al.* Modeling the impact of climate variability on diarrhea-associated diseases in Taiwan (1996–2007). *Sci Total Environ* 2010; 409(1): 43–51.
96. Pascual, M., M. J. Bouma, *et al.* Cholera and climate: revisiting the quantitative evidence. *Microbes and Infection* 2002; 4(2): 237–245.
97. Su, G. L. Correlation of climatic factors and dengue incidence in Metro Manila, Philippines. *Ambio* 2008; 37(4): 292–294.
98. Hii, Y. L., J. Rocklov, *et al.* Climate variability and increase in intensity and magnitude of dengue incidence in Singapore. *Glob Health Action* 2; 2009.
99. UN-ESCAP (United Nations Economic and Social Commission for Asia and the Pacific). Achieving MDGs in Asia: a case for more aid? New York, UN-ESCAP; 2006: 37.
100. Srinivasan, T. N. Poverty and under nutrition in South Asia. *Food Policy* 2000; 25(3): 269–282.
101. Adger, W. N. Social capital, collective action, and adaptation to climate change. *Economic Geography* 2003; 79(4): 387–404.
102. Beg, N., J. C. Morlot, *et al.* Linkages between climate change and sustainable development. *Climate Policy* 2002; 2(2–3): 129–144.

# 21

# Case study: Climate and Health Council

## Engaging health professions in change

*Sue Atkinson, Graeme Maugham and Robin Stott*

### Introduction

There is now almost complete agreement amongst scientists that our climate system is changing and that human activities are the predominant driving force [1]. The effects of climate change are many. The changes to long-term weather and climate systems, water resources (including glaciers, water tables and rivers), flooding, population movement and food security are already having significant adverse health impacts [2, 3], with worse to follow. Climate change is the greatest public health threat of our time and action is needed now.

In 2007, in view of these health concerns, a number of senior doctors, nurses and other health professionals came together to create the Climate and Health Council (CHC). Of significant importance in commencement of the CHC was the support of both recognized experts in the field and the backing of the editors of the *British Medical Journal* (BMJ) and the *Lancet*, both of whom had started writing about climate change some 20 years previously. The editor of the *BMJ* remains to this day one of the strongest supporters and is on the Executive Council of the CHC, as well as being the Vice Chair of the Council.

### Overview of the Climate Health Council

The new CHC came together as a meeting of doctors, nurses and other health professionals recognizing the urgent need to address climate change and to protect health. The CHC's work focuses on the already apparent and predicted health effects of climate change, which can be summarized as, but not limited to:

- The spread of disease, as a warming climate allows disease vectors (such as malaria-carrying mosquitoes) to enter new territories;
- The effects of drought on populations, especially the vulnerable, provoking disease, reducing crop yields and water availability, and so undermining the basic requirements of life;
- Further undermining of health through population displacement due to droughts, food insecurity, permanent flooding or other climate-related mechanisms;

- Direct effects from heatwaves, with an increase in heat-related medical issues, especially in vulnerable groups, such as the elderly;
- With warmer climates, more outdoor activities are likely, which may lead to higher incidences of UV-exposure problems; and
- An increase in health-related issues with the poor who are least able to afford good health care.

Importantly, many of the actions that need to be taken to address climate change will also be of benefit to people's health. These are the 'co-benefits' to health from tackling climate change. Again, these can be summarized as, but are not limited to:

- Promoting more active lifestyles, such as walking and outdoor exercise, to reduce dependence on fossil fuel powered vehicles;
- Promoting healthier diets, which contain less meat and dairy, and through these two above measures, reducing the prevalence of non-communicable diseases (NCDs), such as diabetes, cardiovascular disease, stroke and many cancers;
- Promoting energy efficiency and alternative energy sources in all economies, as a means of reducing air pollution (including $CO_2$ and particulates from burning 'dirty' fuels, such as animal waste in developing countries) and so moving to a global low carbon economy;
- Mitigating mental health illnesses by promoting greater interaction with the environment;
- More responsible resource management, avoiding 'resource wars' and the health issues that result from conflict;
- A more rapid attainment of the UN's Millennium Development Goals (especially Goals 1, 6 and 7 (see Figure 2.1)).

The *Lancet* 'series' of articles on climate change and health showed the health benefits of tackling climate change and, as a series of peer-reviewed articles, demonstrated the 'co-benefits' and showed that 'mitigating strategies will themselves have additional and independent effects on health, most of them beneficial' [4]. The *Lancet* series was supported by a global partnership of funders[1] and was undertaken by an international team of researchers with the aim of informing discussions at the 2009 Copenhagen Conference of Parties (COP) to the UN Framework Convention on Climate Change (COP15). Importantly, they looked at the implications of actions in both high-income and low-income countries. This important series of articles provided the strong 'evidence base' for further action, and the focus of climate change and health impacts.

The CHC is, therefore, dedicated to raising awareness of the adverse health effects of climate change, and to promoting the health co-benefits of tackling these issues simultaneously. In particular, the CHC aims to raise understanding amongst health professionals both within the United Kingdom (UK) and internationally, and to mobilize them to press for action to address climate change and health.

Although the main emphasis of action is in the UK, the CHC has established international contacts and is part of an informal network of health advocacy organizations. Whilst most of the CHC supporters are in the UK, the council also has supporters, most of whom are signatories of its pledge, in 130 countries across Europe and worldwide. It has links with very senior and influential medical professionals and academics worldwide.

This health and policy background leads to the CHC's vision and mission statement.

### *Vision*

We want healthy people and a healthy planet. We want to see a world where climate change is kept in check and has minimal impact on public health. The outcomes we wish to see are:

- No extra deaths caused by climate change;
- The impacts of climate change on health are understood and managed; and
- Climate change is tackled in a way that improves the public's health.

### *Mission statement*

We want health professionals to understand that what is good for the climate is good for health; to understand how climate change affects population health and healthcare systems; and to have the opportunities and information to positively address both issues. To use this awareness to ensure policy makers implement policies that address climate change in an equitable manner so as to give maximum benefit to public health.

People must first call on policy makers and governments to take action. We believe the strongest voices to make this call are those who work within health and health care, who will have to cope with the changes in disease profiles and loss of life that climate change is predicted to cause.

Both individual health professionals and also organizations share health concerns around climate change and both have contributory voices. They must call for action based on a clear understanding of the issues. They must be able to access information when they need it, and that information must be clear, accurate and be presented in an accessible format.

Our approach uses three strategic strands:

- Capacity building;
- Evidence building; and
- Partnerships.

Our initial aim is to mobilize health workers, both in the UK and internationally. The CHC aims to raise awareness amongst health workers about climate change and health, and the co-benefits of addressing the two together, and hence to build the capacity of health workers worldwide to be able to act as advocates for climate change and health.

### *Pledge*

We ask supporters to sign our pledge, a two-part statement asking them to agree to:

- Protect health through active engagement to limit the causes of human-caused climate change; and
- Advocate for the establishment of a consistent and equitable global framework to reduce greenhouse gas emissions (see Box 21.1).

This is backed up by a charter – 'what's good for the climate is good for health' – with five statements which are messages for decision makers from health professionals about the interfaces between climate change and health (see Box 21.2).

## Box 21.1 Climate and Health Council pledge

### *To protect health through active engagement to limit the causes of human-caused climate change*

Tackling climate change and ending poverty are the two most important, urgent priorities to ensure global health, justice and survival for present and future generations. Multiple health benefits will be accrued by individuals and societies who engage in more active, less material dependent lifestyles, thus protecting their local environment and reducing their contribution to climate change.

### *To advocate for the establishment of a consistent and equitable global framework to reduce greenhouse gas emissions*

An equitable framework entails transfer of resources (financial and technological) to poorer nations and should be led and implemented by governments. Such a framework will promote the health of current and future generations, both rich and poor, both locally and globally.

*Source*: CHC.

## Box 21.2 Climate and Health Council charter

### *What's Good for the Climate is Good for Health!*

*Messages to decision makers from the health professions*

A substantial and rapid reduction in greenhouse gas emissions presents an unrivalled opportunity to protect human health around the world. As health professionals, we are in a unique position to help decision makers drive the individual and institutional changes required to prevent disruption of ecosystems, and protect health from climate change. Preventing climate change is good for health because:

1. **CLIMATE CHANGE IS AN AVOIDABLE THREAT TO HEALTH**
   If we continue on current trajectories, climate change and associated environmental threats will destroy the ecosystems on which life depends. Climate change is already causing damage to homes and livelihoods, increasing food insecurity and exacerbating human conflict over natural resources that are fundamental determinants of health – arable land, water and clean air. Although the worst effects are felt in developing countries, no countries are immune to the effects of climate change. Immediate and resolute global action is essential to protect health worldwide.

2. **LOW-CARBON SOCIETIES – THE NEXT GREAT HEALTH ADVANCE**
   Policies that reduce greenhouse gas emissions can result in large health gains with reduction in major killers including heart disease, cancer, obesity, diabetes, road deaths and diseases from air pollution. For example, consuming less food derived from intensively reared livestock,

being more active (e.g. walking or cycling) and relying less on fossil fuel energy, and especially in low-income countries, the mass introduction of low-emission stoves burning local biomass fuels would bring substantial health benefits.

Working together, health professionals and decision makers can promote healthier, more environmentally friendly societies, for example, by promoting the provision of green spaces. A sustainable society is a place where you, your children and your children's children would wish to live.

3. **CLIMATE CHANGE IS INCREASING THE HEALTH DIFFERENTIAL BETWEEN RICH AND POOR. ADDRESSING CLIMATE CHANGE IS AN OPPORTUNITY**
To decrease this differential, and so reduce the inequality and poverty which increases the risk of disease and death for large numbers of people around the world. The poorest countries and the poorest populations within each country experience the worst effects of climate change, whilst the richest countries and populations add far in excess of their fair share of the emissions that contribute to climate change. There is an unprecedented opportunity to reduce global health inequalities through an international agreement based on social justice, whereby national greenhouse gas emissions converge to equal per capita shares within the planet's sustainable and finite limit. Policies to address climate change can bring the greatest health gains to those with the poorest health if they are implemented with health equity and sustainability as central, linked agendas.

4. **HEALTH DEPENDS ON SUSTAINABLE DEVELOPMENT, NOT ON TRADITIONAL GLOBAL ECONOMIC GROWTH**
The pursuit of carbon-emitting economic growth has not and will not provide sustainable economic and social stability – key determinants of health – for much of the world's population now and for the extra two to two-and-a-half billion people to come. In high-income countries, consumerism and overconsumption are associated with ill-health, loss of well-being, stress and dissatisfaction. Sustainable development depends on a sustainable economy: prosperity and fairness without growth. Better health for all – and more equitable opportunity, self-worth, mutual respect and fulfilment – means an acceptable quality of life for all within ecological limits. This includes a significantly reduced level of greenhouse gases in the atmosphere though the development and demographic transition of currently low-emitting populations will entail an increase in their own emissions in the short and medium term, as per point 3 above.

5. **DELAY WILL BE FATAL**
Greenhouse gas emissions must be stabilized as a matter of absolute urgency to avoid reaching the 'tipping point' of one and a half to two degrees centigrade of global warming that is above the global level at the start of the Industrial Revolution. Beyond this, catastrophic consequences for health are increasingly likely. Any delay in controlling emissions will inevitably cause preventable deaths and damage to health and well-being on a massive scale in the next decades.

*Source*: CHC.

Over 6,000 supporters from 130 different countries worldwide have signed the pledge. To ensure we can articulate our message properly, and to support health workers to develop their knowledge and advocacy, we have five key behaviours, which we detail on our website, and which we believe will help any health professional or interested party to deliver the change which is our mission. These are:

*Know* – about the issues and the options you have available;
*Act* – on the information we can provide within your circle of influence;
*Connect* – to others within the profession at a national and international level;
*Persuade* – others to know, act and connect, persuade policy makers, advocate for change;
*Be Creative* – in how you approach the integration of climate change and health policies, in how you advocate, in how you act.

Effective communication underlies all the work of the CHC. In conjunction with a British Academy Film Awards (BAFTA)-winning communications group Magic Lantern, we have developed an interactive social networking website, where ideas can be shared, comments made and supporters may be informed.

The CHC believes strongly in the evidence base for all that it does. The website acts as a major repository for much of the existing evidence about the interfaces and action needed on climate change and health. In the future, the CHC hopes to *build on this evidence.*

The CHC works in *partnership* with other bodies and organizations that share similar concerns and goals about climate change and health, both within the UK, Europe and internationally. For example, in the UK and Europe, the CHC has formed an informal alliance with the NHS Sustainable Development Unit, the Centre for Sustainable Healthcare, Medsin and Medact.[2] The aim is to work collaboratively and complement each other as organizations. The CHC also works very closely internationally with a number of like-minded organizations, such as the Climate and Health Alliance (CHA) in Australia (itself a coalition of bodies with similar aims), Health Care Without Harm (HCWH), the Health and Environment Alliance (HEAL) and with the International Federation of Medical Students' Associations.[3] The CHC has joined these and other organizations to create the 'Global Climate and Health Alliance'. Many of our supporters are medical and nursing students and junior doctors, which provides for an excellent position to influence the next generation of health professionals, who will move into practice, policy and advocacy.

## Successes of the CHC

Over the five years since its establishment, the CHC has been recognized as punching above its weight as a small organization. The CHC has delivered:

1 A 'Spotlight' feature in the *BMJ* on 27 March 2012. This was a special issue on the links between climate change and health, with eight papers from experts covering the science, health risks, politics and policies, resource security, contraction and convergence and identifying what needs to be done [5].
2 Health Summits: at the annual United Nations Conference of Parties – in Cancun, Mexico in 2010 (COP16), in Durban, South Africa in 2011 (COP17), in Doha, Qatar in 2012 (COP18) and again in Warsaw in 2013 (COP19) – organized by the Global Climate and Health Alliance (GCHA) together with the World Medical Association and with support from the WHO, the 2013 conference attracted health and climate experts from

around the world and highlighted the dangerous impacts of climate change on human health and wellbeing. The event established the direction for the international health community to work towards in the run-up to 2015.

3 A focus on simple messaging, in parallel with these Summits. Brief leaflets highlighting 'key facts' have been given to the delegates and negotiators at the COPs. The CHC's medical student members and collaborators have been strikingly effective in developing and using these as useful tools, alongside the health delegates getting the messages across to negotiators and decision makers (example 'leaflets' can be seen in Figures 21.1a–b and 21.2a–b).
4 The CHC website. This has been created to communicate the message, provide evidence and support health workers in their delivery of the message. It has 7,000 views per month from medical institutions and health professionals [6].
5 A pledge, on tackling climate change and health together, which has been signed by over 6,000 individual health professionals internationally, by about 10 universities or faculties and 30 organizations [7].
6 Alliances, where there is a common agenda. Sometimes these have been with what might seem strange 'bed fellows' for an organization focused on improving public health. For example, in 2011, the CHC co-organized a joint conference with the British military. Many commonalities were identified, such as concerns around food security and water shortage, and their health consequences [8, 9].
7 A joint conference, also in 2011, between the CHC and the Royal College of Nursing, calling on nurses to understand the importance of the co-benefits and develop their roles as advocates.
8 The much-acclaimed series of papers in the *Lancet* in October 2009, which was instigated by the CHC [4].
9 Members of the CHC devote time and energy to spreading the word. This is done by talks, meetings, seminars, conferences and presentations to numerous medical, health and student bodies, as well as practitioners and policy makers.
10 Numerous editorials and articles on climate change in prestigious medical journals, including the *BMJ*. Gathering peer-reviewed papers on the CHC website to help advocates and policy makers incorporate evidence-based approaches into policy setting.
11 Raising awareness with professionals about how they can take action within their own lives and work places – for example, linking them to relevant resources from the CHC website, such as energy audit guides for hospitals.
12 An NHS Sustainability Day, in collaboration with others [10], established in 2012. The day provided a focus for action across the UK by healthcare workers in the NHS, drawing attention to the 'waste' of energy in hospitals and other health facilities by undertaking 'energy audits' as a common activity for the day.

## The next steps for the CHC

The CHC is currently developing its application as a charity in its own right, having previously been part of another charity.

The CHC Council has had no regular source of income, and no paid staff, and is dependent on the good will of the executive, board members and occasional interns. It has received occasional one-off grants for particular projects. This is not sustainable in the longer term. The CHC is aiming for more substantial funding and will then fulfil the following strategic objectives, which represent a quantum leap in approach:

(a)

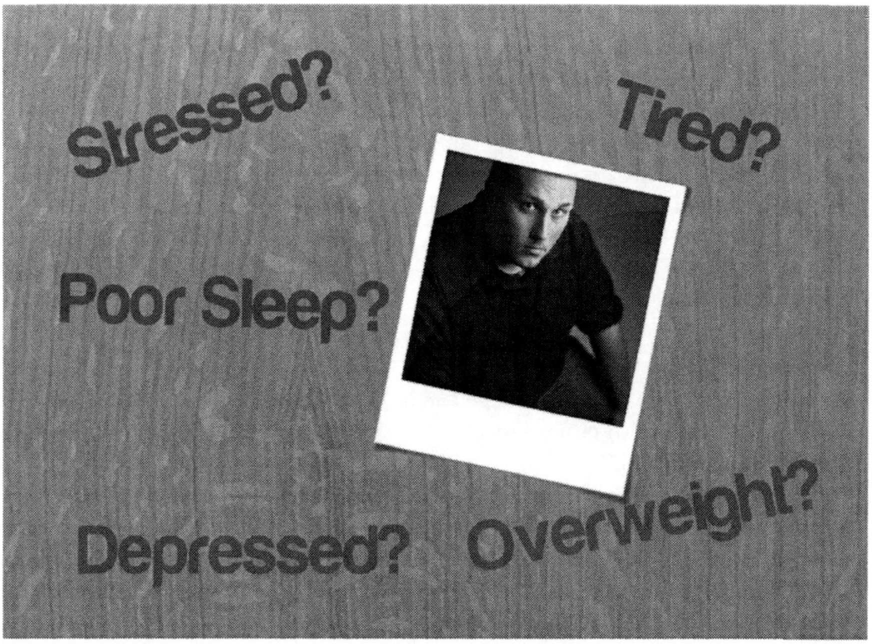


(b)

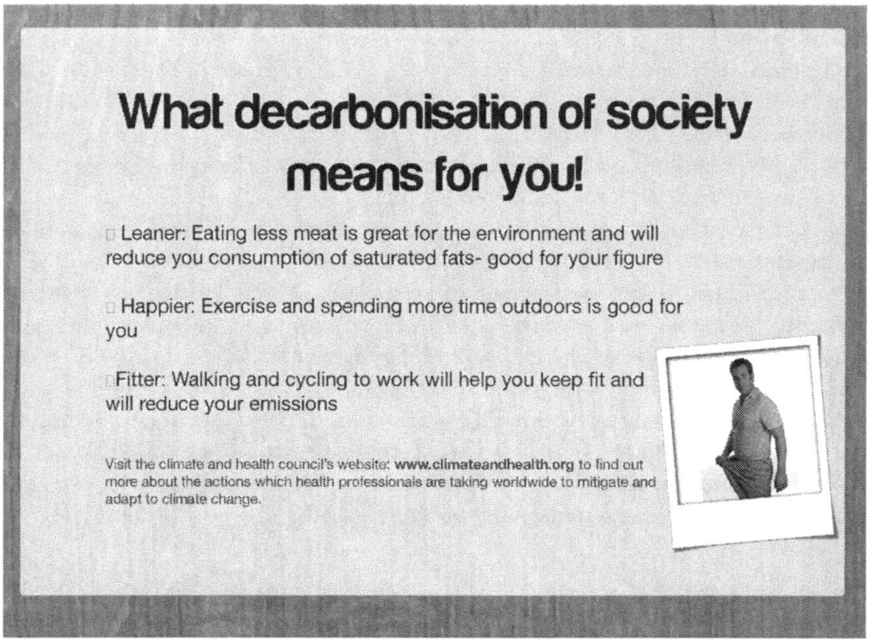


*Figure 21.1a–b* Example 'key facts' leaflet: What decarbonisation of society means for you!
*Source*: CHC.

(a)
(b)
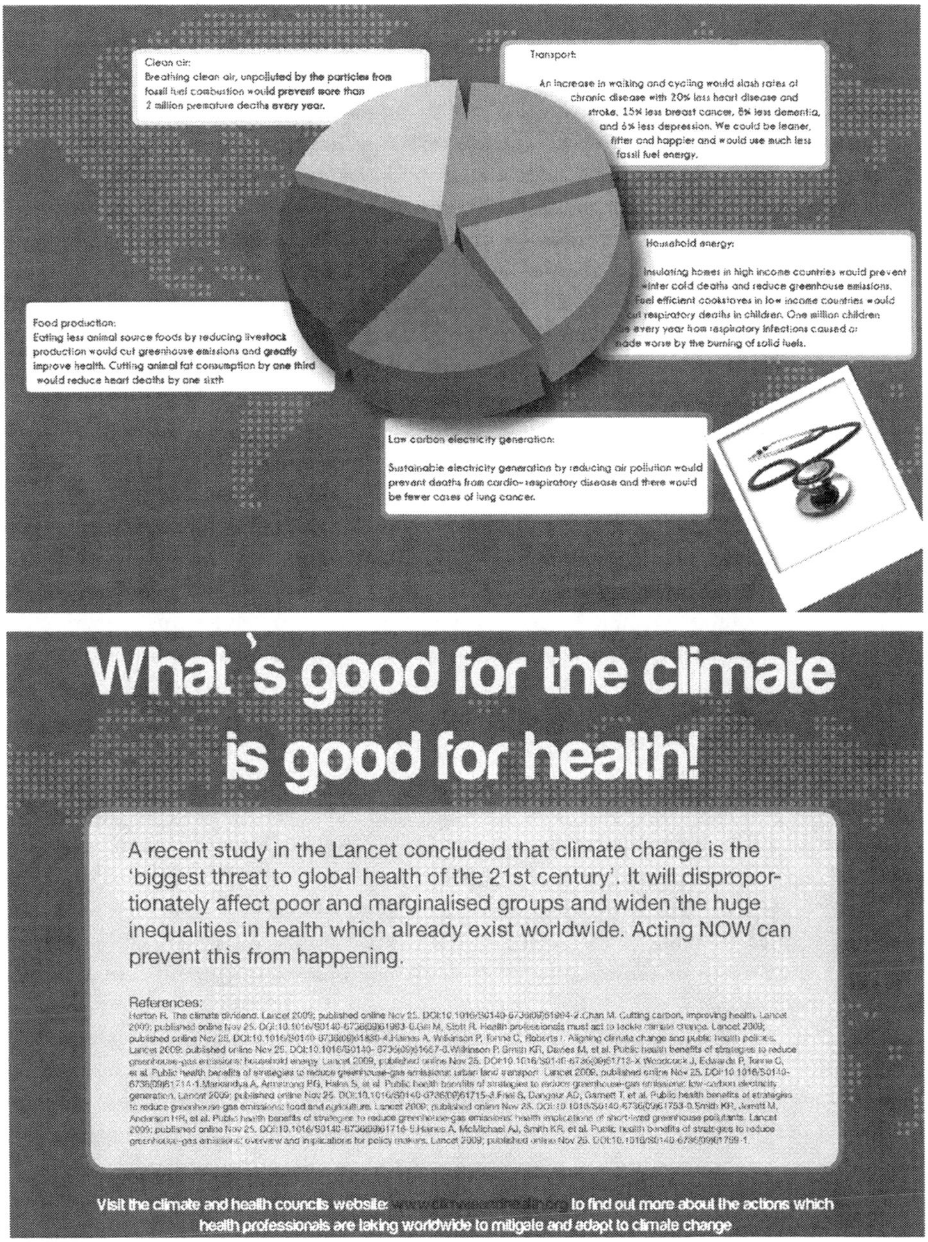


*Figure 21.2a–b* Example 'key facts' leaflet: What's good for the climate is good for health!
*Source*: CHC.

1 Develop an international network of health, climate and sustainability professionals, to enable the flow of information and coordinated advocacy on health and climate policy, engagement and implementation of appropriate change. In particular, the CHC wants to build on its existing global network, by offering greater coordination of the network and

ensuring those involved are better supported and can link with each other. Initial efforts at developing similar councils in other countries have shown this is possible, for example, in Norway, and there are close links with similar bodies that have evolved independently, such as in New Zealand and Australia, but so far growth has been slow.

2 Enable the production of a report to demonstrate the health, environmental and economic case for averting dangerous climate change and adapting and mitigation services to the climate changes locked into global ecosystems. We believe that the Stern Report [11], which clearly identified the financial impact of climate change on global GDP and how tackling it would be the cheaper option in the long term, was a game changer in approaching climate change. More recently, and worryingly, Stern has said 'I got it wrong on climate change – it's far, far worse' [12]. We aim to work in partnership with other organizations to develop a similar report, focusing on the health implications of climate change. And because people need information to make policy, we want to improve on communicating the health dimension of climate change. We think this will support the development of a UK, as well as a global, network of professionals, and will create and inspire case studies for an in-depth report on health and climate change.
3 Communicate case studies to health and sustainability professionals, which demonstrate how health, economic, social and environmental criteria can be positively integrated when developing and delivering policy. We will use this to encourage policy makers to account for, and reduce the negative health outcomes of, climate change. This would be another game changer in how climate change and health inequalities are tackled.

## Conclusion

Climate change is happening and there is now a global industry attempting to address it. This action ranges from technological fixes (new energy sources, better emissions capture) to policy changes and attempts at behaviour change.

The CHC was set up in 2007 to harness the interest and energy of health professionals, to develop their awareness of the interfaces between climate change and health, and to encourage an approach that utilizes the co-benefits of tackling climate change and improving public health.

The CHC has been successful in a number of ways, but has not grown as rapidly as it would have liked, and it has been more difficult than imagined to get the message of health impacts and of the co-benefits across to decision makers. The current economic climate has not helped and provides 'an excuse' for inaction on the part of governments, whereas it should provide a spur to considerations of prevention rather than cure.

The CHC focuses on raising awareness amongst health workers across the globe and enabling them to influence the discourse about climate change to include health, and hence to influence the politicians and decision makers. This still remains a laudable way forward, but many more health workers across the globe need to be recruited as supporters and advocates.

### *What can you do now?*

Go to the CHC website and sign the pledge to be a 'supporter'. Then follow the 'know, act, connect, persuade and be creative' to become part of the CHC capacity worldwide. And for your own action on climate change, follow the Ten Resolutions for Climate and Health [13].

## Acknowledgements

We would like to note our thanks to Professor Ian Roberts and Maya Tickell Painter for developing the CHC leaflets and to Nick Watts for his support with technical issues for the chapter.

## Notes

1 These include the Wellcome Trust, the Royal College of Physicians, the Economic and Social Research Council, the Department of Health, the National Institute for Health Research, the US National Institute of Environmental Health Sciences and the Academy of Medical Sciences, with support from the World Health Organization.
2 Websites for these organizations are as follows: Centre for Sustainable Healthcare – www.sustainablehealthcare.org.uk/; Medsin – www.medsin.org/; Medact – www.medact.org/; and NHS Sustainable Development Unit – http://www.sdu.nhs.uk.
3 Websites for these organizations are as follows: Climate and Health Alliance – http://caha.org.au/; HEAL – www.env-health.org/; HCWH – www.noharm.org/; and The International Federation of Medical Students' Associations – http://www.ifmsa.org/.

## References

1. Rapley C. The Science of Climate Change. *BMJ* 2012; 344: e1026.
2. Costello A, Abbas M, Allen A, *et al.* Managing the Health Effects of Climate Change. Lancet and University College Institute of Global Health Commission. *Lancet* 2009; 373: 1693–733.
3. McMichael AJ, Lindgren E. Climate Change: Present and Future Risks to Health, and Necessary Responses. *J Intern Med* 2011; 270: 401–13.
4. The Lancet. Series on Human Health and Climate Change: Available from: http://www.thelancet.com/climate-change
5. Delamothe T. Climate Change Spotlight: The World on Tilt. *BMJ* 2012; 344: e2207.
6. Climate and Health Council (CHC). Available from: http://www.climateandhealth.org
7. CHC Pledge. Available from: http://www.climateandhealth.org/the_pledge_31.html
8. Tholken H. Politics and Policies. *BMJ* 2012; 344: e1356.
9. Morisetti N. Climate Change and Resource Security. *BMJ* 2012; 344: e1352.
10. NHS Sustainability Day. Available from: http://www.sdu.nhs.uk/news-events/events/84/NHS-Sustainability-Day
11. Stern Report. Available from: http://webarchive.nationalarchives.gov.uk/+/http:/www.hm-treasury.gov.uk/sternreview_index.htm
12. Stewart, H, Elliott, L. Nicholas Stern: 'I got it wrong on climate change – it's far, far worse'. *The Observer*, 26 January 2013. Available from: http://www.guardian.co.uk/environment/2013/jan/27/nicholas-stern-climate-change-davos?utm_source=UK+CHC+Members%2C+not+just+newsletter&utm_campaign=eeb315d32a-CHC_March_Campaign&utm_medium=email
13. Ten Resolutions for Climate and Health (CHC). Available from: http://www.guardian.co.uk/sustainable-business/gallery/2013-resolutions-gallery-health-climate

# 22

# Air pollution

## The public health challenges

*Tze Wai Wong and Andromeda H. S. Wong*

Clean air has become a major public health issue as levels of pollution in many Asian cities climb to unacceptable levels. Hong Kong will be used as a case study to analyse the contributors to air pollution, the harm it poses to health, the possibilities for control and the need for political will.

### Introduction

Air pollution has become a global environmental problem. It hails from a variety of sources, many of them man-made. These include industry, transport vehicles and power stations that run on fossil fuels. Pollutants from these sources not only affect their immediate surroundings, but can also be transported around the planet via atmospheric currents. Thus, the effective control of air pollution must be taken up by governments at local, regional and national levels, and may even require international cooperation.

Because air pollution is ubiquitous, it greatly impacts on human health, particularly in cities where population densities are high. According to the World Health Organization (WHO), roughly 1.3 million deaths worldwide are caused by urban outdoor air pollution every year [1]. For this reason, the WHO has developed a number of *Air Quality Guidelines (AQGs)* that recommend limits in the concentrations of several key air pollutants. These guidelines are meant to aid governments in setting limits for their countries' emissions and planning their developments accordingly.

As our focus is on public health issues in Asia, Hong Kong will be used as a case study to look at the particular problems created by air pollution in fast-growing Asian cities. Hong Kong is a city in southern China, whose history as a British colony has seen it transform from a fishing village to a busy trading port. From the 1960s to the 1970s, it became a base for numerous manufacturing industries. The rapid urban development and population growth associated with this led to environmental problems – it was at this point that the city first began to suffer the effects of air pollution. Today, many of its factories have relocated across the border to mainland China, particularly the neighbouring Pearl River Delta in the Guangdong province, while Hong Kong itself has become a tourist destination and a major financial centre of international importance. However, due to the long-range atmospheric transportation of pollutants around the region, the air pollution problem has persisted. There are also other local sources of pollution, such as road, air and shipping traffic. The resultant impact of air pollution on public health, healthcare costs and even the economy is substantial.

In this chapter, we first introduce the major air pollutants commonly found in ambient air. Next, we examine the air pollution problem throughout history, and describe the link between air pollution and health. We then focus on Hong Kong, describing how it has been tackling its air pollution problem and what lessons it can learn from other polluted cities. Through this process of analysis, we can consider the problem of air pollution holistically and perhaps improve our current strategies for cleaning up our air.

## Major air pollutants

Air pollution can be defined as environmental contamination – by chemical, physical or biological agents – that modifies the atmosphere's natural properties [2], particularly at levels that disrupt the health, safety and comfort of living organisms, or that damage property [3]. Sources for these polluting agents can be natural (such as a forest fire or volcanic eruption) or anthropomorphic (for example, fuel-burning for industry or for motor vehicles). This section introduces the chemical pollutants frequently found in outdoor air, which primarily come from man-made sources and which bear great public health significance [3, 4].

*Carbon monoxide*: Carbon monoxide (CO) is a poisonous gas that is both colourless and odourless. It is formed from the incomplete combustion of carbon – for example, inside an internal combustion engine – and its main source is from vehicular exhaust. Once it is inhaled, CO enters the bloodstream and binds with haemoglobin, the protein necessary for transporting oxygen to each cell in the human body. This reduction of the body's ability to take up oxygen is the reason for its toxicity. At low concentrations, exposure to CO has the greatest effect on people with cardiovascular disease – reducing exercise tolerance, for instance. It can also lead to the impairment of vision, dexterity, and work and learning ability. At very high concentrations, it can be a lethal asphyxiant. Despite its abundance, however, CO can readily be oxidized to become the far less toxic carbon dioxide ($CO_2$) and the use of catalytic converters in motor vehicles has helped to reduce this pollutant's public health impact.

*Sulphur dioxide*: Sulphur dioxide ($SO_2$) is a colourless, pungent, toxic and corrosive gas that, together with other oxides of sulphur, is primarily formed upon the combustion of sulphur-containing fossil fuels. Thus, its sources include power plants and transport vehicles that use high-sulphur coal and diesel, respectively. In the atmosphere, $SO_2$ reacts with oxygen and water, dissolving to form sulphuric acid – a major component of acid rain. The solubility of $SO_2$ is high enough to produce acid even upon contact with the moist tissues of the respiratory tract, thus triggering breathing difficulties and aggravating any existing respiratory diseases like asthma. It also affects the lungs' natural defence mechanisms.

*Nitrogen dioxide*: During fuel combustion at high temperatures, the nitrogen and oxygen in the air can combine to form a range of nitrogen oxides ($NO_x$). These include nitrogen dioxide ($NO_2$), which is a poisonous reddish-brown gas. The primary sources of $NO_2$ are vehicle engines and power plants. As with $SO_2$, nitrogen dioxide can irritate the membranes of the lungs and, where there is an underlying illness, can even cause the bronchi to constrict. It also lowers the body's resistance to diseases such as influenza.

*Ozone*: The highly oxidizing ozone ($O_3$) is a pale blue gas and an important constituent of photochemical smog. However, it is usually not a direct emission from a pollutant source. Rather, it is produced in the atmosphere by the reactions of $NO_x$ with hydrocarbons in sunlight. For this reason, it is known as a 'secondary' air pollutant. Although the 'ozone layer' high up in the stratosphere has a protective effect against ultraviolet radiation, gaseous ozone down in the troposphere is toxic to humans. At high concentrations, it can cause oxidative damage to tissue, causing irritation and inflammation of the lungs and the eyes. Long-term exposure to $O_3$ at ambient levels can increase the lungs' sensitivity to other irritant chemicals, cause lung fibrosis or chronic obstructive pulmonary disease (COPD), and reduce overall *lung function*.

*Particulate matter*: Particulate matter (PM) refers to microscopic solid or liquid particles suspended in the air. It can have varied compositions, such as smoke, dust, sand, soot or other chemicals. Particulates are usually classified by their size: respirable suspended particulates ($PM_{10}$) are those with an aerodynamic diameter of less than ten microns (μm), while fine suspended particulates ($PM_{2.5}$) have a smaller diameter of less than 2.5 μm. While $PM_{10}$ consists of particulates that are small enough to enter the lungs (hence, 'respirable'), particulates classified as $PM_{2.5}$ are sufficiently 'fine' to penetrate all the way to the alveoli, deep within the lungs. Thus, the smaller the particle size, the more dangerous the PM is thought to be. The inhalation of PM can not only exacerbate already existent pulmonary and cardiovascular illnesses, but also increase the risk of developing them. In the long term, exposure to PM can cause lung cancer and premature death. Common sources for PM emissions in an urban environment include industry, power generation and traffic, whereas wood or field burning (e.g. for domestic or agricultural purposes) are likely rural sources.

*Lead*: In its elemental form, lead (Pb) is a toxic and malleable heavy metal that takes on a dull grey appearance upon contact with air. Its frequent application as a fuel additive meant that motorized vehicles that ran on leaded petrol were once an important source of airborne lead, although this practice has now been banned in many countries. Other major sources are chiefly industrial, such as ore smelting and battery recycling. Lead is difficult to expel from the body, and gradually builds up in bone, blood and tissue. It also affects the kidneys and liver, and the central nervous system. In the case of the latter, seizures, behavioural problems and other neurological disorders may result.

Due to their toxicity, the six pollutants above can often be found on lists of key or 'criteria' pollutants that are monitored by governmental bodies, such as the Environmental Protection Agency (EPA) in the United States of America (USA), or the Department for Environment, Food and Rural Affairs (Defra) in the United Kingdom (UK). The WHO has also developed a number of AQGs for $SO_2$, $NO_2$, $O_3$ and PM.

## Important air pollution episodes in history

Air pollution became a problem in London, England, since coal was first used as a fuel in the ninth century. Complaints by citizens of the stench that resulted from coal burning led to the prohibition in 1306 of the use of 'carbone marino' (or 'sea coal') in London's firing kilns by King Edward I of England (r. 1272–1307) [5]. With population growth and a higher demand for fuel, however, the restriction of coal was gradually relaxed. Coal burning became more widespread over the sixteenth and seventeenth centuries. The pollution of air and water, the harm inflicted on people and other living organisms, and the damage to buildings and clothing were recorded in detail. One example was the *Fumifugium, or the Inconvenience of Aer and the Smoake of London Dissipated*, a pamphlet published in 1661. Its author, the writer and diarist John Evelyn (1620–1706), described a horrific vision of London blackened by coal smoke, which prompted King Charles II of England (r. 1660–1685) to request a bill to be put before Parliament. Unfortunately, the bill that Evelyn proposed was dropped, perhaps due to the inconvenience and economic considerations of relocating the polluting industries. Also, medical experts at the time considered smoke to have a protective rather than detrimental effect, as they believed it could ward off infection. In any case, no further government action was taken over the next hundred and fifty years [6].

The problem of air pollution deteriorated further during the Industrial Revolution in the eighteenth to nineteenth centuries, when the urban landscape was filled with factory chimney stacks spewing out black smoke. However, the link between air pollution and health was not understood until after several major incidents, resulting in human and animal illnesses and deaths.

All of these episodes occurred in river valleys, which were readily affected by a meteorological phenomenon known as temperature inversion. Normally, the air at ground level is warmer, and less dense, than the air above it. This layer of warm air will therefore rise and create convection, which will dilute any air pollutants produced at ground level. When a layer of cold, dense air sinks to the bottom of a river valley, this natural convection of air will not occur, resulting in an accumulation of air pollutants at the ground level.

The first such incident recorded was in the Meuse Valley of Belgium in the first week of December 1930, when 63 people and many head of cattle died [7]. Autopsy findings showed signs of inflammatory changes in the major airways of the victims. It was estimated that the concentrations of $SO_2$ ranged from 25 milligrams per cubic metre ($mg/m^3$) to as high as 100 $mg/m^3$. The second incident was the Donora episode in Pennsylvania, USA, in October 1948. It resulted in 20 deaths and about 7,000 illnesses. $SO_2$ concentrations were estimated to range from 1.5–5.5 $mg/m^3$ [8]. The third and most thoroughly studied incident was London's infamous 'Great Smog of 1952', which took place over five days in December of that year [9]. Concentrations of particulates (measured as black smoke) and sulphur dioxide reached very high levels. Subsequent analysis showed a five times increase in death rates that followed the rise in air pollution [10]. Even though the observation was based on grouped data and suffered from ecological fallacy inherent in such studies, it would be difficult to find an alternative explanation to account for the increased *mortality* had it not been caused by air pollution.

The 'Great Smog' incident subsequently led to the UK's Clean Air Act, which was passed by the British Parliament in 1956. With more stringent air pollution control measures, it was thought that air pollutants below the threshold level established at that time would not lead to ill health. By the late 1970s, it was thought that air pollution no longer posed any adverse effects on health. It was not until the 1980s that research on air pollution and health revealed that pollutant concentrations previously thought to be harmless could still demonstrate adverse effects on health.

## Research on the link between air pollution and health

### *Studies of short-term effects of air pollution on health*

Since the 1980s, epidemiologists have used *time series studies* to investigate the effects of short-term changes in air pollution. These studies have shown fairly consistent evidence of adverse effects on health at much lower concentrations of air pollutants than those recorded during the major air pollution episodes mentioned previously. In fact, concentrations in most cities are already sufficient to harm our health. Statistical models have been constructed to show the daily variations in the number of deaths, whether from all causes or due to cardiovascular and respiratory illnesses, and their relationships to daily fluctuations in the concentrations of different air pollutants – particulate matter (PM), sulphur dioxide ($SO_2$) and other gaseous pollutants, such as nitrogen dioxide ($NO_2$) and ozone ($O_3$). Daily admissions of patients suffering from respiratory and cardiovascular illnesses into hospitals were also used as *health outcomes* and their associations were sought with daily changes in air pollutant concentrations using a Poisson regression model. After correcting for the effects of seasonal and other time-dependent variations with health outcomes, the relative possibility of an increase in risk of death or hospital admissions for every unit increase in the concentrations of certain air pollutants can be derived for each air pollutant. While countries differed in the specific *relative risks* derived from such statistical models, the overall result was that concentrations of some air pollutants, notably PM, were consistently related to mortalities and hospital admissions for cardiovascular and respiratory illnesses. In some countries, certain gaseous air pollutants were more prominent risk factors for ill health than others. Notwithstanding the 'ecological' study design of such time series studies, in that variables are measured at a group rather than at an individual level, the consistency of findings in different cities of the world strongly supports the hypothesis that air pollution causes ill health.

The first multi-centre time series study on air pollution and health was the 1993 Air Pollution and Health: European Approach (APHEA) study. The principal investigator was Professor Klea Katsouyanni of the University of Athens. Participants of this study initially came from 15 European cities in 10 different countries, which have a total population of over 25 million people [11].[1] The methodology, including the choice of the statistical model, was standardized. Phase Two of this project was expanded to include 20 countries, covering 32 cities, and an improved, more robust statistical model – the generalized additive model – was adopted. There was a significant increase in the risk of death from all causes (by 0.52 per cent), cardiovascular causes (0.76 per cent) and respiratory causes (0.71 per cent) for every 10 micrograms per cubic metre ($\mu g/m^3$) increase in $PM_{10}$ concentration [12].

A study in the USA, led by Professor Jonathan Samet of the Johns Hopkins Bloomberg School of Public Health, involved an analysis of time series data from a national database on air pollution and health in 100 cities across the country. Data were taken from 1987–2000 for $PM_{10}$ and 1999–2000 for $PM_{2.5}$. Known as the National Morbidity, Mortality and Air Pollution Study (NMMAPS), this was one of the largest multi-centre time series studies reported in literature [13]. The generalized additive model was used. A significant 0.2 per cent increase in all-cause mortality and a 0.24 per cent increase in cardio-respiratory mortality were associated with a 10 $\mu g/m^3$ increase in $PM_{10}$ concentration [14]. For $PM_{2.5}$, the risks were higher (again, per 10 $\mu g/m^3$ concentration increase), at 0.29 per cent and 0.38 per cent for all-cause and cardio-respiratory mortalities, respectively.

Both phases of the APHEA study and the NMMAPS were later combined, together with additional data from 12 Canadian cities, into the Air Pollution and Health: A European and North-American Approach (APHENA) project. This study aimed to determine the combined effects of estimates of air pollutants and also dealt with the heterogeneity of the findings [15].

Since the 1990s, similar time series studies have been conducted in several Asian countries, for example, in China (including Hong Kong), Taiwan and Korea. The Public Health and Air Pollution in Asia (PAPA) study, the largest multi-centre time series study in this continent, was led by Professor Chit-Ming Wong from the University of Hong Kong. It involved three cities in China (Hong Kong, Shanghai and Wuhan) and Bangkok in Thailand, and used hospital admissions and mortality data as health outcomes [16]. The combined excess risks of mortality from all causes, and from cardiovascular and respiratory diseases, ranged from 0.34 to 1.48 per cent for every 10 $\mu g/m^3$ increase in $PM_{10}$, $NO_2$, $SO_2$ and $O_3$ in the four cities. These risks were all statistically significant, except for the association between $O_3$ and respiratory mortalities.

The initial PAPA study was later followed by two more studies, in Chennai and Delhi in India, which also used the same protocol [17]. The results from the PAPA studies, which were comparable to those in the European and American studies, provided much-needed data for health risk assessment in Asia.

Another type of study that demonstrates the short-term effects of air pollution on health outcomes is the *case-crossover study*. This study design removes the time-dependent *confounders* inherent in time series studies by assigning 'cases' (e.g. patients) as their own 'controls' (e.g. healthy people) on days when no 'events' (e.g. hospitalization) occur. Multiple-city studies have found a higher risk of hospital admissions for respiratory illnesses with exposure to $O_3$ and $PM_{10}$ [18].

*Panel studies* examine specific target groups, such as asthmatic children or patients with chronic lung diseases. Typically, they are assessed for respiratory symptoms, history of medication use or lung function, such as the peak expiratory flow rate, on a daily basis, over a defined time period. These results are then examined with corresponding daily changes in air pollutant concentrations [19].

### *Studies of long-term effects of air pollution on health*

Epidemiological studies can also show the harmful effects that long-term exposure to air pollution has on health. For example, scientists frequently conduct *cross-sectional studies* of two or more geographical regions, which have different levels of air pollution. Such studies establish that air pollution has a greater long-term impact on health in highly polluted regions than in less polluted ones. Annual mean concentrations of air pollutants are commonly used to denote long-term exposures to air pollution. Health outcomes include the prevalence of respiratory symptoms and/or illnesses. For young children, lung function tests can also be performed, as the results reflect the health and development of their lungs.

*Cohort studies*, also known as 'follow-up studies', are so called because a group or 'cohort' of people are followed up over a period of time and observed for changes to their health, such as the incidence of a particular disease. Cohort studies can demonstrate a temporal relationship between air pollution and health outcomes (e.g. mortality or changes in lung function). They have also been used to provide better quality evidence for a cause–effect relationship between air pollution and ill health. The earliest cohort study on air pollution and long-term health risk was the Harvard six cities study, led by Professor Douglas Dockery of the Harvard School of Public Health [20]. The American Cancer Society study, led by Dr Arden Pope, is another widely used study for the formulation of *air quality standards*, thanks to its broad geographical coverage and large sample size (with up to 500,000 participants) [21]. As some components of PM, such as the polycyclic aromatic hydrocarbons (PAHs), are known to be carcinogenic, deaths from lung cancer in adults have been studied as one of the health outcomes of air pollution [22]. Besides mortality and *morbidity* studies, the impact of air pollution on children's lung function has been studied extensively in several cohort studies in California, USA [23–25]. There is sufficient evidence for a causal link between long-term exposure to air pollution and children's lung growth.

### Experimental studies

With ample evidence of the harmful effects of air pollution from observational studies, researchers have turned their attention to experimental studies. There are two categories of such studies. The *chamber study* involves releasing a known concentration of an air pollutant to human volunteers under strictly controlled conditions, and measuring the physiological or pathological response to the exposure. Typically, the subjects are studied for the inflammatory responses of their respiratory tract linings, white blood cells and other markers of inflammation in their blood. This can be done by direct observation using a bronchoscope, by taking tissue samples for biopsy or by conducting bronchoalveolar lavage, where fluid is injected into part of the lung and collected again for examination [26].

The other experimental study is known as a *community trial*, a type of *intervention study*. Typically, these studies make use of air pollution control measures that are being implemented in a community by recording the subjects' health status before and after the 'intervention'. The hypothesis is that if the intervention results in a decrease in air pollutant levels, this should result in a demonstrable change in the health of the community. Although such before-and-after intervention studies lack a control group, they can provide strong evidence of a cause–effect relationship between air pollution and health outcomes in the medium to long term (e.g. as measured in months). Following an intervention, for example, it would be difficult to offer an alternative explanation to a significant fall in the death rate or the incidence/prevalence of respiratory or cardiovascular diseases (CVDs), other than the intervention factor.

Two intervention studies have been used by the WHO in developing the recommended guideline concentration of $SO_2$ in its 2005 AQGs [27]. One was a Hong Kong study, led by Professor Anthony Hedley of the University of Hong Kong, while the other study was led by Professor Luke Clancy in Dublin, Ireland [28, 29]. In the Hong Kong study, a mandatory switch to low-sulphur fuel for all vehicles and power plants in 1990 resulted in an average decline of 50 per cent of $SO_2$ concentrations post-intervention. The most polluted areas saw an 80 per cent fall in $SO_2$ concentrations and, while PM levels remained little changed, there was a 41 per cent fall in the sulphate content of respirable particulates. There was a significant decline in the annual trends of mortality from cardiovascular and respiratory causes. The findings suggested a cause–effect relationship between $SO_2$ levels and the various health outcomes studied.

In the Dublin study [28], a ban on coal sales led to a 70 per cent decline in black smoke concentrations and a 34 per cent decline in $SO_2$ levels, which coincided with a significant reduction in deaths due to respiratory disease (by 15.5 per cent) and CVDs (by 10.3 per cent). These findings suggested that the number of deaths can be reduced by limiting the concentrations of particulate matter in the air.

## Air pollution in Hong Kong

### An evolving public health problem

In cities where manufacturing industries flourish, the air quality is likely to deteriorate, prompting the need for data on air pollutant levels and methods for controlling emissions. Such was the case for Hong Kong in the 1970s when industry was at its peak. Chimneys and exhaust fans from buildings in industrial districts, such as Tsuen Wan and Kwun Tong, would constantly spew out a noxious cocktail of toxic gases and fumes. The increased need for power consumption and transport also meant that $SO_2$ became a major air pollutant. Thus, air pollution monitoring in Hong Kong started at this time and was initially performed by the Air Pollution Control Office, under the government's Labour Department. Smoke inspectors patrolled factories for any breach of the law. Air samples were collected for analysis of air pollutants, like $SO_2$ and PM, in the laboratory of the former Industrial Health Division [30].

It was not until 1986 that the Environmental Protection Department (EPD) was established, headed by a Director of Environmental Protection (DEP), with specific responsibilities for enforcing laws against air pollution (the Air Pollution Control Ordinance) and implementing policies in air pollution control. This included the creation of a network of air quality monitoring stations in different districts throughout Hong Kong and the setting of Air Quality Objectives (AQOs) for major air pollutants, including total suspended particulates, respirable suspended particulates, sulphur dioxide, nitrogen dioxide, ozone, lead and carbon monoxide [31].

With China's economic reform that began in 1979, manufacturing industries in Hong Kong took advantage of the cheaper labour market across the border by relocating their factories to mainland China. This gradual but relentless removal of Hong Kong's manufacturing base resulted in a reduction in air pollutant emissions from local factories. At the same time, however, the rapid development of the neighbouring Pearl River Delta as the 'factory of the world' posed a regional air pollution problem to Hong Kong. The pollutant, ozone, is well known to travel long distances, as are fine particulates. The latter often reaches high levels even at the remote air monitoring station of Tap Mun, which is an outlying island in the north-eastern part of Hong Kong that has no vehicular transport.

Besides regional air pollution, there is also the problem of pollution from local sources, predominantly from motor vehicles. Roadside air pollution is an acute problem that affects the lives and health of a large urban population [32]. $PM_{10}$ (70 per cent of which belongs also to $PM_{2.5}$) and $NO_2$ are the predominant air pollutants recorded in roadside air monitoring stations. The continuous urban development on a limited land supply does nothing to improve the situation, as increasingly taller buildings are built on both sides of narrow roads, trapping the air pollutants produced by traffic in so-called 'street canyons' that discourage their natural dispersion.

## *Local research on air pollution and health*

Research on air pollution and health in Hong Kong started in the early 1990s. A cross-sectional study on the respiratory health of school children was conducted before and after the aforementioned government intervention of reducing sulphur content in fuel. The subjects were from two Hong Kong districts: the highly polluted Kwai Tsing and the relatively cleaner Hong Kong Island South [33, 34]. There was a significant decrease in the respiratory symptoms and bronchial hyper-responsiveness among children post-intervention [35, 36]. For the less polluted district, the post-intervention decrease in the crude prevalence ratio of cough and phlegm was 16 per cent and 29 per cent, respectively. For the more polluted district, the decrease was even greater, at 34 per cent and 43 per cent for cough and phlegm, respectively. The prevalence of bronchial hyper-responsiveness decreased from 29 per cent to 16 per cent.

Other cross-sectional studies have also been done. One compared the lung function [37] and physical fitness [38] of school children in districts with different air qualities. Children living in the more polluted district had poorer lung functions than those living in districts with cleaner air. Another study, which focused mainly on indoor air pollution and the prevalence of respiratory illnesses, also compared subjects from two housing estates at different distances to outdoor pollution sources. Children in the district close to the pollution source had three times the prevalence of respiratory illnesses than children living in the district farther away from the source [39].

Time series studies with hospital admissions and mortalities as health outcomes have been conducted since the late 1990s [40–43]. Results were similar to findings reported in other countries, with adverse effects on health being observed for most air pollutants. Newer studies on the harmful effects on health caused by specific components of air pollutants, such as coarse particulates, have also been conducted [44].

Outpatient consultation data were collected prospectively for a time series study on air pollution and community morbidity [45, 46]. Morbidity was measured in terms of consultations to general practitioners (GPs) for upper respiratory tract infections (URTI). The results indicated that high air pollution levels affect not only those with serious illnesses requiring hospitalization, but also the much larger population at risk for minor respiratory illnesses.

Besides epidemiological studies, there have been many studies on atmospheric science, air chemistry, exposure assessment and the toxicology of air pollutants by local academics [47–53].

## *Public perception and awareness of air pollution*

Air pollution is very visible in Hong Kong. Although gaseous air pollutants are invisible by themselves, and particulates are too small to be seen, their combination often forms smog that reduces visibility and gives the sky a grey tinge. The EPD has been reporting on the severity of the problem since the 1990s, using the Air Pollution Index. The index is intended to be a warning system that informs the public of the local air quality on a daily and hourly basis, and cautions them, in the event of high air pollution levels, to avoid outdoor exposure. This system, which is based on methodology designed by the USA Environmental Protection Agency (EPA), relies on a comparison of the prevailing air pollutant concentrations with a set of AQOs recommended by the government.

As a result of the research conducted on air pollution and health, most countries have revised their air quality standards periodically, in the light of new research findings. The USA EPA, for example, is legally obliged to review its National Ambient Air Quality Standards (NAAQS) every five years, as stated in the Clean Air Act. Such a provision is absent in Hong Kong and the updating of the AQOs is dependent entirely on the government's priorities. In fact, the AQOs currently in use in Hong Kong were first formulated in 1987, not long after the EPD was established, and have not been updated since.

An air quality control framework that has no legally required review mechanisms is inherently flawed, as it must be regularly adjusted in concurrence with new scientific findings. We can demonstrate this problem with the following case study. In 1996, the Hong Kong EPD formed a working group to review the AQOs. The group comprised environmental health professionals from the University of Hong Kong and the Chinese University of Hong Kong, as well as representatives from the healthcare professions. After 18 months, the working group produced a report, together with a number of recommendations. After the report was submitted, however, the EPD made no follow-up actions, nor did it call for further meetings with the working group. The underlying motive for the government's backtracking could not be firmly established, but the lack of support by higher-level administration may have been a primary cause. Regardless of the reason, the AQOs are now more than 20 years out of date, rendering the reported API rather meaningless. The percentage of days with officially 'high'

API levels is around 6 per cent of the year; this contrasts with the common, real-life observation of smog for the majority of the year.

In 2008, a study was commissioned by the EPD to create a new, health risk-based air quality reporting system that improves on the current API. The Air Quality Health Index (AQHI) was developed by a multidisciplinary team of academics from three local universities, led by the Chinese University of Hong Kong. It has received much publicity and is scheduled to launch in 2014 [54].

An alternative air pollution indicator that has received media attention is the Hedley Index [55]. Designed by Professor Anthony Hedley of the University of Hong Kong, this index tallies the healthcare costs, in terms of adverse health effects and monetary losses, in real time. The calculations compare the prevailing air pollutant concentrations with the WHO AQGs and the resulting index indicates that air pollution is high on over 90 per cent of days in a year. While this information is of public health importance, by consistently reporting high pollution levels, the public may develop 'warning fatigue' from the Hedley Index. In our view it is therefore not suitable as a tool for regular risk communication, in that it cannot influence people's behaviours on a day-to-day basis. However, it is successful in drawing public attention to the health problem posed by air pollution. The mass media has been active in reporting air pollution as a serious health hazard, and new research findings, both local and overseas, have received wide publicity.

In recent years, many non-governmental organizations (NGOs) have taken an interest in improving air quality in Hong Kong, frequently using their public influence to pressure the government into action. These NGOs include Friends of the Earth, the World Wildlife Fund, Clean the Air, Clean Air Network and Civic Exchange. The latter, a policy think-tank, has organized workshops and seminars for the education of the public on air pollution and commissioned a number of research projects. Civic Exchange has also published several reports on air pollution that deal with different issues, including air pollution in the Pearl River Delta [56, 57]. It has also initiated the Fairwind Charter, a voluntary programme that involves major shipping companies switching to low sulphur fuel when they reach Hong Kong waters. As Hong Kong's container terminal at Kwai Chung remains one of the busiest ports in the world, this programme has significantly reduced the local emissions of $SO_2$ by ocean-going vessels, which have hitherto been using highly polluting bunker fuel.

### *Government efforts in air pollution control*

One of the earliest successful air pollution control measures taken by the Hong Kong EPD was the implementation of a low sulphur fuel policy in 1990. Other methods have included incentives for truck operators to replace their old diesel vehicles with modern ones, which are designed using more stringent emission standards. Public light buses and taxis were also encouraged to switch from the more polluting diesel to the 'cleaner' liquid petroleum gas (LPG). Unfortunately, the benefits of these strategies may have been offset by the rising prevalence of motor vehicles, the use of which has not been limited in any way.

Another major source of air pollution in Hong Kong is from power generation, which uses coal as the dominant fuel because of its low cost. PM and $SO_2$ are major problems for air quality and are expensive to control. Government efforts to reduce emissions from this source include promoting the use of liquid natural gas in local power plants and nuclear energy from the Daya Bay nuclear power station in China.

Another significant development in air pollution control has been the establishment of a joint Hong Kong–Guangdong effort in the reduction of regional emissions and the sharing of air pollution data across the network of air monitoring stations. This offers the public greater transparency over the air quality in the Pearl River Delta. Although the emissions reduction targets have been based on what can practically be done, rather than on what needs to be done, they have resulted in some improvement in air quality. From 2005 to 2012, there was a decline in ambient $PM_{10}$ and $PM_{2.5}$ concentrations (as measured in roof-top air monitoring stations) by 24 per cent and 32 per cent, respectively. Ambient $SO_2$ concentrations fell by 50 per cent. However, ambient $O_3$ rose by 14 per cent, while ambient $NO_2$ concentrations didn't change much. $NO_2$ in roadside stations increased by 24 per cent [58].

In 2009, the EPD commissioned a study to review Hong Kong's AQOs and develop strategies for improving the air quality. The consultancy report recommended a series of short-, medium- and long-term strategies towards the second goal. These included the introduction of low emission or car-free zones, encouraging the use of hybrid or electric vehicles, expanding the current rail network and increasing the use of renewable energy sources for power generation [59]. These recommendations were supported by cost–benefit analyses, which show that the healthcare and social costs of air pollution often outweigh those of implementing the control measures.

However, the new AQOs suggested by the report were disappointingly conservative, and followed the WHO AQG's most lenient targets – either interim target 1 (IT1) or interim target 2 (IT2),[2] if IT1 is already more lax than Hong Kong's existing AQOs. Moreover, this set of AQOs will only be implemented in 2014 – five years after the study report was published. The delay in both the revision of the AQOs and the proactive implementation of air pollution control strategies indicated a lack of commitment by the senior officials of the 2005–2012 administration.

This dismissive attitude may be due to an underlying weakness in the organizational structure of the Environment Bureau, the government policy bureau to which the EPD is accountable. In 2004, the former Environment, Transport and Works Bureau merged with the EPD. Although the latter retained its name, and its head is still known as the Director of Environmental Protection, this post is no longer assigned to environmental science professionals. Instead, an administrative officer is appointed as the DEP, who possesses, amongst other things, the statutory power to grant environmental impact assessment (EIA) permits to developmental projects. Since the merger, public challenges have been raised to the decisions made by the DEP. One such example is the judicial review of the Hong Kong–Zhuhai–Macau bridge project [60], has which received much media attention.

Another shortcoming of the merger is the lack of continuity in the formulation of environmental policies, as the DEP is now a 'rotating' position, with different administrative officers occupying this important post every few years. Moreover, this administrative structure is not conducive to the long-term career prospects of professional officers within the EPD, who are denied the prospect of promotion to the highest management level.

There is scope for optimism, however. The current administration (2012– ) has taken a more proactive role, with the appointments of a Secretary and an Under Secretary for the Environment who are veteran advocates of environmental issues.

## Lessons from other cities

Many other cities have tackled the problem of air pollution control, to varying degrees of success. Hong Kong would do well to learn from some of their experiences. Here, we shall discuss examples from two major cities: London, the British capital once known for its infamous 'fogs'; and Los Angeles, located in San Pedro Bay, which was once nicknamed the 'Bay of Smokes'.

## *London*

The Clean Air Act of 1956 was created in response to the deadly 'Great Smog' in London, which happened four years prior. After this initial enactment, it was updated in 1968 to include the mandatory use of tall chimneys by fuel-burning factories. The larger smoke stacks helped improve the dispersal of pollutants. Following Britain's inclusion in the European Union (EU), further legislation came into play, such as the EU Framework Air Quality Directive of 1996 [61]. Target values have been set for a number of major air pollutants – in the UK, these are known as Air Quality Objectives (AQOs) and have specified dates for achievement.

Apart from national legislation relating to air pollution, control measures specifically for the British capital were established by the Mayor's Air Quality Strategy, first published in 2002. It was directed mainly at road vehicles, setting forth emissions standards for taxis, buses and coaches, as well as two charging schemes for the reduction of traffic (detailed below). Incentives were also provided for the conversion to, or use of, environmentally friendly vehicles that use alternative fuels, such as electric or hybrid cars, or vehicles that run on liquefied petroleum gas (LPG) or compressed natural gas (CNG). Finally, the document proposed a number of energy-saving plans that would help reduce air pollution as well as mitigate the effects of climate change. The Strategy was revised and updated, in 2006 and 2010 [61, 62].

The Congestion Charging (CC) scheme was introduced in 2003 for the purpose of reducing the amount of traffic, and thus the congestion, in central London. The basic idea behind the scheme was a simple one: motorists would be charged for driving their vehicles in a delineated zone within the capital during specific hours of the day. The reinforcement of this scheme was aided by a vast network of cameras that recorded vehicle licence plates and compared them to an up-to-date database of registered and paying drivers [63]. The CC scheme is similar to Singapore's Electronic Road Pricing (ERP) system, which was successfully established in 1998 [64].

The CC scheme ultimately aimed to change travel behaviour by encouraging more people to take alternative methods of transport, including trains, buses and even bicycles. The scheme concurrently raised the money needed to improve public transport from the people who continued to drive. When it was first proposed by Ken Livingstone, then the Mayor of London, the CC scheme faced opposition from many groups but, in a show of political will, the scheme was boldly carried out regardless of the objections. Following implementation, congestion decreased by 26 per cent within the charging zone, while traffic decreased by 15 per cent [61]. This, in turn, reduced emission levels: between 2002 and 2003, emissions of $NO_x$ fell by 12 per cent within the charging zone; those of $PM_{10}$ fell by 11.9 per cent and those of $CO_2$ fell by 19.5 per cent [64]. These reductions are attributed to the CC scheme and do not include the improvements brought about by improved vehicle technology.

The success of the CC scheme prompted the creation of a Low Emission Zone (LEZ), which covered most of Greater London, in 2008. This targeted only highly polluting vehicles, including larger vehicles such as lorries, trucks, buses and coaches, and smaller diesel vehicles like vans, caravans, minibuses and even horse boxes. Cars and motorcycles are excluded. As with the CC, the drivers of the specified diesel vehicles are required to pay a daily charge for each day that they drive within the LEZ, with the charge depending on their vehicle's type and weight. They are exempted from payment, however, if their vehicles comply with the emissions standards – currently updated to the Euro IV standards – for PM. Drivers are thus encouraged to make their vehicles cleaner through measures such as fitting filters to the vehicle exhaust or converting vehicles to run on alternative fuels, such as gas [65].

In 1993, the London Air Quality Network was set up by King's College London, in conjunction with various London Boroughs and Regional Health Authorities [66]. This network has a vast array of more than one hundred air monitoring stations, located all over London, which are classified into six site types: rural, suburban, urban background, roadside, kerbside and industrial. The stations track the concentrations of a variety of air pollutants, including CO, $SO_2$, $NO_2$, $NO_x$, $O_3$, $PM_{10}$ and $PM_{2.5}$. The data these stations provide are vital in assessing not only the current pollution levels around the metropolis, but also the efficacy of the mitigation strategies [67].

## *Los Angeles*

The city of Los Angeles (LA), in California, USA, is another metropolis that has devoted considerable resources to cleaning up its air. The geographical characteristics of California contrive to trap pollutants in air basins, particularly during temperature inversions. It was just such an occurrence that led to LA's first documented case of smog in 1943, where residents complained of respiratory symptoms, eye pain, nausea and even vomiting. Action was taken and the Air Pollution Control Act was signed in 1947. The federal Clean Air Act and California's Ambient Air Quality Standards were first established in the 1960s, while the Air Resources Board (ARB) of California was created in 1967. It remains active today, and is responsible for monitoring air quality, setting and enforcing tighter air quality and emissions standards, and conducting research and providing education on air pollution [68].

The Air Pollution Control Districts, which were originally created for each Californian county following the Air Pollution Control Act, were adjusted in the 1970s to follow topographical rather than legal boundaries, since air pollution was a problem that frequently crossed county borders. Thus, California was split into 15 air basins [69]. One of these, the South Coast Air Basin (SoCAB), covers most of LA County (including the city of LA), all of Orange County, and parts of Riverside and San Bernardino Counties. The South Coast Air Quality Management District (SCAQMD) was formed in 1977 to handle air pollution in SoCAB.

The LA strategy for reducing air pollution focused on developing a tough legal framework that controls emissions and air quality. This framework has to operate concurrently at various levels of authority: at the federal (EPA), state (California ARB), regional (SCAQMD) and local (Southern California Association of Governments or SCAG) levels. For example, regulations for transport vehicles are set by the EPA, while the California ARB handles standards for vehicle fuel. Stationary air pollution sources, like oil refineries and power stations, are made to comply with emissions rules under the SCAQMD Plan, while the SCAG helps to coordinate and carry out the various policies [61].

Another measure, endorsed in 2006, was the San Pedro Bay Ports Clean Air Action Plan. The adjacent ports of Los Angeles and Long Beach – which, combined, constitute the fifth busiest container sea port in the world – cooperated under this plan to reduce marine air pollution. Developed in conjunction with the EPA, California ARB and SCAQMD, the Action Plan targeted emissions from the ocean-going ships and harbour craft. Strategies included setting regulations for cleaner fuel and providing incentives for older diesel engines to be replaced with newer, cleaner ones. Ships in dock are offered 'plug-in' electrical facilities to encourage them to switch off their auxiliary engines. Similar strategies were also applied to the land-based emissions sources, namely, the cargo-handling equipment, trucks and trains that help transport goods to and from the ports. These methods were combined with tighter emissions standards and stricter enforcement [61, 70].

The multifaceted approach used by Los Angeles in tackling its air pollution problem does appear to be successful, with concentrations of the major pollutants – including CO, $NO_2$, $SO_2$, $O_3$, $PM_{10}$ and $PM_{2.5}$ – gradually but steadily falling over the past two decades [71]. Although there is still much to be done before Los Angeles can meet the ultimate goal of 'zero emissions', the air quality there has certainly been improving.

### *Useful strategies*

A common feature of the air quality management systems in London and LA is the comprehensive legal framework, which sets legally binding Air Quality Objectives or Standards that are periodically updated. Mobile emission sources – such as traffic in London and shipping in LA – are addressed using schemes that reduce the existing number of vehicles or promote upgrades to newer and cleaner engines. Other tactics include transport and energy policies that encourage the shift from fossil fuels to renewable or alternative fuels.

Hong Kong could certainly follow the example of these two cities. First, it needs to develop an action plan within a single comprehensive legal framework, incorporating more stringent AQOs. Unlike the standards of London and LA, Hong Kong's existing AQOs are *not* legally binding, and are also relatively lax, not having been adjusted (at the time of writing) since they were first set in 1987. It is therefore not surprising to find that air quality in Hong Kong has taken a turn for the worse, while it has slowly been improving in London and LA.

As a major local source of air pollution, traffic in Hong Kong should be tackled, perhaps by using a congestion pricing system like that in London, in conjunction with policies that promote environmentally friendly vehicles. A further consideration is the 'street canyon' effect, whereby traffic emissions are trapped in the roads by tall buildings on either side. This pollutant dispersal problem is more severe in Hong Kong than in either London or Los Angeles, due to topography, population density and building heights. Although existing 'street canyons' are likely to remain until they are redeveloped, the government should take care not to create more of these when planning new building projects.

Like LA, port activity forms an important part of Hong Kong's economy so the reduction of marine emissions should be another priority. Due to the presence of neighbouring ports, cross-border collaborations would be necessary for regional pollution control policies to succeed.

Although Hong Kong has an air pollution monitoring network, this could be expanded and improved: the 14 existing stations are hardly comparable to London's 100-plus stations, which also represent more types of sampling environment than Hong Kong's two types ('general' and 'roadside'). A more detailed profile of Hong Kong's air pollution situation would assist in the development of future air quality management strategies.

Finally, Hong Kong needs to take the air pollution problem seriously, instead of playing down its importance. This would require more involvement from the public, as well as greater political will from the government. With strong leadership and a positive attitude towards change and improvement, Hong Kong can achieve the high standards of air quality expected from a world-class city.

## Conclusion

Air pollution is a global public health problem that has been growing ever since the beginning of industrialization. The problem is especially serious in rapidly developing regions, such as Asia. The evidence of the harmful effects of air pollution on human health is unequivocal, with numerous studies of different designs coming to similar conclusions, regardless of the geographical region being studied. High levels of air pollutants are frequently linked to mortalities and morbidities due to respiratory and cardiovascular diseases.

Our case study of Hong Kong described the problems it has with both local and regional sources of air pollution – the former is due mostly to traffic and power generation, while the latter is caused by the many industries now found across the border in Guangdong. While the concentrations of air pollutants are being monitored, not enough is being done to reduce them to a level safer for human health, resulting in substantial healthcare costs and economic losses.

Both Hong Kong's existing air pollution warning system, the API, and the standards or AQOs on which it depends, are woefully out of date. Indeed, the AQOs have not been updated at all since they were first established. Although reviews have been conducted and new air quality indices developed, concrete changes have yet to be made, pointing to a lack of political will on the part of the government. Environmental policy makers are not always professionally trained in their area of responsibility, but they do need to become familiarized with the basic science of air pollution and its relation to health.

Another important lesson to learn from the Hong Kong case study is that concerted community efforts, such as the various initiatives by the NGOs, the attention of the media, and applied research by academics and health professionals, are invaluable in pushing governments to action.

There is much that can be done to improve the quality of our air, from measures that directly reduce emissions to strategies that promote environmental friendliness. The conservation of our environment depends on our willingness to change the way we think and act. As a community, we shall have to work in unison for a better environment and a more sustainable way of life.

## Acknowledgements

We would like to thank Mr Benson Yeung, Senior Environmental Protection Officer, Environmental Protection Department, Hong Kong for his valuable comments on the chapter.

## Notes

1 The fifteen cities involved in the project are (in alphabetical order): Amsterdam, Athens, Barcelona, Bratislava, Helsinki, Köln, Kraków, Łódź, London, Lyon, Milan, Paris, Poznań, Rotterdam and Wrocław. The countries are the Netherlands, Greece, Spain, Slovakia, Finland, Germany, Poland, the UK, France and Italy.

2 Interim targets are set by the WHO for developing countries that may not be able to achieve the recommended air quality guidelines. They are designed in a stepwise manner and represent progressive decreases in health risk towards the recommended 'final targets'.

## References

1. World Health Organization. Fact sheet No. 313: Air quality and health (Updated September 2011). Available from: http://www.who.int/mediacentre/factsheets/fs313/en/index.html [Accessed January 2013].
2. World Health Organization. Health topics: Air pollution. World Health Organization, 2013. Available from: http://www.who.int/topics/air_pollution/en/ [Accessed February 2013].
3. Moeller DW. *Environmental Health* (third edition). Cambridge, MA: Harvard University Press, 2005.

4. Blumenthal DS and Ragsdale HL. Chapter 6: Air Pollution. In: *Introduction to Environmental Health* (second edition), Blumenthal DS and Ruttenber AS. New York: Springer, 1995.
5. Plantagenet E. Letter to the Sheriff of Surrey. 1307. Quoted and translated by Sir W. Hawthorne, in Energy and environment, conflict or compromise. Trueman Wood Lecture. *Journal of the Royal Society of Arts*, July 1978.
6. Kessel AS. *Air, the Environment and Public Health.* Cambridge: Cambridge University Press, 2006.
7. Firket J. The cause of the symptoms found in the Meuse Valley during the fog of December 1930. *Bulletin of the Royal Academy of Medicine*, Belgium, 1931; 11: 683–741.
8. Schrenk HH, Heiman H, Clayton GD, *et al.* Air pollution in Donora, PA, epidemiology of the unusual smog episode of October 1948. *US Public Health Bulletin* No. 306. US Government Printing Office, Washington, DC, 1949.
9. Met Office Education Website. Case Study: The Great Smog of 1952. Available from: http://www.metoffice.gov.uk/education/teens/case-studies/great-smog [Accessed February 2013].
10. Beaver H. Interim Report (on London air pollution incident), Committee on Air Pollution: CMD 9011, London: Her Majesty's Stationery Office, 1953.
11. Katsouyanni K, Schwartz J, Spix C, Touloumi G, Zmirou D, Zanobetti A, *et al.* Short-term effects of air pollution on health: a European approach using epidemiologic time series data: the APHEA protocol. *Journal of Epidemiology and Community Health* 1996; 50(Suppl 1): S11–18.
12. Katsouyanni K. APHEA Project: Air Pollution and Health: A European Approach. *Epidemiology* 2006; 17(6S): S19, SS1–02.
13. Samet JM, Zeger SL, Dominici F, Curriero F, Coursac I, Dockery DW, *et al.* National Morbidity, Mortality, and Air Pollution Study. Part II: Morbidity and Mortality from Air Pollution in the United States. Health Effects Institute Report 94-II, Boston, MA, 2000.
14. Dominici F, Peng RD, Zeger SL, Samet JM. Recent developments of the National Morbidity Mortality Air Pollution Study: 1987–2000. *Epidemiology* 2006; 17(6S): S19, SS1–03.
15. Katsouyanni K, Samet JM. Air Pollution and Health: A European and North American Approach (APHENA). Health Effects Institute Report 142, Boston, MA, 2009.
16. Wong CM, Vichit-Vadakan N, Kan H, Qian Z and the PAPA Team. Public Health and Air Pollution in Asia (PAPA): A multicity study of short-term effects of air pollution on mortality. *Environmental Health Perspectives* 2008; 116: 1195–202.
17. Health Effects Institute. Research Report Number 157. Public Health and Air Pollution in Asia (PAPA): Coordinated Studies of Short-Term Exposure to Air Pollution and Daily Mortality in Two Indian Cities. Boston, MA: Health Effects Institute, 2011.
18. Medina-Ramon M, Zanobetti A, Schwartz J. The effect of $O_3$ and $PM_{10}$ on hospital admissions for pneumonia and chronic obstructive pulmonary disease: a national multicity study. *American Journal of Epidemiology* 2006; 763: 579–88.
19. Gent JF, Triche EW, Holford TR, *et al.* Association of low-level ozone and fine particles with respiratory symptoms in children with asthma. *Journal of the American Medical Association* 2003; 290: 1859–67.
20. Dockery DW, Pope CA III, Xu X, Spengler JD, Ware JH, Fay ME, *et al.* An association between air pollution and mortality in six US cities. *New England Journal of Medicine* 1993; 329: 1753–9.
21. Pope CA III, Thun MJ, Namboodiri MM, Dockery DW, Evans JS, Speizer FE, Heath Jr CW. Particulate air pollution as a predictor of mortality in a prospective study of US adults. *American Journal of Respiratory and Critical Care Medicine* 1995; 151: 669–74.
22. Pope CA III, Burnett RT, Thun MJ, Galle EE, Krewski D, Ito K, Thurston GD. Lung cancer, cardiopulmonary mortality, and long-term exposure to fine particulate air pollution. *Journal of the American Medical Association* 2002; 287: 1132–41.
23. Gauderman WJ, McConnell R, Gilliland F, London S, Thomas D, Avol E, *et al.* Association between air pollution and lung function growth in South Californian children. *American Journal of Respiratory and Critical Care Medicine* 2000; 162: 1383–90.
24. Gauderman WJ, Avol E, Gilliland F, Vora H, Thomas D, Berhane K, *et al.* The effects of air pollution on lung development from 10 to 18 years of age. *New England Journal of Medicine* 2004; 351(11): 1057–67.
25. Gauderman WJ, Vora H, McConnell R, Berhane K, Gilliland F, Thomas D, *et al.* Effect of exposure to traffic on lung development from 10 to 18 years of age: a cohort study. *Lancet* 2007; 369(9561): 571–7.

26. Bylin G, Lindvall T, Rehn T, Sundin B. Effects of short-term exposure to ambient nitrogen dioxide concentrations on human bronchial reactivity and lung function. *European Journal of Respiratory Disease* 1985; 66: 205–17.
27. World Health Organization. *Air Quality Guidelines Global Update 2005*. World Health Organization Regional Office for Europe, Copenhagen, Denmark, 2006.
28. Clancy L, Goodman P, Sinclair H, Dockery DW. Effect of air pollution control on death-rates in Dublin, Ireland: an intervention study. *Lancet*, 2002; 360: 1210–14.
29. Hedley AJ, Wong CM, Thach TQ, Ma S, Lam TH, Anderson HR. Cardiorespiratory and all-cause mortality after restrictions on sulphur content of fuel in Hong Kong: an intervention study. *Lancet* 2002; 360: 1646–52.
30. Labour Department, Hong Kong. Annual Departmental Report. Hong Kong Government, 1977.
31. Environmental Protection Department, Hong Kong. Available from: http://www.epd.gov.hk/epd/english/environmentinhk/air/air_quality_objectives/air_quality_objectives.html [Accessed February 2013].
32. Edesess M. Roadside air pollution in Hong Kong: Why is it still so bad? Civic Exchange, Hong Kong, 2011.
33. Ong SG, Liu J, Wong CM, Lam TH, Tam AYC, Daniel L, Hedley AJ. Studies on the respiratory health of primary school children in urban communities of Hong Kong. *Science of the Total Environment* 1991; 106: 123–35.
34. Tam AYC, Wong CM, Lam TH, Ong SG, Peters J, Hedley AJ. Bronchial responsiveness in children exposed to air pollution in Hong Kong. *Chest* 1994; 106: 1056–60.
35. Peters J, Hedley AJ, Wong CM, Lam TH, Ong SG, Liu J, Spiegelhalter DJ. Effects of an ambient air pollution intervention and environmental tobacco smoke on children's respiratory health in Hong Kong. *International Journal of Epidemiology* 1996; 25(4): 821–8.
36. Wong CM, Lam TH, Peters J, Hedley AJ, Ong SG, Tam AYC, *et al.* Comparison between two districts of the effects of an air pollution intervention on bronchial responsiveness in primary school children in Hong Kong. *Journal of Epidemiology and Community Health* 1998; 52(9): 571–8.
37. Yu TS, Wong TW, Wang XR, Song H, Wong SL, Tang JL. Adverse effects of low-level air pollution on respiratory health of school children in Hong Kong. *Journal of Occupational and Environmental Medicine* 2001; 43: 310–6.
38. Yu TS, Wong TW, Liu HJ. Impact of air pollution on cardiopulmonary fitness in schoolchildren. *Journal of Occupational and Environmental Medicine*, 2004; 46: 946–52.
39. Wong TW, Yu TS, Liu HJ, Wong AHS. Household gas cooking: a risk factor for respiratory illnesses in pre-school children. *Archives of Disease in Childhood* 2004; 89: 631–6.
40. Wong TW, Lau TS, Yu TS, Neller A, Wong SL, Tam W, Pang SW. Air pollution and hospital admissions for respiratory and cardiovascular diseases in Hong Kong. *Occupational and Environmental Medicine* 1999; 56(10): 679–83.
41. Wong TW, Tam WS, Yu TS, Wong AHS. Associations between daily mortalities from respiratory and cardiovascular diseases and air pollution in Hong Kong, China. *Occupational and Environmental Medicine* 2002; 59: 30–5.
42. Wong CM, Ma S, Hedley AJ, Lam TH. Does ozone have any effect on daily hospital admissions for circulatory diseases? *Journal of Epidemiology and Community Health* 1999; 53: 580–1.
43. Wong CM, Ma S, Hedley AJ, Lam TH. Effect of air pollution on daily mortality in Hong Kong. *Environmental Health Perspectives* 2001; 109: 335–40.
44. Qiu H, Yu ITS, Tian L, Wang X, Tse LA, Tam W, Wong TW. Effects of coarse particulate matter on emergency hospital admissions for respiratory diseases: a time-series analysis in Hong Kong. *Environmental Health Perspectives* 2012; 120(4): 572–6.
45. Wong TW, Wun YT, Yu TS, Tam WS, Wong CM, Wong AHS. Air pollution and GP consultations for respiratory illnesses. *Journal of Epidemiology and Community Health* 2002; 56: 949–50.
46. Wong TW, Tam W, Yu ITS, Wun YT, Wong AHS, Wong CM. Association between air pollution and general practitioner visits for respiratory diseases in Hong Kong. *Thorax* 2006; 61: 585–91.
47. Yuan Z, Lau AKH, Zhang H, Yu JZ, Louie PKK, Fung JCH. Identifications and spatiotemporal variations of dominant $PM_{10}$ sources over Hong Kong. *Atmospheric Environment* 2006; 40: 1803–15.
48. Huang XF, Yu JZ, Yuan Z, Lau AKH, Louie PKK. Source analysis of high particulate days in Hong Kong. *Atmospheric Environment* 2009; 43: 1196–203.

49. Xiao F, Brajer V, Mead RW. Blowing in the wind: the impact of China's Pearl River Delta on Hong Kong's air quality. *Science of the Total Environment* 2006; 367: 96–111.
50. Ho KF, Lee SC, Chow JC, Watson JG. Characterization of $PM_{10}$ and $PM_{2.5}$ source profiles for fugitive dust in Hong Kong. *Atmospheric Environment* 2003; 37: 1023–32.
51. Lee SC, Ho KF, Chan LY, Zielinska B, Chow JC. Polycyclic aromatic hydrocarbons (PAHs) and carbonyl compounds in urban atmosphere of Hong Kong. *Atmospheric Environment* 2001; 35: 5949–60.
52. Lee SC, Chiu MY, Ho KF, Zou SC, Wang X. Volatile organic compounds (VOCs) in urban atmosphere of Hong Kong. *Chemosphere* 2002; 48: 375–82.
53. So KL, Wang T. On the local and regional influence on ground-level ozone concentrations in Hong Kong. *Environmental Pollution* 2003; 123: 307–17.
54. Wong TW, Tam WWS, Yu ITS, Lau AKH, Pang SW, Wong AHS. Developing a risk-based air quality health index. *Atmospheric Environment* 2013; 76: 52–8.
55. Hedley's environmental index. [Online]. Available from: http://hedleyindex.sph.hku.hk/home.php [Accessed February 2013].
56. Civic Exchange. The air we breathe: a public health dialogue. Report: Public conference on air quality, Hong Kong, 2009.
57. Loh C, Hedley AJ, Wong TW, Ng S, *et al.* A price too high: the health impacts of air pollution in Southern China. Civic Exchange, Hong Kong, 2008.
58. Environmental Protection Department, Hong Kong. Available from: http://www.epd-asg.gov.hk/english/report/files/background%201999_2012e.pdf [Accessed February 2013].
59. Environmental Protection Department, Hong Kong. Review of Air Quality Objectives and development of a long-term air quality strategy for Hong Kong – feasibility study. Final Report, 2009. Available from: http://www.epd.gov.hk/epd/textonly/english/environmentinhk/air/studyrpts/files/Final_ Report_091013.pdf [Accessed February 2013].
60. Kwok D. Hong Kong–Zhuhai–Macau Bridge Judicial Review: Document 1 – Summary of the Case. Hong Kong: Civic Exchange, 2011.
61. Van Rafelghem M, Modini R. Lessons for Hong Kong: Air Quality Management in London and Los Angeles. Hong Kong: Civic Exchange, 2007.
62. Mayor of London. Clearing the Air: The Mayor's Air Quality Strategy (December 2010). London: Greater London Authority, 2010.
63. Transport for London. Congestion Charging. Available from: http://www.tfl.gov.uk/roadusers/congestioncharging/default.aspx [Accessed February 2013].
64. Beevers SD, Carslaw DC. The impact of congestion charging on vehicle emissions in London. *Atmospheric Environment* 2005, 39(1): 1–5.
65. Transport for London. Low Emission Zone. Available from: http://www.tfl.gov.uk/roadusers/lez/default.aspx [Accessed February 2013].
66. Environmental Research Group. The Air Quality Monitoring Team (Leaflet). London: King's College London, 2004.
67. Mittal L, Fuller G. London Air Quality Network: Summary Report 2010. London: Environmental Research Group, King's College London, December 2012.
68. Air Resources Board, California Environmental Protection Agency. Introduction to the California Air Resources Board (Leaflet). Sacramento, CA: Air Resources Board, 2009.
69. Air Resources Board, California Environmental Protection Agency. California Air Basin Map. Last updated March 2011. Available from: http://www.arb.ca.gov/ei/maps/statemap/abmap.htm [Accessed February 2013].
70. The Ports of Long Beach and Los Angeles. San Pedro Bay Ports Clean Air Action Plan. 2000–2013. Available from: http://www.cleanairactionplan.org [Accessed February 2013].
71. United States Environmental Protection Agency. Air Quality Monitoring Information: Air Quality Trends by City, 1990–2010. Last updated January 2012. Available from: http://www.epa.gov/airtrends/factbook.html [Accessed February 2013].

# 23
# Water
## The public health challenges

*Amal K. Mitra*

Water, water, everywhere, . . . Nor any drop to drink.
*(Samuel Taylor Coleridge, 1797–98)*

## Introduction

About 71 per cent of the Earth's surface is water. According to the World Water Council report, around 1.1 billion people (approximately one in every six people) worldwide do not have access to safe drinking water and around 2.6 billion people do not have improved sanitation facilities [1]. Only 46 per cent of people in Africa have access to safe drinking water. Some of the statistics of disparities in access to water resources in different populations are staggering:

- An American taking a 5-minute shower uses up more water than a typical person uses in a whole day in a developing country slum [1].
- A person in the United Kingdom (UK) uses 50 litres of water daily just by flushing toilets, whereas a person in Sub-Saharan Africa only has 5 litres of water to use for everything in a whole day [1].
- Globally several million hours of women's time is spent every day collecting water for domestic use – one of the most basic human needs [1].
- Almost two in every three people who need safe drinking water survive on less than US$2 per day and one in three on less than US$1 per day [1].
- Thousands of students, especially girls, drop out of school each year because of water insecurity or because they have to help fetch water for their families. Investment in drinking water and sanitation (and consequent reduction of diarrhoea) would result in 272 million more attendance days every year [1].

The Millennium Development Goals' (MDGs) target is to, by 2015, halve the proportion of people without sustainable access to safe drinking water and basic sanitation [1]. Achieving this, the MDG would prevent 470,000 diarrhoeal deaths and this would result in an extra 320 million productive working days per year. In economic terms, each dollar invested in water and sanitation would bring back US$3–34 [2].

## Water scarcity

Today, around 700 million people in 43 countries suffer from water scarcity. By 2025, 1.8 billion people will be living in countries or regions with absolute water scarcity and two-thirds of the world's population could be living under stressed water conditions.

Grades of water scarcity can be defined as follows:

a) Absolute scarcity – annual water availability is below 500 $m^3$ per person;
b) Water scarcity – annual water availability is below 1,000 $m^3$ per person;
c) Water stress – annual water availability is below 1,700 $m^3$ per person [3].

If the existing climate situation doesn't change, almost half the world's population will be living in areas of high water stress by 2030 and this includes between 75 million and 250 million people in Africa. In addition, water scarcity in some arid and semi-arid places will displace between 24 million and 700 million people. Sub-Saharan Africa has the largest number of water-stressed countries of any other region [3].

In the UK, authorities define spending of more than 3 per cent of one's income on water as a hardship. Statistics from El Salvador, Jamaica and Nicaragua indicate that the poorest 20 per cent of households spend more than 10 per cent of their total income on water [1]. Americans are the world's biggest water consumers. Every day, Arizona and parts of New Mexico use 300 million gallons more water than they get in renewable supply. The extra water is extracted from underground supplies. By 2020, California will face a shortfall of fresh water as great as the amount it is consuming today [4].

### *What causes water scarcity?*

*Increased demand* – Population growth results in increased water consumption. Today's 5.3 billion population residing in less developed countries is expected to swell to 7.8 billion in 2050. In India alone, the population rate increases by 18 million people annually. By 2040, India's population is expected to be 1.52 billion and India will become the world's most populous country [5]. In that same year, China's population will be 1.45 billion.

*Over-exploitation of groundwater* – Groundwater is the most important source of water supply in developing countries, including Bangladesh. Groundwater is free from disease-producing micro-organisms, which are normally present in large numbers in surface waters, and can be easily abstracted by installation of wells for the development of water supply systems. However, excessive extraction of groundwater may lower the water tables to critical levels and create water scarcity, especially during dry seasons. Dhaka, the capital of Bangladesh, is on average sinking over half an inch a year because of excessive extraction of groundwater [6].

*Urbanization and industrialization* – The influx of a large number of people from rural to urban areas as a result of urbanization and industrialization increases demand for available water, creates more contamination of water bodies and makes people more vulnerable to water scarcity. In a study conducted in Panzhihua, a mining town in China, the level of urbanization increased from 18 per cent in 1965 to 54 per cent in 2005. Due to the rapid industrialization and population growth, there has been an increase in contaminants in water. The amount of coliform count, chemical oxygen demand (COD) and biological oxygen demand (BOD) in the Jinsha River increased and this has caused a significant reduction in the quality of the surface water [7].

*Global warming* – Earth's average surface temperature increased by about 0.8°C (1.4°F) over the last century with about two-thirds of the increase occurring just over the last three decades. This has been caused by the increasing concentrations of greenhouse gases produced by human activities such as increased $CO_2$ emission, deforestation and burning of fossil fuels. Major greenhouse gases include: water vapour – 36 to 70 per cent; $CO_2$ – 9 to 26 per cent; methane – 4 to 9 per cent; and ozone – 3 to 7 per cent. China and the United States make the most $CO_2$ emissions in the world.

*Contamination of water* – Parameters for drinking water quality typically fall under two categories: chemical/physical and microbiological. Chemical/physical parameters include heavy metals, trace organic compounds, total suspended solids (TSS) and turbidity. Chemical parameters tend to pose more of a chronic health risk through buildup of heavy metals although some components like nitrates/nitrites and arsenic can have a more immediate impact. Physical parameters affect the aesthetics and taste of the drinking water and may complicate the removal of microbial pathogens. Microbiological parameters include Coliform bacteria, *E. coli*, and specific pathogenic species of bacteria (such as cholera-causing *Vibrio cholerae*), viruses and protozoan parasites.

## Water regulations in the United States

The United States (US) Federal Water Pollution Control Act, or Clean Water Act (CWA), was introduced in 1972 (originally enacted in 1948) [8]. The CWA set a new national goal 'to restore and maintain the chemical, physical and biological integrity of the Nation's waters'.

*Point sources* – The 1972 CWA introduced the National Pollutant Discharge Elimination System (NPDES), which is a permit system for regulating point sources of pollution. Point sources may not discharge pollutants to surface waters without a permit from NPDES. This system is managed by the United States Environmental Protection Agency (EPA) in partnership with state environmental agencies. The EPA has authorized 46 states to issue permits directly to the discharging facilities.

*Technology-based standards* – The EPA develops these standards for categories of dischargers based on the performance of pollution control technologies. The intent of Congress was to create a 'level-playing field' by establishing a basic national discharge standard for all facilities on an industry-by-industry basis, using the best available technology.

*Water quality standards* – The 1972 Act authorized continued use of the water quality-based approach but in coordination with the technology-based standards. If water quality is still impaired for the particular water body after application of technology-based standards to a permit, then the permit agency may add water quality-based limitations to that permit.

*Nonpoint sources* – Nonpoint source pollutants, such as sediments, nutrients, pesticides, herbicides, fertilizers, animal wastes and other substances that enter the water supply as components of runoff and groundwater, have increased in relative significance and account for more than 50 per cent of the pollution in US waters.

Agricultural stormwater discharges and irrigation return flows were specifically exempted from permit requirements. Congress provided support for research, technical and financial assistance programmes at the US Department of Agriculture to improve runoff management practices on farms.

Stormwater runoff from industrial sources, municipal storm drains and other sources was not specifically addressed in the 1972 Act. However, the courts ruled that stormwater discharges must be covered by the permit programme. The permit agency began to develop regulations for stormwater permit coverage.

*Financing of pollution controls* – Congress created a major public works financing programme for municipal sewage treatment as part of the CWA. In the initial programme, the federal portion of each grant was up to 75 per cent of a facility's capital cost, with the remainder being financed by the state. In subsequent amendments, Congress reduced the federal proportion of the grants. Industrial and other private facilities are required to finance their own treatment improvements.

*Regulation of groundwater use* – The CWA does not directly address groundwater contamination. Groundwater protection provisions are included in the Safe Drinking Water Act (SDWA), Resource Conservation and Recovery Act, and the Superfund Act.

*Regulation of drinking water* – This is under the control of SDWA, which is the principal federal law. Pursuant to the act, the EPA is required to set standards for drinking water quality and oversee all states, localities and water suppliers that implement these standards. The SDWA applies to every public water system in the US. There are currently more than 150,000 public water systems providing water to almost all Americans at some point in their lives; however, the Act does not cover private wells. The SDWA does not govern bottled water. Bottled water is regulated by the Food and Drug Administration (FDA) body under the Federal Food, Drug and Cosmetic Act.

*Primary drinking water regulations* – The SDWA requires the EPA to establish National Primary Drinking Water Regulations (NPDWRs) for contaminants that may cause adverse public health effects. The regulations include both mandatory levels (Maximum Contaminant Levels or MCLs) and non-enforceable health goals (Maximum Contaminant Level Goals or MCLGs) for each included contaminant [8]. For example, MCL for total coliform count is 5 per cent, whereas the MCLG for coliform count is zero; MCL for polychlorinated biphenyls (PCBs) is 0.0005 mg/L; MCL for inorganic mercury is 0.002 mg/L. Future NPDWR standards will apply to non-transient non-community water systems because of concerns for the long-term exposure of a stable population.

*Enforcement* – The NPDES permit is the CWA's principal enforcement tool. The EPA may issue a compliance order or bring a civil suit in the US district court when there is a violation of the terms of a permit. The CWA provides for substantial penalties for permit violators. The CWA also allows individuals to bring a citizen suit in the US district court against persons who violate a permit limit or standard. Individuals may also bring citizen suits against the EPA's administrator (or equivalent state official) for failure to carry out their duties as specified under the CWA.

## Water regulatory legislations in Hong Kong and Singapore

Hong Kong has already started experiencing effects of climate changes on health [9, 10], and key industries and trades could potentially be affected if the predicted 30-centimetre rise in sea level across the Pearl River Delta occurs in the next 20 years. Hong Kong and Singapore are both developed countries in Asia with well-defined legislation and governmental regulatory frameworks to ensure the steady supply of sanitized water to the public. However, based on the differences in their cultures and their demographic distributions, they are facing different challenges and have taken different approaches to solving these problems.

### Hong Kong

In Hong Kong, drinking water is controlled by the Water Supplies Department. The main functions and services of the Water Supplies Department are to: plan and manage water resources and water supply systems, operate and maintain water supply and distribution systems, control the quality of water supply to customers, design and construct waterworks and enforce the waterworks ordinance and regulations [11].

Under the legislative system, the control of waterworks is under the *Waterworks Ordinance* (chapter 102) and *Waterworks Regulations* (chapter 102A). The enactment covers the duties of the water authority, the fire service and the liability for charges. The water pollution control is governed by *The Water Pollution Control Ordinance* (chapter 358), which was enacted in 1980. Other related ordinances and regulations in Hong Kong are summarized in Table 23.1.

All these environmental legislations are regulated by the Environmental Protection Department. A series of guidelines are established for the individual operators, such as restaurants and factories, which aim to reduce water pollution and to improve sewage treatment.

### Singapore

In Singapore, drinking water is regulated by the Public Utilities Board (PUB) under the Ministry of Environment and Water Resources [12]. Singapore has ensured a stable and sustainable supply of water for its people with an integrated water management and four sources of water supply known as the Four National Taps. These sources include: water from local catchment areas, imported water, reclaimed water known as NEWater and desalinated water.

The main functions of the PUB involve the regulation of water supply, sewer layout, drainage provision and developments within the water catchment area. The legislative requirements are set up for construction of facilities, protection of environmental health, control of water supply and discharge, and for occupational safety. The code of practice on sewerage and sanitary works is regulated by the *Sewerage and Drainage Act* (SDA). Sewer Protection Zone requirements have been established to avoid damaging the public sewerage system. Some other water legislations in Singapore are listed in Table 23.1.

### Water resources

Hong Kong and Singapore are both densely populated industrialized cities. They both have a high demand of fresh water supply for the public. With limited sources of local supply from the reservoirs, Hong Kong and Singapore rely on imported water from the Guangdong Province and Johor, respectively. However, their governments have recognized that even the imported water is not a long-lasting solution to the problem and they have to find alternative solutions to ensure a stable and suitable water supply. Hong Kong has signed a water supply agreement with Guangdong that includes different measures to guarantee that the water supplied to Hong Kong achieves certain standards. Similarly, Singapore has signed a series of agreements with the Malaysian government for the rights to obtain water from the assigned rivers in Malaysia.

*Table 23.1* Water regulations of Hong Kong and Singapore

| | *Hong Kong* | *Singapore* |
|---|---|---|
| Area | 1,067 $km^2$ | 700 $km^2$ |
| Regulatory agency | Water Supplies Department | Public Utilities Board (PUB) |
| Related agency | 1. Development Bureau<br>2. Drainage Services Department<br>3. Electrical and Mechanical Services Department<br>4. Marine Department<br>5. Agriculture, Fisheries and Conservation Department<br>6. Environmental Protection Department | 1. National Environmental Agency<br>2. Land Transport Authority<br>3. Fire Safety Bureau<br>4. Singapore Power<br>5. Urban Redevelopment Authority<br>6. National Parks Board |
| Water source | 1. Rainfall water from natural catchment<br>2. Supply from Guangdong<br>3. Sea water (for flushing) | 1. Imported water (from Johor)<br>2. Local catchment (reservoirs)<br>3. NEWater (recycled water)<br>4. Desalinated water |
| Policy | Raw water sources, the water treatment and distribution, the water quality and the water pollution | Physical infrastructure, legislation and enforcement, water pricing, public education, research and technology |
| Main legislation | 1. Waterworks Ordinance (chapter 102)<br>2. Waterworks Regulations (chapter 102A)<br>3. Water Pollution Control Ordinance (chapter 358)<br>4. Water Pollution Control (Sewerage) Regulation (chapter 358AL)<br>5. Water Pollution Control (General) Regulations<br>6. Water Pollution Control (Appeal Board) Regulations<br>7. Water Pollution Control (Sewerage) Regulation, Waste Disposal Ordinance (chapter 354)<br>8. Public Health and Municipal Services Ordinance (chapter 132)<br>9. Dumping At Sea Ordinance (chapter 466)<br>10. Foreshores and Sea Bed (Reclamations) Ordinance (chapter 127)<br>11. Shipping and Port Control Ordinance (chapter 313)<br>12. Merchant Shipping (Prevention and Control of Pollution) Ordinance (chapter 413) | 1. Sewerage and Drainage Act<br>2. Sewerage and Drainage (Trade Effluent) Regulations<br>3. Sewerage Drainage (Sanitary Works) Regulations<br>4. Sewerage Drainage (Surface Water Drainage) Regulations<br>5. Environmental Protection and Management (Trade Effluent) Regulations<br>6. Environmental Public Health (Quality of Piped Drinking Water) Regulations |
| New developments | Pilot plant study on development of desalination facilities in Hong Kong | Environment and Water Industry Development Council to develop the environmental and water industry; has funding to support research |

### *Water pollution control*

Both Hong Kong and Singapore follow the World Health Organization (WHO) standards for controlling bacteriological and chemical contaminants in their water supplied. Hong Kong established water pollution control in four main areas including the establishment of the *Water Pollution Control Ordinance and Regulations*, the constitution of the Harbour Area Treatment Scheme, the management of municipal wastewater and chemical wastes and the implementation of the 'Polluter Pays Policy' [13]. Since the 1980s, under these regulations, the water environment in Hong Kong has gradually improved. The main challenges still include the waste discharge loading from the Pearl River Delta in mainland China.

On the other hand, the main legislation for controlling sewerage in Singapore is *The Sewage and Drainage Act* (SDA) and six related regulations. The Act also provides for penalties for committing offences of water pollution (Table 23.1).

## National water policy in Bangladesh

The government of the People's Republic of Bangladesh adopted a National Water Policy in 1999 [14]. Major challenges identified in Bangladesh include alternating flood and water scarcity during the wet and dry seasons, ever-expanding water needs of a growing economy and population, and massive river sedimentation and river bank erosion. Due to its location as the lowest riparian, Bangladesh has no control over the rivers entering through its borders. The government will endeavour to enter into agreements with co-riparian countries for sharing waters of international rivers. In addition, the government wants to implement the following major initiatives:

1 Comprehensive development and management of the main rivers through a system of barrages and other structural and non-structural measures;
2 Development of water resources of the main rivers for multipurpose use, including irrigation, fisheries, navigation, forestry and aquatic wildlife;
3 De-silting of watercourses to maintain navigation channels and proper drainage;
4 Delineating of water-stress areas;
5 Protection of the water quality and ensuring efficiency of its use;
6 Development of early warning and flood-proofing systems to manage natural disasters; and
7 Designating flood-risk zones and taking appropriate measures.

The National Water Resources Council coordinates all water resources management activities in the country. Bangladesh passed its Water Pollution Control Ordinance in 1970 and the Environment Pollution Control Ordinance (Ordinance No. XIII) in 1977.

## Effect of climate change on water and infectious diseases

A Public Broadcasting Service (PBS) news broadcast in the US reported effects of climate change on the water problem in Bangladesh before the UN global warming conference in 2009 [15]. Bangladesh is probably the most affected country facing the impact of global warming in the world, mainly because of its low-lying areas, frequent occurrences of natural disasters and poor economic conditions. As a consequence, water-borne diseases including diarrhoea, enteric fever, parasitic diseases and mosquito-borne diseases are hyperendemic in the country. To mitigate the consequences of global warming, several innovative measures have been taken in Bangladesh. Some of the solutions suggested by local experts include:

- Use of cell phone technology to inform people of flood warnings;
- Makeshift housing, called cyclone shelters, in boats;
- Floating classrooms using boats;
- Use of flood-resistant rice crops;
- Embankments; and
- Possible use of silt sediments to create new islands.

There is also a growing body of evidence that suggests that climate change will be responsible for the rapidly multiplying rate at which infectious diseases are spreading. Table 23.2 summarizes findings of the effect of climate change on infectious diseases. Vector-borne diseases, which are spread by arthropod species (such as ticks, mosquitoes, flies), are especially sensitive to projected changes in ecological and environmental conditions such as temperature and precipitation [16]. This is because the temperature determines the rate at which insect babies develop into adults, the frequency of their feeding on blood, the rate at which pathogens are acquired and the development of the pathogens themselves inside their vectors. Because these vectors lack thermostatic mechanisms, their body temperature is highly influenced by the ambient temperature [17] (see chapters 19 and 20).

Some diseases that most worry scientists in relation to climate change include malaria, dengue fever, West Nile fever (WNF), cholera, Crimean-Congo haemorrhagic fever, avian influenza, ebola haemorrhagic fever, parasitic infections, Lyme disease and yellow fever. The humid and warm climate in Asia creates perfect conditions for the proliferation of malaria's vectors. A strong association between rising temperatures and increased malaria incidence was observed in the highlands of Kenya [18]. New cases of malaria have been reported in Afghanistan, east Africa and the Indonesia highlands, where previously the malaria vector mosquito had not been able to thrive.

Scientists estimate that dengue fever, another mosquito-borne illness, will continue to emerge in industrialized areas in developing countries in stronger numbers due to warmer global temperatures [19]. In Mexico, the number of dengue cases increased by 600 per cent from 2001 to 2007. Scientists have found that dengue cases in the country have increased by 2.6 per cent for every 1°C increase in weekly maximum temperatures and by 1.9 per cent for every one centimetre increase in weekly precipitation in the period between 1995 and 2005 [20].

Many episodes of WNF occur during or after drought when mosquitoes and birds are brought together in close proximity to available water sources and facilitate the transmission of the disease. Scientists examined 16,298 cases of WNF reported to the Centres for Disease Control and Prevention (CDC) from 2001 to 2005. Warmer temperatures, elevated humidity and heavy precipitation significantly increased the incidence rate of WNF in North America [21].

It has been also suggested in scientific literature that leishmaniasis has emerged in some parts of the Americas as a result of the El Niño/Southern Oscillation (ENSO). In Brazil, researchers observed that there was an increase in visceral leishmaniasis incidences after the El Niño years of 1989 and 1995 [22]. In Bangladesh, attack rates of cholera increased from 0.25 per 1,000 to 10.9 per 1,000, leading to a big epidemic after a devastating cyclone in the southern parts of the country in May 2005 [23].

*Table 23.2* Relation between infectious diseases and climatic changes

| *Author, year* | *Disease* | *Place* | *Methods* | *Major findings* |
|---|---|---|---|---|
| D'Souza *et al.* 2004 [39] | Salmonellosis | Five major cities in Australia, 1991–2001 | Log-linear model between monthly reports of salmonellosis and temperature | A positive correlation between seasonal patterns of salmonellosis and increased temperature. |
| Hales *et al.* 2002 [40] | Dengue fever | Global | Review of global distribution of cases of dengue fever in relation to humidity | With population and climate change projections for 2085, about 5–6 billion people (50–60% of the projected global population) would be at risk of dengue transmission, compared with 3.5 billion people, or 35% of the population, if climate change did not happen. |
| Ludwig *et al.* 2005 [41] | West Nile fever | Camargue, France, 2000 | Cross-sectional study | The aggressiveness of the mosquito vector (*Culex modestus*) was positively correlated with temperature, humidity, rainfall and sunshine during the periods of higher incidence of WNF. |
| Nichols *et al.* 2009 [42] | Infections due to *E. coli, Giardia, Cryptosporidium, Salmonella typhi, S. paratyphi, Campylobacter* | England and Wales, 1910–1999 | Case-crossover study | There was a significant association between excess cumulative rainfall in the previous 7 days and outbreaks ($p = 0.001$). |
| Reacher *et al.* 2004 [43] | Gastroenteritis and psychological distress | Southern England, 2000 | Historical case-control study | With the depth of flooding, a significant increase in risk of gastroenteritis (RR 1.7 [0.9, 3.0] *P* for trend by flood depth = 0.04); adults had a four-times higher risk of psychological distress (RR 4.1 [2.6, 6.4], *P* for trend by flood depth = 0.01). |
| Wang Lu-xi *et al.* 2012 [44] | Typhoid and paratyphoid fever (TPF) | Guizhou, China, 1984–2007 | Cross-sectional study | A strong correlation between incidence of TPF and climate variables, such as monthly average temperature ($r = 0.549$, $p < 0.001$) and precipitation ($r = 0.477$, $p < 0.001$). |
| Xiaodong Liu *et al.* 2011 [45] | Hanta virus haemorrhagic fever | Shenyang, China, 2004–2009 | Cross-sectional study; cross-correlation and autocorrelation analysis | The monthly trends of haemorrhagic fever were significantly associated with temperature, relative humidity, precipitation, air pressure and wind velocity. |

## Industrial and agricultural contamination of water

The common heavy metals and chemicals from industrial and agricultural discharges polluting water include lead, arsenic, mercury, chromium, PCBs, as well as others.

### *Dioxins*

A 22-year study of people in Japan who ate rice oil highly contaminated with PCBs and other dioxin-like compounds showed a 3.4-fold increase (95 per cent confidence intervals, 1.8 to 6.0) in liver cancer. People living near the Seveso herbicide chemical plants in Italy and the herbicide plant workers were heavily exposed to dioxins in 1976 [24]. The people exposed to dioxins developed more of all types of cancers combined than the general population and the number of cancers increased with exposure (dose–response relationship). Polychlorinated dibenzodioxins (PCDD), or simply dioxins, are a group of organic polyhalogenated compounds that are significant environmental pollutants.

There are 75 different PCDD congeners related to dioxin. Congeners that have chlorines in the two, three, seven and eight positions have been found to be significantly toxic. MCL for dioxin is 0.00000003 milligrams per litre (mg/L) or 30 parts per quadrillion and MCGL for dioxin is zero. The major sources of dioxin in drinking water are emissions from waste incineration and other combustion, and discharge from chemical factories. Dioxins and furans can enter the body through breathing contaminated air, drinking contaminated water or eating contaminated food. About 90 per cent of exposure to dioxins and furans is from eating contaminated food, including food cooked with contaminated water. Occupational exposure occurs through a municipal solid waste incinerator, copper smelter, cement kiln or coal-fired power plant. Individuals who burn their household waste or burn wood can be exposed as well. Even forest fires can contribute to the creation of small amounts of dioxins and furans.

Health effects of dioxin poisoning include developmental abnormalities in the enamel of children's teeth, central and peripheral nervous system pathology, thyroid disorders, damage to immune systems, endometriosis and diabetes.

### *Minamata disease*

The Minamata disease is a neurological syndrome caused by severe mercury poisoning. Symptoms include ataxia or lack of muscle coordination, numbness in the hands and feet, general muscle weakness, narrowing of the field of vision, damage to hearing and speech and, in extreme cases, insanity, paralysis, coma and even death. A congenital form of the disease can also affect foetuses in the womb.

It was first detected in the Japanese city of Minamata in 1956 and affected 2,265 victims from March 2001, resulting in 1,784 deaths [25]. Over 10,000 received financial compensation from the Chisso Corporation's chemical factory, which caused methyl mercury poisoning though the industry's wastewater discharge. By 2004, Chisso Corporation had paid US$86 million in compensation and, in the same year, was ordered to clean up its contamination. On 29 March 2010, a settlement was reached to compensate as-yet uncertified victims.

This highly toxic chemical accumulated in shellfish and fish in the Minamata Bay and the Shiranui Sea in Japan, which, when eaten by the local populace, resulted in mercury poisoning. The methyl mercury that caused the Minamata disease is a type of organic mercury which is easily absorbed from the stomach into the blood and carried to the liver and kidney, and then the brain and even the foetus.

## *Vota Dam: a man-made problem*

The Akosombo Dam (also referred to as the Akosombo Hydroelectric Project) is a hydroelectric dam on the Volta River in south-eastern Ghana. The primary purpose of the Akosombo Dam was to provide electricity for the aluminium industry. The Akosombo Dam was called 'the largest single investment in the economic development plans of Ghana'. It benefited from some industrial and economic activities with the addition of lake transportation, increased fishing, new farming activities along the shoreline and tourism [26]. The power generated provided primarily for Ghana, while also supplying power to the neighboring countries of Togo and Benin.

Following the construction of the dam at Akosombo, there has been a steady decline in agricultural productivity along the lake and the associated tributaries. Upstream agricultural systems are losing soil fertility without the periodic flooding that brought nutrients to the soil before the natural river flow was halted by the dam. The nutrient enrichment, in combination with the low water movement, has allowed for the invasion of aquatic weeds (*Cerratophyllum*). The weeds provide the necessary habitat for black-fly, mosquitoes and snails, which are the vectors of water-borne illnesses. Therefore, incidence of some diseases such as schistosomiasis, river blindness and malaria increased as an after-effect of the Volta Dam [26]. In a survey of children from the village of Mepe, Ghana, it was shown that the prevalence of schistosomiasis in children who had visited the Volta Lake at least once was six times higher than those who had never visited the lake (69.9 per cent versus 10.7 per cent) [27].

## *Lead poisoning*

Most of the symptoms of lead poisoning are non-specific and include nausea, vomiting, abdominal pain, diarrhoea, loss of appetite, weakness, lethargy, paresis, convulsions, coma, falling behind in class, retarded growth, blue colouration of gums, anaemia and abnormal behaviour. In most cases, there are no visible symptoms. That is why a blood test remains the only way to detect if someone is suffering from lead poisoning.

Ideally, there should be zero level of lead in the blood. Blood lead level (BLL) of $\geq$ 10 μg/dL is called an elevated level [28] because children show symptoms when BLL is as low as 10 μg/dL. Symptoms from having a high BLL include developmental delays [29], deficits in behavioural functioning [30], decreased stature [31] and diminished hearing acuity [32]. BLLs of $\geq$ 70 μg/dL can cause serious side-effects, such as seizures, coma and death [33]. If BLL is elevated, it should be measured again. If BLL is 45 μg/dL or higher, CDC recommends treatment using a chelating agent in order to remove the lead from the body; however, chelating agents should be used with caution [28].

Lead can enter the human body through air, dust, water or soil. In the air, industrial discharges may contain lead. Such sources of lead include industries or small factories that make battery, cement, ceramics, plastic materials, pharmaceutical products, steel, paint, varnish and glazing materials (see Figure 23.1), or workshops for printing, welding and car repairs. Other common sources of lead were leaded gasoline (before it was banned) and lead-containing house paints (in old houses). Some other less common sources of lead may include imported toys, indigenous medicines and lead-based water pipes.

### Mississippi data

Analysis of secondary data of 42,372 children aged over 5 years in Mississippi from January 1999 to February 2003 shows that the following counties were at high risk (12 per cent or

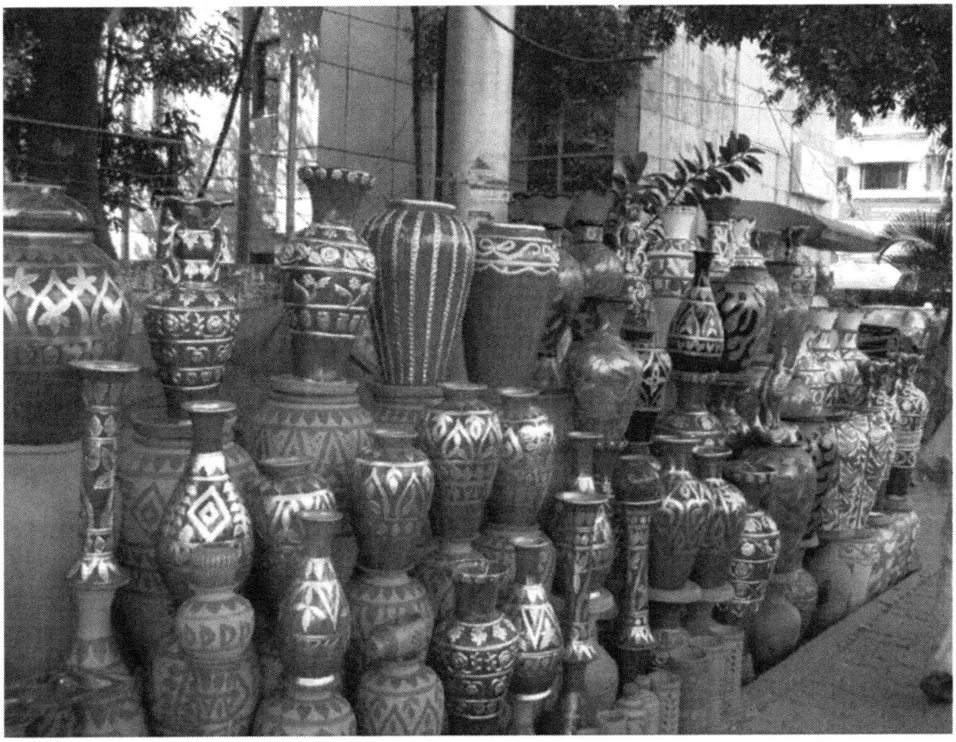

*Figure 23.1* Glazing materials used for potteries may contain lead. This picture was taken in Dhaka, Bangladesh

more children with elevated BLL): Forrest, Oktibbeha, Covington, Coahoma, Greene, Grenada, Pike, Jones and Yazoo (see Figure 23.2).

The proportion of African-Americans with BLL ≥ 10 μg/dL was higher than that of Caucasians (5.6 per cent versus 3.1 per cent). Counties where most of the pre-1950 housing units were located, such as Montgomery, Pike, Adams, Attala, Quitman, Humphreys, Amite, Franklin, Copiah and Webster, had a higher average percentage of children with BLL ≥ 10 μg/dL than the other counties (6.5 per cent versus 4 per cent) [34].

## Bangladesh data

Blood samples collected from 860 school children in six communities during 2007–2009 showed an alarming proportion of children with high BLLs (see Figure 23.3 for blood lead levels in children in urban and rural areas in Bangladesh). In the industrial area of Tongi, about 18 kilometres away from Dhaka city, 104 out of 105 children had high BLLs [35]. Of them, six had BLLs ≥ 45 μg/dL, a level that requires treatment. In another area in Dhaka, where leather tannery factories are located, Jigatola, 91 per cent of 170 school children showed high BLLs. Even in a rural community, Chirirbandar, where no major industries are located, 15 per cent of 197 children had elevated BLLs. According to the CDC guidelines, all these areas were at high risk (12 per cent or more children with high BLLs). These data indicate that an immediate policy is needed for the country to screen blood lead levels of all children aged less than 6 years, as suggested by CDC.

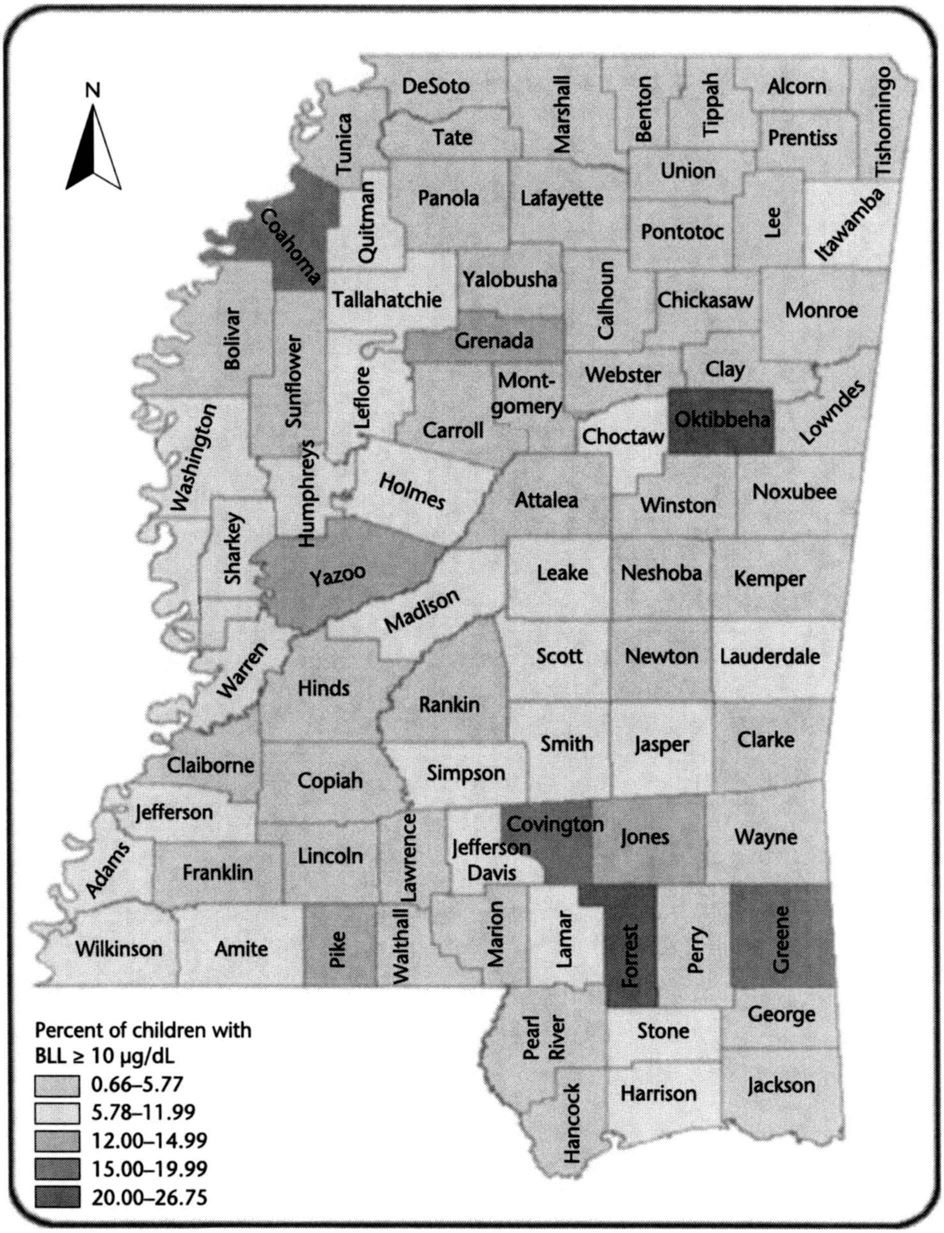


*Figure 23.2* Distribution of children with high blood lead levels in Mississippi, 1999–2003

## *Arsenic poisoning*

The safe level of arsenic in drinking water is 0.01 mg/L; however, the Bangladesh standard is 0.05 mg/L. The food safety limit of arsenic is 1.0 mg/kg. A number of countries including Bangladesh, India, China, Taiwan, Japan, Argentina, Mexico and some parts of the US (Michigan, Minnesota, South Dakota, Oklahoma and Wisconsin) have high concentrations

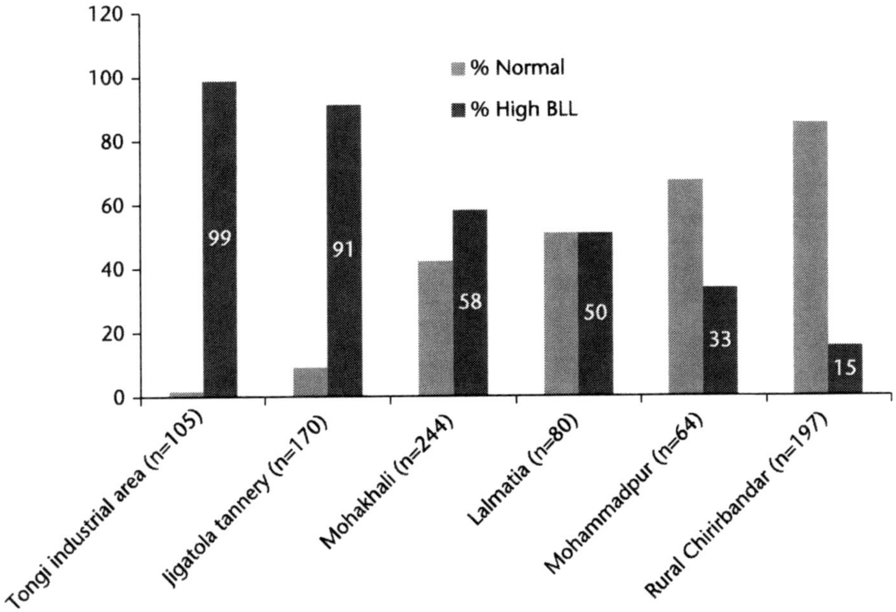


*Figure 23.3* Blood lead levels in children in urban and rural areas in Bangladesh

of arsenic in their water supplies. The case of Bangladesh is especially alarming. About 30 per cent of 10 million shallow tubewells are highly contaminated. A total of 269 out of Bangladesh's 464 administrative units, called *upazilla*, contain high levels of arsenic-contaminated drinking water.

Chronic arsenic poisoning, arsenicosis, can increase the risk of several health hazards such as skin lesions, cancers, restrictive pulmonary disease, peripheral vascular disease (black-foot disease), gangrene, hypertension, non-cirrhotic portal fibrosis, ischemic heart disease and diabetes mellitus. Skin lesions of arsenic poisoning show a typical 'rain-drop appearance' of pigmentation and depigmentation of skin, especially common on the palm, hands and chest (see Figure 23.4). In a sample of 100 hospital patients in southern Bangladesh [36], sites of the skin lesions were predominantly trunk (38 per cent), hands only (18 per cent), both hands and feet (15 per cent), feet only (13 per cent) and chest only (11 per cent). Hyperkeratosis (hardened skin) appears predominantly on the palms and the bottom surface of the foot.

Another study carried out in Bangladesh showed that arsenic has contaminated some of the food chain [37]. Arsenic levels were not high in rice grains but were high in straw. Cattle may have the adverse health effects by eating contaminated straw and humans may be exposed via the plant–animal–human pathway. Also, some vegetables such as potatoes (0.07–1.36 mg/kg), *kachu sak* (*Colocasia antiquorum*; common names include elephant-ear, taro and cocoyam) (0.09–3.99 mg/kg) and *kalmi sak* (*Ipomoea reptoms*; English name is kang kong) (0.1–1.53 mg/kg) had relatively higher concentrations of arsenic. This preliminary study suggested monitoring the arsenic contaminations of the food chain in the country.

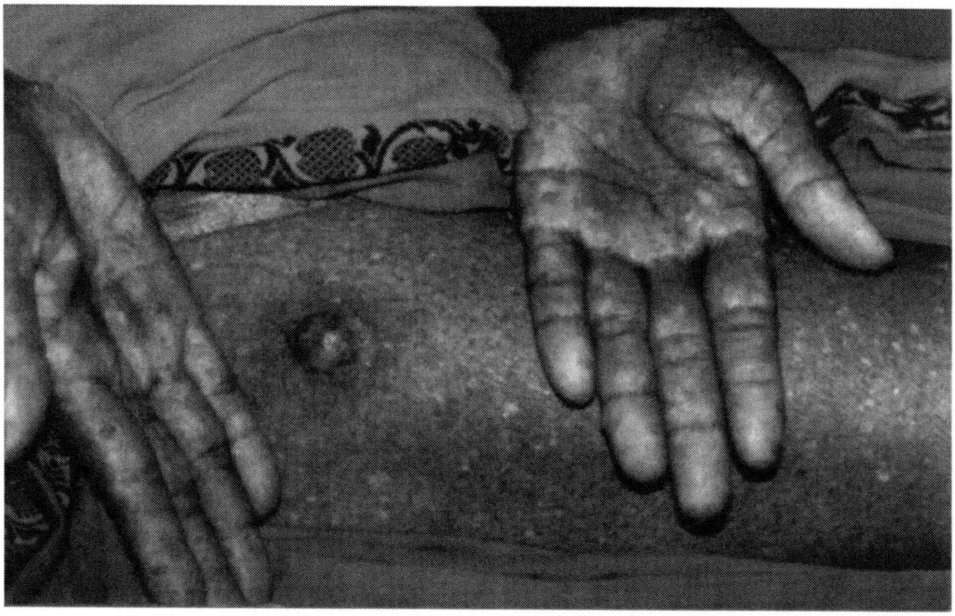

*Figure 23.4* Characteristic rain-drop skin lesions on palms and feet of a 42-year-old woman. She also had a skin noudle, which, on biopsy, showed squamous cell carcinoma

### Methods of arsenic removal

Once contaminated with arsenic, water can be purified by several methods. Use of sono-filter is a popular and low-cost technology – multiple containers with coarse sand, brick chips, wood charcoal and composite iron matrix are used to remove arsenic and other toxic materials from groundwater [38]. Membrane techniques, such as nanofiltration and reverse osmosis are highly efficient in removing arsenic and other contaminants in water. However, these methods involve a high cost and advanced technology. Another method of using cattail plants (*Typha latifolia*) has had around an 89 per cent efficacy in removing arsenic in water after six weeks [46]).

## Conclusion

Providing access to safe drinking water for the vast majority of the population in developing countries is an enormous challenge. Climate changes and global warming, together with rapid population growth, urbanization, over-exploitation of groundwater, bacteriological contamination of surface water and inadequate use of other sources of water, such as rainwater, increase the burden of water scarcity. The CWA sets the standards for monitoring and restoring safe drinking water in the United States. However, many developing countries are not aligned with the Millennium Development Goals' target to halve the proportion of people without sustainable access to safe drinking water and basic sanitation by 2015. According to the World Bank, Singapore, one of Asia's most developed countries, has already achieved a 100 per cent rate in providing a safe and sustainable drinking water supply and improved sanitation facilities in 2008. Provision of adequate water supply in Hong Kong has always been a problem because of the lack of natural lakes and rivers, insufficient groundwater sources and an increasing burden of urban population. About 70 per cent of the water demand in Hong Kong is met by importing water from its neighbouring province. For most other developing countries in the region, such as Bangladesh, India, and many others, providing safe drinking water to most of the population is still a big challenge.

## References

1. United Nations Development Programme. Human Development Report 2006. Beyond scarcity: Power, poverty and the global water crisis. New York; 2006: 2–65.
2. World Health Organization. Costs and benefits of water and sanitation improvements at the global level. Available from: http://www.who.int/water_sanitation_health/wsh0404summary/en/ [Accessed 23 May 2012].
3. United Nations Department of Economic and Social Affairs (UNDESA). International Decade for Action 'Water for Life' 2005–2015. Water Scarcity. Available from: http://www.un.org/waterforlifedecade/scarcity.shtml [Accessed 23 May 2012].
4. Kimball, J. Water scarcity in the US. Available from: http://8020vision.com/2010/06/27/water-scarcity-in-the-us/ [Accessed 12 November 2012].
5. Rogenberg, M. China population: the population growth of the world's largest country. Available from: http://geography.about.com/od/populationgeography/a/chinapopulation.htm [Accessed 23 May 2012].
6. Daily Star. Groundwater loss puts city at risk. Available from: http://www.thedailystar.net/new Design/news-details.php?nid=217458 [Accessed 12 May 2012].
7. Teng, Y, Yang, J, Zuo, R, Wang, J. Impact of urbanization and industrialization upon surface water quality: a pilot study of Panzhihua mining town. *Journal of Earth Science* 2011; 22(5): 658–68.
8. US Environmental Protection Agency. National Pollutant Discharge Elimination System (NPDES). Clean Water Act. Available from: http://cfpub.epa.gov/npdes/cwa.cfm?program_id=45 [Accessed 12 May 2012].
9. Chan, E.Y, Goggins, W.B, Kim, J.J, Griffiths, S.M. A study of intracity variation of temperature-related mortality and socioeconomic status among the Chinese population in Hong Kong. *Journal Epidemiol Community Health* 2012; 66(4): 322–7.
10. Chan, E.Y, Goggins, W.B, Kim, J.J, Griffiths, S, Ma, T.K. Help-seeking behavior during elevated temperature in Chinese population. *Journal Urban Health* 2011; 88(4): 637–50.
11. Water Supplies Department. Principal functions and services. Available from: http://www.wsd.gov.hk/filemanager/en/share/pdf/wsd_leaflet_e.pdf [Accessed 1 May 2012].
12. Public Utilities Board (PUB). Singapore's National Water Agency. Available from: http://www.pub.gov.sg/Pages/default.aspx [Accessed 1 May 2012].
13. Hua, F.L, Tsang, Y.F, Chua, H. Progress of water pollution control in Hong Kong. *Aquatic Ecosystem Health & Management* 2008; 11(2): 225–9.
14. Ministry of Water Resources, Government of the People's Republic of Bangladesh. National Water Policy. Dhaka: 30 January 1999.
15. Public Broadcasting Service. Water world. Available from: http://www.pbs.org/now/shows/543/index.html [Accessed 23 May 2012].
16. Lafferty, K.D. The ecology of climate change and infectious diseases. *Ecology* 2009; 90(4): 888–900.
17. Semenza, J.C, Suk, J.E, Estevez, V, Ebi, K.L, Lindgren, E. Mapping climate change vulnerabilities to infectious diseases in Europe. *Environmental Health Perspectives* 2011; 120: 385–92.
18. Githeko, A.K, Ndegwa, W. Predicting malaria epidemics in the Kenyan highlands using climate data: a tool for decision makers. *Global Change & Human Health* 2001; 2(1): 54–63.
19. Pahomov, L. Reemergence of dengue fever in Argentina as a result of climate change. *Eukaryon* 2011; 7: 87–91.
20. Brunkard, J.M, Cifuentes, E, Rothenberg, S.J. Assessing the roles of temperature, precipitation, and ENSO in dengue re-emergence on the Texas–Mexico border region. *Salud Publica Mex* 2008; 50(3): 227–34.

21. Soverow, J.E, Wellenius, G.A, Fisman, D.N, Mittleman, M.A. Infectious disease in a warming world: how weather influenced West Nile Virus in the United States (2001–2005). *Environmental Health Perspectives* 2009; 117(7): 1049–52.
22. Chaves, L.F, Pascual, M. Climate cycles and forecasts of cutaneous leishmaniasis, a nonstationary vector-borne disease. *PLoS Medicine* 2006; 3: e295.
23. Siddique, A.K, Islam, Q, Akram, K, Mazumder, Y, Mitra, A, Eusof, A. Cholera epidemic and natural disaster: where is the link? *Tropical and Geographic Medicine* 1989; 41: 377–82.
24. Wikipedia. Dioxins and dioxin-like compounds. Available from: http://en.wikipedia.org/wiki/Dioxins_and_dioxin-like_compounds [Accessed 20 April 2012].
25. Ministry of the Environment, Government of Japan. Minamata disease: the history and measures. Available from: http://www.env.go.jp/en/chemi/hs/minamata2002/ [Accessed 20 April 2012].
26. Zakhary, K. Factors affecting the prevalence of schistosomiasis in the Volta region of Ghana. *McGill Journal of Medicine* 2007. Available from: http://www.medicine.mcgill.ca/mjm/v03n02/v03p093/v03p093fs.htm [Accessed 20 April 2012].
27. Jones CR. WHO Report on the Health Component in the Volta Lake Project. Accra, Ghana; 1973.
28. CDC. CDC Lead poisoning prevention and treatment recommendations for refugee children. Available from: http://www.cdc.gov/nceh/lead/Publications/RefugeeToolKit/pdfs/MedicalTechnicalBrief.pdf [Accessed 22 April 2012].
29. Schnaas, L, Rothenberg, S.J, Flores, M.F, Martinez, S, Hernandez, C, Osorio, E, *et al.* Reduced intellectual development in children with prenatal lead exposure. *Environmental Health Perspectives* 2006; 114(5): 791–7.
30. Eubig, P.A, Aguiar, A, Schantz, S.L. Lead and PCBs as risk factors for attention deficit/hyperactivity disorder. *Environmental Health Perspectives* 2010; 118: 1654–67.
31. Frisancho, A.R, Ryan, A.S. Decreased stature associated with moderate blood lead concentrations in Mexican-American children. *American Journal of Clinical Nutrition* 1991; 54(3): 516–19.
32. Staudinger, K.C, Roth, V.S. Occupational lead poisoning. *American Family Medicine* 1998; 57(4): 719–26.
33. Meyer, P.A, Pivetz, T, Dignam, T.A, Homa, D.M, Schoonover, J, Brody, D. Surveillance for elevated blood lead levels among children – United States, 1997–2001. *Morbidity and Mortality Weekly Report* 2003; 52(SS10): 1–21.
34. Mitra, A.K, Downey, J, Ahua, E. Community-based lead outreach and training in Mississippi. Honolulu: Pacific Global Health Conference; 2012.
35. Mitra, A.K, Ahua, E, Saha, P. Prevalence of and risk factors for lead poisoning in young children in Bangladesh. *Journal of Health Population and Nutrition* 2012; 30(4): 404–9.
36. Mitra, A.K, Bose, B.K, Kabir, H, Das, B.K, Hussain, M. Arsenic-related health problems among hospital patients in southern Bangladesh. *Journal of Health Population and Nutrition* 2012; 20: 198–204.
37. Das, H.K, Mitra, A.K, Sengupta, P.K, Hossain, A, Islam, F, Rabbani, G.H. Arsenic concentrations in rice, vegetables, and fish in Bangladesh: a preliminary study. *Environment International* 2004; 30: 383–7.
38. Hussam, A, Munir, A.K.M. SONO water filter: a sustainable solution for arsenic crisis and clean drinking water. Available from: http://chemistry.gmu.edu/faculty/hussam/Arsenic%20Filters/sonofilter_new.pdf [Accessed 1 May 2012].
39. D'Souza, R.M, Becker, N.G, Hall, G, Moodie, K.B. Does ambient temperature affect foodborne disease? *Epidemiology* 2004; 15: 86–92.
40. Hales, S, de Wet, N, Maindonald, J, Woodward, A. Potential effect of population and climate changes on global distribution of dengue fever: an empirical model. *Lancet* 2002; 360: 830–4.
41. Ludwig, A, Bicout, D, Chalvet-Monfray, K, Sabatier, P. Modeling the aggressiveness of the Culex modestus, possible vector of West Nile fever in Camargue, as a function of meteorological data. *Environnement, Risques & Santu* 2005; 4: 109–13.
42. Nichols, G, Lane, C, Asgari, N, Verlander, N.Q, Charlett, A. Rainfall and outbreaks of drinking water related diseases in England and Wales. *Journal of Water and Health* 2009; 7: 1–8.
43. Reacher, M, McKenzie, K, Lane, C, Nichols, T, Kedge, I, Iversen, A, *et al.* Health impacts of flooding in Lewes: a comparison of reported gastrointestinal and other illness and

mental health in flooded and non-flooded households. *Communicable Disease and Public Health* 2004; 7: 39–46.
44. Wang, Lu-xi, Li, Xiu-Jun, Fang, Li-Qun, Wang, Duo-Chun, Cao, Wu-Chun, Kan, Biao. Association between the incidence of typhoid and paratyphoid fever and meteorological variables in Guizhou, China. *Chinese Medical Journal* 2012; 125(3): 455–60.
45. Xiaodong, Liu, Baofa, Jiang, Weidong, Gu, Qiyong, Liu. Temporal trend and climate factors of hemorrhagic fever with renal syndrome epidemic in Shenyang City, China. *BMC Infectious Diseases* 2011; 11: 331.
46. Cattail plants grow in shaded wetlands, such as marshes, swamps and other areas of stagnant water. [Online]. Available from: http://www.blueplanetgreenliving.com/wp-content/uploads/2009/08/cattails-glen.jpg

# 24

# Food security and safety in China and Hong Kong

*Y. Y. Ho and Constance Chan*

## Introduction: safeguarding food safety in Hong Kong

Built from 'barren rock with hardly a house upon it', as described by a British colonist in 1841, Hong Kong transformed from an entrepôt into a global financial centre under British rule. The economy of Hong Kong took off in the 1970s and in the space of some 30 years, Hong Kong's GDP caught up with some developed economies. The economic achievement earned Hong Kong a place as one of the Four Asian Tigers. On 1 July 1997, China resumed sovereignty over Hong Kong and it became a special administrative region of the People's Republic of China. Under the 'one country, two systems' concept, Hong Kong's capitalist political system continues to thrive and the region's free port status maintains. With a land area of only about 1,100 $km^2$, 7 million people call Hong Kong home. While over 90 per cent of the population is of Chinese descent, Hong Kong also houses a sizeable international population.

In terms of culture, Hong Kong is a melting pot of Western and Chinese cultures. Food enjoyment is an important facet of people's daily lives. Hong Kong is widely recognized as a gourmet paradise, with a rich collection of enticing Chinese, Asian and Western cuisines. Hong Kong's economy is largely service-based, with very little local food production. Hong Kong depends almost entirely on imported food, in particular, fresh food from mainland China, and China meets some 50 per cent of Hong Kong's food demand. Due to the globalization of the food trade, food from every corner of the world is also available in Hong Kong. With rising expectations of the community on food safety, food safety management is increasingly difficult and challenging. A food incident that occurs at one corner of the world may spread to another corner in days, if not hours. International collaboration of national food safety authorities holds the key to effective food safety control that travels across international borders. Hong Kong is no exception. The local food safety authority works closely with various food safety authorities, in particular its mainland China counterparts, to ensure that only safe food enters the local market.

This chapter describes risk analysis, the food safety regulatory framework adopted in Hong Kong and how its three components work together. The chapter also uses the incident caused by melamine abuse in milk as a case study to illustrate how food safety can have an immense public health impact. It may also have a long-standing impact on a country's supply of a certain product (in this case, on China's milk supply).

## Establishment of the Centre for Food Safety

Ten years before and after the turn of the bi-millennium, many countries around the world were hit by food safety scares. Bovine spongiform encephalitis (BSE) in the United Kingdom, and dioxins and genetically modified (GM) food scares in Europe, for example, exposed weaknesses in food safety control systems. In response, many countries reorganized their food safety control systems. Locally, following a spate of food incidents that shook the confidence of the community in the government's ability to cope effectively with food safety issues, the Centre for Food Safety (CFS) was established under the Food and Environmental Hygiene Department (FEHD) in May 2006. The establishment of the CFS allows the administration to be more focused on controlling and regulating goods. The CFS has faced and continues to face various food safety challenges. The Sudan dyes in duck eggs incident in 2006, the melamine in dairy products incident in 2008, the salmonella contamination of food in the United States (US) in 2009, dioxin contamination of food in Germany in 2011, radiation contamination of food arising from the Fukushima nuclear power plant incident in Japan in 2011 and plasticizers in Taiwanese drinks in 2011 are some of the more prominent examples. With a stronger staff complement, a better organization structure and enhanced capacity, the CFS rose to the challenges and successfully tackled these incidents. The CFS earned the respect of the local community, as well as the recognition of overseas authorities. In October 2010, the CFS became a World Health Organization (WHO) Collaborating Centre for Risk Analysis of Chemicals in Food. More than ever, the CFS works enthusiastically with international organizations, such as the WHO, and with other countries in the region.

## The risk analysis framework of the Centre for Food Safety

Headed by the Controller, Centre for Food Safety, the CFS adopts the risk analysis framework advocated by WHO and the United Nations Food and Agriculture Organization (FAO) [1]. Under the risk analysis framework, there are three components: risk assessment, risk management and risk communication (see Figure 24.1). The framework covers the food supply chain 'from farm to table', and includes primary production, processing, wholesale and retail. An organization chart can be seen in Figure 24.2.

The CFS has a multidisciplinary team, which includes public health physicians and nurses, veterinarians, health inspectors and professional staff with expertise covering a wide range of food-related disciplines, including food microbiology, nutrition, food science and technology, toxicology, food chemistry and food biotechnology. However, the government cannot work alone in safeguarding food safety. Tripartite collaboration of the government, food industry and consumers is the cornerstone of food safety.

### *Risk assessment*

Under the risk analysis framework, risk assessment forms the scientific basis for risk management and risk communication. In risk assessment, it is necessary to make a clear distinction between the concepts of 'hazard' and 'risk'. A food hazard can be categorized as a biological, chemical or physical hazard, which has the potential to cause harm to humans. Some common examples of hazards are salmonella organisms, environmental pollutants and food additives.

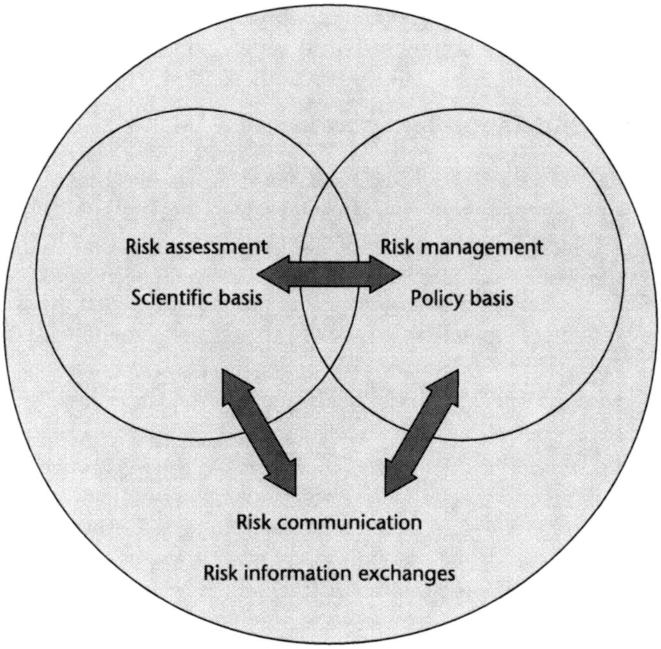


*Figure 24.1* Interaction of the three components of the risk analysis framework [7]

The probability that a hazard can cause harm is termed as its risk. There are four steps in conducting a risk assessment:

1 Hazard identification;
2 Hazard characterization;
3 Exposure assessment; and
4 Risk characterization (see Figure 24.3).

The dosage determines whether a hazard can cause harm. Without exposure, there will be no risk, and an accurate estimation of exposure can better characterize the risk. Through this risk assessment process, hazards associated with food or food ingredients are evaluated and potential risk to the population is assessed, facilitating the formulation of appropriate risk management actions and risk communication messages to protect public health.

Risk assessment remains a weak link under the risk analysis framework, particularly in developing countries. The CFS puts in a lot of effort in building its risk assessment capacity. Exposure assessment is an essential component of the risk assessment process. Accurate estimation of food consumption holds the key to its success. Risk from food depends not only on the nature and level of hazards present in food, but also on the amount of consumption of that particular food.

After its establishment, the CFS conducted the first territory-wide population-based Food Consumption Survey to collect information on the food consumption patterns of the public and published the results in 2010 [2]. With the availability of population food consumption data, the total diet study (TDS) was conducted, which is a specific tool for estimating the dietary exposure to chemicals or nutrients across the total diet. It is recognized

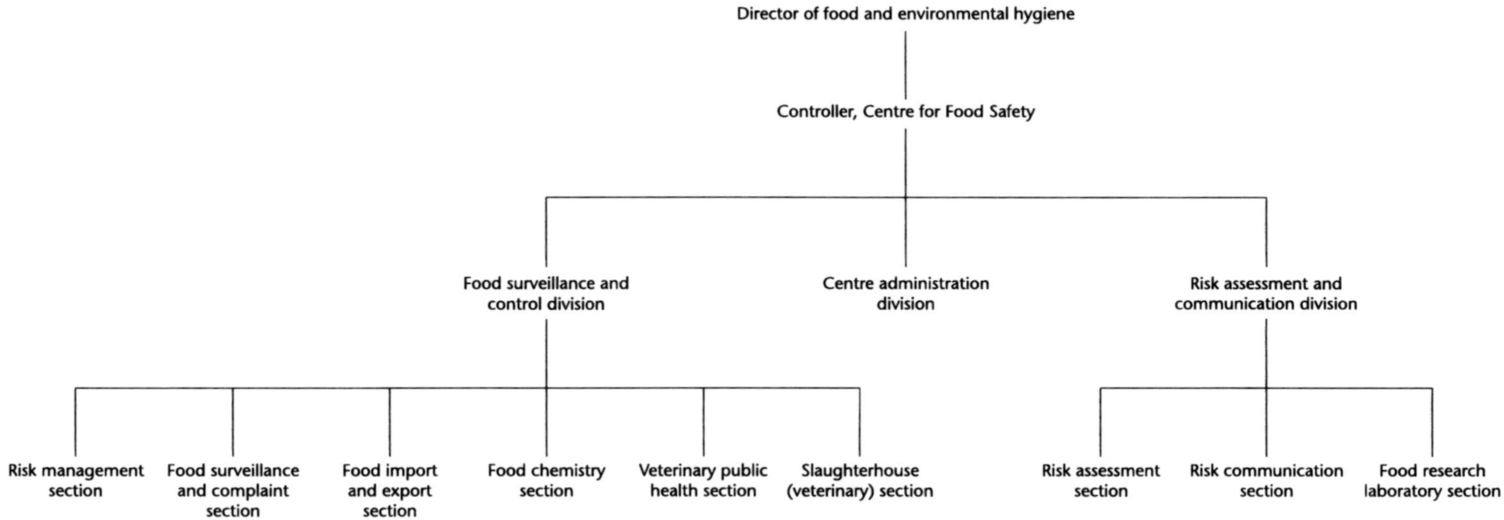


*Figure 24.2* Organizational chart of the Centre for Food Safety [6]

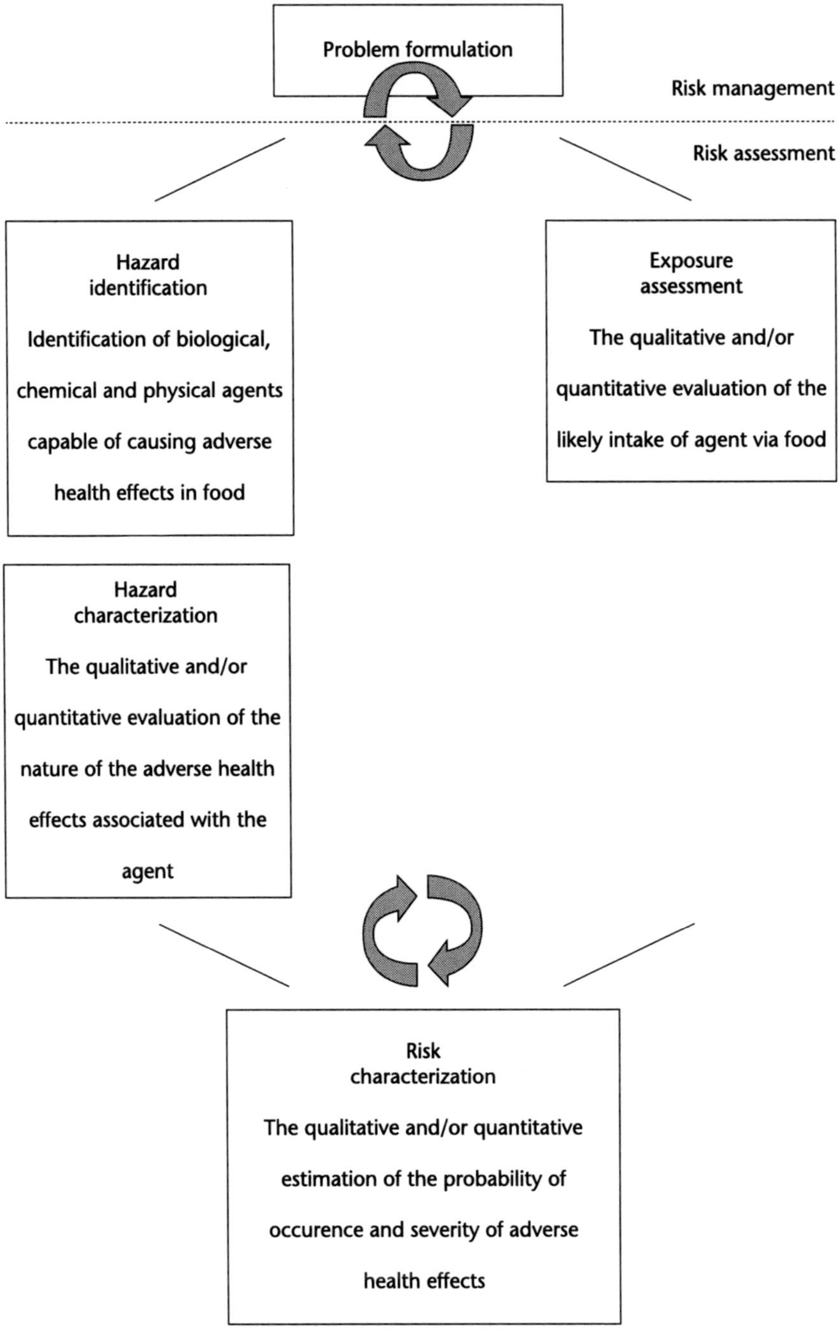


*Figure 24.3* Risk assessment: a scientific process [6]

internationally as the most cost-effective way to estimate the dietary intake of various substances, including contaminants and nutrients, across the total diet for a range of population groups. The TDS aims to find out the magnitude of the risk and the population groups which may be higher risks. While the majority of the contaminants and nutrients studied did not raise any public health concerns, the study did show that 11 per cent of women of childbearing age had dietary exposure to methylmercury, a more toxic form of mercury, exceeding the health-based guidance values (Provisional Tolerable Weekly Intake). Methylmercury exposure during pregnancy is a public health concern due to its potential health risks (e.g. neurotoxicity) to foetuses. Risk managers should take note of these results and conduct risk-based food surveillance work accordingly. As for risk communication, consumers are advised to maintain a balanced and varied diet to avoid excessive exposure to metallic contaminants from a small range of food items. Pregnant women, women planning pregnancy and young children should avoid eating large or predatory fish and types of fish that may contain high levels of methylmercury (e.g. tuna, alfonsino, shark and marlin).

In addition to the TDS, the CFS conducts a number of risk assessment studies every year. These studies, covering various chemical, microbiological and nutritional hazards, were chosen because of their public health significance. For each study, a range of food products is tested and the risk of the population is evaluated. The results of risk assessment studies are translated into useful food safety information for the public in the form of 'Risk in Brief' and risk assessment reports. They are available on the CFS website [3].

## *Risk management*

Risk management is the process of weighing policy alternatives, in consultation with all interested parties; considering risk assessment and other factors relevant for the health protection of consumers and for the promotion of fair trade practices; and, if needed, selecting appropriate prevention and control options. Although the ultimate responsibility of producing safe food lies with the food industry, the food safety authority has an indispensable role to play. In Hong Kong, the major components of risk management work include safety control of imported food, food surveillance, management of food incidents and setting of food standards.

Relying almost entirely on imported food, control at source and monitoring at the border control points are critical factors of import food control. In Hong Kong, the Public Health and Municipal Services Ordinance (Cap. 132) and its subsidiary regulations provide power for the authority to regulate the safety of food. Certain high-risk foods, such as milk, milk products, frozen confections, game, meat and poultry require prior approval of the FEHD. Meat and poultry should come from sources recognized by the FEHD. In addition, administrative arrangements have been established with Chinese authorities for the import of eggs, vegetables and freshwater fish. They have to come from registered farms and processing plants, and be accompanied with health certificates/relevant documents when imported.

The global food supply chain is getting increasingly complex (see Figure 24.4). It is becoming more and more common that a food product may contain ingredients from many different parts of the world. As a result, tracing a food safety problem is not a straightforward exercise. The CFS monitors local and overseas food incidents on a daily basis. The risks of these incidents are evaluated individually to assess their potential impact on local public health. The CFS initiates follow-up actions whenever necessary to safeguard food safety and protect public health.

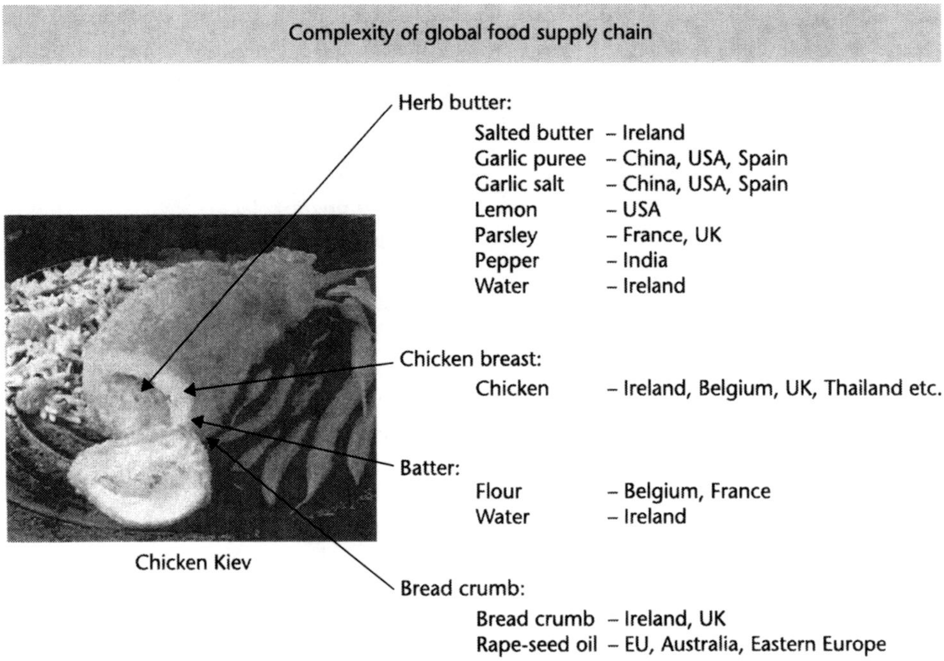


*Figure 24.4* Global food supply chain [5]

Depending on the magnitude of the problem, the CFS carries out risk management measures ranging from strengthening import control, enhancing sample testing and requesting traders to stop selling, to recalling the affected products. Working with international and national authorities, the CFS participates in international food safety information networks, such as the International Food Safety Authorities Network (INFOSAN) established by the WHO and the FAO, as well as the 'Rapid Alert System for Food and Feed' (RASFF) of the European Union. Whenever an international food incident with the possibility of affecting Hong Kong occurs, the CFS will closely liaise with the concerned authorities to keep abreast of the latest developments and to take the most appropriate risk management measures.

As controlling food safety hazards at the source is not always possible, the Food Surveillance Programme remains a key component of the CFS's work to ensure food safety. Inspectors take food samples at import, wholesale and retail levels for microbiological, chemical and radiological testing to ensure that the food is fit for human consumption and complies with the local food safety standards. Each year, a total of about 65,000 food samples are tested under the Food Surveillance Programme (i.e. about nine samples per every 1,000 population). The Food Surveillance Programme is risk based, making reference to previous food surveillance results, local and overseas food incidents, and local food poisoning outbreaks. The Programme covers the following main areas: routine food surveillance, targeted food surveillance, seasonal food surveillance and popular local food items. The CFS reviews the scope and intensity of the Food Surveillance Programme on an annual basis. Targeted surveillance will also be initiated in response to food incidents.

A new Food Safety Ordinance (Chapter 612, Laws of Hong Kong) came into force in 2011, which further gives the CFS the power to safeguard food safety, provides a mandatory registration scheme for food importers and distributors, and sets a requirement for food traders to maintain transaction records. In the event of a food incident, the tracing of food sources becomes more effective. With advances in food technologies and enactment of standards by the Codex Alimentarius Commission, an international food standard setting authority formed by the WHO and the FAO, the CFS updates the food safety regulations and standards, as required, to meet emerging needs.

### *Risk communication*

The importance of risk communication should not be underestimated. It is defined as the interactive exchange of information and opinions throughout the risk analysis process concerning risk, risk-related factors and risk perceptions, among risk assessors, risk managers, consumers, the industry, the academic community and other interested parties, including the explanation of risk assessment findings and the basis of risk management decisions. The CFS believes that the main goal of risk communication is to provide meaningful, relevant and accurate information in clear and understandable terms targeted to relevant audiences, and in a timely manner. To achieve effective communication, the Environmental Protection Agency of the US has identified seven key elements, namely:

1 Involve the public as a partner;
2 Listen to the public's concerns;
3 Be honest, frank and open;
4 Speak clearly with compassion;
5 Meet the needs of the media;
6 Coordinate and collaborate with credible sources; and
7 Plan carefully and evaluate performance.

Taking note of the above key elements, the CFS actively engages the industry and the public, which underlines the importance of a tripartite collaboration among the government, the food industry and consumers. Since the establishment of the CFS, a series of activities have been implemented and channels have been developed to enhance risk communication with the industry and the public. Bilateral dialogues on various food safety issues with members of the trade and general public are conducted through the Trade Consultation Forum and Consumer Liaison Group respectively. For major food safety issues, public consultation exercises are conducted. To establish the CFS as a trustworthy and credible source of information, risk management actions implemented are based on scientific risk assessment under the risk analysis framework.

The CFS assures transparency of the risk analysis process by working with the media. Cultivating a good sense of risk perception is fundamental, while clear and understandable messages are crucial, for effective risk communication. Rapid food alert messages are disseminated through electronic means. Other food safety messages are distributed using traditional channels, such as seminars, exhibitions and various forms of publications and resource materials. During major food incidents, risk management actions are updated on a daily basis and relevant information is made available to the media and the public. An emergency telephone hotline centre is set up to address public concerns and allay their anxieties. The CFS also earns its credibility by working under the steer of the Expert Committee on Food Safety, a consultative committee comprising of local and overseas food experts, academics and members of the trade. The CFS conducts joint studies with the

Consumer Council, a local consumer organization highly regarded by the public. Last but not least, through formative, process and impact evaluation in the form of surveys and focus group discussions, the CFS is ever improving the effectiveness of its work and evaluating its efforts.

## Case study: melamine – a case of blatant abuse

While the standard of food safety has generally been improving in Asia, food safety cannot be taken for granted. In September 2008, an outbreak of urinary tract stones affecting many babies in China was identified. Urinary tract stones are a rare disease in the paediatric age group. Subsequently, a number of milk and milk-containing products tainted with melamine was unveiled in mainland China, Hong Kong and in over 45 countries around the world.

Melamine (also known as tripolycyanamide) is an industrial chemical that is widely used in the production of melamine resins, which are used in glues, paper, textiles and plastics. Although melamine is cheap, it serves no useful function in food. It is not an approved food additive and is not a food ingredient. It is not allowed to be added to food in any quantity. Under Chinese law, the level of protein in milk needs to meet certain concentration requirements. As this requirement is not always attainable, in addition to the pursuit of higher profit, melamine, a rich source of nitrogen, can be added to milk to falsify the level of protein because the laboratory method used for such a test was not specific enough to make a distinction between nitrogen in melamine and nitrogen in milk. It was later found that melamine scrap was added to milk in China to cheat protein measurement in milk and dairy products.

### *Health effects*

Melamine is rather inert and of low acute toxicity. Its addition to milk does not alter the quality of the milk. However, it can cause crystal formation in the urinary tract. In severe cases, these small crystals can form urinary tract calculi, blocking the urinary tract, stopping urine production, causing kidney failure and even leading to death. Melamine has been shown to be carcinogenic in animals but there was inadequate evidence to show that melamine is carcinogenic in humans. Infants are particularly at risk of developing adverse health effects as a result of consuming melamine-tainted milk as melamine-tainted milk may be their sole dietary intake.

The toxic effects of melamine would only develop if its intake exceeds a level known as Tolerable Daily Intake (TDI).[1] In 2007, the US Food and Drug Administration (FDA) derived a TDI of 0.63 mg/kg bw/day for melamine. Based on the Chinese experience, infants and young children are more vulnerable to the effects of melamine. The WHO established a TDI of 0.2 mg/kg bw/day following the incident in 2009.

According to epidemiological information revealed by the Chinese authorities, the incident affected about 300,000 infants and young children in China, resulting in six deaths. Over 99 per cent of the victims were children aged 3 years or below. Affected children might experience symptoms of irritability for unknown reasons, blood in their urine, acute renal failure, urinary stones, high blood pressure or pain in the kidney region.

Most of the infants/children affected were found to have consumed milk formulae contaminated with melamine for three to six months, with the shortest time period of consumption recorded being 15 days. The Sanlu brand was found to be the one having the highest level of melamine (up to 2,563 ppm). Other brands of milk and milk-containing products were also involved, though to a lesser extent. The estimated exposure of infants to adulterated infant formula in China suggested that the exposure ranged from 8.6 to 23.4 mg/kg bw/day, amounting to about 40–120 times the recommended TDI.

### *Public health measures introduced in Hong Kong*

To address various public health and food safety issues arising from the incident in Hong Kong, an Expert Group on Melamine Incident chaired by the Secretary for Food and Health was set up in late September 2008. The Expert Group comprised members from both the public and private sectors: academics, medical, public health, food safety and public communication experts, and government representatives.

When the incident emerged, there was no regulatory standard set for melamine in food globally. Enforcement actions will be hampered without a regulatory standard. Based on the TDI established by the US FDA, Hong Kong, being the first place, set regulatory standards for melamine in food in late September 2008 as an emergency measure. The maximum concentration of melamine allowed in infant foods was 1 mg/kg and 2.5 mg/kg for other food products. Similar regulatory standards were subsequently adopted by various food safety authorities around the world to protect their public's health, particularly infants and young children.

Using the above regulatory limits, the CFS in Hong Kong intensified its food surveillance efforts. A systematic approach was adopted to sample and test milk and milk-containing products, with priorities given to infant formula and food for infants and young children. The results were announced and uploaded onto the CFS's website to enable the public to make informed food choices. Over a period of five months, over 5,000 samples were tested with an unsatisfactory rate of < 1 per cent exceeding the legal limits. The unsatisfactory products included baby food, milk, milk beverages and bakery products. The affected products were recalled and suspended from sale.

A screening service was provided to over 55,000 children. The WHO surveillance case definition was adopted, which defined a case as 'an infant with kidney stones or other kidney problems (e.g. anuria, renal failure) having consumed powdered infant formula produced in China before 6 August 2008, and where other potential causes of kidney stones have been excluded by differential diagnosis' [4]. A total of 15 cases were identified as 'probable' or 'suspected' cases in Hong Kong.

Besides collecting, collating and disseminating daily information on case reports, the Centre for Health Protection (CHP) of the Department of Health (DH) provided a telephone hotline service to answer various enquiries. The CFS also conducted a telephone hotline service to dispense the latest information on results of food samples tested.

### *International collaboration*

The melamine incident is one of the largest blatant food adulteration incidents in modern times, affecting a large number of countries. The WHO played a leading role in information sharing through the WHO/FAO International Food Safety Authorities Network (INFOSAN) (see Box 24.1). It is clear that closer collaboration of national authorities in exchanging information and coordination is beneficial to controlling this type of incident.

## Box 24.1 International Food Safety Authorities Network (INFOSAN)

The International Food Safety Authorities Network (INFOSAN) is a joint initiative between WHO and the FAO. Each member state has a designated INFOSAN emergency contact point for communication between national food safety authorities and the INFOSAN secretariat regarding urgent events.

The network aims to:

- Promote the rapid exchange of information during food safety related events;
- Share information on important food safety related issues of global interest;
- Promote partnership and collaboration between countries; and
- Help countries strengthen their capacity to manage food safety risks.

## Conclusion

As food is increasingly traded around the world, a food incident occurring in one place can quickly affect countries on the other side of the globe. Monitoring food incidents around the world has increasingly been carried out by national food safety authorities on a routine basis. Early response holds the key to successful control of these incidents both at national and international levels.

## Note

1 Tolerable daily intake (TDI) refers to the amount of a contaminant, expressed on a body weight basis, which an individual may ingest daily for a lifetime without causing any appreciable health effect.

## References


1. World Health Organization and Food and Agriculture Organization of the United Nations. Working principles for risk analysis for food safety for application by governments, 1st edn. Rome. WHO, 2007.
2. Food and Environmental Hygiene Department (FEHD). Hong Kong population-based Food Consumption Survey 2005–2007 final report. Hong Kong. FEHD, 2010. Available from: http://cfs.fehd.hksarg/english/programme/programme_firm/files/FCS_final_report.pdf
3. Centre for Food Safety. Government of Hong SAR. Risk Assessment Reports. 2013. Available from: www.cfs.gov.hk
4. World Health Organization. Expert meeting to review toxicological aspects of melamine and cyanuric acid, 1–4 December 2008. Available from: http://www.who.int/foodsafety/fs_management/infosan_events/en/index3.html
5. Adapted with permission from the Food Standards Agency Ireland. Available from: http://www.fsai.ie
6. World Health Organization and Food and Agriculture Organization of the United Nations: Codex Alimentarius Commission Procedural Manual, 12th edn. Rome. WHO and FAO, 2011.
7. Centre for Food Safety: Centre for Food Safety, Hong Kong, Government Logistics Department, 2011.

# 25

# Responding to disasters in low-income countries

*Emily Y. Y. Chan*

## Introduction

Disasters often present severe health consequences for the inhabitants of a community and provide a unique situation for public health actions.

This chapter provides an overview of issues related to disaster and humanitarian crisis in developing countries from a public health perspective. As the study of disaster and humanitarian crisis is multidisciplinary, the chapter starts by describing and defining public health terminologies that are relevant to the study of disasters. The chapter then focuses on delineating the direct and indirect public health impacts of some common natural disasters, the principles of public health need assessments, the fundamentals of disaster health and medical responses and the concept of a five-stage disaster cycle to facilitate disaster health risk analysis and planning. Two case studies are also discussed to describe the impact and illustrate why low-income countries are particularly vulnerable to disasters.

## Overview of disasters

### *Definition of disaster*

The term 'disaster' has many definitions and is dependent on the discipline that studies the subject [1]. The following is a commonly recognized definition:

> A disaster is a result of a vast ecological breakdown in relation between humans and their environment, a serious and sudden onset event (slow such as drought) on such a scale that the stricken community needs extraordinary efforts to cope with it, often with outside help/international aid. [2]

The definition has been recently revised and adopted by the Centre for Research on the Epidemiology of Disasters (CRED):

> A disaster is a situation or event, which overwhelms local capacity, necessitating a request to a national or international level for external assistance; an unforeseen and often sudden event that causes great damage, destruction and human suffering. [3]

Despite the slight difference between the two definitions, both versions contain the following three elements to define disaster: (1) damage involving humans: using phrases such as 'a vast ecological breakdown in relations between humans and their environment' and 'great damage, destruction and human suffering'; (2) characteristics of the event; and (3) the need for external assistance.

### Types of disasters

In general, disasters can be classified into natural or man-made disasters based on their causes and event triggers. However, as man-made disasters include a wide range of categories due to the involvement of different human factors, complex emergencies are usually classified as a separate type of disaster with a distinct set of characteristics. Thus the various types of disasters can be grouped as follows [3]:

*Natural disasters*: Including climatological, hydrological, meteorological, geophysical and biological disasters.
*Man-made disasters*: Including industrial-based, transport-based, biological/chemical-based and others (including famine).
*Complex emergencies*: Conflicts and wars.

Each of these disaster subtypes will have distinct etiology, human impact and response challenges. Relief workers and responders will have to address the specific characteristics of a particular subtype, and therefore is it advisable for them to be knowledgeable about these attributes.

## Disasters and health

### Direct and indirect health impacts of disasters

Depending on the type of disaster and magnitude of the event, different types of disasters may have a specific set of health and public health effects [4, 5, 6]. In general, health impacts can be classified as direct and indirect. Direct health effects include those sustained during a disaster and common examples are mortality, injuries and psychological impact, such as post-traumatic stress disorder. Indirect health effects refer to those attributable to the presence of a crisis and typical examples are malnutrition due to food scarcity, unintentional injuries, transmission of infectious diseases and manifestation of non-communicable diseases (NCDs), as well as social health impacts, such as breakdown of household structure due to death in family members and social networks as a result of population displacements. Damage to the healthcare infrastructure such as hospitals, clinics and communication channels may result in a disruption to services and programmes. Depending on resource availability, the rate of recovery and resilience of the population, the indirect health effects may sustain long after the occurrence of the disaster. Table 25.1 shows some possible public health consequences of disasters [5].

Many factors will affect the magnitude of the impact and damage caused by a disaster. These include, but are not limited to, environmental factors, infrastructure, health service

*Table 25.1* Possible public health consequences of disasters

| *Disaster impact* | *Possible public health consequences* |
|---|---|
| Unexpected number of deaths, injuries or illness in the affected community. | • Exceeds the therapeutic capacities of the local health services and requires external assistance. |
| Destruction of local health infrastructures (such as hospitals), routine health services and preventive activities. | • Leads to long-term health consequences in terms of increased morbidity and mortality.<br>• Leads to the disruption of health care even for those populations who are non-disaster related and who seek care. |
| Causes adverse effects on the environment and the population. | • Leads to an increase of potential risk for communicable diseases and environmental hazards. These might lead to long-term health consequences in terms of increased morbidity, premature death and diminished quality of life. |
| Affects psychological and social behaviour of the stricken community. | • An increase in psychological disturbances (e.g. PTSD, depression, anxiety, panic, neuroses, etc.). |
| Causes shortage of food with severe nutritional consequences (such as starvation). | • Health morbidities and death. |
| Causes large, spontaneous or organized population movements, often to areas where health services cannot cope with the situation. | • Poor sanitation and contaminated water in displaced camps [25] causes an increase in the risk of communicable diseases. |
| Long-term consequences (e.g. nuclear accidents). | • Morbidities and premature death. |

capacity, general baseline health status of the population, burden of disease in the local area and community resilience.

## *Public health impact of disasters*

The health impact and needs of disasters can vary depending on the type of disaster and magnitude of the event. There is currently a major gap in literature regarding an overview of various public health impacts of disaster in the context of low-income countries. Nevertheless, according to Redmond *et al.* [6], the following are some general public health effects of the common types of disasters:

*Effects of floods and high wind*: In general, flood and high wind events do not result in high levels of mortality but may cause a range of morbidities (e.g. typoon, hurricane). However, when compared with other disasters, larger populations tend to be affected due to the extent of the affected area and the post-disaster impact which requires long-term management. For instance, water supplies may be contaminated with sewage and other pollutants potentially leading to the transmission of waterborne diseases. Damage to crops, housing and infrastructure may affect food production and loss of homes and can lead to economic loss.

*Earthquakes*: The major adverse human risk of earthquakes is mortality and morbidity which resulted from the potential collapse of buildings, falling debris and entrapment. Specifically, risks of entrapment mostly lead to hypoxia, hypothermia, gas leaks, smoke, water penetration and electrocution. Survival is linked intimately with immediate actions of survivors and during the first phase of the disaster when the chance of survival is the highest. The number of both injured and killed individuals tends to be high. Earthquakes also destroy transportation and communication systems, and they pose a heavy burden on the health system due to a large amount of injuries that are incurred.

Contrary to floods, water sources are not as likely to be contaminated and there is no evidence that the unburied dead cause the spread of infectious diseases. The risk of disease outbreaks are of less concern than for floods. Even with the low risk of the spread of disease, the burying of the dead is important for cultural and family reasons.

*Tsunamis*: Tsunamis result from earthquakes originating at sea, producing seismic waves and eventually becoming a wall of water that approaches the shore. Most deaths are due to drowning and damage to buildings is attributed to the initial impact and drag. People living close to the sea shore and lowland areas are the most at risk. The number of dead may outnumber the injured in tsunamis.

*Landslides*: Landslides may result from heavy rain and destabilized soil and rocks, particularly in deforested areas. They may follow tsunamis, floods, earthquakes and heavy rains. Crush injury and entrapment are a common cause of mortality and morbidity.

*Volcanic eruptions*: Although these events may be relatively rare compared to other disasters and are considered as specific geographic hazards, residents close to the volcano sites on the highly fertile soil from volcanic ash are often affected. Indirect health impacts from relocation and the loss of homes is likely to have a greater adverse outcome than direct injuries from falling rocks and burns. Special threats to life include ash fall, pyroclastic flows, mud flows, tsunamis and volcanic earthquakes, and toxic gases may be emitted. Volcanic eruptions mainly cause economic loss. Preventive measures can be taken using early warning systems with the help of surveillance systems to detect seismic movements.

## What makes low-income countries particularly vulnerable to disasters?

### *Frequency of disasters*

Globally, with the effect of climate change on the frequencies of meteorological disasters, the number of natural disasters is increasing [7] and low-income countries are usually disproportionately affected (see Chapter 20). Many of the low-income developing countries, especially the large population-based communities in Asia, are subject to seasonal events such as floods, droughts, tropical storms. The pattern of large-scale emergency events and human attributes will leave a smaller window of opportunity between events to prepare for disasters and, as a result, decrease community resiliencies.

### *Baseline health and livelihood status of the population*

Developing countries are usually afflicted by widespread social demographic environmental factors that predispose to a poor baseline health status of the population even during times of non-disaster. Some of these leading factors linked to poor health include physical factors (inadequate sanitation, water, waste disposal and housing) and behavioural factors (sexual behaviour, alcohol abuse and smoking). People in poverty are additionally vulnerable due to a lack of access to health services and information, unsafe environments, and lower levels of literacy and education. As a result of these factors developing countries suffer disproportionally from health and economic losses when compared with developed countries.

## *Demographic and epidemiological transition*

In simple terms, the theory of demographic transition states that 'societies that experience modernization progress from a pre-modern regime of high fertility and high mortality to a post-modern one in which both are low' [8]. An increase in life expectancy and the ageing of populations is leading an epidemiological transition that is shifting the disease profile from communicable diseases to NCDs in many countries. Epidemiological transition is usually referred to as 'the general shift from acute infectious and deficiency diseases characteristic of underdevelopment to chronic non-communicable diseases characteristic of modernization and advanced levels of development' [9]. It can generally be observed when non-communicable, chronic conditions become the predominant disease profile as development evolves. For many low-income countries, this presents a double burden of disease which poses a major public health challenge during disasters. Specifically, in these transition processes, there is a period when a country is still being burdened with communicable diseases, while the spread of non-communicable, chronic health conditions begins to increase. SPHERE [10] standards highlight the need to address the exacerbation of chronic health conditions during disasters. However, due to limited resources, many aid agencies overlook this issue as secondary to more acute problems. As a result, people do not have access to therapies and medicines needed for their well-being, and as a result mortality and morbidity will lead to complications of their conditions.

## *The non-communicable disease (NCD) burden in developing countries*

Globally, communicable diseases are no longer the major cause of mortality as over 60 per cent of all deaths in 2005 were caused by chronic diseases [11]. Although the disease burden in developed countries is mainly from chronic NCDs, more than 80 per cent of the deaths caused by chronic diseases occurred in low-income and middle-income countries [12]. In the twenty-first century, the burden of NCDs in developing countries is an increasing trend as the population ages, urbanization increases and environmental risks increase [11]. The age-standardized death rates for chronic diseases in 15 selected low- and middle-income countries were higher than those in high-income countries [11].

## *Health systems*

The health system plays a key role during disasters, as well as bearing long-term burdens post-disasters. Well-built systems absorb the impact of disasters and respond more efficiently. Therefore, public health related preparedness plans for the health systems are crucial in any disaster management plan and should include supportive policies, allocated resources, risk analysis and contingency plans. Even physical measures such as the reinforcement of health infrastructure and the construction of safer facilities can mitigate the damage during a disaster to ensure that basic services will continue when they are needed most. Unfortunately, due to limited resources, inequitable health care, low provision of public health programmes and low-quality health infrastructure that exist in low-income countries, health systems are rarely prepared for a disaster and have great difficulties managing the event effectively, and therefore often many human lives are lost.

## *Health improvement and health promotion*

Developing countries often fare poorly in their health promotion and improvement programmes as more immediate health needs are prioritized due to resource limitations.

Disaster awareness and disaster health risk literacy in such communities is likely to be limited and will hinder the response [13].

## The public health approach to disaster response

The discipline of public health emphasizes prevention and protection, and aims to reduce health disparities through evidence-based, cost-effective solutions. To address health issues, it adopts a population based, life-course approach. Disaster response is an important element in public health practice since it affects large segments of the population. Disaster risk reduction, mitigation, response and community resilience building programmes can protect large populations from the adverse impacts of disasters. Using disaster epidemiology, disaster responders and public health professionals can establish priorities and guide resource allocation for disaster-affected populations [5, 14]. Following a disaster, essential health services need to meet the needs of the affected population and should include both preventive and curative services that aim to reduce excess morbidity and mortality [10]. Disasters cannot be prevented but their human health impact can be mitigated. Like many other public health programmes, responses to disasters need to be addressed as a long-term sustainable effort. The most important element in a public health approach to disasters and crises is the proactive, preventive and multidisciplinary nature of its response actions. In addition to response, a public health approach to disasters should include risk management with a focus on disaster preparedness and risk reduction to help decrease the vulnerabilities of communities and increase their coping capacity [15]. The public health response to any disaster or crisis has three basic principles [16]. These include: (1) secure the basic resources that human beings require to maintain health; (2) determine the current and likely health threats to the affected community, given the local environment and community's resources, knowledge and enabling health maintaining behaviours; and (3) find and provide resources required to address points 1 and 2.

The SPHERE Project, a voluntary initiative which includes various humanitarian actors – such as international and national NGOs, the International Red Cross and Red Crescent Society, UN agencies, host governments and local affected communities – states that the basic requirements of health include clean water and sanitation, food and nutrition, shelter and clothing, health services and information [10]. According to the SPHERE guidelines, and in line with the organization's aim of 'improv[ing] the quality of assistance to people affected by disaster, and improv[ing] the accountability of states and humanitarian agencies to their constituents, donor and the affected populations', securing these resources is the number one priority immediately following a disaster [10].

Governments should commit to risk reduction and disaster management through a variety of efforts including financial budgeting, policies and legislation, identifying disaster management authorities and resource management [18]. Securing resources for addressing disaster response will rely heavily on the pre-existing commitment of governments and external agencies, therefore planning and preparing for such scenarios is important.

## Application of public health principles in disaster response

The various components of public health practice can be grouped into three widely accepted domains of public health: health protection, health services and health improvement [19]. These domains are commonly applied in general public health practice and can be integrated to disaster response. Epidemiology, biostatistics, clinical trials, and law and ethics are overlapping domains, serving as foundation knowledge in public health practice. Application of this concept to disaster response would look like this:

1 Epidemiology and Biostatistics – Emergency health needs/impact assessment and evaluation: disaster epidemiology;
2 Health Service – Emergency policy analysis and planning, service emergency preparedness and training, disaster response management;
3 Health Protection – Infection control, environmental health risk management, mental health, nutrition, water, shelter, sanitation; and
4 Health Improvement – Coordination, risk communication, resource mobilization, capacity building (e.g. HR development and disaster response team building).

Any intervention during disaster response should be designed using a public health strategy. First, an assessment of the potential health issues in an affected population has to be carried out using a health-needs assessment, which is a systematic method of identifying unmet healthcare needs of a population and making changes to meet those needs [5, 6, 20]. This will determine the health threats and risks in the community, as information will be gathered on the general condition of the population, demographic characteristics and size of the population, current health problems, condition of the environment and security issues, and will identify the special needs of vulnerable groups and detail health system and disaster response capacity [16, 17]. Identifying the causes of morbidity and mortality post-disaster will aid in the design of appropriate health services and programmes. Needs assessments should be prompt, population-based and built upon consensus from all agencies involved to reduce duplicate efforts. Further assessments should be planned to collect data on evolving health needs.

To organize an effective response, a public health intervention may be required and may include one or all of the following factors: public health perspective, understanding health determinants, describing risk factors, adopting the life-course approach, identifying a prevention strategy, balancing population-wide versus individual-based approaches, health disparity, importance of health literacy and social marketing and health priorities.

## Disaster response cycle

An important conceptual framework to guide in disaster-related medical response is the disaster response cycle [21]. In principle, disaster response should be planned and implemented according to the health needs associated with stages of the disaster, taking into account the principles and public health approach discussed previously. Although it is impossible to change the frequency of disasters, it is possible to improve the appropriateness and efficiency of the disaster response to reduce the human impact. Figure 25.1 shows the disaster response cycle. As shown by this figure (25.1), a disaster scenario can be categorized into five phases. The disaster response process should be monitored using a universally accepted guiding framework such as the SPHERE guidelines to ensure effectiveness, accountability and enhancement of response is achieved.

A key driver of emergency preparedness is creating community-based initiatives. Community-based strategies play a vital role in all phases of a disaster including preparedness, protection and response. Contributing actors include community healthcare workers, trained volunteers, local organizations and key players from different sectors (e.g. water, shelter, education, etc.). A community workforce will act as the primary source for disaster management – they will be involved in reducing vulnerabilities, preparedness, prevention

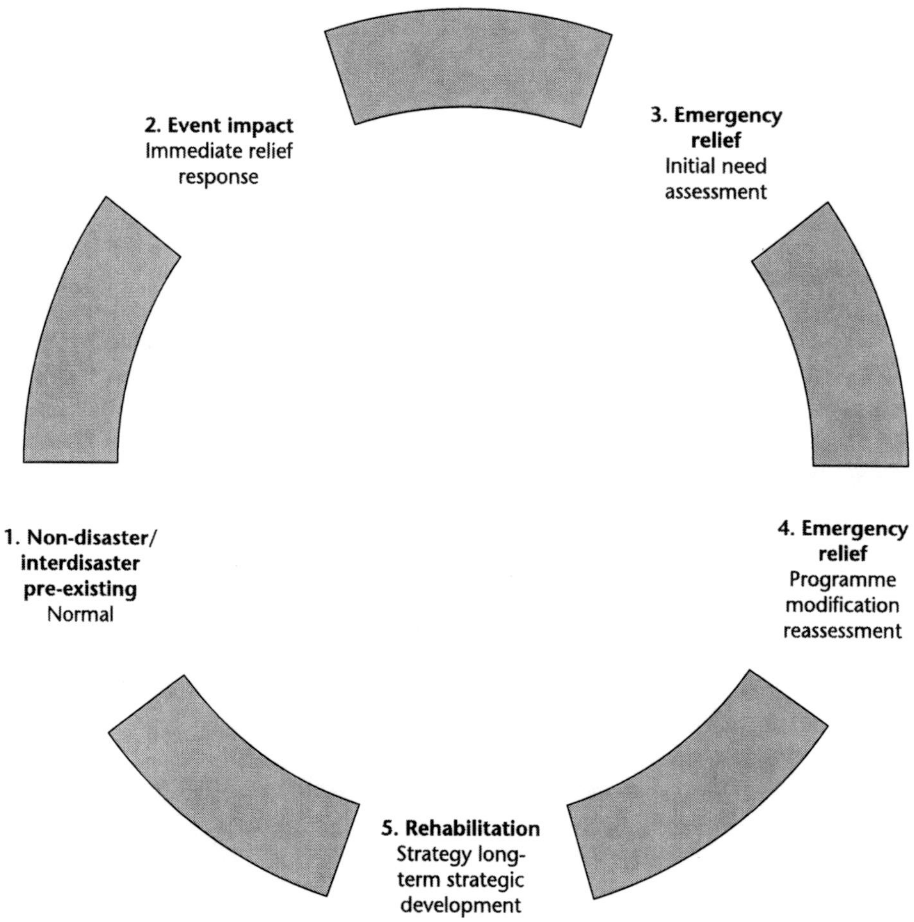


*Figure 25.1* The disaster response cycle [21]

and be the initial responders during emergency response and relief. In addition, the community will be central to post-disaster recovery and a speedy transition to development. See Box 25.1 for a case study on community-based initiatives.

As in any public health initiative, preventive actions are always better than restorative ones and in this view, risk reduction is an integral component of the disaster cycle. During times of non-disaster, various actions can help relieve the burden of future disasters. Since hazard, exposure and vulnerabilities are often higher in low-income settings and management capacity is low, triggers can rather quickly become catastrophic. Having a comprehensive disaster risk reduction plan with emphasis on building individual and community resilience will help mitigate against adverse human health impact. See Box 25.2 for an explanation of risk reduction.

The **first phase** is *non-disaster* or *normal state*. During this phase, disaster preparedness and response of a country or region will be determined by the local health system and medical resources available. In the low-income country, disaster planning may include acute/emergency service but as the pre-disaster services for chronic medical illness will be limited, services

## Box 25.1 Community-based initiatives in action: focus on emergency preparedness

A public health worker was vacationing on the southern coastal region of Sri Lanka when she received warning of the possibly impending tsunami, which happened on 11 April 2011. A magnitude 8.6 earthquake had struck off Aceh province near Indonesia, triggering a tsunami warning throughout the Indian Ocean.

No stranger to the devastation of tsunamis, the community response was unprecedented in its disaster preparedness. Some observations revealed the relevance of community preparedness:

- The situation was much improved from the 2004 tsunami that devastated the country and killed more than 31,000 people.
- On April 11th, the Meteorological Department issued a warning: 'An earthquake near Sumatra Island at 02.08pm (Sri Lanka time) has generated a tsunami that will affect Sri Lanka, those living near and along the Eastern and Southern coastal regions are advised to evacuate to safer places immediately.'
- Apart from SMS alerts sent through the mobile network, local radio and television stations announced the news and mosques rang out instructions. People knew what to expect and they got away as quickly as possible.
- For those who stayed behind, there were small blue boards on the roadside, signifying higher ground to move to in case of a tsunami. Awareness campaigns have been actively implemented throughout the country.
- Community members reacted in a very dynamic manner. Residents who received the SMS alert on their phone had left within the hour and told everyone along the way to do the same. Railroad service was suspended and electricity was limited to reduce the chance of fire. The police and military were dispatched to prevent looting. A group of hotel staff stood by with radio broadcasts of the latest news, the place of worship across the street broadcasted public prayers so that the faithful could pray. Preparedness at the local level ensured an immediate and effective local response to the warning of a tsunami. By all accounts, the country is better prepared than it was and the resiliency of the people can be seen in their quick response and actions.

*Source*: Excerpt from Sri Lanka – A Reflection on Tsunami Watch [23].

for non-communicable or chronic diseases during an emergency will be scare or non-existing. To ensure effective preparedness, health emergency risk reduction, mitigation and disaster preparedness programs will need to be implemented to safeguard the existence of disaster response services for non-communicable and chronic conditions.

The **second phase** of the disaster cycle, *immediate relief*, is characterized by the event itself and the immediate interventions and relief carried out by local response units. At this stage, both government and relief agencies will be strapped for resources due to the immediate surge of emergency needs, mortality cases and the destruction of health infrastructure. In developing countries, which face a double burden of disease, the complex health needs of the population will be great. A poor baseline health profile of the population and limited available resources will have a detrimental effect on the response capacity. Provision of services will be limited to essential life-saving procedures. Except for life-threatening complications of chronic diseases, victims with chronic conditions may be overlooked.

## Box 25.2 Risk reduction

Risk is the likelihood of an adverse outcome. In the context of disaster, risk is defined as 'expected losses of lives, persons injured, property damaged and economic activity disrupted due to a particular hazard for a given area and reference period' [3]. To compute risk, there are a few terminologies to be familiar with.

*Hazard* – A threatening event, or probability of occurrence of a potentially damaging phenomenon within a given time period and area.
*Vulnerability* – The degree of loss (from 0 per cent to 100 per cent) resulting from a potential damaging phenomenon.
*Manageability* – The organizational response to the hazard and the ability of the population to respond to it.

The equation below shows the relationship between the various components of risk: hazard, vulnerability, manageability and exposure:

$$\text{risk} = \text{hazard} \times \text{exposure} \times \text{vulnerability}/\text{manageability}$$ [24].

Risk begins to develop when a triggering event poses a hazard to the environment.

However, a hazard will not become a disaster unless people are affected, i.e. via exposure to the event or the event acting as an agent to the disaster. Given the exposure to the hazard, the degree of impact is dependent on people's vulnerability – the extent to which a community, structure, service or geographic area is likely to be damaged or disrupted by the impact of a particular hazard. This impact can also be mitigated by the manageability capability, which often refers to the organizational response to the hazard and the ability of the population to react. Simple algebraic principles indicate that hazard, exposure and vulnerability must be reduced while manageability must increase in order to reduce risk.

The **third phase** of the disaster cycle, *emergency relief*, highlights the importance of obtaining valid and up-to-date information for further evidence-based interventions. Initial health-needs assessments should be done quickly to aggregate information for appropriate and relevant decision making for interventions and policies in relief.

The **fourth phase** of the disaster cycle, *emergency relief*, focuses on programme modification for interventions and polices in relief based on health-needs assessments data. In low-income countries, the technology and equipment used in post-disaster data collection may not be available. Instead, data collection of post-disaster health needs may need to rely on quick, on-site manual surveys and surveillance tools. It is important to highlight that data should be collected on both acute immediate life-saving needs and chronic medical diseases. Historically, information on chronic diseases is not identified as essential data to collect during needs assessments and it may rule out resource allocation for chronic disease management service provision.

Health-needs assessments often use simple measures such as mortality rather than more relevant determinants that contribute to mortality and morbidity. Oversimplistic indicators are not sufficient to capture all possible solutions to address real needs. Since ill health can be caused by multiple factors, relief operation recommendations drawn from single sector assessments will be inadequate to meet all aspects of underlying health needs. In developing countries, a myriad of underlying issues will hinder good health and these need to be taken into consideration to set up effective programmes.

Due to the target-oriented and short-term nature of most disaster interventions, an exit strategy must be drawn up from the beginning or at least for the **fifth phase** of the disaster cycle, *rehabilitation*. Of note, community participation and collaboration will be essential to the sustainability of post-disaster efforts of a non-acute nature.

## Rapid health assessment

Before implementing any health programmes, the health situation in the affected population has to be assessed to: confirm the emergency; describe the context and nature of the disaster, impact and possible evolution of the emergency; measure its present and potential health impacts; assess the adequacy of existing response capacity and immediate additional needs; and recommend priority actions for immediate response.

### *The importance of needs assessment*

The ability to engage in a needs assessment are essential for those working in disaster relief. A needs assessment is a diagnostic tool for programme planning to determine the current gaps and problems in a given community. In the context of disaster, it helps to set objectives and determine appropriate interventions to meet the needs of that community.

In geographic areas where the intervention or service is unavailable, it helps to determine the feasibility, needs and the reason(s) to provide the intervention or service. In other situations where the intervention or service exists, needs assessment can help to improve the efficiency, quality and coordination of the service.

### *Methods for needs assessment*

Needs assessment can be conducted qualitatively or quantitatively. Generally, qualitative information is collected to identify specific issues before quantitatively assessing the magnitude of the issues.

Examples of qualitative assessment may include literature reviews, focus group discussions, key informant interviews, field observations and site visits. The findings of qualitative studies will help to identify and explain issues that might be relevant to the context. Quantitative assessment consists of short questionnaires and reviews of existing data in health systems. The findings will help to quantify and to prioritize the potential burden in high-risk areas with quantifiable outcomes.

### *Considerations in conducting health-needs assessment*

Before performing a health-needs assessment in a disaster setting, the following should be considered: purpose and goal for the assessment, choice of indicators, applicability, timelines of the programmes and their relevancy to policy translations.

## Box 25.3 Data collection

After the strategy has been decided, obtaining on-the-ground information and conditions becomes the priority. The following ten factors should be addressed when collecting data in a disaster zone:

1 *Understand the profile of the target population*
   - Be informed about the demographic structure, underlying diseases of the target population, access to medical care and the need for long-term care.

2 *Partnerships vs. independence*:
   - How is coordination with different parties being worked out?

3 *Transport and logistics*
   - To have information about different transport routes and their accessibility. Logistics are usually the limiting factor that delays the relief response.

4 *Proximity*

5 *Visibility*

6 *Cultural and local adaptability*
   - Is the intervention locally acceptable? Would people hesitate to use the service because of any cultural differences?

7 *Flexibility*
   - What are some alternative strategies that can be implemented with the available resources?

8 *Resource allocation and donation*
   - Are the supplies suitable and required in the local settings?

9 *Relief workers: working conditions and health problems*
   - Relief workers in the post-disaster situation live under a very stressful environment. It is crucial to have proper procedures to prevent burnout or other health problems.

10 *Rehabilitation needs*

## Programme planning for disaster response

### *Making political decisions*

After collecting information for situation analysis, decisions have to be made to determine a plan for the relief response. Planning is an ongoing process, as situation and implementation often differs from plans made originally. In order to design appropriate response programmes, information will have to be collected at various phases to obtain an updated situation (see Box 25.3 for a summary of data collection).

The considerations to keep in mind when planning for the relief response to a disaster should consist of the following: clear operational principles, needs assessment, target-specific intervention, technical capacity and existing strategy. In addition, sustainability and the long-term implications of the programme activities should be considered during the planning stage of the programme.

### *Urban versus rural disaster response*

As developing countries become more globalized and invest more in the global economy, there is a rapid change in population movements. People are migrating from rural to urban dwellings at an alarming rate and urban environments are rarely prepared for the influx. Slum-like areas which attract people due to working opportunities can be health threats in their own rights due to the suboptimal living conditions that exist in these areas and if disasters occur can exacerbate the health risks.

There is a distinction between urban and rural disaster response, and this differentiation is important. In urban areas where most administration and political decisions are made, disaster response systems are usually more organized, or at least exist in some form. In contrast, rural areas rarely have an existing response system or have one that is fragmented. Technical and human response capacity, as well as resources, will also be concentrated in urban centres, while they will be limited in rural settings. Lastly, while rural areas may have more experience in past disasters, international visibility is low in these areas making a disproportional media focus on urban areas while rural areas are often forgotten [22].

### *Measuring success*

The evaluation and success measurement of medical and public health disaster relief programmes requires the commitment and facilitation of programme stakeholders and policy planners. In addition to good relief programme planning with clear project outcome benchmarks and targets, reporting and accountability structure, technical capacity of staff and participation of field-based stakeholders will be necessary to ensure the accuracy and cooperation of performance tracking and monitoring,

### *Accountability and ethics*

In principle, emphasis on accountability, transparency and community participation are good practice for all health humanitarian actors attending to a disaster. Agencies should disclose and follow standards in their working responsibilities, their accountability principles, their participation within the affected community and the organization ethics they adopt (see Boxes 25.4 and 25.5 for case studies on disasters).

#### Box 25.4 Case study 1: the 2008 Wenchuan earthquake in China

On 12 May 2008, an earthquake measuring 8.0 on the Richter scale occurred in Wenchuan in Sichuan, China. The earthquake, with a death toll of at least 80,000, is considered to be one of the most destructive earthquakes to date. A study of acute relief health needs in the 2008 Sichuan earthquake showed that more than 70 per cent of earthquake survivors had some form of management to their underlying chronic conditions during the emergency phase [26].

Meanwhile, immediate medical and public health needs are often emphasized on physical health outcomes. Yet, through participatory research observation, a number of disaster relief issues were identified. Specifically, the hesitancy of involving external agencies, suboptimal relief organization, inappropriate treatment facilities, forgotten health needs and supplies, health needs of disaster relief workers, concern of treatment cost and logistic arrangement, healthcare entitlement of migrant workers within the disaster areas and mental health needs are all important issues [27].

## Box 25.5 Case study 2: the 2005 Pakistan–Kashmir earthquake

An earthquake struck Pakistan's autonomous state of Kashmir and part of Indian-administrated Kashmir on 8 October 2005. It measured 7.6 on the Richter scale, with the official death toll in Pakistan being 79,000 and nearly 1,400 in Indian-administered Kashmir.

A study indicated that significant differences in demographic and disease profile of users were found between mobile clinic and stationary clinic attendees post-acute emergency in remote setting. Older age, female gender, population living further away from clinics, patients with earthquake-related trauma, wound infection and gastrointestinal conditions were found to be more significantly associated with mobile clinic users. Users of the stationary clinics tended to be younger, living closer to the clinic site and had disease profiles which were predominantly chronic in nature [28].

Studies regarding why disaster medical service providers tended to forget about relief needs of older people indicated that despite the INGOs being inclined to have the technical capacity and resources (such as medicine) to address medical and service needs of older age groups, these INGOs fared the worst among all provider subcategories regarding the provision of age and gender sensitive clinical programmes. Around 80 per cent of the INGOs had the relevant drug supplies, but none of them provided geriatric specific services and mobility aids. On other hand, local (20 per cent) and national (40 per cent) counterparts provided mobility aids and 80 per cent of the local groups reported that they had programmes which were more gender sensitive when compared to those of the INGO (40 per cent) [29].

## Conclusion

Since health emergency risks are more prevalent in low-income countries for the reasons described in this chapter, it is important for low-income countries to undertake appropriate public health preparedness and have measures in place to enable response to disasters. Regardless of whether the disaster response might be in urban or in rural settings, the application of the disaster response cycle during emergency health need assessments, program planning, implementation as well as evaluation will be helpful to ensure relevance, quality and most important of all, accountability to the best benefit of the affected population. Fundamentally, although disasters render enormous health risks particularly in low-income communities, they might also present an opportunity for the civil society, government and global community to engage and work together to maximize the well-being and survival of vulnerable population.

## Acknowledgements

The author wishes to acknowledge the important contribution of her colleagues, Ms Jamie Rodas and Ms PoYi Lee with the earlier stage of this manuscript.

## References

1. Shaluf, I. M., Ahmadun, F. l.-r., Said, A. M. A review of disaster and crisis. *Disaster Prevention and Management* 2003; 12(1), 24–32.
2. Lechat, M. F. *Natural and Man-made Disasters*. London: Oxford University Press, 1984.

3. Centre for Research on the Epidemiology of Disasters (CRED). Glossary EM-DAT 2010. Available at http://www/emdat.be/glossary/9 [Accessed 1 June 2012].
4. Lechat, M. F. Updates: the epidemiology of health effects of disasters. *Epidemiology Reviews* 1990; 12, 192–197.
5. Noji, E. K. *The Public Health Consequences of Disasters*. London: Oxford University Press, 1997.
6. Redmond, A. D., Mahoney, P. F., Ryan, J. M., Macnab, C. *ABC of Conflict and Disaster* (1st edn). London: BMJ Publishing, 2006.
7. EM-DAT. The OFDA/CRED International Disaster Database. CRED, Université catholique de Louvain, Brussels, Belgium, 2010.
8. Lee, R. The demographic transition: three centuries of fundamental change. *Journal of Economic Perspectives* 2003; 17(4), 167–190.
9. Wahdan, M. H. The epidemiological transition. *Eastern Mediterranean Journal* 1996; 2(1), 8–20.
10. The SPHERE Project. Humanitarian Charter and Minimum Standards in Humanitarian Response, 2011. Available at: http://www.sphereproject.org
11. Beaglehole, R., Epping-Jordan, J., Patel, V., Chopra, M., Ebrahim, S., Kidd, M., *et al.* Improving the prevention and management of chronic disease in low-income and middle-income countries: a priority for primary health care. *Lancet* 2011; 372(9642), 940–949.
12. Abegunde, D. O., Mathers, C. D., Adam, T., Ortegon, M., Strong, K. The burden and costs of chronic diseases in low- and middle-income countries. *Lancet* 2007; 370(9603), 1929–1938.
13. The Ottawa Charter for Health Promotion. Paper presented at the First International Conference on Health Promotion, Ottawa, 1986.
14. Binder, S., Sanderson, L. M. The role of the epidemiologist in natural disasters. *Annals of Emergency Medicine* 1987; 16, 1081–1084.
15. Disease Control Priorities Project. Natural Disasters: Coping with the Health Impact, 2007. Available at: http://www.dcp2.org/main/Home.html
16. Bolton, P. Part 3. Direct action: managing disasters and other public health crises. In D. Pencheon, C. Guest, D. Melzer, M. J. A. Gray (eds) *Oxford Handbook of Public Health Practice*. Oxford: Oxford University Press, 2006: 248–256.
17. Landesman, L. Y. *Public Health Management of Disasters. A Practical Guide*. Washington, DC: American Public Health Association, 2001.
18. World Health Organization. Putting it together: stronger public health capacity within disaster management systems. Paper presented at the WHO Conference on the Health Aspects of the Tsunami Disaster in Asia, 2005.
19. Griffiths, S., Jewell, T., Donelly, P. Public health in practice: the three domains of public health. *Public Health* 2005; 119(10), 907–913.
20. Gupa-Sapir, D. Rapid assessment of health needs in mass emergencies: review of current concepts and methods. *World Health Statistics Quarterly* 1999; 44(3), 171–181.
21. Chan, E., Sondorp, E. Medical interventions following natural disasters: missing out on chronic medical needs. *Asia Pacific Journal of Public Health* 2007; 19 (Special), 45–51.
22. Chan, E. Y. Y. A disaster public health education framework to strengthen disaster medical response in Asian urban communities. Paper presented at the Hospital Authority Convention on Collaborative Healthcare, 2011.
23. Rodas, J. Sri Lanka – A Reflection on Tsunami Watch. 2012. Available at: http://ccouc.org/2012/04/26/sri-lanka-a-reflection-on-tsunami-watch/
24. United Nations Disaster Relief Coordinator. *Natural Disasters and Vulnerability Analysis*. Geneva: UNDRO, 1979.
25. Toole, M. J., Waldman, R. J. Prevention of excess mortality in refugee and displaced populations in developing countries. *Journal of the American Medical Association* 1990; 263(64), 3296–3302.
26. Chan, E. Y. Y., Kim, J. J. Chronic health needs immediately after natural disasters in middle income countries: the case of 2008 China Sichuan earthquake. *European Journal of Emergency Medicine* 2011; 18(2), 111–114.
27. Chan, E. Y. Y. The untold stories of Sichuan earthquake. *Lancet* 2008; 372(9636), 359–362.
28. Chan, E. Y. Y., Kim, J. J. Remote mobile health service utilization post 2005 Kashmir–Pakistan earthquake. *European Journal of Emergency Medicine* 2010; 17(3), 158–163.
29. Chan, E. Y. Y., Griffiths, S. Why are older people's health needs forgotten post-natural disaster relief in developing countries? A healthcare provider survey of 2005 Kashmir, Pakistan earthquake. *American Journal of Disaster Medicine* 2009; 4(2), 107–112.

# 26

# Lessons for public health from the 2011 Great East Japan earthquake

*Rosamund J. Southgate*

This case study looks at the Japanese earthquake of 2011, its public health effects, and the response following the earthquake. Analysis of the response provides various public health lessons from which public health professionals and other members of the community can greatly benefit.

## Background on the earthquake

Located on the 'Pacific ring of fire', Japan is prone to frequent earthquakes and tsunamis. It is hailed as the most disaster-prepared country on Earth with state-of-the-art early warning systems, structural defences, evacuation routes, and regular drills for schools, workplaces and incident command systems. However, the events of '3/11' (March 11) were of such a scale that even the most prepared society on the planet was overwhelmed.

On 11 March 2011, a 9.0-Richter scale earthquake hit eastern and central Japan, the tremors lasting for six minutes. The earthquake came from an epicentre 30 kilometres below the Earth's surface and 130 kilometres east of the coastal city of Sendai in the Tohoku region [1]. It was the strongest earthquake ever recorded in Japan [2], so powerful that it moved Japan's largest island, Honshu, by 2.4 metres, as well as shifting the Earth on its axis by 10 to 25 centimetres [3]. The earthquake has become known as the Great East Japan earthquake.

Three minutes after the tremors ceased, a deep-ocean buoy detected significant water movement and tsunami warnings were issued for Japan and other Pacific countries [4].

The earthquake and tsunami together precipitated the third event of the '3/11 triple disaster': three reactors at the Fukushima Daiichi Nuclear Power Plant lost all power and went into meltdown with fires, explosions and radiation that contaminated the land, groundwater and the atmosphere [5].

The destruction caused by the events of 3/11 is staggering. Table 26.1 summarizes the human and material costs of this disaster.

*Table 26.1* Costs of the earthquake, tsunami and nuclear accident of 3/11

| | |
|---|---|
| ***Human cost*** | |
| Killed (or still missing after one year) | 19,100 |
| Injured | 27,100 |
| Number in shelters (at peak) | 440,000 |
| Evacuated from area around the Fukushima nuclear plant | 146,400 |
| ***Material cost*** | |
| Buildings destroyed or damaged | 120,000 |
| Direct economic cost after one year | US$275 billion |

*Sources*: Statistics from [5, 17].

## The aftermath and the response

### *Rescue phase*

The initial response to a disaster is called the 'rescue phase' and involves the actions required to save and preserve life, addressing the immediate public health needs created by the disaster. Actions in the rescue phase included:

*Response coordination*: Local government offices immediately activated their disaster plans and began assessing resources. Within 30 minutes of the earthquake, the national government established the National Disaster Management Headquarters to coordinate the overall response [6].

*Search and rescue (SAR)*: The military and rescue service response included on-the-ground SAR teams, naval ships and helicopters, with international teams giving additional assistance. These efforts resulted in 3,000 people being rescued in the first 48 hours after the earthquake [3]. Figure 26.1 shows rescue helicopters flying over the affected Sendai region.

*Evacuation and shelter*: Homeless survivors headed to pre-designated evacuation shelters in gymnasia and halls. By the end of the first week, 2,400 such shelters were active, supplying water, food and basic health care to nearly 400,000 people [3].

*Access and delivery of survival essentials*: Millions of tonnes of tsunami debris, along with direct damage to roads and bridges, made delivery of survival essentials to the area difficult. The Japanese Self-Defence Force, with assistance from the local US military presence, had cleared many large roads within three days and began delivery of water, blankets and food by air, sea and land. However, fuel shortages meant some evacuation shelters could not be reached for a week.

*Health*: Certain hospitals in every Japanese prefecture are 'disaster-designated hospitals', with stockpiles of medicines and equipment and training to facilitate reception of disaster victims. These hospitals received the injured and many still operated despite structural damage and power outage. In addition, over 190 Disaster Medical Assistance Teams were deployed to give pre-hospital care within the first 48 hours [3, 7]. Common health issues were hypothermia and 'tsunami lung' (direct damage and infection from swallowing tsunami water).

*Nuclear accident*: On the day of the disaster, nearly 150,000 residents within a 20-kilometre radius of the Fukushima Daiichi Plant were evacuated [5]. Fires and radiation leakage

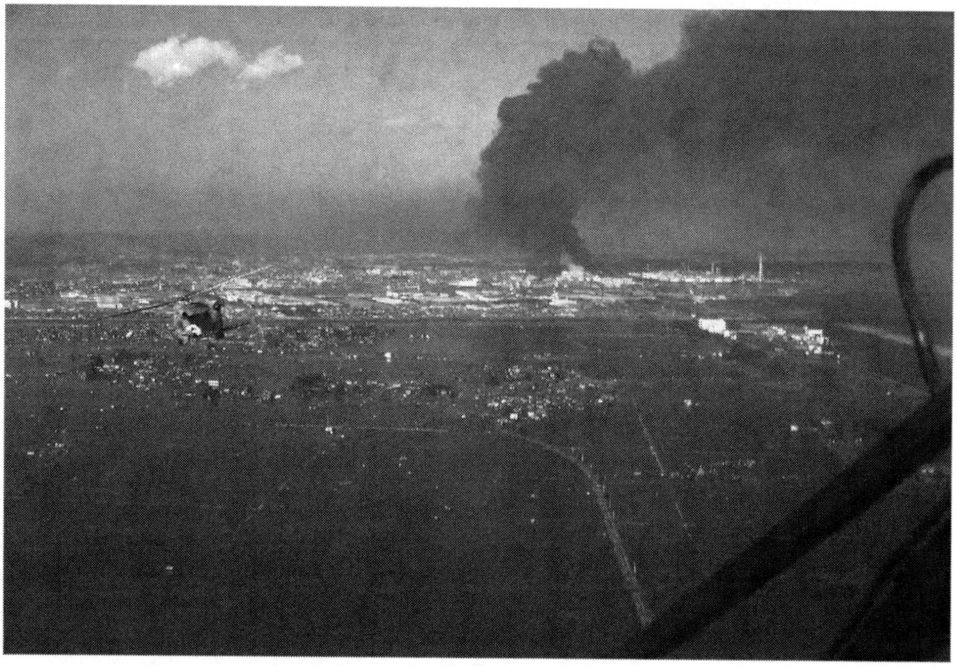

*Figure 26.1* Rescue helicopters flying over the Sendai region [18]

continued uncontrolled for days at the plant [5]. Figure 26.2 shows the fire vehicles at the site trying to extinguish the fire.

## *Relief phase*

Following the initial rescue phase in the first 48 to 72 hours post-disaster, the relief phase aimed to provide longer-term care in a number of sectors. This phase included:

*Response coordination*: Although significant amounts of financial and material aid were donated by governments and groups internationally, the relief response was mainly conducted by Japan through its well-established national, regional and local systems linking all areas of government and public service.

*Healthcare*: 'Disaster-designated hospitals' were quickly mobilized (with many in the worst hit areas suffering structural damage) and were filled to capacity within the first two weeks and began running out of stock. Until transport and access issues were addressed, little outside help was available.

*Shelters and health*: The vast scale of devastation resulted in a prolonged stay in evacuation shelters for a large number of people. Although chronic disease medication was well provisioned, poor diet and lack of physical activity led to poor control of chronic diseases and manifestation of new cases. Public health teams began visiting shelters in the third week following the disaster to provide nutrition and activity solutions plus sorely needed mental health support (this was supported by the Japanese Society of Psychiatry and Neurology). They also undertook disease surveillance. No major outbreaks of infectious

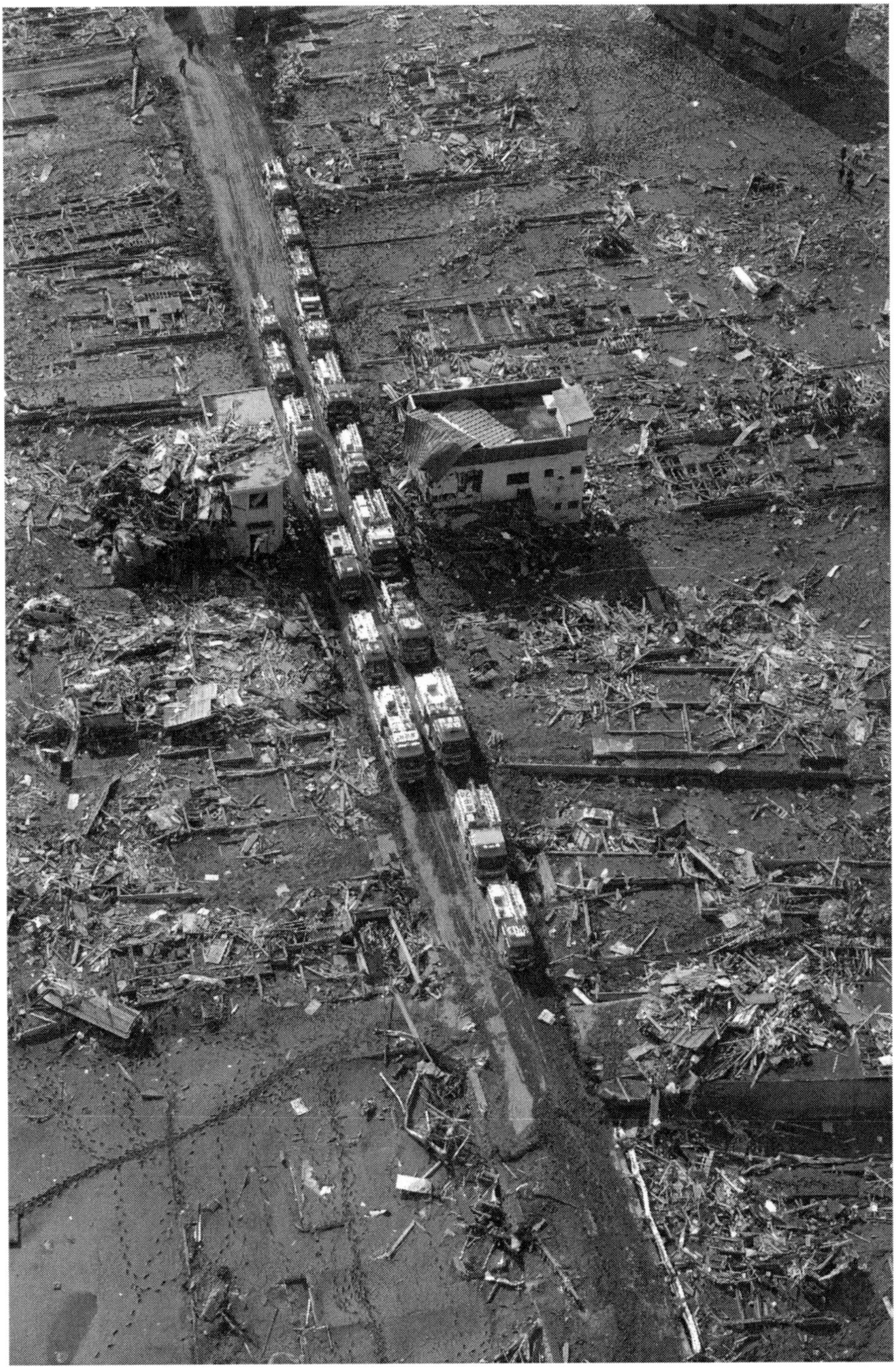

*Figure 26.2* Fire vehicles trying to extinguish the fire [19]

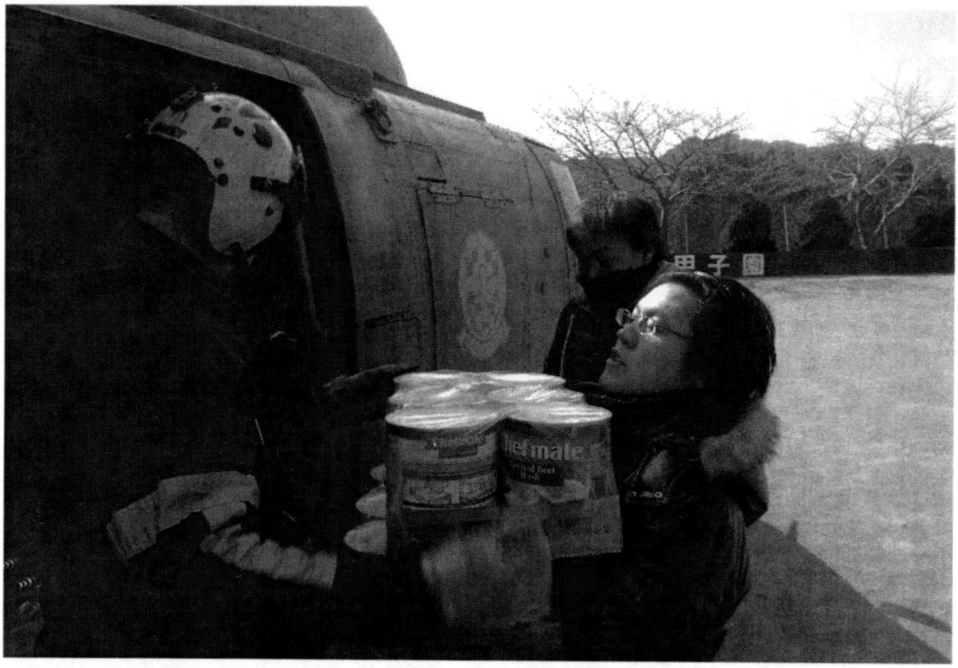

*Figure 26.3* **Sailor gives Japanese woman food during relief efforts [20]**

diseases were seen but poor sanitation in some shelters did lead to small outbreaks of gastroenteritis. Rapid education on carbon monoxide poisoning from using stoves in enclosed spaces was required after several poisonings occurred [3]. Figure 26.3 shows the food relief that was provided.

*Nuclear accident*: As radiation monitoring data became available, further evacuation orders were given for increasingly wider areas around the Fukushima Daiichi Plant. The last order was given a full month after the disaster, when it was discovered that areas up to 30 kilometres from the plant were contaminated with potentially harmful levels of radiation [5]. Worryingly, they had been serving as 'safe' locations, sheltering those who had already been evacuated from closer to the plant [5].

## *Recovery phase*

Once the immediate response to a disaster has ended, the recovery phase begins: this aims to help affected individuals and communities to get their lives back on track. The recovery following 3/11 included:

*Recovery coordination*: The National Recovery plan was published in June 2011. It suggested that the affected areas should be rebuilt with a focus on local communities and a link between communities and nature [8].

*Resettling*: By July 2011, over 20,000 temporary houses had been built. Although authorities tried to house communities together this was not always possible due to the scale of the area affected, thus some communities were divided and unable to provide much-needed emotional and social support to one another. Few temporary housing complexes followed the 'community care' model proposed by architectural researchers using lessons from previous disasters in Japan. Most complexes therefore lacked open space for social gatherings, community centres with support services and transport links to local facilities, and these factors impeded on community and individual recovery [9, 10].

*Family and social support networks*: In 2012, mental health support teams were still visiting shelters, schools and communities, and were careful to work within local cultural norms. However, in addition to the issues of community break-up as discussed above, many families found themselves separated too: during the evacuations, men were accommodated near their hometown to allow them to continue work, while women and children were evacuated to distant prefectures. Although this promotes economic productivity, it can result in prolonged separation of families, breaking up support networks and placing further psychological strain on survivors.

*Support for the elderly*: People aged 65 years and over represented 25 per cent of the population in the three worst-affected prefectures: Tohoku, Iwate and Miyako [11]. When displaced, the elderly were often separated from their family and were accommodated in shelters close to home or in special shelters with higher levels of care. The consequent lack of social support and human interaction has led to problems with mental health and concerns over precipitation of dementia [9]. Physical activity and origami were introduced in shelters to tackle these issues [3].

*Community and culture*: Government and communities alike are realizing the importance of community and culture in recovery. Nearly every building in the coastal village of Kitaura was destroyed and residents were accommodated across many different shelters. Despite their dispersion and losses, the villagers still decided to hold their annual lion dance and festival in November 2011. The festival helped the villagers cope and helped to re-forge community bonds. With a sense of shared purpose, they are determined to rebuild their village together [12].

## Public health lessons

Many aspects of the preparedness and response to 3/11 were impressive, but largely due to the magnitude and severity of the event, it is discerned that many lessons can be learned from such a disaster. Four key points to take away from the events of 3/11 are:

1. Preparedness pays off;
2. Psychosocial health must be considered;
3. Access and transport underline the ability to act; and
4. Public health must become a better advocate for coordinated disaster preparedness and response.

### *Preparedness pays off*

Japan's extensive preparedness activities no doubt saved many lives. The prevalence of earthquake-proof buildings in the country meant that fewer than 300 deaths were attributed to the earthquake. Most buildings withstood the shaking due to the strict building and retrofitting regulations introduced after Japan's Kobe earthquake of 1995, where 5,500 people died immediately as the city's buildings collapsed [6].

Japan also has a good history of putting drills into practice. On the day of 3/11, students at schools and universities took shelter under reinforced desks, communities were evacuated to raised tsunami havens and hospitals quickly cleared lower floors, following drills they have all previously practised every 1 September, which is National Disaster Prevention Day [7, 13, 14]. As well as that, the pre-planning of locations and processes for evacuation meant this procedure was rapidly, and mostly successfully, operationalized.

However, despite everything that being prepared achieved for Japan, there were gaps in preparedness and, due to this, livelihoods and lives were lost. For example, there was evidence of early warning but a late reaction by individuals. In some coastal areas, more than one in ten people who received the tsunami early warning text messages delayed their evacuation to do something else first and consequently were killed by the tsunami [6]. Better community awareness and education may have prevented this.

As well as that, certain risks were taken with the risk assessments. The Japanese government's investigation into the Fukushima Daiichi nuclear accident revealed that experts' risk assessments predicted tsunamis taller than a ten-metre sea wall at the plant but the power company *and* its regulators had chosen not to act [5].

Plans were also in place so that evacuation shelters were supplied with food and water but prolonged stays had not been well prepared for. High-energy foods remained the staple with no provision for those with high blood pressure or diabetes. Space and motivation for physical activity were also lacking. Public health nutritionists were eventually brought in but not before adverse impacts on long-term conditions had already occurred [3, 6].

Public health professionals can do a lot to help individuals, communities and countries reduce the impact of disasters but, as these examples show, preparedness must be robustly considered, coordinated and communicated.

### *Psychosocial health must be considered*

Mental wellbeing is a significant aspect of health and psychosocial support is as much a requirement in recovery from disasters as physical care. It is important to provide mental, as well as physical, activity in shelters, particularly for elderly people, and they themselves should be involved in planning the layout and functions of these shelters.

Support from family and community networks is important for psychosocial health also. Although it can be difficult to plan emergency resettlement and evacuation, recognition of the human need for social support is essential. The role of beacons of hope – signs of return to normalcy – can aid recovery significantly and should be actively encouraged in recovering communities. Kitaura village's lion dance, for example, and the significant effort put in by the Japanese and US forces to quickly reopen Sendai airport [15] were both signs of return to normalcy for the stricken city.

### *Access and transport underline the ability to act*

Supply of water, blankets and food to shelters and survivors, re-stocking of hospitals, transport of patients and many other essential public health activities and other actions were delayed due to blocked roads and lack of fuel [3, 6, 12]. This issue was also encountered after the 2005 Indian Ocean tsunami [16] and is a consequence of the vast amounts of debris tsunamis leave.

Although debris clearance is a massive undertaking, requiring significant input of limited resources, it must be remembered that the majority of both immediate and down-the-line response activities are dependent on gaining access to the affected communities. More focus earlier in the response phase is needed and greater use of resources offered by other countries (especially the military) should be undertaken.

### *Public health must become a better advocate for coordinated disaster preparedness and response*

Disasters can impact on all aspects of people's wellbeing and life, and so too can disaster preparedness and response activities. Public health specialists are in the unique position of being trained to recognize these impacts and the mandate to demand the protection of wellbeing and, ultimately, life.

Many of the above lessons-to-be-learned require improved coordination between certain people. For instance better coordination is needed between the following groups:

- *Engineers and healthcare planners* to ensure hospitals are built in appropriate locations, are easy to access in a disaster and can withstand local hazards.
- *Public health and shelter coordinators* to ensure exercise, healthy diets and opportunities for social interaction and community participation are planned and appropriately delivered.
- *Expert hazard assessors and risk managers* to match the predictions of hazards with mitigation activities (e.g. revising the height of sea wall defences and ensuring earthquake *and* tsunami drills in schools in at-risk areas).
- *Industry, academia and public health professionals* to use industry's technical know-how, academia's knowledge and public health's on-the-ground experience to improve the ability to predict and model disasters.

Without better-coordinated action in the above areas, lives will be endangered. Wherever the disaster is, public health professionals have a right and a responsibility to intervene. It is important to become better advocates for coordinated disaster preparedness and response, and demand action where neglect is evident. Public health professionals, along with various other groups, should aim to keep improving disaster rescue, relief and recovery.

## References


1. USGS (United States Geological Survey). Magnitude 9.0 – Near the East Coast of Honshu, Japan. 2011. Available at: http://earthquake.usgs.gov/earthquakes/eqinthenews/2011/usc0001xgp/
2. USGS. USGS Updates Magnitude of Japan's 2011 Tohoku Earthquake to 9.0. 2011. Available at: http://earthquake.usgs.gov/earthquakes/eqinthenews/2011/usc0001xgp/
3. WPRO (World Health Organization Regional Office for the Western Pacific). The Great East Japan Earthquake: A Story of Devastating Natural Disaster, A Tale of Human Compassion. Geneva: WHO, 2011.
4. NOAA (National Oceanic and Atmospheric Administration). Factsheet: The Tōhoku, Japan Earthquake and Tsunami of March 11, 2011. Available at: http://www.tsunami.gov/events/11Mar2011factsheet.php
5. NAIIC (National Diet of Japan Fukushima Nuclear Accident Independent Investigation Commission). The Official Report of the Fukushima Nuclear Accident Independent Investigation Commission – Executive Summary. Tokyo: National Diet of Japan, 2012.
6. Sakamoto M. Emergency Response in the Great Hanshin–Awaji Earthquake and the Great East Japan Earthquake: Lessons and Improvements. Paper presented at the United Nations' University Research Workshop on Human Security and Natural Disasters, Tokyo, February 2012.
7. Norris J. Japan Earthquake and Tsunami One Year Later – Lingering Impacts and Lessons, 2012. Available at:http://www.ucsf.edu/news/2012/03/11714/japan-earthquake-and-tsunami-one-year-later-lingering-impacts-and-lessons

8. Reconstruction Design Council in Response to the Great East Japan Earthquake. Towards Reconstruction: Hope Beyond the Disaster, Report to the Prime Minister, 25 June 2011, Tokyo: Cabinet Secretariat.
9. Otani J. Ageing Society and Post-Disaster Community Security. Paper presented at the United Nations' University Research Workshop on Human Security and Natural Disasters, Tokyo, February 2012.
10. Nishio A. Community Building in Temporary Housing: Recovery Process of the Great East Japan Earthquake. Paper presented at the Second Joint World Conference on Social Work and Social Development, Stockholm, July 2012.
11. Japanese Statistics Bureau. *Japan Statistical Yearbook 2012.* Chapter 2: Population and households. 2–9 Population of three age groups by prefecture. Tokyo: Statistics Bureau.
12. Fukushima A. Natural Disasters: Addressing Vulnerability, Coping Capacity and Impact Reduction through Human Security. Paper presented at the United Nations' University Research Workshop on Human Security and Natural Disasters, Tokyo, February 2012.
13. Birmingham L. Japan's Earthquake Warning System Explained. *Time World,* 18 March 2012. Available at: http://www.time.com/time/world/article/0,8599,2059780,00.html
14. Parker B. Why Did the 2011 Japan Tsunami Kill So Many People? *Huffington Post,* 11 March 2012. Available at: http://www.huffingtonpost.com/bruce-parker/japan-tsunami_b_1335737.html
15. Mutzabaugh B. Sendai: Airport's Remarkable Reopening Aided by U.S. Military. *USA Today* – Travel, 15 April 2011. Available at: http://travel.usatoday.com/flights/post/2011/04/sendai-airport-reopens/155985/1
16. Da Silva J. for the Disaster Emergency Committee. *Lessons from Aceh. Key Considerations in Post-Disaster Reconstruction.* Rugby: Practical Action Publishing, 2010.
17. Daniell J. CATDAT Situation Report 50: One Year Summary of Losses in the Japanese Earthquake/ Tsunami of March 11th 2011. 2012. Available at: http://earthquake-report.com/
18. US Navy photo. Helicopter flies over Sendai. 2011. Available at: http://en.wikinews.org/w/index.php?title=File:SH60B_helicopter_flies_over_Sendai.jpg&filetimestamp=20110316141528
19. McCord D. Mass Communication Specialist 3rd Class. Tsunami fire vehicles. 2011. Available at: http://en.wikipedia.org/wiki/File:2011TsunamiFireVehicles.jpg
20. Conant J. Naval Air Crewman 2nd Class. Sailor/California native gives Japanese woman food during relief efforts. 2011. Available at: http://www.flickr.com/photos/usnavy/5540310550/

# 27

# Public health roles in response to the 2011 Thailand flooding

*Phitaya Charupoonphol*

## Introduction: overview of the flooding

In 2011, Thailand faced the worst flooding it had seen in 50 years. Floodwaters swamped more than two-thirds of the country, submerging rice fields and shutting down hundreds of factories. Severe flooding started at the end of July and spread through the provinces of northern, north-eastern and central Thailand along the Mekong and Chao Phraya river basins. In October, floodwaters reached the mouth of the Chao Phraya and inundated parts of Bangkok. Flooding persisted in some areas until mid-January 2012, and resulted in a total of 815 deaths and 13.6 million people affected (see Figure 27.1). Sixty-five of Thailand's 76 provinces were declared flood disaster zones and over 20,000 square kilometres of farm-land were damaged (see Figures 27.2 and 27.3). The disaster has been described as 'the worst flooding yet in terms of the amount of water and people affected' (see Table 27.1). The World Bank ranked it the world's fourth costliest disaster, surpassed only by the 2011 earthquake and tsunami in Japan, the 1995 Kobe earthquake and Hurricane Katrina in 2005 [1].

The latest damage estimation as reported by the Federation of Thai Industry is at least 185 billion baht, and includes 65 billion baht damage to Thai industry, agriculture and housing in the communities and suburb villages (see Figure 27.4). A large part of the damage stems from the effect on manufacturing industry, with 930 factories in 28 provinces affected. The flooding was estimated to result in a loss of 0.6 to 0.9 per cent in terms of economic growth. Disruption included closing schools early and letting go of workers from flooded factories. Not all factories are expected to reopen, causing a significant long-term job loss in central Thailand [2] (see Box 27.1).

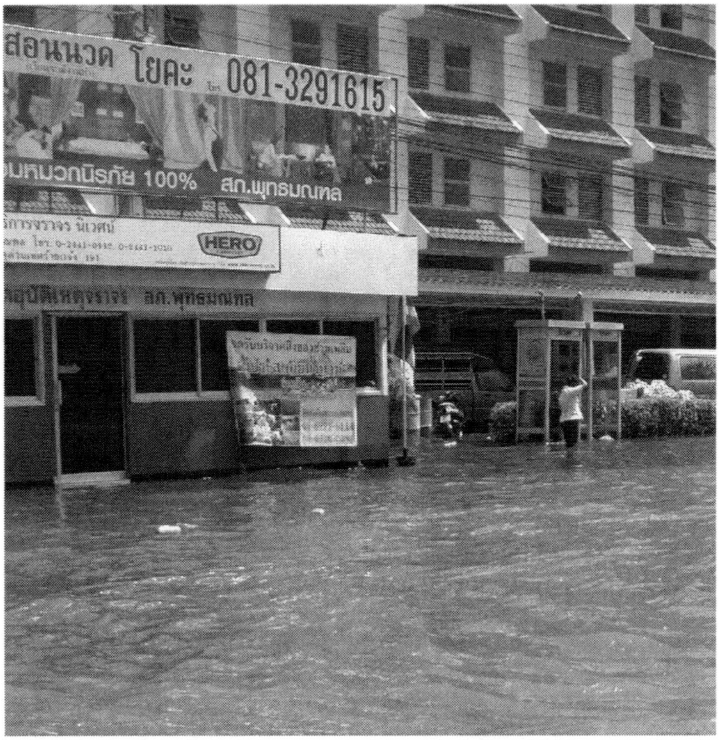


*Figure 27.1* Severe flooding spread through the provinces of northern, north-eastern and central Thailand

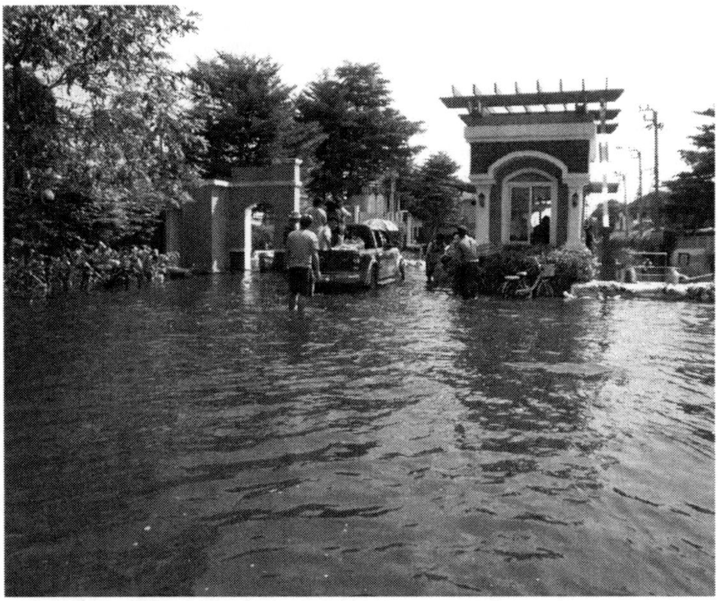

*Figure 27.2* Transportation was cut off in the heart of Bangkok

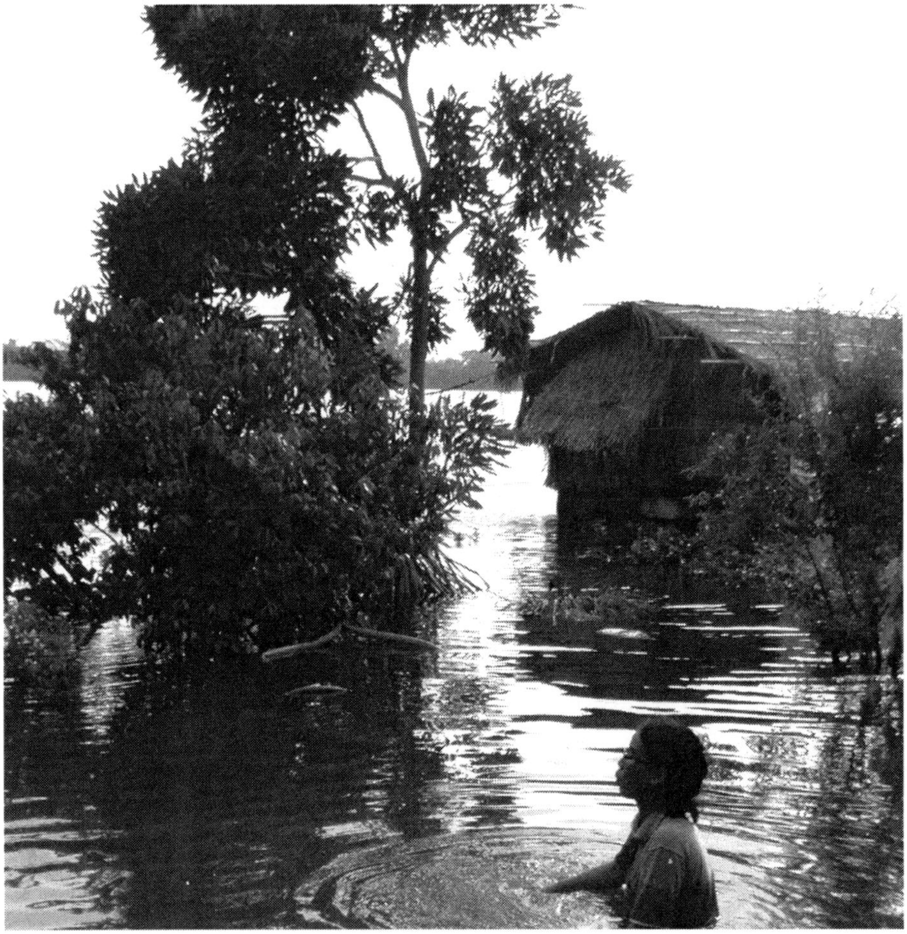

*Figure 27.3* Sixty-five provinces of Thailand were declared flood disaster zones, including rural communities

*Table 27.1* Natural disasters through the years in Thailand

| *Disaster* | *Date* | *Killed* |
|---|---|---|
| Wind storm | 27 Oct 1962 | 769 |
| Flood | 18 Nov 1988 | 664 |
| Wave/surge | Jun 1955 | 500 |
| Wind storm | 3 Nov 1989 | 458 |
| Flood | 3 Jan 1975 | 239 |
| Flood | 8 Sep 1995 | 231 |
| Flood | 28 Oct 1995 | 200 |
| Flood | 11 Aug 2001 | 104 |
| Epidemic | Oct 1977 | 100 |
| Flood | Aug 1978 | 96 |

*(Continued overleaf)*

*Table 27.1* Continued

| *Disaster* | *Date* | *Affected* |
|---|---|---|
| Drought | Jan 1999 | 6,000,000 |
| Flood | Jun 1996 | 5,000,000 |
| Flood | 8 Sep 1995 | 4,280,984 |
| Flood | 3 Jan 1975 | 3,000,093 |
| Flood | Jul 2000 | 2,500,000 |
| Drought | Mar 1991 | 2,500,000 |
| Wind storm | 17 Aug 1991 | 1,894,238 |
| Flood | Aug 1978 | 1,628,400 |
| Flood | 18 Nov 1988 | 1,114,819 |
| Flood | Aug 1983 | 1,000,000 |
| Flood | July 2011–Jan 2012 | 13,600,000 |
| Flood | Oct 2010–Nov 2010 | 7,000,000 |

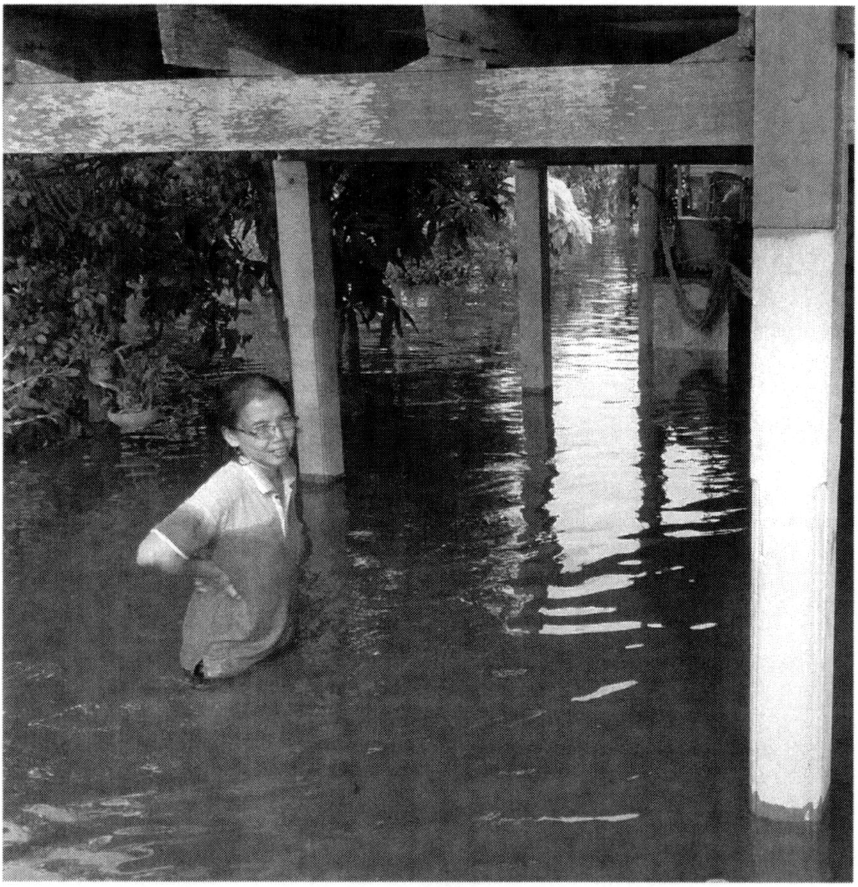

*Figure 27.4* The highest level of flooding the country has ever experienced

## Box 27.1 Case study: how are businesses affected by the flood?

Thailand is the world's second largest producer of hard disk drives accounting for approximately 25 per cent of the world's production. Many of the factories that make hard disk drives have been flooded, including Western Digital, leading to the prediction of a worldwide shortage of hard disk drives in the future.

Western Digital was able to save one of their plants that was flooded on 15 October 2011 and used it as a backup plant from 30 November 2011. Some operations were expected to take longer to recover, whilst other plants were still under two feet of water as of 2 December 2011. Western Digital's flood-related costs were estimated to be US$225–275 million; however, an insurance claim of US$50 million for property damage and another claim for business interruption will help lower the net impact.

The economies of other countries besides Thailand will be significantly impacted by the flood as well. The country that will be hardest hit is Japan [3]. Japanese firms with plants in Thailand include Toyota, Honda, Hitachi and Canon. One analyst predicted the profits of one firm, Toyota, may be cut by ¥200 billion (US$2.5 billion). Worker incomes in Thailand and Japan are also impacted.

Thailand accounts for about 30 per cent of global trade in rice and 25 per cent of the main crops are not expected to survive after the flooding. On the other side of the world, rice farmers in Arkansas, that usually account for 42 per cent of the US output, were also flooded early this year and were then faced with a drought, which meant their crops were reduced by 32 per cent according to the USDA [3].

These two critical episodes have certainly caused worldwide impacts on rice production and prices, and in Thailand, where rice farmers are typically short of reserved capital. This means that Thailand farmers have lost both their investments in the current crop and have to wait for the floodwaters to recede prior to planting new ones, which all results in financial hardship.

## Mitigation measures and plans

### *Flood management in Thailand*

Thailand is a Southeast Asian country with a population of 69 million. It is situated in the Indo-Chinese Peninsula, sharing borders with Myanmar, Laos, Cambodia and Malaysia. Physio-graphically, the country may be divided into four regions: the North (mountainous), Central Plain (Cho Phraya River Basin), the Eastern Uplands and the Southern Peninsula.

Thailand has a tropical climate. The climate seasons are based on two major wind systems, the north-east and south-west monsoons. The former, the dry cool period, occurs from mid-October to mid-February due to winds flowing from the north-east. The latter, the wet period, occurs from mid-May to mid-September. In addition to monsoons, Thailand is also subjected to tropical storms from the South China Sea, the Western Pacific, the Gulf of Thailand and the Andaman Sea. They are born as typhoons, tropical storms and tropical depression.

Floods in Thailand are normally caused by tropical storms and depression, and rarely by typhoons. Other causes that aggravate floods include insufficient capacity of rivers and canals, poor drainage and sewerage systems in populated areas, destruction of forests, poor management of land and inadequacy of reservoirs. In the Bangkok metropolitan area, flooding is

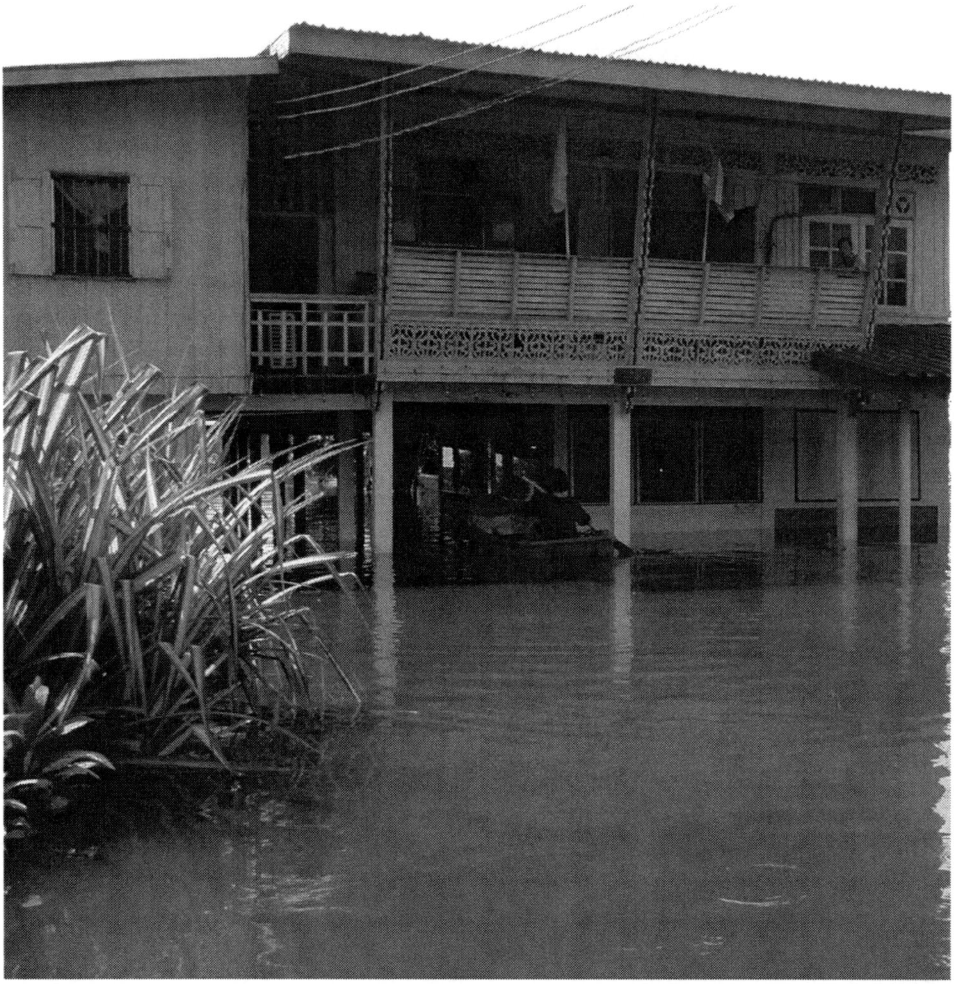

*Figure 27.5* Some of the hardest hit areas were around Bangkok

caused by downpours of heavy rain leading to rivers overflowing onto the flood plain of the Chao Phraya River and, along with the tidal effect, this contributes to land subsidence due to groundwater (see Figure 27.5).

Drainage control systems, including multiple dams, irrigation canals and flood detention basins, have been implemented but are inadequate to prevent flood damage, especially in rural areas. A system of drainage tunnels was implemented from 2001 to prevent flooding in Bangkok, which has seen only minor flooding since the major flood of 1995. Other regions, however, have experienced severe flooding as recently as 2010 [4].

## *Disaster management in Thailand*

According to the Civil Defence Act 1979, disaster management covers both natural and man-made disasters. Thailand's disaster management system is divided into three levels of responsibility:

1 *Policy and strategic response*: Disaster policy and strategy is conducted in cooperation with government policy and the National Economic and Social Development Plan. The National Safety Committee of Thailand (NSCT) is responsible for policy and strategic response relating to emergencies classified as accidents. The Civil Defence Committee (CDC) is responsible for policy and strategy regarding disaster, rear security and damage control. The National Security Council (NSC) is responsible for policy and strategy in relation to national security, i.e. warfare.
2 *Policy implementation*: The Civil Defence Secretariat is responsible for implementing the policies which the said committees have assigned. This includes drafting guidelines for operational units and dictating practical procedures for each type of disaster, including floods, storms, fires and droughts.
3 *Disaster mitigation*: According to the Civil Defence Act 1979, local authorities are responsible for creating preparedness plans for disasters, whereas mitigation in each administrative area remains the responsibility of the preparation unit. However, due to budget constraints and reduction of government equipment costs in local administrative areas, Thailand has improved its disaster mitigation system on a regional basis by setting up units at three operational levels: emergency, main and support. These are responsible for their designated areas in Bangkok and the provinces.

## Master disaster management plan

The Civil Defence Secretariat is responsible for identifying disaster prevention measures and policies, and formulating the National Civil Defence Plan (NCDP). This plan serves as the master plan for all agencies concerned and provides guidelines for the management of disasters. The Civil Defence Secretariat also provides equipment, technical assistance and training courses for local agencies and the public, and coordinates with agencies that are in charge of disaster relief and rescue operations.

According to the Civil Defence Act 1979, functional agencies are responsible for formulating their own disaster management plans. These plans are reviewed and updated every three years for approval by the NCDP. Thailand has now established a Geographic Information System (GIS) to manage disaster-related information. Currently, there is a database system for chemical risk areas, flood- and mudslide-prone areas, and concerned agencies and experts.

## Disaster management in the non-health sector

According to the Civil Defence Act 1979, the disaster management system comprises three levels. They work together to manage the referral system and problem-solve in particular situations:

*National*: It is the responsibility of the National Civil Defence Committee (NCDC) to coordinate all activities relevant to civil defence and disaster management. The NCDC is chaired by the Minister of Interior, with members from government agencies from all over the country. The NSCT was established in 1982 due to a rise in road accidents and handles man-made disaster management only. The National Disaster Warning Centre was established under the Order of the Office of the Prime Minister. Its major task is to detect earthquakes and to analyse seismic data to determine the possibility of a tsunami before issuing notifications to the public, authorities and rescue teams.

*Regional*: Twelve Regional Disaster Prevention and Mitigation Centres have been established to render technical assistance and auxiliary services to local CDCs. Each of these centres is headed by a director reporting to the Director-General of the Department of Disaster Prevention and Mitigation (DDPM).

*Local*: The main actors are the local CDCs at provincial, district and local levels.

### *Disaster management in the health sector*

Currently, there is no single department devoted to Emergency and Humanitarian Action/Health Action in Crises (EHA/HAC) in the Ministry of Public Health (MOPH). The MOPH's EHA-related activities are spread across various divisions of the MOPH and, therefore, there is no clear focal point in the health sector, but despite this, the MOPH responds to crises effectively. A team of officials from various divisions respond to emergencies. The Narenthorn Centre is a division under the office of the permanent secretary of the MOPH and provides emergency medical services (EMS) throughout the country. In addition, the MOPH has recognized that an 'appropriate structure' is necessary to address emergencies based on various national-level committees to control epidemic, pandemic and other potential hazards [5].

## Public health roles in response to the 2011 flooding

### *The public health system*

During the flood, the MOPH adjusted its medical and public health services, including disease surveillance and control systems, to cope with the emergency situation. It did the following:

1 Mobilized medical teams, nurses and medical equipment to assist health facilities of affected provinces. www.mobile medical units were set up to provide both physical and mental healthcare services to flood victims. Temporary shelters were provided for victims that remained at home.
2 Initiated supplemental disease surveillance to quickly find patients who might need care in the shelters and in the community, and to monitor the health situation in affected populations.
3 Dispatched rapid response teams to investigate reported outbreaks, implement prevention and control measures, and ensure food safety and safe drinking water in the shelters and the community [6].

In retrospect, the MOPH found that disease outbreak and other health threats related to the flood were not as high as anticipated. Thailand's disease surveillance data showed that the most common illnesses that affected populations were athlete's foot, upper respiratory tract infection, conjunctivitis and food poisoning. These illnesses were mostly found in the shelters and were quickly managed. Overall, rates for these conditions were not too different from the seasonal occurrences in previous years. Most deaths associated with the flood were due to accidents, especially drowning and electrocutions. Importantly, no major disease outbreaks were detected. Despite its impacts on health, the flood crisis has presented the MOPH with an opportunity to strengthen its collaboration with all related agencies and its health system, while also innovating new and better approaches which could be used as the basis for disaster preparedness, response and recovery for future events (see Table 27.2).

*Table 27.2* The surveillance status

*Event-based surveillance: Network of Surveillance and Rapid Response Team (SRRT) notified and conducted the investigation of 38 events as follows**

| *Diseases* | *1–9 Oct.* | *10–16 Oct.* | *17–23 Oct.* | *24–30 Oct.* | *1–6 Nov.* | *7–13 Nov.* | *14–20 Nov.* | *21–27 Nov.* | *28 Nov.–4 Dec.* | *Total* |
|---|---|---|---|---|---|---|---|---|---|---|
| Food poisoning/ diarrhoea | 1 (99) | 3 (1, 37, 48) | 3 (10, 21, 30) | 3 (5, 25, 40) | 6 (3, 6, 8, 11, 19, 26) | 0 | 3 (5, 15, 19) | 2 (141, 58) | 2 (62, 15) | 23 (704) |
| Leptospirosis | 0 | 0 | 1 (1) | 1 (1) | 1 (7) | 1 (1) | 1 (1) | 0 | 0 | 7 (12) |
| Chicken pox | 0 | 0 | 0 | 0 | 1 (3) | 1 (1) | 0 | 0 | 0 | 3 (7) |
| Chemical intoxication | 0 | 1 | 1 (3) | 1 | 0 | 0 | 0 | 0 | 0 | 2 |
| Conjunctivitis | 0 | 0 | 1 (21) | 0 | 0 | 1 (15) | 0 | 0 | 0 | 2 (36) |
| Measles | 0 | 0 | 1 (2) | 0 | 0 | 0 | 0 | 0 | 0 | 1 (2) |

*Note*: * Number of cases in each event is in parentheses.

### Flood victims requiring attention

Public health offices in provinces where the flood had subsided were ordered to start their post-flood rehabilitation, which included the improvement of water systems, disease prevention and mental health care. In provinces that still had floods, mobile medical teams were dispatched to help victims. The top five diseases found among flood victims were athlete's foot, influenza, muscle ache, headache and stress. The MOPH instructed its officials and village health volunteers to take care of flood victims' mental health conditions after a number were diagnosed with depression [7]. Anxiety and stress are common reactions to a crisis. During the first two to four weeks, common symptoms include headaches, exhaustion, loss of appetite, sleep deprivation and fear. Support from family and friends for anxiety victims is important.

Volunteer support from staff from mental health institutions was deployed in two ways: taking care of flood victims sheltering at evacuation centres and visiting those stranded in their homes (see Box 27.2 for one example of how volunteer staff can help – making an emergency DIY toilet).

## Box 27.2 Making a DIY emergency toilet in a flood crisis

A toilet is a necessary convenience for human beings, even in a flood crisis. When a toilet is unavailable, people should discharge into plastic bags and spread calcium hydroxide or liquid chlorine 2 per cent into the bag and then wrap it tightly. If you cannot get calcium hydroxide and liquid chlorine 2 per cent, just wrap the bag tightly.

A simple, private toilet can be made quickly and easily in a crisis situation by following the steps outlined below.

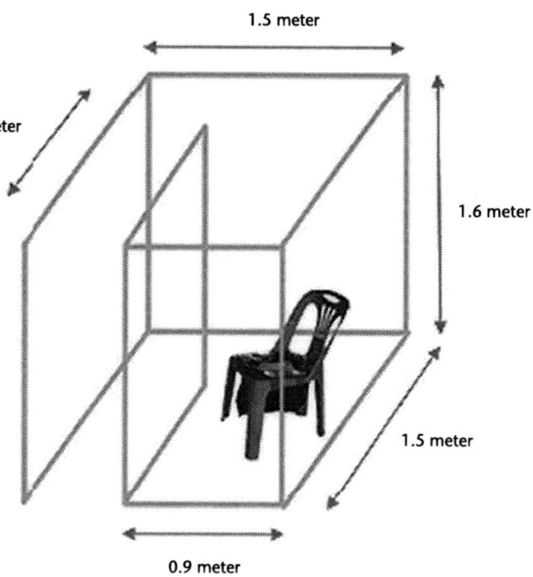


### Materials

1. A plastic chair
2. Plastic bag
3. Cardboard/inner tube
4. Adhesive tape
5. PVC pipes
6. Plastic canvas
7. Rope

### How to make an emergency toilet

First, make a hole in the seat by cutting into the middle of it. To make the seat more comfortable, cut pieces of cardboard or inner tube in round shapes the same size as the seat and place on the seat.

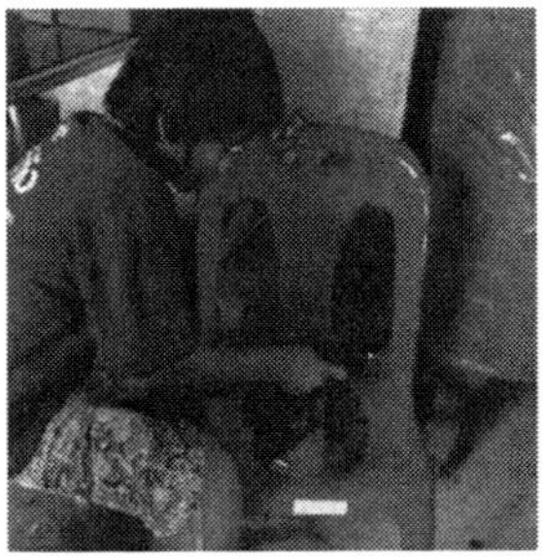
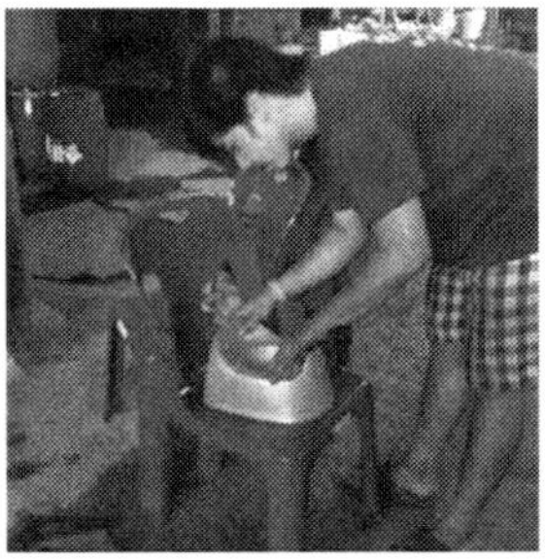
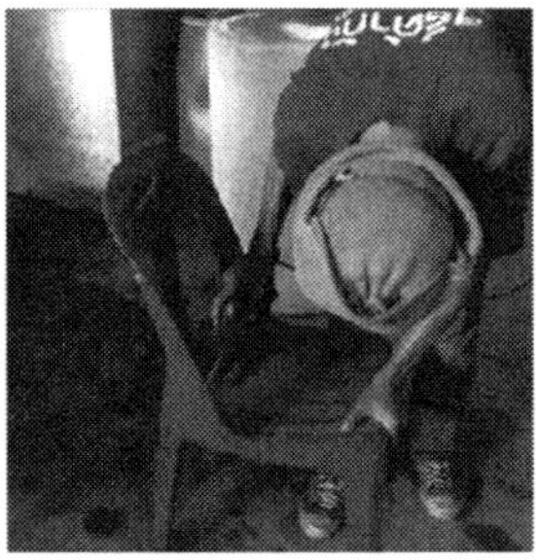

Then, put a plastic bag in the hole of the seat and adhere it to the chair by adhesive tape. Make sure that the bag is firmly stuck to the chair.

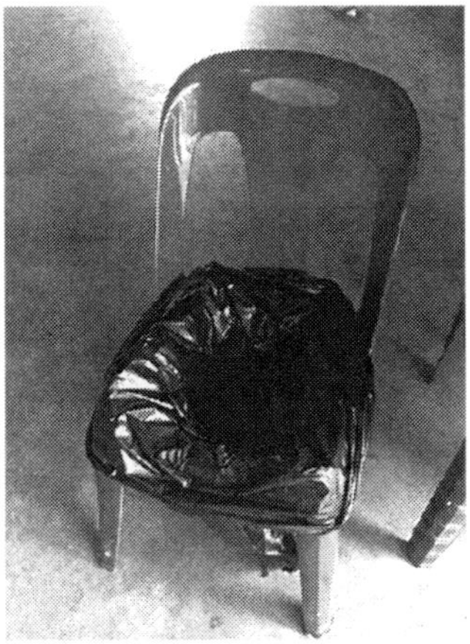

Next, make a cubicle by structuring the PVC pipes as pictured below.
Finally, wrap a plastic canvas to the formed PVC pipes and adhere it to the pipes by rope or adhesive tape.

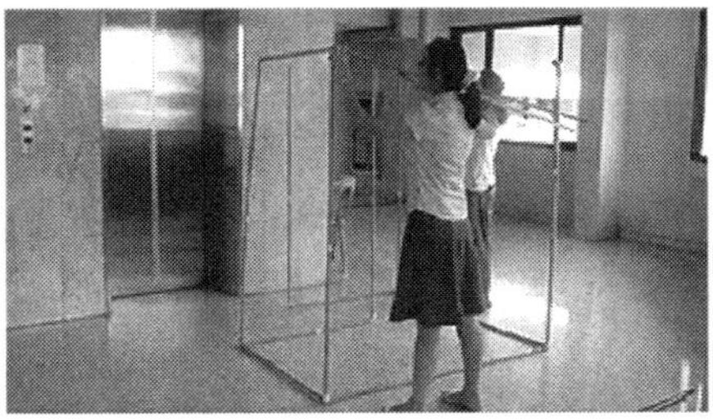
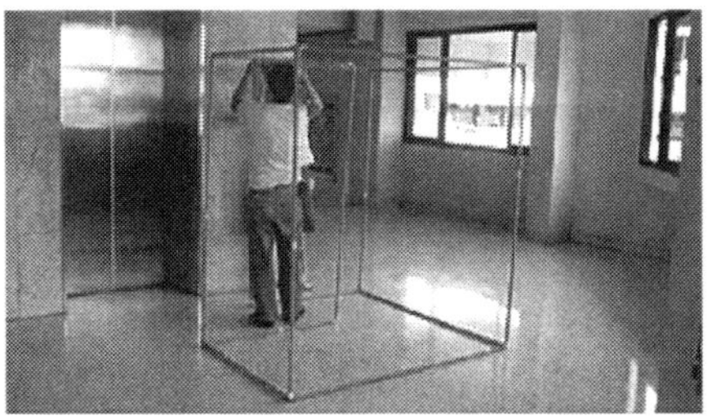

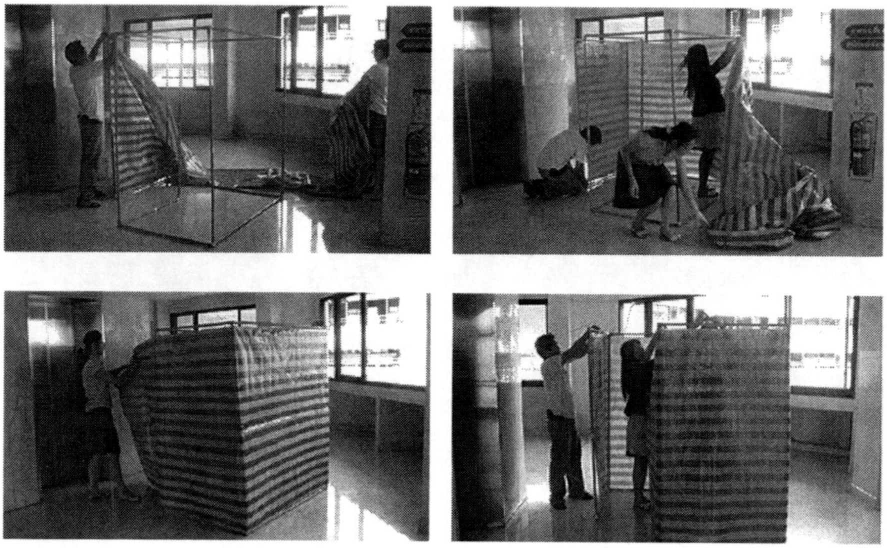

## *Health services system during flooding*

The health service system was divided into three main systems, including the most important medical emergency service system and the outpatient service system, particularly the setting up of field hospitals around flood areas. Also, an inpatient service system was initiated in affected hospitals and unaffected community hospitals. At the time of the main flood, a field hospital was established. The patients were able to access medical services through these avenues and some were referred to the surrounding network hospital for proper management. The major services at the affected hospitals included emergency room services, outpatient services, hospitalized patient services and provision of social support by hospital teams and the community.

## *Referral system*

The referral centre coordinated with the hospital network to refer patients. The system aimed to: support the services of the primary care unit for the fieldwork and sharing of information about patients who may be affected by the flood; prepare patients' current medical information; limit the number of patients in the hospital for affected patients; and prepare patients who may need to be transported. The outpatient, monitoring and screening for diseases information was reported to the management team. It was necessary to put intensive care patients (ICU-RCU-NICU-SNB-patients with mechanical ventilators) in the same ward to create space in case patients needed to be transferred. Working with the home-visit health promotion team to follow up patients with chronic diseases, it was essential for the referral centre to know which hospitals had the capacity to take care of the referred patients. The emergency resuscitation team could work on dry or flooded areas.

## *Management of hospital personnel*

Medical personnel who escaped the flooding were prepared to work with the community hospital that was established to support a new centre for patient care. The management team was concerned with ensuring the safety of patients remaining in hospital, ensuring proper personnel management and maintaining infrastructure, such as electricity, water, telephone, radio communications and wastewater treatment.

### *Preparation of rehabilitation*

The Hospital Board Committee established a hospital rehabilitation plan with two phases:

- *During the flood* – activities included surveillance of disease outbreaks, sanitary care and providing healthcare services for emergency/outpatients/inpatients; and
- *After the flood* – there were plans to hasten the recovery of the hospital by focusing on the restoration of critical systems, such as wastewater treatment, electrical, medical and medical equipment, elevator, telephone and repair utility of hospital buildings.

Two weeks after the flood, the hospital could resume its services. It reopened with a capacity for 300 and later expanded to accommodate the increasing volume of patients. To aid with its restoration and amendments, the government and private sectors called for donations and volunteers.

### *Management of flood prevention*

Strategic planning, in terms of how to cope and actively prevent disasters, should be prepared. The flood prevention committee should consist of a director, the involved deputy directors, a head of the environment unit and a chief of general administration. The committee should plan, prepare and train the possibly affected people, maintenance technicians and supervisors on how to cope with floods. The role of the committee should include the collection of information and useful data, and an analysis of the situation. Incident Command System (ICS), principle of public health emergency management, risk evaluation and management, communication, line of command, triage in disaster setting, treatment, crisis resource management (CRM), workshop discussions and dry-run scenarios are all components that need to be included in strategic planning for management of floods and other disasters.

### *Establishment of the command centre for flooding prevention*

The command centre was responsible for evaluating the real-time water level, monitoring the impact of services from flood conditions, coordinating the transportation for transfers, moving people away from flood areas, moving patients in critical conditions, launching flood protection policies, issuing warnings and strengthening the flood protection system [8].

### *Plans for flood conditions*

The hospital has a programme for flood conditions with cooperation from the hospital administrative board. The provision of health care was divided into two groups: general illnesses and chronic illnesses. Management plans, including resource management (personnel, vehicles, drugs and medical supplies), were initiated to provide support to the public by the Office of the Royal Household and other agencies. The emergency medical services system was set up in response to the public to address the situation both within the province and in neighbouring provinces [6].

The above plan was used to minimize the effect on the public utility of the hospital and to protect the power supply in terms of ascertaining the electric power backup system, fuel, gas and water pumps, as well as other tools, needed to prepare the backup generators in case of emergency.

## The public health role in disaster mitigation, preparedness, response and recovery: a summary

The public health role in disaster mitigation, preparedness, response and recovery includes [9]:

- Identifying community resources applicable to the physical, social and psychosocial effects of a disaster;
- Identifying groups most at risk (i.e. children, the elderly, homeless, chronically ill, homebound, physically or mentally disabled);
- Providing disaster education both prior to (i.e. what to expect in a disaster) and post (i.e. how to deal with the effects) the event;
- Taking responsibility for the health of a community following a disaster;
- Using such resources as assessment, epidemiology and data analysis to make and implement recommendations for limiting morbidity and mortality following a disaster;
- Cooperating and collaborating with other partners to ensure that primary health, public health and mental health issues are adequately addressed in disaster planning;
- Preventing diseases by providing health advisories on injury prevention, food and water safety, and vector control. This includes water-borne diseases from flood water (e.g. dysentery due to enterotoxigenic *Escherichia coli*, *Shigella*, hepatitis A, leptospirosis and giardiasis) and risk of disease from eating or drinking anything contaminated with flood water or spoiled from lack of refrigeration:
  - Water-borne skin infection, anxiety and stress due to flooding
  - Vector (snake, insect and rodent) control
  - Surveillance for injuries, increases in vector populations, infectious diseases, drinking water sources, and disruption of sewer and solid waste collection systems;
- Initiating injury prevention and surveillance programmes – injury prevention from exposure to fires, explosions from gas leaks, downed live wires, hazardous waste, contamination and debris;
- Conducting a needs assessment on the public health infrastructure (e.g. water, sewage and electricity), and on health, medical and pharmaceutical services and supplies. Some areas need to cut off electricity services to prevent electrical injuries;
- Assuring that health services continue post-impact, and including acute, continuity of care, primary care and emergency care;
- Communicating with government officials about the public health effects of potential disasters and providing expert assistance during and after disasters. Communication needs to happen with, and information needs to be shared between, the following:
  - Those providing medical care (hospitals and their emergency departments, community providers, and other public health and social service agencies)
  - First responders (fire, police, EMS) and other responders (national guard)
  - Local and regional laboratories
  - Officials, mayors, governor(s)
  - Partners (Thai Red Cross, public works)

  - Health-related agencies
  - The media
  - The general public;
- Developing and advocating public policies designed to reduce the public health impact of potential disasters;
- Collaborating with other health and human service professionals to rigorously evaluate intervention outcomes. Once a disaster strikes, these agencies need to coordinate the development of an action plan to address community health needs:
  - Ensure the continuity of healthcare services (acute emergency care, primary care and preventive care)
  - Ensure that essential facilities will be able to function post-impact (hospitals, health departments, physicians' offices, storage sites for healthcare supplies, dispatch centres, paging services and ambulance stations).

Public health considerations in recovery and reconstruction include to:

- Organize community-wide programmes for delivery of health care and public health services, including special needs shelters;
- Provide community education to enhance public awareness (i.e. injury control), aid community adjustment, form the basis for future disaster mitigation and educate the community about the likely health risks and how to deal with them; and
- Access health needs in the community (see Figure 27.6).

Three phases that happened post-impact in the affected community are:

- *Emergency phase* – focuses on saving lives through search and rescue, first aid, emergency medical assistance and overall disaster assessment. Efforts are immediately begun to repair critical facilities, restore communications and transportation networks, and, in some cases, evacuate residents from areas still vulnerable to further disaster (see Figure 27.7);
- *Transition or recovery phase* – people return to work, damaged buildings and infrastructure are repaired, and other actions that allow the community to return to normalcy as soon as possible are initiated. Victims begin their emotional recovery and may experience depression and post-traumatic stress disorder. External assistance is provided in the form of cash and credit. Construction projects and job creation are the most appropriate types of aid:
  - Traditionally, four stages of recovery have been categorized. These include emergency response, including debris removal and provision of temporary housing; restoration of public services, including electricity, water and telephone; replacement and reconstruction of capital stock; and initiation of improvements and developmental reconstruction that stimulate economic growth and local development;
- *Reconstruction phase* – characterized by physical reordering of communications, utilities, roads and the general physical environment. Residents repair or rebuild their housing and agricultural activities resume (see Figure 27.8).

## The Philosophy of Sufficiency Economy and flood management

The Philosophy of Sufficiency Economy, bestowed by His Majesty, the King Bhumibol Adulyadej, to the people of Thailand in 1974, was reiterated after the economic crisis

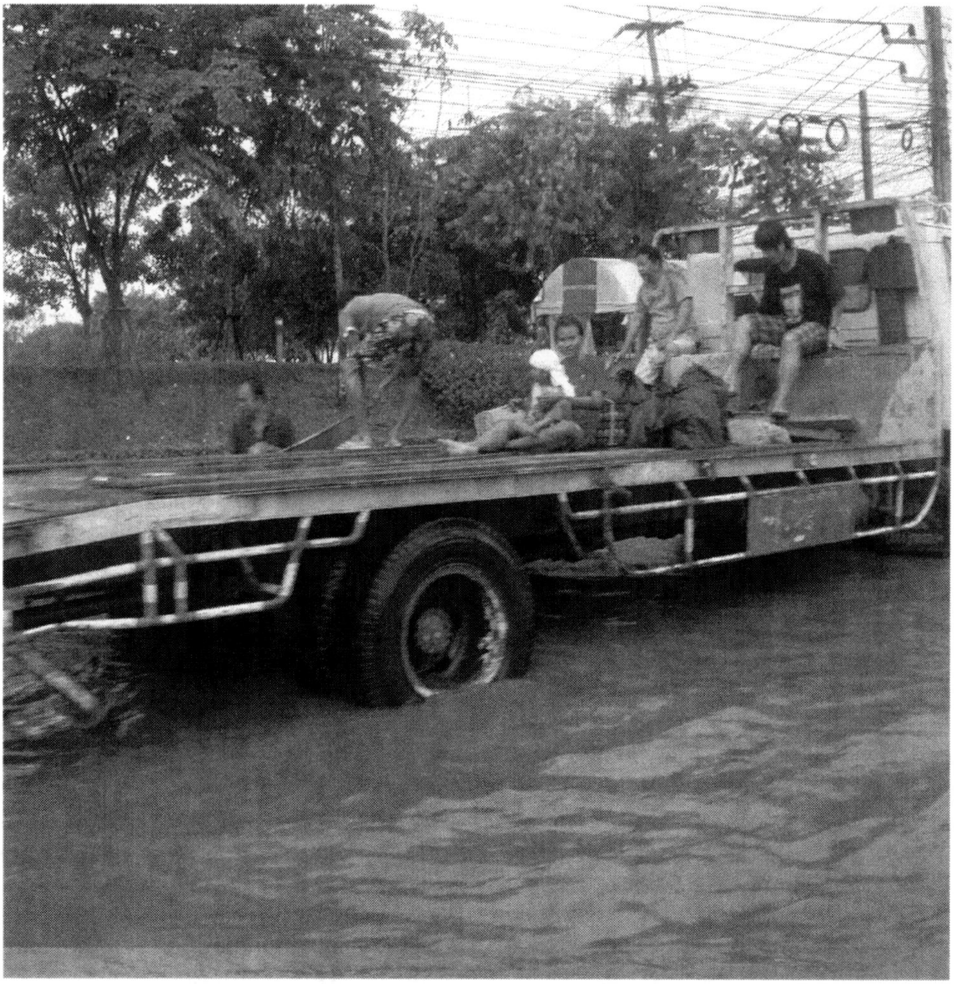

*Figure 27.6* Community participation was the key to survival

in 1997, emphasizing a more balanced, holistic and sustainable development approach [10]. This has been widely adopted by individual, community, business, household and government levels.

The Philosophy of Sufficiency Economy is that:

> Economic development must be done step by step. It should begin with the strengthening of our economic foundation by assuring that the majority of our population has enough to live on. Once reasonable progress has been achieved, one should then embark on the next steps, by pursuing more advanced levels of economic development.

There are three pillars of sufficiency economy: moderation, reasonableness and risk management.

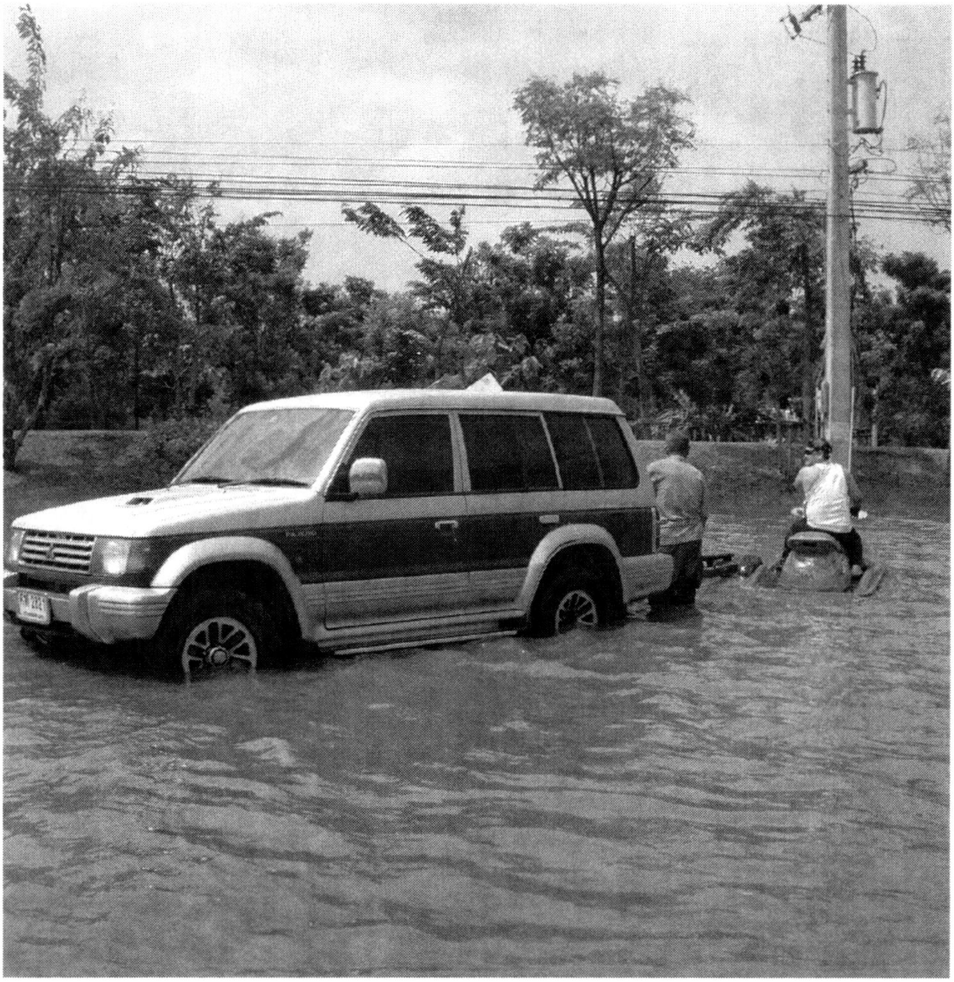

*Figure 27.7* The road was cut off by flooding in suburban areas

## *Flood management*

His Majesty has devoted a lot of time to seeking solutions to flood problems in Thailand. His concern for the people has led to various methodologies, including:

- *Dike construction* – in applying this ancient practice to modern flood prevention, the dikes should be built to a size suitable for the job and at an appropriate distance from the bank of the canals. This will prevent water overflowing the banks from undermining the dikes;
- *Water diversion ditches* – for diverting all or part of the floodwaters. Ditches or canals are built to link with existing waterways so that floodwaters are drained away. Alternatively, these diversion ditches can be linked directly to the sea;
- *Watercourse improvement* – to help floodwaters drain out effectively or the water to flow more rapidly. The idea is to excavate the canal bed to make water flow more quickly;

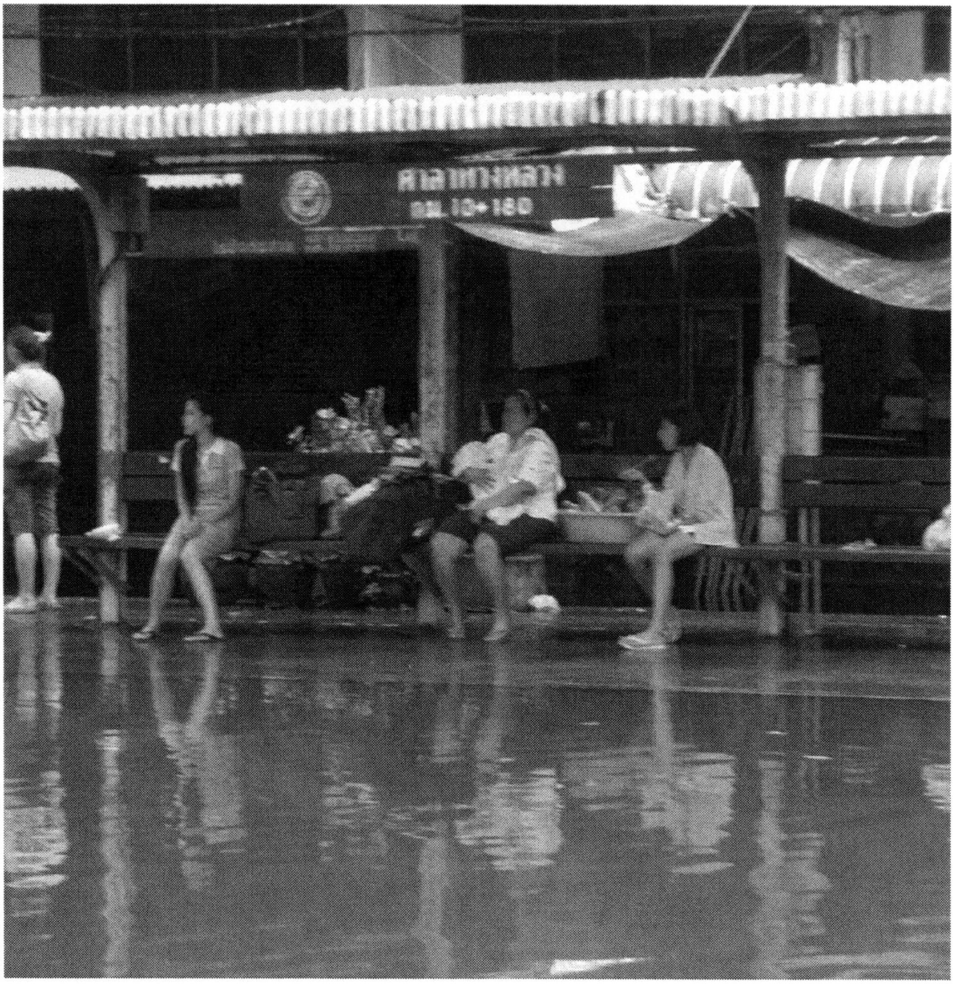

*Figure 27.8* The roads were under water for weeks

smooth the banks to reduce obstacles to water flow; and remove weeds, water hyacinth and other objects that impede water flow. In addition, if a waterway has many curves, new straight courses for water to flow more efficiently can be dug; and

- *Reservoir construction* – the reservoirs are to keep the water out of areas frequently inundated by heavy flooding.

His Majesty devised a flood management system for Bangkok called Kaem Ling (Monkey's Cheeks). 'A monkey will, if you throw a banana, open its mouth and swallow the banana whole and keep it in his cheek. A monkey can keep almost an entire bunch of bananas inside its cheeks. Only later will the monkey take the bananas out, chew and swallow them.' Three principles to which the Kaem Ling Project has successfully adhered include: identifying sites

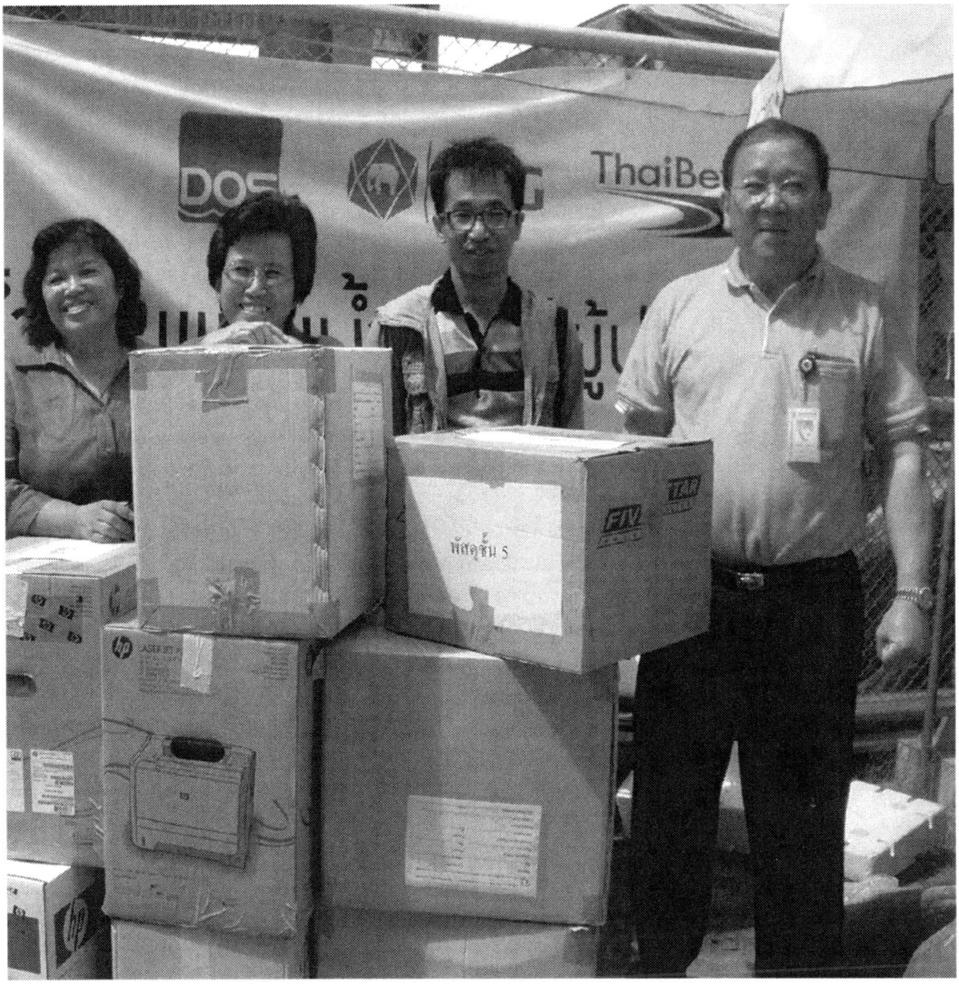

*Figure 27.9* Several organizations, including the Mahidol University team, helped to pack supplies of food to give to the flood victims

to serve as storage reservoirs and divert water into them, building waterways leading to the water storage reservoirs and continually draining water out of these reservoirs.

## *Flood preparedness*

This includes using environmental health management systems, such as dumping garbage in the correct places, and concentrating on food and drinking water.

*Drinking water supply*: During floods, the water treatment plant facility in Bangkok was able to protect the water so tap water was safe to consume. The metropolitan waterworks authority certified the tap water quality by assigning the Faculty of Public Health at the

Mahidol University to monitor and verify those results with water quality standards (see Figure 27.9). The Faculty of Public Health provided drinking water to the community and certified the quality of the water. Two steps of activated carbon, cationic resin, ceramic filter and UV disinfection were installed and supplied about 1,000 litres/day with low cost and maintenance.

*Potential of technology and social media in flooding response*: Social media is perhaps the most important channel of communication during a crisis. University students developed a Facebook page to provide information on ensuring the safety of pets during the flood crisis. Users could find more information about the flood situation from the flood-related professionals on their Facebook pages and Twitter posts.

In the light of coordination issues, it is undeniable that the government, civil society organizations, NGOs, citizen volunteer groups and the private sector are keen to use technology. The government has a greater role ahead to lead these numerous stakeholders to assess, build and increase the technology capacity of the country. The following examples of social media were used during the 2011 flood crisis:

- Facebook page, 'Nam Kheun Hai Reeb Bok' ('inform quickly when the water comes'): www.facebook.com/room2680 – this gathered flood situation updates and led to the sharing of updates by specific groups. An example is www.facebook.com/Muslim Thai Flood; and
- Roo Su Flood (Fighting Flood with Knowledge) is a popular YouTube animation. In less than a week, the first episode, which seeks to educate people about how the flood happened, got over 700,000 hits, while the Facebook page attracted over 75,000 fans. Roo Su Flood's fourth episode, telling people how to prepare and deal with the flood, got more than 80,000 views in just a few days.

## Conclusion

Floods are human disasters which may cause mild to severe impacts on a country's security and its people. Appropriate preparedness and network establishment of all responsible concerning agencies can particularly remedy and help prevent a severe disaster, saving financial costs and, more importantly, people's lives.

## Note

All figures come from the Faculty of Public Health, Mahidol University and are reproduced here with permission.

## References

1. The World Bank. The World Bank Supports Thailand's Post-Floods Recovery Effort. 13 December 2011. [Online]. Available from: http://www.worldbank.org/en/news/2011/12/13/world-bank-supports-thailands-post-floods-recovery-effort [Accessed 25 January 2012].
2. 24/7 Emergency Operation Center for Flood, Storm and Landslide. Flood, storm and landslide situation report in Thai. 7 November 2011. [Online]. Available from: http://disaster.go.th/dpm/flood/news/ news_thai/EOCReport6NOV.pdf [Accessed 7 November 2011].
3. Wikipedia. 2011 Thailand Floods. [Online]. Available from: http://en.wikipedia.org/wiki/2011_Thailand_floods – cite_note-Businessweek-75

4. Bureau of Epidemiology. Report on the operation of the flooding relief. 2011.
5. Department of Medical Services. Master plan for public health service during flood. 2011.
6. Department of Health Service Support. Report on the operation of the flooding relief. 2011.
7. Department of Mental Health. Mental disorders during flood. 2011.
8. Bureau of Epidemiology. Report on the surveillance system of the flooding relief. 2011.
9. Malilay, J. Floods. In E. Noji (ed.) *The Public Health Consequences of Disasters*. Oxford University Press: New York, 1997, pp. 287–301.
10. Chaipattana Foundation, 2012.

## Bibliography

Becker, K., Ohl, C.A., and McCormick, N. (1999). Morbidity and mortality associated with Hurricane Floyd – North Carolina, September–October 1999. *Morbidity and Mortality Weekly Report*, 49, 369–72.

Bronstert, A. (2003). Floods and climate change: interactions and impacts. *Risk Analysis*, 23, 545–57.

Bureau of Epidemiology. (2011). Report on diseases under epidemiological surveillance system, 2011.

Cairncross, S., O'Neill, D., McCoy, A., and Sethi, D. (2003). Health, environment and the burden of disease: a guidance note, DFID, London.

Department of Disease Control. (2011). Report on the operations of the flooding disease control.

Department of Disease Control. (2011). Statistics on major communicable diseases, during flood.

Department of Health. (2011). Situation of domestic water supply and health impact. Food and Water Sanitation Division.

Department of Mental Health, Thailand Ministry of Public Health. Project of an organization of Mental Health Center (MHC) for Thai tsunami disaster. http://www.dmh.go.th/english/tsunami/project1.asp [Accessed June 19, 2006].

Department of Mental Health, Thailand Ministry of Public Health. Project of continuous provision of mental intervention and rehabilitation for tsunami victims. http://www.dmh.go.th/english/tsunami/project2.asp [Accessed June 19, 2006].

Few, R. (2003). Flooding, vulnerability and coping strategies: local responses to a global threat. *Progress in Development Studies*, 3, 43–58.

Flood drainage to complete in December. *The Nation*. 26 October 2011. http://www. nationmulti-media.com/national/Flood-drainage-to-complete-in-December-30168608.html

Flood, storm and landslide situation report in Thai. 24/7 Emergency Operation Center for Flood, Storm and Landslide. 7 November 2011. http://disaster.go.th/dpm/flood/news/news_thai/EOCReport6NOV.pdf [Retrieved 7 November 2011].

Flood, storm and landslide situation report in Thai. 24/7 Emergency Operation Center for Flood, Storm and Landslide. 17 January 2012. http://disaster.go.th/dpm/flood/news/news_thai/EOCReport17JAN.pdf [Retrieved 25 January 2012].

French, J., Ing, R., Von Allmen, S., and Wood, R. (1983). Mortality from flash floods: a review of national weather service reports, 1969–81. *Public Health Rep*, 98, 584–8.

Guha-Sapir, D. (1991). Rapid assessment of health needs in mass emergencies: review of current concepts and methods. *World Health Statistics Quarterly* – Rapport Trimestriel de Statistiques Sanitaires Mondiales, 44, 171–81.

Handmer, J.W. and Smith, D.I. (1983). Health hazards of floods: hospital admissions for Lismore. *Australian Geographical Studies*, 21, 221–30.

Hulme, M. (2003). Abrupt climate change: can society cope?, Tyndall Working Paper 30. Tyndall Centre for Climate Change Research, Norwich, UK.

Kovats, R.S., Ebi, K.L., and Menne, B. (2003). Methods of assessing human health vulnerability and public health adaptation to climate change, WHO/WMO/Health Canada, Copenhagen.

McCluskey, J. (2001). Water supply, health and vulnerability in floods. *Waterlines*, 19, 14–17.

Mason, Margie (3 November 2011). Trash, sewage boost disease risk in Bangkok floods, MSNBC. http://www.msnbc.msn.com/id/45144879/ns/health/t/trash-sewage-boost-disease-risk-bangkok-floods/

NSW Health. (2000). Disaster mental health response handbook. NSW Health, North Sydney.

PAHO. (2000). Principles of disaster mitigation in health facilities. Pan American Health Organization, Washington, DC.

PAHO. (2001). Editorial: protecting the Health Services Network. *Disaster Preparedness and Mitigation in the Americas*, 84, 1, 7.
PAHO. (2003). Protecting new health facilities from natural disaster: guidelines for the promotion of disaster mitigation. Pan American Health Organization, The World Bank Group, Washington, DC.
Tapsell, S.M., Penning-Rowsell, E.C., Tunstall, S.M., and Wilson, T.L. (2002). Vulnerability to flooding: health and social dimensions. *Philos Transact Ser A Math Phys Eng Sci*, 360, 1511–25.
The World Bank Supports Thailand's Post-Floods Recovery Effort. World Bank. 13 December 2011. http://www.worldbank.org/en/news/2011/12/13/world-bank-supports-thailands-post-floods-recovery-effort [Retrieved 25 January 2012].
Western Digital's flood-hit Thailand ops to hurt company. Reuters. 17 October 2011. http://www.reuters.com/article/2011/10/17/us-westerndigital-idUSTRE79G3E520111017 [Retrieved 29 October 2011].
WHO (2002). Floods: climate change and adaptation strategies for human health. Report on a WHO meeting. 30 June–2 July 2002, London, World Health Organization Regional Office for Europe, Denmark.

# 28
# Occupational health

*Weihong Chen and Tangchun Wu*

## Introduction

Occupational health is an important branch of public health devoted to the prevention of occupational disease and injury, and to the promotion of work capacity and working quality of life. It is a cross-disciplinary field concerned with protecting the safety, health and welfare of people engaged in work or employment. Since 1950, the International Labour Organization (ILO) and the World Health Organization (WHO) have shared a common definition of occupational health for all. It was adopted by the Joint ILO/WHO Committee on Occupational Health at its first session in 1950 and was revised at its twelfth session in 1995 [1]. The definition of occupational health states that it should aim for the promotion and maintenance of the highest degree of physical, mental and social wellbeing of workers in all occupations; the prevention amongst workers of departure from health caused by their working conditions; the protection of workers in their employment from risks resulting from factors adverse to health; the placing and maintenance of the worker in an occupational environment adapted to his physiological and psychological capabilities; or the adaptation of work to man and of each man to his job [1, 2].

The basic tasks of occupational health are the recognition, evaluation, prevention and control of harmful occupational working conditions. Here, working conditions refers to the working environment and all aspects of an employee's terms and conditions of employment. Normally, it includes three parts: (1) *the production process* starting from raw materials through to the finished production. This process could be changed depending on the production technology, machinery and equipment, and kind of materials and processes; (2) *the labour process*, which includes labour organization, layout of production equipment, operators' posture and form of labour; and (3) *the working environment*, which can be identified as the place of work. The environment includes the indoor environment of a factory or office building, or a car or truck and the surrounding atmospheric environment, as well as the natural environment of any outdoor work.

## Overview of occupational hazards

Occupational hazards or occupationally harmful factors are various adverse factors that might damage the health and affect the ability of people to work in their working environments [3]. Occupational hazards can be divided into three categories as outlined below.

### *Occupational hazards from the production process*

During the production process, the main hazards are chemical, physical and biological. Such hazards and their possibly adverse health effects are summarized in Table 28.1. A mixture or combination of many types of occupational hazards often occurs in one workplace.

*Chemical hazards*: During the production process, raw materials, intermediate products, finished products and by-products or waste are possible chemical hazards. Chemicals stay in the air in the form of dust, smoke, mist, vapour or gas. They enter the body mainly through the respiratory tract, and also through the skin and the digestive tract. Their adverse effects depend on the volatility, solubility and particle size of the chemical solids. Some chemicals may form toxic metabolites during the metabolic processes and induce secondary poisoning.

*Table 28.1* Occupational hazards and their main adverse health effects

| *Occupational hazards* | *Examples in workplace* | *Main adverse health effects* |
|---|---|---|
| ***Chemical hazards***<br>Metals and metalloids<br>Irritant gases<br>Asphyxiating gases<br>Organic solvents<br>Particulate matter | Chemical toxins and industrial dust<br>Lead, manganese, arsenic, chromium<br>Chlorine, ammonia, sulfur dioxide, nitrogen oxides<br>Carbon monoxide, hydrogen sulfide, hydrogen cyanide, methane<br>Benzene, n-hexane, carbon disulfide<br>Silica, coal mine dust, asbestos | Poisoning, irritation, tumour, allergy, neurasthenia syndrome<br>Chemical pulmonary oedema, skin and mucous membrane irritation<br>Asphyxia and tumour<br>Hematopoietic system damage, nervous system damage, skin disease<br>Pneumoconiosis, lung cancer, cardiovascular disease, respiratory diseases (COPD, asthma, *et al.*) |
| ***Physical hazards***<br>Noise<br>Vibration<br>Heat and cold<br>Barometric pressure<br>Non-ionizing radiation<br>Ionizing radiation<br>Other | Steady-state noise and impulse noise<br>Smelting, summer open-air jobs<br>Ultraviolet, infrared, radio frequency radiation<br>X-ray, $\gamma$-ray | Noise-induced hearing loss<br>Vibration disease<br>Heat stroke and frostbite<br>Decompression sickness<br>Neurasthenia syndrome, keratitis, cataracts<br>Tumour, radiation sickness |
| ***Biological hazards***<br>Infectious microorganisms<br>Animals and plants<br>Chemical hazards of biological origin | Pathogenic bacteria and virus<br>Animal hair, mulberry caterpillar, pollen<br>Botulinum toxins, ricin, saxitoxin | Infectious diseases (tuberculosis, hepatitis, *et al.*)<br>Poisoning, allergy, infectious diseases<br>Poisoning, allergy |

*Physical hazards*: Physical hazards are a common source of injuries. They are perhaps unavoidable in certain industries, such as construction and smelting. The main physical hazards include: (1) abnormal weather conditions: high and low temperatures, and high humidity; (2) abnormal pressure: high or low pressure; (3) noise and vibrations; (4) non-ionizing radiation: visible light, ultraviolet light, infrared light, radio frequency radiation or lasers; and (5) ionizing radiation, such as X-ray, γ-ray.

*Biological hazards*: Biological factors include infectious microorganisms, plant or animal toxins, and animals. Infectious pathogenic microorganisms are important occupational hazards mainly affecting healthcare workers in hospitals. Microorganisms, especially pathogenic microorganisms or parasites, can occur in the production of raw materials and in their surrounding environment. The main biological factors include: bacteria, such as *Mycobacterium tuberculosis*, *Bacillus anthracis* and Brucella; viruses, such as the avian influenza virus, hepatitis C and tick-borne encephalitis virus; and mould, such as sugar cane mould and so on. Microorganisms may cause allergic reactions or diseases, such as viral hepatitis and Lyme disease. Plants may produce toxins, and animals may attack and transmit infections to zookeepers or postal delivery workers.

### Occupational hazards in the labour process

The labour process can be defined as the sum of the various operations by which workers need to complete a task in the production process. It mainly relates to labour intensity, and organization and work methods. These include where and how workers sit or stand, whether they use personal protective equipment or not, and the circumstances under which they take a break. This process can have a harmful effect on health in various ways: (1) if the labour organization and system are irrational, the systems for work and breaks will be unreasonable; (2) if there is a psychological nature to occupational stress, such as in the case of motor vehicle drivers; (3) if the intensity of labour is too great or the job demands are too high, as when, for example, the workload does not match the workers' physiological conditions; (4) if unsuitable physical motions cause acute or chronic injury; and (5) if bad positions, postures or use of unreasonable tools are demanded.

### Occupational hazards in the working environment

The working environment refers to the environment in which workers perform operations, such as in the observation or management of production activities. It takes into account the layout of the buildings, health protection, safety conditions and facilities in the workplace. Commonly, working environmental hazards include: (1) the surrounding natural environment, such as solar radiation during the hot season, low pressure in a plateau environment, high temperatures and humidity occurring deep underground; (2) unreasonable factory buildings or internal layout, such as factory buildings that do not comply with occupational health standards, and have poor ventilation, inadequate lighting and confined spaces, or combine toxic and non-toxic sections in a workshop; and (3) environmental pollution caused by unreasonable production processes or mismanagement.

## Occupations and health

Labour is necessary for human survival and development. It should be coordinated with health so that they complement and promote each other, not work against each other. Good working conditions can promote health, while poor working conditions can cause damage to health. Apart from a small number of genetic diseases, the vast majority of occupational diseases, work-related diseases, and the occurrence and development of early health damage are the results of the interaction between environmental factors and the body itself. It is estimated that about 70 per cent to 95 per cent of the risk for chronic diseases may be attributed to the influence of environmental exposure [4, 5]. The workforce can provide a research base for clarifying the impact of the environment and genetic characteristics on human health. This is due to several factors as outlined below:

1 The target system or organs for study will be decided by the chemical and physical properties of potential occupational hazards;
2 Various occupational groups have a relatively specific incidence spectrum of disease;
3 The level of exposure to occupational hazards can be accurately measured or calculated. For example, cumulative exposure is equal to the exposed concentration (or strength) multiplied by the duration of exposure. The dose–response relationship describes the change in effect on an organism caused by differing levels of exposure (or doses) to a stressor (usually a chemical) after a certain exposure time. The relationship between exposure and adverse health effects can be estimated; and
4 The health status of workers can be dynamically observed and analysed through regular medical examinations.

The study of occupational groups will not only help in the research of occupational diseases, but will also help further clarify the occurrence and mechanism of other environment-related diseases that pose heavy economic burdens. The extent of damage caused by environmentally harmful factors is also determined by the individual's characteristics, including gender, age, health status, nutritional status and genes. Adverse health effects on different workers vary within the same occupational environment. Healthy worker effect (HWE) is a phenomenon initially observed in studies of occupational diseases. Workers usually exhibit lower morbidity or mortality than the general population because the severely and chronically ill are ordinarily excluded from employment [6]. This should be taken into account in studies on occupational health and occupational medicine. However, health-related damage among workers includes work-related injuries, occupational diseases (including occupational poisoning), work-related diseases, as well as early health damage possibly occurring due to the lack of preventive measures, and to technical limitations.

### *Work-related injuries*

Work-related injuries mainly refer to health damage resulting from work. For example, some workers suffer from sprains or strains when handling equipment at work. Common causes of work-related injuries are poor ergonomics, manual handling of heavy loads, misuse or failure of equipment, exposure to general hazards, inadequate safety training and inappropriate clothing. Falls, which are common work-related injuries, are a persistent hazard found in all occupational settings. A fall can occur during the simple act of walking or climbing a ladder or maintaining a circuit high above the ground. According to data from the United States (US) Bureau of Labor Statistics, 605 workers were killed and an estimated 212,760 were seriously injured by falls in 2009 [7]. General hazards in a work environment include electricity, explosive materials, fire, flammable gases, heat, high-pressure gases and liquids, powerful or sharp moving machinery, radiation and toxic materials. The prevention and control of accidents should be a joint responsibility of those in production safety supervision and in the health sector. Attention should be paid to security risk assessment, safety training, control banding, personal protective equipment, safety guards, mechanisms on machinery and safety barriers.

## *Occupational diseases*

When the effect of occupational hazards on workers exceeds the body's ability to cope with them and compensatory functional or organic pathological changes occur, disease appears as an occupational disease. The incidence of occupational diseases depends on three main factors: the properties of occupational hazards, the concentration and intensity of occupational hazards and the health status of the individual.

### Properties of occupational hazards

These determine whether adverse health effects happen or not, as well as the severity of the occupational health damage. On one hand, the properties refer to the basic structure and chemical properties of occupational hazards [8]. For example, in the various types of chromium works, the carcinogenic role of hexavalent chromium is the greatest. Another example is the various crystal structures of quartz. The order of ability for causing fibrosis and silicosis is crystalline quartz > aphanitic quartz > amorphous quartz. On the other hand, the physical properties of the hazard also affect its toxicity. Gaseous chemical substances easily diffuse in the air, for example, and the rate of diffusion is determined not only by the initial concentration of the chemicals, but also by the proportion of the gaseous chemicals and the environmental airflow (wind speed). Health damage caused by solid material is associated with its dispersion. For example, the proportion of carbon disulfide ($CS_2$) steam is 2.60 and is heavier than air. It sinks easily and its distribution in the air shows a gradient. Those working in low-lying locations are prone to poisoning. However, if the initial concentration of $CS_2$ is less than 1 mg/L, this phenomenon is not obvious. The proportion of carbon monoxide (CO) is 0.96, close to the proportion of air, so it is rapidly diffused in the air. The adverse health effects of solid substances are related to their dispersability (the extent to which the material is pulverized). Amongst different kinds of asbestos, diameter sizes from large to small are as follows: anthophyllite > amosite > chrysotile > crocidolite. The diameter of crocidolite is smallest, and fibrosis and carcinogenicity of crocidolite is also the strongest among the different kinds of asbestos. The melting point of chemicals also affects their action. During lead and zinc smelting, the boiling point of zinc is 907°C and the boiling point of lead is 1620°C. When heated to melting point, zinc evaporates into the air before lead does and forms zinc oxide dust. Thus workers will develop zinc poisoning before they develop lead poisoning.

### Concentration and intensity of occupational hazards

The number of biological factors that enter the body cannot be estimated. However, damage to health from physical and chemical hazards is related to their intensity or number. When most occupational diseases are diagnosed, a calculation of the number or intensity of the occupational hazards should be made. The exposed dose (dose, D) is the exposure concentration or intensity (concentration, C) multiplied by the exposure duration (time, T), which can be expressed as $D = CT$.

To protect workers, many countries such as the USA, China and most European countries require limits on the exposure to workplace occupational hazards [9]. In the USA, there is a legal limit for the exposure of an employee to a chemical substance or physical agent [10]. For chemicals, regulation is usually expressed in milligrams per cubic metre ($mg/m^3$). Units of measure for physical agents, such as noise, are specific to the agent. Exposure limits for chemicals refer to the highest levels of chemicals in the air that can be tolerated without harmful health effects. Some harmful substances accumulate in the body. Exposure to these substances can cause occupational injuries or diseases that develop only after long-term exposure to small quantities of the substance. Some substances do not accumulate in the body; however, they can cause functional changes that can later cause them to build up in the body. When it is not possible to measure exposure levels, contact time or duration of exposure can be used to estimate workers' exposure or risk of injury. Careful enquiry about the amount of time and the manner in which a worker has been exposed to an occupational hazard can provide very practical information in the diagnosis of occupational disease.

## Individual health status

Although the dose (or strength)–effect relationship is subject to a general rule [11], individual differences among employees lead to different degrees of injury to health for workers in the same operating environment. Despite an exposure to similar levels of chemicals in the air, some workers are prone to poisoning, while others are not. Increasingly, current research is finding that individual genetic characteristics may play an important role in this phenomenon. For example, those susceptible to aniline chemicals tend to have congenital defects of glucose-6-phosphate dehydrogenase. In recent years, an association between lead poisoning and ALAD genotype polymorphism has been found, as has another association between the susceptibility to benzene poisoning and genotype polymorphism of P450 metabolic enzyme. Results have shown that workers with AA+GA genotype had a significantly higher level of DNA damage than those with GG genotype at aryl hydrocarbon receptor (receptor of polycyclic aromatic hydrocarbons) gene in coke-oven workers [12]. In addition, the toxic effect of chemicals on women is different from that in men. For example, women workers are more sensitive to some chemicals, such as arsenic, benzene and carbon monoxide during pregnancy [13].

In both animal experiments and in human health examinations, it has been observed that some organs and systems are very sensitive to particular chemicals and can be easily injured. For example, amino and nitro compounds of benzene damage the erythrocytes and the liver [8]. Benzene can inhibit the hematopoietic system and cadmium induces kidney damage. The affinity of these chemicals for their target organs provides a theoretical basis for occupation contraindications. Many individual factors (e.g. the status of health and nutrition, lifestyle, exercise, age and genes) could interact with occupational hazards and induce different outcomes in the body, which should be taken into consideration.

Based on the common understanding of their nature, occupational diseases have five distinct characteristics:

1 *The specificity of the cause*: Occupational disease develops only after exposure to occupational hazards. Work history, exposure to occupational hazards and workplace monitoring are necessary to diagnose occupational diseases. The incidence or development of occupational diseases can be decreased after controlling these hazards. For example, hydrogen sulphide poisoning, caused by exposure to hydrogen sulphide in the petroleum industry, is one of the most common occupational poisonings in China [14].

2 *The etiology of most of diseases can be detected*: Occupational hazards and levels of exposure can be determined. Normally, damage to health is related to exposure dose or strength. There is a positive dose–response or exposure–response relationship between occupational hazard exposure and adverse health effects. For example, a clear dose–response relationship exists between cumulative crystalline silica dust exposure and risk of silicosis [15.]
3 *Different clinical characteristics exist in different exposed populations*: There are different incident clusters of particular diseases among different groups exposed to occupational hazards. Clinical characteristics of the same disease vary in workers resulting from different exposure levels and from differences among individuals. For example, for workers exposed to high levels of benzene, the common clinical symptom is narcotic symptoms of the nervous system, such as drowsiness, fatigue, rapid heartbeat, confusion or unconsciousness. But workers with long-term exposure to low levels of benzene may have clinical symptoms of aplastic anaemia.
4 *The earlier diseases are diagnosed, the better the prognosis will be*: Treatment alone of patients who remain exposed to an occupational hazard is useless.
5 *There is no specific treatment for most occupational diseases*: It is therefore important to improve preventive measures and protect workers from harm. For example, pneumoconiosis is the most serious occupational disease in China. A report from the Chinese Ministry of Health showed that a total of 676,541 pneumoconiosis cases were diagnosed from 1949 to 2010. The pulmonary fibrosis of pneumoconiosis is still irreversible [14]. The best ways to eliminate pneumoconiosis include effective dust control measures, health surveillance and management, and strengthening of personal protection and health education.

Protecting the health of workers, productivity and economic development are the goals of prevention and control of occupational diseases. A diagnosis of an occupational disease should be supported by adequate material including occupational history, a survey of occupational hygiene in the workplace, corresponding clinical symptoms and all necessary laboratory tests results. Furthermore, to obtain an accurate diagnosis of an occupational disease, similar diseases caused by non-occupational factors should be excluded and a comprehensive analysis should be conducted. The diagnosis principle of occupational diseases is as follows:

1 *Occupational history*: This is an important premise for the diagnosis of an occupational disease. The patient's occupational history should be recorded in detail, including the nature of the current employment, length of service and type of exposure to occupational hazards, operating methods, protective measures in use and previous work history. This information will be helpful in coming to an initial decision about the possibility and severity of the occupational disease caused by occupational hazards.
2 *Workplace survey*: This is an important basis for the diagnosis of occupational diseases. A job site survey would reveal useful information about the production process, the labour process, the strength of the occupational hazards and the preventive measures taken. This information is not only useful for the diagnosis of occupational diseases, but also for a risk assessment for those working under the same conditions, and could prompt a thorough evaluation of exposure levels and control measures for hazards in the workplace.
3 *Symptoms and signs*: The clinical symptoms of occupational diseases are complex and diverse. Different clinical symptoms could be induced by the same occupational hazard in different pathogenic conditions. In addition, the same symptoms could be a result

of different pathogenic conditions. Non-occupational factors can also lead to the same clinical symptoms as occupational factors. Therefore, in the process of clinical data collection and analysis, it is necessary to pay attention to the common points of different occupational diseases, and various special and atypical clinical manifestations. It is also important to exclude similar diseases caused by other occupational hazards, and to identify occupational diseases and non-occupational diseases. Generally, a causal relationship is clear in acute occupational poisoning. But a causal relationship is difficult to determine in chronic occupational poisoning. A diagnostic analysis should be carried out to compare the clinical symptoms of occupational disease with the toxic effects of the occupational hazard and its exposure levels.

4 *Laboratory tests*: The results of laboratory tests are essential for the diagnosis of occupational diseases. Normally, there are three categories of biomarkers: exposure, effect and susceptibility. Exposure biomarkers refer to the measurable exogenous substances in the body, their metabolites, or the product of an interaction between exogenous substances or metabolites and their target molecules or cells. For example, urinary lead and blood lead are biomarkers for lead exposure. Blood benzene and urinary phenol are biomarkers for benzene exposure. Effect biomarkers are measurable biochemical, physiologic, behavioural or other alterations in the body. These alterations are associated with an established or possible health impairment or disease caused by occupational hazards. These biomarkers include the index reflects poison effect (for example, excessive urinary δ-aminolevulinic acid (δ-ALA)reflects lead poisoning) and index reflecting tissues and organic impairment induced by occupational hazards (for example, as part of routine blood and urine tests, liver function and kidney function tests could indicate health damage). Susceptibility biomarkers are an indicator of an inherent or acquired ability for the body to respond to exposure to a specific chemical substance. The main biomarkers are some key metabolic enzymes and DNA damage repair genes. Gene polymorphism is often used as one of the susceptibility biomarkers. For example, AhR genetic 1661 point A/A+G/A, ERCC2 (rs50871 and rs50872)are very useful.

A practical diagnosis needs a comprehensive analysis, including the principles above. Incomplete information, especially the neglect of occupational history and workplace survey data, will result in misdiagnosis. To avoid misdiagnosis, symptomatic treatment and dynamic observation will be very helpful.

## *Work-related diseases*

Work-related diseases are different from occupational diseases. Occupational diseases are the legally defined diseases caused only by specific occupational hazards. They are registered in a statutory list of occupational diseases. Work-related diseases, on the other hand, are multi-factorial diseases [16]. They are not only related to work, but also occur in non-occupational populations. Some people develop these diseases without an occupational history. When work-related diseases occur in workers, the diseases will be in an aggravated, accelerative or recurrent condition and the ability to work will be significantly diminished due to the exposure to occupational hazards. The range of work-related diseases is greater than that of occupational diseases, which leads to an increasingly heavy economic burden. The ILO is especially concerned with controlling work-related diseases. The goal is to protect and promote the health of workers, and to promote economic development. Common work-related diseases are:

1 *Somatopsychic illness*, such as mental anxiety, depression and neurasthenia syndrome caused by heavy workloads; various types of occupational stress; night work; eating disorders; excessive alcohol consumption; smoking and others. Sometimes psychological effects and organ dysfunction occur due to the fear of a harmful occupational factor. The results of an investigation on 1,077 train drivers in China found that rates of depression in male train drivers (50.23 per cent) was significantly higher than that in male adults (17 per cent) [17].
2 *Chronic non-specific respiratory diseases*, including chronic bronchitis, emphysema and bronchial asthma, which are multi-factorial diseases [18]. Smoking, ambient air pollution and respiratory recurrent infections are often the main causes. Patients may develop severe chronic non-specific respiratory diseases even if air pollutants are below permitted limits. For example, occupational exposure to ozone and oxides of nitrogen has been reported to cause chronic bronchitis among workers [18].
3 *Other disorders*, including hypertension, peptic ulcers and back pain, are often associated with particular kinds of work. For example, exposure to carbon disulfide may exacerbate the progress of atherosclerosis.

### *Earlier health damage*

The effect of occupational hazards on human health can be manifested at the molecular, cellular, tissue, organ, individual and population levels. The effect of harmful occupational factors on the body's biological macromolecules (DNA, proteins, etc.) is a key step to health damage caused by occupational hazards. Most occupational hazards enter the body through the respiratory tract, directly or through metabolism, causing a series of reactions, including oxidative stress, inflammatory and immune responses, which are the body's positive and important defence reactions. However, if the body produces too weak or too strong a reaction to a hazard, it may be harmful and may signal early health damage. More importantly, if hazards are too strong or the reaction of the body is not appropriate, a variety of early health damages (decline in lung function, intensification of atherosclerosis or decline in heart rate variability) or various diseases (chronic obstructive pulmonary, coronary heart disease) can occur. A molecular epidemiology study of steel workers observed that coke-oven exposure resulted in a dose-dependent increase in levels of DNA damage and micronuclei rate. DNA damage and micronuclei could be considered as early damage for workers exposed to carcinogens [19]. Early health damage caused by occupational hazards can develop into two completely opposite outcomes: health or disease. Emphasis on early health damage caused by occupational hazards could help to prevent occupational diseases.

## Characteristics of occupational hazards and health injuries in Asia and Africa

Occupational health and safety practices vary among nations which have different approaches to legislation, regulation, enforcement and incentives for compliance. In the European Union, for example, some member states promote occupational safety and health by providing public monies, such as subsidies, grants or financing, while others have created tax incentives for occupational health and safety investments. In Asian countries, for example, in the People's Republic of China (PRC), the Ministry of Health is responsible for occupational disease prevention and the State Administration of Work Safety is responsible for safety issues at work. At the provincial and municipal level, there are health supervisors for occupational health and local bureaus of work safety for safety. The Occupational Disease Control Act of PRC came into force on 1 May 2002 and the Work Safety Act of PRC on 1 November 2002 [20]. The Occupational Disease Control Act is under revision. The prevention of occupational disease is still in its initial stage compared with developed countries, such as the USA or Germany.

Most countries in Asia and Africa are developing countries. From the report of the ILO, more than 1.1 million people die as a direct result of occupational accidents or work-related diseases each year in Asia and the Pacific [21]. The most affected groups are the poorest, least protected, least informed and least trained workers. Health hazards in the workplace are as old as work itself, but at the same time they continue to change and evolve with the changing nature of work and the changing composition of the workforce. Many hazardous industries and jobs have been 'exported' from developed countries to developing countries. In addition, many hazardous jobs are done by migrant or temporary workers, who suffer an increased risk of injury and illness as a result of their precarious work status [22].

There are several distinct characteristics of occupational hazards in developing countries in Asia. First, the traditional occupational hazards and health injuries, such as pneumoconiosis, acute and chronic poisoning and hearing loss, still account for the majority of occupational diseases [23]. New types of occupational injuries caused by new technologies and materials, such as nano dust, are increasing. There is growing concern about new occupational hazards, for instance, adverse ergonomic design, forced posture and psychological stress related to work. Second, the issues of pesticide poisoning and agricultural occupational health have received little attention. Few studies have been carried out, and few occupational standards have been established in this field [23]. Third, the occupational health of floating populations and how to protect the health of migrant workers still needs to be addressed. Fourth, work-related diseases have become more complex with the diversification of employment patterns [23]. And lastly, the relationship between exposure to low concentration, long-term multi-factor occupational hazards and health injuries is a new research topic.

It is estimated that over 2 million people worldwide die annually of occupational injuries and work-related diseases [24]. And it is estimated that 160 million people suffer from work-related diseases and 270 million people suffer fatal and non-fatal work-related accidents per year [24]. The WHO's World Health Report 2002 indicates that 1.5 per cent of the global burden in terms of disability-adjusted life years result from only a selected subset of occupational risks [25]. In developing countries, the aforementioned risks reach a proportion that is estimated to be 10 to 20 times higher than in established market economies. At present, rapid changes in working life are affecting both the health of workers and the environment. This is particularly the case in the African region where the introduction of new technologies, new chemical substances and materials has led to new occupational and work-related diseases and injuries, while traditional hazards, such as high dust or noise levels in the workplace, have not been dealt with adequately. This leads to an increased burden of occupational diseases and injuries. An additional problem in the African region is the high prevalence and incidence of HIV/AIDS. The HIV/AIDS pandemic is eroding the human resource capacity by reducing the labour force in all sectors and posing a major burden on basic healthcare systems.

Occupational accidents and occupational diseases have an impact not only on the lives of individual workers, but also on the productivity and profitability of their enterprises and, ultimately, on the welfare of the whole society. How to intervene effectively to reduce the risk of workplace hazards is receiving increased attention in developing countries. Governments, workers and employers urgently need to increase their efforts to prevent accidents and diseases in the workplace in Asia and Africa. Currently, many reforms are taking place: countries are setting up information systems; training their health personnel, labour inspectors and other relevant actors; and developing policies and guidelines. A large group of international collaborators from different regions are supporting those activities.

## Three levels of prevention for occupational hazards

In order to protect and promote the health of occupational groups, occupational damage can be controlled via three preventive measures: primary prevention, secondary prevention and tertiary prevention.

### *Primary prevention*

Primary prevention is also called etiologic prevention and involves eliminating or controlling the effects and damage caused by occupational hazards by reducing or eliminating the exposure opportunities of workers. This can be done by improving production technology and production equipment, and by using protective equipment to confine or isolate occupational hazards and by using personal protective equipment rationally. The main strategies include:

- An improvement in production technology and production equipment made in order to control the concentration or strength of hazards. The concentration or strength of occupational hazards should be lower than occupational exposure limits for hazardous agents in the workplace. For instance, industrial dust has been partly controlled by wet work and ventilation systems in coal mines [26].
- Use of non-toxic or less-toxic chemical substances instead of highly toxic materials. For example, benzene is a solvent of viscose used in the leather industry. In primary prevention, ethanol, which has low toxicity, is substituted for benzene, which has high toxicity.
- Use of personal protective equipment and comprehensive healthcare measures [27].

### *Secondary prevention*

Secondary prevention is the early detection of physical injury caused by occupational hazards. Although primary prevention is the ideal method, the costs are high. Moreover, under current conditions, it is often difficult to achieve the ideal arrangements. Some hazards still occur and cause health damage so secondary prevention is necessary. The main method of secondary prevention consists in regular monitoring of occupational hazards and the organization of periodic medical examinations for exposed workers. In this way lesions or injuries can be detected in their early stages and can be treated in a timely fashion. A timetable of regular medical examination can be determined according to the following principles: latency and severity of disease, exposure duration and concentration or intensity of occupational hazards, and susceptibility of the exposed people. Physical examinations should combine both routine examination and the specific and sensitive detection indicators. For instance, pulmonary ventilation function examination or X-ray pulmonary radiography are indicators of functional and pathological changes for dust workers [27]. In another example, the micronucleus rate can be recognized as an early detector of occupational carcinogens, such as radiation, polycyclic aromatic hydrocarbons, as well as others.

### *Tertiary prevention*

Tertiary prevention is useful in preventing occupational hazards. It refers to the measures that actively treat and promote rehabilitation for patients suffering from occupational diseases. Its principles are:

- Exposed patients should be removed from the original job and receive reasonable treatments.
- The occurrence of a new occupational case is a sentinel health event to prompt a thorough evaluation of exposure levels of specific hazards and control measures in the workplace. The production environment and process should be improved accordingly.
- Steps should be taken to promote the recovery of patients and prevent complications. Other than in a few types of occupational poisonings, which have special antidotes, the majority of occupational diseases have no specific treatment and are regularly treated according to their symptoms. For example, there is no effective method of treating pulmonary fibrosis caused by dust exposure and industrial noise-induced hearing loss.

Overall, the key points of all three levels of prevention are to prevent hazards at their source, to provide early detection and early treatment, to promote recovery, to prevent complications and to improve quality of life. Primary prevention is the most important because it prevents workers from damage at the source of the occupational hazard. Secondary and tertiary prevention are extensions and supplements of primary prevention, all of which constitute the system of occupational health and occupational medicine.

## Conclusion

The objectives of occupational health are to identify and evaluate occupational hazards in the workplace, to prevent and control occupational hazards produced by working conditions, and to maintain and promote the highest degree of physical, mental and social wellbeing of workers in all occupations. Adverse health effects caused by occupational hazards include work-related injuries, occupational diseases, work-related diseases, as well as early health damage possibly caused by a lack of preventive measures, and to technical limitations. Three levels of prevention are useful in obstructing occupational hazards and reversing adverse health effects in the workplace.

## References


1. Stellman JM. *Encyclopaedia of Occupational Health and Safety.* 4th edn. International Labour Office. Geneva, 1998.
2. Coppee GH. Occupational health services and practice. Available from: http://www.ilo.org/safework_bookshelf/english?content&nd=857170174
3. NIOSH Workplace Safety and Health Topics. National Institute of Occupational Safety and Health. Available from: http://www.cdc.gov/niosh/topics/machine/ [Accessed 11 July 2012].
4. Anand P, Kunnumakara AB, Sundaram C, Harikumar KB, Tharakan ST, Lai OS, *et al.* Cancer is a preventable disease that requires major lifestyle changes. *Pharm Res.* 2008; 25(9): 2097–2116.
5. Bhatnagar A. Environmental cardiology, studying mechanistic links between pollution and heart disease. *Circulation Res.* 2006; 99: 692–705.
6. Li C, Sung F. A review of the healthy worker effect in occupational epidemiology. *Occup. Med.* 1999; 49(4): 225–229.

7. Fall Injuries Prevention in the Workplace. NIOSH Workplace Safety and Health Topic. National Institute for Occupational Safety and Health. Available from: http://www.cdc.gov/niosh/topics/falls/ [Accessed 12 July 2012].
8. Levy BS, Wagner GR, Rest KM, Weeks JL. Occupational disease and injury. American Public Health Association. Washington, DC, 2005.
9. American Conference of Governmental Industrial Hygienists. *Threshold Limit Values and Biological Exposure Indices for Substances in Workroom*. Cincinnati, OH: ACGIH, 2009.
10. Occupational Safety and Health Administration (OSHA) Permissible Exposure Limits (PELs). Available from: http://www.osha.gov/dsg/topics/pel/index.html
11. Crump KS, Hoel DG, Langley CH, Peto R. Fundamental carcinogenic processes and their implications for low dose risk assessment. *Cancer Research*. 1976; 36(9_Part1): 2973–2979.
12. Chen Y, Bai Y, Yuan J, Chen W, Sun J, Wang H, *et al*. Association of polymorphisms in AhR, CYP1A1, GSTM1 and GSTT1 genes with levels of DNA damage in peripheral blood lymphocytes among coke-oven workers. *Cancer Epidemiol Biomarkers Prev*. 2006; 15(9): 1703–1707.
13. Bureau for Workers' Activities. Male and female reproductive health hazards in the workplace. International Labour Office. Geneva, 1996; 27–36.
14. Chinese Annual Health Statistical Report in 2010. Beijing: Ministry of Health of the People's Republic of China, 2011.
15. Chen W, Zhuang Z, Attfield MD, Chen BT, Gao P, Harrison JC, *et al*. Exposure to silica and silicosis among tin miners in China: exposure–response analyses and risk assessment. *Occup Environ Med*. 2001; 58: 31–37.
16. Levy BS, Wegman DH (eds). *Occupational Health: Recognizing and Preventing Work Related Disease and Injury*. 4th edn. Philadelphia, PA: Lippincott Williams & Wilkins, 2000.
17. Chen M, Liu B, Ge M, Ren N, Zhu D. Occupational stress and its influential factors analysis for train drivers. *Chinese J Prevent Med*. 2012; 13(3): 187–191.
18. National Institute for Occupational Safety and Health. *Work-related Lung Disease Surveillance Report, 2002*. Cincinnati, OH: NIOSH, 2003.
19. Yang X, Zheng J, Bai Y, Tian F, Yuan J, Sun J, *et al*. Using lymphocytes and plasma Hsp70 as biomarkers for assessing coke oven exposure among steel workers. *Environ Health Perspect*. 2007; 115: 1573–1577.
20. Shou Y, Lu R, Lin J, Xu Y, Zhu Y, Schweigert M. The Occupational Disease Prevention and Control Act of the People's Republic of China: an awareness assessment among workers at foreign-invested enterprises. *New Solut*. 2011; 21(1): 103–116.
21. Occupational Safety and Health in Asia and the Pacific. International Labour Organization. 2008. Available from: http://www.ilo.org/asia/whatwedo/projects/WCMS_099347/lang--en/index.htm
22. Eijkemans G. WHO and ILO. Joint Effort on Occupational Health and Safety in Africa. *African Newsletters on Occupational Health and Safety*. 2004; 14: 28–29.
23. Sun G, Wu T, Niu Q. *Occupational Health and Occupational Medicine*. 7th edn. Beijing: People's Health Publishing House, 2012; 15–16.
24. Occupational safety and health. International Labour Organization. Available from: http://www.ilo.org/global/standards/subjects-covered-by-international-labor-standards/occupational-safety-and-health/lang--en/index.htm
25. Mathers CD, Vos T, Lopez AD, Salomon J, Ezzati M (eds). *National Burden of Disease Studies: A Practical Guide*. Edition 2.0. Global Program on Evidence for Health Policy. Geneva: World Health Organization, 2001.
26. Kissell FN. *Handbook for Dust Control in Mining*. IC 9465. (DHHS [NIOSH] Publication No. 2003–147). Washington, DC: NIOSH, 2003; 36–70.
27. McCunney J, *et al*. (eds). *A Practical Approach to Occupational and Environmental Medicine*. Philadelphia, PA: Lippincott Williams & Wilkins, 2003.

# Part V
# Health improvement

# Introduction to Part V: health improvement

*Siân M. Griffiths*

## Prevention rather than cure: the challenge of non-communicable diseases

Chronic non-communicable diseases (NCDs), such as diabetes, hypertension, cardiovascular disease and cancer are reaching global epidemic proportions even amongst younger populations, and now not only in developed countries but also in low- and middle-income countries. For example, the longer-term pathology of chronic heart disease – related to lack of exercise and fat/sugar/salt-loaded diets – places a burden on society and its healthcare systems, causing early mortality and long-term morbidity in the community. The current relentless epidemic of obesity shows we have yet to be truly effective in our efforts to halt the rising tide of NCDs. The solution lies not only in individuals making changes to their lifestyles but in actions taken by local communities, national governments and global communities. Approaches described in the Alma Ata declaration of 1978 have been refined through iteration of the Ottawa and Bangkok charters and most recently the Health in All Policies (HiAPs) approach. This approach emphasizes that, since health is determined to a large extent by factors outside the health arena, an effective health policy must involve all relevant policy areas, in particular social and regional policy, taxation, environment, education and research. In 2013, the World Health Assembly (WHA) agreed a global action plan for the prevention and control of non-communicable diseases 2013–2020 [1]. Based on the vision of creating a world free of the avoidable burden of NCDs, targets based on the overarching principles of values and global public health approaches have been established, as summarized in Figure V.1.

Against this background, in Chapter 29 Thow and colleagues describe the burden of NCDs in the Asia-Pacific region and provide examples of successful upstream intervention projects implemented to modify the common risk factors of tobacco consumption, physical inactivity and poor diets. Regionally the prevalence of cardiovascular risk factors and cardiovascular disease (CVD) are highest among the lowest socio-economic groups. And patterns of disease differ. For example, in Japan, South Korea, China, Hong Kong, Taiwan and Thailand rates of strokes are higher than those of coronary heart disease – and considerably higher than rates observed in most Western countries. This is in part due to high salt intakes in these countries, often in the form of sauces and other preserved foods. The most significant

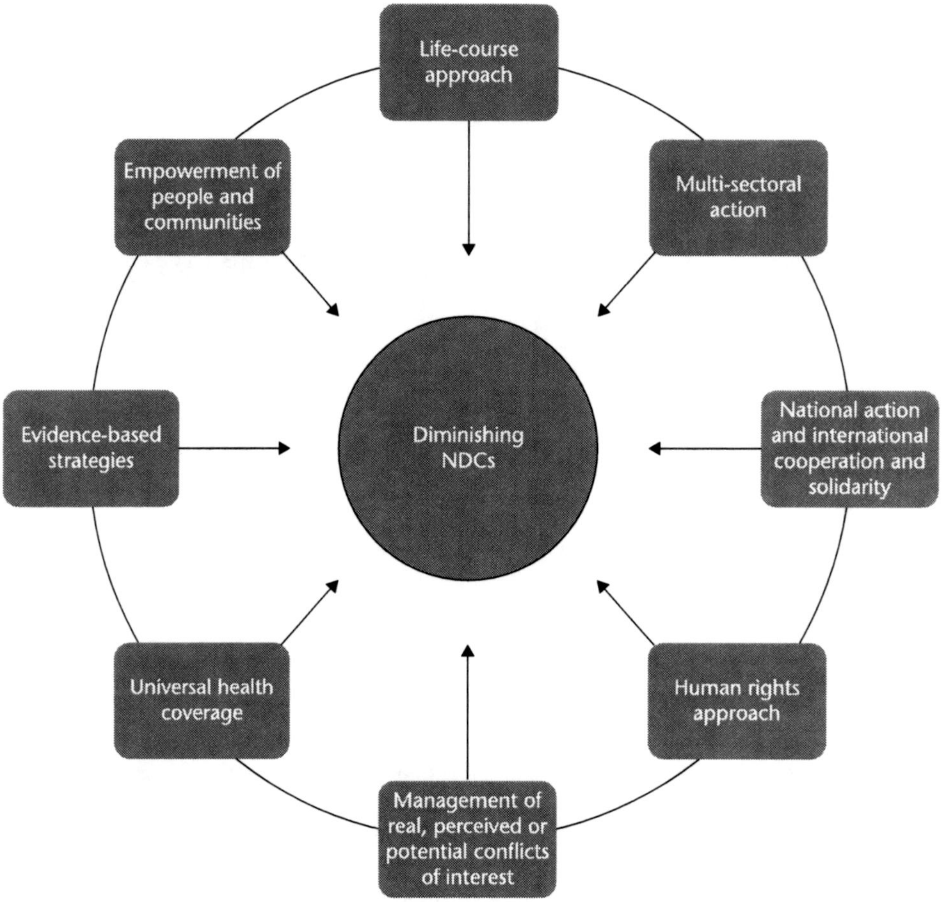


*Figure V.1* **Overarching and global public health approaches to diminish NCDs**

shift over recent decades has been seen in Pacific Island countries, as reflected by their high rates of diet-related NCDs and high levels of mortality from CVD. These increasing rates can be mapped onto the nutrition transition, which is characterized by decreased consumption of traditional staple foods such as starchy roots, pulses and cereals, and other plant foods, and accompanied by increased consumption of animal products (mainly milk, cheese and meat), refined cereals (such as white rice) and vegetable oils. Rising consumption of processed foods, including soft drinks, is part of this dietary transition, and has contributed to increased intakes of fat, salt and sugar. The authors provide a series of successful case studies as exemplars for the rest of the region, showing that a combination of strategies that improve food availability through policies, settings-based approaches and consumer education can support healthy diets and contribute towards disease prevention. Such approaches are immensely important when considering the burden of NCDs.

In Chapter 30 Zabetian and colleagues describe the threat of the often silent epidemic of diabetes in Asia where elevated glucose levels are often asymptomatic and can remain undetected unless screened for or discovered once disabling diabetes-related complications develop.

The burden is compounded not only by earlier onset and co-morbidity but also by increasing longevity. Most populations in Asia are ageing, due to the rapid socio-economic and nutrition transitions in the region. A high proportion of older people will be affected by diabetes and, in Asia, many are as yet unaware of this. More than 60 per cent of people with undiagnosed diabetes in the world are living in the Southeast Asia and Western Pacific regions, and approximately 50 per cent of diabetes cases in Southeast Asia are undiagnosed. Overall, Asian populations experience greater diabetes complication burdens than European/Caucasian populations. For example, the age of the first myocardial infarction is ten years earlier among south Asians and Asians have a higher likelihood of progression to end-stage renal disease (ESRD) than Caucasians. The onset of complications exponentially increases the economic burdens experienced by individuals and families. Like other NCDs, diabetes is a multi-factorial condition where genetic and environmental influences combine to increase its risk. Different populations exhibit different combinations of risk factors and experience varying interactions between risk factors. The authors stress the urgency for action to meet the challenge of providing equitable, accessible, appropriate and affordable long-term care.

Whilst good community based services are important in management of diabetes and other NCDs, so too is the role of NGOs. In Chapter 31, Ma and Yeung provide a case study of the work of a non-government organization (NGO) in Hong Kong and describe how, working closely with the government, health services and the professions, programmes and other community outreach initiatives can be developed to help raise the awareness of diabetes and its implications. Diabetes Hongkong was founded as a charitable organization by a group of healthcare professionals and volunteers, with the mission to serve all people with diabetes and their families, promote social awareness and concern towards diabetes, and strive for optimal care and prevention of the disease. Their main activities are public education; providing social and medical support for people with diabetes and their families; continuing education and training for healthcare professionals involved in the delivery of diabetes care; advocacy for all people with diabetes and their families in Hong Kong; liaising with other national and international diabetes associations for exchange of information and experiences in diabetes care; and encouraging research and safeguarding standards of care in the management of diabetes. As such, they demonstrate the powerful role that the NGO sector can play in engaging communities.

Diabetes is amongst the NCDs that have been increasing in mainland China, where around 260 million patients have been diagnosed with an NCD, and as the population ages the numbers continue to grow. The third national survey of causes of death showed that among urban and rural areas the top four causes of death are cerebrovascular disease, cancer, respiratory disease and heart disease, and the prevalence difference between the urban and rural regions is narrowing. In 2010, 85 per cent of the total deaths and 75 per cent of the total number of premature deaths were caused by NCDs. With the increased exposure to the risk factors, the number of patients with major NCDs both in urban and rural areas has changed significantly. From 1998 to 2008, the number of patients with diabetes and hypertension increased by 1.98 times and 2.31 times, respectively. The next two decades may well see a doubling or tripling of these figures, especially given the significant levels of predisposing factors in the population, including 30 per cent being obese or overweight, 28.1 per cent smoking tobacco, 30.6 per cent taking inadequate physical activity and 38.2 per cent having high-blood pressure. In 2010, nearly 600 million Chinese people over the age of 40 had at least one risk factor for an NCD. In Chapter 32, Li and colleagues discuss the ecological causation of the current epidemic – a combination of individual behaviour, genetic predisposition and environmental factors, affected by the political and socio-economic environment.

They discuss the attributes of different strategies which can be employed, whether to focus on high-risk individuals specifically or on population-wide interventions, and describe the policies, surveillance systems and intervention strategies promulgated by the government, as well as initiatives at the grassroots level.

One of the biggest challenges faced by China is the numbers, particularly men, who smoke. How to promote tobacco cessation to reduce the number of smokers and decrease the associated disease burden is a huge challenge. With an estimated 301 million smokers, smoking-related illness kills more than 1 million Chinese citizens each year. One in three of the world's smokers is a Chinese male, and tobacco production and cigarette consumption continues to rise. China, along with many other countries, has signed the Framework Convention for Tobacco Control (FCTC). However its implementation remains patchy and challenging for many reasons including the income from tobacco growing, sales and taxation.

Another massive – and often forgotten – burden of disease across the region is related to mental health. In Chapter 33, Samuel Wong describes the burden of disease that can be attributed to neuropsychiatric disorders, highlighting that the majority of this burden comes from common mental disorders including chronic major depression, alcohol use, substance abuse, dementia and schizophrenia. It is estimated that one in four people will develop one or more mental or behavioural disorders during their lifetime and major depression, one of the most common mental disorders, is expected to be second only to CVD by the year 2020, accounting for 5.7 per cent of DALYs worldwide. Mental health problems can account for up to 40 per cent of consultations in primary care. Asia is one of the regions cited by the WHO as having both a lack of resources and of treatments for mental health disorders especially in the community. Mental disorders often go under-treated and place a heavy burden on families. Major depression is the most common mental disorder and has been shown to be related to significant disability, particularly since relationships exist between common chronic conditions, such as CVDs and diabetes, and depression. Medical conditions can also affect the risk of mental disorders and mental disorders can affect other clinical conditions, as well as affecting the treatment adherence and patients' outcomes of chronic physical conditions. This complex set of interactions underlines the need for mental health promotion, that is, activities to address and intervene on the determinants of mental health by creating the individual, social and environmental conditions that enable optimal psychological development. In addition to paucity of resources for mental health and under-diagnosis of conditions, stigma is a common problem. All too often vulnerable groups such as the long-term mentally ill are excluded from health promotion campaigns – a double jeopardy since persons with mental illness are about twice as likely to smoke as other persons.

Mackay and colleagues in Chapter 34 provide a case study of tobacco control measures put in place over the last 40 years in Hong Kong to achieve the current low rates of tobacco smoking in the SAR. Advocacy has played a key role and, from the early 1980s onwards, the influential NGO – the Hong Kong Council on Smoking and Health – helped to lobby the government, promoted policy and legislative changes, as well as campaigned in schools. They successfully promoted the understanding that running health promotion campaigns was in itself insufficient and that introducing comprehensive tobacco control policies and legislation was essential. Political, economic, environment and trade components were needed in their campaigning, as well as tackling the tobacco industry head on. Their efforts have resulted in one of the lowest smoking rates in the world, achieved by working at all levels of society and across government. The authors argue that a new paradigm is needed to address the health epidemics of the twenty-first century, one that embraces international treaties for public health, uses laws and fiscal means, recognizes the crucial role of government, addresses a wide range of issues from corporate criminality to poverty alleviation, forms new partnerships and sets targets. Political mapping of obstacles, including the role of tobacco in the development agenda, is also needed. Mackay *et al.*'s case study clearly demonstrates that legislation is a key component of any strategy to promote population health change.

This is further demonstrated by the case study in Chapter 35 by Mercurio who describes the experience of the *Tobacco Plain Packaging Bill 2011* and other legislation in Australia introduced in early 2012 to prohibit the use of tobacco industry trademarks, logos, colours, brand imagery or promotional text on tobacco product packaging other than brand names and product names in a prescribed standard font style and position. In addition, graphic health warnings are to be displayed and packaging to be generally standardized. The purpose of this move is to discourage smoking and implement Australia's obligations under the WHO FCTC. Tobacco consumption in Australia has declined by approximately one-third since 1990 and currently, 17 per cent of Australia's population smokes, which is lower than most comparable countries. This legislation represents a further effort to reduce the impact of tobacco company strategies to promote smoking, as they will no longer be able to use their trademarks or brand logos on cigarette packages. Mercurio describes the legal challenges being brought by the tobacco companies against plain packaging. Globally public health colleagues watch with interest for the outcome, and many are already exploring the potential introduction of plain packaging to their own countries if the Australian experience is shown to be both legal and effective in reducing tobacco-related harm.

Smoking is also one of the principal risk factors in the aetiology of cancer, being responsible for 22 per cent of global cancer deaths and 7.1 per cent of global lung cancer deaths. Tobacco control exemplifies the need to combine primary prevention preventing the onset of disease by reducing risk factors in the population either through changes in behaviour and lifestyle, or through changes in the environment supported by appropriate public policies and health education – with secondary prevention halting the progress of an established but possibly asymptomatic disease to provide early diagnosis and treatment backed up by counselling, health education and effective treatment. In Chapter 36, Wong and Chor provide two case studies of common Asian cancers for which screening practice across the region varies. Colorectal cancer (CRC) and breast cancer have emerged as leading causes of cancer mortality in the region. In the past decades, Asia-Pacific countries such as China, South Korea, Japan and Singapore have witnessed a two- to three-fold rise in incidence of CRC and have been gradually catching up with the figures in Western countries. The incidence of breast cancer was previously very low in the Asia-Pacific region but increased substantially in the past two decades. The highest rise was observed in Korea, China and Japan, especially among middle-aged women. The authors discuss the case for and against screening, concluding that as both CRC and breast cancer are rising rapidly in the region – and are the causes of a significant number of deaths – it is important to implement well-developed screening programmes for these cancers as they become available. They recognize that this is a complex area with controversies and challenges that require consistent, thorough reviews to support multifaceted strategies designed at the patient, community and governmental levels.

## Reference

1. World Health Organization. Draft action plan for the prevention and control of noncommunicable diseases 2013–2020 (13.2.). In Sixty-sixth World Health Assembly: daily notes on proceedings. 2013. [Online]. Available from: http://www.who.int/mediacentre/events/2013/wha66/journal/en/

# 29

# Policy for the prevention of diet-related non-communicable diseases in the Asia-Pacific region

*Anne Marie Thow, Shauna Downs and Stephen Leeder*

## Introduction

The 2011 United Nations High Level meeting on non-communicable diseases (NCDs) was convened due to the growing international alarm about the threat to health, development and economies posed by these diseases. The political statement issued on behalf of over 110 participant nations resolved to develop effective programmes to prevent and control NCDs. Later, the final report of the Rio+20 Conference on Sustainable Development also highlighted that NCDs are a challenge to sustainable development.

The causes of NCDs in the Asia-Pacific region are potentially modifiable – tobacco, physical inactivity and poor diets are common risk factors for several of the major NCDs, including diabetes, cardiovascular disease and some cancers. Diet-related NCDs in particular remain a significant challenge due to the nutrition transition occurring in the region.

In this chapter, we describe the emerging epidemic of diet-related NCDs in the Asia-Pacific region and identify strategies for prevention. Some parts of this region have shown leadership in using policy to prevent diet-related NCDs, and inspiration can be drawn from these achievements for wider national and international application.

## Epidemiology of diet-related NCDs in the Asia-Pacific region

Diet-related NCDs include cardiovascular disease, diabetes and some cancers – mainly breast, colorectal and prostate [1]. Mortality from cardiovascular disease and diabetes in the Asia-Pacific region ranges from relatively low in the higher-income countries (such as Australia, Japan, New Zealand and Singapore) through to extremely high rates in Pacific Island nations (see Figure 29.1). Although mortality rates for the higher-income countries are relatively low, diet-related NCDs still comprise a considerable proportion of the burden of disease due to the chronic nature of morbidity (see Figure 29.2). The increasing incidence and subsequent prevalence of diet-related NCDs among low socio-economic population groups is widening health inequities within and among countries in the Asia-Pacific region [1].

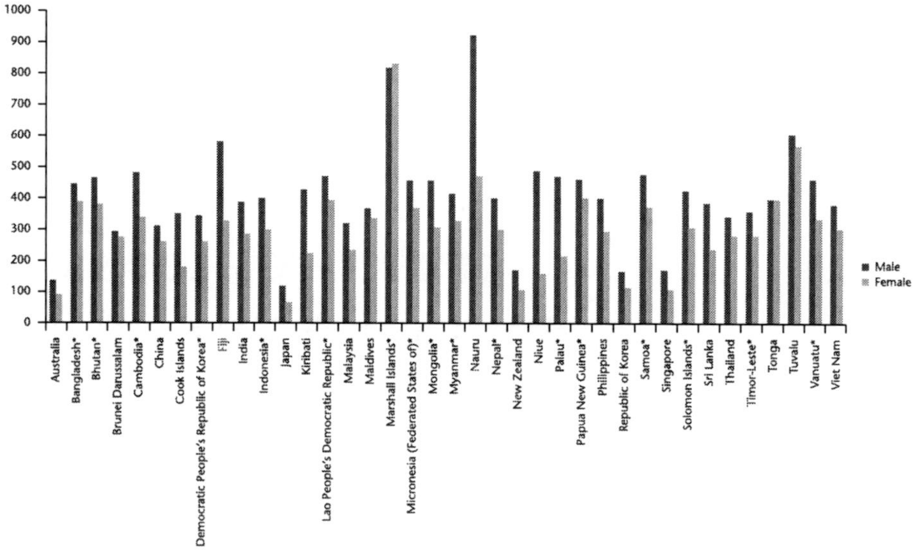


*Figure 29.1* Cardiovascular diseases and diabetes, deaths per 100,000 (age-standardized estimate) [109]

*Note*: * Country data not available. Global Health Observatory Data Repository presents estimate based on a combination of country life tables, cause of death models, regional cause of death patterns, and WHO and UNAIDS programme estimates for some major causes (not including chronic diseases).

Urbanization is strongly associated with diet-related NCDs in both Asia and the Pacific due to changes in diets and physical activity patterns due to an urban lifestyle, greater food availability and changing work patterns [2, 3].

In the Pacific Islands, cardiovascular disease (CVD) is the main cause of death in most countries [2, 4]. It accounts for more than a quarter of all mortality in the South-East Asia Region (SEAR) [5], and in fact around half the world's cases of CVD occur in the region [6]. The prevalence of cardiovascular risk factors and CVD are highest among the lowest socio-economic groups regionally [5]. In Japan, South Korea, China, Hong Kong, Taiwan and Thailand, rates of strokes are higher than coronary heart disease – and considerably higher than rates observed in most Western countries [7]. This is likely due to high salt intakes, often in the form of sauces and other preserved foods in these countries [8].

The prevalence of diabetes across the region has risen considerably over the past 40 years [9]. Diabetes rates more than tripled in Indonesia, South Korea, Thailand and India between 1970 and 1989, and 1990 and 2005, and doubled in Singapore and Taiwan [10]. Very high prevalence rates of diabetes – up to 40 per cent – have been reported in some Pacific Island countries, including Nauru [9].

High prevalence rates of risk factors for diet-related NCDs, such as elevated cholesterol, hypertension and impaired glucose tolerance, have also been reported in the Asia-Pacific region. Cholesterol levels are strongly associated with CVD risk, and are on average higher in Australia and New Zealand (around 5.5 mmol/l) than in Asia (around 4.9 mmol/l) [11]. The reported prevalence of hypertension ranges from less than 10 per cent in Fiji to around 25 per cent in Indonesia, Taiwan, Thailand, China, South Korea, Australia and New Zealand, to nearly 50 per cent in Mongolia [12]. As well as that, it is estimated that 66 per cent of some

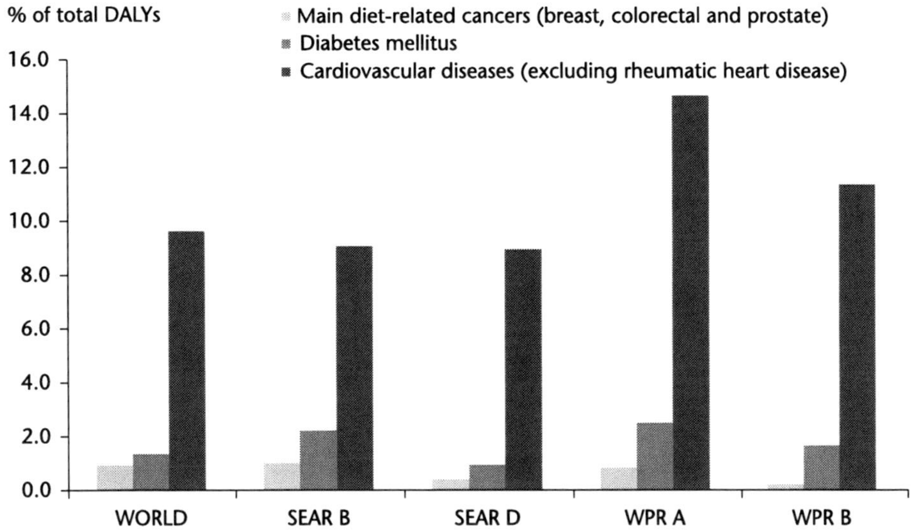


*Figure 29.2* DALYs as a percent of total by cause, countries grouped by WHO subregion, estimates for 2004 [109]

*Notes*: SEAR B: Indonesia, Sri Lanka, Thailand.
SEAR D: Bangladesh, Bhutan, Democratic People's Republic of Korea, India, Maldives, Myanmar, Nepal, Timor-Leste.
WPR A: Australia, Brunei Darussalam, Japan, New Zealand, Singapore.
WPR B: Cambodia, China, Cook Islands, Fiji, Kiribati, Lao People's Democratic Republic, Malaysia, Marshall Islands, Micronesia (Federated States of), Mongolia, Nauru, Niue, Palau, Papua New Guinea, Philippines, Republic of Korea, Samoa, Solomon Islands, Tonga, Tuvalu, Vanuatu, Vietnam.

subtypes of CVD can be attributed to high blood pressure in the region [12]. In Southeast Asia, the estimated prevalence of diabetes was over 5 per cent, and for impaired glucose tolerance was 6–7 per cent in 2007 [1, 3]. In 2000, more than half of global diabetes deaths occurred in the Asia-Pacific region, indicating a disproportionately high burden in the region [1].

Diet-related NCDs are all also associated with a high body mass index (BMI) [13]. The proportion of overweight adults has increased very rapidly in China, whilst in India, the shift is most pronounced among urban residents and high-income rural residents [14]. Prevalence of overweight and obese children in Shanghai and Heilongjiang, China, was 32.5 per cent for males and 17.6 per cent for females in 2005, compared to less than 2 per cent just 20 years earlier [15].

In addition, the risks associated with diet-related NCDs are not limited to one generation – an intergenerational and epigenetic effect may be at play. These high rates of diet-related NCDs, and the recent rapid increases seen in the region, may in part be due to adverse nutrition in utero development and early childhood [16]. Studies have shown that this may lead to a predisposition to NCDs later in life and at lower levels of BMI than seen in higher-income countries [5, 17, 18].

A significant part of the social and economic burden of diet-related NCDs stems from morbidity and ongoing treatment costs, exacerbated by improved healthcare technology and availability [5, 19]. The economic costs related to CVD and diabetes represent 4 to 8 per cent of the economy in China [20]. Thailand has experienced a five-fold increase in the rate of hospitalizations for heart disease and diabetes from the mid-1990s to the mid-2000s [21]. At the household level, healthcare costs associated with ischaemic heart disease in Malaysia have been shown to lead to considerable out-of-pocket expenditures – and in some cases catastrophic health spending – as well as social costs for patients and their families [22]. Comorbidities are becoming more prevalent and can also significantly increase the cost of treatment. A study in Taiwan found that for patients with end-stage renal disease, also having diabetes more than tripled the cost of their health care [23]. A World Bank study in three Pacific countries in 2000 found that the cost of treating NCDs comprised between 39 per cent and 58 per cent of total health expenditure [24]. In Pacific Island countries, costs are further increased by the high costs of drugs and laboratory tests [25].

Effects of high BMI on mortality are apparent at younger ages in the South-East Asian region as compared to what is observed globally [5]. In China, diabetes prevalence among 35–44-year olds increased by 88 per cent from 1994 to 2000, and the prevalence in south Indians younger than 44 years increased from 25 per cent in 2000 to 35.7 per cent in 2006 [3]. Social and economic costs are compounded when parents of young children and primary income earners suffer from chronic diseases [26].

A further contributor to rising costs is that people are often unaware that they have a diet-related NCD, particularly in the early stages, thus they are denied benefits of early intervention. For example, in 2004, less than half of the people with high blood pressure in China were aware of their condition [19]. Similarly, two-thirds of those with diabetes in China in 2003 were undiagnosed [9, 27]. In the early stages of diet-related NCDs, intervention can be effective in slowing the progression of complications and reducing the need for surgery and protracted hospital stays [1].

## The nutrition transition in the Asia-Pacific region

The nutrition transition in the Asia-Pacific region has been characterized by decreased consumption of traditional staples such as starchy roots, pulses and cereals, and other plant foods, accompanied by increased consumption of animal products (mainly milk, cheese and meat), refined cereals (such as white rice) and vegetable oils. Food supply statistics reflect this change, with availability of transition foods, such as meat, rising across the region (see Figure 29.3). Rising consumption of processed foods, such as soft drinks, has accompanied this dietary transition, and contributed to increased intakes of fat, salt and sugar [17, 28, 29, 30]. These dietary changes are associated with cancers, CVD and diabetes in the Asia-Pacific region [31–34].

While there are differences among countries in dietary patterns and their subsequent nutrition transitions, and indeed among sub-populations within countries to a certain extent, these dietary changes stem from shared causal factors. Popkin and colleagues [35] describe 'technological clashes with human biology' as a critical underpinning factor for this. This includes such aspects as:

- preferences for sweet foods intersecting with increased availability of cheap caloric sweeteners and processed foods;
- unlinked thirst and hunger/satiety mechanisms intersecting with the global introduction (and heavy marketing) of new kinds of caloric beverages; and
- innate preferences for fatty foods intersecting with increased availability and affordability of edible oils due to high-yield oilseeds and cheap removal of oils.

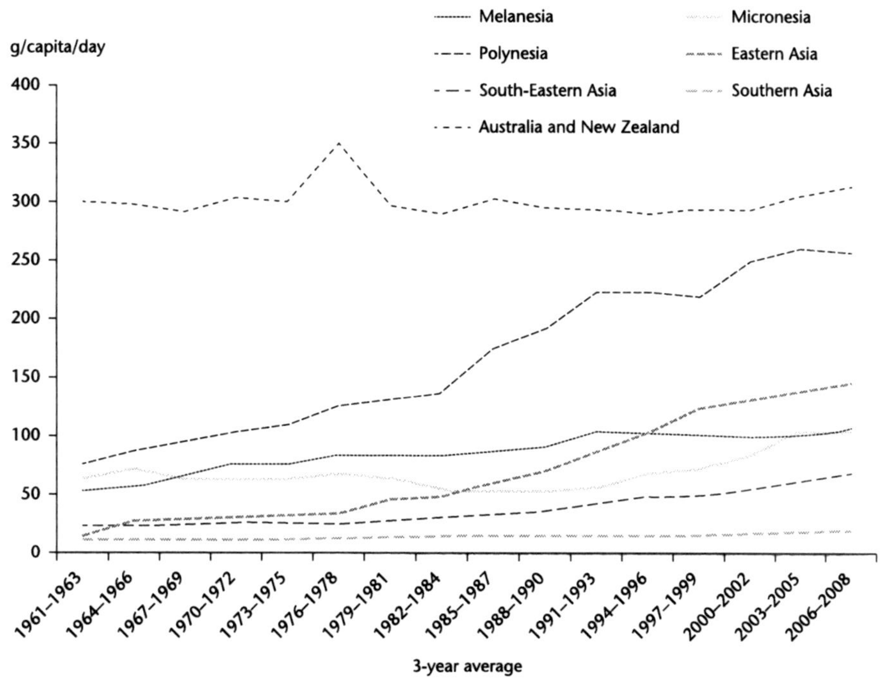


*Figure 29.3* Meat availability (food supply) data by region, 1961–2008, grams/capita/day [110]

These technological and personal factors are reinforced by social change and increased demand for convenience foods, rising incomes and food industry strategies to promote consumption of high value (usually highly processed) foods [36–38].

The most significant shift has been seen in Pacific Island countries, reflected by their extremely high rates of diet-related NCDs [39]. Imported foods, including refined cereals and cheap fatty meats, have replaced traditional diets across the region, and the availability of starchy root crops, the traditional staple, has declined (see Figure 29.4).

Pacific Island economies are extremely open and trade has played a major role in the dietary transition in these countries. This openness has contributed to urbanization, economic development, decreased investment in local agriculture, export promotion, food industry investment and the growth of food and development aid, which have all increased the availability and affordability of meat and highly processed foods, and contributed to decreased access to traditional staples [40–42]. High intakes of cheap fatty imported meat are of particular concern [43].

In Asian countries, the shift to refined carbohydrates from traditional types of rice and other staple foods, and increased consumption of animal products, has accompanied economic development, modernization and rapid urbanization [3, 14, 17]. Intakes of trans fatty acids, which significantly increases CVD risk, are very high in the region, particularly in South Asia due to the consumption of *vanaspati*, a hydrogenated fat [44].

International trade and investment has also contributed to the nutrition transition happening in Asia, through increasing availability and affordability of processed foods, sugar and fat [21]. Urbanization has meant that urban populations consume more diverse diets

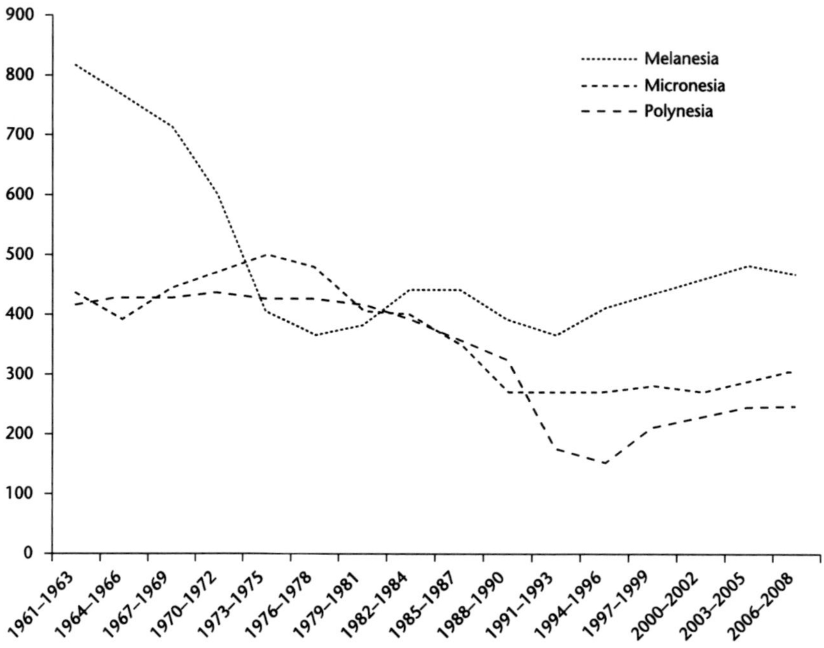


*Figure 29.4* Starchy root availability (food supply) data by region, 1961–2008, grams/capita/day [110]

than rural populations, but with higher intakes of transition foods (e.g. fatty meats and processed foods) [3].

Despite a common perception that diet-related NCDs and consumption of transitional foods are a problem mainly of the wealthy, these dietary changes are now also common among the lower-middle class and the poor [5]. Poor diets, leading to an increased overweight population, are becoming a greater burden for the poor than for the rich in China, with subsequent large increases in hypertension, stroke and adult-onset diabetes [19]. Similarly in India, poor diets and becoming overweight are growing problems amongst rural and middle-income populations [44, 45].

A dual burden of malnutrition – the coexistence of over- and under-nutrition – is increasingly apparent within countries in Asia [17, 32]. This has even been observed within households in China, Indonesia, Vietnam and Bangladesh [46, 47].

## Preventing diet-related NCDs in the Asia-Pacific region: the need for a policy approach

The nutrition transitions that are occurring in the region have not occurred unremarked: they have provoked profound concern among many citizens, in government and in the affected communities. As the burden of diet-related NCDs has risen, countries in the Asia-Pacific region have acted to introduce policies and programmes to improve diets. Key programmatic approaches include education, community intervention and settings-based interventions.

Education to improve knowledge of a healthy diet has included social marketing campaigns, community-based interventions and tailored programmes delivered by healthcare providers [48]. For example, Malaysia has implemented a multi-centre nutrition education programme, as well as an annual healthy lifestyle campaign [47]. In China, community education programmes have been developed to reduce hypertension through improving nutrition and physical activity, and targeted health education has been effective in reducing stroke incidence [49]. Settings-based approaches, such as increasing the healthfulness of foods sold in school canteens or removing vending machines from workplaces, are also effective in improving diets [48, 50]. Thailand and Singapore have been leaders in school-based obesity prevention programmes and school-based interventions have also been found to be effective in India [51]. India has also implemented workplace interventions with exercise, nutrition education and changes to cafeteria menus [48].

However, these behaviour-focused interventions have had limited success in preventing diet-related NCDs at a population level [52]. Given the socio-cultural and environmental drivers of dietary change, these interventions need to be accompanied by policy change to make affordable healthy food available in the Asia-Pacific region [53–55]. In order to be effective, this policy change needs to span multiple sectors, including agriculture, manufacturing, retail, education, culture, trade and economics [56–58].

As healthcare costs widen, and individual-focused interventions yield little change in dietary behaviours at a population level, there is growing interest for the Asia-Pacific region to use policy to create incentives for healthy diets [59, 60]. Countries in the Asia-Pacific region have implemented innovative policies to improve the food supply, and have demonstrated that policy change is possible and effective. Examples of successful policy change from the region, presented as case studies here, offer an opportunity to build on existing successes.

### *Case study 1: promoting healthy traditional diets in Pohnpei*

At the end of World War II, the population of Pohnpei, part of the Federated States of Micronesia, had virtually no NCDs [4, 24]. In less than 50 years, the diabetes prevalence had risen to 43 per cent and obesity was widespread in adults [24]. During this time, imported foods replaced traditional healthy foods, including high nutrient local root crops and bananas. Diets shifted to imported, refined, less nutritious foods, such as white rice, fatty meats, canned meat products and soft drinks [61].

In 2006, the Let's Go Local campaign commenced with a focus to promote healthy traditional foods. The campaign used a wide range of strategies, including policy change, education and community intervention [24, 62]. Policy change included the proclamation of *karat* (a highly nutritious local variety) as the Pohnpei State Banana, and this led to the manufacturing of national *karat* postal stamps, the conservation of rare carotenoid-rich plants in gene bank collections, support for small-scale local food processing and development of charcoal ovens for preparing healthy traditional foods. An awareness campaign was conducted, which included posters with messages promoting yellow-fleshed fruit and vegetables as a good source of vitamin A and other health benefits, the production of a 'Going Yellow' video and Go Local billboards displayed across the island. Community interventions included community meetings, school activities, agriculture workshops and cooking classes.

The intervention led to significant dietary improvements, as well as to positive changes in attitudes towards local food. Consumption of imported low-nutrient value foods decreased, including refined rice (average daily rice consumption from 846 g/person in 2005 to 544 g/person in 2007; $p = 0.0002$), while dietary diversity and consumption of healthy traditional staple foods and vegetables increased significantly, as did pro-vitamin A carotenoid intake (from 227 μg/person in 2005 to 475 μg/person in 2007; $p = 0.02$) [62].

## *Case study 2: trans fat policy in Korea*

While South Korea has undergone major socio-economic, dietary and epidemiological transitions from the 1970s [63, 64], the change in obesity and diet-related NCDs has been less than in other Asian countries [65]. One of the reasons that rates of diet-related NCDs remain low in South Korea is because relatively early in the economic transition, the government implemented policies and programmes to prevent nutrition-related chronic diseases and obesity, for example, the 1995 National Health Promotion Act [66]. Initiatives included large-scale nutrition education programmes in schools, involving dietitians devising school meals, workplace health examinations, and nutrition education, counselling and cooking training [48]. These policies and programmes have all included promotion of traditional diets, therefore vegetable consumption in South Korea is among the highest in Asia and the 'vegetable-centred' traditional dietary culture is still dominant today [65].

As of 2007, packaged foods in Korea have been required to include nutrition labels under the Food Labelling Standard. As part of the labelling standards, it is now also mandatory to include trans fat content on Korean food labels, and for products containing less than 0.2g of trans fat per serving, a declaration of 'trans fat-free' can be made. Since implementation, the content of trans fat has decreased markedly in virtually all products suggesting that partially hydrogenated vegetable oils (PHVOs) were being replaced with alternative oils [67].

However, not all is entirely well. The large increase observed in the saturated fat content of bakery products suggests that PHVOs were substituted with palm stearin, which is high in saturated fat. Because the removal of trans fat means an increase of saturated fat in some products, it is important to monitor progress in terms of product reformulation. Although there will be public health benefits from replacing trans fats with saturated fat, these benefits would be substantially greater if these replacements are with oils high in polyunsaturated fats [68].

Korea has demonstrated the capacity to influence diets through ongoing policy support for a healthy food supply. As part of this initiative, the country has also drafted nutrition standards for high-calorie foods with low nutritional values [69]. The Korean Food and Drug Administration plans to continue focusing on improving diets by developing action plans to deal with the food environment, food processing, school lunches and education [66].

## *Case study 3: salt intervention in Japan*

Japanese salt intakes have traditionally been high as compared to other populations [70]. In response to one of the highest mortality rates from stroke in the world in the 1950s, the Japanese government initiated a public health education campaign aimed at reducing salt intakes [70, 71]. Throughout the 1970s, salt intakes declined from 13.5 g/day to 12.1 g/day [70, 72], and in the north of Japan, where intakes were much higher than in the rest of the country, they fell from 18 g/day to 14 g/day [70, 73]. Coinciding with the decline in salt intakes, was a fall in blood pressure and an 80 per cent reduction in stroke mortality [74–76]. The trend towards decreasing salt intakes continued until the mid-1980s, when it levelled off and even increased slightly [71], suggesting the need for sustained government engagement in order for health promotion campaigns aimed at reducing salt to have lasting effects.

Between the late 1970s and 1980s, the government launched two health promotion initiatives to improve the health of Japanese society [77]. These were followed by the 'Japan Health 21' national health promotion initiative in 2000, which is supported by the 'Health Promotion' law [78]. The Japanese Health Promotion Law stipulates that each municipality should develop health promotion plans under the auspices of 'Japan Health 21' [79]. The government has since implemented a national monitoring system for health and nutrition, disseminated resources, improved the food environment, increased nutrition education and invested in human resources such as dietitians [77].

Among other dietary indicators, the initiative primarily set a target to reduce salt intakes to less than 10 g/day [77]; although this exceeds the Japanese Society of Hypertension recommendations, it was likely chosen as an achievable target in recognition that dietary salt reduction is a gradual process that should be done progressively over time. The mid-term evaluation did indicate a reduction in salt intakes, especially among males aged 50 to 59 years [77]. Overall salt intake decreased by 2.3 g/day from baseline to the mid-term evaluation [77]. However, measurement differed for both time points, and although salt intake decreased, it remains far above the target set out by the Japanese Society of Hypertension of 6 g/day [80]. Nevertheless, local communities continue to initiate programmes in Japan to reduce salt intakes [81]. Although additional progress remains necessary in Japan, it is comforting to know that salt intakes have been nearly halved since the 1950s [82].

### *Case study 4: soft drink taxes in Pacific Island countries*

In response to their high burden of NCDs, Samoa, Nauru and French Polynesia were among the first countries in the world to implement health-promoting taxes on food products associated with obesity and NCDs. These Pacific Island countries have implemented taxes as a way to reduce consumption of sugary drinks, obesity and type 2 diabetes. International evidence suggests that they can be an effective measure to reduce soft drink consumption and NCDs [83].

In Samoa, a tax was introduced by the Minister of Finance to both raise revenue and improve health outcomes for the community [84]. The tax increased the price of soft drinks such that they became more expensive than bottled water (which is not subject to the tax) so it is therefore an appropriate alternative to soft drink consumption given consumers' limited access to safe water [85].

In Nauru, a 'sugar levy' of 30 per cent on imported sugar, confectionery, carbonated soft drinks, cordials, flavoured milks and drink mixes was implemented in 2007 to 'discourage excessive consumption of sugar' [86]. After the levy was introduced, the retail price of 375-ml cans of soft drink increased by 20 per cent, although this did not make them more expensive than bottled water (locally produced desalinated water delivered to households is much cheaper) [85].

In 2002, the French Polynesian government introduced taxes on sweetened drinks, beer, confectionery and ice cream to fund the establishment of *Établissement pour la prévention*, a prevention fund [85]. These taxes were proposed in response to the growing concern about poor nutrition and NCDs, and because the government wanted to enact preventive health interventions, as well as fund hospitals. The taxes gained widespread support from government ministers because the range of activities supported by the fund included public health, education, youth and culture, sport, family and road safety. The taxes contributed to soft drinks being more expensive than water.

## Challenges: competing agendas and the globalized food industry

Despite the innovative policies and programmes that have been implemented in the Asia-Pacific region to prevent diet-related NCDs, the burden of diet-related diseases remains significant and implementation of policies remains patchy [87–89]. As per the recommendations discussed above, there is a need to scale-up existing interventions and to address the underlying drivers of food supply change on a more widespread basis.

However, policy change to improve the food supply faces challenges on a number of fronts. First, there is an ongoing tension within governments around the world between supporting economic growth through the profitability of the food industry, and supporting health through promoting the consumption of traditional and unprocessed foods (which tend not to be of economic high-value) [90]. Second, it is always difficult for staff within one branch or portfolio of government to influence policy in another. But this is accentuated when proposals come from health, which is often of a lower status in governments [91, 92]. The prevailing economic paradigm, reinforced by multilateral institutions such as the International Monetary Fund, seeks to reduce government interference in markets, including in the form of public health intervention [40, 93, 94]. Third, the food industry is heavily invested in the current food supply and actively seeks to maintain the status quo. The industry is thus likely to oppose the systemic change to the food supply needed to improve diets [95]. This occurs at a national level through lobbying of governments [96]. But with the globalization of the food industry, policies to improve the healthfulness of the food supply affect trade in food and are thus open for challenge within multilateral trade forums [97, 98].

In this section, we present two case studies of challenges to policies designed to prevent diet-related NCDs in the Asia-Pacific region.

### *Case study 5: Turkey tail ban overturned in Samoa*

In 2007, the government of Samoa implemented a ban on the importation of turkey tails (an exceptionally fatty meat remnant with poor marketability in the USA from which it was principally imported) to help curb the rise in diseases such as diabetes, high blood pressure, and heart and kidney failure [99]. The ban had an immediate effect on the availability of turkey tails and imports ceased from August 2007 [100]. Analysis of import statistics following the ban showed no noticeable replacement with other meat products, suggesting that the ban had been effective in reducing the supply of fatty meats in Samoa. A consumer survey conducted by the Nutrition Department in the Ministry of Health (n = 56) found that respondents were aware of the ban and that around 50 per cent supported the policy as a means to improve diets and health. All but one respondent reported being regular consumers of turkey tails prior to the ban [100].

In 2011, Samoa completed its accession to the World Trade Organization (WTO). One of the requirements stipulated by the working party, which included the USA, was the removal of the turkey tail ban [101]. During negotiations, members of the working party raised concerns regarding the ban due to its focus on just a single food to address the complex condition of NCDs, which have several causes, particularly in the context of the availability of other high-fat food [101]. The lack of clear criteria for selecting this product over other similar products available to consumers was also highlighted as a concern.

The government of Samoa agreed to implement less trade-restrictive measures and revoke the current prohibition order on the importation of turkey tails. As a two-year interim measure, the Food and Drugs Act 1967 would be amended to give power to the Minister of Health to make an order prohibiting the wholesale and retail sale of a product/good or class of products/goods in Samoa, and the sale of turkey tails and turkey tail products remained prohibited. In addition, an import duty of 300 per cent would be applied to turkey tail products entering Samoa.

The new measures would allow time to develop and implement a nation-wide programme promoting healthier diet and lifestyle choices to combat the spread of obesity and diabetes. At the end of this period, the ban on domestic sales of turkey tails and turkey tail products would be eliminated and replaced with an import duty of 100 per cent or other tax regulation, as well as with the recommendations from a study in conformity with the WTO Agreement [101]. At the time of writing, the results of the study were not yet available.

### *Case study 6: labelling legislation delayed in Thailand*

In 2006, in response to concerns regarding poor diets, childhood obesity and diet-related NCDs, the Ministry of Health in Thailand proposed labelling snack foods with 'traffic light' labels. Traffic light labelling had been developed by the UK Food Standards Agency early in 2006 and evidence was emerging that pictorial front-of-pack labels could assist consumers in choosing healthy foods [102]. The Thai proposal was to include the words: 'Children Should Take Less' in red text on the packaging, as well as traffic-light coloured symbols for energy, sugar, fat and sodium content to the packaging of snack foods commonly consumed by children [103]. The foods initially selected were: potato chips, corn chips, rice crisps, biscuits and 'stuffed wafers'.

As this measure would affect imported snack foods, and Thailand is a member of the WTO, the Thai Food Commission advised the Ministry of Health to notify the WTO Committee on Technical Barriers to Trade [103]. In response to this, the USA raised concerns regarding the proposed measure [104], some of which were:

- Unclear criteria used to add or remove foods to or from the list of applicable foods, and the reasons for inclusion of the categories stated;
- The scientific basis for the ranges set forth in the proposal for colour grades;
- Availability of consumer data showing that consumers would not be misled by this information on the labelling;
- 'Demonization' of the foods on the list (the US representative argued that this food could be part of a healthy diet if eaten with moderation); and
- The merits of putting colour codes on the label as colour grading for the same food could change based on package size – an inconsistency that could be confusing to the consumer.

The proposed legislation was amended in September 2007 to remove the traffic light labelling requirement and change the message to 'Should consume less, and take exercise for better health' [105, 106].

A subsequent consumer survey conducted by the Thai Food and Drug Administration found widespread support for the nutrition labelling, but also that the existing nutrition fact tables were difficult to understand [106]. In 2011, the Thai Food and Drug Administration passed a regulation on a 'Guideline Daily Amounts' (thumbnail) nutrition labelling system [107]. This front-of-pack labelling system provides simple nutrition information and has been accompanied by a consumer education campaign [106].

## Conclusion

The challenge of diet-related NCDs in the Asia-Pacific region is significant for the health sector, but has powerful socio-cultural and economic dimensions and determinants. The nutrition transition is well established in the region, and food supply has shifted away from traditional foods towards foods high in sugar, fat and salt. As a result, effective intervention requires supportive policies from across government sectors.

Case studies show that policy change in the Asia-Pacific region to prevent diet-related NCDs is both possible and effective. A combination of strategies that improve food availability through policies, settings-based approaches and consumer education can support healthy diets and prevent disease. In particular, policy-based intervention can address the underlying drivers of dietary change and demonstrates high-level support for healthy diets which can lead to further institutional and attitudinal change.

Challenges to scaling-up implementation of policies to improve the food supply are considerable and include reshaping current incentives for production and consumption, in the face of an industry that is well developed in line with existing incentives [108]. Overcoming these challenges will require investment in policy coherence between government sectors, as well as a consideration of the economic costs that changes to the food industry pose. To support the development of public policy for healthy eating across sectors, countries need to consider not only the implications of international trade agreements for domestic policy space, but also keep in mind the potential for the health sector to play an active role in this process.

## References


1. SEARO and WPRO (2008). Health in Asia and the Pacific Manila, World Health Organization – Western Pacific and South-East Asia.
2. Taylor, R. (2008). History of public health in Pacific Island countries. *Public Health in Asia and the Pacific.* M. J. Lewis and K. L. MacPherson. London, Routledge.
3. Ramachandran, A., R. C. Wan Ma, *et al.* (2010). Diabetes in Asia. *The Lancet* 375(9712): 408–418.
4. Coyne, T. (2000). *Lifestyle Diseases in Pacific Communities.* Noumea, Secretariat of the Pacific Community.
5. Dhillon, P. K., P. Jeemon, *et al.* (2012). Status of epidemiology in the WHO South-East Asia region: burden of disease, determinants of health and epidemiological research, workforce and training capacity. *International Journal of Epidemiology* 41(3): 847–860.
6. Woodward, M., A. Martiniuk, *et al.* (2008). Elevated total cholesterol: its prevalence and population-attributable fraction for mortality from coronary heart disease and ischaemic stroke in the Asia-Pacific region. *European Journal of Cardiovascular Prevention & Rehabilitation* 15(4): 397–401.
7. Ueshima, H., A. Sekikawa, *et al.* (2008). Cardiovascular disease and risk factors in Asia. *Circulation* 118(25): 2702–2709.
8. Takachi, R., M. Inoue, *et al.* (2010). Consumption of sodium and salted foods in relation to cancer and cardiovascular disease: the Japan Public Health Center-based Prospective Study. *American Journal of Clinical Nutrition* 91(2): 456–464.
9. Chan, J. N., V. Malik, *et al.* (2009). Diabetes in Asia: epidemiology, risk factors, and pathophysiology. *Journal of the American Medical Association* 301(20): 2129–2140.
10. Yoon, K.-H., J.-H. Lee, *et al.* (2006). Epidemic obesity and type 2 diabetes in Asia. *The Lancet* 368(9548): 1681–1688.
11. Asia Pacific Cohort Studies Collaboration (2003). Cholesterol, coronary heart disease, and stroke in the Asia Pacific region. *International Journal of Epidemiology* 32(4): 563–572.
12. Martiniuk, A. L., C. M. Lee, *et al.* (2007). Hypertension: its prevalence and population-attributable fraction for mortality from cardiovascular disease in the Asia-Pacific region. *Journal of Hypertension* 25(1): 73–79
13. Lee, C. M. Y., S. Colagiuri, *et al.* (2011). The burden of cardiovascular disease associated with high body mass index in the Asia-Pacific region. *Obesity Reviews* 12(5): e454–e459.
14. Popkin, B. M., S. Horton, *et al.* (2001). Trends in diet, nutritional status, and diet-related noncommunicable diseases in China and India: the economic costs of the nutrition transition. *Nutrition Reviews* 59(12): 379–390.

15. Ji, C. Y. and T. O. Cheng (2008). Prevalence and geographic distribution of childhood obesity in China in 2005. *International Journal of Cardiology* 131(1): 1–8.
16. Lewis, M. J. and K. L. MacPherson (2012). Health transitions and the double disease burden in Asian and Pacific countries: some introductory observations. *Health Transitions and the Double Disease Burden in Asia and the Pacific.* M. J. Lewis and K. L. MacPherson. London, Routledge: 279–301.
17. Misra, A., N. Singhal, *et al.* (2011). Nutrition transition in India: secular trends in dietary intake and their relationship to diet-related non-communicable diseases. *Journal of Diabetes* 3(4): 278–292.
18. Popkin, B. M. (2012). The nutrition transition is speeding up: a global perspective. *Nutritional Health.* N. J. Temple, T. Wilson and J. D. R. Jacobs. Totowa, NJ, Humana Press: 85–99.
19. Liu, Y., K. Rao, *et al.* (2008). China's health system performance. *The Lancet* 372(9653): 1914–1923.
20. Popkin, B. M. (2008). Will China's nutrition transition overwhelm its health care system and slow economic growth? *Health Affairs* 27(4): 1064–1076.
21. James, W. P. T., N. Rojroongwasinkul, *et al.* (2010). Food imports and dietary change: a perspective from Thailand. *Trade, Food, Diet and Health: Perspectives and Policy Options.* C. Hawkes, C. Blouin, S. Henson, N. Drager and L. Dubé. Oxford, Wiley-Blackwell: 147–168.
22. Sukeri, S. (2012). The economic and social impact of ischaemic heart disease on households in Malaysia. PhD. School of Public Health, University of Sydney.
23. Yang, W.-C., S.-J. Hwang, *et al.* (2001). The impact of diabetes on economic costs in dialysis patients: experiences in Taiwan. *Diabetes Research and Clinical Practice* 54, Supplement 1(0): 47–54.
24. Cheng, M. H. (2010). Asia-Pacific faces diabetes challenge. *The Lancet* 375(9733): 2207–2210.
25. Foliaki, S. and N. Pearce (2003). Prevention and control of diabetes in Pacific people. *BMJ* 327(7412): 437–439.
26. Leeder, S., S. Raymond, *et al.* (2004). *A Race against Time: The Challenge of Cardiovascular Disease in Developing Economies.* New York, Columbia University Press.
27. Wong K. C. and Z. Wang. (2006) Prevalence of type 2 diabetes mellitus of Chinese populations in Mainland China, Hong Kong, and Taiwan. *Diabetes Research and Clinical Practice* 73: 126–134.
28. Gibson, J. (1998). Urban demand for food, beverages, betelnut and tobacco in Papua New Guinea. *Papua New Guinea Journal of Agriculture, Forestry and Fisheries* 41(2): 37–42.
29. Hughes, R. G. and M. A. Lawrence (2005). Globalization, food and health in Pacific Island countries. *Asia Pacific Journal of Clinical Nutrition* 14(4): 298–306.
30. Astrup, A., J. Dyerberg, *et al.* (2008). Nutrition transition and its relationship to the development of obesity and related chronic diseases. *Obesity Reviews* 9(s 1): 48–52.
31. Hughes, R. G. (2003). Diet, food supply and obesity in the Pacific. Suva, World Health Organization Regional Office for the Western Pacific.
32. Schmidhuber, J. and P. Shetty (2005). The nutrition transition to 2030: why developing countries are likely to bear the major burden. *Acta Agriculturae Scand Section C* 2: 150–166.
33. Hu, F. B. (2011). Globalization of diabetes. *Diabetes Care* 34(6): 1249–1257.
34. Hu, E. A., A. Pan, *et al.* (2012). White rice consumption and risk of type 2 diabetes: meta-analysis and systematic review. *BMJ* 344: e1454.
35. Popkin, B. M., L. S. Adair, *et al.* (2012). Global nutrition transition and the pandemic of obesity in developing countries. *Nutrition Reviews* 70(1): 3–21.
36. Schmidhuber, J. and P. Shetty (2005). Nutrition transition, obesity and noncommunicable diseases: drivers, outlook and concerns. *SCN News* 29: 13–19.
37. Witkowski, T. H. (2007). Food marketing and obesity in developing countries: analysis, ethics and public policy. *Journal of Macromarketing* 27(2): 126–137.
38. Popkin, B. M. (2011). Contemporary nutritional transition: determinants of diet and its impact on body composition. *Proceedings of the Nutrition Society* 70(01): 82–91.
39. Taylor, R. (2012). The double disease burden in Pacific Island states (except Papua New Guinea). *Health Transitions and the Double Disease Burden in Asia and the Pacific.* M. J. Lewis and K. L. MacPherson. London, Routledge: 279–301.
40. Thow, A. M. and W. Snowdon (2010). The effect of trade and trade policy on diet and health in the Pacific Islands. *Trade, Food, Diet and Health: Perspectives and Policy Options.* C. Hawkes, C. Blouin, S. Henson, N. Drager and L. Dubé. Oxford, Wiley-Blackwell: 147–168.
41. Dancause, K. N., C. Dehuff, *et al.* (2011). Behavioral changes associated with economic development in the South Pacific: health transition in Vanuatu. *American Journal of Human Biology* 23(3): 366–376.

42. Thow, A. M., P. Heywood, *et al.* (2011). Trade and the nutrition transition: strengthening policy for health in the Pacific. *Ecology of Food and Nutrition* 50(1): 18–42.
43. Gewertz, D. B. and F. Errington (2009). Pacific Island flaps. *Cheap Meat: Flap Food Nations in the Pacific Islands*. Berkeley, University of California Press.
44. Misra, A., L. Khurana, *et al.* (2009). South Asian diets and insulin resistance. *British Journal of Nutrition* 101(4): 465–473.
45. Kinra, S., L. J. Bowen, *et al.* (2010). Sociodemographic patterning of non-communicable disease risk factors in rural India: a cross sectional study. *BMJ* 341: c4974.
46. Doak, C. M., L. S. Adair, *et al.* (2005). The dual burden household and the nutrition transition paradox. *International Journal of Obesity* 29(1): 129–136.
47. Jehn, M. and A. Brewis (2009). Paradoxical malnutrition in mother–child pairs: Untangling the phenomenon of over- and under-nutrition in underdeveloped economies. *Economics & Human Biology* 7(1): 28–35.
48. Doak, C. (2002). Large-scale interventions and programmes addressing nutrition-related chronic diseases and obesity: examples from 14 countries. *Public Health Nutrition* 5(1A): 275–277.
49. Fang, X.-H., R. A. Kronmal, *et al.* (1999). Prevention of stroke in urban China. *Stroke* 30(3): 495–501.
50. Neumark-Sztainer, D., S. A. French, *et al.* (2005). School lunch and snacking patterns among high school students: associations with school food environment and policies. *International Journal of Behavioral Nutrition and Physical Activity* 2(1): 14.
51. Singhal, N., A. Misra, *et al.* (2010). Effects of controlled school-based multi-component model of nutrition and lifestyle interventions on behavior modification, anthropometry and metabolic risk profile of urban Asian Indian adolescents in North India. *Eur J Clin Nutr* 64(4): 364–373.
52. Swinburn, B. A., G. Sacks, *et al.* (2011). The global obesity pandemic: shaped by global drivers and local environments. *The Lancet* 378(9793): 804–814.
53. Hossain, P., B. Kawar, *et al.* (2007). Obesity and diabetes in the developing world – a growing challenge. *New England Journal of Medicine* 356(3): 213–215.
54. Dans, A., N. Ng, *et al.* (2011). The rise of chronic non-communicable diseases in Southeast Asia: time for action. *The Lancet* 377(9766): 680–689.
55. Hu, F. B., Y. Liu, *et al.* (2011). Preventing chronic diseases by promoting healthy diet and lifestyle: public policy implications for China. *Obesity Reviews* 12(7): 552–559.
56. Adeyi, O., O. Smith, *et al.* (2007). *Public Policy and the Challenge of Chronic Noncommunicable Diseases*. Washington, DC, World Bank.
57. Meiro-Lorenzo, M., T. L. Villafana, *et al.* (2011). Effective responses to non-communicable disease: embracing action beyond the health sector. Washington, DC, World Bank.
58. United Nations General Assembly (2011). Political declaration of the High-level Meeting of the General Assembly on the Prevention and Control of Non-communicable Diseases. New York, United Nations.
59. WHO (2007). Report Meeting of Ministers of Health for the Pacific Island Countries. *Reports*. Manila, World Health Organization Regional Office for the Western Pacific.
60. SEARO (2011). Health and Development Challenges of Noncommunicable Diseases in the South-East Asia Region. Jakarta, Indonesia, World Health Organization Regional Office for South-East Asia.
61. Corsi, A., L. Englberger, *et al.* (2008). A participatory assessment of dietary patterns and food behavior in Pohnpei, Federated States of Micronesia. *Asia Pacific Journal of Clinical Nutrition* 17(2): 309–316.
62. Englberger, L., H. Kuhnlein, *et al.* (2010). Pohnpei, FSM case study in a global health project documents its local food resources and successfully promotes local food for health. *Pacific Health Dialogue* 16(1): 129–136.
63. Jang, M. and D. Berry (2011). Overweight, obesity, and metabolic syndrome in adults and children in South Korea: a review of the literature. *Clinical Nursing Research* 20(3): 276–291.
64. Lee, S.-K. and J. Sobal (2003). Socio-economic, dietary, activity, nutrition and body weight transitions in South Korea. *Public Health Nutrition* 6(07): 665–674.
65. Lee, M.-J., B. M. Popkin, *et al.* (2002). The unique aspects of the nutrition transition in South Korea: the retention of healthful elements in their traditional diet. *Public Health Nutrition* 5(1a): 197–203.
66. Park, H. K. (2008). Nutrition policy in South Korea. *Asia Pac J Clin Nutr* 17(Suppl 1): 343–345.

67. Lee, J. H., P. Adhikari, *et al.* (2010). Trans fatty acids content and fatty acid profiles in the selected food products from Korea between 2005 and 2008. *J Food Sci* 75(7): c647–652.
68. Mozaffarian, D. and R. Clarke (2009). Quantitative effects on cardiovascular risk factors and coronary heart disease risk of replacing partially hydrogenated vegetable oils with other fats and oils. *Eur J Clin Nutr* 63 Suppl 2: S22–33.
69. Korea Food and Drug Administration (2009). Nutrition Standards for High-Calorie Foods with Low Nutritional Value.
70. He, F. J. and G. A. MacGregor (2009). A comprehensive review on salt and health and current experience of worldwide salt reduction programmes. *J Hum Hypertens* 23(6): 363–384.
71. Elliott, P. and I. Brown (2007). Sodium intakes around the world: background document prepared for the Forum and Technical meeting on Reducing Salt Intake in Populations (Paris, 5–7 October 2006). Geneva, WHO.
72. Cappuccio, F. P., S. Capewell, *et al.* (2011). Policy options to reduce population salt intake. *BMJ* 343: d4995.
73. Anderson, C. A., L. J. Appel, *et al.* (2010). Dietary sources of sodium in China, Japan, the United Kingdom, and the United States, women and men aged 40 to 59 years: the INTERMAP study. *J Am Diet Assoc* 110(5): 736–745.
74. Tanaka, H., Y. Tanaka, *et al.* (1982). Secular trends in mortality for cerebrovascular diseases in Japan, 1960 to 1979. *Stroke* 13(5): 574–581.
75. Sasaki, S. (2011). The value of the National Health and Nutrition Survey in Japan. *The Lancet* 378(9798): 1205–1206.
76. Sasaki N., (1979). The salt factor in apoplexy and hypertension: epidemiological studies in Japan. *Prophylactic Approach to Hypertensive Diseases*. Y. Yamori. New York, Raven Press: 467–474.
77. Udagawa, K., M. Miyoshi, *et al.* (2008). Mid-term evaluation of 'Health Japan 21': focus area for the nutrition and diet. *Asia Pac J Clin Nutr* 17(Suppl 2): 445–452.
78. Shibaike, N., O. Utsunomiya, *et al.* (2002). 5. Action by Ministry of Health, Labor and Welfare National Health Promotion in the 21st century 'Health Japan 21'. *Intern Med* 41(1): 70–71.
79. Government of Japan (2002). Health Promotion Law. Public Law 103, 154 Congress.
80. Kawano, Y., T. Tsuchihashi, *et al.* (2007). Report of the Working Group for Dietary Salt Reduction of the Japanese Society of Hypertension: (2) Assessment of salt intake in the management of hypertension. *Hypertens Res* 30(10): 887–893.
81. Omori, A. (2012). Taking salt off the menu: community projects aim to achieve healthier diets. *Daily Yomiuri online*.
82. Katanoda, K. and Y. Matsumura (2002). National Nutrition Survey in Japan – its methodological transition and current findings. *J Nutr Sci Vitaminol (Tokyo)* 48(5): 423–432.
83. Mytton, O. T., D. Clarke, M. Rayner. (2012) Taxing unhealthy food and drinks to improve health. *BMJ* 344: e2931.
84. Hang, N. L. (2006). *2006/07 Budget Address*. Apia, Government of Samoa.
85. Thow, A. M., C. Quested, *et al.* (2011). Taxing soft drinks in the Pacific: implementation lessons for improving health. *Health Promotion International* 26(1): 55–64.
86. Minister for Finance (2007). Republic of Nauru 2007–08 Budget. Nauru, Government of Nauru.
87. Zhai, F., D. Fu, *et al.* (2002). What is China doing in policy-making to push back the negative aspects of the nutrition transition? *Public Health Nutrition* 5(1a): 269–273.
88. Leowski, J. and A. Krishnan (2009). Capacity to control noncommunicable diseases in the countries of South-East Asia. *Health Policy (Amsterdam, Netherlands)* 92(1): 43–48.
89. Thow, A. M., W. Snowdon, *et al.* (2011). The role of policy in improving diets: experiences from the Pacific Obesity Prevention in Communities food policy project. *Obesity Reviews* 12: 68–74.
90. Story, M., M. W. Hamm, *et al.* (2009). Food systems and public health: linkages to achieve healthier diets and healthier communities. *Journal of Hunger & Environmental Nutrition* 4(3–4): 219–224.
91. Baum, F. (1999). Social capital: is it good for your health? Issues for a public health agenda. *Journal of Epidemiology and Community Health* 53: 195–196.
92. Labonté, R. and T. Schrecker (2007). Globalization and social determinants of health: promoting health equity in global governance (part 3 of 3). *Globalization and Health* 3(7).
93. Szreter, S. (2003). The population health approach in historical perspective. *American Journal of Public Health* 93(3): 421–431.
94. Thomas, C. and M. Weber (2004). The politics of global health governance: Whatever happened to 'Health for All by the Year 2000'? *Global Governance* 10: 187–205.

95. Dunn, S. (2011). The modern food industry and public health: a Galbraithian perspective. *Journal of Post Keynesian Economics* 33(3): 491–516.
96. Cohen, D. (2011). Will industry influence derail UN summit? *BMJ* 343: d5328.
97. Stuckler, D., M. McKee, *et al.* (2012). Manufacturing epidemics: the role of global producers in increased consumption of unhealthy commodities including processed foods, alcohol, and tobacco. *PLoS Med* 9(6): e1001235.
98. Thow, A. M. (2009). Trade liberalisation and the nutrition transition: mapping the pathways for public health nutritionists. *Public Health Nutrition* 12: 2150–2158.
99. Leota, T. L. A. (2007). Prohibition order on the importation of turkey tails, Pursuant to Section 49 of the Customs Act 1977. Ministry for Revenue, Government of Samoa, Published in *The Samoa Observer*, 20 September 2007.
100. Thow, A. M., B. Swinburn, *et al.* (2010). Trade and food policy: case studies from three Pacific Island Countries. *Food Policy* 35: 556–564.
101. World Trade Organization (2011). Report of the working party on the accession of Samoa to the World Trade Organization. Geneva, WTO.
102. Lobstein, T. and S. Davies (2009). Defining and labelling 'healthy' and 'unhealthy' food. *Public Health Nutrition* 12(03): 331–340.
103. WTO (2006). Notification to Committee on Technical Barriers to Trade. Geneva, World Trade Organization.
104. WTO (2007). Minutes of the meeting of 21 March 2007, Committee on Technical Barriers to Trade. Geneva, World Trade Organization.
105. WTO (2007). Notification to Committee on Technical Barriers to Trade, addendum. Geneva, World Trade Organization.
106. Parinyasiri, T. (2010). Nutrition labeling and claims in Thailand update. ILSI Seminar and Workshop on nutrition labeling, claims and communication strategies for the consumers.
107. Sirikeratikul, S. and O. Vasquez (2011). *Thai FDA's New Guideline Daily Amounts (GDA) Labeling*. Washington, DC, United States Department of Agriculture Foreign Agricultural Service.
108. Hawkes, C. (2012). Food policies for healthy populations and healthy economies. *British Medical Journal* 344: e2801.
109. World Health Organization. Global Health Observatory Data Repository. Available at: http://apps.who.int/gho/data/?region=searo# [Accessed 7 October 2012].
110. United Nations Food and Agriculture Organization. FAOSTAT. Available at: http://faostat3.fao.org/home/index.html#HOME [Accessed 5 October 2012].

# 30

# The challenge of non-communicable diseases in Asia

## The case of diabetes

*Azadeh Zabetian, Mary Beth Weber, Lisa R. Staimez, Roopa Shivashankar, K. M. Venkat Narayan and Mohammed K. Ali*

### Introduction

Chronic non-communicable diseases (NCDs or 'chronic diseases') include cardiovascular diseases (CVD), diabetes, cancers and chronic respiratory diseases. Cumulatively, these diseases threaten the health and economies of individuals, families, communities and, in fact, entire populations. Chronic diseases account for 60 per cent of all deaths worldwide and 80 per cent of these occur in low- and middle-income countries (LMIC) [1–3]. In Asia, major demographic, economic, socio-cultural and nutrition transitions over the past four decades have been associated with a meteoric rise in chronic disease burdens and projections suggest that Asia will continue to be the epicentre of cardio-metabolic burdens in the decades to come.

Diabetes mellitus is a prototypical NCD and is biochemically characterized by a relative deficiency of insulin (either insufficient secretion from the pancreas and/or inadequate sensitivity of the body's tissues to insulin), which results in elevated blood glucose levels. This complex metabolic disorder exemplifies a number of features that are common across NCDs. First, NCDs are considered 'silent epidemics' [3], for example, elevated glucose levels seen in diabetes are asymptomatic and can remain undetected [4] unless screened for or discovered once disabling diabetes-related complications develop [5, 6]. Second, NCDs tend to be multi-factorial, such that genetic composition increases vulnerability to the effects of environmental triggers (dietary, activity and other lifestyle factors such as tobacco exposure) [7]. Third, NCDs are long-standing, progressive and costly. For example, diabetes is associated with diminished functional capacity, increased physical and psychosocial morbidity, occurrence of comorbidities and complications and higher utilization of health services. Furthermore, individuals with diabetes have higher medical costs plus opportunity costs [8] associated with self-care and disability [9], as well as premature mortality (life expectancy is shortened by approximately 7 to 15 years) [10, 11] compared to those without diabetes.

In this chapter, diabetes is used as an example to discuss the challenges of addressing NCDs in Asia. After concisely conveying the existing data regarding the epidemiology of diabetes and its risk factors, a synopsis of the prevention and treatment approaches is provided, as well as a discussion of the challenges of translating proven approaches into policies and practice in Asia. The chapter mainly focuses on type 2 diabetes, which is the most common type of diabetes accounting for 90 to 95 per cent of all diabetes cases in the world [12].

## Epidemiology of diabetes/pre-diabetes

Most countries in Asia have experienced population ageing in recent years, which is due to the rapid socio-economic, health, and nutrition transitions in the region [13]. Increased life expectancy is associated with the emergence of chronic diseases like diabetes, as seen in Asia, which is experiencing a rapid growth in diabetes [14, 15]. For example, it is projected that China, India, Bangladesh, Indonesia and Pakistan will be among the top ten countries in the world in terms of the number of people affected by diabetes by 2030 [12]. Understanding the distribution and determinants of diabetes is helpful to conceptualize the avenues needed for prevention and control responses.

The prevalence of diabetes varies across Asia. This may be because the region is comprised of a number of different populations that are heterogeneous in terms of demographic and economic transition, socio-economic status and cultures. Also, the prevalence data are derived from epidemiological studies that have used different research methods (e.g. sampling, outcome assessment and analytical methods), and surveyed populations differ in terms of their age–sex distributions and level of representativeness of their populations; therefore, results are not easily comparable across studies and countries. Organizations that have successfully pooled data from various countries, such as the International Diabetes Federation (IDF), highlight that almost one-fifth of all people with diabetes in the world are from the Southeast Asia region (71.4 million adults) [12]. China and India have the highest absolute number of people with diabetes in the world, 92 million and 63 million, respectively [12]. This is largely due to large population size in these two countries but might also be related to environmental and genetic influences.

Although limited in their representativeness and comparability, there are a number of individual studies reporting diabetes prevalence in Asian countries (see Table 30.1). A recent study from four states of India estimated a countrywide diabetes prevalence of 6.2 per cent [16] and data from China showed national prevalence of around 9.7 per cent [17]. Limited epidemiological data from the Philippines suggested that 8 per cent of the population is affected by diabetes [18]. Similar prevalence rates are estimated for other Southeast Asian countries: Thailand (6.8–11.9 per cent), Hong Kong (9 per cent) and Taiwan (9–11 per cent) [18]. In Japan, the prevalence of diabetes ranged widely with 4–12 per cent of the population aged ≥ 40 years being affected [19]. Meanwhile, older data have shown that diabetes prevalence rates in Pakistan (9.3 per cent in males and 11.1 per cent in females) [20] and Sri Lanka (10.9 per cent) [21] are also similar. Lower diabetes prevalence was observed in Vietnam (two studies reporting 1.4 per cent and 3.8 per cent) [22, 23] and Indonesia (two studies reporting 1.63 per cent and 5.7 per cent) [24, 25].

Trend data are useful for monitoring burdens, evaluating the effects of interventions and for health planning. To convey diabetes prevalence data that provides an impression of trends in the region, estimates from the Global Burden of Disease (GBD) study [26] were used. These estimates are derived through comprehensive data compilation from published and unpublished evidence all over the world with the application of uniform analytical methods

*Table 30.1* Diabetes prevalence in individual studies from countries in Asia

| *Country* | *Year* | *Sample size* | *Sample* | *Age range* | *% of women* | *Diabetes diagnostic method* | *Criteria* | *Prevalence of diabetes (%)* | *Adjustment for age* |
|---|---|---|---|---|---|---|---|---|---|
| India [16] | 2011 | 13,055 | Three states (Tamilnadu, Maharashtra and Jharkhand) and one union territory (Chandigarh) | ≥20 | M/W | FPG/OGTT | WHO 1999 | 6.2 | No |
| China [17] | 2010 | 46,239 | 14 provinces and municipalities | ≥20 | M/W | FPG/OGTT | WHO 1999 | 9.7 (10.6 M/8.8 W) | Yes |
| Thailand [124] | 2004 | 37,138 | National | ≥15 | M/W | FPG | ≥7mmol/l | 6.7 | Yes |
| Vietnam [23] | 2001 | 2,932 | Ho Chi Minh, screening program | ≥15 | 74.4 | FPG | ADA | 3.8 | Yes |
| Sri Lanka [21] | 2005–2006 | 4,532 | National | ≥18 | M/W | FPG/OGTT | ADA1997, WHO | 10.9 | No |
| Bangladesh [125] | 2005 | 836 | Remote rural areas of Northern Bangladesh | ≥25 | M/W | OGTT | WHO | 7.2 (95% CI 5.4–9.0) | No |
| Nepal [126] | 2007 | 740 | Semi-urban | 21–94 | 60 | Not reported | Not reported | 9.5 | No |
| Singapore [127] | 2004 | 4,168 | National | 18–74 | M/W | FPG/OGTT | WHO 1985 | 8.2 (8.9 M/ 7.6 W) | No |
| Taiwan [128] | 2004 | 1,475,975 | Taiwan National Health Insurance Research Database | ≥20 | M/W | Insurance claims data (diagnostic code of diabetes) self-reported previous physician diagnosis | Not reported | 6.5 M/6.6 W | Yes |
| Indonesia [25] | 2009 | 24,417 | National/urban | >15 | M/W | OGTT | WHO 1999 and ADA 2003 | 5.7 | No |

*Abbreviations*
FPG: Fasting Plasma Glucose
OGTT: Oral Glucose Tolerance Test
M: men/W: women
WHO 1999: World Health Organization definition for diabetes in 1999 [129]
WHO 1985: World Health Organization definition for diabetes in 1985 [130]
ADA 1997: American Diabetes Association definition for diabetes in 1997 [131]
ADA 2003: American Diabetes Association definition for diabetes in 2003 [132]

*Table 30.2* Country-specific trends of diabetes prevalence during 1980–2008

| *Country* | *2008 prevalence %* | | *Trend since 1980* |
|---|---|---|---|
| | *Males* | *Females* | |
| ***Asia-Pacific high income*** | | | |
| Japan | 7.2 | 4.7 | Upward |
| South Korea | 6.8 | 5.3 | Downward |
| Singapore | 7.5 | 5.4 | Downward |
| ***East Asia*** | | | |
| China | 9.6 | 9.4 | Stable |
| Hong Kong SAR | 10.5 | 9.2 | Stable |
| North Korea | 7.7 | 7.5 | Downward |
| Taiwan | 8.2 | 7.7 | Downward |
| ***South Asia*** | | | |
| Bangladesh | 9.2 | 9.9 | Upward |
| India | 11.1 | 10.8 | Upward |
| Nepal | 9.8 | 9.3 | Upward |
| Pakistan | 11.7 | 14.1 | Upward |
| ***Southeast Asia*** | | | |
| Indonesia | 6.6 | 7.1 | Downward |
| Malaysia | 11.6 | 11.2 | Upward |
| Philippines | 6.5 | 6.6 | Downward |
| Sri Lanka | 9.3 | 8.6 | Upward |
| Thailand | 7.3 | 7.1 | Stable |
| Vietnam | 7.5 | 7.9 | Stable |

*Source*: Adopted from Weber *et al.* [31] and the Global Burden of Disease Study [26].

that can account for changing age distributions, year, level of urbanization and national incomes across countries over time (see Table 30.2). The data showed that diabetes prevalence in the sub-region of south Asian countries has consistently increased since 1980. Other countries with rising diabetes prevalence include Japan, Malaysia and Sri Lanka. Individually published studies from these countries reaffirmed that diabetes prevalence has increased since 1980 [14, 27–30]. The GBD study also noted that population growth and ageing are the main driving factors for these observed trends [26].

Other important themes emerging from the GBD data are that: diabetes prevalence has flattened and even decreased over the last three decades among high-income Asia-Pacific countries (e.g. South Korea, Singapore and Taiwan), despite the fact that all of these countries have ageing populations; and increases in diabetes prevalence have tended to be more prominent among the lower-income or fast-transitioning countries of the region. These observed patterns might be due to natural plateauing of the epidemic, the implementation of effective interventions or policies in high-income countries, demographic changes (mortality, birth, immigration), or may be associated with data irregularities [31]. Crucially, a high proportion of those affected by diabetes in Asia are as yet unaware of this. The IDF noted that more than 60 per cent of people with undiagnosed diabetes in the world are living in the Southeast Asia and Western Pacific regions [12]. Estimates suggest that approximately 50 per cent of diabetes cases in Southeast Asia are undiagnosed [32]. Estimates for the proportion of the undiagnosed diabetes among populations of Western Pacific countries such as China (68.6 per cent undiagnosed) and Hong Kong, as well as Taiwan (52.6 per cent) were similar [33].

There are also sizeable populations with pre-diabetes – impaired glucose tolerance (IGT) and/or impaired fasting glucose (IFG) – in Asia, signifying a large pool of people that are susceptible to developing diabetes and diabetes-related complications [14]. For example, over half of the Asian Indian population with pre-diabetes enrolled in the Indian Diabetes Prevention Programme developed diabetes within three years of the follow-up (55 per cent conversion rate) [34]. In terms of IGT, Malaysia (18.4 per cent), China (13.5 per cent) and Hong Kong (13.5 per cent) are recognized among the countries with the highest prevalence of pre-diabetes [35]. Meanwhile, low prevalence of pre-diabetes was reported in rural Pakistan (IFG prevalence: 4.2 per cent in males and 2.3 per cent in females) [36], Vietnam (IFG prevalence: 2.5 per cent) [23] and in a community-based survey on a South Indian population (4.1 per cent, IGT and 7.1 per cent, IFG) [37]. It is unclear whether the observed prevalence in these countries implies faster conversion to frank diabetes without a detectable precursor phase or that there is insufficient testing for pre-diabetes, which requires oral glucose tolerance testing to accurately detect. The alarmingly high rates of pre-diabetes and undiagnosed diabetes in Asia highlight the critical need for timely and efficient methods of early detection across the region.

## Complications of diabetes

Diabetes is associated with seriously disabling, and even fatal, microvascular (chronic kidney disease, retinopathy and limb disease, which includes foot ulcers and neuropathy) and macrovascular complications (heart disease, stroke, peripheral vascular disease). The duration of diabetes and control of cardio-metabolic parameters (glycemia, blood pressure, lipids) predict the progression to complications. Asian populations experience greater diabetes complication burdens than European/Caucasian populations [38]. For example, the age of the first myocardial infarction is ten years earlier among South Asians and Asians have a higher likelihood of progression to end-stage renal disease (ESRD) than Caucasians [39, 40] (see Table 30.3). Onset of complications exponentially increases the economic burdens experienced by individuals and families.

Data on prevalence of diabetes complications in the region are scarce. The patterns observed to date suggest that the distribution of macrovascular complications varies by ethnicity. South Asians, Pacific Islanders and Korean populations, for example, experience a higher prevalence of coronary heart disease [41, 42], while the prevalence of stroke, a leading cardiovascular cause of death in the region, is significantly higher among the Chinese and Japanese Asians [31, 40–42].

On the other hand, renal disease, a microvascular complication of diabetes, is highly prevalent among people with diabetes throughout the region [40, 43] (see Table 30.3). The Developing Education on Microalbuminuria for Awareness of Renal and cardiovascular risk in Diabetes (DEMAND) study (2003) found that two-thirds of patients had some form of albuminuria (44 per cent with microalbuminuria and 12 per cent with macroalbuminuria) in Asia [39]. The highest prevalence and incidence of ESRD in the region was found among Malays with diabetes [44, 45]. This group also revealed as having the highest mortality rates due to heart failure, which might be owed to the powerful association between renal function and coronary heart disease [40]. Data on CVD-related mortality rates among diabetes patients, which require follow-up of large cohorts, are not yet available in the Asian context.

Diabetes retinopathy has different stages and can be sight-threatening in its progressive stages, leading to blindness. The prevalence of diabetes retinopathy is about 30 per cent in Asians with type 2 diabetes [14], mostly observed in its advanced stages. In Asians who are newly diagnosed with diabetes, both background and sight-threatening retinopathy were two

*Table 30.3* Diabetes quality of care outcome indicators measured in multinational studies in Asia

| *Author and year* | *Sample size* | *Countries* | *Study setting* | *Participant information* | | | | *Complications** | | *QOC indicators* | | |
|---|---|---|---|---|---|---|---|---|---|---|---|---|
| | | | | *Age (yrs)** | *Gender (Male %)*** | *Duration (yrs)* | *BMI (kg/m²)** | *Macro vascular* | *Micro vascular* | *HbA1c (%)**** | *SBP (mmHg)**** | *LDLc (mg/dl)**** |
| Chuang (2002) [102] | 24,317 | Bangladesh, People's Republic of China, India, Indonesia, Malaysia, Philippines, Singapore, South Korea, Sri Lanka, Taiwan, Thailand and Vietnam | Sp | 57.7 ±12.2 | 44 | 9.2 ± 6.8 | 24.4±4.0 | + | +++ | 8.6±2.0 | >140 = 27% | |
| Wu (2005) [118][a] | 6,482 | China, Hong Kong, Indonesia, Malaysia, Pakistan, Philippines, Singapore, South Korea, Taiwan and Thailand | Sp | 61.1 | 42 | 6.9 | 25.5 | | | 7.8 | 142.7 | |
| Eppens (2006) [133][b] | 331 | Western Australia, China, China–Hong Kong, Indonesia, Japan, South Korea, Malaysia, Philippines, Singapore, Taiwan and Thailand | Sp | Median: 14.9 | Median: 45 | Median: 2.3 | Overweight 41%[c] | | + | Median: 7 | BP> 95th percentile for age/sex = 24% | Median: 112.1 |
| Chuang (2006) [47] | 8,054 | Indonesia, Malaysia, Philippines, Singapore, South Korea, Taiwan, Thailand and Vietnam | Pri | 60 | | 6 | 24.59 | + | +++ | 7.9 | | 146.8 |
| Mohamed (2008) [48][d] | 15,549 | China, Indonesia, Korea, Malaysia, Philippines, Singapore, Taiwan, Thailand and Vietnam | Pri | 59.2±12.0 | 41 | 8±5.9 | 24.9±3.9 | + | +++ | 8.0±2.0 | 133.0±19 | |

| | | | | | | | | | | | | |
|---|---|---|---|---|---|---|---|---|---|---|---|---|
| Pan (2008) [119] | 8,561 | People's Republic of China, Hong Kong, Indonesia, the Republic of Korea, Malaysia, Singapore, the Republic of China and Thailand | Pri | 60 | 49 | 7.3±6.2 | 24.7±3.9 | ++ | +++ | 7.8±1.8 | 133±18 | |
| Chan (2009) [94][e] | 5,886 | Korea, China, Indonesia, India, Hong Kong, Taiwan, Malaysia and Thailand | Sp | 55 | | 8.3 | | ++ | +++ | 7.7 | <130 and <80 = 24 | <100 = 37% |

*Abbreviations*
Yrs: years; SD: Standard Deviation; BMI: Body Mass Index; QOC: Quality of Care; HbA1c: Glycosylated Haemoglobin; SBP: Systolic Blood Pressure; LDLc: Low Density Lipoprotein Cholesterol; Sp: Specialist centre; Pri: Primary health care

*Notes*: * Micro-vascular: Includes micro-vascular diabetes complications (retinopathy, nephropathy, neuropathy and diabetes foot complications)
Macro-vascular: Includes cardiovascular diseases (coronary artery diseases, myocardial infarction, angina), cerebro-vascular diseases (stroke and transient ischemic attacks) and peripheral vascular diseases
+: <10% of population has ≥ 1of the complications
++: 10–25% of population has ≥ 1of the complications
+++: >25% of population has at least ≥ 1 of the complications
** Values are provided either mean±SD or just mean unless specified in the box
*** Values are in percentage unless specified
[a] Excluded patient with known macroalbuminuria
[b] Only patients with onset of type 2 diabetes ≤18 years
[c] BMI cut off was defined based on the Cole *et al.* study [134]
[d] Comparison of two cross-sectional study Diab-Asia 1998 and 2003. 2003 values are reported here. 1998 values are reported in Chuang (2002) [102]
[e] Only Asia component of larger study presented

times more prevalent than in their European counterparts [46]. This may have to do with the duration of exposure to elevated glucose levels before diagnosis (i.e. longer period of being undiagnosed).

Diabetes is also known to be a leading cause of limb complications. Several multinational studies showed that diabetic neuropathy is very common in Asia, with prevalence estimates ranging from 27 to 32.6 per cent in different populations (see Table 30.3). Although low prevalence of peripheral vascular complications as well as low incidence of lower extremity amputations (lower extremity amputations rates: 0.6–0.9 per cent in multi-country studies [47, 48]) has been shown in the region, the total number of people with diabetes-related foot complications is relatively high in Asia due to the large population sizes.

Asia had the second highest number of deaths related to diabetes worldwide (1.16 million deaths in 2011) [12]. In terms of major causes of mortality among Asian people with diabetes, longitudinal studies with a median 5.4 years of follow-up from China, Japan, Korea and Southeast Asia show that diabetes is associated with 62 per cent higher all-cause mortality (95 per cent confidence intervals: 1.44, 1.83), 95 per cent higher fatal cardiovascular disease (95 per cent CI: 1.62, 2.35) and 48 per cent higher non-cardiovascular disease mortality (95 per cent CI: 1.26, 1.75) [42]. The major causes of mortality among Asian people with diabetes may be changing as prevalence of diabetes and patterns in quality of care have evolved over the last two decades [40].

## Risk factors of diabetes

Like other NCDs, diabetes is a multi-factorial condition where genetic and environmental influences combine to increase its risk. Different populations exhibit different combinations of risk factors and experience varying interactions between risk factors. To convey the epidemiology of diabetes in Asia more clearly, the discussion on risk factors will be divided into groups of risk factors that we have control over (modifiable) and those that we cannot change ('non-modifiable'). Better understanding of the prominent diabetes risk factors in Asia will help to design effective preventive strategies and therefore lessen the burdens of this disease.

### *Non-modifiable risk factors*

#### Age

Risk of diabetes increases with age due to concomitant increases in weight and physical inactivity leading to insulin resistance. However, young to middle-aged adults experience a disproportionate burden of diabetes in some Asian countries [49]. Factors such as childhood obesity and gestational diabetes may contribute to the increasing epidemic of young-onset diabetes (diagnosed < 35 years) [40]. In addition, the variety of mechanisms of the pathogenesis of diabetes may influence the age of onset – in a study across four countries (China, India, Japan, Singapore), the prevalence of IFG did not increase with age, however IGT prevalence did increase in the elderly [50].

#### Family history

Family history of diabetes is another strong, independent risk factor for diabetes, representing the culmination of genetic, environmental and behavioural impacts of previous generations and the early-life home environment [51]. Family history of two parents with diabetes has been associated with over an eight-fold increase in diabetes incidence compared to individuals with no family history of diabetes [52]. Family history may be more important than other risk factors such as age or body mass index (BMI) among Asian populations with a high propensity to develop diabetes [27].

### Genetic risk factors

Building upon research initially limited to European populations, Genome-Wide Association (GWA) studies in Asian populations have elucidated additional culprit genes associated with diabetes such as the potassium voltage-gated channel, KQT-like subfamily, member 1 (KCNQ1) [53, 54]. While genetic discoveries highlight the role of beta cell function in pathogenesis [53], the heterogeneity of discovered genes suggests that type 2 diabetes is a result of defects in different molecular pathways. A focused study on phenotypically homogenous subgroups of individuals may be a useful approach in unravelling the aetiology of the disease [55]. Approximately 14 per cent of the diabetes disease burden is explained by genes alone [56, 57] and, in general, variations in genes associated with type 2 diabetes are consistent and largely similar across race/ethnic populations.

## *Potentially modifiable risk factors*

### Adiposity and abdominal obesity

Excess adiposity (fat deposition in the body) promotes stress and inflammation within the body's cells and causes them to become insulin resistant, thereby increasing the risk of diabetes [58]. BMI is a common and easy-to-measure indicator of excess weight and obesity and is used to identify individuals at risk of diabetes and cardiovascular disease. The World Health Organization (WHO) examined ethnic variation in BMI and disease risk and concluded that Asians, in particular, have a greater percentage body fat for any given BMI level compared to other ethnic groups and that Asians are at a higher risk of cardio-metabolic diseases at lower BMI levels than the existing WHO cut-off points for being overweight ($\geq$ 25 kg/m$^2$) and obesity ($\geq$ 30 kg/m$^2$) [59]. As such, WHO recommends the following classification among Asian groups: 18.5–22.9 kg/m$^2$ for normal weight, 23.0–27.5 kg/m$^2$ for overweight and 27.5 kg/m$^2$ or higher for obesity [60].

Another important factor in how adiposity influences diabetes risk relates to where the body fat is deposited. Fat can be located beneath the skin (subcutaneous fat) or around internal organs (visceral fat). Fat concentrated around the abdominal organs (abdominal obesity), in particular, influences glucose metabolism and diabetes, independent of the overall obesity defined by BMI [61–64]. Metabolically active visceral adiposity in the abdominal cavity can lead to insulin resistance and increased glucose intolerance [65–67]. Asian groups exhibit a higher prevalence of abdominal obesity and stronger associations of abdominal obesity and diabetes compared to those of European descent [14, 40, 68]. However, heterogeneity exists among Asian groups, suggesting that across Asian populations, different forms of fat distribution may differentially impact the risk of diabetes [69].

### Diet and physical activity

Across Asia, there is great variation in quantity and quality of diets, cultural norms, food environments and food security which results in diverse differences of how strongly diets impact diabetes risk. Many parts of Asia are undergoing nutritional transitions associated with economic development, yet individual countries are at different stages of transition based on the country's levels of urbanization, policies, trade and culture [70]. It has been noted that higher consumption of animal fat, refined carbohydrates and sweeteners are associated with increased prevalence of chronic diseases [71–73]. Along with poorer diet quality, there have also been transitions toward less physically demanding occupations in China, India and elsewhere in Asia [72]. Cars are replacing bicycles as the primary mode of transportation as the rapid uptake of technologies in developing countries shifts occupations from agriculture to manufacturing and services [40, 74]. Decreased physical activity is associated with an increased diabetes risk due to the effects that lack of physical activity have on muscle and lipid metabolism (fatty acid-induced insulin resistance, reduced glucose uptake), independent of visceral fat [75].

### Migration and urbanization

Demographic and environmental features of migration and urbanization are important potentially modifiable risk factors for diabetes. Urbanization and internal rural to urban migration have led to decreased physical activity, increased proportion of high-energy foods in the diet, increased BMI and central adiposity and new alternative environmental impacts on health [76]. Like intra-country migration, studies of inter-country migration have also documented similar trends [77]. Japanese Americans living in Hawaii and Los Angeles exhibit a higher incidence of diabetes, increased insulin resistance, increased cholesterol and increased triglyceride levels as compared to the native Japanese living in Japan [78]. Japanese Americans appear to consume a significantly greater percentage of daily calories from animal protein and weigh more than their counterparts in Japan [31, 79]. Furthermore, the Chinese population in China have reported doing more vigorous activity, sleeping and walking more hours and sitting less hours than the Chinese population in North America [80]. More research is needed to understand the interaction of environments with heritable factors and how environments may be modified to improve metabolic profiles.

## Diabetes prevention

### *Evidence from efficacy trials*

Lifestyle intervention programmes seek to prevent diabetes by teaching participants about diet change, benefits of increased physical activity and/or weight loss. There is strong evidence from large, randomized trials that lifestyle intervention programmes can prevent, or at least delay, diabetes in high-risk populations (e.g. those with pre-diabetes). Lifestyle intervention trials done in Finland and the United States have shown benefits for diabetes risk reduction in higher-BMI populations. In Asia, three such trials were conducted, specifically in China, India and Japan.

The first trial testing the effectiveness of lifestyle programmes for diabetes prevention was the Da Qing IGT and Diabetes Study in China [81]. Thirty-three clinics (with a total of 577 participants) were randomized to provide one-on-one, physician-led training to people with IGT on one of the following: adopting a low-fat diet rich in vegetables, with reductions in simple sugar and alcohol; increasing physical activity; improving diet and increasing physical activity; or no active intervention (control arm). After six years of follow-up, compared to participants in the control arm, individuals in each of the three lifestyle groups exhibited significant relative risk reductions in diabetes incidence: 31 per cent in the diet group, 42 per cent in the exercise group and 42 per cent in the diet and exercise group [81]. The results were similar in all participants, regardless of baseline weight. The positive effects of the lifestyle interventions were long-lasting, albeit attenuated. After 20 years of follow-up, the cumulative incidence of diabetes was 43 per cent lower in the intervention group (all lifestyle education groups combined) compared to the control group and, adjusting for clinic and age, intervention participants had an average of 3.6 more diabetes-free years compared to those in the control arm [82].

The Indian Diabetes Prevention Programme (IDPP) randomized 531 Asian Indian adults with IGT to receive either: standard lifestyle advice; lifestyle education; metformin, a glucose lowering drug prescribed at 250 mg twice daily; or lifestyle education plus metformin [34]. Participants receiving lifestyle education were advised to exercise at least 30 minutes per day and follow a healthier diet by reducing total calories, fat and refined carbohydrates and increasing fibre consumption. Compared to the control arm, there were significant reductions in diabetes incidence in the lifestyle arm, metformin arm and lifestyle plus metformin arm of 28.5 per cent, 28.2 per cent and 26.4 per cent, respectively, at the end of a three-year follow-up period. There was no significant loss of weight or waist circumference in any of the study arms. Further analysis showed that the IDPP lifestyle intervention programme was cost-effective for diabetes prevention in India [83].

In Japan, 458 men with IGT were randomized to receive either a standard lifestyle intervention or a more intensive lifestyle education programme, with both programmes advising participants to improve their diets and increase physical activity [84]. Participants in the intensive lifestyle programme were told to work towards a goal BMI of 22 $kg/m^2$, while participants in the standard lifestyle arm were asked to maintain a BMI of 24 $kg/m^2$ or less. The four-year cumulative incidence of diabetes was 3 per cent for participants in the intensive lifestyle arm compared to 9.3 per cent among participants in the standard lifestyle arm, a 67.5 per cent relative risk reduction [84].

### *Evidence from translational research*

Translational research seeks to bridge the gap between efficacy trials and the delivery of interventions in real-life communities by identifying models of delivery and testing their effectiveness, acceptability and sustainability [85]. In Asia, the Japan Diabetes Prevention Program tested delivering lifestyle education to patients with IGT through existing clinic resources and found significant decreases in BMI and body weight, as well as increases in insulin sensitivity. Intervention participants also had a non-significant 53 per cent relative risk reduction in diabetes incidence compared to the control group [86]. In India, the Diabetes Community Lifestyle Improvement Program (D-CLIP) is a randomized, controlled translation study testing a step-wise intervention: a culturally tailored lifestyle curriculum (based on the US DPP) [87], as well as metformin for participants whose blood glucose remained persistently elevated after four months [88]. This study incorporates cost-effectiveness and qualitative assessments to measure programme sustainability and acceptability.

## Diabetes control

Evidence has shown that managing glucose and other CVD risk factors and regular preventive screenings are beneficial for delaying the onset or impacts of the debilitating complications (eye, renal, cardiovascular and neurological) associated with diabetes [89–91]. Evaluating the extent to which people with diabetes are able to manage their condition and delay disease progression can be accomplished at the clinical level where data from those accessing the care is audited. Though population data from surveys tend to be more representative, the data can only be used to evaluate patients with known diabetes. For patients with as-yet undiagnosed diabetes, surveys stimulate detection and appropriate referral for therapy, but evaluating these patients does not provide an accurate or appropriate impression of control.

Both process and outcome variables are now widely accepted as appropriate indicators of diabetes management [91–93]. However, not all indicators are widely available in patient record systems, registries or even through surveys. The recommended indicators for assessing the quality of diabetes management and its comparison across international health systems are summarized in Table 30.4 [93]. Also, based on evidence, clinical guidelines are developed and put into practice, which provide the thresholds/targets that serve as benchmarks for evaluation.

## *Current status of quality of diabetes care in Asia*

In Asia, the published literature reporting on achievements of diabetes care processes is limited to the International Diabetes Management Practice Study (IDMPS) that uses standardized methods across sites [94]. This study surveyed diabetes patients attending specialist clinics in 17 countries (of which eight were Asian countries) and found that 36 per cent of diabetes patients in Asia had no glycosylated haemoglobin (HbA1c; a measure of glucose control over three to six months) test, 13 per cent were not tested for lipids, 26 per cent were not screened for microalbuminuria and 26 per cent had not had retinal examinations. Also audit reports from individual clinics in the region expounded similar statistics: just 20

*Table 30.4* Diabetes quality of care measures proposed for use in health system comparisons

| *Area* | *Indicator name* | *ADA recommendations* |
|---|---|---|
| Processes of diabetes care | Annual glycosylated haemoglobin ($HbA_1c$) testing | 2–4 times annually |
| | Annual LDL cholesterol (LDLc) testing | At least once annually |
| | Annual blood pressure testing | Annually and at routine visits |
| | Annual screening for nephropathy | At least once annually |
| | Annual eye examination | At least once annually |
| Proximal outcomes | $HbA_1c$ control | ≤ 7.0% individualize based on patient profile |
| | LDL cholesterol control | <2.6 mmol/l (100mg/dl); <1.8mmol/l (70 mg/dl) if overt CVD |
| | BP control | 130/80 mmHg (sitting) |
| Distal outcomes | Kidney disease in persons with diabetes | |
| | Cardiovascular mortality in patients with diabetes | |
| | Lower-extremity amputation rates | |

*Source*: Adopted from Nicolucci *et al.* [93] and the American Diabetes Association Standards of Care, 2012 [91].

per cent to 50 per cent of patients in diabetes clinics had ≥ 1 annual test for HbA1c [95–97]. The frequency of blood lipid testing was relatively better, with 57 per cent of patients with diabetes reporting annual testing [95–98]. Dilated eye examination was uncommon in most reports and as low as 5 per cent in Sri Lankan clinics [99–101]. More than 50 per cent of patients reported receiving annual urinary protein examination, though their test results were not reported clearly.

The DiabCare-Asia study is a multi-country survey of diabetes clinics and was conducted in two waves – 1998 [102] and 2003 [48] (see Table 30.3). Glycemic control was similar at the two survey time-points, implying little or no improvements in diabetes care over time. Later, the IDMPS study [94] reported better levels of glycemic control across eight countries in Asia. However, since the sample populations and methods of assessment differ, these data do not necessarily imply actual improvements in diabetes care. Most clinic-based studies reported higher mean HbA1c's in the region (8–11 per cent) and this was irrespective of the clinic type (primary or specialist) or patient demographic characteristics [95, 99, 103–112]. Though a few studies reported mean HbA1c of 7.4 per cent [98, 113, 114], none reported mean values below the target control of ≤ 7 per cent.

Though Low Density Lipoprotein cholesterol (LDLc) was not measured in the DiabCare-Asia study (see Table 30.3), other multinational studies in Asia reported a mean LDLc of 142 mg/dl among people with diabetes in 2001 [47] and found that one-third of patients with diabetes had LDLc less than the target value of 100 mg/dl [94]. Mean LDLc values varied between 120 and 150 mg/dl [95, 103, 104, 111, 114–116] and studies from Thailand [98] and Malaysia [117] reported mean LDLc < 100mg/dl among people with diabetes. Only a quarter of the diabetes population achieved American Diabetes Association (ADA) recommended targets for blood pressure control (< 130 mmHg for systolic blood pressure and < 80 mm Hg for diastolic blood pressure) [93] and mean systolic blood pressure varied between 130 and 140 mm Hg [48, 118, 119] in these populations.

In summary, data from multiple countries provide a sense of generalization in terms of their themes (especially where standardized tools have been used). The current evidence on quality of diabetes care in Asia is inadequate to inform policy decisions and interventions. Nationally representative data are available from only four countries in the region: China [120], Malaysia (public and private clinics) [75, 105], the Philippines [106] and Thailand (national diabetes registry involving eleven hospitals and medical colleges) [121]. This limited available data show that glycemic and other CVD risk factors control are poorly achieved for people with diabetes in the region.

A large proportion of the world's diabetes patients live in India and China [40]. As such, there is a great need for monitoring the quality of care provided for individuals with diabetes and an increasing accountability among providers and patients. Registries, audits and population assessments that use standardized tools and targets will be beneficial in evaluating the effects of quality improvement programmes.

## Challenges and future directions

Chronic NCDs, especially diabetes, impose huge health and economic burdens in Asia. In this chapter, we have provided an overview of the spectrum of issues related to diabetes, from its key risk factors and trends to policy-level interventions aimed at minimizing the effects of the growth in diabetes. To conclude, below is a summary of the major challenges related to diabetes in Asia, as well as some recommendations.

*Table 30.5* Economic development and health expenditure among some countries in Asia during the past decade

| *Country* | *Total population, millions (2011 estimate)* | *% of urban (2010)* | *Cumulative GDP growth from 2000–2010 (%)* | *Health expenditure (% of government expenditure) 2000* | *Health expenditure (% of government expenditure) 2010* |
|---|---|---|---|---|---|
| ***Asia-Pacific high income*** | | | | | |
| Japan | 127 | 67 | 157.2 | 16 | 18.4 |
| Singapore | 5 | 100 | 252.5 | 6.21 | 8.02 |
| ***East Asia*** | | | | | |
| China | 1,343 | 47 | 3676.6 | 11.5 | 12.07 |
| Hong Kong | 7 | 100 | 239.8 | Not reported | Not reported |
| ***South Asia*** | | | | | |
| Bangladesh | 161 | 28 | 239.8 | 7.56 | 7.36 |
| India | 1,205 | 30 | 390.1 | 3.93 | 3.56 |
| Nepal | 29 | 19 | 420.2 | 7.74 | 7.92 |
| Pakistan | 190 | 36 | 289.3 | 2.35 | 3.63 |
| ***Southeast Asia*** | | | | | |
| Philippines | 103 | 49 | | 7.02 | 7.55 |
| Malaysia | 29 | 72 | 300.3 | 6.23 | 9.21 |
| Indonesia | 248 | 44 | 526.6 | 4.53 | 7.75 |
| Sri Lanka | 21 | 14 | 385.9 | 6.88 | 5.77 |
| Thailand | 67 | 34 | 283.9 | 9.95 | 12.7 |

*Source*: Google Public Data 2010.

1 *Data that are critical for informing appropriate healthcare planning and response strategies are lacking in most Asian countries.* Planning and investing in surveillance systems for chronic diseases may have important benefits for the region. In particular, regular and representative population-based data that are comparable across different countries of the region are useful in monitoring trends, evaluating prevention and control efforts and identifying residual gaps.

2 *Most Asian countries have large rural populations, which are sometimes larger than their urban populations* (see Table 30.5). However, population-based research on diabetes tends to be localized in major urban areas in Asia. Therefore, there is a lack of high-quality data regarding rural diabetes. A recent systematic review suggested a five-fold increase in rural diabetes prevalence in low- and middle-income countries (LMICs) over the past two decades [122]. Surveillance data in such regions will help to actually monitor trends, design and implement appropriate preventive and control responses and will also aid in monitoring the impacts of interventions. In addition, evaluating the quality of care among diabetes patients would increase the level of accountability among care providers and help to establish a culture of auditing.

3 *Diabetes and its related outcomes are preventable with appropriate interventions.* However, there is a spectrum of risk and a high proportion of people with undiagnosed diabetes and pre-diabetes. Therefore, any efforts to address diabetes should be comprehensive and consist of: programmes aimed at increasing awareness, early detection guidelines and programmes,

referrals for lifestyle modification or effective diabetes management, appropriate human resources and infrastructure, adequate access and financing mechanisms and empowered, motivated end-users (i.e. those affected). Weaving these components into systems that reinforce positive preventive and care behaviours will help to increase the efficiency and effectiveness of such programmes.

4 *Lifestyle and self-management behaviours are complex and are influenced by a menagerie of factors including culture, religion, community views and norms, availability of food and accessibility of safe, suitable locations for physical activity.* Asia is a large, multicultural region, so intervention programmes need to be context- and culture-specific. Furthermore, diabetes programmes in Asia should address the unique risk profile of Asian populations (diabetes onset at younger ages and lower BMIs), the ongoing nutritional transitions and changes in activity patterns, and must be cost-effective and designed with sustainable financing mechanisms in mind.

5 *Despite major economic developments across Asia and gross domestic product (GDP) growth, social concerns have not been given comparable attention by governments, as evidenced by the very modest increases in resource allocation to the health sector.* The inadequacy of government-funded healthcare facilities prompts large proportions of Asia's populations to opt for out-of-pocket payments for health services which deplete household incomes, resulting in significant opportunity costs (e.g. diverting resources from children's education opportunities), widening of health disparities and increasing the risk of catastrophic health expenditures. Though there will be a lag in experiencing the economic effects of diabetes in the region (lower productivity and increased premature mortality among the economically active), advocacy that conveys the projected economic costs of chronic diseases may stimulate decision-makers to consider placing greater emphasis on social development, particularly health and education.

6 *Historically, health systems in most LMICs have been designed to respond to acute health conditions.* Going forward, integrating services to incorporate chronic disease care may offer efficient care delivery models but will require the redesigning of systems, the generation of capacity (health care and administrative) and evidence of sustainability (cost-effectiveness and acceptability) [123]. With this growth in systems, a parallel focus on developing research capacity, especially in health services, will develop a culture of evaluation, evidence-based decision-making and auditing. As the sophistication of methods evolves, countries in Asia may benefit from large-scale policy and programme evaluations and identify the highest return on investments in terms of health gains and reduction in health disparities. Compelling evidence is helpful in securing political will and increases the likelihood of success of prevention and control strategies.

## References


1. Mathers C. D., Lopez A. D., Murray C. J. L. The Burden of Disease and Mortality by Condition: Data, Methods, and Results for 2001. In: Lopez AD, Mathers CD, Ezzati M, Jamison DT, Murray CJL, editors. *Global Burden of Disease and Risk Factors*. New York: Oxford University Press; 2006.
2. International Diabetes Federation. The human, social and economic impact of diabetes. Brussels 2007 [February 2008]; Available from: http://www.idf.org/home/index.cfm?node=41
3. Economic Intelligence Unit. The silent epidemic: An economic study of diabetes in developed and developing countries. New York, London, Hong Kong: *The Economist* June 2007.
4. Aschner Pablo. Diabetes trends in Latin America. *Diabetes/Metabolism Research and Reviews*. 2002; 18(S3): S27–S31.
5. Chaturvedi N. The burden of diabetes and its complications: trends and implications for intervention. *Diabetes Res Clin Pract*. 2007; 76(Suppl 1): S3–S12.

6. Danaei G., Lawes C. M., Vander Hoorn S., Murray C. J., Ezzati M. Global and regional mortality from ischaemic heart disease and stroke attributable to higher-than-optimum blood glucose concentration: comparative risk assessment. *Lancet*. 2006; 368(9548): 1651–9.
7. Ordovas J. M., Shen J. Gene–environment interactions and susceptibility to metabolic syndrome and other chronic diseases. *Journal of Periodontology*. 2008; 79(8 Suppl): 1508–13.
8. Narayan K. M. Venkat, Gregg Edward W., Fagot-Campagna Anne, Engelgau Michael M., Vinicor Frank. Diabetes – a common, growing, serious, costly, and potentially preventable public health problem. *Diabetes Research and Clinical Practice*. 2000; 50(Supplement 2): S77–S84.
9. Gregg Edward W., Brown Arleen M. Cognitive and physical disabilities and aging-related complications of diabetes. *Clinical Diabetes*. 2003, 21: 113–18.
10. Morgan C. L., Currie C. J., Peters J. R. Relationship between diabetes and mortality: a population study using record linkage. *Diabetes Care*. 2000; 23(8): 1103–7.
11. Franco Oscar H., Steyerberg Ewout W., Hu Frank B., Mackenbach Johan, Nusselder Wilma. Associations of diabetes mellitus with total life expectancy and life expectancy with and without cardiovascular disease. *Arch Intern Med*. 2007; 167(11): 1145–51.
12. International Diabetes Federation 2011. *The Diabetes Atlas*. Brussels, Belgium: Int. Diabetes Fed. 5th ed. Available from: http://www.idf.org/diabetesatlas/ [database on the Internet].
13. Monteiro C. A., Moura E. C., Conde W. L., Popkin B. M. Socioeconomic status and obesity in adult populations of developing countries: a review. *Bulletin of the World Health Organization*. 2004; 82(12): 940–6.
14. Ramachandran A., Ma R. C., Snehalatha C. Diabetes in Asia. *Lancet*. 2010; 375(9712): 408–18.
15. Chinese Academy of Social Sciences; Indian National Science Academy; Indonesian Academy of Sciences; National Research Council of the U.S. National Academies; Science Council of Japan. *Preparing for the Challenges of Population Aging in Asia: Strengthening the Scientific Basis of Policy Development*. Washington (DC): The National Academies Collection: Reports funded by National Institutes of Health; 2011.
16. Anjana R. M., Pradeepa R., Deepa M., Datta M., Sudha V., Unnikrishnan R., *et al*. Prevalence of diabetes and prediabetes (impaired fasting glucose and/or impaired glucose tolerance) in urban and rural India: phase I results of the Indian Council of Medical Research-INdia DIABetes (ICMR-INDIAB) study. *Diabetologia*. 2011; 54(12): 3022–7.
17. Yang W., Lu J., Weng J., Jia W., Ji L., Xiao J., *et al*. Prevalence of diabetes among men and women in China. *New England Journal of Medicine*. 2010; 362(12): 1090–101.
18. Cockram C. S. The epidemiology of diabetes mellitus in the Asia-Pacific region. *Hong Kong Medical Journal* = Xianggang yi xue za zhi / Hong Kong Academy of Medicine. 2000; 6(1): 43–52.
19. Akazawa Y. Prevalence and incidence of diabetes mellitus by WHO criteria. *Diabetes Res Clin Pract*. 1994; 24(Suppl): S23–S7.
20. Shera A. S., Jawad F., Maqsood A. Prevalence of diabetes in Pakistan. *Diabetes Res Clin Pract*. 2007; 76(2): 219–22.
21. Katulanda P., Constantine G. R., Mahesh J. G., Sheriff R., Seneviratne R. D., Wijeratne S., *et al*. Prevalence and projections of diabetes and pre-diabetes in adults in Sri Lanka – Sri Lanka Diabetes, Cardiovascular Study (SLDCS). *Diabetic Medicine: A Journal of the British Diabetic Association*. 2008; 25(9): 1062–9.
22. Quoc P. S., Charles M. A., Cuong N. H., Lieu L. H., Tuan N. A., Thomas M., *et al*. Blood glucose distribution and prevalence of diabetes in Hanoi (Vietnam). *American Journal of Epidemiology*. 1994; 139(7): 713–22.
23. Duc Son L. N., Kusama K., Hung N. T., Loan T. T., Chuyen N. V., Kunii D., *et al*. Prevalence and risk factors for diabetes in Ho Chi Minh City, Vietnam. *Diabetic Medicine: A Journal of the British Diabetic Association*. 2004; 21(4): 371–6.
24. Sutanegara D., Budhiarta A. A. The epidemiology and management of diabetes mellitus in Indonesia. *Diabetes Res Clin Pract*. 2000; 50(Suppl 2): S9–S16.
25. Mihardja L., Delima, Manz H. S., Ghani L., Soegondo S. Prevalence and determinants of diabetes mellitus and impaired glucose tolerance in Indonesia (a part of basic health research/Riskesdas). *Acta Medica Indonesiana*. 2009; 41(4): 169–74.
26. Danaei G., Finucane M. M., Lu Y., Singh G. M., Cowan M. J., Paciorek C. J., *et al*. National, regional, and global trends in fasting plasma glucose and diabetes prevalence since 1980: systematic analysis of health examination surveys and epidemiological studies with 370 country-years and 2.7 million participants. *Lancet*. 2011; 378(9785): 31–40.

27. Jayawardena R., Ranasinghe P., Byrne N. M., Soares M. J., Katulanda P., Hills A. P. Prevalence and trends of the diabetes epidemic in South Asia: a systematic review and meta-analysis. *BMC Public Health*. 2012; 12(1): 380.
28. Ohmura T., Ueda K., Kiyohara Y., Kato I., Iwamoto H., Nakayama K., *et al.* Prevalence of type 2 (non-insulin-dependent) diabetes mellitus and impaired glucose tolerance in the Japanese general population: the Hisayama Study. *Diabetologia*. 1993; 36(11): 1198–203.
29. Sekikawa A., Eguchi H., Tominaga M., Igarashi K., Abe T., Manaka H., *et al.* Prevalence of type 2 diabetes mellitus and impaired glucose tolerance in a rural area of Japan. The Funagata diabetes study. *Journal of Diabetes and its Complications*. 2000; 14(2): 78–83.
30. Kitazawa Y., Murakami K., Goto Y., Hamazaki S. Prevalence of diabetes mellitus detected by 75 g GTT in Tokyo. *Tohoku Journal of Experimental Medicine*. 1983; 141(Suppl): 229–34.
31. Weber M. B., Oza-Frank R., Staimez L. R., Ali M. K., Narayan K. M. Type 2 diabetes in Asians: prevalence, risk factors, and effectiveness of behavioral intervention at individual and population levels. *Annual Review of Nutrition*. 2012; 32: 417–39.
32. Nyamdorj R., Pitkaniemi J., Tuomilehto J., Hammar N., Stehouwer C. D., Lam T. H., *et al.* Ethnic comparison of the association of undiagnosed diabetes with obesity. *Int J Obes (Lond)*. 2010; 34(2): 332–9.
33. Wong K. C., Wang Z. Prevalence of type 2 diabetes mellitus of Chinese populations in Mainland China, Hong Kong, and Taiwan. *Diabetes Research and Clinical Practice*. 2006; 73(2): 126–34.
34. Ramachandran A., Snehalatha C., Mary S., Mukesh B., Bhaskar A. D., Vijay V. The Indian Diabetes Prevention Programme shows that lifestyle modification and metformin prevent type 2 diabetes in Asian Indian subjects with impaired glucose tolerance (IDPP-1). *Diabetologia*. 2006; 49(2): 289–97.
35. Brown T. T., Cole S. R., Li X., Kingsley L. A., Palella F. J., Riddler S. A., *et al.* Antiretroviral therapy and the prevalence and incidence of diabetes mellitus in the multicenter AIDS cohort study. *Archives of Internal Medicine*. 2005; 165(10): 1179–84.
36. Basit A., Hydrie M. Z., Ahmed K., Hakeem R. Prevalence of diabetes, impaired fasting glucose and associated risk factors in a rural area of Baluchistan province according to new ADA criteria. *JPMA Journal of the Pakistan Medical Association*. 2002; 52(8): 357–60.
37. Menon V. U., Kumar K. V., Gilchrist A., Sugathan T. N., Sundaram K. R., Nair V., *et al.* Prevalence of known and undetected diabetes and associated risk factors in central Kerala – ADEPS. *Diabetes Research and Clinical Practice*. 2006; 74(3): 289–94.
38. Chowdhury T. A., Lasker S. S. Complications and cardiovascular risk factors in South Asians and Europeans with early-onset type 2 diabetes. *QJM*: monthly journal of the Association of Physicians. 2002; 95(4): 241–6.
39. Parving H. H., Lewis J. B., Ravid M., Remuzzi G., Hunsicker L. G. Prevalence and risk factors for microalbuminuria in a referred cohort of type II diabetic patients: a global perspective. *Kidney International*. 2006; 69(11): 2057–63.
40. Chan J. C., Malik V., Jia W., Kadowaki T., Yajnik C. S., Yoon K. H., *et al.* Diabetes in Asia: epidemiology, risk factors, and pathophysiology. *JAMA*. 2009; 301(20): 2129–40.
41. Joshi P., Islam S., Pais P., Reddy S., Dorairaj P., Kazmi K., *et al.* Risk factors for early myocardial infarction in South Asians compared with individuals in other countries. *JAMA*. 2007; 297(3): 286–94.
42. Woodward M., Zhang X., Barzi F., Pan W., Ueshima H., Rodgers A., *et al.* The effects of diabetes on the risks of major cardiovascular diseases and death in the Asia-Pacific region. *Diabetes Care*. 2003; 26(2): 360–6.
43. Luk A. O., So W. Y., Ma R. C., Kong A. P., Ozaki R., Ng V. S., *et al.* Metabolic syndrome predicts new onset of chronic kidney disease in 5,829 patients with type 2 diabetes: a 5-year prospective analysis of the Hong Kong Diabetes Registry. *Diabetes Care*. 2008; 31(12): 2357–61.
44. Liu W. J., Hooi L. S. Patients with end stage renal disease: a registry at Sultanah Aminah Hospital, Johor Bahru, Malaysia. *Medical Journal of Malaysia*. 2007; 62(3): 197–200.
45. Yoon K. H., Lee J. H., Kim J. W., Cho J. H., Choi Y. H., Ko S. H., *et al.* Epidemic obesity and type 2 diabetes in Asia. *Lancet*. 2006; 368(9548): 1681–8.
46. Raymond N. T., Varadhan L., Reynold D. R., Bush K., Sankaranarayanan S., Bellary S., *et al.* Higher prevalence of retinopathy in diabetic patients of South Asian ethnicity compared with white Europeans in the community: a cross-sectional study. *Diabetes Care*. 2009; 32(3): 410–15.

47. Chuang L. M., Soegondo S., Soewondo P., Young-Seol K., Mohamed M., Dalisay E., *et al.* Comparisons of the outcomes on control, type of management and complications status in early onset and late onset type 2 diabetes in Asia. *Diabetes Res Clin Pract.* 2006; 71(2): 146–55.
48. Mohamed M. An audit on diabetes management in Asian patients treated by specialists: the DiabCare-Asia 1998 and 2003 studies. *Curr Med Res Opin.* 2008; 24(2): 507–14.
49. Chan J. C., Chan S. P., Deerochanawong C., Go R. T., Lee K. O., Ma R. C., *et al.* Diabetic dyslipidaemia in Asian populations in the Western Pacific Region: what we know and don't know. *Diabetes Research and Clinical Practice.* 2011; 94(1): 1–13.
50. Qiao Q., Hu G., Tuomilehto J., Nakagami T., Balkau B., Borch-Johnsen K., *et al.* Age- and sex-specific prevalence of diabetes and impaired glucose regulation in 11 Asian cohorts. *Diabetes Care.* 2003; 26(6): 1770–80.
51. Annis A. M., Caulder M. S., Cook M. L., Duquette D. Family history, diabetes, and other demographic and risk factors among participants of the National Health and Nutrition Examination Survey 1999–2002. *Preventing Chronic Disease.* 2005; 2(2): A19.
52. Goldfine A. B., Bouche C., Parker R. A., Kim C., Kerivan A., Soeldner J. S., *et al.* Insulin resistance is a poor predictor of type 2 diabetes in individuals with no family history of disease. *Proceedings of the National Academy of Sciences of the United States of America.* 2003; 100(5): 2724–9.
53. Elbein S. C. Genetics factors contributing to type 2 diabetes across ethnicities. *Journal of Diabetes Science and Technology.* 2009; 3(4): 685–9.
54. Gibson Greg. *It Takes a Genome: How a Clash Between Our Genes and Modern Life Is Making Us Sick.* Upper Saddle River, NJ: FT Press Science. 2009.
55. O'Rahilly S., Barroso I., Wareham N. J. Genetic factors in type 2 diabetes: the end of the beginning? *Science.* 2005; 307(5708): 370–3.
56. Chung J. O., Cho D. H., Chung D. J., Chung M. Y. Plasma C-peptide level is inversely associated with family history of type 2 diabetes in Korean type 2 diabetic patients. *Endocrine Journal.* 2010; 57(10): 931–8.
57. Stolerman E. S., Florez J. C. Genomics of type 2 diabetes mellitus: implications for the clinician. *Nature Reviews Endocrinology.* 2009; 5(8): 429–36.
58. Samuel V. T., Petersen K. F., Shulman G. I. Lipid-induced insulin resistance: unravelling the mechanism. *Lancet.* 2010; 375(9733): 2267–77.
59. Amati F., Dube J. J., Coen P. M., Stefanovic-Racic M., Toledo F. G., Goodpaster B. H. Physical inactivity and obesity underlie the insulin resistance of aging. *Diabetes Care.* 2009; 32(8): 1547–9.
60. World Health Organization. Appropriate body-mass index for Asian populations and its implications for policy and intervention strategies. *Lancet.* 2004; 363(9403): 157–63.
61. Report of the expert committee on the diagnosis and classification of diabetes mellitus. *Diabetes Care.* 2003; 26(Suppl 1): S5–S20.
62. Balkau B., Deanfield J. E., Despres J. P., Bassand J. P., Fox K. A., Smith S. C., Jr., *et al.* International Day for the Evaluation of Abdominal Obesity (IDEA): a study of waist circumference, cardiovascular disease, and diabetes mellitus in 168,000 primary care patients in 63 countries. *Circulation.* 2007; 116(17): 1942–51.
63. Boffetta P., McLerran D., Chen Y., Inoue M., Sinha R., He J., *et al.* Body mass index and diabetes in Asia: a cross-sectional pooled analysis of 900,000 individuals in the Asia cohort consortium. *PLoS One.* 2011; 6(6): e19930.
64. Kissebah A. H., Vydelingum N., Murray R., Evans D. J., Hartz A. J., Kalkhoff R. K., *et al.* Relation of body fat distribution to metabolic complications of obesity. *Journal of Clinical Endocrinology and Metabolism.* 1982; 54(2): 254–60.
65. Boyko E. J., Fujimoto W. Y., Leonetti D. L., Newell-Morris L. Visceral adiposity and risk of type 2 diabetes: a prospective study among Japanese Americans. *Diabetes Care.* 2000; 23(4): 465–71.
66. Indulekha K., Anjana R. M., Surendar J., Mohan V. Association of visceral and subcutaneous fat with glucose intolerance, insulin resistance, adipocytokines and inflammatory markers in Asian Indians (CURES-113). *Clinical Biochemistry.* 2011; 44(4): 281–7.
67. Montague C. T., O'Rahilly S. The perils of portliness: causes and consequences of visceral adiposity. *Diabetes.* 2000; 49(6): 883–8.
68. Shah A., Hernandez A., Mathur D., Budoff M. J., Kanaya A. M. Adipokines and body fat composition in South Asians: results of the Metabolic Syndrome and Atherosclerosis in South Asians Living in America (MASALA) study. *Int J Obes (Lond).* 2012; 36(6): 810–16.

69. Gao H., Salim A., Lee J., Tai E. S., van Dam R. M. Can body fat distribution, adiponectin levels and inflammation explain differences in insulin resistance between ethnic Chinese, Malays and Asian Indians? *Int J Obes (Lond).* 2012; 36(8): 1086–93.
70. Cuong T. Q., Dibley M. J., Bowe S., Hanh T. T., Loan T. T. Obesity in adults: an emerging problem in urban areas of Ho Chi Minh City, Vietnam. *European Journal of Clinical Nutrition.* 2007; 61(5): 673–81.
71. Misra A., Sharma R., Gulati S., Joshi S. R., Sharma V., Ghafoorunissa, *et al.* Consensus dietary guidelines for healthy living and prevention of obesity, the metabolic syndrome, diabetes, and related disorders in Asian Indians. *Diabetes Technology & Therapeutics.* 2011; 13(6): 683–94.
72. Hu F. B. Globalization of diabetes: the role of diet, lifestyle, and genes. *Diabetes Care.* 2011; 34(6): 1249–57.
73. Vessby B., Uusitupa M., Hermansen K., Riccardi G., Rivellese A. A., Tapsell L. C., *et al.* Substituting dietary saturated for monounsaturated fat impairs insulin sensitivity in healthy men and women: The KANWU Study. *Diabetologia.* 2001; 44(3): 312–19.
74. Mafauzy M. Diabetes control and complications in public hospitals in Malaysia. *Medical Journal of Malaysia.* 2006; 61(4): 477–83.
75. Zierath J. R., Krook A., Wallberg-Henriksson H. Insulin action and insulin resistance in human skeletal muscle. *Diabetologia.* 2000; 43(7): 821–35.
76. Ramachandran A., Snehalatha C., Shetty A. S., Nanditha A. Trends in prevalence of diabetes in Asian countries. *World Journal of Diabetes.* 2012; 3(6): 110–17.
77. Misra A., Ganda O. P. Migration and its impact on adiposity and type 2 diabetes. *Nutrition.* 2007; 23(9): 696–708.
78. Nakanishi S., Okubo M., Yoneda M., Jitsuiki K., Yamane K., Kohno N. A comparison between Japanese-Americans living in Hawaii and Los Angeles and native Japanese: the impact of lifestyle westernization on diabetes mellitus. *Biomedicine & Pharmacotherapy.* 2004; 58(10): 571–7.
79. Fujimoto W. Y., Hershon K., Kinyoun J., Stolov W., Weinberg C., Ishiwata K., *et al.* Type II diabetes mellitus in Seattle and Tokyo. *Tohoku Journal of Experimental Medicine.* 1983; 141(Suppl): 133–9.
80. Lee M. M., Wu-Williams A., Whittemore A. S., Zheng S., Gallagher R., Teh C. Z., *et al.* Comparison of dietary habits, physical activity and body size among Chinese in North America and China. *International Journal of Epidemiology.* 1994; 23(5): 984–90.
81. Pan X. R., Li G. W., Hu Y. H., Wang J. X., Yang W. Y., An Z. X., *et al.* Effects of diet and exercise in preventing NIDDM in people with impaired glucose tolerance. The Da Qing IGT and Diabetes Study. *Diabetes Care.* 1997; 20(4): 537–44.
82. Li G., Zhang P., Wang J., Gregg E. W., Yang W., Gong Q., *et al.* The long-term effect of lifestyle interventions to prevent diabetes in the China Da Qing Diabetes Prevention Study: a 20-year follow-up study. *Lancet.* 2008; 371(9626): 1783–9.
83. Ramachandran A., Snehalatha C., Yamuna A., Mary S., Ping Z. Cost-effectiveness of the interventions in the primary prevention of diabetes among Asian Indians: within-trial results of the Indian Diabetes Prevention Programme (IDPP). *Diabetes Care.* 2007; 30(10): 2548–52.
84. Kosaka K., Noda M., Kuzuya T. Prevention of type 2 diabetes by lifestyle intervention: a Japanese trial in IGT males. *Diabetes Res Clin Pract.* 2005; 67(2): 152–62.
85. Ogilvie D., Craig P., Griffin S., Macintyre S., Wareham N. J. A translational framework for public health research. *BMC Public Health.* 2009; 9: 116.
86. Sakane N., Sato J., Tsushita K., Tsujii S., Kotani K., Tsuzaki K., *et al.* Prevention of type 2 diabetes in a primary healthcare setting: three-year results of lifestyle intervention in Japanese subjects with impaired glucose tolerance. *BMC Public Health.* 2011; 11(1): 40.
87. Knowler W. C., Barrett-Connor E., Fowler S. E., Hamman R. F., Lachin J. M., Walker E. A., *et al.* Reduction in the incidence of type 2 diabetes with lifestyle intervention or metformin. *N Engl J Med.* 2002; 346(6): 393–403.
88. Weber M. B., Ranjani H., Meyers G. C., Mohan V., Narayan K. M. A model of translational research for diabetes prevention in low- and middle-income countries: The Diabetes Community Lifestyle Improvement Program (D-CLIP) trial. *Primary Care Diabetes.* 2012; 6(1): 3–9.
89. Collins R., Armitage J., Parish S., Sleigh P., Peto R. MRC/BHF Heart Protection Study of cholesterol-lowering with simvastatin in 5963 people with diabetes: a randomised placebo-controlled trial. *Lancet.* 2003; 361(9374): 2005–16.
90. Chalmers J., Joshi R., Patel A. Advances in reducing the burden of vascular disease in type 2 diabetes. *Clin Exp Pharmacol Physiol.* 2008; 35(4): 434–7.

91. Standards of Medical Care in Diabetes – 2010. *Diabetes Care*. 2010; 33(Suppl 1): S11–S61.
92. Fleming B. B., Greenfield S., Engelgau M. M., Pogach L. M., Clauser S. B., Parrott M. A. The Diabetes Quality Improvement Project: moving science into health policy to gain an edge on the diabetes epidemic. *Diabetes Care*. 2001; 24(10): 1815–20.
93. Nicolucci A., Greenfield S., Mattke S. Selecting indicators for the quality of diabetes care at the health systems level in OECD countries. *Int J Qual Health Care*. 2006; 18(Suppl 1): 26–30.
94. Chan J. C. N., Gagliardino J. J., Baik S. H., Chantelot J. M., Ferreira S. R. G., Hancu N., *et al.* Multifaceted determinants for achieving glycemic control the international diabetes management practice study (IDMPS). *Diabetes Care*. 2009; 32(2): 227–33.
95. Chetthakul T., Pongchaiyakul C., Tandhanand S. Improvement of diabetic care at Maharat Nakhon Ratchasima Hospital (the study of DiabCare-Asia from 1997 to 2003). *J Med Assoc Thai*. 2006; 89(1): 56–62.
96. Lee T. W., Chan S. C., Chua W. T., Harbinder K., Khoo Y. L., Ow Yeang Y. L., *et al.* Audit of diabetes mellitus in general practice. *Med J Malaysia*. 2004; 59(3): 317–22.
97. Habib S. S., Aslam M. Risk factors, knowledge and health status in diabetic patients. *Saudi Med J*. 2003; 24(11): 1219–24.
98. Tan F., Chan G., Wong J. S., Rozario F. Standard of care for type 2 diabetic patients in a public hospital general medical clinic: report of a self-audit. *Med J Malaysia*. 2008; 63(3): 224–8.
99. Jayawardena M. H., Idampitiya C., Jayawarna C., Wanigasuriya K., Thomson G. A., Fernando D. J. An audit of standards of care at a Sri Lankan diabetic clinic. *Diabetes Res Clin Pract*. 2007; 75(2): 249–51.
100. Fernando D. J., Perera S. D. The work of a diabetes clinic: an audit. *Ceylon Med J*. 1994; 39(3): 138–9.
101. Idampitiya C., Lenora D., Lau S., Thomson G. A., Fernando D. J. Improving the quality of diabetes care in a Sri Lankan diabetes clinic through a diabetes nurse educator. *Diabetes Res Clin Pract*. 2008; 80(1): e25–6.
102. Chuang L. M., Tsai S. T., Huang B. Y., Tai T. Y. The status of diabetes control in Asia – a cross-sectional survey of 24,317 patients with diabetes mellitus in 1998. *Diabet Med*. 2002; 19(12): 978–85.
103. Ismail I. S., Nazaimoon W., Mohamad W., Letchuman R., Singaraveloo M., Hew F. L., *et al.* Ethnicity and glycaemic control are major determinants of diabetic dyslipidaemia in Malaysia. *Diabet Med*. 2001; 18(6): 501–8.
104. Eid M., Mafauzy M., Faridah A. R. Non-achievement of clinical targets in patients with type 2 diabetes mellitus. *Med J Malaysia*. 2004; 59(2): 177–84.
105. Mafauzy M. Diabetes control and complications in private primary healthcare in Malaysia. *Med J Malaysia*. 2005; 60(2): 212–17.
106. Lantion-Ang L. C. Epidemiology of diabetes mellitus in Western pacific region: focus on Philippines. *Diabetes Res Clin Pract*. 2000; 50(Suppl 2): S29–S34.
107. Nitiyanant W., Chetthakul T., Sang-A-kad P., Therakiatkumjorn C., Kunsuikmengrai K., Yeo J. P. A survey study on diabetes management and complication status in primary care setting in Thailand. *J Med Assoc Thai*. 2007; 90(1): 65–71.
108. Ramachandran A., Snehalatha C., Sasikala R., Satyavani K., Vijay V. Vascular complications in young Asian Indian patients with type 1 diabetes mellitus. *Diabetes Res Clin Pract*. 2000; 48(1): 51–6.
109. Mohan V., Meera R., Premalatha G., Deepa R., Miranda P., Rema M. Frequency of proteinuria in type 2 diabetes mellitus seen at a diabetes centre in southern India. *Postgrad Med J*. 2000; 76(899): 569–73.
110. Rahman Afridi M. M., Khan M. N. Role of health education in the management of diabetes mellitus. *Journal of the College of Physicians and Surgeons Pakistan*. 2003; 13(10): 558–61.
111. Basit A., Hydrie M. Z., Hakeem R., Ahmedani M. Y., Masood Q. Frequency of chronic complications of type II diabetes. *J Coll Physicians Surg Pak*. 2004; 14(2): 79–83.
112. Mahmood K., Aamir A. H. Glycemic control status in patients with type-2 diabetes. *J Coll Physicians Surg Pak*. 2005; 15(6): 323–5.
113. Wong J. S., Rahimah N. Glycaemic control of diabetic patients in an urban primary health care setting in Sarawak: the Tanah Puteh Health Centre experience. *Med J Malaysia*. 2004; 59(3): 411–17.
114. Wong J. S., Tan F., Lee P. Y. The state of lipid control in patients with diabetes in a public health care centre. *Asia Pac J Public Health*. 2007; 19(3): 16–21.

115. Chan G. C., Ghazali O., Khoo E. M. Management of type 2 diabetes mellitus: Is it in accordance with the guidelines? *Medical Journal of Malaysia*. 2005; 60(5): 578–84.
116. Taweepolcharoen N., Sumrithe S., Kunentrasai N., Phraisuwanna S. Diabetes control in a university primary care setting in Thailand. *Quality in Primary Care*. 2006; 14(4): 219–23.
117. Worawongprapa O. Glycemic control in diabetes with metabolic syndrome in community hospital. *J Med Assoc Thai*. 2008; 91(5): 641–7.
118. Wu A. Y., Kong N. C., de Leon F. A., Pan C. Y., Tai T. Y., Yeung V. T., *et al*. An alarmingly high prevalence of diabetic nephropathy in Asian type 2 diabetic patients: the MicroAlbuminuria Prevalence (MAP) Study. *Diabetologia*. 2005; 48(1): 17–26.
119. Pan C. Y., Ho L. T., Soegondo S., Prodjosudjadi W., Suwanwalaikorn S., Lim S. C., *et al*. Prevalence of albuminuria and cardiovascular risk profile in a referred cohort of patients with type 2 diabetes: an Asian perspective. *Diabetes Technol Ther*. 2008; 10(5): 397–403.
120. Guo X. H., Yuan L., Lou Q. Q., Shen L., Sun Z. L., Zhao F., *et al*. A nationwide survey of diabetes education, self-management and glycemic control in patients with type 2 diabetes in China. *Chin Med J (Engl)*. 2012; 125(23): 4175–80.
121. Leelawattana R., Pratipanawatr T., Bunnag P., Kosachunhanun N., Suwanwalaikorn S., Krittiyawong S., *et al*. Thailand diabetes registry project: prevalence of vascular complications in long-standing type 2 diabetes. *J Med Assoc Thai*. 2006; 89(Suppl 1): S54–S9.
122. Hwang C. K., Han P. V., Zabetian A., Ali M. K., Narayan K. M. Rural diabetes prevalence quintuples over twenty-five years in low- and middle-income countries: a systematic review and meta-analysis. *Diabetes Research and Clinical Practice*. 2012; 96(3): 271–85.
123. Narayan K. M. Venkat, Zhang P., Kanaya A. M., Williams D. E., Engelgau M. M., Imperatore G., *et al*. Diabetes: the pandemic and potential solutions. In: Jamison DT, Breman JG, Measham AR, Alleyne G, Claeson M, Evans DB, *et al*., editors. *Disease Control Priorities in Developing Countries*, 2nd ed. New York: Oxford University Press; 2006, tables 30.3 and 4.
124. Aekplakorn W., Abbott-Klafter J., Premgamone A., Dhanamun B., Chaikittiporn C., Chongsuvivatwong V., *et al*. Prevalence and management of diabetes and associated risk factors by regions of Thailand: Third National Health Examination Survey 2004. *Diabetes Care*. 2007; 30(8): 2007–12.
125. Akhter Afroza, Fatema Kaniz, Afroz Afsana, Bhowmik Bishwajit, Ali Liaquat, Hussain Akhtar. Prevalence of diabetes mellitus and its associated risk indicators in a rural Bangladeshi population. *Open Diabetes Journal*. 2011, 4: 6–13.
126. Ono K., Limbu Y. R., Rai S. K., Kurokawa M., Yanagida J., Rai G., *et al*. The prevalence of type 2 diabetes mellitus and impaired fasting glucose in semi-urban population of Nepal. *Nepal Medical College Journal: NMCJ*. 2007; 9(3): 154–6.
127. Ministry of Health. WHO Global Infobase: National Health Survey 2004, Singapore. World Health Organization Website. Available from: http://www.who.int/infobase/.2005 (Accessed March 31, 2009). [database on the Internet].
128. Chang C. H., Shau W. Y., Jiang Y. D., Li H. Y., Chang T. J., Sheu W. H., *et al*. Type 2 diabetes prevalence and incidence among adults in Taiwan during 1999–2004: a national health insurance data set study. *Diabetic Medicine*. 2010; 27(6): 636–43.
129. World Health Organization: Definition, diagnosis and classification of diabetes mellitus and its complications: Report of a WHO Consultation. Part 1. Diagnosis and classification of diabetes mellitus. Geneva: World Health Organization; 1999.
130. Diabetes mellitus. Report of a WHO Study Group. World Health Organization technical report series. 1985; 727: 1–113.
131. Report of the Expert Committee on the Diagnosis and Classification of Diabetes Mellitus. *Diabetes Care*. 1997; 20(7): 1183–97.
132. Diagnosis and classification of diabetes mellitus. *Diabetes Care*. 2004; 27(Suppl 1): S5–S10.
133. Eppens M. C., Craig M. E., Jones T. W., Silink M., Ong S., Ping Y. J. Type 2 diabetes in youth from the Western Pacific region: glycaemic control, diabetes care and complications. *Curr Med Res Opin*. 2006; 22(5): 1013–20.
134. Cole T. J., Flegal K. M., Nicholls D., Jackson A. A. Body mass index cut-offs to define thinness in children and adolescents: international survey. *BMJ* (Clinical research ed). 2007; 335(7612): 194.

# 31

# Community outreach to prevent diabetes in Hong Kong

## Diabetes Hongkong as a case study

*Ronald C. W. Ma and Vincent T. F. Yeung*

## Introduction

There is an epidemic of diabetes in Asia [1, 2, 3]. According to the International Diabetes Federation, there are an estimated 132 million individuals with diabetes living in the Western Pacific region, making this the area with the largest number of diabetes sufferers [4]. In Hong Kong, it is estimated that there are approximately half a million adults with diabetes [4]. As well as that, an epidemiology study done in Hong Kong found that around 60 per cent of adults affected with diabetes were undiagnosed [5]. The majority of diabetes patients in Hong Kong are under care in the public sector and 97 per cent of these patients have type 2 diabetes [6]. Diabetes not only inflicts one in five adults aged 55 to 64 years [5], but also affects a rising number of young adults, putting them at increased risk of diabetic complications. According to the Centre for Health Protection of the Department of Health, diabetes accounts for more than 24,000 inpatient discharges and deaths each year, and is one of the major causes of morbidity and mortality in the territory [7]. Diabetes remains one of the leading causes of blindness and currently accounts for approximately 50 per cent of patients entering dialysis programmes each year [8]. In this chapter, we outline the causes that contribute to the epidemic of diabetes in Hong Kong and discuss the importance of health literacy in the prevention of diabetes. We then use Diabetes Hongkong as a case study to analyse how a non-government organization can develop programmes and other community outreach initiatives to help raise the awareness of diabetes and combat the prevalence of the disease.

## Contributing causes to the epidemic of diabetes in Hong Kong

Factors that drive the increasing prevalence of diabetes in Hong Kong are similar to factors amongst other populations and include an ageing population, sedentary lifestyle and unhealthy diet [2, 9]. Increasing obesity, especially central obesity (increased waist circumference), has become an important problem and childhood obesity is also becomingly increasingly common

[10]. According to the Student Health Service (SHS), the proportion of primary school children who are overweight and obese has been increasing steadily in Hong Kong, from 16.4 per cent in 1997/1998 to 22.2 per cent in 2008/2009 [11]. Other factors that contribute to obesity, especially among the younger generation, include the increased intake of energy-dense food and sugar-sweetened beverages, and reduced physical activity [12]. It has also been found that lack of sleep is associated with increased obesity in adults, as well as in children [13, 14].

## Importance of health literacy in the prevention of diabetes

It is increasingly recognized that health literacy is a key determinant of health. This is particularly important for non-communicable diseases (NCDs) such as diabetes, for which sedentary lifestyles and dietary patterns are important modifiable risk factors. Differences in the levels of health literacy, especially between different social and economic groups, play an important role in health inequalities among different populations. For example, a lack of education and a low socio-economic position has been found to be associated with increased risk of diabetes [15]. For patients with diabetes, education on self-management of the disease is recognized as one of the cornerstones for prevention of diabetes-related complications or adverse outcomes [16, 17]. More importantly, though, is the prevention of diabetes among the large population of at-risk individuals. Randomized clinical trials have demonstrated that lifestyle modification is an effective means to reduce the risk of diabetes, as well as diabetes-related complications among at-risk individuals with impaired glucose tolerance or elevated fasting glucose [18, 19]. Primary prevention of diabetes has been shown to be highly cost-effective compared to treatment of diabetes or related complications [20].

## The role of Diabetes Hongkong

In order to fulfil the need to increase public awareness of diabetes, Diabetes Hongkong was founded as a charitable organization by a group of healthcare professionals and volunteers, with the mission to serve all people with diabetes and their families, promote social awareness and concern about diabetes, and strive for optimal care and prevention of the disease (see Figure 31.1). Since its establishment in 1996, Diabetes Hongkong has grown to become the largest non-governmental organization in Hong Kong promoting the prevention of diabetes and organizing programmes to raise diabetes awareness. Approximately 10 per cent of its members are healthcare professionals and patients with diabetes account for more than 70 per cent of its members. The remaining members comprise family members of patients with diabetes, volunteers or other members of the general public. Diabetes Hongkong is a Member Association of the International Diabetes Federation (IDF), which is an umbrella organization of over 200 national diabetes associations in 160 countries, representing the interests of the growing number of people with diabetes and those at risk. Since its establishment, Diabetes Hongkong has been working closely with government authorities, local universities, hospitals, patient self-help groups, pharmaceutical companies and other related associations in the fight against diabetes. Diabetes Hongkong aims to:

1 Promote public awareness and improve understanding of diabetes via public education;
2 Provide social and medical support for people with diabetes and their families;
3 Provide continuing education and training for healthcare professionals involved in the delivery of diabetes care;

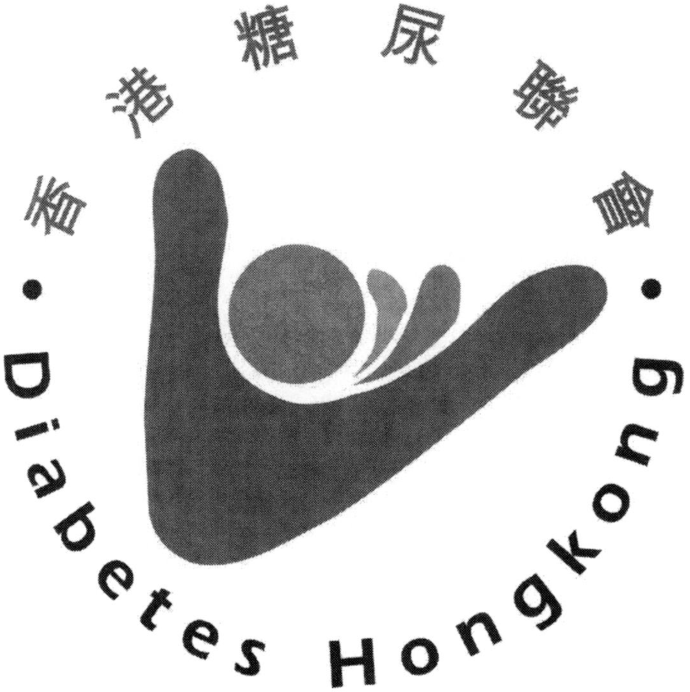


*Figure 31.1* The logo of Diabetes Hongkong, which highlights the spirit of collaboration for better care and education. The map of Hong Kong is displayed in the central globe, while digits of different colours, representing different groups, including patients, family members and healthcare professionals, join together to support the development of diabetes services in Hong Kong

*Source*: Diabetes Hongkong.

4 Act as an advocate for all people with diabetes and their families in Hong Kong;
5 Liaise with other national and international diabetes associations for exchange of information and experiences in diabetes care; and
6 Encourage research and safeguard standards of care in the management of diabetes.

## Diabetes Hongkong and community outreach

In order to improve awareness of diabetes and its complications, community education is an important aspect of Diabetes Hongkong's work. Since its establishment, Diabetes Hongkong has been conducting regular educational activities in local community centres, other public venues and schools. Accessible to the public and free of charge, four to six seminars by health-care professionals are organized every year to empower patients with skills in diabetes management and promote the prevention of the disease. Over the last few years, a wellness promotion campaign has also been developed in order to empower employees at corporations and companies to become aware of the dangers of diabetes and related NCDs, and to teach them about lifestyle measures to reduce the risk of diabetes. Between 2011 and 2012 alone, more than 15 community outreach events were conducted, reaching an audience of over 2,600 adults.

A diabetes complication screening service for patients with diabetes was initiated in 2000. In addition to fundus photography and screening for microalbuminuria, diabetes education is also provided by the centre nurse to reinforce to patients the importance of self-management.

## School-Based Education Programme for the prevention of obesity and diabetes in children

Childhood obesity is becoming an increasingly common problem in Asia. According to statistics of the SHS, the prevalence of overweight including obesity (defined as more than 120 per cent median weight for height) among primary school students increased from 16.4 per cent in the 1997/1998 school year to 22.2 per cent in the 2008/2009 school year [11]. The promotion of the awareness and knowledge of diabetes through education is one of the best ways to prevent diabetes. This is particularly effective if started early, for example with school children and young people. Diabetes Hongkong initiated a School-Based Education Programme in primary schools in 2009, with the aim of developing an outreach programme to educate school children, teachers and parents about the hazards of overweight and obesity. Research suggests that targeting primary school children is much more likely to have a beneficial impact compared to secondary schools, which is probably too late in terms of shaping their perspective on health and self-care. The programme's objectives include to:

- Enhance the understanding and awareness about diabetes amongst school children;
- Highlight the importance of regular exercise and healthy diet for preventing diabetes and other chronic diseases; and
- Raise the awareness about diabetes to parents, teachers and social workers, and to equip them with the skills and knowledge to help children adopt a healthy lifestyle.

The programme was developed by a committee consisting of endocrinologists, paediatricians, dietitians, diabetes nurse educators and other professionals, and was conducted by a nursing professional with volunteer support from health workers and patients with diabetes. Through a wide range of educational activities carried out in school campuses, such as talks/workshops, exhibitions, video clips, interactive game stations and quiz competitions, the programme disseminates health information to school children in a fun and interactive way, mainly through experiential learning (see Figure 31.2a–c). Educational leaflets and materials on nutrition, exercise, obesity and diabetes are also provided to the participants and their families. A structured Intervention Programme for overweight children was also developed and its impact following a short period of intensive education (28 hours over seven sessions) has been examined.

Between May 2009 and April 2011, the entire programme was conducted in 36 community primary schools in Hong Kong, with participation from 22,207 school children. A survey conducted among 4,135 participants identified several common misconceptions about healthy living. There was very poor knowledge of what are healthy versus unhealthy food items, and 70 per cent of children regarded diabetes as predominantly a disease of the liver. A repeat evaluation indicated there was significant improvement in the children's knowledge after completing the programme.

In the six-month pilot Intervention Programme, which comprised of health-related activities, as well as dietary consultations by dietitians and physical education workshops to help children incorporate regular daily exercise into their usual school routine, 21 overweight children were recruited (mean age $9.9 \pm 1.4$ yrs, BMI $25.0 \pm 3.7$ kg/m$^2$, body fat $39.6 \pm 10.0$ per cent). There was significant improvement in dietary patterns, with increased intake of

(a)

(b)

(c)

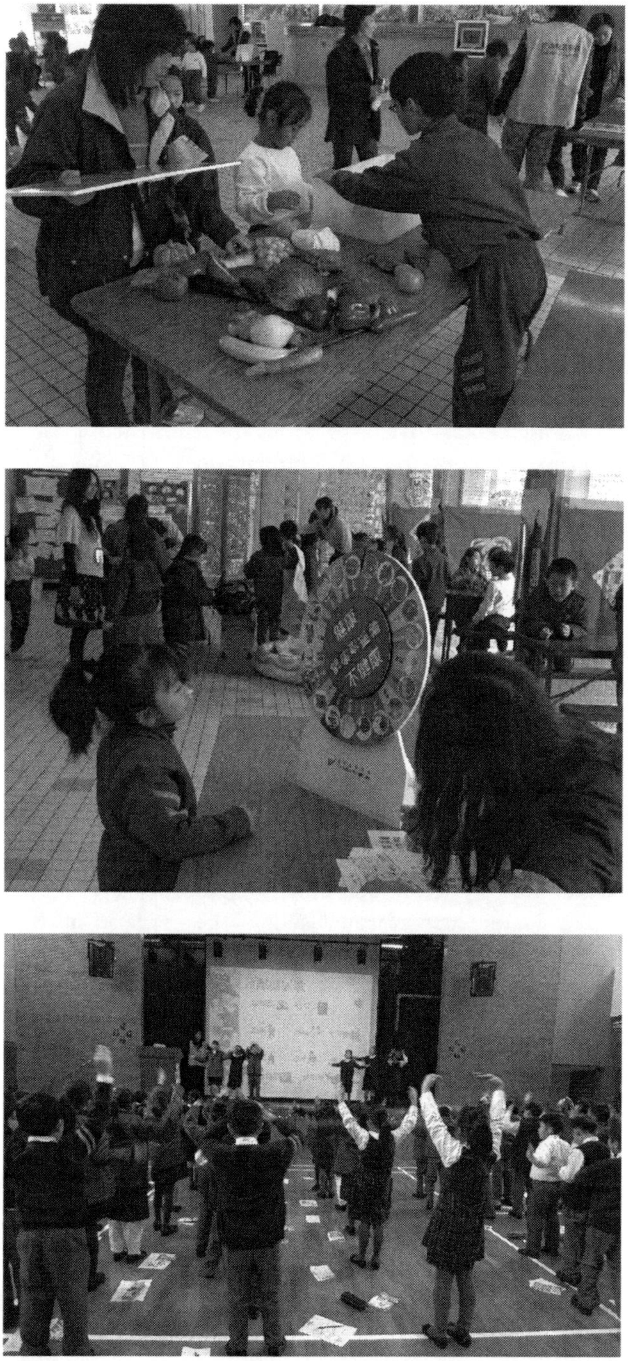

*Figure 31.2a–c* The School-Based Education Programme is designed to provide educational information about healthy lifestyles to primary school children through experiential learning

*Source*: Diabetes Hongkong.

fruits and vegetables, reduced intake of sugar-sweetened beverages and more children starting to eat breakfast. There was also evidence of reduced BMI, total body fat and body fat percentage after 28 weeks ($p < 0.01$). The level of participation and support from parents and teachers was good. The initial results suggest that a school-based education programme is effective in bringing about healthy behavioural changes in young children and is consistent with the results observed in the HEALTHY Study in the USA [21].

Given the positive response from schools and the encouraging findings, the educational programme is now being expanded to more primary schools in Hong Kong in order to provide much-needed healthcare education to children at this critical stage of their personal development. Following the completion of the first phase of the programme in April 2011, it has been incorporated as one of the key activities of Diabetes Hongkong and has been conducted in another 14 schools over the last 12 months, reaching an additional 10,335 students. To date, the programme has been successfully conducted in a total of 54 primary schools across Hong Kong, reaching a total of 39,744 students. These outreach activities complement the 'EatSmart@school.hk' campaign led by the Department of Health in Hong Kong, which is also being conducted in local schools to encourage schools to introduce healthier school meals.

Of course as with any programme or initiative, there are various challenges. The challenges identified in conducting school-based education have to be addressed to constantly improve these programmes. Some of these include:

- Varying enthusiasm of teachers to incorporate extra classes into the busy school curriculum;
- The need to fit the programme and activities into usual school routine;
- Level of health literacy and science literacy of primary school students;
- Delivery of information by health professionals versus teachers;
- How to engage the students in the learning experience;
- How to reinforce the message after the period of interaction;
- How to involve the teachers and parents as much as possible;
- How to target the messages to particular at-risk individuals without stigmatizing the students;
- The logistics of delivering the workshops in allocated periods; and
- How to incorporate health literacy into the training of teachers.

## The Diabetes Hongkong Healthy Run

The Diabetes Hongkong Healthy Run was initiated in 2004 by Dr Tsang Man Wo, a past president of Diabetes Hongkong, to promote regular exercise as an important means for the prevention of diabetes in at-risk individuals. Good weight management and regular exercise has been shown to be effective in improving diabetes control, as well as lowering the risk for diabetes and other serious complications [18, 19, 22]. When the programme was launched, individuals with risk factors for diabetes were invited to take part in either a programme of exercise intervention with regular long-distance running or to receive dietary education. Participants who increased their physical activity were noted to have improvements in body weight and metabolic indices.

Over the years, the programme has been expanded to include the general public and has evolved into a much larger annual event, also receiving support from the local health authorities. In 2012, in addition to the regular ten-kilometre event, a five-kilometre fun run was organized, attracting 1,500 participants. Other media activities around this annual event also serve to promote the importance of physical activity to the general public.

## Other outreach education activities

In addition to the community education programme, school-based education programme and Healthy Run, Diabetes Hongkong undertakes other activities that serve to promote awareness of diabetes and its related complications. Since its first issue in February 1998, the Diabetes Hongkong newsletter, which is now published three times annually, has served as a regular channel to provide useful, practical information to patients and the public alike on topics related to diabetes. The newsletter currently has a circulation of over 7,000 copies per issue and is distributed to members and local diabetes centres, as well as to public libraries, university libraries and overseas diabetes organizations.

The World Diabetes Day (WDD), which is celebrated on 14 November every year provides another focal point for diabetes educational activities. The WDD was founded in 1991 by the International Diabetes Federation and the World Health Organization (WHO) in response to growing concerns about the escalating health threats of diabetes. The WDD campaign is led by the International Diabetes Federation and its member associations, and aims to draw public attention to issues relating to the disease. The WDD became an official United Nations Day in 2007, following the passage of the United Nations Resolution 61/225, which recognizes that diabetes is a chronic, debilitating and costly disease associated with severe complications, which poses severe risks for families, member states and the entire world, as well as posing serious challenges to the achievement of internationally agreed development goals, including the Millennium Development Goals.

In addition to an annual 'Walk for Diabetes', Diabetes Hongkong also organizes various activities around this day. This includes media sharing in radio programmes, as well as the publication of educational articles in local newspapers to raise public awareness about the disease and its complications, as well as the impact it has on the lives of people affected by it.

## Conclusion

Diabetes has become an important global health problem. With increasing prevalence and earlier onset, the potential health burden associated with diabetes and its complications is of grave concern. Strategies to reduce the impact of diabetes need to address several factors, as well as target different populations. Early detection, structured intervention and regular screening for diabetic complications can help to reduce the risk of long-term ramifications. Nevertheless, primary prevention of diabetes is an important and cost-effective strategy to reduce the burden of the disease. In addition to health authorities, government agencies and healthcare providers, non-government and professional organizations also have an important role to play in promoting public education about the hazards of diabetes and other NCDs by reaching out to local communities and through the dissemination of practical information. The United Nations High-level Meeting on Non-Communicable Diseases held on 19–20 September 2011 in New York represents a milestone in the history of the global diabetes and NCDs epidemic. Hopefully, through this watershed event, governments globally will be committed to bring about progress in national policies and plans, essential medicines and technologies, prevention strategies, health systems strengthening, resourcing and partnerships to implement elements of the United Nations Declaration on NCDs. Partnerships between governments and the diabetes community will be an important component of this multi-sectoral NCD partnership. The outreach activities of Diabetes Hongkong provide a useful example of how professional organizations can operate effectively at the local level to help accelerate progress on diabetes and other NCDs.

## Acknowledgements

We would like to acknowledge the generous support of numerous donors and organizations towards the work of Diabetes Hongkong. In particular, we would like to acknowledge support from the Chow Tai Fok Charity Foundation, the 'Love Ideas, Love HK' campaign of the Li Ka Shing Foundation, Goldman Sachs (Asia) Charitable Contributions Committee and Operation Santa Claus. We thank the SK Yee Medical Foundation for supporting the establishment of the diabetes complication screening service, and donations from the Sedan Chair Charities Fund which has helped support this service for patients with diabetes. We thank past presidents, council members and members of the different subcommittees of Diabetes Hongkong, who have contributed much to the work described above. The Diabetes Hongkong School Education Program was initiated with a generous donation from the Air Cargo Community Charity Golf Tournament held in December 2008. We would like to thank other members of the Diabetes Hongkong School Education Project Committee: Mr Pedro Ching, Dr Hong Chen, Ms Jo Jo Kwan, Ms Chin San Law, Ms Flavia U and Dr Jenny Leung. We would like to express our sincere thanks to the dedicated staff at Diabetes Hongkong, in particular, Ms Gladdie Chu, the Executive Officer and Ms Eva Li, the centre nurse, who was responsible for coordinating the School Education Project. We would also like to thank all our volunteers who have helped with our various activities in the community. For further information about Diabetes Hongkong, please visit the official website: http://www.diabetes-hk.org

## References

1. Chan, J. C., V. Malik, *et al.* Diabetes in Asia: epidemiology, risk factors, and pathophysiology. *JAMA* 2009; 301(20): 2129–40.
2. Ma, R. C. and P. C. Tong. Epidemiology of Type 2 Diabetes. *Textbook of Diabetes.* R. Holt, B. Goldstein, A. Flyvbjerg and C. S. Cockram, Chichester. Wiley-Blackwell, 2010: 45–68.
3. Ramachandran, A., R. C. Ma, *et al.* Diabetes in Asia. *Lancet* 2010; 375(9712): 408–18.
4. International Diabetes Federation. *Diabetes Atlas*, 2011.
5. Lam, T. H., L. J. Liu, *et al.* Fibrinogen, other cardiovascular risk factors and diabetes mellitus in Hong Kong: a community with high prevalence of Type 2 diabetes mellitus and impaired glucose tolerance. *Diabet Med* 2000; 17(11): 798–806.
6. Chan, J. C. N. Heterogeneity of diabetes mellitus and diabetes care in Hong Kong Chinese. *Hong Kong Medical Journal* 2000; 6: 77–84.
7. Centre for Health Protection, Department of Health. *Diabetes Mellitus.* Hong Kong, 2012.
8. Ho, Y. W., K. F. Chau, *et al.* Hong Kong Renal Registry Report 2010. *Hong Kong Journal of Nephrology* 2010; 12(2): 81–98.
9. Chan, J. C. and C. S. Cockram. Epidemiology of Diabetes Mellitus in China. *The Epidemiology of Diabetes Mellitus.* J.-M. Ekoe, M. Rewers, R. Williams and P. Zimmet. Chichester, John Wiley, 2008: 179–206.
10. Ko, G. T., R. Ozaki, *et al.* The problem of obesity among adolescents in Hong Kong: a comparison using various diagnostic criteria. *BMC Pediatr* 2008; 8: 10.
11. Student Health Service. Department of Health, 2010.
12. Ko, G. T., W. Y. So, *et al.* Risk associations of obesity with sugar-sweetened beverages and lifestyle factors in Chinese: the 'Better Health for Better Hong Kong' health promotion campaign. *Eur J Clin Nutr* 2010; 64(12): 1386–92.

13. Ko, G. T., J. C. Chan, *et al.* Association between sleeping hours, working hours and obesity in Hong Kong Chinese: the 'better health for better Hong Kong' health promotion campaign. *Int J Obes (Lond)* 2007; 31(2): 254–60.
14. Wing, Y. K., S. X. Li, *et al.* The effect of weekend and holiday sleep compensation on childhood overweight and obesity. *Pediatrics* 2009; 124(5): e994–e1000.
15. Agardh, E., P. Allebeck, *et al.* Type 2 diabetes incidence and socio-economic position: a systematic review and meta-analysis. *Int J Epidemiol* 2011; 40(3): 804–18.
16. Davies, M. J., S. Heller, *et al.* Effectiveness of the diabetes education and self management for ongoing and newly diagnosed (DESMOND) programme for people with newly diagnosed type 2 diabetes: cluster randomised controlled trial. *BMJ* 2008; 336(7642): 491–5.
17. Snoek, F. and A. Visser. Improving quality of life in diabetes: how effective is education? *Patient Educ Couns* 2003; 51(1): 1–3.
18. Gong, Q., E. W. Gregg, *et al.* Long-term effects of a randomised trial of a 6-year lifestyle intervention in impaired glucose tolerance on diabetes-related microvascular complications: the China Da Qing Diabetes Prevention Outcome Study. *Diabetologia* 2011; 54(2): 300–7.
19. Pan, X. R., G. W. Li, *et al.* Effects of diet and exercise in preventing NIDDM in people with impaired glucose tolerance. *Diabetes Care* 1997; 20: 537–44.
20. Narayan, K. M., P. Zhang, *et al.* How should developing countries manage diabetes? *CMAJ* 2006; 175(7): 733.
21. Foster, G. D., B. Linder, *et al.* A school-based intervention for diabetes risk reduction. *N Engl J Med* 2010; 363(5): 443–53.
22. Rejeski, W. J., E. H. Ip, *et al.* Lifestyle change and mobility in obese adults with type 2 diabetes. *N Engl J Med* 2012; 366(13): 1209–17.

# 32

# Challenges of non-communicable diseases in China

*Liming Li, Jun Lv and Johnny Yu Jiang*

## Introduction

More than 30 years of reform and development have resulted in China's health services and the health status of its population improving significantly. The key health indicators, particularly in the urban areas in the east of the country, are close to the level of developed countries or moderately developed countries. Whilst still a burden particularly amongst poorer rural communities infectious diseases are being effectively controlled, with a significant reduction in annual incidence from 6,000/100,000 in 1950 to 471.33/100,000 in 2011 [1]. Substantial progress has been made in improving life expectancy and decreasing mortality rates for children under 5 [2]. However, industrialization and urbanization, rapid lifestyle changes and an increasingly ageing population have led to chronic non-communicable diseases (NCDs) – particularly the big four cardiovascular diseases, cancers, chronic respiratory diseases and type 2 diabetes – becoming major threats to public health in China [3]. This chapter describes the burden of disease attributable to NCDs in China. It describes both the predisposing factors and the initiatives being undertaken to stem the rising tide of the epidemic, which is affecting urban and rural areas, and all strata of society.

## NCDs in China

In 2008, an estimated 56 million people died as a result of an NCD, accounting for 63 per cent of all deaths globally [4] and this figure is expected to rise to 75 per cent in 2030 [5]. In 2008, about one-quarter of the global NCD-related deaths occurred in the working population under the age of 60 and, in 2010, 80 per cent of chronic disease deaths occurred in low- and middle-income countries [6]. These types of diseases are now the world's number one killer and hinder social development, undermine the realization of the Millennium Development Goals (MDGs) and increase social injustice.

Around 260 million patients have been diagnosed with an NCD in China and the number is growing fast [7]. The third national survey on causes of death showed that among urban and rural areas, the top four causes of death are cerebrovascular disease, cancer, respiratory disease and heart disease, and the prevalence difference between the urban and rural regions is narrowing. In China, 85 per cent of the total deaths in 2010 were caused by NCDs [8] and 3.71 million premature deaths were due to NCDs, accounting for 75 per cent of the total number of premature deaths. The age distribution of chronic disease patients tends to be younger than in the West, with 45 per cent of patients dying before the age of 70. Predetermining factors such as a poor diet, high-blood pressure, tobacco use, high cholesterol and fasting blood glucose, and exposure to ambient and household air pollution are now the main public health challenges for policy makers [9].

The common NCDs share the characteristics of a long duration, growing epidemic, expensive costs and a high chance of morbidity or mortality. The medical costs of NCDs were estimated to be RMB1.4762 trillion (US$210 billion) in 2005, and the burden of disease caused by NCDs increased from 54 per cent in 1993 to 63 per cent in 2005 [10] to 69 per cent in 2009 [11]. Reducing cardiovascular mortality by 1 per cent per year between 2010 and 2040 could generate an economic value equivalent of 68 per cent of China's real GDP in 2010 or over US$10.7 trillion [12]. These diseases not only seriously affect the Chinese people's life and health, but have also become a huge burden on social and economic development.

The World Health Organization (WHO) NCD 2011 report data show that deaths caused by high blood pressure, smoking, high blood glucose, as well as overweight and obesity, respectively accounted for 13 per cent (7 million deaths), 9 per cent (6 million deaths), 6 per cent and 5 per cent (5.3 million deaths) of the annual total deaths [13].

In China, 28.1 per cent of the population smoke tobacco, 30.6 per cent do not get enough physical activity, 38.2 per cent have high blood pressure, 25.2 per cent have high blood glucose (including 9.7 per cent diabetes and 15.5 per cent for pre-diabetes), 33.5 per cent have high cholesterol, 25.4 per cent are overweight and 5.7 per cent are obese [14, 15, 16]. Problems related to NCDs caused by dietary changes, chronic infection and oral diseases also cannot be ignored. It is estimated that over 50 per cent of the NCD burden is preventable by modifying health and biological factors, such as changing diets to reduce fat, salt and sugar; stopping tobacco smoking; and promoting physical activity [12]. With the increased exposure to the risk factors, the number of patients with major NCDs both in urban and rural areas has changed significantly. From 1998 to 2008, the number of patients with diabetes and hypertension increased by 1.98 times and 2.31 times, respectively, while cerebrovascular diseases and cancer had an increase of 66 per cent and 91.6 per cent, respectively. The next two decades may well see a doubling or tripling of these figures [17]. In 2010, nearly 600 million Chinese people over the age of 40 had at least one risk factor for an NCD. It is predicted that, by 2030, among the population aged 40 years and above, there will be 54 million patients with cardiovascular disease (CVD), 55 million patients with chronic obstructive pulmonary disease (COPD), 64 million diabetic patients and 7.4 million lung cancer patients [18]. For common NCDs, such as ischaemic heart disease and lung cancer, the population mortality rates have been declining in most Western countries, but are increasing in China as a result of adverse changes in lifestyle, diet and tobacco use [19–21]. NCDs account for over 80 per cent of annual deaths and contribute to 68.6 per cent of the country's disease burden [19]. For each major NCD in China, there is still a large unexplained variation in the age-specific rates between different populations and different regions [22–24] suggesting that some important non-genetic causes remain to be discovered. In addition to behavioural and environmental factors, genetic factors and gene–environment interactions are likely to play important roles in disease causation [25–27]. In order to address the NCD prevalence in China, a large blood-based prospective study, the China Kadoorie Biobank (CKB, known previously as the Kadoorie Study of Chronic Diseases in China [KSCDC]), was launched in 2004 with the goal of recruiting 0.5 million people and assessing their health for at least two decades [28].

The current burden of disease reflects the past level of exposure to risk factors and the future burden of disease will depend on the current level of exposure. As risks of NCDs continue to increase, the problems caused by NCDs will become more and more serious if measures are not taken. Tobacco cessation is one of the most tangible ways in which the disease burden could be reduced. With an estimated 301 million smokers, smoking-related illness kills more than 1 million Chinese citizens each year. One in three of the world's smokers is a Chinese man and tobacco production and cigarette consumption continue to rise [29]. Both individual measures, such as education and cessation support, as well as strategies to increase accessibility, such as increasing price, are under consideration since China signed the WHO Framework Convention on Tobacco Control (FCTC) [30]. In March 2011, the Ministry of Health (MOH) issued a set of rules on implementation of the regulations [31]. In June 2011, the Ministry of Education and the MOH jointly released guidelines for schools, making them smoke-free, and in the same year the State Administration of Radio, Film and Television issued a notification to stop tobacco advertising in film and on television, and limiting scenes with smoking particularly by adolescents. These steps are all significant but, as with all policies, the challenge is in their implementation.

Another key contributor to the epidemiological time bomb of NCDs in China is the changing diet in both urban and rural areas. In the past 20 years, food supply has increased and diets are richer in fats and sugars, and lower in cereals. Fast food outlets in urban areas, and obesity and overweight, are increasing problems particularly amongst children. The government is promoting educational and primary care initiatives to increase dietary literacy and physical activity. Active campaigns [32] on consumption in rural areas have been launched and techniques such as social marketing are being initiated at local levels. Alcohol consumption is also a contributor to the increasing rates of NCDs, including hypertension and CVD, and is a consequence of the expansion of production, as well as consumption, which has accompanied economic growth [33]. Steps are now being taken to raise awareness of the potential risks of alcohol and to try and reduce alcohol-related harm.

## The causal chain and risk factors for NCDs

The causal chain and risk factors for major NCDs, such as heart disease, stroke, cancer, chronic respiratory diseases and diabetes, can be seen in Figure 32.1. Unhealthy diets and excessive energy intakes, physical inactivity and smoking are the most common – and the most important – modifiable risk factors for NCDs. These behaviours contribute to the four NCDs (cancer, heart disease and stroke, type 2 diabetes and pulmonary diseases, such as asthma) that cause over 50 per cent of all deaths worldwide [34]. These risk factors, so-called intermediate factors in the chronic disease process, can further lead to high blood pressure, high blood glucose, dyslipidemia, and overweight and obesity. They are often referred to as 'direct' causes or 'closer' causes, meaning they are closer to the disease outcome in the etiology chain and also refer to a relatively clear etiology in the medical profession. The narrower the population with 'closer' causes is, the smaller the chance of prevention.

The remote end of the cause chain – the cause of causes – includes the fundamental socio-economic, cultural, political and environmental factors relating to diseases. Although the causal relationship between remote risk factors and diseases may not be very clear, the available evidence is sufficient to support that further action is required. An intervention process where such factors are improved will protect more people, and thus have a higher chance to prevent chronic diseases and reduce the overall burden of disease.

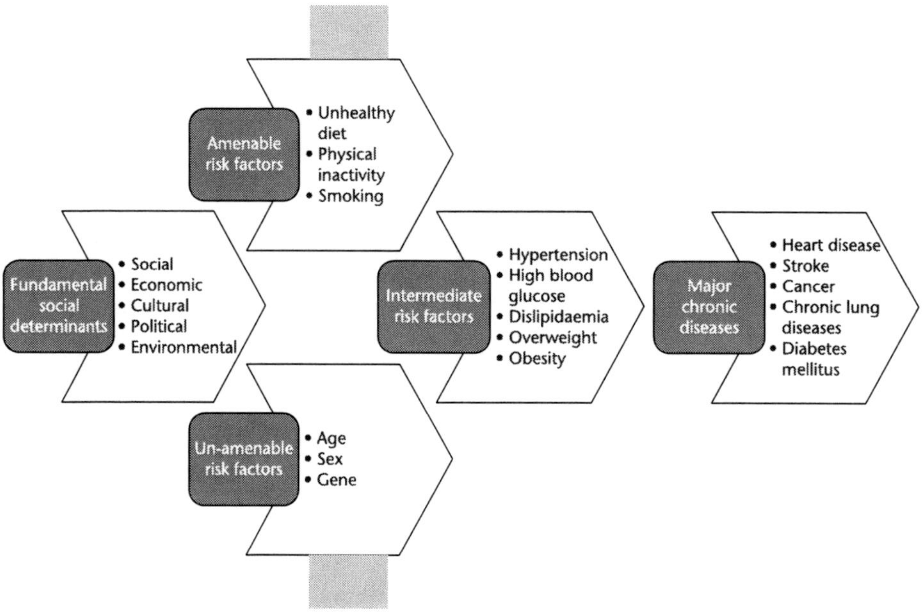


*Figure 32.1* The causal chain and risk factors for major NCDs

As mentioned above, unhealthy diets, physical inactivity and smoking are the three most important risk factors for major NCDs. Some people still think that the disease risk of the individual depends on his/her choice of unhealthy behaviours and inherent genetic susceptibility. However, an individual's behaviour is very complex and affected by an interaction of many factors on different levels. Choosing a healthy lifestyle not only depends on an individual's knowledge and attitudes, but also on his/her social, economic and political environments. Story and Edwards *et al.* [35, 36] studied the influencing factors of dietary habits and physical activity, and concluded that the main factors for individual health behaviour or lifestyle choices are the individual's own factors, the social environment, the workplace environment, the natural environment, the built environment, the macro-economic policy and the cultural environment.

The WHO concurs: its definition of the social determinants of health (SDH) is that besides those factors directly leading to diseases, the conditions in which people are born, grow, live, work and age, including the health system, and the health risk factors of the living and working environments within different social structures and conditions (including poverty and social exclusion), also contribute to the prevalence of diseases. Tarlov [37] calls this the social environmental characteristics, which could reflect different statuses of class, power and wealth in the social structure.

Due to the uneven distribution of these social determinants, people in and between societies have different opportunities to enjoy good health. Different populations in different environments have different material conditions, psychosocial support and possible behavioural choices, which exposes them to different risks for diseases and, finally, leads to health inequities.

## Key strategies for dealing with NCDs

To cope with the challenges of NCDs, effective strategies need:

- Government engagement;
- Expert guidance;
- Social mobilization;
- Multi-sector participation;
- Participation of the whole population; and
- The creation of a health-promoting and maintaining environment.

Different strategic approaches can be considered, which can be complementary and are not mutually exclusive.

### *High-risk strategy*

Recalling chronic disease prevention practices in recent decades, it is not difficult to see that a high-risk strategy has attracted more attention and preference. In addition to being compatible with the existing healthcare system with its biomedical model of disease-orientation, a high-risk strategy possesses many other advantages including:

- Only high-risk individuals will receive the intervention causing no unnecessary interference to other low-risk individuals;
- Due to the obvious need of some individual health problems, both the high-risk individuals and doctors will be willing to accept targeted interventions to solve the problem;
- Implementation of interventions for high-risk individuals creates a clear input and output with significant health gains; and
- Healthcare resources are limited and utilizing a high-risk strategy for resource utilization may be more cost-effective.

Although these advantages exist, in reality, a high-risk strategy often pays more attention to research. The practice of high-risk prevention strategies focuses more on the 'disease', emphasizing early screening and treatment of the disease rather than addressing upstream factors.

### *Whole-population strategy*

When common diseases exist in a population, a large number of people will be exposed to some of the same fundamental causes. A widespread problem requires a wide-coverage strategy, which means implementing a whole-population prevention strategy. The goal of the whole-population strategy is to make the entire population's exposure (such as blood pressure) move towards the direction of low risk by changing the exposure situation. For many common NCDs, the majority of patients come from a low-risk population rather than from a high-risk group and thus a population approach is appropriate.

If the overall level of the public's awareness about NCDs and associated risk factors is poor, health education should benefit the public in the early stages of chronic disease prevention. Health education is very important, as is primary care monitoring (of blood pressure, for example), but social and political measures are also needed to help solve the fundamental problems and policies, and legal, economic and environmental measures are needed to create the conditions in which to be healthy and to remove obstacles that hinder individuals adopting healthy behaviours.

Limitations of the whole-population strategy include:

- Even though the strategy has benefits for the whole population, for most individuals, the impact of prevention will not be immediately obvious or be particularly significant. Also, it is often not well perceived and understood so it is difficult for individuals, as well as medical staff and policy makers, to have the impetus for action; and
- As the whole-population approach only has a few benefits for most individuals, any associated risks cancel out the benefits, and thus more stringent safety approaches are required.

### *Integrating the high-risk and population-based strategies*

Whole-population and high-risk strategies are both very important for the prevention and treatment of NCDs, and have different advantages and limitations. The high-risk strategy has a clear target and effectiveness with strong operability, and can be easily understood and accepted. The whole-population strategy often uses more basic, low-cost interventions and is a way to achieve good health for the whole population. Chronic disease prevention and control should combine the two strategies. Measures for the entire population include the use of policies, laws and regulations (such as smoking bans in public places); economic measures (such as increases in tobacco excise tax); improvement of the built environment (such as the repair of walking paths and cycle tracks, designing of green spaces, increase in sports venues, and renovating stairwells in high buildings, thereby increasing the individual's level of physical activity) and so on. Interventions should be carried out in communities, especially in schools and workplaces, which are the best places for direct interventions for young people and adults. Measures for individuals could include screening to detect high-risk individuals and clinical prevention (such as high-risk individuals combining taking aspirin with beta blockers, diuretics and statins to prevent cardiovascular events).

This strategic approach takes measures to integrate therapy management for different diseases based on their common risk factors. For example, effective tobacco control, healthy diets and active sports could reduce 50 per cent of the deaths related to CVD, cancer, diabetes and chronic respiratory diseases. Disease management training for patients with various diseases can also help reduce their risk behaviours and effectively control diseases.

### *Environmental support intervention for individuals*

In the past, emphasis was placed on an individual's choice of unhealthy behaviour or inherent genetic susceptibility being at the root of the cause of their NCD. For nearly half a century, prevention and control of NCDs mainly focused on interventions to impact on an individual's behaviour. However, this viewpoint of 'blaming the victim' was widely criticized at the end of the twentieth century. Many public health workers have come to the realization that a close relationship between human health and the natural and social environment exists. If the environmental effects of shaping individual behaviour are ignored, the prevention effects of strategies relying solely on health education for individuals to change their lifestyle are very limited. Different environmental factors can affect an individual's behaviour and thus indirectly increase the individual's risk of disease. These factors include the availability of healthy and unhealthy commodities, price and the availability of sports venues in communities.

In addition, a number of environmental factors can directly increase the risk of chronic disease. For example, excessive or high concentrations of harmful gases, particulate matter or allergens in the air may increase the risk of COPD, asthma, lung cancer and other respiratory diseases, and, at the same time, promote the risk of death in patients with CVD. Usually environmental factors cannot be changed by the individual, highlighting the importance of support from the government and from society to create a health-promoting environment. In addition, because people in different socio-economic groups may be exposed to different environmental influences, the chance of people living a healthy lifestyle is unequal. In general, the more socio-economically disadvantaged, the less environmental support to lead a healthy life. In such an environment, an individual will have greater resistance to changing behaviours. For example, lower socio-economic groups often have a limited choice and less control of choices about dietary nutrition, living conditions, education and health care, and if they are already suffering from an NCD, this will put an even heavier burden on their family. In these situations, it is unfair to attribute their health problems to themselves alone.

According to the Sydney Resolution [38], a healthy environment should at least include the following aspects:

- A healthy living environment: rational urban planning; smoke-free; suitable for outdoor walking, cycling and sport; pollution-free greenbelt and safe;
- Healthy food availability: everyone can afford to buy healthy food;
- Healthy business activities: business activities should not harm people's health and should promote people to choose a healthy lifestyle;
- Health-conscious public policy: forming social and economic policies, laws and regulations to promote health; and
- Healthy society: solving problems on health equity and being concerned about disadvantaged socio-economic groups.

As such, health is the product of many sectors in society – politics, economy, culture, education, media, transportation, construction and the natural environment. Therefore, government-led, multi-sectoral participation and collaboration is essential to create healthy supportive environments and the health aspects of all policies (HiAP) are an important consideration [39].

## *Life-course approach*

The factors affecting our health start before our conception and the health of the foetus in the womb can affect the development of NCDs in later life. The risks of developing disease and disability accumulate with age and are influenced by social and physical factors at all stages of life (see Figure 32.2).

A life-course approach addresses cumulative adverse effects on people's lives by fostering health from gestation through to old age. There are also critical periods such as early childhood and adolescence when environmental exposures may do more harm to health than at other times. Being healthy before conception, adopting a healthy lifestyle during the antenatal period and ensuring healthy opportunities for children at all stages of development are important for future prevention of NCDs. Social, behavioural and environmental factors all impact on the potential for a healthy future and continue to do so throughout the life course to old age [40].

Understanding the importance of the life-course approach has led to different initiatives to promote: preconception care, optimum care in pregnancy, efforts to ensure safe delivery,

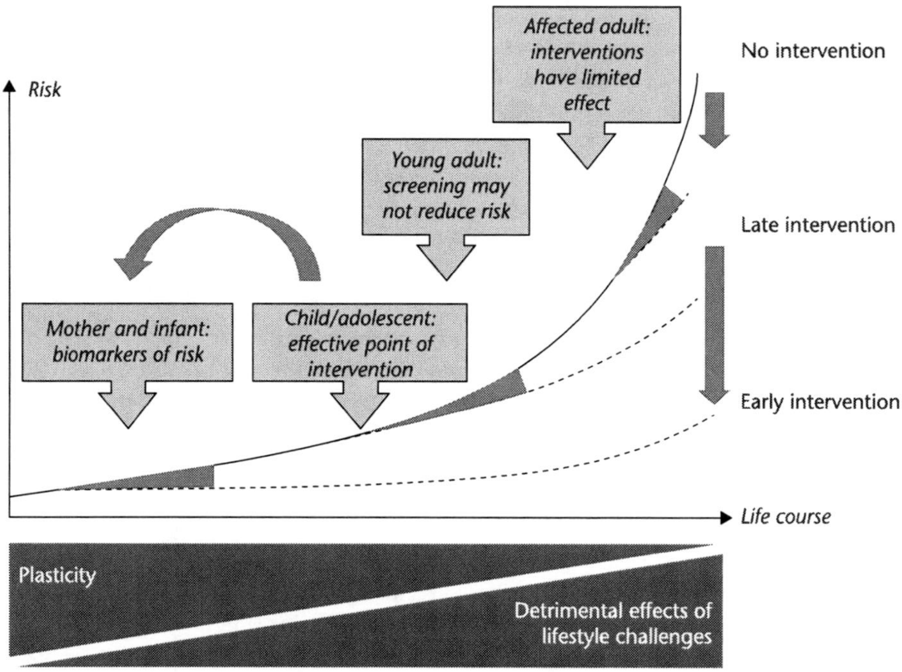


*Figure 32.2* Life-course view of NCDs

*Source*: [40] and Professor Mark Hanson.

as well as focus on vulnerable children and adolescents, and developing interventions tailored to promoting and maintaining health in middle and older age.

## Current approaches to the prevention and control of NCDs in China

### *Organization and networks*

Prevention and control practice for NCDs in China dates back to 1958. Before the 1990s, this practice mainly depended on experts' opinions and clinical treatment in major hospitals. In 1994, the Division of Chronic Non-communicable Disease Control and Management (now the Division of Chronic Disease Control and Nutrition Management) was established under the Department of Disease Control of the MOH. This signalled that the prevention and control of NCDs were being incorporated into government policy. In 2002, the Chinese Centre for Disease Control and Prevention (China CDC) (including the Centre for Chronic Non-communicable Disease Control and Prevention) was established, and this accelerated the establishment of counterpart local CDCs. In 2008, the proportions of institutional settings with Divisions of Chronic Disease Control and Prevention in provincial, city and county CDCs were 100 per cent, 62.8 per cent and 43.7 per cent, respectively [41].

Whilst 29.8 per cent of the city CDCs and 41.3 per cent of the county CDCs have no specific sector for chronic disease control and prevention, there are some institutes that take on the relevant responsibilities, mainly the Health Education Institute, the Endemic Disease Prevention Institute and the Planned Immunity Institute. In the cities, 7.4 per cent of the CDCs and 15 per cent of the CDCs in the counties still have no specific sectors to do the work on chronic disease control and prevention. Apart from the CDCs, China's major chronic disease network consists of the National Cancer Prevention Research Office established in 1969 (renamed to the Cancer Prevention Research Office of the MOH in 1978), the National Cerebrovascular Disease Prevention Research Officeestablished in 1987, the National Cancer Registration Centre established in 2002, the Cardiovascular Disease Prevention Research Centre of MOH established in 2003, and the National Cancer and the National Cardiovascular Disease Centres established recently. Moreover, national organizations, associations and societies, such as the Chinese League for Prevention and Control of Hypertension, the Chinese Association on Tobacco Control, the Chinese Anti-Cancer Association, the Cancer Foundation of China, the Chinese Society of Respiratory Diseases and the Chinese Society of Cardiology also play important roles.

## *Types of prevention and control practice*

### Survey and surveillance

Epidemiological surveys and surveillance are important components of NCD prevention and control practice, and provide critical basic data for developing strategies and measures. Since the 1950s, China has launched three national surveys on nutrition (1959, 1982 and 1992), three national surveys on hypertension (1959, 1979–1980 and 1991), two surveys on diabetes (1984 and 1995), one survey on nutrition and health status (2002), three national retrospective surveys on cancer (1973, 1990 and 2006) and four national population surveys on tobacco use (1984, 1996, 2002 and 2010; the 2010 one is part of the General Agreement on Trade in Services programme on global adult smoking).

Under the leadership of the MOH, the Chinese Academy of Prevention Medicine (now China CDC) set up a typical Chinese disease surveillance point (DSP) system in 1990. In 2004, a national surveillance system on NCDs and their risk factors was set up in the China CDC. National NCD surveillance was conducted every three years. Overall, public health workers do a good job on mortality surveillance among NCDs in China, but insufficient surveillance is being done on incidence and risk factors.

### Practice activities

In the past, the practice of prevention and control of NCDs in China contributed to the exploration of community-based comprehensive prevention and control strategies, proper skills, training and implementation mechanisms, and accumulated experiences and lessons in the field. Those practices included examples such as the community-based prevention and control of cardio-cerebrovascular disease in the Beijing Shougang Corporation from 1969, the prevention and control of the four major NCDs (malignant tumour, coronary heart disease, stroke and hypertension) in Tianjin from 1984, a health promotion sub-project of the disease prevention project supported by the World Bank loan (Health VII project) from 1995, and the comprehensive prevention and control model on community NCDs from 1997. The practice of the prevention and control of NCDs on a national level has been strengthened in the last ten years.

## *Examples of prevention and control practice*

In this section, we outline examples of prevention and control programmes focusing on NCDs, intermediate risk factors for major NCDs and behavioural risk factors for NCDs.

### Focusing on NCDs

The local public health special funds subsidized by central government finance on early diagnosis and treatment program (2006–2008) covered 31 provinces and 118 study sites, and were concerned with cervical cancer, breast cancer, oesophageal cancer, gastric cancer, liver cancer, colorectal carcinoma and nasopharyngeal carcinoma. This programme explored screening methods and suitable models of service provision, and accomplished the purpose of early detection, early diagnosis and early treatment of cancer.

### Focusing on intermediate risk factors for major NCDs

The National Community Program on hypertension standardized Management Program (from 2005) was carried out in 1,800 Community Health Centres (CHCs) in 20 regions, and explored the popularizing of the 'Guidelines for hypertension prevention and control' and the launching of the community standardized management on hypertension.

The local comprehensive prevention and control program subsidized by central government finance (from 2006) has been expanded to 30 communities of 31 provinces (municipalities directly under the central government, autonomous regions), covering a population of 1.25 million. This programme focused the factors of 'maintain[ing] a healthy weight' and 'control[ling] hypertension', implemented intervention programmes for high-risk populations and patients, adopted health and disease management strategies, and utilized community service sectors as its platform.

An example of good practice in China, Hangzhou was one of three study sites for the Community Interventions for Health (CIH) project. The CIH project is the action research-arm of the Oxford Health Alliance (OxHA), and is designed to develop and showcase sustainable interventions in addressing unhealthy diets, tobacco use and lack of physical activity, as well as demonstrating their effectiveness in preventing disease in a practical and scientifically rigorous way. The project in China addresses both chronic disease risk factors and barriers hindering change in order to find better ways to navigate policy change, find sustainable funding and build community capacity for NCD prevention and control, and to develop systems of surveillance and evaluation that are scientifically sound. A two-year intervention pilot study was carried out in neighbourhoods, schools, workplaces and health centres. Focusing on high-risk communities, the projects use four strategies for change: community coalition building, health education, media and structural change. Its long-term aim is to create environments and policies that reduce exposure to the three main risk factors for the four leading chronic diseases [42].

### Focusing on behavioural risk factors of NCDs

The National Healthy Lifestyle Initiative (2007–2015) themed on 'Harmonious life, Healthy Chinese' is aimed at improving people's ability to choose health consciousness and healthy lifestyles, creating a long-term, sustainable, supporting environment. The first strand is the 'Health One Two One', which introduces the 6 steps on diet, 4 methods on physical activities and '1,000 footsteps', and develops a series of health measurements. At present, 28 provinces have launched this initiative.

In addition, the MOH has begun to advocate that counties (cities and districts) set up and apply national-level and provincial-level comprehensive prevention and control demonstration areas. The evaluation rules were integrated with modern advanced elements on NCD prevention and control, based on traditional practice. For instance, a steering group headed by a major government leader is responsible for the work of demonstration areas, which includes:

- The establishing of a coordinated working system involving multiple sectors;
- Releasing government policies on chronic disease prevention, planning disease control and related matters;
- Increasing the coverage of fitness promoting environments/places and health education activities' rooms within local communities;
- Offering courses on NCD and health education in kindergartens, primary and secondary schools, and via seminars;
- Implementing group gymnastics at workplaces;
- Advocating food processing and sale companies to label nutritional ingredients in food; and
- Creating smoke-free workplaces.

It is worth mentioning that the government has also tightened the extent to which cities can modify the natural environment; promoted urban landscape building and building of urban green spaces, fitness paths and centres, and sports facilities; developed the public transportation networks; and revised the local regulations on tobacco control in public areas. These activities were undertaken in cooperation with the Olympic Games; the Asian Games; and the World Expo in Beijing, Shanghai, Guangzhou and Hangzhou, and create a supporting environment for healthy lifestyles for citizens, which seem to have a greater influence than the practices within the health system.

In the panel session on NCDs during the Global Health Policy Summit 2012, it was concluded that there is a need for citizens to take ownership over their own health and become engaged – structured self-management innovations will be key to achieving value and productivity in health systems. As well as that, the Ministries of Health and Finance must work together as the economic case for tackling NCDs is beyond question and structural barriers must not inhibit progress [43].

In May 2012, to effectively solve the existing problems relating to NCDs, 15 ministries including the MOH, the State Development and Reform Commission, the Ministry of Finance and others jointly issued the 'NCDs prevention and control work plan of China (2012–2015)', which is the first national comprehensive plan for NCDs in the country. This plan incorporates the 'Twelfth Five-Year Plan' and acts as a milestone showing the promise of the political declaration of NCD prevention and control made by the Chinese government during the 2011 United Nations High-Level Meeting on Non-Communicable Diseases. Moreover, the MOH has developed many professional guidelines, including diagnosis and treatment guidelines for malignant tumours, heart diseases, stroke, diabetes, COPDs; prevention and control guidelines for intermediate risk factors of hypertension, dyslipidemia, overweight and obesity; and lifestyle risk factor guidelines for quitting smoking, as well as dietary ones (including snacks). Meanwhile, two publications have also been published: the *Chinese Expert Consensus for Chronic Disease Prevention and Control* and the *NCD Prevention and Control Core Information*.

## Conclusion

As this chapter has shown, NCDs pose a major threat to the future prosperity of China as they can increase the burden of disease, as well as social and economic costs. Prevention is therefore of the utmost importance with support from the government at all levels, civil society, the health-care system, local communities and individuals themselves. A Delphi study of the Subcommittee of NCDs [44], an expert committee on disease control and prevention established by the MOH in 2010, found general agreement that progress was being made in addressing this challenge, for example the establishment of the national surveillance system for mortality which is better established than the surveillance for behavioural risk factors and morbidity. There had also been an increase in national intervention demonstration programmes. However, the study also highlighted that, as in most other countries, investment in the prevention of NCDs was inadequate and underfunded. The coming ten years are a critical time for China in the prevention and control of the threat posed to the country's prosperity by the growing burden of NCDs. More attention is required to develop sustainable multi-sectoral mechanisms, rather than just having a piecemeal programmatic approach, to ensure the health of future generations.

## References


1. Ministry of Health of P.R. China. (2011) *National notifiable communicable diseases overview 2011.* Beijing: Ministry of Health of P.R. China.
2. The Lancet. Towards better health for people in China. *Lancet* 2013; 381(9882): 1959.
3. The Lancet. China's major health challenge: control of chronic diseases. *Lancet* 2011; 378: 457.
4. World Bank. (2009). *World development indicators.* Washington, DC: International Bank for Reconstruction and Development, World Bank.
5. World Health Organization. (2008). *The global burden of disease: 2004 update.* Geneva: World Health Organization.
6. World Health Organization. (2011). *Global status report on noncommunicable diseases 2010.* Geneva: World Health Organization.
7. Ministry of Health of P.R. China. (2012). *NCDs prevention and control work plan of China (2012–2015).* Beijing: Ministry of Health of P.R. China.
8. China National Center for Cardiovascular Diseases. (2010). *Report on cardiovascular disease in China, 2010.* Beijing: China National Center for Cardiovascular Diseases.
9. Yang GH, Wang Y, Zeng YX, Gao GF, *et al.* Rapid health transition in China, 1990–2010: findings from the Global Burden of Disease study 2010. *Lancet* 2013; 381(9882): 1987–2015.
10. Ministry of Health of P.R. China. (2011). *Report on chronic disease in China, 2011.* Beijing: Ministry of Health of P.R. China.
11. World Health Organization, *Burden of disease study*, 2009.
12. World Bank. Toward a Healthy and Harmonious Life in China: Stemming the Rising Tide of Non-communicable Diseases. [Online]. Available from: http://www.worldbank.org/en/news/feature/2011/07/26/toward-health-harmonious-life-china-stemming-rising-tide-of-non-communicable-diseases
13. World Health Organization. (2009). *Global health risks: mortality and burden of disease attributable to selected major risks.* Geneva: World Health Organization.
14. World Health Organization. (2010). *WHO report on the global tobacco epidemic (China report), 2010.* Geneva: World Health Organization.
15. World Health Organization. (2010). *Noncommunicable diseases country profiles 2011: WHO global report.* Geneva: World Health Organization.
16. Yang WY, Lu JM, Weng JP, *et al.* (2010). Prevalence of diabetes among men and women in China. *N Engl J Med* 362: 1090–101.
17. World Bank. (2011). *Growing 'epidemic' of heart attacks, strokes, cancer, diabetes threatens China's economic and social well-being.* World Bank.
18. Chinese Center for Disease Control and Prevention (China CDC). (2007). *China national NCD risk factor surveillance, 2007.* Beijing: China CDC.

19. Yang G, Kong L, Zhao W, *et al.* Emergence of chronic non-communicable diseases in China. *Lancet* 2008; 372: 1697–705.
20. Yang G, Fan L, Tan J, *et al.* Smoking in China: findings of the 1996 National Prevalence Survey. *JAMA* 1999; 282: 1247–53.
21. Wang H, Du S, Zhai F, Popkin BM. Trends in the distribution of body mass index among Chinese adults, aged 20–45 years (1989–2000). *Int J Obes* 2007; 31: 272–28.
22. Li JY, Liu BQ, Li GY, Chen ZJ, Sun XI, Rong SD. Atlas of cancer mortality in the People's Republic of China. An aid for cancer control and research. *Int J Epidemiol* 1981; 10: 127–33.
23. Chen JS, Campbell TC, Li JY, Peto R. (eds). *Diet, lifestyle and mortality in China: a study of the characteristics of 65 Chinese counties.* Oxford: Oxford University Press; 1990.
24. Chen JS, Peto R, Pan WH, Liu B, Campbell TC. (eds). *Mortality, biochemistry, diet and lifestyle in rural China: geographic study of the characteristics of 69 counties in mainland China and 16 areas in Taiwan.* Oxford: Oxford University Press; 2006.
25. Collins FS, Green ED, Guttmacher AE, Guyer MS. A vision for the future of genomics research. *Nature* 2003; 422: 835–47.
26. Davey Smith G, Ebrahim S, Lewis S, Hansell AL, Palmer LJ, Burton PR. Genetic epidemiology and public health: hope, hype, and future prospects. *Lancet* 2005; 366: 1484–98.
27. Hunter DJ. Gene–environment interactions in human diseases. *Nat Rev Genet* 2005; 6: 287–98.
28. Chen Z, Chen J, Collins R, *et al.* China Kadoorie Biobank of 0.5 million people: survey methods, baseline characteristics and long-term follow-up. *International Journal of Epidemiology* 2011; 40(6): 1652–66.
29. Yang GH, Kong LZ, Zhao WH, Wan X, *et al.* Emergence of chronic non-communicable diseases in China. *Lancet* 2008; 372(9650): 1697–705.
30. Mackay J, Ritthiphakdee B, Reddy KS. Tobacco control in Asia. *Lancet* 2013; 381(9877): 1581–7.
31. World Health Organization Framework Convention on Tobacco Control. China tightens rules on smoking in public places and indirect advertising. World Health Organization.
32. Centers for Disease Control and Prevention. Shaking the Salt Habit: Sodium – Hypertension Control in China. Centers for Disease Control and Prevention, USA.
33. World Health Organization. (2013). Alcohol and alcohol-related harm in China: policy changes needed. *Bulletin of the World Health Organization* 91: 270–6.
34. 3Four50. [Online]. Available from: http://www.3four50.com/
35. Story M, Kaphingst KM, Robinson-O'Brien R, *et al.* Creating healthy food and eating environments: policy and environmental approaches [J]. *Annual Review of Public Health* 2008; 29(1): 253–72.
36. Edwards P and Tsouros A. Promoting physical activity and active living in urban environments: the role of local governments. 2006. [Online]. Available from: http://www.euro.who.int/__data/assets/pdf_file/0009/98424/E89498.pdf
37. Tarlov A. Social determinants of health: the sociobiological translation. In Blane D, Brunner E, Wilkinson R (eds). *Health and social organization.* London: Routledge; 1996: 71–93.
38. The Sydney Resolution. Healthy People in Healthy Places on a Healthy Planet. Oxford Health Alliance, 27 February 2008. Available from: http://www.3four50.com/v2/index.php?page=sydney_challenge
39. Hanson M, Godfrey KM, Lillycrop KA, Burdge GC, Cluckman PD. Developmental plasticity and developmental origins of non-communicable disease: theoretical considerations and epigenetic mechanisms. *Progress in Biophysics and Molecular Biology* 2011; 106(1): 272–80.
40. World Health Organization. The implications for training of embracing: a life course approach to health. 2000. [Online]. Available from: www.who.int/ageing/publications/lifecourse/alc;lifecourse_training_en
41. Yin XJ, Shi XM, Si X, *et al.* Assessment of capacity for chronic noncommunicable diseases prevention and control of the Center for Disease Control and Prevention Organizations in China. *Chin J Epidemiol* 2010; 31(10): 1125–9.
42. O'Connor Duffany K, Finegood DT, Matthews D, McKee M, Narayan KMV, Puska P, *et al.* Community Interventions for Health (CIH): a novel approach to tackling the worldwide epidemic of chronic disease. *CVD Prevent Control* 2011; 6(2): 47–56.

43. Global Health Policy Forum. Global Health Policy Summit 2012: report of the inaugural meeting 1 August 2012, London. Report of the Global Health Policy Summit 2012. [Online]. Available from: https://workspace.imperial.ac.uk/global-health-innovation/Public/GHPS_2012_Summit_Report.pdf
44. Lv J, Liu M, Jiang Y, Li LM. Prevention and control of major non-communicable diseases in China from 1990 to 2009: results of a two-round Delphi survey. Global Health Action 2013. [Online]. Available from: http://dx.doi.org/10.3402/gha.v6i0.20004

# 33

# Mental health as a public health concern

*Samuel Y. S. Wong*

> Mental health and mental well being are fundamental to the quality of life and productivity of individuals, families, communities and nations, enabling people to experience life as meaningful and to be creative and active citizens. [1]

## Introduction: mental health problem as a public health problem

The World Health Organization (WHO) defines mental health as 'a state of well-being in which every individual realizes his or her own potential, can cope with the normal stresses of life, can work productively and fruitfully, and is able to make a contribution to her or his community' [2]. However, it is mental disorders that are often the subject of research and investigation rather than mental health, especially among clinical researchers and epidemiologists who study the epidemiology of common mental disorders, the burden associated with mental disorders, as well as deciding on the need for treatment of those suffering from mental disorders among clinicians.

At present, there are two well-established systems and classification of mental disorders with the two different systems having converged in the more recent revisions. Chapter V of the International Classification of Disease (tenth edition) published by the WHO describes the classification of mental and behavioural disorders and has categorized all mental disorders into ten main groups [3]. Another classification system, the Diagnostic and Statistical Manual for Mental Disorders (DSM), published by the American Psychiatric Association, describes the diagnostic criteria for more than 290 mental disorders. Recently, the DSM-5 Task Force for the DSM-V5 Diagnostic and Statistical Manual for Mental Disorders V [4] (published May 2013) has further revised the definition of the term 'Mental Disorder' and defined it as:

> A Mental Disorder is a health condition characterized by significant dysfunction in an individual's cognitions, emotions, or behaviours that reflects a disturbance in the psychological, biological, or developmental process underlying mental functioning. Some disorders may not be diagnosable until they have caused significant distress or impairment of performance.

A mental disorder is not merely an expectable or culturally sanctioned response to a specific event such as the death of a loved one. Neither culturally deviant behaviour (e.g. political, religious, or sexual) nor a conflict that is primarily between the individual and society is a mental disorder unless the deviance or conflict results from a dysfunction in the individual, as described above [4].

## The magnitude of the public health problem

### *Epidemiology and burden of mental health problems*

It has been established that around 14 per cent of the global burden of disease can be attributed to neuropsychiatric disorders [5], with the majority of this burden coming from common mental disorders that include chronic major depression, alcohol use, substance abuse, dementia and schizophrenia, and one in four people will develop one or more mental or behavioural disorders during their lifetime [6]. One of the methods that can be used to measure the burden associated with disability from diseases is the Disability Adjusted Life Years (DALYs). This is measured as the sum of years lived with the disability and years of life lost associated with a given condition, and is often used as a measure of disease burden in mental health related disorders. Mental and neurological disorders were shown to account for 13 per cent of the total DALYs lost due to all diseases and injuries worldwide [7]. Major depression, one of the most common mental disorders, is expected to be second only to cardiovascular disease, which is predicted to be the leading cause of DALYs by the year 2020. It alone will account for 5.7 per cent of DALYs worldwide.

Although a previous survey conducted by the WHO in 2004 [8] reported the 12-month prevalence of any mental disorder in China (Beijing and Shanghai) to be 9.1 per cent and 4.3 per cent respectively, a more recent report on an epidemiological survey by Phillips *et al.* in 2009 [9] in four provinces in China reported a much higher prevalence of mental disorders, with the one-month prevalence of any mental disorder being 17.5 per cent, while the prevalence of mood disorders being around 6 per cent, anxiety disorders being 5.6 per cent with psychotic disorders being 1 per cent.

In addition to disability, mental disorders are also associated with an increased risk of mortality, in particular, the impact of mental disorders on the occurrence of intentional injury and non-intentional injury. A systematic review [10] showed that mental disorders (depression, schizophrenia and other psychoses, and alcohol-use and substance-use disorders) are important immediate risk factors for suicide, with the median prevalence of mental disorders reaching 91 per cent among those who committed suicide, with similar reported findings observed in India [11] and China [12].

One of the problems in Asia with respect to mental health and mental disorders is that they often go under-treated. Indeed, Asia is one of the regions cited by the WHO as the area with both a lack of resources and treatments for mental health disorders especially in the community. In a recent publication series by *The Lancet* [13], the authors highlighted the lack of infrastructure, resources including drugs and mental health professionals, as well as a lack of integrated health policies aiming to improve mental health in many parts of the world especially among middle- and low-income countries in Africa and Asia.

### *Non-communicable diseases and mental health problems*

The WHO defines health as 'a state of complete physical, mental and social well being and not merely the absence of diseases or infirmity' [14]. Thus, we need to know that good health also includes good mental health functioning. Physical, mental and social functioning are interrelated, and evidence shows that physical illness can increase the risk of having mental illnesses and vice versa. This is especially important when non-communicable diseases (NCDs) are becoming the leading cause of death and morbidity worldwide [15]. For example, it has been shown that major depression is a risk factor for the development and progression of both physical and social disability [16, 17] while disability increases a person's risk for developing major depression among older adults [18, 19].

### *Depression and cardiovascular and cerebrovascular diseases*

The relationship between depression and cardiovascular diseases is bidirectional and seems to occur in both Western and Asian countries. For example, in Hong Kong, among first time stroke patients [20], it has been shown that 17 per cent were diagnosed with post-stroke depression. Similarly, in China, among a sample of Chinese elderly living in a rural community [21], and using a structured and validated questionnaire that measured clinically relevant depressive symptoms, it has been shown that up to 62 per cent could be classified as suffering from clinically relevant depressive symptoms. For acute coronary syndrome, a study conducted in China [22] among more than 600 patients with coronary diseases showed that 46 per cent had clinically relevant depressive symptoms although some of these symptoms improved when the cardiac conditions improved. Similarly, a cohort study conducted in Korea showed [23] that the presence of heart disease was significantly associated with incidence of late-life depression in the community-dwelling elderly. In Hong Kong, it has also been shown in a large cohort of Chinese elderly that the presence of peripheral vascular disease [24] was associated with increased odds of having clinically relevant depressive symptoms.

Population-based studies have shown that the presence of depression and anxiety is associated with an increased risk of coronary heart disease including angina and myocardial infarction [25]. Similarly, population-based studies have demonstrated that depression is also related to an increased risk of stroke [26, 27], independent of other risk factors for cardiovascular diseases.

Among patients who suffer from a non-fatal myocardial infarction, the presence of depression among those patients is consistently shown to increase the risk of adverse outcomes, including the recurrence of cardiac events and both cardiovascular specific events. It has also been shown that all these can cause mortality [25]. In addition, the presence of myocardial infarction also increases the incidence of depression [28]. In terms of strokes, evidence shows that there is a significant and strong relationship between the presence of a stroke and a subsequent development of depression [29, 30, 31]. Similarly, the coexistence of depression among stroke survivors is associated with poorer outcomes and increased mortality [32, 33].

### *Depression and diabetes mellitus*

Although the prospective relationship between depression and diabetes mellitus is not established, there is ample evidence for the coexistence of depression among people with diabetes mellitus. A meta-analysis of 20 controlled studies shows that the odds of having depression among people with diabetes mellitus is about 2.0 [34].

In Hong Kong, an epidemiological study [35] showed that the prevalence of depression among elderly Chinese who suffered from diabetes mellitus was higher with a prevalence of

26 per cent. Similarly, in Malaysia, a study [36] of more than 500 diabetic outpatients found that the prevalence of depressive symptoms was around 31 per cent.

Evidence shows that people who are affected with diabetes mellitus and co-morbid depression have a poorer compliance of diabetic medication [37], poorer self-care [38, 39] and have poorer glycemic control when compared to people with diabetes mellitus but without co-morbid depression or anxiety [40]. Moreover, it has been consistently shown that people suffering from diabetes mellitus and also with co-morbid depression or anxiety are also associated with an increased risk of diabetes complications [41], as well as increased mortality [42].

According to Prince *et al.* [5], several mechanisms can account for the association between mental disorders (i.e. depression) and chronic medical conditions. Mental disorders can affect the occurrence of medical conditions by:

- Sharing common genetic or environmental risk factors;
- Being associated with unhealthy behaviours such as cigarette smoking, alcohol consumption, poor diet and reduced physical activity; and
- Exerting their biological effects, such as the effects on serotonin metabolism, cortisol metabolism, inflammatory process and cell-mediated immunity.

Medical conditions can also affect the occurrence of mental disorders by:

- Direct effects of disease process on the brain including infections, cerebrovascular diseases, diabetes, substance abuse with impact on cognitive impairment, and mood and behavioural disturbance; and
- The psychological burden exerted by the presence of chronic conditions, including the difficulty in adjusting to the illness, functional decline, changes in social environment and relationships due to the presence of illnesses, and adverse symptoms associated with illnesses, such as the presence of pain, disability and side effects from medications.

Mental conditions can affect the treatment adherence and patients' outcomes of chronic physical conditions by:

- Delaying help-seeking, detection and treatment of chronic conditions;
- Receiving poorer quality of medical care due to the presence of coexisting mental conditions; and
- Affecting the adherence of medical regimens and the compliance of behavioural modification and health promoting activities suggested by healthcare or public health providers.

Figure 33.1 shows the co-morbidity of major depression and other chronic conditions.

## Preventing mental disorders

There are three types of prevention methods in mental health [46]:

1. Universal, for a whole population in a group with all levels of risk;
2. Selective, for select individuals with demonstrated increased risk of developing illness; and
3. Indicated, addressing high-risk individuals with pre-morbid signs and symptoms.

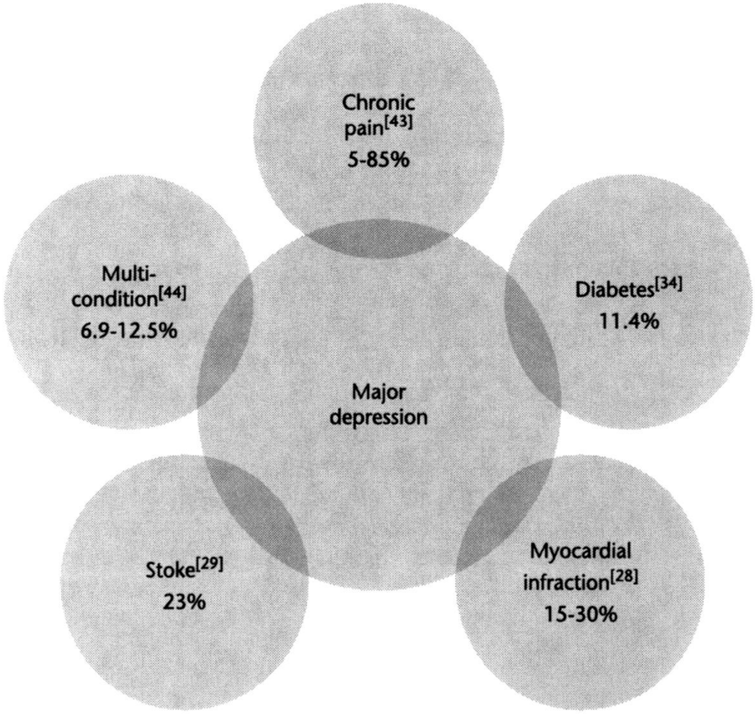


*Figure 33.1* Co-morbidity of major depression and other chronic conditions [28, 29, 34, 43, 44]

Although universal mental health preventive intervention is the ultimate goal, it is suggested that the most cost-effective goal is to identify a population at sufficiently high risk to justify the expense of intervention, as well as to shorten the duration of the persistence of the early symptoms, and to stop the progression of severity so that the person does not meet the diagnostic levels of mental problems and does not suffer from the associated impact on their social and occupational functioning [47]. Evidence from a meta-analysis showed that well-designed indicated interventions were effective and could reduce the incidence of common mental disorders, such as depression and anxiety disorders [48]. These studies also showed that these interventions were likely to be more cost-effective than alternative approaches [49, 50].

Recently, the WHO has advocated for integrating mental health into primary care, which can be considered a selective approach for preventive intervention. Indeed, mental health problems are commonly encountered in primary care and many people who are seen in the primary care settings are at a higher risk for the development of mental disorders when compared to the risk for the general population. For example, studies showed that a mental health problem can account for up to 40 per cent of consultations and is the sole reason for attending in 20–25 per cent of consultations in the UK [51]. In addition to being a common presentation in primary care, the strong association between the presence of mental disorders or problems among people with physical health conditions is also one of the reasons that can explain the high prevalence of mental health problems in primary care.

There are several advantages for integrating mental health into primary care to provide preventive interventions in primary care [52]. These are summarized below:

- Since multi-morbidity (the presence of two or more chronic conditions in a person) is a common phenomenon in primary care, providing preventive interventions in the primary care setting may improve early detection and treatment of mental health problems, especially for people with multiple chronic conditions who are at a higher risk for developing mental health problems. The generalist primary care providers can also address mental, physical and social aspects of care at the same time, addressing mental health symptoms in the context of social life stress and distress in patients using the bio-psycho-social model rather than strictly adhering to the medical model.
- Medically unexplained symptoms (MUS) are one of the common presentations in primary care and people affected by MUS are often frequent attendees of primary care. Many of these patients also suffer from mental health problems and it makes primary care the ideal setting to treat their co-morbid mental health problems.
- Many people are unwilling to talk about their mental health problems and are often worried about the stigma of being diagnosed or treated for mental illness. This makes many people affected unwilling to seek psychiatric care or refuse to be referred to psychiatrists or psychologists. Since patients often have continuing relationships with their primary care providers, or a continuing longitudinal relationship with a particular primary care group or practice team, treating mental health problems in primary care may make it less stigmatizing for patients and the long-term relationship with primary care providers may make patients more willing to disclose their mental health issues to their primary care providers.

### *An example of an integrated primary care mental health programme: the stepped care approach for depression*

As the demand for psychological intervention often exceeds the supply of mental health services, the use of a stepped care approach for mental health problems is one of the solutions to the imbalance in supply and demand for mental health services. The stepped care model may be the most cost-effective model in this system where the effectiveness of interventions is maximized while making the best use of available resources [54–56].

People have various degrees and severity of depressive symptoms so not all of them will need the same type or intensity of mental health interventions. For people with very mild or sub-threshold depressive symptoms, some of their symptoms may disappear without any intervention, and watchful waiting and monitoring by primary care providers may be the best intervention for them. In addition, some of these patients might be able to be helped by simple self-help interventions, such as reading a self-help book or watching a video on psycho-education of depression (Steps 1–2). For those with mild to moderate symptoms, patients may benefit from a brief telephone psycho-education or problem-solving treatment conducted by a paraprofessional or mental health professional (Step 2). Others with more severe symptoms may require more intensive individual or group problem-solving treatment or psychological treatment, or the initiation of medications (Step 3). Those with even more severe symptoms (moderate to severe) may require even more intensive individual psychological treatment with pharmacotherapy by medical doctors (mental health workers and psychiatrists working together with primary care providers). Among those with atypical psychological problems, resistant depression or persisting depression despite medical and psychological treatment or with immediate risk to life, a specialized mental health team, including psychiatrists and crisis intervention, may be needed with more complex interventions (Step 4). The stepped care model seems to be a logical approach from both clinical, public health and economic perspectives (see Figure 33.2 for the NICE stepped care approach for depression management).

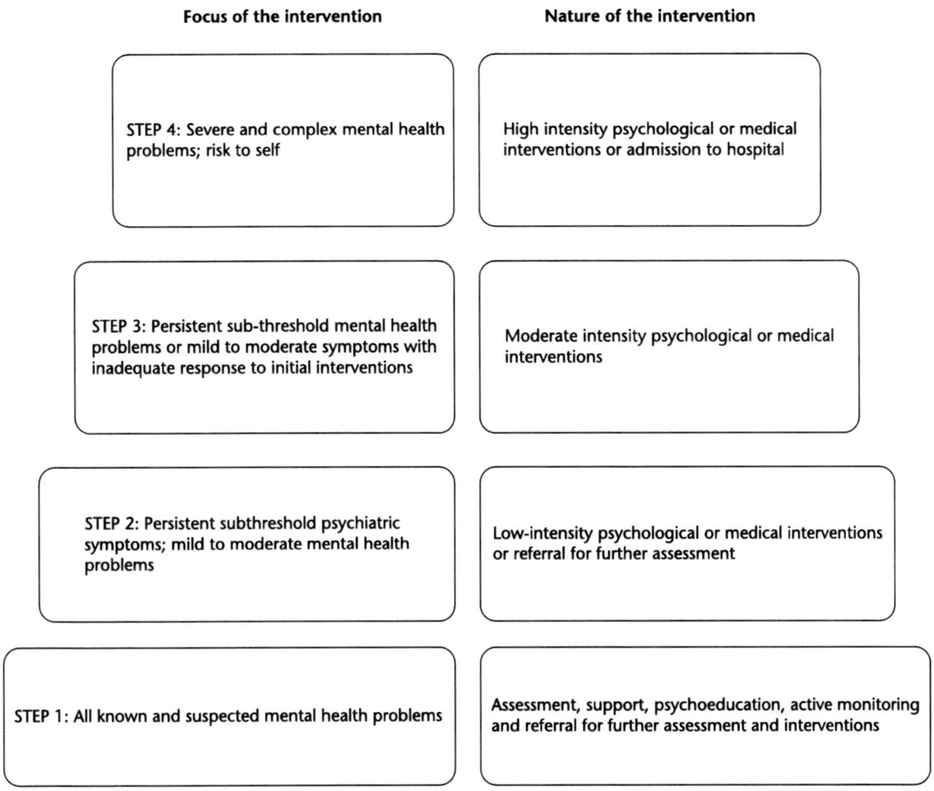


*Figure 33.2* NICE stepped care approach for depression management (modified) [53]

## *Collaborative care approach for managing depression*

Collaborative care for depression is a complex intervention that involves a multidisciplinary team approach with case management for depression. The majority of evidence for the effectiveness of a collaborative care approach for managing depression comes from the USA where a number of clinical trials have been conducted. Some of the better-known ones are the IMPACT [57] and Pathways projects [53, 58]. These studies demonstrated the superiority of the collaborative approach for depression when compared to usual care in the improvement of depression outcomes while the Pathways project specifically looked into the effectiveness of a collaborative care approach among people with coexisting chronic medical illness.

One of the key features of a collaborative approach for managing depression is the use of a case manager with the support of a liaison/consultant psychiatrist and the involvement of family doctors/primary care doctors. The case managers in these studies are usually trained nurses with specific training in case management and psychological interventions. The case managers are very important in the collaborative care approach for depression as they act as coordinators with the responsibility to work closely with patients (provide interpersonal continuity of care) to advise and supervise the appropriate interventions, monitor the patient's symptoms and problems with adjustment of interventions, as well as directly deliver some of the lower intensity psychological interventions. In these interventions, a

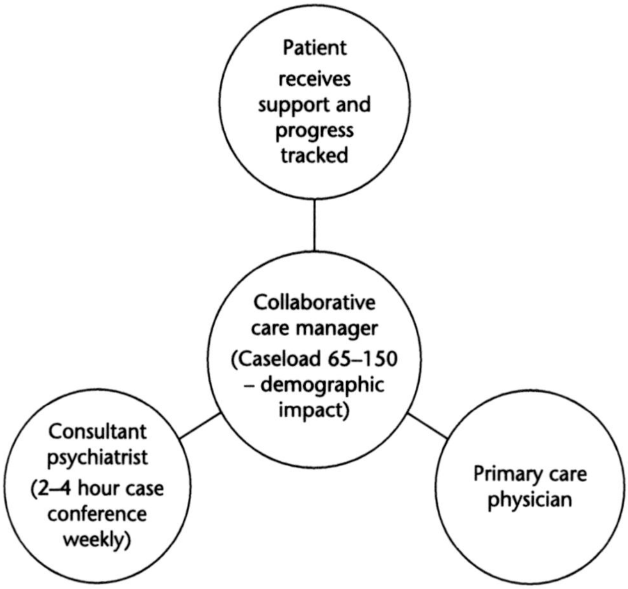


*Figure 33.3* Impact model [53]

combination of both face-to-face and telephone contact, differing in frequency, were usually used (see Figure 33.3).

## Promoting mental health

Mental health promotion refers to interventions or strategies aimed at promoting mental well-being or positive mental health by increasing psychological well-being, competence and resilience. Mental health promotion activities address and intervene on the determinants of mental health by creating the individual, social and environmental conditions that enable optimal psychological development [59, 60]. It should be noted that although mental health promotion aims at increasing positive mental health, this is often associated with the secondary outcome of decreasing the incidence of mental health disorders in the community as positive mental health is considered a powerful protective factor against the occurrence of mental disorders. Often the prevention of mental disorders and positive mental health are described as two overlapping and related components of a single concept of mental health [61] (see Figure 33.4).

## Social, environmental and economic determinants of mental health

People living in poor social environments and those with lower socio-economic statuses are found to have increased risk for poor mental health, depression as well as lower self-perceived well-being [62]. Other factors such as war and displacement, racial discrimination and unstable employment and income have also been shown to be related to higher levels

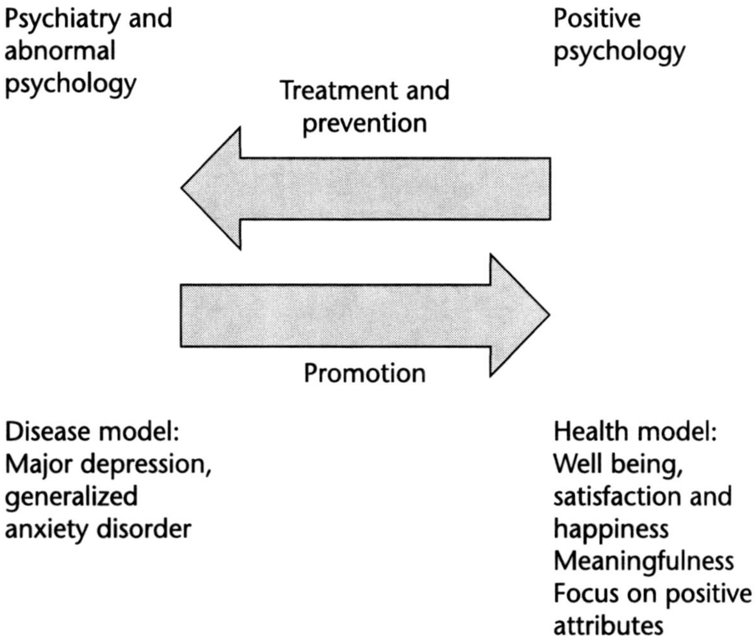


*Figure 33.4* Mental health promotion and mental health problem treatment and prevention

of psychological symptoms and psychiatric disorders [63]. For example, the health of migrant factory workers in China (see Box 33.1) has been an important research area due to the large migrant population in China, especially migrants who move from poorer areas to more urbanized ones. The association of being a migrant worker and mental health has been studied by Mou *et al.* in 2010 [64]. The researchers found that the prevalence of depressive symptoms was high with a prevalence of 21 per cent among more than 4,000 migrant workers and factors, such as mobility, job arrangement and self-rated health, were associated with clinically relevant depressive symptoms (see Table 33.1 for a summary of evidence-based social, environmental and economic determinants of mental health).

*Table 33.1* Some examples of social and environmental determinants of mental health

| *Risk factors* | *Protective factors* |
|---|---|
| Poor socio-economic status | Social support |
| War and displacement | Good community network |
| Racial discrimination | Positive interpersonal relationships |
| Unstable employment | Economic stability |
| Unstable income | Social justice |
| Social disadvantage | |

*Source*: [60, 62–64].

### Box 33.1 Suicide in the workplace – a case study among migrant workers in Foxconn, China

Between January and May 2010, 13 young workers at two Foxconn production facilities in southern China attempted to commit, or committed, suicide. Foxconn is the world's largest contract electronics manufacturer with customers that included Apple, HP, Dell, IBM, Samsung, Nokia, Hitachi and other electronic giants. However, within a short period of time in 2010, 13 young workers at two production facilities in Shenzhen attempted suicide, with ten dying and three sustaining significant injuries.

What factors might have been related to this dramatic incidence of suicide at Foxconn? Management at the company claimed the deaths were primarily related to the immaturity and rather feeble state of mind of the young rural migrants. However, researchers [45] have identified several social factors that might have been related to the suicides at Foxconn, including working conditions, management style and wage policies. Migrant workers at the company work and live on the campuses provided. A significant proportion of a worker's monthly total wage is from doing overtime and employees experience long hours of repetitive work for a low income that hardly makes ends meet. Moreover, the management style at Foxconn, it has been suggested, is 'military-like'. For example, one plant has recruited more than 1,000 security guards to keep internal order with guards standing by 24 hours a day at checkpoints in both factory building and dormitory, and all employees, whether going to the toilet or canteen, must be checked. Reports in the media about detention, abuse and use of violence by security were not uncommon. Many workers rarely stop working except to sleep or eat. This has made workers suffer tremendous stress with limited resources and free time which may have increased the risk for depression and suicide.

Most of the migrant workers came from rural China to work in factories within urban cities, such as Shenzhen, often wishing to make money to improve their rural family's living conditions. There is often a huge discrepancy between these migrant workers' high expectations and the harsh reality of their lives in the factories. The pressure of being away from home with little support and care from their work environment and society may have contributed to emotional problems among this group.

## *Recommendations for the future of mental health in Asia*

Mental health problems are common and they tend to occur more frequently among people with multiple or coexisting chronic conditions. With the increasing burden of non-communicable diseases both in developing and developed countries in Asia, the traditional disease-specific approach (i.e. managing mental health problems separately from other chronic conditions) may not be feasible due to limited healthcare costs, especially in developing countries. The development of integrated primary care services that include the holistic management of both mental health and other chronic conditions of individuals may be the most feasible and cost-effective way to deal with the increasing burden of mental health problems.

## Conclusion: summary points

- Mental health problems are prevalent in the community with the most common problem being major depression.
- Many mental health problems are associated with significant disability and morbidity.
- There is a high co-morbidity and multi-morbidity of mental health problems with other chronic medical conditions, making it important to manage these problems together.
- Integrated primary mental health care is an effective way to deal with the increasing burden of mental health problems especially in the community settings, although resources are specifically lacking in developing countries in Asia and Africa.
- The stepped care and collaborative care approaches for common mental health problems could be a cost-effective way to manage mental health problems.

### *Sample self-reflective exercises*

- What is the difference between mental health and mental health problems? What is the relationship between the two concepts?
- What are the reasons for integrating mental health care into primary care? Describe one model that has been shown to be cost-effective.
- What are the mechanisms that can explain the high co-morbidity between chronic medical conditions and mental health problems?

## References


1. WHO. Mental health: facing the challenges, building solutions. Report from the WHO European Ministerial Conference. Copenhagen: WHO Regional Office for Europe, 2005.
2. WHO. Mental health: a state of well-being. Available at: http://www.who.int/features/factfiles/mental_health/en/index.html [Accessed 5 November 2012].
3. WHO. International Statistical Classification of Diseases and Related Health Problems, 10th revision. Geneva: World Health Organization; 1992–94.
4. American Psychiatric Association. DSM-V Development: Definition of a mental disorder. Available at: http://www.dsm5.org/Pages/Default.aspx [Accessed 5 November 2012].
5. Prince M, Patel V, Saxena S, *et al.* No health without mental health. *Lancet* 2007; 370: 859–77.
6. WHO. The world health report 2001: Mental health: new understanding, new hope. World Health Organization; 2001.
7. WHO. The world health report 2004: Changing history. World Health Organization; 2004.
8. The WHO World Mental Health Survey Consortium. Prevalence, severity, and unmet need for treatment of mental disorders in the World Health Organization World Mental Health Surveys. *JAMA* 2004; 291: 2581–90.
9. Phillips MR, Zhang J, Shi Q, *et al.* Prevalence, treatment, and associated disability of mental disorders in four provinces in China during 2001–5: an epidemiological survey. *Lancet* 2009; 373: 2041–53.
10. Cavanagh JT, Carson AJ, Sharpe M, Lawrie SM. Psychological autopsy studies of suicide: a systematic review. *Psychol Med* 2003; 33(3): 395–405.
11. Vijayakumar L, Rajkumar S. Are risk factors for suicide universal? A case-control study in India. *Acta Psychiatr Scand* 1999; 99(6): 407–11.
12. Phillips MR, Yang G, Zhang Y, *et al.* Risk factors for suicide in China: a national cross-sectional psychological autopsy study. *Lancet* 2002; 360: 1728–36.
13. Saxena S, Thornicroft G, Knapp M, Whiteford H. Resources for mental health: scarcity, inequity, and inefficiency. *Lancet* 2007; 370: 878–89.

14. WHO. Basic Documents. 43rd edition. Geneva: World Health Organization; 2001: 1.
15. Mathers CD, Loncar D. Projections of global mortality and burden of disease from 2002 to 2030. *PLoS Med* 2006; 3(11): e442.
16. Bruce ML, Seeman TE, Merrill SS, Blazer DG. The impact of depressive symptomatology on physical disability: MacArthur Studies of Successful Aging. *Am J Public Health* 1994; 84(11): 1796–9.
17. Penninx BW, Guralnik JM, Ferrucci L, *et al.* Depressive symptoms and physical decline in community-dwelling older persons. *JAMA* 1998; 279(21): 1720–6.
18. Cole MG, Dendukuri N. Risk factors for depression among elderly community subjects: a systematic review and meta-analysis. *Am J Psychiatry* 2003; 160(6): 1147–56.
19. Braam AW, Prince MJ, Beekman AT, *et al.* Physical health and depressive symptoms in older Europeans. Results from EURODEP. *Br J Psychiatry* 2005; 187: 35–42.
20. Wai-Kwong Tang WK, Ungvari GS, Chiu HFK, *et al.* Psychiatric morbidity in first time stroke patients in Hong Kong: a pilot study in a rehabilitation unit. *Australian and New Zealand Journal of Psychiatry* 2002; 36: 544–9.
21. Fuh JL, Liu HC, Wang SJ. Poststroke depression among the Chinese elderly in a rural community. *Stroke* 1997; 28: 1126–9.
22. Ma W, Hu D, Liu G, *et al.* Predictors of quality of life in Chinese patients with acute coronary syndrome. *Asian Cardiovasc Thorac Ann* 2010; 18: 469–75.
23. Kim JM, Stewart R, Kim SW, *et al.* Vascular risk factors and incident late-life depression in a Korean population. *British Journal of Psychiatry* 2006; 189: 26–30.
24. Wong SYS, Woo J, Hong AWL, *et al.* Clinically relevant depressive symptoms and peripheral arterial disease in elderly men and women. Results from a large cohort study in Southern China. *Journal of Psychosomatic Research* 2007; 63: 471–6.
25. Hemingway H, Marmot M. Evidence-based cardiology: psychosocial factors in the aetiology and prognosis of coronary heart disease. Systematic review of prospective cohort studies. *BMJ* 1999; 318: 1460–7.
26. Larson SL, Owens PL, Ford D, Eaton W. Depressive disorder, dysthymia, risk of stroke: thirteen year follow-up from the Baltimore epidemiologic catchment area study. *Stroke* 2001; 32(9): 1979–83.
27. Ohira T, Iso H, Satoh S, *et al.* Prospective study of depressive symptoms and risk of stroke among Japanese. *Stroke* 2001; 32(4): 903–8.
28. Strik JJ, Lousberg R, Cheriex EC, Honig A. One year cumulative incidence of depression following myocardial infarction and impact on cardiac outcome. *J Psychosom Res* 2004; 56(1): 59–66.
29. Aben I, Lodder J, Honig A, *et al.* Focal or generalized vascular brain damage and vulnerability to depression after stroke: a 1 year prospective study. *Int Psychogeriatr* 2006; 18(1): 19–35.
30. Kim JM, Stewart R, Kim SW, *et al.* Vascular risk factors and incident late-life depression in a Korean population. *Br J Psychiatry* 2006; 189: 26–30.
31. Whyte EM, Mulsant BH, Vanderbilt J, *et al.* Depression after stroke: a prospective epidemiological study. *J Am Geriatr Soc* 2004; 52(5): 774–8.
32. Chemerinski E, Robinson RG, Kosier JT. Improved recovery in activities of daily living associated with remission of poststroke depression. *Stroke* 2001; 32(1): 113–17.
33. Morris PL, Robinson RG, Andrzejewski P, *et al.* Association of depression with 10-year poststroke mortality. *Am J Psychiatry* 1993; 150(1): 124–9.
34. Anderson RJ, Freedland KE, Clouse RE, Lustman PJ. The prevalence of comorbid depression in adults with diabetes: a meta-analysis. *Diabetes Care* 2001; 24(6): 1069–78.
35. Chou KL, Chi I. Prevalence of depression among elderly Chinese with diabetes. *Int J Geriatr Psychiatry* 2005; 20: 570–5.
36. Chong SA, Subramaniam M, Chan YH, *et al.* Depressive symptoms and diabetes mellitus in an Asian multiracial population. *Asian Journal of Psychiatry* 2009; 2: 66–70.
37. Ciechanowski PS, Katon WJ, Russo JE. Depression and diabetes: impact of depressive symptoms on adherence, function, and costs. *Arch Intern Med* 2000; 160(21): 3278–85.
38. Lin EH, Katon W, Von KM, *et al.* Relationship of depression and diabetes self-care, medication adherence, and preventive care. *Diabetes Care* 2004; 27(9): 2154–60.
39. McKeller JD, Humphreys K, Piette JD. Depression increases diabetes symptoms by complicating patients' self-care adherence. *Diabetes Educ* 2004; 30(3): 485–92.
40. Lustman PJ, Anderson RJ, Freedland KE, *et al.* Depression and poor glycemic control: a meta-analytic review of the literature. *Diabetes Care* 2000; 23(7): 934–42.

41. De Groot M, Anderson R, Freedland KE, *et al.* Association of depression and diabetes complications: a meta-analysis. *Psychosom Med* 2001; 63(4): 619–30.
42. Katon WJ, Rutter C, Simon G, *et al.* The association of comorbid depression with mortality in patients with type 2 diabetes. *Diabetes Care* 2005; 28(11): 2668–72.
43. Kessler RC, Zhao S, Blazer DG, Swartz M. Prevalence, correlates, and course of minor depression and major depression in the National Comorbidity Survey. *J Affect Disord* 1997; 45(1–2): 19–30.
44. Bair MJ, Robinson RL, Katon W, Kroenke K. Depression and pain comorbidity: a literature review. INTERMED 2003; 163(20): 2433–45.
45. Chan J, Ngai P. Suicide as protest for the new generation of Chinese migrant workers: Foxconn, global capital and the state. *Asia-Pacific Journal* 2010; 37(2): 10.
46. Mrazek PJ, Haggerty RJ (eds). *Reducing risks for mental disorders: frontiers for preventive intervention research.* Washington, DC: National Academy Press; 1994.
47. Haggerty M, *Medicine I: reducing risks for mental disorders.* Washington, DC, National Academy Press; 1994.
48. Cuijpers P, Van Straten A, Smit F. Preventing the incidence of new cases of mental disorders: a meta-analytic review. *J Nerv Ment Dis* 2005; 193(2): 119–25.
49. Simt F, Ederveen A, Cuijpers P, *et al.* Opportunities for cost-effective prevention of late-life depression: an epidemiological approach. *Arch Gen Psychiatry* 2006; 63(3): 290–6.
50. Van't Veer-Tazelaar PJ, van Marwijk HW, van Oppen P, *et al.* Stepped-care prevention of anxiety and depression in later life: a randomized controlled trial. *Arch Gen Psychiatry* 2009; 66(3): 297–304.
51. Goldberg D, Huxley P. *Common mental disorders: a bio-social model.* London: Routledge, 1992.
52. Lester H, Glasby J, Tylee A. Integrated primary mental health care: threat of opportunity in the new NHS? *Br J Gen Pract* 2004; 54(501): 285–91.
53. Primary Care Commissioning. Collaborative Care Report Phase 1. NHS; 2010.
54. Haaga DA. Introduction to the special section on stepped care models in psychotherapy. *J Consult Clin Psychol* 2000; 68(4): 547–8.
55. Hunkeler EM, Katon W, Tang L, *et al.* Long-term outcomes from the IMPACT randomised trial for depressed elderly patients in primary care. *BMJ* 2006; 332: 259–63.
56. Van't Veer-Tazelaar PJ, van Marwijk HW, van Oppen P, *et al.* Prevention of anxiety and depression in the age group of 75 years and over: a randomized controlled trial testing the feasibility and effectiveness of a generic stepped care programme among elderly community residents at high risk of developing anxiety and depression versus usual care. *BMC Public Health* 2006; 6: 186–94.
57. Unutzer J, Katon W, Callahan CM, *et al.* Collaborative care management of late-life depression in the primary care setting: a randomized controlled trial. *JAMA* 2002; 288(22): 2836–45.
58. Katon WJ, Von Korff M, Lin EH, *et al.* The Pathways study: a randomised controlled trial of collaborative care in patients with diabetes and depression. *Arch Gen Psychiatry* 2004; 61(10): 1042–9.
59. Hosman C, Jane-Llopis E. Political challenges 2: mental health. In: *The evidence of health promotion effectiveness: shaping public health in a new Europe.* Brussels, ECSC-EC-EAEC; 1999, pp. 29–31.
60. Hosman C, Jane-Llopis E, Saxena S (eds). *Prevention of mental disorders: effective interventions and policy options.* Oxford, Oxford University Press; 2005.
61. Detels R, *et al* (eds). *Oxford textbook of public health.* 3rd edn. Oxford, Oxford University Press; 2002.
62. Patel V, Jane-Llopis E. Poverty, social exclusion and disadvantages groups. In: Hosman C, Jane-Llopis E, Saxena S (eds) *Prevention of mental disorders: effective interventions and policy options.* Oxford, Oxford University Press; 2005.
63. Musisi S, Mollica R, Weiss M. Supporting refugees and victims of war. In: Hosman C, Jane-Llopis E, Saxena S (eds) *Prevention of mental disorders: effective interventions and policy options.* Oxford, Oxford University Press; 2005.
64. Mou J. Health of migrant factory workers in Shenzhen, China: mobility, self-reported health and healthcare utilisation. PhD thesis. Chinese University of Hong Kong; 2010.

# 34

# Controlling the tobacco epidemic

## Lessons from Hong Kong

*Judith Mackay, T. H. Lam and Sophia S. C. Chan*

### Introduction

This chapter uses tobacco control in Hong Kong as an example of public health policy development, the support of civil society and the role of advocacy, and suggests that these actions are ubiquitous in public health in Asia and worldwide. The chapter examines the history of tobacco control in Hong Kong and draws out principles as to how this has led to the present low smoking prevalence rates, the players involved, factors that have been influential, obstacles, lessons learned and the next steps which need to be taken, leading to an eventual end-game scenario for tobacco use.

### The history of tobacco control in Hong Kong

#### *An early start*

Hong Kong initiated tobacco control measures in the 1970s (see Table 34.1). The then British colonial government benefited from the experience of tobacco control measures in the United Kingdom and could also observe such measures being introduced in Singapore. Key tobacco control advocates were also active from the early 1980s [1] and the Hong Kong Council on Smoking and Health (the first government-funded council in Asia) was established in 1987, with one of the authors, Judith Mackay, its founding Executive Director. International non-governmental organizations (NGOs), such as the Union for International Cancer Control (UICC), in conjunction with the Hong Kong Anti-Cancer Society, ran tobacco control meetings and workshops, for example the 1981 conference on 'Cancer Education in Schools' and the 1983 seminar on 'Smoking and its Effects on Health'.

#### *The next stage*

After the initial introduction of health education in schools, the government and civil society soon realized that this alone was insufficient to deal with the growing tobacco pandemic, and that it could only be reduced by introducing comprehensive tobacco control policies and

*Table 34.1* Key events in tobacco control, Hong Kong

| | |
|---|---|
| ***1970s*** | |
| Late 1970s | Government introduces health education against smoking. |
| ***1980s*** | |
| 1982 | First tobacco control law: Smoking (Public Health) Ordinance No. 58 (followed by 4 further amendments in 1983–1987).<br>Smoking partially banned in public transport, some public places and places of entertainment.<br>All cigarette packets to carry single health warning and tar group designation.<br>All cigarette advertisements to carry health warning and tar group (with a few exemptions). |
| 1983 | Establishment of no-smoking areas in schools, hospitals, clinics and food business premises, and public waiting areas of government offices. |
| 1983 | Tobacco Institute of HK established by the tobacco companies (dissolved in 2005). |
| 1983 | HK Anti-Cancer Society and HK Government Education Department seminar on 'Smoking and its Effects on Health'. |
| 1984+ | First celebration of annual no-smoking day. |
| 1980s | HK Fire Services Department estimate about 33% of all fires are caused by careless smoking. |
| 1987 | Smokeless Tobacco Products (Prohibition) Regulations: ban on manufacture, importation and sale of smokeless tobacco (first in Asia). |
| 1987 | HK Council on Smoking and Health (COSH) established, the first government-funded council in Asia. |
| 1988 | Public opinion surveys on various aspects of tobacco used to influence government, employers and public opinion. |
| ***1990s*** | |
| 1990 | Tobacco advertising on TV and radio banned. |
| 1990s | NGO anti-smoking groups established:<br>Asian Consultancy on Tobacco Control (1990)<br>ASH (Action on Smoking and Health) (1993)<br>PASS (People Acting for a Smokeless Society) (1994–2000)<br>Clear the Air (1997). |
| 1994 | World Health Organization (WHO) Tobacco or Health medal awarded to Cathay Pacific Airways for becoming 100% smoke-free. |
| 1995 | Survey reports recognition of cigarette brand names and logos by young children (Peters *et al.* 1995: 150–5) [2]. |
| 1995 | Education Department launched Anti-smoking teaching kit. |
| 1995 | First survey on economic effects of smoking (Tsang 1995: 482) [3]. |
| 1996 | Ban on smoking in government premises. |
| 1997 | Smoking (Public Health) (Amendment) Ordinance 1997 (implemented in stages)<br>– Extension of advertising bans<br>– Bans cigarette vending machines<br>– Bans smoking in public areas in department stores, shopping malls, supermarkets, banks<br>– No smoking areas of one-third of seats in restaurants over 200 seats<br>– Bans on packets containing less than 20 cigarettes<br>– Lowering maximum tar level from 20 mg to 17 mg<br>– Banning terms like 'mild' unless < 9 mg tar. |

(*Continued overleaf*)

*Table 34.1* Continued

| | |
|---|---|
| 1998 | HK Children's Charter: 'The Right to Freedom from the Harm of Tobacco' launched by COSH. |
| 1999 | First smoking cessation clinic in Ruttonjee Hospital (pilot project funded by COSH and led by the University of HK). |
| ***2000s*** | |
| 2001 | Tobacco Control Office established in the Department of Health.<br>Department of Health established a smoking cessation hotline. |
| 2006 | WHO Framework Convention on Tobacco Control (WHO FCTC) comes into effect |
| 2006 | Smoking (Public Health) Ordinance 2006: smoking ban in indoor workplaces and restaurants, but a major loophole is that the onus is on the smoker not the venue management. |
| 2007 | Six pictorial warnings cover at least 50% of principal pack surfaces. |
| 2009 | Tobacco excise tax 50% increase in annual budget. |
| 2009 | Ban on smoking in bars, karaokes, saunas, massage parlours (delayed implementation of 2007 law). |
| ***2010s*** | |
| 2010 | Budget: ban on imported duty-free cigarettes (only 19 sticks allowed). |
| 2011 | Budget: tobacco tax increase brings excise tax to 69% of retail price on certain brands. |
| 2012 | WHO Collaborating Centre for Smoking Cessation and Treatment of Tobacco Dependence opened in the Department of Health. |
| 2012 | Health organizations announce an end-game goal of < 5% smoking prevalence by 2022. |

legislation; addressing political, economic, environment and trade components; and tackling the tobacco industry head-on. This political awareness was crucial.

Even before the stricter tobacco control measures, such as legislation for smoke-free areas, packet warnings, bans on advertising or tobacco taxation policy were implemented, Hong Kong was at an advantage. The first government general household survey in 1982 showed low female smoking prevalence rates (5.6 per cent), mirroring female prevalence rates in most of Asia. In contrast, male prevalence rates (39.7 per cent) followed the rates of Western, high-income countries and were lower than the Asian average of 50–60 per cent.

The key events described in Table 34.1 have led to a reduction in male prevalence rates and maintained the low female prevalence rates (see Figure 34.1). Hong Kong now has the lowest prevalence rates in Asia (see Table 34.2) and among the lowest in the world (see Figures 34.2 and 34.3). By 2010, the female smoking prevalence rates had declined to 3 per cent and the male rates to 19.9 per cent, with an overall prevalence of 11.1 per cent. However, this should not give rise to any complacency as there is particular concern about an increase in smoking among girls in Asia.

## *Compliance*

Overall, there has been strong compliance with legislation such as smoke-free areas, especially with that designed to protect children and non-smokers, who are the majority of

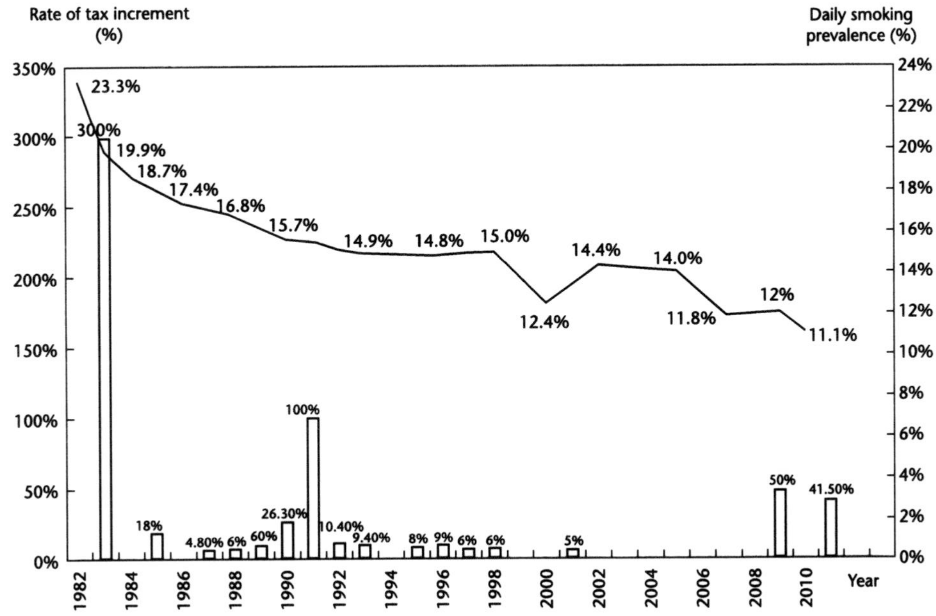


*Figure 34.1* Tobacco tax and smoking prevalence in Hong Kong, 1982–2010 [4]

the population. New forms of transport that were smoke-free from inception, such as the Mass Transit Railway (MTR), had excellent compliance. More difficult were venues such as certain bars, amusement game centres and cooked food stalls in some districts, partly because the legal onus lies on smokers, not on the premises' managers or licensees, and the Tobacco Control Office in the Department of Health had, and still has, an insufficient number of enforcement officers. The tobacco industry has complied with the letter of the laws as they came into effect, such as advertising bans and packet warnings, but constantly seeks new ways of advertising, marketing and promotion, requiring perpetual updating and strengthening of the laws.

*Table 34.2* Daily cigarette use in selected Asian countries, 2011 or most recent data

| *Smoking prevalence, %* | *Total* | *Male* | *Female* |
|---|---|---|---|
| China | 28.1 | 52.9 | 2.4 |
| Republic Korea | 27.7 | 47.7 | 7.3 |
| Japan | 23.4 | 38.2 | 10.9 |
| Thailand | 20.2 | 39.1 | 2.2 |
| Vietnam | 15.6 | 31.0 | 1.0 |
| Singapore | 13.0 | 22.8 | 3.6 |
| Hong Kong | 10.7 | 19.1 | 3.1 |

*Sources*: [5, 6].

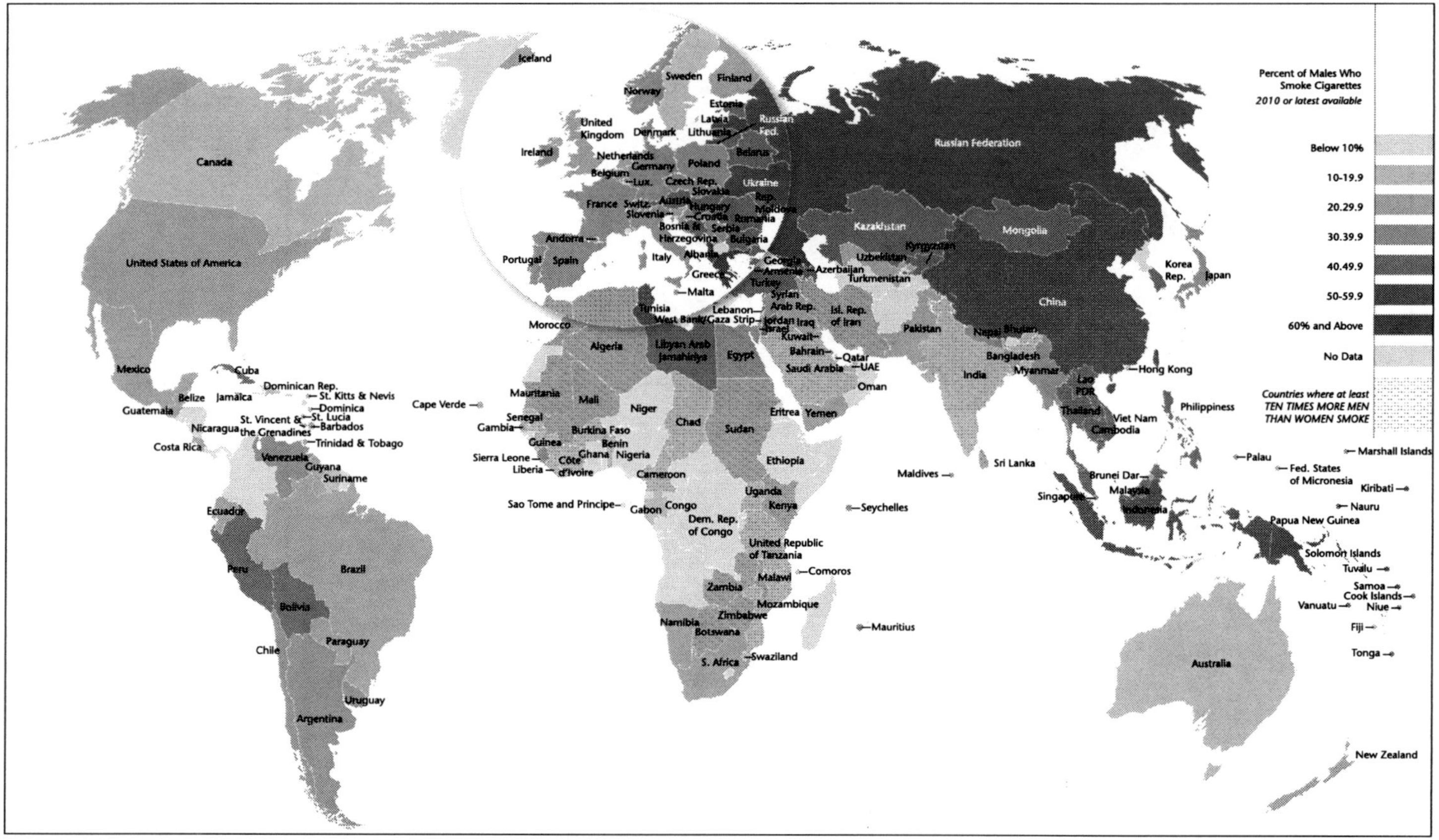


*Figure 34.2* Prevalence of male cigarette smoking by country, 2010 or later [7]

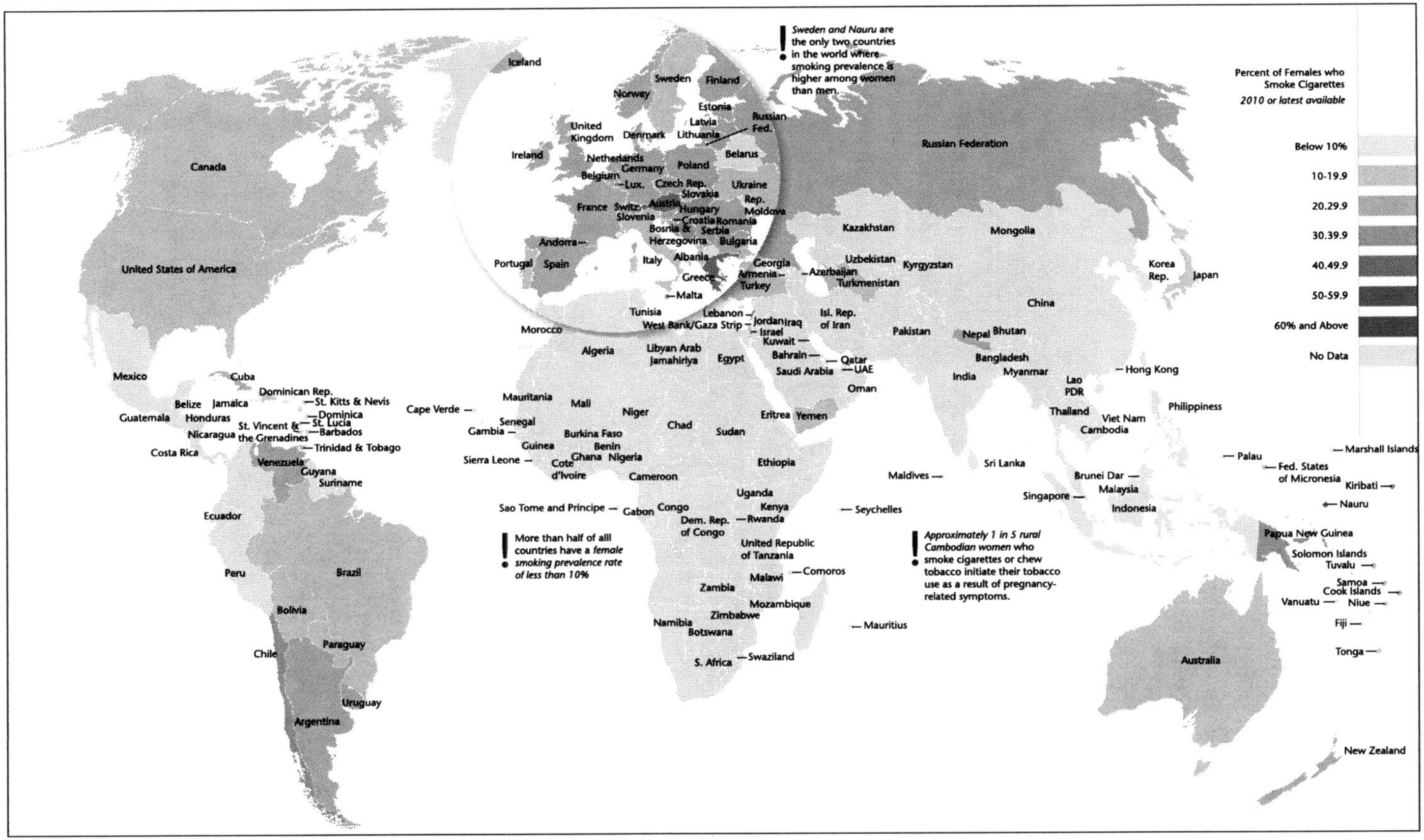


*Figure 34.3* Prevalence of female cigarette smoking by country, 2010 or later [8]

## Key support for tobacco control in Hong Kong

### Research

Local research was crucial in providing Hong Kong data to the decision makers. University departments and other health organizations conducted high-quality research on smoking prevalence and related factors in adults, youth and children; effective cessation intervention; adverse health effects of active smoking and environmental tobacco smoke [9, 10]; public opinion; and the economic aspects of tobacco. The involvement of respected academic institutions in utilizing their research for tobacco control advocacy added great weight to the political lobbying.

### Medical and allied health schools

Medical and allied health schools incorporated tobacco issues into the curriculum. The University of Hong Kong School of Nursing and the School of Public Health started the first smoking cessation counsellor training in the year 2000 and have so far trained over 2,000 healthcare professionals throughout Hong Kong and China. This pioneer effort has also built capacity among nurses and created a new role for them from 2002, staffing most smoking cessation clinics/services in Hong Kong. Academic courses in tobacco control are integrated into the medical and nursing curricula. The University of Hong Kong introduced tobacco control into the medical curriculum in 1994 [11] and, in recent years, medical students have been involved in campaigns on smoke-free legislation, tobacco tax increases and the banning of retail tobacco display, which have received wide media coverage. The Chinese University of Hong Kong's public health curricula emphasized the need for action at global, local and individual levels, as well as the need to encourage students to participate in local advocacy with the NGO sector on various issues, such as increasing tobacco taxes.

### Government

In the early days, government officials and some Legislative Council members were very supportive of tobacco control measures. The government was robust in standing up to the tobacco industry and many measures passed relatively easily. The political will with regard to tobacco control in Hong Kong is still much stronger than in many jurisdictions, but the legislative process has become more protracted, involving exhaustive political processes, consultation and debate before legislation can be passed. Few policy makers, including those for example, in the Legislative Council in Hong Kong, have the scientific background to enable them to evaluate claims and counterclaims or interpret the quality of evidence. Often governments believe that scientific evidence is but one aspect of designing policy, and that they must listen to all opinions, including anti-public-health opinions of the vested interests of the tobacco, retailing, catering, advertising and allied industries, as well as public opinion (which may be uninformed, for example on the effect of tax increases in preventing youth smoking).

### World Health Organization (WHO)

The WHO has assisted Hong Kong (and other jurisdictions) in numerous ways, with targeted advice and guidelines, five-yearly Western Pacific Region Action Plans on Tobacco or Health from 1990 and the continuing celebration of World No-Tobacco Day since 1988 [12]. Of considerable importance and influence is the WHO Framework Convention on Tobacco Control (WHO FCTC), WHO's first health treaty, which came into force in China (including Hong Kong and Macau) in 2006, placing Hong Kong under international obligation to follow the WHO FCTC and its Guidelines. Of the 177 countries now Parties to this treaty, the Western Pacific Region is currently still the only WHO region where all countries have ratified the WHO FCTC [13]. The WHO FCTC has led to increased resources, for example, from the Bloomberg Initiative [14] and the Bill and Melinda Gates Foundation [15] in low- and middle-income countries. The reporting system required under the Convention is an impetus to countries to implement the measures.

WHO MPOWER (**M**onitor tobacco use and prevention policies, **P**rotect people from tobacco smoke, **O**ffer help to quit tobacco use, **W**arn about the dangers of tobacco, **E**nforce bans on tobacco advertising, promotion and sponsorship and **R**aise taxes on tobacco) was a tool developed by the WHO to provide a detailed roadmap for effective solutions, complementing the WHO FCTC. Using the WHO MPOWER's practical measures, WHO issues biennial Global Tobacco Control Reports, which unfortunately cannot separately include Hong Kong statistics, as Hong Kong is not a United Nations member state.

### *Civil society*

Hong Kong also benefited from having a long history of highly visible tobacco control individuals and key non-governmental organizations supporting tobacco control (see Table 34.1), such as the Hong Kong Council on Smoking and Health. The advocates and organizations had international links and were able to channel information, such as global best practices on tobacco control, to decision makers in Hong Kong. The medical associations, the Hong Kong Academy of Medicine and its affiliated colleges, have given unanimous support to tobacco control. Coalitions of organizations and individuals spoke with a more powerful voice than they would have been able to do individually.

### *Advocacy and lobbying*

Public health advocacy and lobbying has been, and is, a fundamental component of advancing public health. None of the early public health professionals received any formal training in public health advocacy, but rose to the challenge and learned how to lobby finance ministers, how to make a submission to the Legislature, how to raise awareness and solicit support of the public and the media, and how to debate with the tobacco industry and their supporters – the latter often best performed by civil society rather than by governments. Zen poet Ryokan (1758–1831) said, 'In this one bowl, there is rice from a thousand households,' which exemplifies the multifaceted and complementary relationship between government and civil society, and the often inseparable yet unmeasurable role each has to play in the success of health policy development.

### *Media*

After the media realized the ban on tobacco advertising in 1990 would not hurt their business, the media have, in general, been very supportive of tobacco control measures. Some media still like to present 'both-sides-of-the-argument' and invite, and report on, anti-public-health comments from the tobacco industry and related sectors.

## Lessons learned

### *The specific role of government*

Only governments can mandate public health legislation, such as smoke-free areas, packet warnings and bans on all tobacco promotion, remove business operating licences for non-compliance with laws such as sales to minors, implement taxation policy and ratify UN treaties, such as the WHO FCTC – although this all works best when supported by civil society. Therefore it is worth repeating that political lobbying must be high on the agenda of anyone hoping to influence public health policy.

### *A step-by-step approach is no longer enough*

The Hong Kong government adopted an incremental approach to achieve the stated policy objective of discouraging smoking and minimizing public exposure to tobacco smoking [16]. This cautious step-by-step method may have been appropriate in the last century but today the magnitude of the epidemic demands far more robust and accelerated measures, especially in view of obligations under the WHO FCTC. WHO recommends strong, comprehensive policies of simultaneous legislation, taxation, publicity, monitoring, evaluation, education and law enforcement, based on proven, tested and effective tobacco control interventions, based on decades of global experience.

### *Employers*

Employers, including government as an employer, have a role and a responsibility to provide a safe, healthy, smoke-free environment for employees. Tobacco has been rightly perceived in Hong Kong as an occupational health and safety issue, and lobbying for smoke-free restaurants and bars was therefore framed principally as worker protection, an approach reinforced by research studies on hospitality workers [17, 18, 19] and policy guidelines from UN agencies [20, 21]. It has been imperative to redress the argument put forward by the tobacco and hospitality industries that such legislation will cause economic harm and job losses. Employers need information on tobacco-attributable health costs, time off work, early retirement and premature death, risk of fires, damage to fabric and litter, and the reassurance that creating smoke-free workplaces will not harm their business.

### *Economic arguments*

At every level – government, business, individual – it has been crucial to master and present the health economic arguments, as one of the biggest misconceptions perpetrated by the tobacco industry and its supporters is that tobacco control, for example the creation of smoke-free areas or bans on tobacco promotion, will cause economic harm. Global experience has shown this is simply not true. Tobacco control is not an issue of health OR wealth, but rather of health AND wealth.

### *Mainstream public health*

Tobacco control action globally has moved away from being individualistic and ad hoc to becoming part of mainstream public health, as evidenced by the WHO FCTC [22] and the

United Nations Summit on Non-Communicable Diseases in 2011 [23]. One new challenge is the integration of tobacco control within the framework of NCD prevention and the development agenda. This has involved the need for systematic planning, such as identifying objectives and strategies, political mapping of key decision makers, the strengths and weaknesses of the opposition, media advocacy objectives and messages, the framing of issues, mobilization of support and allies, and whether or not to form formal coalitions [24].

### *Mistakes*

Mistakes were made, as in many countries, in that the early laws had loopholes and were neither sufficiently specific nor comprehensive. For example, the early bans on promotion only covered tobacco advertising, and not sponsorship and other marketing and promotion by the tobacco companies, and had to be revised and strengthened. The early packet warnings were only 10 per cent in area and had no graphic element. There was an early focus on traditional school-based education in Hong Kong, which is now known not to reduce youth uptake. Early attempts at educational messages were underfunded (in comparison to the slick advertisements of the tobacco industry), clumsy, technical and difficult to understand by the general public, or were soft, positive or humorous, which is now understood to be less effective at changing tobacco use behaviour. Effective messages must be clear and simple, such as the current 'Tobacco kills more than one in two smokers', to have effect [25].

The most recent legislative mistake in Hong Kong was to put the legal onus on the smoker in the ban on smoking in restaurants and bars, an error that still has not been corrected. Thus, owners and managers have little incentive in maintaining smoke-free premises and some even try to capture business from others by secretively allowing smokers to smoke in smoke-free premises.

### *Obstacles to tobacco control*

In Hong Kong, obstacles to tobacco control are surprisingly similar to those in most other parts of the world. They include the tobacco industry, with its huge influence and financial might, promotion of smoking, denial of health evidence, opposition to tobacco control measures, economic disinformation, attacks on individuals, organizations and WHO, and legal challenges and litigation against governments. Other obstacles are the preoccupation of governments with other events or diseases that cause far fewer deaths than tobacco, such as SARS, Avian flu or financial crises; a focus on curative medicine, not prevention; tobacco tax revenue but not the debit seen; and misperceived economic losses if tobacco control measures are taken.

Public health professionals in Australia have coined the term 'The Scream Test' as an unofficial indication as to what works and what does not: the tobacco industry 'screams' at tax increases, promotion bans, the creation of smoke-free areas and, latterly, at plain packaging – a good indication that these are highly effective. The industry welcomes traditional health education in schools and bans on sales to minors, a good indication that these are ineffective in reducing smoking rates.

## The next steps

### *MPOWER*

No matter how much a country or region has achieved in tobacco control, it always seems there is more work ahead. Under the framework and guidance of MPOWER, a 'checklist' for the next steps for Hong Kong (and for many other jurisdictions that have already undertaken a raft of tobacco control measures) will include:

**M**onitor: continue to monitor tobacco prevalence, health and economic effects, the tobacco industry, and also evaluate which strategies and policies are the most effective. The next challenge is to translate these data into policy and action.

**P**rotect people from tobacco smoke by making all public areas tobacco-free, including outdoor areas of restaurants and pubs, and increasing enforcement. The legal onus in hospitality venues should be on managers/licensees to enforce the ban, or face a warning and then lose their operating licence if they don't comply. Introduce a ban on smoking in cars carrying children.

**O**ffer help to quit tobacco use by increasing free, available, accessible quitting facilities and assistance. All health professionals should be more actively engaged in providing smoking cessation advice. Tobacco control should be integrated into all relevant professional teaching curricula. Quit hotline numbers should be on all tobacco packs.

**W**arn about the dangers of tobacco by devoting more resources to social marketing campaigns, which have been underutilized and under-resourced in Asia. Continue to pre-test and evaluate campaigns to determine the most effective strategies to reduce tobacco use. Extend the area of pictorial warning to more than 75 per cent and change these every two years under the authorization of the Department of Health. Ban point-of-sale advertising, including counter display, in all retail outlets, moving cigarettes under the counter as in Thailand and Australia. License all retailers, whether shops or news-stands, and retailers should lose their licence if they display point-of-sale cigarettes, including news-stand decoration or counter displays in cigarette colours or images (or if they sell to children). Introduce plain packaging, consisting only of pictorial warnings and the brand name in a standardized, plain print, without tobacco logos, colours and designs, as has been pioneered in Australia [26].

**E**nforce bans on tobacco advertising, promotion and sponsorship. At the moment, these are fairly comprehensive in Hong Kong, but as the industry is constantly finding other ways to promote their products, vigilance is needed to make sure all forms of promotion are banned, for example, paid product placement in movies [27], which has been shown to influence youth [28].

**R**aise taxes on tobacco which, according to WHO, is the single most effective way to encourage tobacco users to quit and prevent youth from starting to smoke [29]. Increase tobacco excise tax to at least 75 per cent of retail price. Develop a sound and planned five-year tobacco tax policy plan, taking inflation into account. Designate any increase in tax revenue for health promotion and tobacco control rather than simply absorbing the revenue into the general tax fund. Strengthen policies against illicit trade, in accordance with the first protocol of the WHO FCTC [30].

### *Additional action regarding the tobacco industry*

> It is horrific to think that an industry known for its dirty tricks and dirty laundry could be allowed to trump what is clearly in the public's best interests.
>
> *(WHO Director-General Margaret Chan, 2011 [31])*

All jurisdictions need to be vigilant that the tobacco industry has no part in developing public health policies. WHO has erected a 'firewall' between itself and the tobacco industry to avoid undue influence by tobacco companies. Article 5.3 of the WHO FCTC, which applies to all sectors of government, states: 'In setting and implementing their public health policies with respect to tobacco control, Parties shall act to protect these policies from commercial and other vested interests of the tobacco industry in accordance with national law.' The Guidelines for Implementation of Article 5.3, Item 4.10 state: 'Parties should not allow any official or employee of government or of any semi/quasi-governmental body to accept payments, gifts or services, monetary or in-kind, from the tobacco industry.' [32]

## Conclusion

It usually takes at least a century from identification to eradication of epidemics, such as smallpox and polio. Some, such as tuberculosis and malaria, are still not eradicated after centuries. So perhaps it is not surprising that it is taking so long to eradicate tobacco use, a human-made epidemic in which the harmfulness of tobacco is established beyond doubt, especially when the public health approach is so different from that used to combat communicable diseases. The epidemic is completely preventable through political will and proven tools exist to reduce this epidemic.

A new paradigm is needed for addressing the health epidemics of the twenty-first century and their risk factors; embracing international treaties for public health; using laws and fiscal means to reduce the epidemic; recognizing the crucial role of government; addressing an extraordinary range of issues from corporate criminality to poverty alleviation; forming new partnerships; political mapping of obstacles; including tobacco in the development agenda; and the undeniable need to set targets. This paradigm will be equally appropriate for other non-communicable diseases and their risk factors, such as a taxation policy on alcohol, dealing with the fast food and drink industries, and public health policies to reduce obesity.

Health organizations in Hong Kong have set an 'end-game' target of less than 5 per cent smoking prevalence by February 2022, hoping to be the first jurisdiction in the world to achieve this target. Whether they will or not will depend on political will. This epidemic will not be solved in the corridors of hospitals, but in the corridors of power.

## Acknowledgements

We would like to thank the Tobacco Control Office, Department of Health, Hong Kong SAR; the HK Council on Smoking and Health; and James Middleton, Chair, Clear the Air, for their comments and contribution to this chapter.

We would also like to thank the American Cancer Society and World Lung Foundation for permission to reproduce the maps from *The Tobacco Atlas*. The Hong Kong Council on Smoking and Health kindly supplied Figure 34.1.

## References

1. Mackay, J.M. and Barnes, G.T. Effect of strong government measures against tobacco in Hong Kong, *BMJ* 1986; 292: 1435–7. Available at: http://www.bmj.com/content/292/6533/1435 [Accessed 1 January 2013].
2. Peters, J., Betson, C.L., Hedley, A.J. *et al.* Recognition of cigarette brand names and logos by young children in Hong Kong, *Tobacco Control* 1995; 4: 150–5. Available at: http://tobaccocontrol.bmj.com/content/4/2/150.full.pdf+html [Accessed 1 January 2013].
3. Tsang, H.F. Cigarette smoking in Hong Kong – how many it kills and how much it costs. *Hong Kong Practitioner* 1995; 17(10): 482–9.

4. Tobacco tax and smoking prevalence in Hong Kong, 1982–2010. Hong Kong Council on Smoking and Health, 2012.
5. World Health Organization. WHO report on the global tobacco epidemic 2011: warning about the danger of tobacco. Geneva: World Health Organization. Available at: http://www.who.int/tobacco/global_report/2011/en/ [Accessed 1 January 2013].
6. Social Surveys Section. Thematic household survey report No. 36. Hong Kong: Census and Statistics Department, 2008.
7. Eriksen, M., Mackay, J., Ross, H. *The Tobacco Atlas*. Fourth Ed. Atlanta, GA: American Cancer Society; New York, NY: World Lung Foundation; 2012. Available at: tobaccoatlas.org.
8. Eriksen, M., Mackay, J., Ross, H. *The Tobacco Atlas*. Fourth Ed. Atlanta, GA: American Cancer Society; New York, NY: World Lung Foundation; 2012. Available at: tobaccoatlas.org.
9. Kwok, M.K., Schooling, C.M., Ho, L.M., Leung, S.S.L., Mak, K.H, McGhee, S.M., *et al.* Early life second-hand smoke exposure and serious infectious morbidity during the first 8 years: evidence from Hong Kong's 'Children of 1997' birth cohort. *Tobacco Control* 2008; 17: 263–70. Available at: http://tobaccocontrol.bmj.com/cgi/content/abstract/17/4/263?etoc [Accessed 1 January 2013].
10. Ding, D., Fung, J.W.H., Zhang, Q., Yip, G.W.K., Chan, C.-K., Yu, C.-M. Effect of household passive smoking exposure on the risk of ischaemic heart disease in never-smoke female patients in Hong Kong, *Tobacco Control* 2009; 18: 354–7. Available at: http://tobaccocontrol.bmj.com/content/18/5/354.full [Accessed 1 January 2013].
11. Chung, T.W.H., Lam, T.H., Cheng, Y.H. Knowledge and attitudes about smoking in medical students before and after a tobacco seminar. *Medical Education* 1996; 30(4): 90–5.
12. World Health Organization. The MPOWER measures. 2008. Available at: http://www.who.int/tobacco/mpower/package/en/ [Accessed 1 January 2013].
13. WHO Framework Convention on Tobacco Control. Parties to the WHO Framework Convention on Tobacco Control, 2012. Available at: http://www.who.int/fctc/signatories_parties/en/index.html [Accessed 1 January 2013].
14. Tobacco Control Grants. Bloomberg Initiative to reduce tobacco use grants program. Available at: http://www.tobaccocontrolgrants.org/ [Accessed 1 January 2013].
15. Bill and Melinda Gates Foundation. Topics: Tobacco overview. 2012. Available at: http://www.gatesfoundation.org/topics/Pages/tobacco.aspx. [Accessed 1 January 2013].
16. Tobacco Control Consultation Taskforce. Proposed legislative amendments to Smoking (Public Health) Ordinance (Cap 371). 2001. Available at: http://www.fhb.gov.hk/download/press_and_publications/consultation/Smoke/Pamphlet.pdf [Accessed 1 January 2013].
17. Allwright, S., Gillian, P., Greiner, B., Mullally, B., Pursell, L., Kelly, A., *et al.* Legislation for smoke-free workplaces and health of bar workers in Ireland: before and after study. *BMJ* 2005; 331(7525): 1117. Available at: http://www.bmj.com/content/331/7525/1117 [Accessed 1 January 2013].
18. Ferrante, D., Linetzky, B., Virgolini, M., Apelberg, B. Reduction in hospital admissions for acute coronary syndrome after the successful implementation of 100% smoke-free legislation in Argentina: a comparison with partial smoking restrictions. *Tobacco Control* 2012; 21(4): 402–6. Available at: http://tobaccocontrol.bmj.com/content/21/4/402.full [Accessed 1 January 2013].
19. Issa, J.S., Abe, T.M.O., Pereira, A.C., Megid, M.C., Shimabukuro, C.E., Valentin, L.S.O., *et al.* The effect of Sao Paulo's smoke-free legislation on carbon monoxide concentration in hospitality venues and their workers. *Tobacco Control* 2011; 20(2): 156–62. Available at: http://tobaccocontrol.bmj.com/content/20/2/156.full [Accessed 1 January 2013].
20. World Health Organization. Regional action plan for the tobacco-free initiative in the Western Pacific (2010–2014). Geneva: World Health Organization; 2009. Available at: http://www.wpro.who.int/tobacco/documents/RAP_ENGLISH/en/index.html [Accessed 1 January 2013].
21. The World Bank. Smoke-free workplaces at a glance. 2011. Available at: http://siteresources.worldbank.org/INTPHAAG/Resources/AAGSmokeFreeWorkplaces.pdf [Accessed 1 January 2013].
22. WHO Framework Convention on Tobacco Control. Documentation. 2009. Available at: http://apps.who.int/gb/fctc/ [Accessed 1 January 2013].
23. United Nations. United Nations political declaration of the high-level meeting of the General Assembly on the prevention and control of non-communicable diseases. 2011. Available at: http://www.un.org/en/ga/ncdmeeting2011/pdf/NCD_draft_political_declaration.pdf [Accessed 1 January 2013].

24. Chapman, S. Advocacy for public health: A primer. *J Epidemiol Community Health* 2004; 58(5): 361–5. Available at: http://jech.bmj.com/content/58/5/361.full [Accessed 1 January 2013].
25. Lam, T.H. Absolute risk of tobacco deaths: one in two smokers will be killed by smoking. *Archives of Internal Medicine* 2012; 172(11): 845–6. Available at: http://archinte.jamanetwork.com/article.aspx?articleid=1182209 [Accessed 1 January 2013].
26. Tobacco Plain Packaging Act 2011. (Australia). Available at: http://www.comlaw.gov.au/Details/C2011A00148 [Accessed 14 December 2012].
27. World Health Organization. Smoke-free movies: from evidence to action. Geneva: World Health Organization; 2011. Available at: http://whqlibdoc.who.int/publications/2009/9789241597937_eng.pdf [Accessed 1 January 2013].
28. US Surgeon General's report. Preventing tobacco use among youth and young adults. 2012. Available at: http://www.surgeongeneral.gov/library/reports/preventing-youth-tobacco-use/ [Accessed 1 January 2013].
29. World Health Organization. Tobacco control economics. 2012. Available at: http://www.who.int/tobacco/economics/en/ [Accessed 1 January 2013].
30. WHO Framework Convention on Tobacco Control. Protocol to eliminate illicit trade in tobacco products. 2012. Available at: http://apps.who.int/gb/fctc/PDF/cop5/FCTC_COP5%281%29-en.pdf [Accessed 1 January 2013].
31. AFP. WHO chief slams tobacco industry tactics. 2011. Available at: http://www.heraldsun.com.au/news/breaking-news/who-chief-slams-tobacco-industry-tactics/story-e6frf7jx-1226163323603 [Accessed 1 January 2013].
32. World Health Organization. Guidelines for implementation of article 5.3 of the WHO Framework Convention on Tobacco Control. 2010. Available at: http://www.who.int/fctc/guidelines/article_5_3.pdf [Accessed 1 January 2013].

# 35

# Public health law case study

## Plain packaging of tobacco products

*Bryan Mercurio*

### Introduction

In April 2010, then Prime Minister of Australia, Julia Gillard, announced Australia's intention to require tobacco to be sold in 'plain packaging' [1]. Australia followed this announcement with the introduction of the *Tobacco Plain Packaging Bill 2011* (Cth) and other legislation on 6 July 2011 which, among other things, prohibits the use of tobacco industry trademarks, logos, colours, brand imagery or promotional text on tobacco product packaging other than brand names and product names in a prescribed standard font style and position and in a 'drab dark brown' colour package. In addition, the graphic health warnings displayed on the front of the package have to be increased from 30 per cent to 75 per cent (graphic health warnings already must cover 90 per cent of the back of cigarette packages) [2, 3, 4, 5]. In short, Australia's legislation (which entered into force on 1 December 2012) prohibits the use of company branding and logos, and generally standardizes the appearance of all tobacco packaging while also enlarging the mandatory health warnings appearing on tobacco packaging.

Aimed at discouraging smoking initiation and relapse, encouraging cessation of smoking, reducing exposure to second-hand smoke and implementing Australia's obligations under the World Health Organization (WHO) Framework Convention on Tobacco Control [6], this ground-breaking legislation aims to prevent tobacco companies from using their trademarks or any brand logos on cigarette packages. Public health advocates have universally applauded Australia's legislation, while the tobacco industry has not only derided it but also sought to attack it on three separate legal fronts: domestically under a constitutional challenge, and internationally under international investment law and international trade law. For these reasons, the legislation for plain packaging of tobacco products serves as a useful case study of the inevitable intersection – and perhaps clash – of public health law and international economic law.

In this chapter, I first aim to briefly discuss the restrictive nature of tobacco marketing and advertising while also highlighting the importance of the tobacco package to the industry in the next section. Then I briefly review the three legal challenges to the legislation and conclude with a prediction on the likely effect of plain packaging legislation on the tobacco industry.

## Twenty-first-century tobacco marketing

Despite some of the health risks associated with tobacco being widely known among the medical community in the 1950s, Australia was not at the forefront of curtailing or controlling the advertising and marketing of tobacco. For instance, by the time Australia introduced a voluntary tobacco advertising code for television, the United Kingdom (UK) had already banned tobacco advertising on television in 1965, while the United States (US) had already required compulsory health warning labels on cigarette packets.

By the time Australia strengthened and extended the voluntary advertising code for radio in 1971, both the UK and US banned cigarette advertising on radio and television. Australia finally introduced mandatory health warnings for radio and television tobacco advertisements in 1972 before banning such advertising in 1976. It also first introduced health warnings on cigarette packaging in 1973 and, since that time, the warnings have progressively taken a more prominent place on the packaging. For instance, in 1995, Australia required health warnings printed in black on a white background to cover at least 25 per cent of the front of a cigarette pack while additional health information and the information line telephone number covered 33 per cent of the back of the pack, as well as one side panel containing information explaining the tar, nicotine and carbon monoxide content of that brand. The restrictions were strengthened in 2006 when Australia required all packs to contain pictorial warnings covering 30 per cent of the front and 90 per cent of the back of the pack.

In 1999, Australia banned tobacco advertising in newspapers and magazines and since that time it has extended the ban to, among other things, paid product placement, cinema, any type of tickets, outdoor advertising on billboards or public transport and sporting/cultural events [7]. Tobacco can still be legally marketed through direct mail, the Internet and at the point of sale (although over the past decade several Australian states have introduced measures to restrict and curb such advertising) [8].

Like numerous other jurisdictions (including ones as diverse as in Brazil, Costa Rica, Hong Kong, Iceland, Israel, New Zealand, Singapore and Uruguay), Australia prohibits smoking in enclosed dining areas, enclosed public places and almost all enclosed workplaces. In 1997, it also became one of the first countries to ban smoking in bars, pubs, clubs and casinos. Tobacco is highly taxed in Australia and correspondingly cigarettes are relatively expensive, with a pack of 25 retailing for approximately AU$16.

Unsurprisingly, these measures have resulted in a steady reduction in the smoking rate in Australia. Tobacco consumption in the country has declined by approximately one-third since 1990 [9]. Currently, 17 per cent of Australia's population smokes, which is lower than most comparable countries [9]. The measures, no doubt coupled with the corresponding decline in smoking rates, led one employee of British American Tobacco Australia to state in an internal CD Rom (created in 2001) that 'Australia has one of the darkest markets in the world' in terms of manufacturing and marketing tobacco products [10]. One prominent reason for Australia's leadership in the international tobacco control movement has been its strong anti-tobacco lobby. In this regards, a Philip Morris report dating back to 1992 states:

> Australia has one of the best organised, best financed, most politically savvy and well connected anti-smoking movements in the world. They are aggressive and have been able to use the levers of power very effectively to propose and pass draconian legislation . . . . The implications of Australian anti-smoking activity are significant outside Australia because Australia serves as a seedbed for anti-smoking programmes around the world [11].

A parallel development in the fight against smoking has been the WHO's Framework Convention on Tobacco Control, a ground-breaking piece of international negotiation which targets both the supply and demand for tobacco products.[1] Article 11 of the Convention deals with the packaging and labelling of tobacco products, and *inter alia*, requires that health warnings in written or pictorial format be '50 per cent or more of the principal display areas but shall be no less than 30 per cent of the principal display areas'. Moreover, Article 13 of the Convention, entitled 'Tobacco advertising, promotion and sponsorship', recognizes that a 'comprehensive ban on advertising, promotion and sponsorship would reduce the consumption of tobacco products' (Article 13.1) and states that '[e]ach Party shall, in accordance with its constitution or constitutional principles, undertake a comprehensive ban of all tobacco advertising, promotion and sponsorship' (Article 13.2) [12]. While some may contend that the presence of Article 11 excludes packaging from the ambit of Article 13, the Convention defines 'tobacco advertising and promotion' broadly and in a manner in which does not necessarily exclude packaging from Article 13. The definition of 'tobacco advertising and promotion is 'any form of commercial communication, recommendation or action with the aim, effect or likely effect of promoting a tobacco product or tobacco use either directly or indirectly'.

At a minimum, the Framework Convention on Tobacco Control adds further legitimacy to jurisdictional efforts to reduce smoking rates and curtail the uptake of smoking among youths.

## Legal challenges

As mentioned in the previous section, several tobacco companies are challenging Australia's plain packaging legislation domestically and in two international forums. While the legal arguments are different in each of the three challenges, the crux of each case remains the same: the industry is claiming that their property has been expropriated (i.e. taken), that these measures that Australia wants to take will not reduce smoking rates and that the measures will make it hard for the companies to differentiate their brands from those of other tobacco brands and products.

One of the three challenges to Australia's plain packaging legislation has already been decided with a 6–1 majority decision of the High Court of Australia determining that the plain packaging legislation is not inconsistent with the Australian Constitution. In the related cases of *British American Tobacco Australasia Limited and Ors v. The Commonwealth of Australia*, HCA Case S389/2011 and *JT International SA v. Commonwealth of Australia*, HCA Case S409/2011, British American Tobacco and other industry leaders challenged the legislation as a violation of Section 51(xxxi) of the Australian Constitution, which grants the Commonwealth of Australia the power to make laws with respect to 'the acquisition of property on just terms from any State or person for any purpose in respect of which the Parliament has power to make laws'. In so deciding, the High Court found that other products also attract restrictions and regulations and that the plain packaging legislation is but the latest in a long line of tobacco control measures. For instance, Justice Kiefel wrote that 'many kinds of products have been subjected to regulation in order to prevent or reduce the likelihood of harm', before specifically pointing to labelling for medicines, poisonous substances and even some food products in order 'to protect and promote public health'. Meanwhile, Justice Crennan noted that the objects of the legislation are to 'improve public health and to give effect to certain obligations that Australia has as a party to the [WHO] Framework Convention on Tobacco Control'. In a strong conclusion, Justice Hayne and Bell stated that warning labels 'affect no acquisition of property'. In its analysis relating specifically to the trademark issues, several of the justices reiterated the basic justification of IPRs, that of a balance between creators/owners and users. In this regard, Justice French emphasized the public policy approach to IP legislation while Justice Gummow stated that the relevant Australian legislation does not confer 'a liberty to use registered trademarks free from restraints found in other statutes'.

In totality, the High Court did not accept the argument that the restrictions placed on the packaging of tobacco products amounted to an acquisition of property on less than just terms as it did not find there had been any acquisition of property. Justice Hayne and Bell concluded that the legislation 'is not a law by which the Commonwealth acquires any interest in property, however slight or insubstantial it may be . . . [the legislation] is not a law with respect to the acquisition of property'. This ruling is not surprising given the long history of the High Court interpreting Section 51 of the Australian Constitution widely in a manner which limits the protection of property rights[2] by requiring that an acquisition of property confer a proprietary benefit or interest on the Commonwealth. Of course, the plaintiffs could have foreseen such reasoning and argued that the Commonwealth would benefit through reduced health expenditure resulting from a reduction in smoking rates. Such an argument, however, would have involved admitting that the plain packaging legislation would achieve its desired objectives and thus directly contradict their position in the pending investment and trade dispute settlement forums.

The two remaining challenges to the legislation are ongoing and yet undecided, one under international investment law and another under international trade law. In both claims, public health plays a large role in determining the validity of Australia's measures. More specifically, in both forums, Australia's health-related justification for implementing plain packaging of tobacco products will come under attack. If Australia cannot demonstrate that its measures are likely to result in a reduction of smoking rates and in the take-up of smoking among young adults, then it is likely that the measures will be found inconsistent with the investment and trade rules, respectively. On the other hand, if Australia can demonstrate the link between the measures and a reduction of smoking rates and in the take-up of smoking among young adults, then it stands a good chance of defeating both claims.

The legal challenge under international investment law is being brought by Philip Morris under a bilateral investment treaty (BIT) between Australia and Hong Kong signed in 1993. This treaty, like the majority of BITs, provides for investor–state dispute settlement which allows an 'investor' to bring an arbitral claim directly against the state. In its claim, Philip Morris is alleging numerous breaches of the treaty. For instance, Philip Morris is claiming that the Australian measures 'impair[s] by *unreasonable or discriminatory measures* the management, maintenance, use, enjoyment, extension, sale and, should it so happen, liquidation of [its] investments [in Australia]' (Article 2.2 of the Hong Kong–Australia BIT). Philip Morris is also alleging a breach of 'fair and equitable treatment' (Article 2.2 of the Hong Kong–Australia BIT), which involves the claim that the measures wither lack of fairness and proportionality of the legislation, the legitimate expectations of the investor or contain inconsistencies with the relevant international framework (i.e. WTO and other relevant intellectual property-related treaties, such as the Paris Convention). Philip Morris is also claiming that the measures result in a de facto 'expropriation' of its investment, as the measures allegedly deprive Philip Morris of the usage, enjoyment and/or rights of ownership (Article 6 of the Hong Kong–Australia BIT).

In the first two claims, in order to have any chance of success, Philip Morris must seek to discredit the seemingly 'legitimate purpose', 'proportionality' and 'fairness' of the measures. In attempting to do so, Philip Morris argues that the measures mandating plain packaging and an increase in the size of graphic health warnings are 'unreasonable' in that there is 'no credible evidence that [the measures] will reduce smoking prevalence . . . its contribution to public health is purely speculative and there is, in fact, evidence that it will have a negative effect in this regard' [13, 14].[3] Philip Morris also asserts the benefits (if any) of the legislation are 'entirely disproportionate to the harm it will cause' to the investments of Philip Morris [13]. More specifically, Philip Morris argues that Australia's measures will result in the commoditization of tobacco products in Australia, which in turn will lead to a sharp reduction in the price for which they are sold and an increase in the availability of illicit products (such as counterfeit and illegally imported cigarettes) [13].[4] Correspondingly, Philip Morris argues the goodwill generated by its intellectual property will be 'substantially destroyed', the effect of which will be 'devastating' on its investments in Australia [13].

A substantial part of Australia's defence will be centred around its measure on the basis of available evidence. Australia will stress that its legislation applies to both local and foreign investors – in other words, that there is not any intent to discriminate against foreign producers – and that the relevant laws and regulations are firmly based in public health policy. Australia stands a fair chance of successfully defending its measures for a number of reasons. First, based on existing jurisprudence it is extremely doubtful that the plain packaging legislation amounts to 'intentional discrimination on the basis of foreign nationality'.[5] Moreover, in terms of the claim of a breach of the 'unreasonable or discriminatory' standard, Australia will argue that the measures do not meet the level of action required for a breach. Traditionally, arbitral tribunals view this standard as being aimed at measures which lack a 'rational decision making process'[6] and are thus 'manifested in their arbitrariness' [15] as opposed to simply being a means for the investor to initiate a substantive review of the host country's public policy. For instance, the tribunal in *Saluka Czech Republic* stated that the standard is about disciplining conduct which 'manifestly violate[s] the requirements of consistency, transparency, even-handedness and non-discrimination'.[7] Moreover, and despite Philip Morris' claims to the contrary, credible evidence does seem to exist linking plain packaging and the reduction in brand logos to a reduction in smoking rates [16, 17, 18, 19, 20]. For instance, Wakefield found that when compared with current cigarette packaging, 'plain packs with increasingly fewer brand design elements are perceived increasingly unfavourably in terms of smokers' appraisals of the packs, the smokers who might smoke such packs, and the inferred experience of smoking a cigarette from these packs'. Further studies concluded by Wakefield and others repeated these findings and also found that increasing the size of the graphic pictorial health warning results in even less appeal for young adults and would-be smokers [16, 21, 22, 23]. Thus, by removing brand image associations, there is expected to be a corresponding reduction in the appeal of smoking to young adults.

In order to be successful in its claim of a breach of 'fair and equitable' treatment, Philip Morris must present evidence demonstrating manifestly unfair or inequitable conduct – that is, conduct which 'cannot be rationally supported by recourse to a legitimate and otherwise non-discriminatory public policy goal'.[8] This will be difficult as there does not appear to be anything 'manifestly unfair' about the Australian measures; on the contrary, evidence compiled over the last several decades supports public policy measures to limit the prevalence of smoking among all segments of the population, of which would include graphic health warnings and restrictions on advertising and packaging of tobacco products. More specifically, while Philip Morris claims that the measures are maintained without credible evidence,[9] Australia could point to several studies indicating a direct link between graphic health warnings and packaging restrictions to a reduction in the attractiveness of tobacco to potential smokers [16, 21, 22, 23]. In the context of a similar Philip Morris claim against Uruguay, Weiler bluntly states: 'The very fact that [Philip Morris] has launched this claim demonstrates its perception of the effectiveness of the measures at issue. That is why [its] propaganda consistently includes allegations that these measures only change consumption patterns – by shifting market share to contraband and counterfeit brands – rather than reducing consumption or uptake overall' [15].

In its claim of an unlawful expropriation, Philip Morris argues that the plain packaging legislation will result in the 'effective extinguishment' of its intellectual property rights (IPRs) [13] and an 'undermining of the economic rationale of its investments and substantial destruction of the value of (Philip Morris in Australia)' [13]. Philip Morris further argues that consumers will be unable to distinguish between competitor products, and therefore competition will become 'primarily based on price' and tobacco products will effectively become an 'undifferentiated commodity' [13]. In totality, Philip Morris is arguing that the effective extinguishment and loss of value is equivalent to a permanent and substantial deprivation of IPRs and goodwill and thus an expropriation under Article 6 of the Hong Kong–Australia BIT. As with Philip Morris' other claims, it also stresses that there is 'no credible evidence that plain packaging legislation will have the claimed effect of enhanced public health (indeed there is evidence to suggest that it may have the opposite effect)' [13].

Australia will defend its measures by arguing that the legislation does not prevent Philip Morris from acquiring and maintaining its trademarks, nor from using them in all circumstances [24]. Instead, the measures merely regulate the use of trademarks on tobacco products. Australia will also argue that it is not the intention of the measures to expropriate but solely to promote health and protect the health of its citizens. While intent is not necessary in order to establish expropriation, several commentators believe it is a relevant consideration [24, 25, 26].[10] Likewise, Australia would also deem relevant the fact that its response is proportionate to the health risks associated with smoking and in line with the WHO Framework Convention on Tobacco Control [24].

Ultimately, the claim may come down to whether Philip Morris, as an investor, could be deemed to have had a 'legitimate expectation' that such measures would not be introduced in Australia at the time it made its investment [26]. Weighing against Philip Morris in this regard is the fact that Philip Morris Asia did not become the sole shareholder (that is, 'invest') in Philip Morris (Australia) until approximately one year following the Australian government's announcement that it would legislate for plain packaging of tobacco products [1]. As investors making the claim of indirect expropriation rarely succeed,[11] especially in cases where non-discriminatory regulatory measures involve the public interest [27], Philip Morris' claim of an unlawful expropriation is unlikely to be successful.

The third legal challenge against Australia's plain packaging legislation is taking place at the World Trade Organization (WTO), where Ukraine, the Dominican Republic and Honduras have all filed complaints alleging breaches of the General Agreement on Tariffs and Trade (GATT), Agreement on Trade-Related Aspects of Intellectual Property Rights (TRIPS) and the Agreement on Technical Barriers to Trade (TBT). Interestingly, none of the three complainants have any trade in tobacco products with Australia and it is thought that the tobacco industry is funding and providing technical assistance in these matters. The WTO litigation is complex and time does not permit a thorough review of all aspects of the claims.[12] While the complainants' case has arguable merit, it is likely to fail.

Taking some of the TRIPS-based claims as an example, the complainants are essentially arguing that the TRIPS Agreement contains a right to 'use' a trademark. They base this claim on Article 15(4) of TRIPS, which states: 'The nature of the goods or services to which a trademark is to be applied shall in no case form an obstacle to registration of the trademark.' In order to be successful under Article 15(4) (and the similarly worded Article 7 of the Paris

Convention),[13] the complainants have to equate 'registration' with 'use' as Australia has prohibited the registration of any tobacco trademark. While one report authored by the lawyers representing Philip Morris in its investment claim against Uruguay asserts that use is 'inexplicably linked with registration' [28] and another report produced by leading IP scholar Daniel Gervais for Japan Tobacco International repeatedly claims that the 'spirit' of the Agreement is to permit 'use' [29], it is extremely doubtful as to whether Article 15(4) of TRIPS or Article 7 of the Paris Convention contains a right to 'use' a mark [29, 30, 31, 32, 33, 34].[14]

Even if the complainants establish their case, Article 17 of TRIPS grants members considerable discretion to provide for 'limited exceptions to the rights conferred by a trademark, such as fair use of descriptive terms, provided that such exceptions take account of the legitimate interests of the owner of the trademark and of third parties'. Thus, TRIPS allows members to make use of exceptions where measures would otherwise be inconsistent with other provisions of TRIPS. While it will be argued that plain packaging is not a 'limited' exception nor does it 'take account of the legitimate interests' of the trademark owner [28], this argument is likely to fail as it is widely recognized that TRIPS provides negative rights, that is, TRIPS merely grants trademark owners the right to *prevent* others from using their trademarks as opposed to providing a positive right to the trademark owner to *use* the trademark [35, 36].

The complainants have also claimed a breach of Article 20 of TRIPS, which prohibits members from placing 'unjustifiable encumbrances' on the use of a trademark. There is little doubt that the Australian measures encumber the use of trademarks on tobacco packaging. The issue, however, is whether the encumbrance is justifiable when set in the context of public health policies and the stated aims of the measures.[15] To some commentators, the legitimate interests of the rights holder are irrelevant to the test under Article 20 (in contrast to Article 17) and thus the consistency of plain packaging turns merely on whether it is a 'justifiable' encumbrance in light of the stated public health rationale [30, 36]. This is debatable, but support can be found in Articles 8 of TRIPS, which, *inter alia*, provides that members may take 'measures necessary to protect public health' [30, 37], as well as in the Doha Declaration on TRIPS and Public Health, which stresses the right of members to protect public health [30].

## Concluding analysis

To the surprise, and perhaps consternation, of many in the wider field of public health, plain packaging of tobacco products impinges upon not only domestic law but also the distinct fields of both international investment law and international trade law. In doing so, this issue reveals the significant overlap that exists between public health and several fields of law.

Taking a broader look at the issues, it is clear that if, as expected, Australia successfully defends its measures in the investment arbitration and at the WTO, it will serve as a test case for both other nations considering adopting similar measures (such jurisdictions include India, the European Union, New Zealand, United Kingdom and Norway) [38, 39] as well as for the industry. Australia is a relatively small market and the industry may use it to 'prove' that plain packaging is not effective in reducing smoking or take-up rates. It could try to 'prove' this by sacrificing profits and drastically reducing the price of tobacco products in Australia in an effort to maintain the allegiance of smokers and increase total sales. But this strategy could be countered, as the government could simply raise taxes or set a minimum price on tobacco, which may deter smokers or potential smokers. Of course, such a government response would feed into the long-term aims of the industry, as it could then be argued that the tax rise/minimum pricing and not the plain packaging was the effective deterrent.

Expectations also play in the favour of the industry, as some expect plain packaging to immediately and dramatically reduce smoking rates. This is an unrealistic and unreasonable demand: 40 years of data indicate progressively more restrictive public policy measures contribute to the slow and steady decline in smoking rates. There is nothing to indicate that plain packaging could rapidly accelerate the trend. Moreover, the aim of plain packaging to reduce the appeal of smoking, particularly in young adults and potential future smokers, will take years to capture full effect. It is unlikely anything short of a ban on the sale of tobacco products would immediately and dramatically reduce smoking rates.

On the other hand, industry success in either the investment or trade forum would cause considerable discontent not only in Australia but also in the worldwide public health community. The international economic law system would (whether fairly or unjustifiably) be castigated, which could potentially cause long-term and irreversible damage. To some extent, such criticism in the international investment environment would be unwarranted as the more modern BITs contain explicit language relating to health measures that provide an extra layer of protection against the finding of an inconsistency with the relevant treaty; Australia's BITs do not contain such language. Moreover, what is lost in all of the legal wrangling over plain packaging is the fact that if Australia was so concerned about the harmful effects of smoking, it could simply ban its sale and consumption of tobacco products and there would be little avenue for recourse by the industry to any international tribunal.

## Notes

1 See Articles 6–14 for provisions relating to the reduction in demand and Articles 15–17 for provisions targeting supply.

2 See, e.g., *Phonographic Performance Company of Australia Limited v Commonwealth of Australia* [2012] HCA 8 (28 March 2012); *Grain Pool of WA v Commonwealth* (2000) 202 CLR 479; *Nintendo Co Ltd v Centronics Systems Pty Ltd* (1994) 181 CLR 134.

3 The JTI Response further questions the objectiveness of the Australian government 'Expert Advisory Group', noting that several members of the group are the authors of studies for which the government relies in support of plain packaging.

4 See also Parliamentary Secretary briefing B09/4084, 22 September 2009, authored by Ian Goss, IP Australia; document released under Freedom of Information requests (138 of 1660). JTI Response, at paras 5.20–5.24, 5.28.

5 *EDF (Services) Limited v Romania (Award)*, ICSID Case No. ARB/05/13, 8 October 2009, para 303.

6 See, e.g. *LG&E Energy Corp. v Argentine Republic (Decision on Liability)*, ICSID Case No. ARB/02/01, 3 October 2006, at para 158: 'It is apparent from the Bilateral Treaty that Argentina and the United States wanted to prohibit themselves from implementing measures that affect the investments of nationals of the other Party without engaging in a *rational decision-making process*. Such process would include a consideration of the effect of a measure on foreign investments and a balance of the interests of the State with any burden imposed on such investments' (emphasis added).

7 *Saluka Investment BV (the Netherlands) v The Czech Republic (Partial Award)*, Permanent Court of Arbitration, 17 March 2006, at para 307.

8 See, e.g. *International Thunderbird Gaming Corporation v Mexico (Award)*, Ad Hoc UNCITRAL Arbitral Tribunal, 26 January 2006, para 194.

9 Commentators questioning the perceived positive effects of plain packaging include: Michael L. Capella, Charles R. Taylor, and Cynthia Webster, 'The effect of cigarette advertising bans on consumption: a meta-analysis' *Journal of Advertising*, vol. 37, no. 2 (Summer 2008), pp. 7–18; Allan Main, 'Plain packaging of cigarettes: economics and unintended consequences' blog entry, 20 August 2012, http://sciblogs.co.nz/guestwork/2012/08/20/plain-packaging-of-cigarettes-economics-and-unintended-consequences/; Patrick Basham and John Luik, 'Why the plain packaging consultation is deeply flawed' Institute of Economic Affairs, 9 July 2012, http://www.iea.org.uk/blog/why-the-plain-packagingconsultation-is-deeply-flawed

10 Also see, *Siemens v Argentina (Award)*, ICSID Arbitral Tribunal, Case No. ARB/02/8, 6 February 2007, at para 270.
11 See contra, *Siemens v Argentina*, above n. 10; *Compania de Aguas del Aconquija, S.A. & Vivendi Universal v Argentine Republic*, ICSID Case No. ARB/97/3, 20 August 2007.
12 For instance, Ukraine has claimed breaches of Articles 1, 1.1, 2.1, 3.1, 15, 16, 20 and 27 of TRIPS; Article 2.1 and 2.2 of the TBT Agreement; and Article III:4 of the GATT.
13 The Paris Convention is incorporated into the TRIPS Agreement via Article 2.
14 Moreover, while the panel in EC–Trademarks and GIs did state that a trademark owner had an 'interest in using its trademark in connection with the relevant goods and service', the panel went on to stress that the TRIPS Agreement 'does not generally provide for the grant of positive rights to exploit or use certain subject matter'. Likewise, it is doubtful that 'registration' under Article 6 *quinquies* of the Paris Convention can be equated with 'use'.
15 IP Australia advised the government in 2009 that plain packaging of cigarettes would breach Article 20 of the TRIPS Agreement. See Parliamentary Secretary briefing B09/4084, 22 September 2009, authored by Ian Goss, IP Australia; document released under Freedom of Information requests (138 of 1660).

## References

1. Prime Minister of Australia. Anti-Smoking Action. Press Release; 29 April 2010.
2. Parliament of the Commonwealth of Australia. Tobacco Plain Packaging Bill 2011 (Cth).
3. Parliament of the Commonwealth of Australia. Trade Marks Amendment (Tobacco Plain Packaging) Bill 2011 (Cth).
4. Parliament of the Commonwealth of Australia. Trade Practices (Consumer Product Information Standards) (Tobacco) Regulations 2004 (Cth).
5. Parliament of the Commonwealth of Australia, House of Representatives. Tobacco Plain Packaging Bill 2011: Explanatory Memorandum; 6 July 2011.
6. Parliament of the Commonwealth of Australia. Tobacco Plain Packaging Bill 2011 (Cth), cl 3(1).
7. National Archives of Australia. Tobacco advertising ban in Australia – Fact sheet 252. Available from: http://www.naa.gov.au/collection/fact-sheets/fs252.aspx
8. Tobacco Products Regulation Act (SA) 2004.
9. Scollo, MM, Winstanley, MH (eds). *Tobacco in Australia: Facts and Issues*. 3rd edn. Victoria: Cancer Council; 2008, chapters 1–2. Available from: www.tobaccoinaustralia.org.au
10. Chapman, S, Byrne F, Carter SM. Australia is one of the darkest markets in the world: the global importance of Australian tobacco control. *Tobacco Control* 2003; 12(iii): 1–3. Available from: http://legacy.library.ucsf.edu/tid/fgw48e00
11. Philip Morris. Corporate Affairs plan: Philip Morris (Australia) Limited. 19 October 1992, Bates No. 2023240608/0627, available from: http://legacy.library.ucsf.edu/tid/fgw48e00 (cited in Chapman *et al.* Australia is one of the darkest markets in the world: the global importance of Australian tobacco control. *Tobacco Control* 2003; 12(iii): 1–3).
12. World Health Organization. Framework Convention on Tobacco Control; 2003.
13. Allens Arthur Robinson. Notice of Claim Under the Australia/Hong Kong Agreements for the Promotion and Protection of Investment. 15 July 2011: paras 10a, 10b (in the context of the FET claim), paras 33–35, para 44–45 (in the context of the claim of 'unreasonable or arbitrary' conduct). Available under Freedom of Information from: www.dfat.gov.au/foi/downloads/dfat-foi-11-20550.pdf
14. Japan Tobacco International. JTI's response to the Australian Government's Consultation Paper on the Tobacco Plain Packaging Bill 2011 Exposure Draft. 2 June 2011, paras 3.3–3.18, 4.7–4.9. Available from: www.jti.com/download_file/705/585/
15. Weiler, T. Philip Morris vs. Uruguay: An analysis of tobacco control measures in the context of international investment law. Report #1 for Physicians for a Smoke Free Canada: 18–22.
16. Germain, D, Wakefield, M, Durkin, S. Adolescents' perceptions of cigarette brand image: does plain packaging make a difference? *Journal of Adolescent Health* 2010; 46: 385.
17. Hammond, D, Parkinson, C. The impact of cigarette package design on perceptions of risk. *Journal of Public Health* 2009; 1.
18. Freeman, B, Chapman, S, Rimmer, M. The case for the plain packaging of tobacco products. *Addiction* 2008; 103: 580.

19. Scheffels, J. A difference that makes a difference: young adult smokers' accounts of cigarette brands and package design. *Tobacco Control* 2008; 17: 118.
20. Wakefield, M, Germain D, Durkin, S. How does increasingly plainer cigarette packaging influence adult smokers' perceptions about brand image? An experimental study. *Tobacco Control* 2008; 17: 416.
21. Wakefield, M, Germain, D, Durkin, S, Hammond, D, Goldberg, M, Borland, R. Do larger pictorial health warnings diminish the need for plain packaging of cigarettes? *Addiction* 2012, 107(6): 1159–1167.
22. Hoek, J, Wong, C, Gendall, P, Louviere, J, Cong, K. Effects of dissuasive packaging on young adult smokers. *Tobacco Control* 2011, 20(3): 183–188.
23. Moodie, C, Mackintosh, AM, Hastings, G, Ford, A. Young adult smokers' perceptions of plain packaging: a pilot naturalistic study. *Tobacco Control* 2011, 20(5): 367–373.
24. Voon, T, Mitchell, A. Time to quit? Assessing international investment claims against plain tobacco packaging in Australia. *Journal of International Economic Law* 2011; 14(3): 532–533. University of Melbourne Legal Studies Research Paper No. 560.
25. Reinisch, A. Legality of expropriations, in August Reinisch (ed.) *Standards of Investment Protection*. Oxford: Oxford University Press; 2008: 446–447.
26. Hoffmann, A. Indirect expropriation, in August Reinisch (ed.) *Standards of Investment Protection*. Oxford: Oxford University Press; 2008: 161–162.
27. Schreuer, C. Introduction: interrelationships of standards, in August Reinisch (ed.) *Standards of Investment Protection*. Oxford: Oxford University Press; 2008: 1–2.
28. Lalive LLP. Why plain packaging is in violation of WTO Members' international obligations under TRIPS and the Paris Convention. 23 July 2009: paras 17, 27–31. Available from: www.plainpackaging.com/downloads/LALIVE_Analysis_23_July_2009.pdf
29. Gervais, D. Analysis of the compatibility of certain tobacco product packaging rules with the TRIPS Agreement and the Paris Convention. Report produced for Japan Tobacco International, 30 November 2010: paras 30, 57, 65–68.
30. Voon, T, Mitchell, A. Implications of WTO law for plain packaging of tobacco products, in Mitchell, A, Voon, T, Liberman, L (eds) *Public Health and Plain Packaging of Cigarettes: Legal Issues*. Cheltenham: Edward Elgar; 2012: 7, 11–14. Available from: www.ssrn.com
31. Correa, C. *Trade Related Aspects of Intellectual Property Rights: A Commentary on the TRIPS Agreement*. Oxford: Oxford University Press; 2007: 182.
32. WTO Panel Report. European Communities – Protection of Trademarks and Geographical Indications for Agricultural Products and Foodstuffs. WT/DS290/R. Adopted on 20 April 2005: paras 7.246, 7.610–7.611.
33. Davison, M. The legitimacy of plain packaging under international intellectual property law: why there is no right to use a trademark under either the Paris Convention or the TRIPS Agreement, in Mitchell, M, Voon, T, Liberman J (eds) *Public Health and Plain Packaging of Cigarettes: Legal Issues*. Cheltenham: Edward Elgar; 2012: 2–3. Available from www.ssrn.com [Accessed 12 July 2012].
34. Stern, S, Draubins, O. Generic packaging – a bridge (over the bodies of IP rights) too far? *Australian Intellectual Property Law Bulletin* 2011; 23(146): 151.
35. Appellate Body Report. United States – Section 211 Omnibus Appropriations Act of 1998. WT/DS176/AB/R. Adopted on 1 February 2002: para 186.
36. De Carvalho, NP. *The TRIPS Regime of Trademarks and Designs*. 2nd edn. The Hague: Kluwer Law International; 2011: 384, 441–442.
37. Mitchell, M. Australia's move to the plain packaging of cigarettes and its WTO compatibility. *Asian Journal of WTO & International Health Law and Policy* 2010; 5(405): 418–421.
38. United Kingdom Government. Healthy Lives, Healthy People: A Tobacco Control Plan for England. 9 March 2011: paras 3.6–3.7.
39. European Commission. Public consultation on the possible revision of the Tobacco Products Directive (2001/37/EC). July 2011: part 6.3.

# 36

# Screening for cancer

## Colorectal cancer and breast cancer in Hong Kong as case studies

*Martin Wong and Josette Chor*

### Introduction

This chapter will look at the increase of colorectal and breast cancer in the Asia-Pacific region and briefly discuss cancer trends in the region and globally. Since colorectal cancer (CRC) and breast cancer are rising so drastically in the region, this chapter will then use these two cancers as examples to discuss cancer screening programmes. The chapter will highlight screening experiences of these cancers in Hong Kong, look at controversies associated with population-based screening, summarize the significant challenges in designing and implementing screening programmes and make predictions on future perspectives.

### Epidemiology of cancers in the Asia-Pacific region

Cancer has become the major cause of death in the Asia-Pacific countries [1] and its incidence continued to rise in the past decade. Worldwide, the number of deaths from cancer was 7.6 million in 2008, accounting for 13 per cent of all mortalities. This figure has been projected to reach 13.1 million by 2030. In the United States (US), the economic burden of cancer is substantial, with a *prevalence cost* estimated to be US$124.5 billion in 2010 and $157.8 billion in 2020. The highest costs were due to breast cancer (US$16.5 billion) and colorectal cancer (US$14.1 billion) [2].

In the Asia-Pacific region, there were a total of 3 million new cases of cancer in 2010 and from these, more than 2 million patients died. It has been estimated that the incidence of all cancers will increase to 7.1 million in the region by 2020 if the current prevention and treatment strategies do not change [3]. Ageing populations and the adoption of Westernized lifestyles have been recognized as major causative factors of this increasing trend. In addition, 30 per cent of cancer mortality is related to five leading behavioural and dietary risks. These are: obesity, low intake of fruit and vegetables, lack of physical exercise, smoking tobacco and consumption of alcohol [4]. Smoking is the principal risk factor for cancer resulting in 22 per cent of global cancer deaths and 7.1 per cent of global lung cancer deaths.

In the Asia-Pacific countries, a wide variation in cancer incidence and types exists. However, there is a clear epidemiological trend for some cancers declining whilst others are increasing. According to a recent review [1], rates of stomach cancer have previously been high in Far East countries but low in Southeast Asian countries [5]. Rates of liver cancer are high in Northeast Asian countries including China, Japan, Korea and Mongolia. Although both the stomach and liver have been leading sites of malignancy in the past, the incidence rates for cancers in those areas have been dramatically declining since the end of the 1990s [6].

On the other hand, CRC and breast cancer have emerged as leading causes of cancer mortality in the region (see Figure 36.1a and b). CRC is currently the third most common

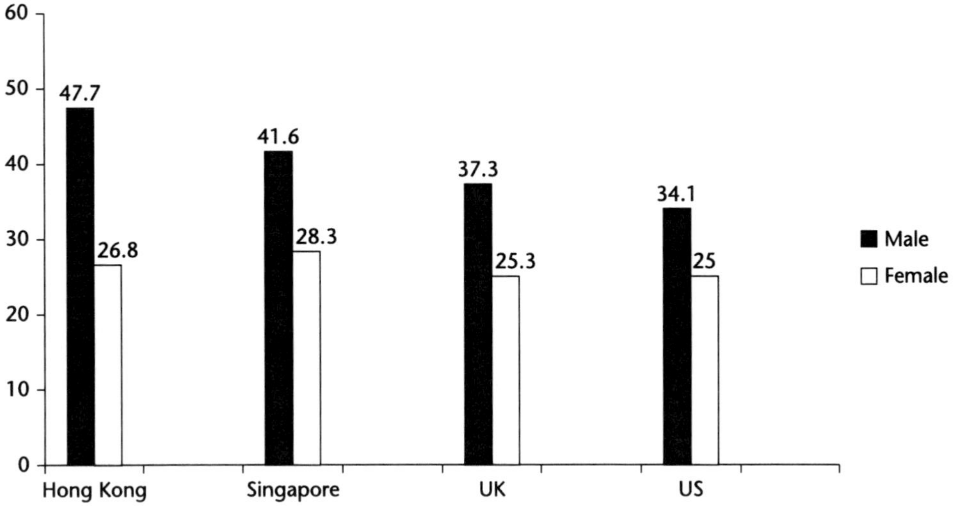


*Figure 36.1a* Comparison of age-standardized incidence of colorectal cancer (CRC) in Hong Kong, Singapore, the UK and the US in 2008 (per 100,000 population)

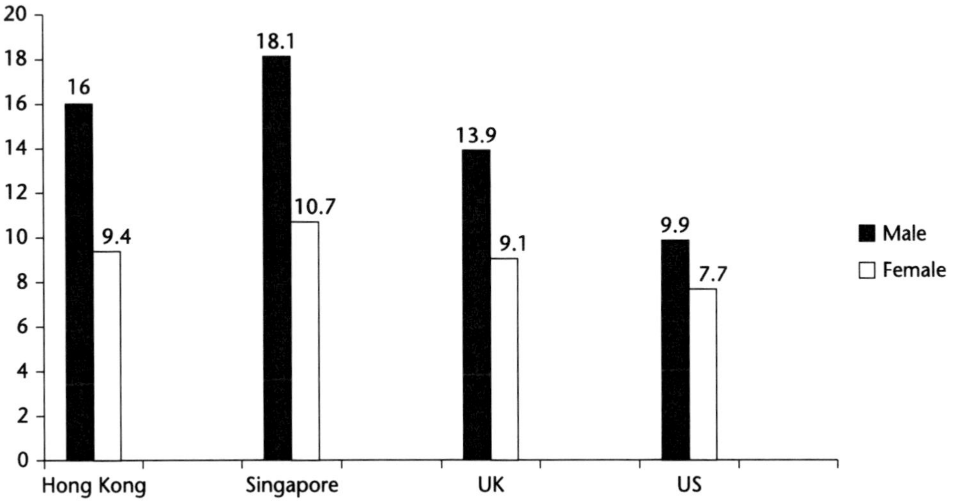


*Figure 36.1b* Comparison of age-standardized mortality of colorectal cancer (CRC) in Hong Kong, Singapore, the UK and the US in 2008 (per 100,000 population)

cancer in men and the second most common in women worldwide, accounting for approximately 10 per cent of all cancers. It leads to 8 per cent of all cancer mortalities in the world and it is the fourth most common cause of death from cancer [7]. In the past decades, Asia-Pacific countries such as China, South Korea, Japan and Singapore have witnessed a two- to three-fold rise in incidence of CRC [8], and have been gradually catching up with the figures in Western countries, such as the US and the United Kingdom (UK). The direct medical cost for the care of colorectal neoplasia was estimated to be US$1,941 for low risk polyps and US$45,115 for stage IV CRC in the initial year of care, bringing a substantial global public health burden to the healthcare systems [9] (see Table 36.1).

The incidence of breast cancer was previously very low in the Asia-Pacific region but increased substantially in the past two decades [10]. The highest rise was observed in Korea, China and Japan, especially among middle-aged women [11]. According to GLOBOCAN, breast cancer was the most prevalent cancer among women, with an estimated 1.38 million new cancer cases being diagnosed in 2008, and incidence rates ranging from 19.3 to 89.7 per 100,000. This was evident especially in more developed countries in the Asia-Pacific region (see Table 36.2).

*Table 36.1* The age-standardized incidence and mortality rates of colorectal cancer (CRC) in Hong Kong, Singapore, the UK and the US in 2008

| | *Hong Kong** | | *Singapore [4, 12, 20]* | | *UK [4, 12, 20]* | | *US [4, 12, 20]* | |
|---|---|---|---|---|---|---|---|---|
| | *M* | *F* | *M* | *F* | *M* | *F* | *M* | *F* |
| Age-standardized incidence rate (per 100,000 population) | 39.9 | 26.8 | 41.6 | 28.3 | 37.3 | 25.3 | 34.1 | 25.0 |
| Age-standardized mortality rate (per 100,000 population) | 16.0 | 9.4 | 18.1 | 10.7 | 13.9 | 9.1 | 9.9 | 7.7 |

*Sources*: [4, 12, 20].
*Note*: * The age-standardized rates for Hong Kong are calculated using the same age-standardization method adopted by GLOBOCAN 2008, in which the age-standardized rates are calculated using ten age-groups based on the World Standard population modified by Doll *et al.* (1966) from that proposed by Segi (1960) [109, 110].

*Table 36.2* The age-standardized incidence and mortality rates of breast cancer in Hong Kong, Singapore, the UK and the US in 2008

| | *Hong Kong** | *Singapore [4, 12, 20]* | *UK [4, 12, 20]* | *US [4, 12, 20]* |
|---|---|---|---|---|
| Age-standardized incidence rate (per 100,000 population) | 47.7 | 59.9 | 89.1 | 76.0 |
| Age-standardized mortality rate (per 100,000 population) | 8.5 | 13.6 | 18.6 | 14.7 |

*Sources*: [4, 12, 20].
*Note*: * The age-standardized rates for Hong Kong are calculated using the same age-standardization method adopted by GLOBOCAN 2008, in which the age-standardized rates are calculated using ten age-groups based on the World Standard population modified by Doll *et al.* (1966) from that proposed by Segi (1960) [109, 110].

## Guiding principles for cancer screening

'Screening' is defined as testing people who are as yet asymptomatic to indicate their likelihood of having a particular disease [12]. The concept of screening implies that early detection will lead to better prognosis, as treatment will be more effective if started before the disease becomes clinically manifested than later treatment when disease is symptomatic. However, not all diseases are appropriate for screening. The traditional criteria devised by Wilson and Jungner are a widely recognized framework for appraising disease entities that are suitable for screening [13]. The first criterion states that the condition in question should pose an important health problem – this usually refers to common diseases in the community, which, if left unmanaged, could lead to serious health consequences. Common life-threatening conditions such as breast cancer and CRC meet this criterion as they do potentially lead to serious and irreversible consequences. Other criteria state that the disease should be in a recognizably early stage and that its natural history is well known. Adequate facilities for the diagnosis and treatment of abnormalities detected should be provided and the screening tests should have high levels of accuracy and be suitable and acceptable to the population. Determined by the natural history of the disease, screening should be repeated at regular intervals and its anticipated benefits should be higher than its potential harm. At the population level, screening programmes should have good profiles of feasibility, which measure their cost-effectiveness, the subsequent diagnosis and treatment of individuals who test positive and the numbers of cases detected. The effectiveness of the programme in reducing morbidity and mortality from the disease is equally crucial and its cost should be balanced against the benefit it provides. It is important to remember that screening might also cause harm, including the psychological stress of being given a falsely positive result or false reassurance in the event of a false negative result or due to the relative invasiveness of some screening tests [14].

## Screening statistics, recommendations and supporting evidence

Early detection of cancers through screening programmes for secondary prevention is one of the most important public health strategies [1]. The local situation of colorectal and breast cancer in Hong Kong will be described, followed by recommendations for screening from international authorities, as well as a discussion of the major controversies that exist for both cancers.

### *Colorectal cancer (CRC)*

Similar as in other Asia-Pacific countries, CRC is becoming a significant health threat to the Hong Kong population. It is the second most common cause of cancer in both males and females. There were 4,335 newly diagnosed cases, accounting for 16.7 per cent of all new cancer cases in Hong Kong in 2009 [15]. Its crude and age-standardized incidence rates were 62.2 and 39.2 per 100,000 persons, respectively, in 2009 and more than 1,700 people died of CRC that same year. The age-standardized mortality rates were 25.1 and 15 per 100,000, respectively.

Three landmark randomized controlled studies have shown that CRC screening using Faecal Occult Blood Testing (FOBT) is effective in reducing cancer mortality by 15–33 per cent [16–18]. A 25 per cent relative risk reduction in CRC mortality was found for those attending at least one round of FOBT screening, according to a systematic review conducted in 2007 [19]. Screening colonoscopy studies have demonstrated that 0.5–1 per cent of patients will have CRC detected and 5–10 per cent of patients will have advanced neoplasia detected. The risk of colonoscopy in experienced hands is low with 0.3 per cent rate of serious adverse events [20]. Guidelines from the US Preventive Services Task Force (USPSTF), the European Nations, the Asia-Pacific Consensus statements and other authorities recommended FOBT as one of the first-line screening modalities, especially in resource-limited regions [21–24]. It is commonly agreed that average-risk people aged 50 years and above should undergo an annual FOBT, flexible sigmoidoscopy every five years or a colonoscopy every ten years. This screening recommendation has also been suggested by the more recent guidelines from the American Cancer Society, Multi-Society Task Force on CRC and the American College of Radiology [24–26].

Tests that primarily detect cancer in the early stages include sensitive guaiac-based FOBT or faecal immunochemical tests. Tests that detect both cancer and pre-malignant lesions like adenomatous polyps include sigmoidoscopy and colonoscopy [27]. Many experts have the opinion that colonoscopy is not an ideal screening test for the general public since it is costly, bears risks and is relatively invasive [27]. The evidence for effectiveness of colonoscopy in CRC programmes is also indirect, as only case control studies showed that colonoscopic screening reduced mortality [28–30]. However, colonoscopy has the capability to detect and remove adenomas and, as previously mentioned, studies on screening colonoscopy have shown positive results. The procedure, if performed at ten-year intervals, is cost-effective relative to other screening programmes [27]. In the absence of other more effective tests, colonoscopy has been the predominant form of first-line screening tests in the US [27].

### *Breast cancer*

Breast cancer is the most common malignancy and the third cause of cancer mortality among females [15] in Hong Kong. In 2009, there were 2,945 new cases registered and 555 people died from breast cancer, accounting for 24 per cent and 10.8 per cent of the cases, respectively. The age-standardized and crude rates of breast cancer were 54.9 and 79.9 per 100,000 women, respectively. The crude mortality rate was 15 per 100,000 females and the age-standardized mortality rate was 9.8 per 100,000 world-standardized population. Both the incidence and mortality rates increased sharply in the past decade and it has been estimated that the age-standardized incidence rate will increase by 1.7 per cent per year. The cumulative risk of developing cancer is one in 23 (0 to 74 years) and the potential years of life lost at age 75 is 7,035, as estimated in 2004 [31]. When compared with other Asian countries such as Japan and Korea, the incidence rate of breast cancer in Hong Kong was intermediate to high [20]. The breast cancer incidence in Taiwan and China has increased 50–100 per cent in the past 20 years [32]. Moreover, most patients with breast cancer in Asia were of younger age. In Taiwan, 50 per cent of these patients were younger than 50 years and 29.3 per cent were under the age of 40 [33]. In Singapore, 13.6 per cent of women with breast cancer were below the age of 40. Incidence rates also nearly doubled over the ten-year time period in Korea with peaks in the 40 and above age group [34]. Furthermore, breast cancers tend to be diagnosed at a later stage in Asia [33, 35]. In Taiwan, 80.3 per cent of tumours were larger than 2 cm [36]. In Singapore, 21.5 per cent of patients have locally advanced or metastatic breast cancer [33]. In India, nearly 70 per cent of women in India presented with stage III or IV disease compared with 10 per cent in the US [37]. A study from Malaysia found that most women who presented with advanced disease were symptomatic patients [38].

The major risk factors for breast cancer include family history, personal history of ovarian problems, endometrial cancer, advanced age, reproductive and hormonal history, physical inactivity and alcohol consumption [39–41]. These factors were similar between Asian and Western populations. The risk of developing breast cancer increases with greater degrees of relatedness with the affected family members, the number of relatives who have had breast cancer and the age at which the relatives developed breast cancer (the younger they were, the higher the chance of development of breast cancer in the patients). In addition, germline mutations in BRCA 1/2 genes are associated with an approximately 40–80 per cent lifetime risk of breast cancer [42, 43] and, globally, half the women with a BRCA1 mutation develop breast cancer by the age of 50 [44].

## Controversies of screening

### *Colorectal cancer (CRC)*

Whether we should screen for CRC in average-risk subjects aged 50 years or above and which modality is more preferred as the first-line screening tool are no longer controversial topics. The major controversies of CRC screening now include age-to-start screening, age-to-stop screening and the appropriate interval to do next screening after a negative screening colonoscopy [27]. Also, there are debates regarding whether higher risk individuals should be screened using different test modalities or at an earlier age. Additional factors include the affordability of the tests, as well as the organizational consequences such as whether there are adequate services to treat patients who have cancers detected.

#### Age-to-start screening – sex and race

Although current guidelines unanimously suggest 50 years as an age cut-off for screening, women are at a lower age-adjusted risk than men [45], generally lagging approximately seven to ten years behind. In addition, black people have a higher risk of CRC and age-adjusted rates of advanced neoplasia than Caucasians from a multicentre study in the US [46]. It has been suggested that for women screening should start after menopause when the risks at developing the cancers start to increase. It is also suggested that black people should initiate screening before the age of 50, at say 45 years. However, this recommendation needs screening customization and there are concerns for complicating the decision-making process.

#### Age-to-stop screening

The current guidelines recommend people aged 50 to 75 years to undergo routine CRC screening. The USPSTF does not recommend screening for individuals aged between 75 and 85 years and advises against screening for people aged 85 years and above, who have had previous screening tests done. This is based on a decision model where the gain from screening is lower than the anticipated risks for people older than 75 years [25]. Nevertheless, since the rates of advanced neoplasm and cancer increase with age, it has been suggested that screening decision should be made not solely on chronological age, but depending on comorbidities and patient preferences.

#### Intervals after a negative colonoscopy

The recommended interval of waiting ten years after a negative colonoscopy is based on indirect evidence. The risk of developing CRC after a negative examination is significantly lowered and this risk reduction could persist for more than ten years. A retrospective cohort study conducted in Canada showed that people who had a negative result from colonoscopy had a standardized incidence ratio for CRC of 0.59 at two years, 0.55 at five years and 0.28 at ten years relative to the estimated rates of CRC in the province [47]. The controversy arises as 0.3–0.9 per cent of patients with adenomas detected at baseline colonoscopy who had had a polypectomy were found to have interval cancers within three to five years. Thus there is still a risk of interval cancer developing despite a negative colonoscopy exam. The ten-year interval recommendation is nevertheless supported by two studies. A subset of patients who had no cancer at baseline were screened by colonoscopy. A five-year follow up of these patients found that only 2.4 per cent had advanced cancer at five years and there were no new cases of CRC [48]. Similarly, a prospective cohort study that looked at 1,200 patients who had a repeated colonoscopy after having a negative screening colonoscopy found that there were no individuals with cancer at a mean follow-up of 5.3 years. A total of 16 per cent had adenoma but only 1.3 per cent had one or more advanced adenomas, defined as tubular adenomas sized at least 1 cm in diameter, polyps with villous histological features or high-grade dysplasia [49]. Therefore, the suggested ten-year interval after having a negative colonoscopy sounds to be a reasonable rationale based on current evidence.

### Higher risk individuals – should they be screened differently?

Risk factors for CRC have been well established. These include older age [50–52], being male [50, 52], currently smoking [53–56], family history of CRC in first-degree relatives [50], obesity [57], certain ethnic groups in Asia like Chinese, Japanese and Korean [8, 58], as well as unhealthy dietary habits such as a high consumption of red meat, fish, processed food and animal fats [53–56]. The Asia-Pacific Working Group (APWG) on colorectal cancer has developed a validated clinical score to predict the risk for colorectal advanced neoplasia for the Asian population [59]. The working group conducted a study in 11 Asian cities involving 2,752 asymptomatic patients undergoing colonoscopy and from this the Asia-Pacific Colorectal Screening (APCS) scoring system was devised. Based on age, gender, family history of CRC and smoking, the system enables risk stratification using elementary clinical information to classify the subjects into three tiers: low (scores 0–1), moderate (2–3) and high (4–7). The high-risk individuals have a fourfold increased risk for colorectal neoplasia. This tool provides the option of risk stratification to optimize the cost-effectiveness of screening. It has been proposed that in countries with a high prevalence of CRC, those with higher risk scores could potentially be offered colonoscopy as the first-line screening option whilst FOBT could be offered as a screening test to average-risk individuals.

Recent evidence showed that patients with non-alcoholic fatty liver disease (NAFLD) were subject to a higher risk of developing CRC and that colorectal neoplasia were found more frequently in a proximal colon [60]. It has therefore been suggested that colonoscopy should be conducted more frequently in people with NAFLD, starting screening at a younger age (e.g. at 40 years old). Similar arguments could be extended to people with multiple risk factors; however, further studies are needed to establish the effectiveness of screening among various high-risk groups at earlier age cut-offs.

## *Breast cancer*

### Overview of the breast screening situation in Asia

There is no organized mammography screening in Hong Kong although the country has the highest incidence rate in Asia. In Hong Kong, a previous study in women aged 65 or above with a positive family history of breast cancer found that only 25.93 per cent of women have ever had a mammogram [61]. This figure is not significantly different from the mammography screening rate in the general population. Both are surprisingly low for a developed country. Korea, Japan and Singapore are the only countries in Asia with population-based breast cancer screening by mammography. The participation rate ranges from 12.4–41.7 per cent [62–64].

Taiwan has adopted a two-stage approach to breast cancer screening. The rationale behind this is the low incidence of breast cancer in the country and therefore mammography is only provided to the high-risk population for cost-effectiveness reasons. Annual mammographic screening is offered to high-risk populations who had or have first-degree relatives with breast cancer. This approach was estimated to result in a 33 per cent reduction of breast cancer mortality but this only covered 5 per cent of breast cancer incidence in Taiwan [65].

## Acceptance of breast screening

Asian women have misconceptions about breast cancer and breast screening practice, which include a lack of knowledge about the risk of cancer, perceived risk, cancer symptoms and treatment options [66–68]. The level of acceptance of mammography varies in different countries due to differences in culture, perception and health literacy rates. Most studies showed that women who are more knowledgeable about breast cancer and breast screening are more likely to have mammography. Asian women are influenced by cultural influences, such as paternalism, seeking alternative and traditional medicine and ignorance of women's health problems. Past unpleasant experiences, fear of the test and perceived costs are also barriers.

## Economic evaluation

A study in Japan has shown that the cost per life year saved was US$18,200. This was less cost-effective than in Europe, as compared to Australia, but more cost-effective than in the US [69]. A Taiwan study has divided the target group into a general population and a high-risk population. The costs per life year saved were US$72,480 and US$4,851, respectively [9] with annual screening [70].

Since there is no organized screening in Hong Kong, studies using a theoretical cost-effectiveness analysis model in a hypothetical situation only used data from opportunistic screening. Using this approach, it was found that breast cancer screening was the least cost-effective method in screening when compared with cervical cancer and CRC screening [71]. The most cost-effective scenario for mammographic screening was biennial screening for women aged 50 to 74 years with US$3,088/DALY averted. Another study showed the incremental cost-effectiveness ratio was US$61,600/QALY saved and US$64,400 per life year saved [72]. It was estimated that US$801,230 is required to avoid one cancer death [73].

Whether a screening programme is cost-effective depends on the societal willingness to accept the pay level. However, little is known about the willingness for people to pay and there is no QALY league table for health services of priority in Asia. More work is needed to determine the most effective population-based approach and the factor of it being a woman's choice has to be considered when making decisions at a policy level.

## Experiences of screening: barriers and challenges

### *Colorectal cancer (CRC)*

#### Low levels of screening participation and compliance

Studies from Japan, France and England showed that participation or compliance rates in CRC screening using FOBT remained low, ranging from 17–61 per cent [74–76]. A recent cost-effectiveness simulation model showed that if compliance with diagnostic follow-up was increased by 20 per cent, mortality could be reduced by 9.3 per cent; and if initial screening compliance could be enhanced by 50 per cent, cancer deaths would be reduced by 50.4 per cent [77]. The bowel cancer screening FOBT pilot conducted between 2000 and 2005 in England evaluated the uptake rate of an unhydrated guaiac based test with six sample collection spots and found that the crude uptake rate was 61.8 per cent, 57 per cent and 58.7 per cent in the first, second and third rounds, respectively [78]. The research identified that men, those of younger age, those who resided in deprived areas and those who were from regions with a higher proportion of residents from the Indian subcontinent were less likely to be compliant for the FOBT uptake. Another study performed from a French population showed that only 34.7 per cent participated in the screening programme [79] and that the factors associated with non-participation included being male and having a higher rate of social deprivation. The uptake rate was also found to be lower among the youngest and the eldest people.

#### Perceptual barriers to screening

Perceptions of screening also create barriers to successful screening programmes. One of the most popular frameworks to explain health-seeking behaviour is the Health Belief Model (HBM), which focuses on the attitudes and behaviors of individuals [80, 81]. This model postulates that the motivation to change health behaviour is influenced by perceived susceptibility, perceived severity, perceived benefit, perceived barriers and cues to action. The HBM proposes that a higher level of perceived susceptibility, severity and benefit increases readiness to take action, whereas this readiness is only enhanced when the barriers to undertake the behaviour are removed and the ability to take action is present. There are at least three levels of barriers which are determinants of CRC screening, and these are patient-related, physician-driven and healthcare system-based.

***Patient factors:*** A population-based telephone survey involving more than 1,000 randomly selected Chinese residents in Hong Kong aged between 30 and 65 years showed that only 10 per cent had undertaken a CRC screening test [82]. These participants were found to have a low knowledge of CRC symptoms and risk factors. Their perceived health status, psychological constructs and perception of access barriers to CRC testing were all high. Interestingly, those with higher perceived severity for CRC were less likely to undergo screening, implying a psychological aversion to face the adverse consequence of a higher-than-average positive screening result [82].

Worldwide, a substantial body of evidence points towards a low level of knowledge of CRC. The APWG in colorectal cancer conducted a multinational survey in various Asia-Pacific regions and found that the median symptom and risk factor knowledge scores of the population ranged from zero to four out of nine (with zero signifying the lowest level of knowledge and nine signifying the highest level of knowledge), with many regions scoring zero [83]. Another survey among moderate risk patients in West Malaysia reported that only 4.1 per cent had good knowledge of CRC and its screening programme [84]. Other studies on CRC knowledge among indigenous Western Australians [85], Iranians [86], American Indians [87], and ethnically diverse population in Australia [88] and Hong Kong [89] consistently found a low level of knowledge of CRC, including awareness of its symptoms and risk factors, as well as an understanding of the importance of CRC screening.

Prominent psychological barriers of CRC screening included concerns about pain, discomfort, unpleasantness associated with CRC testing and fear of follow-up procedures. Lack of insurance coverage is also a significant barrier, as there is an absence of incentive to undertake screening when no symptoms exist. Financial cost and lack of time commitment are the major access barriers to undertake CRC screening tests [82]. Other studies have reported that embarrassment associated with CRC screening has been a particularly important obstacle to undergo a screening test [90–92]. In addition, persistent compliance to CRC screening requires high levels of health awareness over time and this continuity of screening is much needed for overall programme success.

***Physician and health system-driven factors:*** Physician recommendation has been identified as the most influential factor determining the undertaking of screening tests [93–95]. It has been shown that patients who received a physician recommendation for CRC screening were 23 times more likely to undergo CRC screening tests [82]. However, given their busy clinical schedules, physicians might encounter difficulties in discussing CRC screening when it is not a patient's agenda in a clinic consultation. Also daily consultations are usually for giving a variety of possible anticipatory, opportunistic advice for patients and therefore CRC screening might not be perceived as the first priority. Some physicians also reported insufficient training and some doubted the relevance of training in this area. Physicians are also concerned about practical and administrative obstacles for screening procedures in their practice [96].

The Cancer Expert Working Group on Cancer Prevention and Screening (CEWG) of Hong Kong reports that the lack of readiness and capacity for designing and implementing a CRC screening programme have been perceived as important system-driven factors to delay the introduction of a screening programme [97]. The working group based their opinion on local statistics and overseas experience and assumed 50 per cent coverage and an FOBT positivity rate of 1.77 per cent. It was estimated that this uptake would result in demands for laboratory analysis of 900,000 FOBT samples and 16,000 colonoscopies for follow-up of those screened positive. The resources required, including colonoscopic capacity, laboratory services and further management, such as counselling, treatment and follow-up, have been regarded as prohibitive. There is also concern over the longer waiting time and delay in treatment among symptomatic cases once population-based cases are detected. However, these decisions are not being made with the rigorous analysis applied in other countries such as the UK where QALY analysis shows that the screening programme is cost-effective [98].

## *Breast cancer*

### Informed decision

Recently, there have been debates about the bias existing in the information provided in the leaflets given to women invited for breast cancer screening. Separate articles published in the *Lancet* and *British Medical Journal* both urged that balanced information must be presented to healthy individuals to facilitate the informed decision-making process [99, 100]. This is extremely important, especially because whilst many agencies are enthusiastic about cancer screening, some women perceive screening as an expression of paternalism [101]. Previous studies in the UK and other European countries have found that the information in leaflets given by various screening programmes has been biased in favour of screening and underplayed its risks [102, 103]. Although the need for balanced information was stressed by health professionals, little was known about what kind of information was needed to make an informed decision from the women's perspective in Asia.

## Lack of evidence

In Western countries, there has been a long, ongoing debate about whether mammographic screening imposes more benefits by saving lives or does more harm by over-diagnosis and over-treatment. A review in the *Lancet* [104] in 2012 seems to have helped us close the chapter on this debate. Based on a meta-analysis of 11 randomized trials, the review concluded that the relative risk of breast cancer mortality for women invited for screening as compared with controls was 0.80 (95 per cent CI 0.73–0.89), which is a relative risk reduction of 20 per cent. The conclusion drawn was that for every 10,000 UK women aged 50 invited for screening in the next 20 years, 43 deaths from breast cancer would be prevented and 129 cases of breast cancer, invasive and non-invasive, would be over-diagnosed; that is one breast cancer death prevented for about every three over-diagnosed cases identified and treated. Of the roughly 307,000 women aged 50 to 52 who are invited to begin screening every year, just over 1 per cent would have an over-diagnosed cancer.

In 2010, a report by the Cancer Expert Working Group in Hong Kong stated that

> there was *insufficient evidence* to recommend for or against routine mammography screening for the general female population in Hong Kong. The Working Group agreed that there should be more research on the effectiveness of breast screening among Hong Kong women, as well as their attitude.

Studies including a randomized controlled trial would help us find the most appropriate and cost-effective solution for our locality.

## New imaging modalities

Full-Field Digital Mammography (FFDM) is now being considered in most countries. It offers population-based, mammographic screening using Screen-Film Mammography (SFM) to combat the problem of archiving and image storage. With FFDM, the radiation dose can be reduced by up to 50 per cent. The potential advantages of FFDM include better image quality, more accurate and less manpower consuming computer aided analysis, telemammography and more efficient data archiving [105].

Ultrasound has always been suggested by clinicians as an alternative in breast cancer screening for its better detection rate in young women and non-radioactive modalities. However, there have been no randomized studies comparing the differences in breast cancer detection by mammogram and ultrasound.

## Looking forward: increasing capacity via concerted efforts

### *Colorectal cancer (CRC)*

To combat the public health challenges of the rapid increase in incidence and mortality of CRC in the Asia-Pacific region, strategies designed at the patient, community and governmental levels to enhance screening will need to be multifaceted. They will also require a multidisciplinary approach with involvement from major stakeholders including physicians, patients, policy-makers and health educators.

To facilitate CRC screening for the general public and to decrease the factors hindering CRC screening the following need to be addressed:

1 *Lack of knowledge on CRC symptoms and risk factors of the general public*: more intervention in terms of educational initiatives, such as [82] public awareness campaigns, educational seminars, workshops and exhibitions to improve the overall awareness of CRC screening.
2 *Low persistent compliance with screening programmes*: recent initiatives for designing and implementing community-based, adherence-promoting programmes should be more targeted. Specific interventions targeting different factors to enhance screening compliance have been met with variable degrees of success [106]. It therefore seems worthwhile that more incentives are built into compliance-enhancing programmes, including reminder letters, one-to-one phone calls, personalized mailed interventions with telephone follow-ups and computer or video-based interventions with client-tailored messages [107].
3 *Psychological barriers*: it has been suggested that community members such as ex-bowel cancer patients could act as lay health advisers and establish a network of peer educators so that counselling programmes could be conducted to relieve the psychological concerns of those with a family history of positive cancers. Sharing groups and information exchange sessions organized by lay health advisers from existing community networks have been proven effective to provide satisfactory emotional and instrumental support [108]. The social welfare sector therefore plays a crucial role and should involve the elderly centres in the district which are often excellent hubs for provision of sharing and counselling services.
4 *Constraints on physician practice and consultation time*: physicians should be provided with more time and incentives to refer appropriate patients for CRC screening during their consultations. Since the time and efforts involved in explaining screening might not be affordable in some clinics, resource centres specializing in handling screening referrals could be set up near to the practice.
5 *Governmental commitments and resource injection*: in order for population-based screening programmes to succeed, the government should have a vision to foresee the positive longer-term effectiveness of cancer screening. This involves injecting more resources to build programme infrastructure and facilities, as well as to train more healthcare professionals to acquire the knowledge and skills of CRC screening tests. It is worthwhile for the government to consider risk stratification models based on validated tools like the APCS scores to optimize the efficiency of screening resources by targeting individuals at high risks of developing CRC. This could then be evaluated for their feasibility and cost-effectiveness to work out the best model for CRC screening programmes, tailor-made to local needs. Since one of the major concerns for implementing population-based CRC screening programmes in the Asia-Pacific countries includes the capacity of health

services, such as the availability of colonoscopists, training programmes for primary care physicians to conduct CRC screening tests in their surgeries should be a prioritized policy agenda. In addition, a central population register should be established to ensure accessibility to screening services and continuity of screening programmes.*

### *Breast cancer*

Epidemiology suggests that the increasing incidence of breast cancer is a pressing issue in many Asian countries. However, we need to know more about how Asian women accept the breast screening programme, as well as the feasibility of establishing a population-wide system. Most previous studies done in Asia have been either unrepresentative of populations receiving opportunistic screening or from modelling. Moreover, we also need data on the evaluation of the existing population-based screening programmes in countries such as Singapore, Japan and Korea.

As both CRC and breast cancer are rising so rapidly in the Asia-Pacific region, and are the cause of a significant number of deaths, it is of the utmost importance to implement well-developed screening programmes for these cancers as they become available. As seen in the case of Hong Kong, screening programmes for CRC and breast cancer are able to be implemented; however, they do come with their own sets of controversies (such as age to start/stop, screening for higher-risk individuals, acceptance and the economics involved) and challenges (such as a low level of compliance, health-system driven factors and challenges of new imaging modalities). Without consistent, thorough reviews that lead to multifaceted strategies designed at the patient, community and governmental levels, screening for CRC and breast cancer could continue to pose barriers in the Asia-Pacific region.

## References


1. Yoo K-Y. Cancer Prevention in the Asia Pacific Region. *Asian Pacific J Cancer Prev* 2010; 11, 839–44.
2. Yabroff KR, Lund J, Kepka D, Mariotto A. Economic burden of cancer in the United States: estimates, projections, and future research. *Cancer Epidemiol Biomarkers Prev* 2011; 20(10), 2006–14.
3. Mackay J, Jernal A, Lee NC, *et al. The cancer atlas.* Atlanta, GA, American Cancer Society, 44, 2006.
4. The World Health Organization. Available at: http://www.who.int/mediacentre/factsheets/fs297/en/ [Accessed 28 July 2012].
5. Shin HR, Masuyer E, Ferlay J, *et al.* Cancer in Asia – incidence rates based on data in cancer incidence in five continents IX (1998–2002). *Asian Pac J Cancer Prev* 2010; 11, 11–16.
6. Ngoan LT, Yoshimura T. Pattern and time trends of stomach cancer in Asia from 1950–99. *Asian Pac J Cancer Prev* 2002; 3, 47–54.
7. Ferlay J, Shin HR, Bray F, Forman D, Mathers C, Parkin DM. Estimates of worldwide burden of cancer in 2008: GLOBOCAN 2008. *Int J Cancer* 2010; 127: 2893–917.
8. Sung JJY, Lau JYW, Goh KL, Leung WK, for the Asia Pacific Working Group on Colorectal Cancer. Increasing incidence of colorectal cancer in Asia: implications for screening. *Lancet Oncol* 2005; 6: 871–6.
9. Wong CK, Lam CL, Poon JT, *et al.* Direct medical costs of care for Chinese patients with colorectal neoplasia: a health care service provider perspective. *J Eval Clin Pract* 2011; Nov. 23. doi: 10.1111/j.1365-2753.2011.01776.x.
10. Yoo KY, Kim Y, Park SK, *et al.* Lifestyle, genetic susceptibility and future trends of breast cancer in Korea. *Asian Pac J Cancer Prev* 2006; 7, 679–82.


* ACRC screening pilot programme has been set up in January 2014.

11. Bray F, McCarron P, Parkin DM. The changing global patterns of female breast cancer incidence and mortality. *Breast Cancer Res* 2004; 6, 229–39.
12. GLOBOCAN 2008. Cancer fact sheet. Available at: http://globocan.iarc.fr/factsheets/cancers/breast.asp [Accessed 28 July 2012].
13. Wilson JMG, Jungner G. Principles and practice of screening for disease. Public Health Paper no. 34. Geneva: WHO; 1968.
14. Independent UK Panel on Breast Cancer Screening. The benefits and harms of breast cancer screening: an independent review. *Lancet* 2012; 380(9855), 1778–86.
15. Hong Kong Cancer Registry. Available at: http://www3.ha.org.hk/cancereg/statistics.html [Accessed 14 July 2012].
16. Hardcastle JD, Chamberlain JO, Robinson MH, *et al.* Randomised controlled trial of faecal-occult-blood screening for colorectal cancer. *Lancet* 1996; 348: 1472–7.
17. Jorgensen OD, Kronborg O, Fenger C. A randomised study of screening for colorectal cancer using faecal occult blood testing: results after 13 years and seven biennial screening rounds. *Gut* 2002; 50: 29–32.
18. Mandel JS, Church TR, Ederer F, *et al.* Colorectal cancer mortality: effectiveness of biennial screening for fecal occult blood. *J Natl Cancer Inst* 1999; 91: 434–7.
19. Hewitson P, Glasziou P, Irwig L, Towler B, Watson E. Screening for colorectal cancer using the faecal occult blood test, Hemoccult. *Cochrane Database Syst Rev* 2007 Jan 24; (1): CD001216.
20. Curado MP, Edwards B, Shin, HR, Storm H, Ferlay J, Boyle P. *Cancer Incidence in Five Continents*, Vol. IX. IARC Scientific Publications No. 160, Lyon, IARC; 2007.
21. Pignone M, Rich M, Teutsch SM, Berg AO, Lohr KN. Screening for colorectal cancer in adults at average risk: a summary of the evidence for the U.S. Preventive Services Task Force. *Ann Intern Med* 2002; 137: 132–41.
22. Levin B, Lieberman AD, McFarland B *et al.* Screening and surveillance for the early detection of colorectal cancer and adenomatous polyps, 2008: a joint guideline from the American Cancer Society, the U.S. Multi-Society Task Force on Colorectal Cancer, and the American College of Radiology. *CA Cancer J Clin* 2008; 58: 130–60.
23. Sung JJ, Lau JY, Young GP, *et al.* Asia Pacific consensus recommendations for colorectal cancer screening. *Gut* 2008; 57: 1166–76.
24. Recommendations on cancer screening in the European Union. Advisory Committee on Cancer Prevention. *Eur J Cancer* 2000; 36: 1473–8.
25. Whitlock EP, Lin JS, Liles E *et al.* Screening for colorectal cancer: a targeted, updated systematic review for the U.S. Preventive Services Task Force. *Ann Intern Med* 2008; 149: 658.
26. US Preventive Services Task Force. Screening for colorectal cancer: US Preventive Services Task Force recommendation statement. *Ann Intern Med* 2008; 149: 627–37.
27. Lieberman D. Colon cancer screening and surveillance controversies. *Curr Opin Gastroenterol* 2009; 25: 422–7.
28. Muller AD, Sonnenberg A. Prevention of colorectal cancer by flexible sigmoidoscopy and polypectomy: a case-control study of 32,702 veterans. *Ann Intern Med* 1995; 123: 904–10.
29. Singh H, Turner D, Xue L *et al.* Risk of developing colorectal cancer following a negative colonoscopy examination. Evidence for a 10-year interval between colonoscopies. *JAMA* 2006; 295: 2366–73.
30. Baxter NN, Goldwasser MA, Paszat LF *et al.* Association of colonoscopy and death from colorectal cancer: a population-based, case-control study. *Ann Intern Med* 2009; 150: 1–8.
31. Breast cancer. 2006. Available from: http://www.chp.gov.hk
32. Huang CS, Chang KJ, Shen CY. Breast cancer screening in Taiwan and China. *Breast Dis* 2001; 13: 41–8.
33. Tan SM. How relevant is breast cancer screening in the Asia/Pacific region? *Breast* 2007; 16(2): 113–19.
34. Lee JH, Yim SH, Won YJ, Jung KW, Son BH, Lee HD, *et al.* Population-based breast cancer statistics in Korea during 1993–2002: incidence, mortality, and survival. *J Korean Med Sci* 2007; 22(Suppl): S11–S16.
35. Agarwal G, Pradeep PV, Aggarwal V, Yip CH, Cheung PS. Spectrum of breast cancer in Asian women. *World J Surg* 2007; 31(5): 1031–40.

36. Chie WCCKJ. Factors related to tumor size of breast cancer at treatment in Taiwan. Preventive Medicine 1994; 23(1): 91–7.
37. Green MRV. Epidemiology, screening and diagnosis of breast cancer in the Asia-Pacific region: Current perspectives and important considerations. *Asia Pacific Journal of Clinical Oncology* 2008; 4(Suppl 3): S5–S13.
38. Taib NA, Yip CH, Ibrahim M, Ng CJ, Farizah H. Breast cancer in Malaysia: are our women getting the right message? 10 year-experience in a single institution in Malaysia. *Asian Pacific Journal of Cancer Prevention* 2007; 8(1): 141–5.
39. Tao SC, Yu MC, Ross RK, Xiu KW. Risk factors for breast cancer in Chinese women of Beijing. *Int J Cancer* 1988; 42(4): 495–8.
40. Yuan JM, Yu MC, Ross RK, Gao YT, Henderson BE. Risk factors for breast cancer in Chinese women in Shanghai. *Cancer Res* 1988; 48(7): 1949–53.
41. Genetics of Breast and Ovarian Cancer (PDQ). National Cancer Institute, U.S. National Institutes of Health; 2008.
42. Saslow D, Boetes C, Burke W *et al.* American Cancer Society guidelines for breast screening with MRI as an adjunct to mammography. *CA Cancer J Clin* 2007; 57(2): 75–89.
43. Genetics of Breast and Ovarian Cancer (PDQ). National Cancer Institute, U.S. National Institutes of Health; 2008.
44. Easton DF, Ford D, Bishop DT. Breast and ovarian cancer incidence in BRCA1-mutation carriers. Breast Cancer Linkage Consortium. *Am J Hum Genet* 1995; 56(1): 265–71.
45. Jemal A, Siegel R, Ward E *et al.* Cancer statistics 2008. *CA Cancer J Clin* 2008; 58: 71–96.
46. Lieberman D, Holub J, Moravec M *et al.* Prevalence of colon polyps detected by colonoscopy screening in asymptomatic black and white patients. *JAMA* 2008; 300: 1417–22.
47. Regula J, Rupinski M, Kraszewska E *et al.* Colonoscopy in colorectal-cancer screening for detection of advanced neoplasia. *N Engl J Med* 2006; 355: 1863–72.
48. Liebermann DA, Weiss DG, Harford WV *et al.* Five-year colon surveillance after screening colonoscopy. *Gastroenterology* 2007; 133: 1077–85.
49. Imperiale TF, Glowinski EA, Lin-Cooper C *et al.* Five-year risk of colorectal neoplasia after negative screening colonoscopy. *N Engl J Med* 2008; 359: 1218–24.
50. Lin OS, Kozarek RA, Schembre DB, *et al.* Risk stratification for colon neoplasia: screening strategies using colonoscopy and computerized tomographic colonography. *Gastroenterology* 2006; 131: 1011e19.
51. Driver JA, Gaziano JM, Gelber RP, *et al.* Development of a risk score for colorectal cancer in men. *Am J Med* 2007; 120: 257e63.
52. Imperiale TF, Wagner DR, Lin CY, *et al.* Using risk for advanced proximal colonic neoplasia to tailor endoscopic screening for colorectal cancer. *Ann Intern Med* 2003; 139: 959e65.
53. Ho JW, Lam TH, Tse CW, *et al.* Smoking, drinking and colorectal cancer in Hong Kong Chinese: a case control study. *Int J Cancer* 2004; 109: 587e97.
54. Otani T, Iwasaki M, Yamamoto S, *et al.* Alcohol consumption, smoking, and subsequent risk of colorectal cancer in middle-aged and elderly Japanese men and women: Japan Public Health Center-based prospective study. *Cancer Epidemiol Biomarkers Prev* 2003; 12: 1492e500.
55. Toyomura K, Yamaguchi K, Kawamoto H, *et al.* Relation of cigarette smoking and alcohol use to colorectal adenomas by subsite: the Self-Defense Forces health study. *Cancer Sci* 2004; 95: 72e6.
56. Tsong WH, Koh WP, Yuan JM, *et al.* Cigarettes and alcohol in relation to colorectal cancer: the Singapore Chinese Health Study. *Br J Cancer* 2007; 96: 821e7.
57. Frezza EE, Wachtel MS, Chiriva-Internati M. Influence of obesity on the risk of developing colon cancer. *Gut* 2006; 55: 285e91.
58. Leung WK, Ho KY, Kim WH, *et al.* Colorectal neoplasia in Asia: a multicenter colonoscopy survey in symptomatic patients. *Gastrointest Endosc* 2006; 64: 751e9.
59. Yeoh KG, Ho KY, Chiu HM *et al.* for the Asia Pacific Working Group on Colorectal Cancer. The Asia-Pacific Colorectal Screening score: a validated tool that stratifies risk for colorectal advanced neoplasia in asymptomatic Asian subjects. *Gut* 2011. doi:10.1136/gut.2010.221168.
60. Wong VW, Wong GL, Tsang SW *et al.* High prevalence of colorectal neoplasm in patients with non-alcoholic steatohepatitis. *Gut* 2011; 60: 829–36.
61. Chor JSY, Leung JCS, Chan DCS, Griffiths S, Leung PC. Breast cancer screening practice of elderly in Hong Kong worth re-evaluation of health promotion policy. *Journal of Public Health* 2008; 30(1): 110–11.

62. Ng EH, Ng FC, Tan PH, Low SC, Chiang G, Tan KP, *et al.* Results of intermediate measures from a population-based, randomized trial of mammographic screening prevalence and detection of breast carcinoma among Asian women: the Singapore Breast Screening Project. *Cancer* 1998; 82(8): 1521–8.
63. Morimoto T, Nagao T, Okazaki K, Kira M, Nakagawa Y, Tangoku A. Current status of breast cancer screening in the world. *Breast Cancer* 2009; 16(1): 2–9.
64. Anderson G, Jun M, Choi K. Breast cancer screening for Korean women must consider traditional risks as well as two genetic risk factors: genetic polymorphisms and inheritable gene mutations. *Cancer Nurs* 2007; 30(3): 213–22.
65. Huang CS, Chang KJ, Shen CY. Breast cancer screening in Taiwan and China. *Breast Dis* 2001; 13: 41–8.
66. Chong PN, Krishnan M, Hong CY, Swah TS. Knowledge and practice of breast cancer screening amongst public health nurses in Singapore. *Singapore Med J* 2002; 43(10): 509–16.
67. Seah M, Tan SM. Am I breast cancer smart? Assessing breast cancer knowledge among health professionals. *Singapore Med J* 2007; 48(2): 158–62.
68. Sim HL, Seah M, Tan SM. Breast cancer knowledge and screening practices: A survey of 1,000 Asian women. *Singapore Med J* 2009; 50(2): 132–8.
69. Brown ML, Fintor L. Cost-effectiveness of breast cancer screening: preliminary results of a systematic review of the literature. *Breast Cancer Res Treat* 1993; 25(2): 113–18.
70. Lai MS, Yen MF, Kuo HS, Koong SL, Chen TH, Duffy SW. Efficacy of breast-cancer screening for female relatives of breast-cancer-index cases: Taiwan multicentre cancer screening (TAMCAS). *Int J Cancer* 1998; 78(1): 21–6.
71. Woo PP, Kim JJ, Leung GM. What is the most cost-effective population-based cancer screening program for Chinese women? *J Clin Oncol* 2007; 25(6): 617–24.
72. Wong IO, Kuntz KM, Cowling BJ, Lam CL, Leung GM. Cost effectiveness of mammography screening for Chinese women. *Cancer* 2007; 110(4): 885–95.
73. Lam CLK. The price of cancer screening. *Hong Kong Practitioner* 2004; 26(3): 142–5.
74. Goulard H, Boussac-Zarebska M, Ancelle-Park R *et al.* Evaluation epidemiologique du depistage du cancer du colon et du rectum. Premières campagnes du programme pilote français. Available from: http://www.invs.sante.fr/publications/2007/cancer_colon_rectum/cancer_colon_rectum.pdf [Accessed 25 July 2012].
75. Saito H. Colorectal cancer screening using immunochemical faecal occult blood testing in Japan. *J Med Screen* 2006; 13: S6–7.
76. Weller D, Coleman D, Robertson R *et al.* The UK colorectal cancer screening pilot: results of the second round of screening in England. *Br J Cancer* 2007; 97: 1601–5.
77. Subramanian S, Bobashev G, Morris RJ. Modeling the cost-effectiveness of colorectal cancer screening: policy guidance based on patient preferences and compliance. *Cancer Epidemiol Biomarkers Prev* 2009; 18: 1971–8.
78. Moss SM, Campbell C, Melia J, *et al.* Performance measures in three rounds of the English bowel cancer screening pilot. *Gut* 2012; 61: 101–7.
79. Pornet C, Dejardin O, Morlais F, Bouvier V, Launoy G. Socioeconomic determinants for compliance to colorectal cancer screening. A multilevel analysis. *J Epidemiol Community Health* 2010; 64: 318–24.
80. Rosenstock IM, Strecher VJ, Becker MH. Social learning theory and the Health Belief Model. *Health Educ Q* 1988; 15: 175–83.
81. Champion VL. Instrument development for health belief model constructs. *Adv Nurs Sci* 1984; 6: 73–8.
82. Sung JJ, Choi SY, Chan FK, Ching JY, Lau JT, Griffiths S. Obstacles to colorectal cancer screening in Chinese: a study based on the health belief model. *Am J Gastroenterol* 2008; 103: 974–81.
83. Koo JH, Leong RWL, Ching J *et al*, for the Asia-Pacific Working Group in Colorectal Cancer. Knowledge of, attitudes toward, and barriers to participation of colorectal cancer screening tests in the Asia-Pacific region: a multicenter study. *Gastroinest Endosc* 2012; 76: 126–35.
84. Harmy MY, Norwati D, Noor NM, Amry AR. Knowledge and attitude of colorectal cancer screening among moderate risk patients in West Malaysia. *Asian Pacific J Cancer Prev* 2011; 12: 1957–60.
85. Christou A, Thompson SC. Colorectal cancer screening knowledge, attitudes and behavioural intention among Indigenous Western Australians. *BMC Public Health* 2012; 12: 528.

86. Salimzadeh H, Delavari A, Montazeri A, Mirzazadeh A. Knowledge and practice of Iranians toward colorectal cancer, and barriers to screening. *Int J Prev Med* 2012; 3: 29–35.
87. Sanderson PR, Weinstein N, Teufel-Shone N, Martinez ME. Assessing colorectal cancer screening knowledge at tribal fairs. *Prev Chronic Dis* 2011; 8: 1–10.
88. Javanparast S, Ward PR, Carter SM, Wilson CJ. Barriers to and facilitators of colorectal cancer screening in different population subgroups in Adelaide, South Australia. *MJA* 2012; 196: 521–3.
89. Tam TKW, Ng KK, Lau CM, Lai TC, Lai WY, Tsang LCY. Fecal occult blood screening: knowledge, attitudes, and practice in four Hong Kong primary care clinics. *Hong Kong Med J* 2011; 17: 350–7.
90. Rawl SM, Menon U, Champion VL *et al.* Colorectal cancer screening beliefs: focus groups with first-degree relatives. *Cancer Practice* 2000; 8: 32–7.
91. McCaffery K, Borril J, Williamson S *et al.* Declining the offer of flexible sigmoidoscopy screening for bowel cancer: a qualitative investigation of the decision-making process. *Social Science and Medicine* 2001; 53: 679–91.
92. Lewis SF, Jensen NM. Screening sigmoidoscopy: factors associated with utilization. *Journal of General Internal Medicine* 1996; 11: 542–4.
93. Paskett ED, D'Agostino R, Tatum C, *et al.* Colorectal cancer screening practices among low-income women. *Clin J Women's Health* 2000; 1: 3–9.
94. Hawley ST, Earp JA, O'Malley M, *et al.* The role of physician recommendation in women's mammography use: is it a 2-stage process? *Med Care* 2000; 38: 392–403.
95. Klabunde CN, Vernon SW, Nadel MR, Breen N, Seeff LC, Brown ML. Barriers to colorectal cancer screening: a comparison of reports from primary care physicians and average-risk adults. *Med Care* 2005; 43: 939–44.
96. Aubin-Auger I, Mercier A, Lebeau J, *et al.* Obstacles to colorectal screening in general practice: a qualitative study of GPs and patients. *Fam Pract* 2011; 28: 670–6.
97. Cancer Expert Working Group on Cancer Prevention and Screening. Recommendations on Colorectal Cancer Screening. Available: Centre for Health Protection, Hong Kong Government.
98. Sharp L, Tilson L, Whyte S, O'Ceilleachair A, Walsh C, Usher C, *et al.* Cost-effectiveness of population-based screening for colorectal cancer: a comparison of guaiac-based faecal occult blood testing, faecal immunochemical testing and flexible sigmoidoscopy. *Br J Cancer* 2012; 106: 805–16.
99. The trouble with screening. *Lancet* 2009; 373(9671): 1223.
100. Gotzsche PC, Hartling OJ, Nielsen M, Brodersen J, Jorgensen KJ. Breast screening: the facts – or maybe not. *BMJ* 2009; 338: b86.
101. Osterlie W, Solbjor M, Skolbekken JA, Hofvind S, Saetnan AR, Forsmo S. Challenges of informed choice in organised screening. *J Med Ethics* 2008; 34(9): e5.
102. Giordano L, Rowinski M, Gaudenzi G, Segnan N. What information do breast cancer screening programmes provide to Italian women? *Eur J Public Health* 2005; 15(1): 66–9.
103. Nekhlyudov L, Li R, Fletcher SW. Informed decision making before initiating screening mammography: does it occur and does it make a difference? *Health Expect* 2008; 11(4): 366–75.
104. Independent UK Panel on Breast Cancer Screening. The benefits and harms of breast cancer screening. An independent review. *Lancet* 2012; 380: 1778–86.
105. Fischer U, Hermann KP, Baum F. Digital mammography: current state and future aspects. *Eur Radiol* 2006; 16(1): 38–44.
106. Gimeno García AZ. Factors influencing colorectal cancer screening participation. *Gastroenterol Res Pract* 2012; 483417. Epub 2011 Dec 1.
107. Lairson DR, Chang YC, Bettencourt JL, Vernon SW, Greisinger A. Estimating development cost for a tailored interactive computer program to enhance colorectal cancer screening compliance. *J Am Med Inform Assoc* 2006; 13(5): 476–84.
108. Ueland AS, Hornung PA, Greenwald B. Colorectal cancer prevention and screening: A Health Belief Model-based research study to increase disease awareness. *Gastroenterol Nurs* 2006; 29: 357–63.
109. Doll R, Payne P, Waterhouse J, International Union Against Cancer, Cancer incidence in five continents: a technical report, New York: International Union Against Cancer/Springer Verlag, 1966.
110. Segi M, Fujisaku S, Kurihare M, Narai Y, Sasajima K. The age-adjusted death rates for neoplasms in some selected sites in 23 countries in 1954–1955 and their geographical correlation. *Tohoku Journal of Experimental Medicine* 1960; 72: 93–103.

# Part VI

# Health services

# Introduction to Part VI: health services

*Eng Kiong Yeoh and Siân M. Griffiths*

Health policy and management is a multidisciplinary field of inquiry and practice concerned with the delivery, quality and costs of health care for individuals and populations. How health services are provided impacts on the health of the population, as well as on their health seeking behaviours. This part will use case studies to illustrate the issues which arise when shaping and reforming systems.

There are many opportunities for synergy at a local level between public health (population) and primary care (individual) approaches to be shared within primary care organizations. This can be seen in the provision of services for children. In Chapter 37 Abraham describes the public health approach to global child health. She uses three common areas of practice to highlight the diversity of the challenges across Asia – vaccination and immunization, under- and over-nutrition, and substance misuse. Over 12.5 million children and adolescents in Asia do not have access to immunization services and it is estimated that about 500,000 children younger than 5 years of age die from vaccine-preventable diseases in Asia each year. The importance of vaccines in protecting children's health is demonstrated through the case study of rotavirus. An estimated 45 per cent of deaths due to rotavirus gastroenteritis can be avoided through vaccination, which is now recommended as part of routine schedules by WHO. The chapter goes on to discuss the double challenge of obesity and undernutrition which coexist in developing regions in South Asia and the Asia-Pacific region, and the existence of both reflects the wide socio-economic disparities in the region. Asia has undergone a considerable socio-economic transition over the last 30 years, which has resulted in increased food availability, improved health care and transportation. Urbanization has contributed to obesity by lowering the amount of energy expended in labour, for example bicycles being replaced by cars as the primary mode of transport, and an increase in sedentary activities, such as watching TV and playing video games. Urbanization has also led to dietary changes, such as an increase in calories consumed in meals, total fat consumption and meals eaten outside of the home, as well as fast-food intake. Obesity is particularly problematic in Asia as the risks for diabetes, CVDs and metabolic syndrome occur at a lower body mass index (BMI) among Asian populations.

Drug use and abuse, the third illustration, is increasing, particularly among teens in Asia, and at increasingly younger ages. Risk factors include individual, family, community and school issues. Addressing supply and demand issues, emphasizing the importance of resisting substance use, and treating drug dependence and its related complications are important parts of the management of drug and alcohol use. NGOs are often involved not only in primary prevention through education but also through advocacy for service delivery, as well as providing support for families.

MacRae *et al.* provide a case study in Chapter 38 from their work with Save the Children in China where they have been working with frontline healthcare workers and communities to bridge the 'policy to practice' divide in the field of maternal and child health. Critical to their approach has been an engagement from local authorities who manage migrant and rural communities. They describe two programmes of work which successfully demonstrated how NGOs – working in partnership with local governments – can achieve change. The first example was a successful programme to train village primary healthcare providers in rural areas of the Yunan province using innovative training programmes to introduce the national Integrated Management of Childhood Illness (IMCI). The second example is the improvement in school health clinics and hygiene facilities. This project provided training for school health teachers and health centre staff to establish children's records and to give them health checks. An important element was integration of health education into the school curriculum. Parents were also mobilized to support and reinforce the health and hygiene messages that children were learning in schools. Evaluation of the project in Shanghai between October 2008 and September 2011 showed improved access to hygiene facilities, as well as improved health outcomes for the children and as a result the Shanghai Municipal Education Commission issued a policy allocating special funds for health promotion in schools for migrant children.

Chapter 39 on gender and women's health provides case studies that once again highlight the interrelationship between health and socio-political and cultural factors. The impact of gender on health and the important role of social and economic factors of health, such as residential area, access to education and health, and economic wellbeing, are increasingly well recognized. Carmen Wong and Josette Chor describe how gendered roles form the spheres of influence in families and communities. The unequal power relationships can hinder access to education and employment, and eventually result in discrimination which consequently impacts on an individual's access to health care. They highlight that in order to achieve better health and attain gender equity, discrimination based on a person's biological sex has to be eliminated in the provision of opportunities, resources and access to services. Over half a million women worldwide still die from treatable and preventable complications of pregnancy and childbirth each year despite global efforts such as the safe motherhood initiative, which has increased the coverage of antenatal care by 20 per cent and skilled birth attendants at birth by 39 per cent in developing countries. Overall, in the Asia-Pacific region, the lifetime risk of maternal death is still relatively high at one in 260, as compared with one in 39 in Sub-Saharan Africa and one in 1,700 in central and Eastern Europe. Current progress has, in part, been attributed to improvements in education and physical accessibility to health services, as well as the increasing use of contraceptives by women of reproductive age, and improved distribution and access to antiretroviral medication for HIV positive women. The authors provide two case studies to illustrate the links between gender, disadvantage and socio-cultural environments. The first describes the difficulties facing women who are New Immigrants from Mainland China in Hong Kong and the second examines the success of the Self-Employed Women's Association (SEWA) in India. SEWA recognized that to improve women's health it was necessary to strengthen women's economic status, decision-making ability, maternal and child health, and education and housing on both an individual and a community level. As a result, women were able to access and afford healthcare services, build up supportive social networks and remain in employment when faced with challenges to their reproductive and caregiver roles. This demonstration of the impact of empowering women is particularly relevant in Southeast Asia where the gender wage gap can be as high as 38 per cent, as in Korea, and over 30 per cent in Japan, despite legislation to ensure equal pay for equal work regardless of gender.

Development of gender and culturally sensitive healthcare programmes and services from conceptualization, planning and implementation are key to reducing gender inequality and to improving health for women, and through them their children and their communities. Primary care services have an important role to play in providing services for women and children, as they provide ongoing care at a community level. As such they are often closely integrated with public health services. In many situations, primary care clinicians and their teams are indeed the main provider of public health services and increasing attention is being paid to effective and efficient models for integrating personal health care and public health, and organizing primary care on the principle of ongoing care for individuals in the context of an identified population. Primary health care has been defined by the WHO as 'essential health care made universally accessible to individuals and families in the community by means acceptable to them, through their full participation and at a cost that the community and country can afford' [1]. As such, principles of population-based universal access and equity underlie primary care policies and the importance of primary care as the basis for health services is constantly reiterated. For example, when launching the WHO report 'Now More Than Ever', Margaret Chan, Director General of the WHO said:

> Countries with solid health infrastructures and efficient mechanisms for reaching vulnerable populations will be in the best position to cope with threats to health security . . . . If we want to reach the health-related Goals, we must return to the values, principles, and approaches of primary health care. [2]

This approach is based on evidence provided by researchers such as Barbara Starfield whose research found that primary care produces better population health outcomes, reduces the rate of avoidable mortality, improves continuity and access to health care, results in higher patient satisfaction, and reduces health-related disparities at a lower overall cost for health care.

The integration of family medicine with population-based approaches is increasingly recognized as providing best quality care to patients in the community setting. Support for this approach comes from many researchers including Dahrouge and colleagues who found that in the Canadian healthcare system – where the primary care system is well developed – improved health outcomes for chronic disease management [3] were linked to cost savings through reductions in hospitalizations, professional visits, emergency room visits. Increased productivity and higher continuity of care was associated with lower resource utilization and reduced healthcare costs [3]. Others have not necessarily found savings but have clearly demonstrated that primary care improves the quality of patient care. Kringos *et al.* [4] opine that since primary care and public health share similar goals of health improvement, they are uniquely positioned to play critical and complementary roles in tackling the complex health problems on a shared platform particularly in creating intersectoral partnerships at community level. For example, primary care contributes to NCD prevention and control through primary prevention of risk factors (promotion of physical activity, discouragement of smoking initiation), secondary prevention of complications resulting from existing risk factors, and tertiary prevention (rehabilitation and prevention of future complications resulting from stroke or uncontrolled diabetes). In using this terminology, one can equate primary care as family medicine or general practice and public health as population health. Population health outcomes have been found to be better in countries that have a strong primary care structure and robust mechanisms to support coordination and comprehensiveness. Stronger systems are associated with lower rates of avoidable admissions to hospital and fewer potential years of life lost for most of the conditions that were studied in Europe. These systems are supported by van Weel and colleagues [5] who argue that:

> The future of primary care, and health care in general, will depend on how effectively primary practices achieve this community-oriented primary care approach and contribute to equity and social cohesion. Current efforts to revitalise primary health care worldwide should go hand in hand with attention to the social determinants of health. Just as social determinants approach to improving health equity must involve health care so must programmes to control priority public health conditions include attention to the social determinants of health.

The need to redefine primary care and link it to public health impact has been reflected by many including Frenk [6] who has argued that:

> We should be able to launch a fundamental shift from the rigid pyramidal structures that have prevailed in the health sector to adaptable networks that improve access to all levels of care. [6]

He places emphasis on the breadth of interactions outside the health services, focusing on the networks which extend the reach of comprehensive care into schools, workplaces, recreational areas and homes of those who live with a chronic condition. He postulates that the vision is to assure that high-quality services are provided on the basis of a defined population, through proactive strategies, favouring continuity of care, guaranteeing an explicit set of entitlements and assuring universal social protection in health.

Primary care strategies need to be context specific, in particular with reference to income and resources. Across the Asia-Pacific region this thinking is challenging given the high levels of out-of-pocket spending in health care particularly for primary care. In Hong Kong, whilst 80 per cent of hospital care is in the public sector, three-quarters of primary care is provided in the private sector which is fragmented and exists within a laissez-faire market with low levels of professional regulation and very little population-based data. Public health services, such as immunization and other child health services, are still provided in the clinics organized by the government with little or no communication with private doctors. Although it is the aspiration of the policy makers to create a system in which primary care and having a GP is the norm, the public have yet to adopt behaviours conducive to developing this model. Other countries have shown that promoting models of primary care services requires both bottom-up and top-down approaches, as exemplified by the massive efforts in mainland China to refocus and reinvigorate primary care. This has been a central plank of the healthcare reform agenda over the last decade or so. The healthcare system at the national and local levels has significantly invested in community health centres and community-based systems to provide universal access to primary care, to emphasize prevention, to enable choice between Western and traditional medicines and to strengthen programmes within local communities. This is described in Chapter 40 by Wang and Wang who focus on describing the past, present and future of primary care development in China in terms of policy, organization and management within the context of China's healthcare reforms.

Primary care was first established as the cornerstone of China's healthcare system under the centrally planned economy after 1949. It had a significant impact and was considered to be an exemplary model for other countries during that era. The national health policy laid heavy emphasis on preventive health services and on mass mobilization health campaigns for the whole population. This included the role of 'barefoot doctors' who were responsible for the provision of door-to-door healthcare services, focusing predominantly on prevention at population level. Patients were referred to healthcare sectors at higher levels by the barefoot doctors based on the severity of the patient's disease or condition. Thus until the late 1970s, China's primary care contributed to the rapid improvement in the population's health status. When the planned economy ended at the end of the 1970s, overall investment in public health and primary care services fell. In tune with the widespread and rapid economic reforms, a market-oriented healthcare initiative introduced market liberalization and privatization into the healthcare system. This resulted in a pattern of providing curative care, which was more profitable, and largely neglecting the less-profitable health promotion and disease prevention services. In rural areas, as the collective way of financing rural health care was abandoned, the prevention-focused Rural Cooperative Medical Scheme (RCMS) was almost dismantled and the barefoot doctors lost their regular source of income as under-trained fee-for-service village doctors became the source of primary care, making most of their income through drug prescriptions and dispensing activities with less incentive to provide preventive healthcare services. Due to rising public dissatisfaction at the unaffordable health care and inappropriate high demands on hospitals in healthcare delivery, the Community Health Service (CHS) has been introduced and is referred to as primary care. Since 1999, the concept of general practice and general practitioners as primary care providers working in the community is being promoted as part of the reform programme which aims to provide universally accessible services at affordable prices to its 1.3 billion population. The challenges lie in the huge disparities between urban and rural areas, with a shortage of appropriately trained healthcare workers.

The CHS plays an additional important role as the basis and first point of contact for the public health system. In any Community Health Centre (CHC), you will be able to see evidence not only of integration between primary and secondary services but between Western-derived biomedicine medicine (BM) and Traditional Chinese Medicine (TCM). Traditional, Complementary and Alternative Medicine (TCAM) is defined by the WHO as 'a broad domain of healing resources that encompasses all health systems, modalities and practices, and their accompanying theories and beliefs, other than those intrinsic to the politically dominant health system of a particular society or culture in a given historical period'. In many Asian countries, TCAM is an integral part of the healthcare ecology, being deeply rooted in the social and cultural fabric of the community. The WHO produced the Traditional Medicine Strategy 2002–2005, which specified the goals of increasing governmental support for TCAM amongst member states, and promoting the integration of TCAM into national healthcare systems. In Chapter 41 Chung uses Hong Kong as a case study to describe how TCM coexists with Western medicine. At the time of reunification with mainland China in 1997, TCM was formally included in the healthcare system. Since then, the three major developments in TCM have been the formal regulation and registration of TCM practitioners by the Chinese Medicine Council of Hong Kong (CMCHK), the establishment of full-time undergraduate training of TCM practitioners in three local universities, the implementation of compulsory Continuing Medical Education (CME) and the introduction of TCM services into the public healthcare system. However, whilst formal regulation and tertiary education have enabled the TCM sector to become professional, these measures alone have failed to integrate TCM with Western medicine. There is currently no mutual recognition of practice and barriers, such as not being able to formally refer and share patient information, which hinders closer working relationships. However, as Chung argues, a society that offers both modalities of care publicly might well wish to promote a greater understanding of TCM amongst the whole clinician community since the public utilize both types of care. The notion of integration – between hospital and community care; between preventive and curative care; between TCM and Western medicine; between health and social care; between formal and informal care – is important for the future development of effective community-based services.

The second section of Part VI on health services examines health systems in different Asian settings. The World Health Organization (WHO) defines a health system as all organizations, people and actions whose primary intent is to promote, restore and maintain health, and includes efforts to influence the determinants of health as well as more direct health improving activities. The WHO health system framework consists of six building blocks: (i) service delivery, (ii) health workforce, (iii) information, (iv) medical produces, vaccines and technologies, (v) financing and (vi) leadership and governance, which are interconnected and should function in concert to be effective.

The WHO health system framework is grounded in systems theory, and the six building blocks are the components or subsystem of a health system, which are interrelated. Outputs of any one of the subsystems affect other components of the system and impact on the output of the whole system. Health systems function in the wider environment of human social–political–economic systems, influenced and receiving inputs from this macro-system and providing outputs to it. Systems theory provides a conceptual basis for understanding and studying health systems and how they function to achieve the goal of improving health. Studying the relationships of the subsystems, the six building blocks and how outputs of each subsystem affect the others and impact the output of the total system, will lead to a better understanding of how health systems function and how they can be more effective. The framework can be applied for comparative analysis of health systems to assess their performance, what has been achieved and how they have improved health.

This section comprises five chapters, examining the subsystems of service delivery, health workforce, financing, leadership and governance. The first four chapters discuss and analyse the achievements and challenges of health systems in Asia. Starting with an overview of the achievements and challenges of health systems in the whole of Asia, the subsequent three cover Taiwan, Thailand and the Philippines and provide a contrast of a high-income, upper middle-income and lower middle-income economy in Asia at varying stages of their evolution to universal health coverage. Taiwan implemented its National Health Insurance Scheme in 1995 which covered 99.5 per cent of the whole population in 2011. Thailand has more recently introduced a universal coverage scheme in 2001 which covered 75 per cent of the population in 2010. In 1995, the Philippines committed to achieve universal health care within 15 years. These four chapters highlight the impact of socio-economic development on health and on investments in health systems infrastructure as well as the organization and functioning of health systems and how they have contributed to health, the outputs. Health provides the resource to society, for socio-economic development completing a virtuous cycle, in a demonstration of 'system theory in action'.

Asia is a diversified region in terms of economic development, socio-demographic structure and policy environment. This is reflected in the heterogeneity and stages of development of the health systems. For instance, the public share of total health expenditure (THE) was

12 per cent for Myanmar and 37 per cent for Cambodia in 2010. In recent decades, there has been rapid socio-economic development in the Asia-Pacific region with corresponding changes in their health systems. Yeoh and his colleagues in Chapter 42 give an overview of the achievements and challenges of health systems in Asia. They start with discussing the dramatic improvements in socio-economic conditions in Asia and how these in concert with investments in health systems have improved the health of the population in Asia. They analyse infant and maternal mortality and investments in health systems infrastructure in the context of four levels of economic development, high, upper-middle, lower-middle and low income. This is followed by an analysis and discussion of the effects of economic success and the challenges this creates for health systems. The demographic profile of an ageing population and the epidemiological transition of an increasing prevalence of chronic, non-communicable diseases, present challenges for the health systems. Asia is facing challenges of the increasing demand from a more affluent and educated society for more and better health care. Substantial investments in the health system infrastructure are required and how these are to be financed are issues the different Asian economies need to address.

The next chapter is on the health financing system in Taiwan, a high-income country in Asia. Chiang begins by giving readers a contextual framework for the introduction of the national health insurance (NHI). He describes how the historical and political environment has been the key determinant of the evolution of NHI from the laissez-faire market to the present health financing system in Taiwan. In Asia, Taiwan is one of a few governments utilizing social health insurance as a tool for financing healthcare. Chiang describes how the distinctive characteristics of NHI have contributed to the success of NHI in improving the accessibility, quality and equity of health services. He reviews the trends in national health expenditure by dismantling the sources and types of service providers and studying the relationship with healthcare reforms. Chiang concludes his chapter with the observation that NHI has adversely affected Taiwan's 'medical ecology' – medical centres and hospitals have grown at incredible pace and the insured population has overused health services. This has led to rapid cost escalation and creates a daunting challenge to the financial sustainability of the social insurance system. He concludes that Taiwan NHI has an unfinished reform agenda and advocates a system perspective as he notes 'everything is connected to everything else'. Systems theory would have predicted the impact of 'financing' one of the six building blocks (subsystems) of health systems on the other building blocks 'service delivery' and 'medical products and technology'.

Health workforce is the second building block of a health system. Health professionals engage with patients and the community in delivering health care and in actions that improve health. The attributes of a well-performing health workforce are: availability, competence, responsiveness and productivity. Chapter 44 examines the management of health human resources in the Philippines, a lower middle-income country which has a mixed health system of public and private financing and provision, which has committed to universal health coverage in 1995, to be achieved over a period of 20 years. Herrera discusses the quality and quantity dimensions of a well-performing workforce. The numbers and composition of health professionals is a function of 'production' and 'separation', through retirement, employment change, migration and death. Other than having sufficient numbers and composition of a well-performing health workforce, they also have to be fairly distributed. In examining the stocks and trends in production capacity and employment she notes the 'absence of a comprehensive registry or database' and estimates have to be made from multiple sources. One source of government data registered only 36,500 nurses across all regions. Contrasting estimates are in 2008, around 400,000 licensed nurses were not gainfully employed. There was a total disconnect between production of nurses and absorptive capacity of the system. She discusses the phenomenon of scarcity coexisting with excess. Regional mal-distribution, urban–rural divide and the diverse capabilities and capacities of local governments in a decentralized system are contributing factors to the phenomenon and to the inequitable distribution of health human resources in the Philippines. A phenomenal rate of migration of nurses to other countries is another unfortunate characteristic of the system. A staggering 85 per cent, more than 300,000, of the country's nurses chose to work abroad in 2003. The issues of the work-force in the Philippines are a unique case study of the interconnectedness of the six building blocks, the subsystems, and the disastrous consequences if they are in 'disconnect'.

Medical tourism is one of the health policies that a number of governments use to generate trade in health care and revenue for the economy. The governments in Singapore, South Korea, Malaysia and Thailand encourage the service providers, particularly the private sector, to attract patients from other countries, supported by establishing enabling policies. In Chapter 45 Supakankunti shares the Thai experience in medical tourism in an upper middle-income country. She first describes the background of economic development and the achievements in the health system, leading to the implementation of the national universal coverage scheme in 2001 in Thailand. Then, she discusses the definition, the development and the roles of health policy on medical tourism initiated by the Thai government – Thai Medical Hub Policy – and the impact of the growth of medical tourism on the movements of healthcare professionals from the public to the private sector, and from rural to urban locations. In concluding the chapter, she identifies the strengths and weakness of the policy.

How does one study and compare health systems? The final chapter gives readers one perspective. Phua and Lin discuss the concepts and different definitions of a health system. The primary goal of a health system should focus on health improvement of the population. The conceptualization and framework of the health system developed by the WHO provides a basis of understanding how a health system functions effectively and how the performance may be assessed. The authors elaborate on how the functions of health systems, health financing, provision of health services, regulation and stewardship influence performance. Factors within and outside the health system are interrelated. The second section of the chapter discusses the three main issues of governance faced by the health sector: (1) allocation of funds, (2) efficiency of health programmes, and (3) equitable distribution of the benefit of health services. The concepts of equity and approaches, motion of technical and allocated efficiency and resource allocation issues are further elaborated and discussed.

## References


1. World Health Organization. The World Health Report 2008 – Primary Health Care (Now More Than Ever). [Online]. Available from: http://www.who.int/whr/2008/en/
2. Lancet. Margaret Chan puts primary health care centre stage at WHO. *Lancet* 2008; 371(9627): 1811.
3. Dahrouge, S, Devlin, RA, Hogg, B, Russell, G, Coyle, D, Fergusson, D. The Economic Impact of Improvements in Primary Healthcare Performance PHC. [Online]. Available from: http://bit.ly/KJVjE6
4. Kringos, SD, Boerma, WGW, Hutchinson, A, van der Zee, J, Groenewegen, PP. The breadth of primary care: a systematic literature review of its core dimensions. *BMC Health Services Research* 2010; 10: 65.
5. van Weel, C, de Maeseneer, J, Roberts, R. Integration of personal and community health care. *Lancet* 2008; 372(9642): 871–2.
6. Frenk, J. Reinventing primary health care: the need for systems integration. *Lancet* 2009; 374(9684): 170–3.

# 37

# Child and teen health in Southeast Asia

*Anisha Abraham*

## Introduction

Child health encompasses a child's state of physical, mental, intellectual, social and emotional well-being, not just the absence of disease or infirmity in a child. Healthy children live in families, environments and communities that provide them with the opportunity to reach their fullest developmental potential [1]. Good health in childhood builds a strong foundation for health and well-being in adulthood. Ensuring healthy growth and development of children and adolescents should be an important public health priority globally and in Asia. Child health can be optimized by developing policies to promote health, prevent disease and foster equity for children and young people within a framework of sustainable development [2].

According to the most recent 2012 UNICEF report, there has been substantial progress made towards achieving the Millennium Development Goal 4 in improving child health and reducing child and adolescent mortality [3] (see Chapter 2). For example, the worldwide number of under-5 deaths was 6.9 million in 2011, a decline of 41 per cent from 12 million in 1990. In addition, under-5 mortality rates have been reduced by over 50 per cent in Eastern, Southeastern and Western Asia. However, high mortality rates persist in Central and Southern Asia [4]. There were 61 deaths per 1,000 children under 5 years in Central Asia and 42 deaths per 1,000 children in Southern India. India, China and Pakistan are among the top five countries in the world with the highest child mortality rates [5].

Globally, the leading causes of death among children under age 5 are pneumonia, preterm birth complications, diarrhoea, intra-partum related complications and malaria [6]. By comparison, the chief causes of death in people aged 10 to 24 years are road traffic accidents, self-inflicted injuries, violence, lower respiratory infections, tuberculosis and HIV [7]. Chronic health conditions for children and teens include asthma, obesity, HIV and diabetes, as well as disabilities and mental health disorders, such as dyslexia, autism and depression.

The causes of child and teen morbidity and mortality globally and in Asia are largely preventable [8]. For example, the main causes of death in newborns are preterm births and intra-partum complications, which could be minimized by quality care during pregnancy, safe delivery by a skilled birth attendant, strong neonatal care and early initiation of exclusive breastfeeding. From one month to 5 years of age, the chief causes of death are pneumonia, diarrhoea, malaria and measles. Addressing major risk factors, such as malnutrition, are important steps to preventing pneumonia and diarrhoea, as are vaccinations and breastfeeding [9]. Overall, using health promotion, disease prevention, education and surveillance improves health. In addition, strong social policies, comprehensive community support and educational investment are important for optimal child and adolescent health.

In this chapter, we will illustrate some of the public health challenges faced by children in Asia by focusing on the strategies for screening, treatment and prevention in three areas: vaccination, overnutrition and obesity, and substance addiction in childhood and adolescence.

## Birth through adolescence

The first years of life are the most important in setting the stage for optimal health and development. Challenges to health in newborn and childhood periods include infections, such as pneumonia and malaria. During the adolescent years, mental health and sexual/reproductive health related problems become more important.

Physical, intellectual, emotional and social maturity are important markers of a child's overall health and well-being. During the life course from birth through to adolescence, monitoring of growth and developmental milestones at regular intervals is recommended. An example of this is the United States (US) Bright Futures by the American Academy of Pediatrics routine health evaluations at two weeks, one month, two months, four months, six months, one year, 15/18 months, two years and then annually [10]. Checking body length/height, weight, head circumference and blood pressure, as well as discussing the child's growth, nutrition and oral health and providing routine vaccinations, are all part of routine standardized monitoring to detect health problems at an early stage [10].

Community health centres and schools in Asia provide good opportunities for early detection of nutritional issues, such as being overweight or underweight. Checking for abnormalities, such as anaemia and lead (based on community needs), can be very useful. Later in the life span, screening adolescents for high-risk behaviours, such as drug and alcohol use, and suicide and depression, should be incorporated into practice. In general, routine health visits and screening often do not occur on a regular basis in many developing Asian countries given limitations in care, staffing and financial costs. As such, young people in Asia are at a higher risk for problems affecting growth and development.

## Overview of vaccination practices in Asia

Vaccines prevent diseases in people who receive them and protect those who contact unvaccinated infected individuals. In 1796, Edward Jenner successfully used cowpox material to create immunity to smallpox and made the practice of vaccination widespread [11]. In the 1930s, antitoxins/vaccines against diphtheria, tetanus, anthrax, cholera, plague, typhoid and tuberculosis were developed. Since the mid-twentieth century, methods for growing viruses have led to the development of a number of immunizations against more common childhood diseases, such as polio, measles, mumps and rubella [9]. Vaccinations introduce a part, killed or weakened disease organism to the body and cause an immune response without causing symptoms of the disease.

In general, a newborn baby's immunity conferred by his or her mother is short lived. If a baby or child is not vaccinated and exposed to certain pathogens, they may not be strong enough to fight the disease. Immunizing a sufficient proportion of children and decreasing the spread of infection helps not only to protect the individual but also the health of the community, especially those who are not immunized, a concept known as community or herd immunity [12]. Childhood vaccination has substantially reduced the morbidity and mortality from infectious diseases in much of the developed world. For some of the most deadly childhood diseases, such as measles, polio, diphtheria, tetanus, pertussis, pneumonia due to *Haemophilus influenzae* type B and *Streptococcus pneumoniae* and diarrhoea due to rotavirus, vaccines are available and can protect children from illness and death [13]. Worldwide vaccination campaigns have almost eliminated polio and yearly influenza vaccination campaigns have reduced the significant impact of the seasonal influenza infection [14, 15].

Over 12.5 million children and adolescents in Asia do not have access to immunization services. It is estimated that about 500,000 children younger than 5 years of age die from vaccine-preventable diseases in Asia each year. Childhood immunization schemes in developed countries usually include coverage against poliomyelitis, diphtheria, measles, mumps, rubella, tetanus, haemophilus influenza B, hepatitis B and whooping cough, as well as providing the option for rotavirus, chickenpox, influenza, human papilloma virus and hepatitis A [16].

In the South-East Asia region, childhood immunizations policies generally follow at least the World Health Organization (WHO)-recommended schedules against six diseases: measles, polio, diphtheria, pertussis, tetanus and tuberculosis. In addition, hepatitis B has been incorporated into some schemes. However, vaccines against hepatitis A, haemophilus influenza and some diarrhoeal diseases have been available but not used extensively in the public health programmes of many developing Asian countries because of cost and resource limitations [16].

The cost of fully immunizing a child with the six basic vaccinations ranges from US$20 to US$25 [16]. The best systems incorporate free services and easy accessibility to immunizations. Schemes in Southeast Asia are variable as some are fully subsidized and include several vaccinations, such as in Hong Kong, while others, such as in Cambodia, are less comprehensive. Very few countries in Asia, such as India and Indonesia, produce significant quantities of routine vaccines. Countries that do not produce vaccines, either purchase from vaccine manufacturers or from international systems, such as the UNICEF Supply Division [16].

Comprehensive immunization schemes should include methods for evaluating vaccine delivery, monitoring outbreaks and revaluating community vaccination needs. For example, in Hong Kong, it is legally required by the Quarantine and Prevention of Disease Ordinance that doctors report vaccine-preventable diseases, such as measles, to the Child Health Bureau [14]. Migrant status, for example, can affect immunization uptake. Research conducted on mothers from mainland China delivering in Hong Kong demonstrate that maternal mainland status was a significant factor in delayed immunization uptake for children [17]. There are, therefore, many barriers to comprehensive vaccination schemes in Southeast Asia, particularly in low-income countries, including costs, availability and acceptability as illustrated by the examples of rotavirus, pertussis and human papilloma virus vaccines summarized below.

### *Rotavirus*

Rotavirus vaccine is an example of an immunization that has clear benefits in reducing disease burden with minimal side effects. Rotavirus is a leading cause of severe diarrhoea among infants and young children. Each year, more than 600,000 children in the world die from rotavirus and nearly every child in Southeast Asia will probably suffer an episode of rotavirus diarrhoea before the age of 5 [18]. Although the severity of rotavirus infections differs in developed and developing countries, rates of infection are similar. Clean water supplies and good hygiene have little effect on transmission. The vaccine for rotavirus has been proven to be effective in reducing the disease burden and transmission, especially in poorer countries where most of the deaths from the disease occur [18].

In 2006, two vaccines against rotavirus A infection were shown to be safe and effective for children. Both are taken orally and contain the disabled live virus. A review estimated that vaccination against rotavirus would prevent about 45 per cent of deaths due to rotavirus gastroenteritis. Thus, the WHO recommended that the rotavirus vaccine be included in all national immunization programmes [19]. By the end of 2011, the rotavirus vaccine was introduced in 31 Asian countries. Collaboration between the WHO and Centres for Disease Control (CDCs) funded by the Global Alliance for Vaccine Initiative has helped to improve subsidization of vaccines. However, gaps in service and availability exist throughout Asia and demonstrate the challenges of optimizing funding and supply of vaccine despite its clear benefits for children. For example, Hong Kong still does not have rotavirus included on its list of immunizations covered by the government for children [14].

### *Pertussis*

Pertussis (whooping cough) is a viral infection characterized by a sudden onset of high fever, headache, malaise, non-productive cough, sore throat and rhinitis. In the very young, frail elderly and those with serious medical conditions, infection can cause complications, including pneumonia and death. In 1974, Japan had a successful pertussis vaccination programme with 80 per cent of Japanese children vaccinated. Unfortunately, unfounded rumours spread that the vaccine was not safe. By 1976, only 10 per cent of infants were vaccinated. In 1979, a major epidemic led to 13,000 cases and 41 deaths. In response, in 1981, the government began a high-profile campaign in support of vaccinating with acellular pertussis vaccine and the number of cases of infection dropped again. The brief pertussis epidemic in Japan illustrates the need for sustained vaccination campaigns, as well as the importance of community education regarding the benefits and risks of specific immunizations [20].

### *Human papillomavirus*

Human papillomavirus, or HPV, is part of a large family of viruses of which some are sexually transmitted. Certain forms of HPV cause genital warts while other types are the main causes of cervical cancer, associated with anal, penile, throat and mouth cancers. Nearly 80 per cent of women have been infected with genital HPV by the time they are 50 years old in the US. A quadrivalent vaccine against the four common types of HPV (including against types causing genital warts) and a bivalent vaccine against two types of HPV have been approved. The vaccine is 100 per cent effective against precursors of cervical cancer when given prior to sexual activity. The target age for the vaccine is 11 to 12 years [21]. The vaccine has also been approved for males. Data have shown that when a vaccine is given to both girls and boys, rather than to girls alone, the uptake is higher [22].

In the United Kingdom (UK), for example, the rubella immunization programme was aimed at schoolgirls, healthcare workers and susceptible adult women. The weaknesses of this approach became clear in 1993 and 1996, when an increase in rubella was associated with unimmunized males. In 1998, the measles, mumps and rubella vaccines were introduced in the UK for all children aged 12 to 15 months. Vaccinating males helped significantly in rubella eradication efforts [23].

The HPV vaccine was introduced in 43 countries in Asia by the end of 2011. Interest in giving the vaccine has varied largely because of the association with an infection that is sexually transmitted and uptake has been low in many Asian countries for this reason. For example, a recent survey conducted in Hong Kong among mothers found that only 4 per cent of the respondents had their daughters vaccinated, 38 per cent said they were considering letting their daughters have the vaccination and the remaining 59 per cent said their daughters did not have the vaccination [24]. Given the likelihood for suboptimal vaccine coverage among women owing to vaccine refusal, cost and weaknesses in the vaccine delivery system, an HPV vaccine policy including men and women may become necessary to adequately control the disease. Thus, the example of HPV illustrates the need for a gender-neutral policy to enhance use of a vaccine.

### *The future of vaccines*

What is the future of vaccines? Issues that are being addressed include creating single-dose vaccines that can be used after birth as opposed to multiple dose vaccines; developing vaccines that do not need refrigeration or even injection to improve ease of delivery especially in poor remote areas; and utilizing technology, such as the use of mobile phone applications, to improve tracking of vaccinations needed or administered. Finally, new vaccines are being developed against diseases such as herpes simplex, HIV, malaria, chlamydia and dengue. Unfortunately, combination and newly developed vaccines are relatively expensive which may prevent their introduction in many Asian countries with large populations and limited financial resources [9].

## Overnutrition and obesity

The WHO predicts that, by 2015, approximately 2 to 3 billion adults will be overweight and more than 700 million will be obese in the world. In 2010, around 43 million children under 5 were overweight, of which close to 35 million were living in developing countries and 8 million in developed countries. In Asian countries, the prevalence of obesity and overweight children and adults has increased exponentially in the past few decades. For example, an estimated 215 million people in China are overweight or obese [25]. According to the Chinese Ministry of Education, 8 per cent of 10–12-year-olds in China's cities are considered obese and an additional 15 per cent are overweight [26].

Obesity in childhood and adolescence is largely associated with obesity in adulthood [27]. In fact, obese children will have a risk as high as 80 per cent of developing adulthood obesity. Obesity has negative health impacts in childhood and later in life. Affected children experience adverse outcomes, such as breathing difficulties, increased risk of fractures, hypertension, early markers of cardiovascular disease (CVD), insulin resistance and psychological effects [28].

### *Complications of obesity*

Obesity has been identified as a significant cause of disability and premature deaths. Obesity increases the risk of many diseases, including CVDs, hypertension, hyperlipidemia and diabetes mellitus [29]. Obesity not only causes ill health, but also leads to significant economic burdens in a society. Direct economic costs of obesity are assessed in several developed countries in the range of 2 to 7 per cent of total healthcare costs while less is known about the direct economic costs in developing countries [30]. There are also other, non-financial costs to consider, such as reduced quality of life and productivity loss attributed to medical leave [31].

Systematic national data on prevalence of obesity vary. Some countries, such as Vietnam and Indonesia, are in the early stages of assessment while others, such as Japan, Singapore, Malaysia and Hong Kong, have more sophisticated data collection.

### *The paradox of obesity*

Obesity can be classified as overnutrition or a form of malnutrition caused by excessive intake of calories and nutrients. Undernutrition, on the other hand, is a lack of calories and nutrition which leads to stunting, nutrient deficiencies and other problems [32]. Childhood underweight is the leading cause of global burden of disease. Deaths attributable to undernutrition encompass 53 per cent of all childhood deaths in the world [33]. In the past, obesity had been restricted to developed, high-income countries but now, it is an increasing issue in poor and middle-income nations as well [34].

Both obesity and undernutrition coexist in developing regions in South Asia and the Asia-Pacific region mainly due to wide socio-economic disparities. It is estimated that by the year 2015, non-communicable diseases (NCDs) associated with overnutrition will surpass undernutrition as the leading causes of death in low-income communities [35]. The Philippines is an example of an Asian country with both undernutrition and overnutrition. Among adults, the prevalence of being underweight is 13.2 per cent while the prevalence of being overweight is 20.2 per cent [36].

Obesity is also an example of a multi-factorial disease that arises through the interaction of multiple genetic and environmental factors. In some countries, children are initially underweight and as adults are overweight. This has been attributed to the 'thrifty phenotype' in which a low birth weight followed by a rapid childhood weight gain promotes the development of obesity [37].

### *Causes of obesity*

Asia has undergone a considerable socio-economic transition over the last 30 years, which has resulted in increased food availability, improved health care and transportation [34]. Urbanization has contributed to obesity by lowering the amount of energy expended in labour, replacing bicycles with automobiles as the primary mode of transport, and increasing sedentary activities, such as watching TV and playing video games. Urbanization has also led to dietary changes, such as an increase in calories consumed in meals, total fat consumption and meals eaten outside of the home, as well as fast-food intake [38]. Among Chinese children, for example, there has been an increase in dietary fat and high-energy consumption and less time spent on moderate/vigorous physical activities [39].

### *Diagnosis and screening*

Obesity is particularly problematic in Asia as the risks for diabetes, CVDs and metabolic syndrome occur at a lower body mass index (BMI) among Asian populations. In addition, many Asians, especially south Asians, have a higher total and central fat composition for a given body weight when compared with matched Caucasian, non-Asians. Diagnosing the BMI in a child is based on BMI and percentiles for age as opposed to BMI in adults. Generally a BMI of over 90 per cent for age is considered overweight and 99 per cent is obese for a child or adolescent under 18 years of age. For Asian adults, a BMI of 23 is considered overweight and 25 is obese as compared to 28 and 30 in non-Asian adults [29].

### *Treatment and prevention*

Obtaining an evidence base for treatment of obesity in children and teens has proven very difficult. For example, over the last 25 years, there have been very few published randomized control trials of obesity management targeting adolescents. On an individual level, recommendations for how to address obesity in children and adolescents include using motivational and behavioural counselling to cut back on sweetened beverages and TV and computer time, as well as to increase activity level and consumption of fresh fruits and vegetables. In certain cases, very low energy diets, pharmacological and bariatric surgery have been used for adolescents with co-morbidities, such as severe hypertension and diabetes. Bariatric surgery, in particular, has been shown to be a very effective means of addressing obesity-related complications but is also extremely expensive and requires extensive follow-up [40, 41].

Primary preventions that have a community or public health approach are the measures that are most likely to be successful in addressing obesity. Community-based settings can take into account local needs, offer accessibility required for long-term programmes and have facilities for multidisciplinary group interventions. School-based interventions using increased physical activity, reduced TV watching, improved availability of healthy food choices in cafeterias and a reduced intake of carbonated drinks have been shown to be successful for the short to medium term [40, 41].

Some countries, including Pakistan, Singapore, India and China, have initiated successful national programmes related to obesity and nutrition. National programmes have also been initiated for prevention of NCDs. Singapore's 'Fit and Trim' programme in school children has led to a remarkable drop in prevalence of obesity from 16.6 per cent in 1992 to 14.6 per cent in 2000 among children aged 11–12 years, and from 15.5 per cent to 13.1 per cent among adolescents aged 15–16 years [42]. The Ministry of Health in Malaysia has laid down guidelines for reduction of overweight and obesity in children and adolescents which include: reduction in energy intake by use of conventional food, improving physical activity and thus energy expenditure, behaviour modification associated with eating habits and activity pattern, and involvement of the family in the process of change. Guidelines are also provided to parents to promote healthy eating amongst children and for improving their physical activity levels [43] (see Chapter 29).

Consideration has been given in some countries to higher taxes on unhealthy foods, improved nutrition labelling and better access to physical fitness [40, 41]. On a community and governmental level, however, many developing Asian countries lack proper urban planning and the density of the population is high in cities and towns. Overall serious governmental action is required to reduce the health related problems and economic healthcare cost of obesity in childhood and adolescence [44].

## Substance abuse

Increasingly, morbidity and mortality trends for young people in developing nations are paralleling those in the industrialized world. Trends in adolescent morbidity and mortality have shifted over the past decade from predominately infectious to social etiologies. Unintentional injury, for example, is currently the main cause of death of young people in nearly every region of the world, with homicide, war and suicide following behind [45].

With the era of technology and increased availability of computers and phones, children and teens are also faced with new forms of morbidity, such as Internet addiction. A study conducted among incoming university students in Hong Kong showed that 99.4 per cent of students had used the Internet with an average of 2.8 hours/day and 14.9 per cent reported heavy Internet use (> 4 hours/day). Heavy users were less likely to socialize face-to-face and were more likely to skip school, engage in online chatting and games, and meet strangers from the Internet [46].

Globally, up to 1 in 5 of children and teens suffer from a disabling mental illness. The WHO suggests that by 2020, teen psychiatric disorders will increase by more than 50 per cent worldwide to become one of the five leading causes of disability among adolescents. The WHO estimates that 5 in 10 leading causes of disability in those aged 15 to 44 are psychiatric conditions, such as alcohol use disorder and depression [47]. One of the most common mental health disorders among young people is depression. Of significant concern is that depression among young people is often combined with substance abuse, such as cannabis, methamphetamines and alcohol, which puts teens at an even greater risk for suicide [45].

### *What is substance abuse?*

Use of alcohol, tobacco and illicit drugs continues to be a major international health concern. Drug abuse is defined as the use of drugs that are illegal or harmful to oneself and cause significant adverse consequences, such as accidents or injuries, legal problems or risky behaviours. Substance dependence is continued substance abuse despite significant substance-related problems. This usually includes tolerance of the drug, as well as withdrawal [48]. Early onset of substance use is associated with a greater risk of alcohol-related car crashes, physical fights and other injuries. In addition, substance-abusing teens are at greater risk for unprotected sexual activity, depression, suicidal ideation and poor school performance [40, 41].

In utero, exposure to drugs and alcohol leads to sub-optimal foetal development and subsequent health problems, such as foetal alcohol syndrome [49]. In adolescence, heavy drug use during times of critical brain development may cause permanent changes in the way the brain works and responds to rewards and consequences. Researchers using an imaging machine (MRI) to scan brains of binge drinking teenagers consuming four to five or more drinks in a few hours at one sitting, at least one time during the previous three months, found that the white matter in their brains was abnormal when compared with the white matter of teens that did not binge drink. Thus binge drinking could be affecting thinking, learning and memory. Adolescent brains may be more vulnerable to effects of even small doses of drugs and alcohol, and more regular drinking can have more severe consequences, such as high blood pressure and liver disease [50].

### *Incidence and prevalence of drug and alcohol abuse*

At least 15.3 million people have drug-use disorders worldwide, and this includes children and adolescents. In 2012, 3.4 to 6.6 per cent of the world's population aged 15 to 64 used psychoactive substances, such as cannabis, amphetamines, cocaine, opioids and non-prescribed psychoactive prescription medication [51]. Globally, cannabis is the most commonly used drug followed by amphetamine-type stimulants, then cocaine and opioids. Opioids are ranked on top in terms of harm associated with use. The use of psychoactive substances causes significant health and social problems for users, and also for others in their families and communities. The WHO estimated that 0.7 per cent of the global burden of disease is due to cocaine and opioid use, with the social cost of illicit substance use being in the region of 2 per cent of GDP in those countries that have measured it. Alarmingly, only 12 to 30 per cent of problem drug users in the world receive treatment each year [47].

The harmful use of alcohol is a global problem which compromises both individual and social development. Alcohol use results in 2.5 million deaths each year and accounts for 9 per cent of all deaths in people aged 15 to 25. Alcohol is the world's third largest risk factor for premature mortality, disability and loss of health, and is the leading risk factor in the Western Pacific [52].

Harmful drinking is a major determinant for disorders, such as alcohol dependence, as well as CVD and cirrhosis of the liver. The harmful use of alcohol is also associated with several infectious diseases like HIV/AIDS, tuberculosis and sexually transmitted infections (STIs). A significant proportion of the disease burden attributable to harmful drinking arises from unintentional and intentional injuries, including those due to road traffic accidents, violence and suicides.

Socio-demographic trends, such as the population's gender and age balance, and the rate of urbanization and socio-economic factors, such as levels of disposable income, inequality and unemployment, as well as peer group and ease of obtaining alcohol, play a role in its use. A study conducted among university students in Hong Kong showed that, by the second year of school, the proportion of respondents who reported ever drinking increased from 71.8 per cent to 86.6 per cent among men and 53.0 per cent to 80.6 per cent among women, and the prevalence of binge drinking in the preceding month doubled among males (11.6 per cent to 21.7 per cent) and nearly tripled among females (2.8 per cent to 7.9 per cent). Students with 'some' or 'many' friends who used alcohol frequently were three times more likely to binge drink. Results suggest that students in Hong Kong binge drink primarily for mood enhancement and for socializing purposes. In addition, the uptake of heavy drinking among Hong Kong university students appears to be associated with a number of specific factors including discounted alcohol rates for students at pubs, the wide accessibility of alcohol, lax enforcement of the drinking age, and the reduction in alcohol taxes on wine and beer [53].

### *Types of substances used*

Opioids continue to be the dominant drug type accounting for treatment demand in Asia. The use of stimulants is increasing overall in the region as well. In Japan and the Republic of Korea, crystalline methamphetamine is the most commonly used drug. In China, opioids, mainly heroin, are the primary drug of concern, followed by amphetamines [52]. In Hong Kong, youth substance abuse is increasing and the age of first use is decreasing. For example, among students aged 12 or below, 4.6 per cent indicated that they had abused drugs. According to recent government reports, ketamine is the most common drug used by teens in Hong Kong [54]. In developing Asian countries, there are limited data about youth substance use, however, international organizations, such as the WHO and the United Nations Drug Control Programme, have begun to promote scientific studies to collect information. One study by WHO/UNDCP aiming to examine the use of drugs among young people in specific sites in Thailand, the Philippines and Vietnam found variations in the rate and types of drugs used. In the Philippines, between 2–7 per cent of young people reported using a variety of illicit substances, such as cannabis, injections, heroin, cocaine, mandrax and ecstasy compared to 2–2.1 per cent of youth in Thailand reporting the use of illicit substances, such as amphetamines, cannabis, hallucinogens, versus 3 per cent of youth in Vietnam using substances, mainly heroin and injections. Use of alcohol and tobacco products was common in all countries particularly among young males [55].

## Drug-related complications

Drug use, notably injecting drug use, is a significant vector for spreading HIV, and hepatitis B and C. UNODC estimates that approximately 20 per cent of drug users worldwide have HIV, 46.7 per cent have hepatitis C and 14.6 per cent have hepatitis B. These viruses can cause or exacerbate a range of symptoms and ailments with potentially fatal outcomes, and, in general, add to the global burden of disease [51].

UNODC estimates suggest that about 12 per cent of illicit drug users, which includes adults and young adults, develop drug dependency and become 'problem' drug users [55]. Drug-dependent people require treatment, which may place a financial burden on the individuals and their families, or on society at large.

## Risk factors for drug use

Individual risk factors for substance abuse include childhood trauma, abuse and poor self-esteem, as well as a lack of social bonding and sensation seeking. During teen years, anti-social behaviour, hyperactivity and having mental problems play an important role. Substance abuse and depression coexist in 25 per cent of adolescents. Family factors include parental history of drug use and family conflicts. In addition, failure at school and lack of commitment to school, relationship problems and drug-using friends all contribute to children and adolescents abusing alcohol and drugs. Finally, other factors that influence drug and alcohol use include laws and attitudes in the social environment, peer group, and the availability and accessibility of alcohol as demonstrated by the example of university students in Hong Kong [56].

## Treatment

Individual screening in primary care and school-based settings may be useful to identify people who are experiencing substance-related problems, and to provide information about the associated risks and problems [57]. Screening is beneficial in reducing high-risk activities for teens, but is not common practice in Asia. In a health study of 7,371 primary care patients in Hong Kong, only 29 per cent of the patients reported being asked about their use of alcohol or drugs in the past year [58]. Screening tools can include self-report tools, such as interviews and self-administered questionnaires. Biological markers, such as serum drug testing and urine testing, may also be useful in specific situations when voluntary consent is given, but is less useful in school-based or community-wide practices. Treatment should include behavioural counselling to change motivation and need for drug use [56]. In chronic users, treatment may also include pharmacological methods to reduce withdrawal and coexisting depression and anxiety.

## Prevention

Effective drug prevention initiatives should aim to change behaviour among children and teens. Interventions should be evidence based, developmentally appropriate and interactive. Prevention programmes should also be long term with repeated interventions (i.e. booster programmes) to reinforce the original prevention goals. Ideally, programmes should be initiated before drug use commences. It has been shown that prevention programmes should address all forms of drug use, including the use of legal drugs, such as tobacco and alcohol; the use of illegal drugs, such as marijuana or heroin; and the inappropriate use of legally obtained substances, such as inhalants, prescription medications or over-the-counter drugs [51]. Peer education programmes may have some benefits in addressing substance use and other risk behaviours as demonstrated by the university peer health programme in Shantou, China [59].

Research findings have shown that scare tactics and blaming adolescents for their weaknesses do not work in addressing substance use. In addition, reducing supply cannot alone solve the problem as demand continues to exist. In contrast, family-based interventions and reduction of both supply and demand do work. Other useful interventions are involvement of teens in the process of formulating services, development of policies involving stakeholders in different sectors, and use of resources devoted to primary, secondary and tertiary prevention [60].

The aforementioned WHO/UNDCP study recommends facilitating economic development, mobilizing community groups, teaching teens through awareness campaigns and peer education not to succumb to substance use, strengthening social support groups, reducing liquor and tobacco outlets, and increasing deterrence of illegal drug trafficking to address substance use in selected developing countries in Southeast Asia [54]. As evidenced by research in tackling child and adolescent obesity, multi-tiered community-based approaches and governmental involvement are necessary in addressing the growing problem of youth substance use.

## Conclusion

According to the WHO, an estimated two-thirds of children globally could be saved from death through simple interventions, such as better nutrition and skilled birth attendance [1]. Other interventions to promote optimal health include providing vaccinations, performing newborn/child examinations and screening for obesity. Strong social policies and comprehensive community support are essential for optimal child health.

Childhood vaccination has substantially reduced the morbidity and mortality from infectious diseases in much of the developed world and will continue to be a priority in public health in Asia despite multiple challenges including cost, supply and public acceptance.

Overweight and obesity have reached epidemic proportions in many Asian countries. These countries also face an increasing burden of obesity-related disorders, such as diabetes, hypertension and CVDs, which develop at a younger age than in Western populations. The major causative factors are related to lifestyle changes occurring because of rapid socio-economic transition. Asian populations show several differences in genetic factors when compared with the Caucasian population, and they also have lower cut points for environmental risk factors. National programmes targeting public awareness, education and improved structural facilities to promote healthy lifestyles are integral to alleviating the economic and healthcare burden of obesity-related disorders.

Drug use and abuse is increasing, particularly among teens in Asia, and at increasingly younger ages. Risk factors include individual, family, community and school issues. Common drugs used in Asia are opioids and stimulants although drug-use patterns are very specific to each country and region. Overall, addressing supply and demand issues, emphasizing the importance of resisting substance use, and treating drug dependence and its related complications are important parts of the management of drug and alcohol use.

## References

1. World Health Organization. What are the key health dangers for children? 2012. Available from: http://www.who.int/features/qa/13/en/index.html [Accessed 10 November 2012].

2. Ministry of Health and Long-Term Care. Child Health. 2012. Available from: http://www.mhp.gov.on.ca/en/healthy-communities/public-health/guidance-docs/ChildHealth.PDF0 [Accessed 10 December 2012].
3. You D., New J., Wardlaw T. *et al.* Levels and Trends in Child Mortality Report 2012. Estimates Developed by the UN Inter-agency Group for Child Mortality Estimation. UN Interagency Report, 2012.
4. Hill K., You D., Inoue M., *et al.* Child mortality estimation: accelerated progress in reducing global child mortality, 1990–2010. *PLoS Medicine* 2012; 9(8) e1001303.
5. Unicef. Child Mortality Report 2012. Available from: http://www.childinfo.org/files/Child_Mortality_Report_2012.pdf
6. Liu L., Johnson H., Cousens S., *et al.* Global, regional, and national causes of child mortality: an updated systematic analysis for 2010 with time trends since 2000. *Lancet* 2012; 379: 2151–61.
7. Patton C., *et al.* Global patterns of mortality in young people: a systematic analysis of population health data. *Lancet* 2009; 374(9693): 881–92.
8. Bryce J., *et al.* WHO estimates of the causes of death in children. *Lancet* 2005; 365(9465): 1147–52.
9. College of Physicians of Philadelphia. History of Vaccines. 2012. Available from: http://www.historyofvaccines.org/content/timelines/all [Accessed 10 November 2012].
10. American Academy of Pediatrics. Bright Futures. Available from: http://brightfutures.aap.org/ [Accessed 15 December 2012].
11. Riedel S. Edward Jenner and the history of smallpox and vaccination. *Proc Bayl Univ Med Cent* 2005; 18(1): 21–5.
12. CDC. Vaccines and Immunizations. 2011. Available from: http://www.cdc.gov/vaccines/about/terms/glossary.htm#commimmunity
13. World Health Organization. Children: Reducing Mortality. WHO Media Centre. Available from: http://www.who.int/mediacentre/factsheets/fs178/en/
14. Government of Hong Kong. Hong Kong Vaccination Schedule. 2012. Available from: http://www.fhs.gov.hk/english/main_ser/child_health/child_health_recommend.htm [Accessed 10 November 2012].
15. World Health Organization. Immunization Monitoring. 2012. Available from: http://www.who.int/immunization_monitoring/en [Accessed 10 November 2012].
16. WHO Task Force for Development of a Regional Vaccine Policy World Health Organization Regional Office for South-East Asia. 2011. Vaccines in South East Asia.
17. Fong H. Responding to the Public Health Burden of Births to Mainland Migrant Mothers in Hong Kong. Abstract. 13th World Congress on Public Health. 2012.
18. CDC. Rotavirus Vaccine. 2012. Available from: http://www.cdc.gov/rotavirus/about/index.html [Accessed 15 December 2012].
19. World Health Organization. Rotavirus. 2011. Available from: http://www.who.int/nuvi/rotavirus/en/
20. Baker J. The pertussis vaccine controversy in Great Britain, 1974–1986. *Vaccine* 2003; 21: 4003–11.
21. Hamborsky J., McIntyre L. Centers for Disease Control and Prevention of Vaccine-Preventable Diseases. Human Papillomavirus. 11th ed. Washington, DC: Public Health Foundation, 2009.
22. Giuliano A., Salmon D. The Case for a Gender-Neutral (Universal) Human Papillomavirus Vaccination Policy in the United States: Point Cancer Epidemiol Biomarkers 2008; 17, 805. Available from: http://cebp.aacrjournals.org/content/17/4/805.long – target-1, http://cebp.aacrjournals.org/content/17/4/805.long – target-2
23. Mammas I.N., Spandidos D.A. Vaccination against human papillomavirus in childhood: the next rubella analogue? *J Buon* 2012; 17(2): 389–90. Available from: http://www.ncbi.nlm.nih.gov/pubmed/22740223
24. International Planned Parenthood Federation. Family Planning Association of Hong Kong Survey on HPV and Cervical Cancer Screening. 2009. Available from: http://www.ippfeseaor.org/en/News/Country+highlights/FPAHKPublicSurvey.htm [Accessed 10 November 2012].
25. World Health Organization. WHO Facts on Obesity. 2012. Available from: http://www.who.int/features/factfiles/obesity/en/ [Accessed 15 November 2012].
26. MacLeod C. Obesity of China's kids stuns officials. *USA Today.* 2007. Available from: http://usatoday30.usatoday.com/news/world/2007-01-08-chinese-obesity_x.htm

27. Serdula M.K., Ivery D., Coates R.J., *et al.* Do obese children become obese adults? A review of the literature. *Prev Med* 1993; 22(2): 167–77.
28. Guo S.S., Chumlea W.C. Tracking of body mass index in children in relation to overweight in adulthood. *Am J Clin Nutr* 1999; 70(1): 145S–8S.
29. World Health Organization. Obesity and Overweight Fact Sheet No. 311. 2006.
30. World Health Organization. The World Health Report 2002: Reducing Risks, Promoting Healthy Life. Geneva, 2002.
31. World Health Organization. Report of a Joint WHO/FAO. WHO Technical Report Series No. 916. Diet, Nutrition and the Prevention of Chronic Diseases. 2003. Available from: http://whqlibdoc.who.int/trs/who_TRS_916.pdf [Accessed 12 November 2012].
32. Blair M., Stewart-Brown S., Waterson T., *et al.* *Child Public Health.* Oxford: Oxford University Press, 2003.
33. Caulfield L., *et al.* Undernutrition as an underlying cause of child deaths associated with diarrhea, pneumonia, malaria, and measles. *Am J Clin Nutr* 2004; 80, (1): 193–8.
34. Ramachandran A., Snehalatha C. Rising burden of obesity in Asia. *Journal of Obesity* 2010. Article ID 868573, doi:10.1155/2010/868573.
35. Tanumihardjo S., *et al.* Poverty, obesity, and malnutrition: an international perspective recognizing the paradox. *Journal of the American Dietetic Association* 2007; 107(11): 1966–972.
36. Villavieja G.M. 1998 updating of nutritional status of Filipino children at the provincial level. *Philippine Journal of Nutrition* 2001; 48: 1–14.
37. Prentice A.M. The emerging epidemic of obesity in developing countries. *International Journal of Epidemiology* 2006; 35(1): 93–9.
38. Jacobsen K. *Introduction to Global Child Health.* Sudbury, MA: Jones and Bartlett Publishers, 2008: 55–90, 203–207.
39. Li Y., Zhai F. Determinants of childhood overweight and obesity in China. *British Journal of Nutrition* 2007; 97(1): 210–15.
40. Steinbeck K. Obesity in adolescents. In Brown R., Bennett D. (eds) *Adolescent Medicine: State of the Art Reviews. International Health Issues in Adolescents.* Elk Grove Village, IL: American Academy of Pediatrics 2009: 900–14.
41. Hassan, A. *et al.* Adolescent substance abuse around the world. In Brown R, Bennett D. (eds) *Adolescent Medicine: State of the Art Reviews. International Health Issues in Adolescents.* Elk Grove Village, IL: American Academy of Pediatrics 2009: 915–29.
42. Toh C.M., Cutter J., Chew S.K. School based intervention has reduced obesity in Singapore. *British Medical Journal* 2002; 324(7334): 427.
43. Sidik S.M., Ahmad R. Childhood obesity: contributing factors, consequences and intervention. *Malaysian Journal of Nutrition* 2004; 10(1): 13–22.
44. Kumanyika S.K., Obarzanek S., Obarzanek E. Population-based prevention of obesity: the need for comprehensive promotion of healthful eating, physical activity, and energy balance: a scientific statement from American Heart Association Council on Epidemiology and Prevention. Interdisciplinary Committee for Prevention. *Circulation* 2008; 118(4): 428–64.
45. Blum R., Nelson-Mmari K. The health of young people in a global context. *Journal of Adolescent Health* 2004; 35(5): 402–18.
46. Lau C.H., Griffiths S., Chow K.W., *et al.* Heavy Internet use and correlations with interpersonal behaviours among university entrants in Hong Kong. *Asia-Pacific Journal of Public Health* 2008; 134–40.
47. World Health Organization. Substance Abuse Facts. 2012. Available from: http://www.who.int/substance_abuse/facts [Accessed 10 November 2012].
48. World Health Organization. Dependence Syndrome. 2012. Available from: http://www.who.int/substance_abuse/terminology/definition1/en/
49. A.D.A.M. Medical Encyclopaedia. Fetal alcohol syndrome. 2012. Available from: http://www.ncbi.nlm.nih.gov/pubmedhealth/PMH0001909/
50. Weinberger D., Elvevag B., Giedd J. The Adolescent Brain: A Work in Progress for the National Campaign to Prevent Teen Pregnancy. 2005.
51. United Nations Office on Drugs and Crime. World Drug Report 2012. Available from: http://www.unodc.org/unodc/en/data-and-analysis/WDR-2012.html [Accessed 10 March 2013].
52. SEARO. Substance Abuse in Asia. 2012. Available from: http://www.searo.who.int/en/Section1174/Section1199/Section2278_12023.htm [Accessed 10 November 2012].

53. Kim J.H., Chan K., Chow J., *et al.* University binge drinking patterns and changes in patterns of alcohol consumption among Chinese undergraduates in a Hong Kong university. *J of American College Health* 2009; 58(3): 255–65.
54. The Government of the Hong Kong SAR. Narcotics Division, Security Bureau. Introduction. 2013. Available from: http://cs-crda.nd.gov.hk/en/introduction.asp
55. WHO/UNDCP. Substance Abuse in South East Asia Knowledge, Attitudes, Practices and Opportunities for Intervention. 2003. Available from: http://whqlibdoc.who.int/publications/2003/9241590793.pdf [Accessed 15 December 2012].
56. Greydanus D.E., Patel D.R. The adolescent and substance abuse: current concepts. *Current Problems in Pediatric and Adolescent Health Care* 2005; 35: 78–98.
57. Gray K.M. *et al.* Advances in diagnosis of adolescent substance abuse. *Adolescent Medicine Clinics* 2006; 17(2): 411–25.
58. Lau J.T.F., Kim J.H., Tsui H.Y. Prevalence, health outcomes and patterns of psychotropic substance use in a Chinese population in Hong Kong. *Substance Use & Misuse* 2005; 40(2): 187–209.
59. Li L.P., Chow K.W., Griffiths S., *et al.* University-based peer health education in China: the Shantou experience. *Journal of American College Health* 2009; 57(5): 549–51.
60. Shek D.T. Tackling adolescent substance abuse in Hong Kong: where we should and should not go. *Scientific World Journal* 2007; 7: 2021–30.

# 38

# Non-governmental organizations and health

## A case study on Save the Children, China

*Pia MacRae, Ruikan Yang, Linghui Jiang and Jinping Guo*

### Introduction

Civil society[1] has played a key role in public health in many countries, including those with strong public provision of health services. Historically, the Chinese government[2] limited the space for the emergence of an independent civil society. Today this is changing with a greater encouragement of citizens and civil society actors in various areas of policy, as well as local governments engaging in pragmatic partnerships at the grassroots level. While China has seen the emergence of civil society players in health [1] (notably in the area of HIV/AIDS [2, 3, 4]), the space has not yet been clearly defined.

The government remains the key service provider for health in China. Alongside government structures, there is a parallel service network of mass organizations and government-organized, non-governmental organizations (known as 'GONGOs'[3]), which typically operate through vertical hierarchies. GONGOs are organized by the government in China. Their work mainly focuses on the development of civil society in terms of education, children, women and other aspects. They operate in a top-down way oriented by the government.

However, non-state actors are also increasingly getting both indirect and direct recognition.[4] In China, apart from GONGOs, there are some grassroots non-governmental organizations (NGOs) that are nowadays playing more and more important roles.

This case study will discuss the potential role that NGOs can play in promoting public health in China through the lens of one international NGO's (INGO) experience. As was made clear through the response to the HIV/AIDS epidemic, NGOs can play a unique role in empowering and giving a voice to under-represented groups;[5] however, we would also like to argue that they can play an important role in demonstrating models of service provision and advocating for policy change.

Save the Children (SC), an INGO working in 120 countries to bring about immediate and lasting change for children, has demonstrated this through building on existing programmatic approaches used in education and child protection to establish a value-added role as a civil society organization within the health system in China. This suggests that there is a role outside the field of HIV/AIDS, where the 'taboo' nature of the challenge, the behavioural element to preventive measures and the existence of international response tools made it a catalyst for the emergence of public health NGOs in China. Besides various INGOs working in China, some local NGOs include the Chi Heng Foundation, the Beijing Dongzhen Nalan Culture Communication Centre, CHAIN – China HIV/AIDS Information Network, the Beijing Zhiaixing Information and Counselling Centre, and the Beijing Loving Source Education and Research Centre, as well as others.

## Overview of Save the Children

SC has been operating in China since the late 1980s. Early programmatic work primarily focused on education and child protection,[6] typically delivered in partnership with government partners. Evaluations and informal feedback[7] suggest partners identify particular value of the organization because of its 'international ideas', the participatory style of training and communications, professional management processes and, finally, flexibility of approach [5].

In 2009, SC China programmes made a strategic decision to move into health programming.[8] While China is well on track to achieve the Millennium Development Goals (MDGs) 4 and 5[9] (see Chapter 2), the impressive headline national data mask ongoing challenges: government and health analysts recognize that current strategies and systems are having less impact on the remaining high child mortality rates among the bottom wealth quintile and that significant gaps are emerging in health outcomes.

In the poorest areas in China, including most of the western provinces and among some ethnic minority populations, a combination of factors have limited access and utilization of services due to complex factors, such as long distances, limited financial support and shortage of qualified doctors, resulting in slow changes in maternal and child health status. The result is similar for poor rural-to-city migrants, who are unable to register in the cities and therefore face a lack of entitlement to services, which are otherwise available to residents. They may also have substandard living conditions (with poor hygiene facilities and cramped living accommodation) and demanding employment, which increases their health vulnerability and frequent moves make check-ups and continuity of health care difficult (see Chapter 3). Most of the living conditions of migrants are not good. For example, it is very common for a migrant family with three or four people to live in a small, damp and dark room with mould. At the same time, migrants also need to work hard to earn a living, but without good living conditions, they get sick very easily. When they get sick, with no access to health services, their health situation becomes more and more vulnerable.

Expanding on methodologies that SC had pioneered in other areas of work in China, including combining internationally tested guidelines for practice with a participatory approach, SC began to work with frontline healthcare workers and communities to bridge the 'policy to practice' divide in the field of maternal and child health. Critical to the approach was an engagement of encouragement from local authorities, who manage migrant and rural communities, to look for the strengths and resources of these groups.[10] Two examples from a much wider portfolio of work are shared below. The first one discusses how SC has helped build skills amongst rural doctors and the second demonstrates how SC has been working with children affected by migration.

## Save the Children case study 1: demonstrating models of service provision

China's challenges in the health sector in moving from policy to practice include a lack of policy flexibility, capacity and reach of the health system, and the quality of delivery of care. The Integrated Management of Childhood Illnesses (IMCI), a key Ministry of Health tool for managing paediatric health, is an internationally evidence-based health intervention (see Figure 38.1). However, in practice, training of doctors had been too short for its implementation and had failed to equip trainees to put their newly learnt skills into practice. Furthermore, once trained, there was no follow-up supervisory mechanism or requirement for continuous professional development and updating (see Figure 38.2). In addition, primary healthcare providers at village level had not been included in national IMCI training programmes.

With the Yunnan Provincial Health Bureau, SC China trained village doctors from 16 prefectures and cities on the case management skills for sick children under 5, including assessment, classification and treatment, checking immunization and feeding, and providing follow-up care. They became local trainers and delivered training workshops (see Figure 38.3) for village-level healthcare providers to increase their case management skills and improve the quality of services at the grassroots level (see Figure 38.4).

With increased support from the local health system, such as supportive supervision visits in the workplace, increased availability of medical equipment and drugs, and improved case recording forms, the majority of the 55 trained healthcare providers at the village level have been applying IMCI in their practice. According to the most recent supervision visit to the 55 trained village-level healthcare providers, over 80 per cent can correctly assess a sick child,

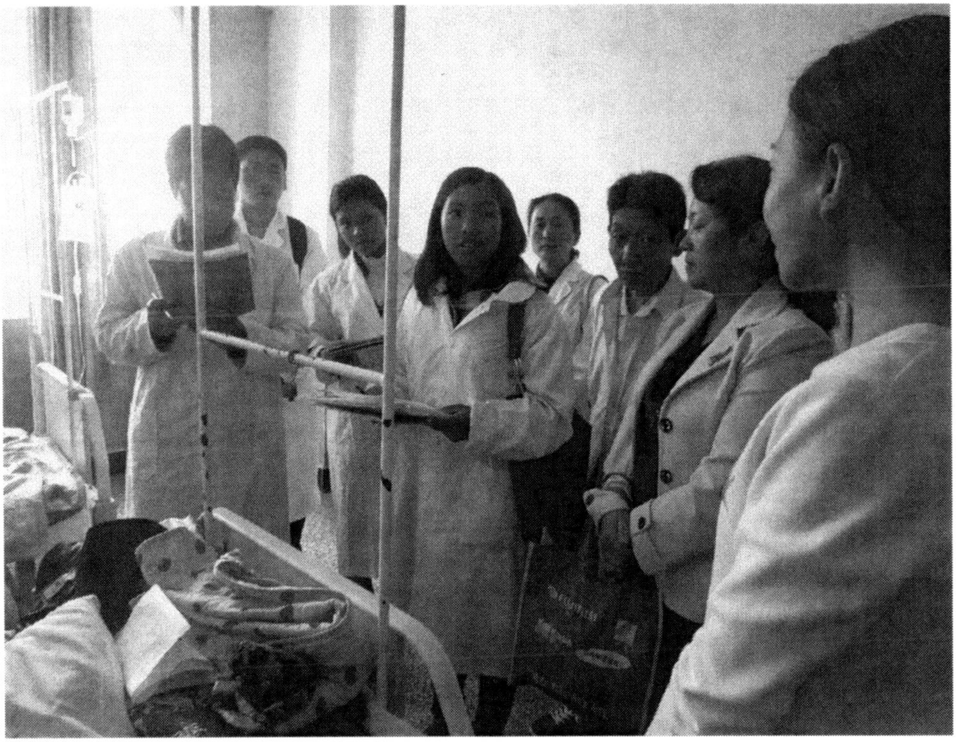

*Figure 38.1* Local trainer facilitating a small group working on their assignment in the IMCI training workshop

*Source*: Save the Children.

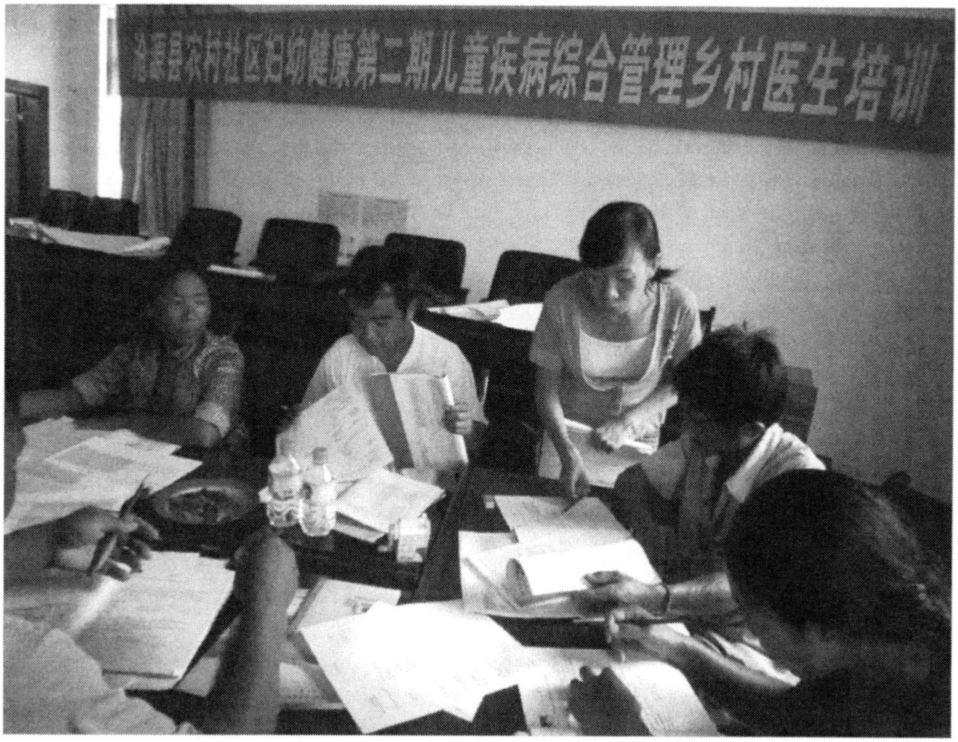
县农村社区妇幼健康第二期儿童疾病综合管理乡村医生培训

*Figure 38.2* Local trainer refreshing the IMCI procedure
*Source*: Save the Children

70 per cent can correctly classify a sick child and more than 60 per cent can apply the IMCI recommended treatment.

To our knowledge, this was the first effort to introduce IMCI at the village level in China, making it functional and so promoting health equity by strengthening primary health care and improving the quality of care in rural areas.

Evaluation suggests that the key to the success of the intervention has been the combination of two main approaches:

1 Building on internationally established good practice, such as extending the length of training courses, making the training more problem based and learner centred, as well as introducing follow-up supervision; and
2 Adapting training approaches and materials, including using staff who could deliver lectures in local languages, adapting the training model and contextualizing the content.[11]

## Save the Children case study 2: advocating for policy change

The second example of how an INGO can work with local systems comes from our work with the migrant community in Shanghai. Building on existing programmatic work, one of SC China programme's first health entry points was through the promotion of school health

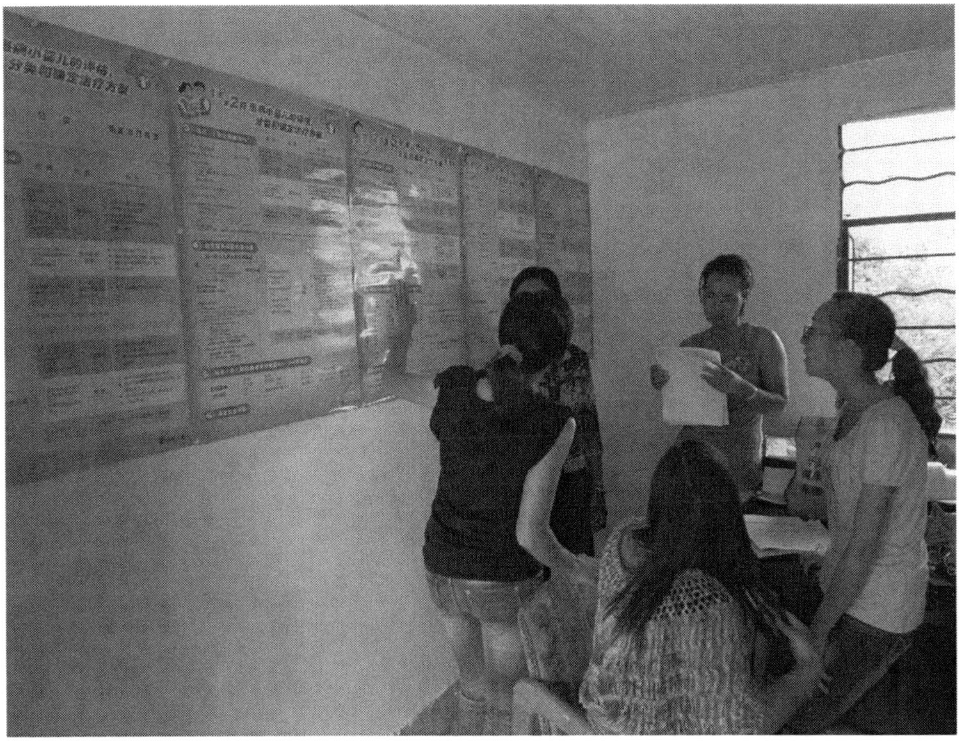

*Figure 38.3* Participants reporting their IMCI cases during the clinical practice session of an IMCI training workshop

*Source*: Save the Children.

and nutrition. This intervention allowed SC staff to build on their considerable experience in supporting a more participatory and child-focused teaching methodology.

Projects were established in both rural and urban settings (including in Yunnan,[12] Tibet[13] and Shanghai[14]), with the objective of providing baseline data on the health status of primary school children. The next steps in all areas were to improve school health clinics and hygiene facilities, to provide training for school health teachers and health centre staff, to establish children's records and to give them health checks. An important element was to integrate health education into the school curriculum. Parents were also mobilized to support and reinforce the health and hygiene messages that children were learning in schools.

Part of the official management of China's unprecedented domestic migration has been conducted through China's longstanding *hukou* (household registration) system (see Chapter 3). Migrant parents must choose either to leave their children at home with grandparents or other caregivers, or to put them into private 'migrant schools', which until recently were largely unregulated.[15] If migrant parents choose to leave their children at their home of origin, children then become left-behind children. The problems left-behind children face include a lack of parental support and care, lack of qualified family education, being isolated and lonely with old grandparents, and no mental wellbeing and psychological support. However, if children move with their parents to the cities, then they become migrant children. Unable to get access to education in public-funded primary schools in urban settings, they instead attend migrant

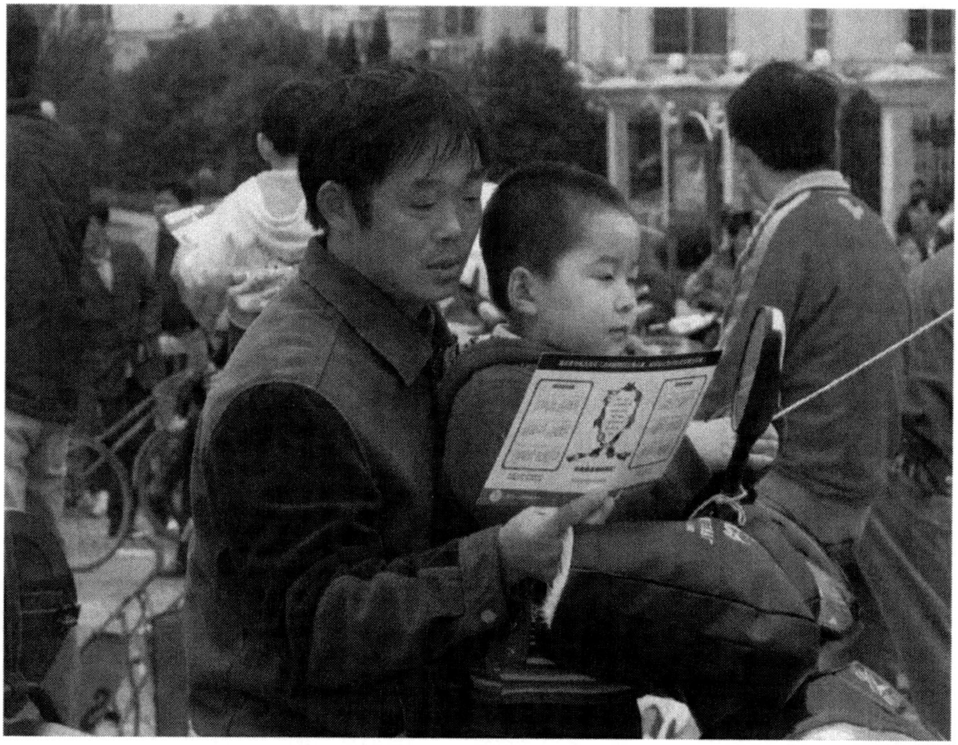

*Figure 38.4* **A local supervisor is observing the IMCI case management process by a trained village-level healthcare provider**

*Source*: Save the Children.

schools. Usually the teaching quality and teaching skills of migrant teachers is not as good. The children's living conditions are poor, crowded, damp and not hygienic. In addition, parents are often too busy making a living to care for their children, not to mention to care about their study, knowledge learning, or even doing parental education.

Evaluation of the project in Shanghai between October 2008 and September 2011 showed improved access to hygiene facilities, as well as improved health outcomes for the children. Improved access to hygiene facilities meant that all project schools were equipped with health facilities, such as vision charts, weight and height measurement, and first-aid kits.

One of the most striking results was that over 80 per cent of migrant students improved their anaemia statuses. As a result of these findings, we were able to work with our partner, the Shanghai Welfare and Population Foundation, to submit a proposal to the Shanghai Political Consultative Conference for improving health services in schools for migrant children based on our pilot projects. The Shanghai Political Consultative Conference along with the People's Congress meeting are two important conferences for government decision-making and are held annually at different levels to discuss the country's strategies, laws and regulations, as well as current issues. All proposals have to be submitted through members of the Conference. Once the proposal has been received, the city government will discuss it with the relevant government departments and give feedback to the members and occasionally to the wider public.

This resulted in the Shanghai Municipal Education Commission issuing a policy[16] [6] allocating special funds for health promotion in schools for migrant children. The policy includes setting up clinics (with standard equipment) at 162[17] elementary schools, training a healthcare teacher from each school and providing physical examinations for all students of elementary migrant schools starting from the new school year in 2011.

## Conclusion

Save the Children's experiences have encouraged us to take a positive assessment of the role that INGOs can play in supporting the public health agenda in China. Our case studies suggest that focusing on empowerment and giving a voice to under-represented groups, demonstrating models of service provision and advocating for policy change are fruitful entry points for NGOs to support the Chinese public health system. Furthermore, our collaboration with government partners indicates that the role of NGOs is increasingly recognized by state policy makers and implementers.

## Notes

1 Civil society actors in health include professional associations and specialized charities, whose mandates range from research to the promotion of public health messages and advocacy.
2 In this chapter, China and Chinese refers to the People's Republic of China.
3 Examples of GONGOs in the health field include: the Chinese Medical Association (CMA), the Chinese Preventative Medical Association (CPMA), the Chinese Medical Doctor Association (CMDA), the Chinese Maternal and Child Health Association and the Women's Federation, which touches on women's health issues.
4 For instance, a recent speech by the Minister of Health suggested that their future planning was assuming the emergence of independent civil society actors (14 February 2011). Similarly, Article 7 of the People's Republic of China on Prevention and Treatment of Infectious Diseases Law states that: 'Units and individuals that have remarkable achievements in or contributions to the work of prevention and treating infectious diseases shall be commended or awarded.' See AsianLII at http://www.asianlii.org/cn/legis/cen/laws/patoidl487/
5 We will not seek to make the case again for empowering the community and giving a voice to under-represented groups, given the existing body of experience from the HIV/AIDS groups, though these approaches have been fundamental to Save the Children's health promotion work in China, both in rural and urban migrant communities. Child-led research to give a voice to the children: *Listen, secrets – issues and research by children affected by the HIV/AIDS in Xinjiang and Yunnan, China. (2006)*; capacity building for health promoters in rural communities in Longchuan county of Yunnan: *The final evaluation report of community-based maternal and child health promotion project in Longchuan County of Yunnan (2011)*; setting up community health activity centres for promotion of knowledge and information sharing between villagers in rural and urban migrant communities.
6 One of the key reference points for strategic shaping of the programme has been the UN Convention on the Rights of the Child, which China ratified in 1992.
7 For instance, SC's 2010 evaluation report on improving school health and hygiene for migrant children quotes a teacher from a Huaao school stating: 'I have changed the approach of how I communicate with my daughter; things have been different since then. I think I have changed and so then, my communication style has changed'; and a quote from Taijing school: 'I was getting easily angry when children were not listening to me in class. With the training, I learnt that a healthy way to be is to calm myself down and then talk to the children. This is really useful.'
8 Other INGOs working in health in China include Médecins Sans Frontières (MSF) and Path. There are also international foundations operating in China which have funded Chinese civil society organizations, notably the Gates Foundation (through the China–Gates AIDS Project), the Global Fund and the Ford Foundation.

9 MDG's goal 4: reduce child mortality (target: reduce, by two-thirds, the under-5 mortality rate, between 1990 and 2015); MDG's goal 5: improve maternal health (target: reduce, by three-quarters, the maternal mortality ratio, by 2015).

10 Often officials and official written communications focus on the negative aspects of these groups.

11 Local trainers were recruited and trained to deliver the workshops to grassroots-level healthcare providers in their local dialect: training aids were locally made and reference was made to relevant Chinese regulations.

12 Since 2009, support was given to nine elementary schools in Yunnan in health education. In 2011, we provided training for 580 teachers, covering the design of school health curriculum, nutritious diets and first aid, and organized onsite health activities.

13 In 2011, SC helped four schools in Tibet to construct seven deep wells, one toilet and a waste treatment system.

14 In 2011, SC supported 22 privately run migrant elementary schools in Shanghai to conduct health education. A total of 130 healthcare teachers and schools leaders from project schools participated in the training. The training covered the responsibilities of healthcare teachers, prevention of common childhood diseases, planned immunization, use and management of school clinics, child mental health and first aid.

15 Even when regulated, they usually provide education at a lower standard to 'mainstream' schools, with students more likely to leave school following completion of the *chuzhong* (the final compulsory stage of middle school), or they progress to vocational training. Most migrant schools are run at low costs, are located in the outskirts of cities and have a poor quality of teaching, as well as underdeveloped teaching facilities and hygiene practices. However, migrant schools are not the direct cause of students with higher potential leaving school after the free compulsory education stage that is junior secondary school. It is the issue of their *hukou* which excludes migrant children from sitting a *gaokao* (university entrance examination) because the eligibility to take a *gaokao* is based upon having a local *hukou*. This may, therefore, discourage many migrant children to pursue further education at senior secondary level. Also, families of migrant school children are mostly poor and thus cannot afford the tuition fees arising from senior secondary education. As a consequence, migrant children, who still have intention of residing in cities, are mostly forced to turn to vocational education after graduating from junior secondary or to seek employment.

16 Shanghai Municipal Education Commission issued the Notice on Strengthening Sanitation Management of Privately-Run Elementary Schools Enrolling Migrant Children in 2011 in June 2011.

17 Four schools were subsequently closed resulting in the total reach being 158 schools, with a student population of around 132,800.

## References

1. Schwartz, J., Shieh, S. *State and Society Responses to Social Welfare Needs in China – Serving the People*, Routledge, 2009.
2. Kaufman, J. The role of NGOs in China's AIDS crisis, in *State and Society Responses to Social Welfare Needs in China–Serving the People*, J. Schwartz, S. Shieh (eds), Routledge, 2009.
3. Chen, H.T., Liao, Q. A pilot study of the NGO-based relational intervention model for HIV prevention among drug users in China, *AIDS Education and Prevention* 2005; 17(6): 503–14.
4. Multisectoral Responses to Mobile Population's HIV Vulnerability – Examples from People's Republic of China, Thailand and Viet Nam, UNDP South East Asia HIV and Development Programme, 2003.
5. Save the Children China Programme. Improving school health and hygiene for migrant children in Beijing, 2010.
6. Notice on Strengthening Sanitation Management of Privately-Run Elementary Schools Enrolling Migrant Children 2011, China: Shanghai Municipal Education Commission. Multisectoral Responses to Mobile Population's HIV Vulnerability – Examples from People's Republic of China, Thailand and Viet Nam, UNDP South East Asia HIV and Development Programme, 2003.

# 39

# Providing services for women's health

*Carmen Wong and Josette Chor*

Women have the right to the enjoyment of the highest attainable standard of physical and mental health. The enjoyment of this right is vital to their life and wellbeing and their ability to participate in all areas of public and private life. Health is a state of complete physical, mental and social wellbeing and not merely the absence of disease or infirmity. Women's health involves their emotional, social and physical wellbeing and is determined by the social, political and economic context of their lives, as well as biology.

(*Beijing Platform for Action, 1995 [1]*)

## Introduction

Men and women have fundamental biological differences and this can be reflected in their vulnerability to certain illness and a differing pattern of health. Early efforts in improving women's health have largely focused on the reproductive function of women. However, the scope of health issues of women has been increasingly recognized to extend from biological to gendered roles, which lie deep-seated within communities and societies.

## Gender as a social determinant of health

Sex defines men and women in terms of their biological differences whereas gender is a social construct that can be dynamic, relational, hierarchical and institutional, and thus is a key determinant of health. Gendered roles form the spheres of influence in families and communities, and can manifest as unequal power relationships, hinder access to education and employment, and result in discrimination which consequently impacts on an individual's access to health care and their ability to attain good physical and mental health.

When fairness and justice in the distribution of the responsibilities and benefits of men and women are compromised, disparities in health can result. In order to achieve better health and attain gender equity, discrimination has to be eliminated in the provision of opportunities, resources and access to services, based on a person's biological sex.

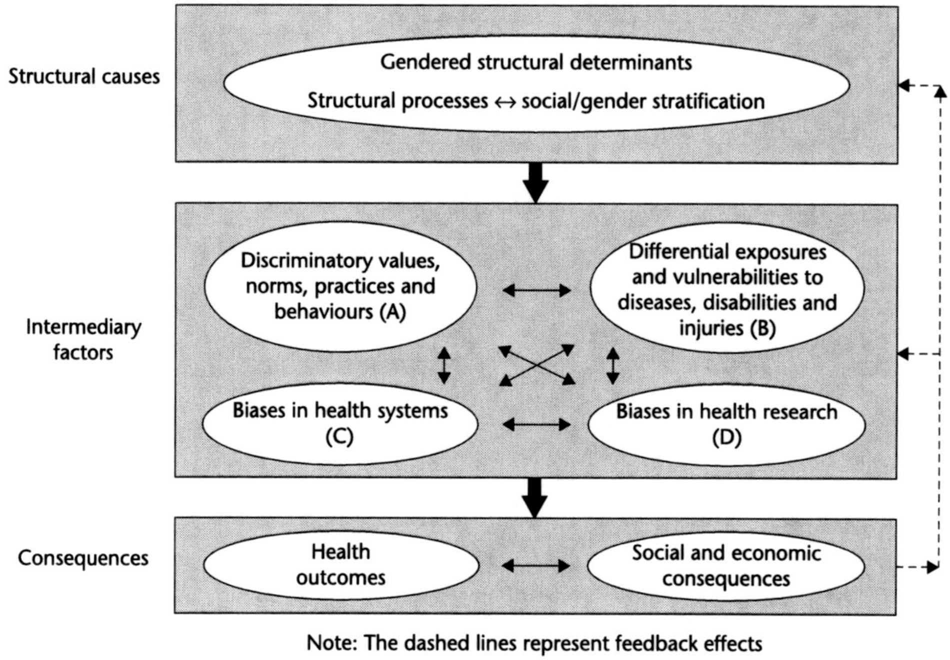


*Figure 39.1* Framework for the role of gender as a social determinant of health [2]

In providing services for women's health, it is important to understand gender as a social determinant of health (see Figure 39.1). There should be an awareness of gender in structural societal processes, such as education and work, as well as the interacting complexities of cultural norms and behaviours, biases of healthcare services provision and access, and the inherent biases in academic research ranging from available funding to subject recruitment. These factors all impact on the focus, direction and goals of women's health service provision.

## Tackling reproductive health

The impact of their reproductive role has long been recognized as a determinant of women's health, and key changes in women's health status have largely been developed by increasing and improving maternal health services over the past few decades particularly with efforts to tackle the United Nations Millennium Development Goals (MDGs) (Chapter 2). However, over half a million women worldwide still die from treatable and preventable complications of pregnancy and childbirth each year despite various global efforts, such as the Safe Motherhood initiative launched in 1987, which had increased the coverage of antenatal care by 20 per cent [4] and of skilled attendant at birth by 39 per cent [5] in developing countries by 2007. Of concern is the growing discrepancy between developed and developing countries in the maternal mortality ratio (MMR), a measure of the risk of death once a woman is pregnant (the number of deaths per 100,000 live births) despite improvements over the past decades. For example, although the global MMR has fallen from 400 in 1990 to 210 in 2010, developing countries in the Asia-Pacific region, such as Bangladesh, Indonesia and Nepal (that have MMRs of 240, 220 and 170, respectively), continue to contrast markedly with more developed neighbours, such as China, Australia, Japan and Singapore (MMRs of 37, 7, 5 and 3 respectively) [6].

Overall, in the Asia-Pacific region, the lifetime risk of maternal death is still relatively high at one in 260, as compared with one in 39 in Sub-Saharan Africa and one in 1,700 in Central and Eastern Europe and the Commonwealth of Independent States. In parts of Asia, there has been little change in the past two decades and maternal health has seen the least progress of all the MDGs [7]. The fifth MDG (MDG5) seeks to improve maternal health, with a target of reducing the MMR by 75 per cent between 1990 and 2015. Of the ten countries that had achieved this MDG by 2010, four were in the Asia-Pacific region: Bhutan (82 per cent), Islamic Republic of Iran (81 per cent), Nepal (78 per cent) and Vietnam (76 per cent).

Overall, despite the global decline in MMR over the last two decades, further work is needed in tackling other determinants of maternal mortality and morbidity so as to define indicators and predictors of improvement. Current progress has, in part, been attributed to improvements in education and physical accessibility to health services, as well as the increasing use of contraceptives by women of reproductive age, and improved distribution and access to antiretroviral medication for HIV positive women [8]. It is important that concerns on the quality of care, as well as political and funding priorities and commitments are addressed to enhance efforts [9].

Gender has increasingly been recognized as a factor that impacts health and plays an important role in social and economic factors of health, such as residential area, access to education and health, and economic wellbeing [8]. Discrepancies in health have been shown to exist in most countries and across all ages. Even in the most developed countries, women and girls in poorer households have shown lower use of healthcare resources and higher rates of mortality. Healthcare services for women need to be tailored and be responsive to the individual and community needs, as well as increase the scope of services offered and reduce the barriers to access [10]. Even within local regions with advanced healthcare systems, challenges exist that require the input of governmental policies and an integrated approach. In the quest to achieve MDG5 by 2015, increased efforts in addressing unmet needs, adopting an early interventional approach in adolescence, as well as further political drive to enhance funding, are priorities [8].

## *Case study 1: tackling reproductive health – new immigrants from mainland China (NIMC)*

In most countries, new immigrants would be defined as people coming from other countries and usually from other ethnic groups. However, because of the 'one country, two systems' policy (see Chapter 3), Chinese people from mainland China have no right of abode in Hong Kong. Due to the proximity of the two places, there is an increasing number of cross-border marriages and births from mainland mothers. These people comprise the main source of new immigrants in Hong Kong. Although they live in the same country and share the same ethnicity with the Hong Kong people, they have difficulties in adapting to the local society because of differences in their social systems, culture and language. In 2011, there were 171,322 new immigrants from mainland China (NIMC) in Hong Kong, attributing to 2.5 per cent of the whole population [11].

### Socio-demographics

Most of the NIMC are women who enter Hong Kong to reunite with their families. The sex ratio was 460 males per 1,000 females in 2011, which was much lower than the ratio in Hong

Kong's entire population (939/1,000). Most of the NIMC are of reproductive age. Women in the age group 25 to 44 years constitute 40.7 per cent of all NIMC. Therefore, the demand for maternal and child health services is relatively higher than it is for the general population.

According to data from the Immigration Department in 2011, 65.6 per cent of the NIMC found it difficult to adapt to life in Hong Kong and 10.5 per cent needed support in medical services [11]. The proportion of NIMC using Cantonese as their main language was 75.8 per cent, which was much lower than the 91.5 per cent in the whole population. Language barriers may pose adjustment problems and decrease access to health care [11, 12].

The educational attainment of NIMC who are aged 15 or above is much lower than in the whole population. The proportion of NIMC attaining lower secondary school education or below was 56.0 per cent compared with 40.9 per cent in the whole population. NIMC also have much lower median monthly household incomes than the whole population ($14,070 versus $20,500) and tend to live in the Kowloon district of Hong Kong, further posing a problem in the planning and distribution of resources in social and health services to meet the needs of this vulnerable group.

## Reproductive services

Female new immigrants are often much younger than their husbands. The median age difference of these couples was 8.0 years, which was much higher than couples in the whole population (3.6 years). This may in part explain the reported family disputes or domestic violence in these families, whilst other factors may include husband has low education level, unemployment, presence of extramarital affairs, alcohol abuse or mental illness [13].

Women from mainland China have very different views towards reproduction, contraception and abortion. According to a study done by the Hong Kong Family Planning Association, female NIMC want more children [14]. They have much poorer levels of knowledge about contraception when compared with local women. Also, more NIMC women thought contraception was a wife's responsibility rather than a couple's mutual responsibility. Women from mainland China were more inclined to adhere to traditional Chinese beliefs that men are superior to women and women should not reject husbands' requests for sexual intercourse. Abortion is more common in NIMC than in local women (39 per cent versus 25.4 per cent). Poor knowledge about contraception and the one child policy in China are contributing factors as well. All these differences in women's perception and sexual practice require targeted health education and promotion towards NIMC.

## Maternity services

The maternal mortality rate has remained very low in the past 20 years. There was only one registered maternal death in 2010, making the maternal mortality rate to be 1.1 per 100,000 registered live births [15]. The combination of high-quality healthcare services and guaranteed Hong Kong residency for newborns led to an influx of mainland mothers seeking maternal care. In 2011, there were 95,500 live births in Hong Kong, of which 43,982 were born to mainland mothers [16]. The rapid increase in the demand for maternity services caused huge discontentment among local women, which resulted in the government taking action to stop mainland mothers from coming to Hong Kong to deliver their babies.

Despite free maternal healthcare services provided in Hong Kong, the birth rate among Hong Kong women has been decreasing. Women born in 1945 had an average of 1.28 children by the age of 30, while women born in 1976 only had 0.48 children when they reached the same age [17]. One reason is the increasing age of marriage. The median age at first marriage for women in 2011 was 28.9 and the median age for women at first childbirth was 30.0 [18, 19]. This has led to an increase in complicated pregnancies, the need for more specialized obstetrics service and an increase in couples with infertility problems. One in six couples have been estimated to at some point suffer from subfertility [20]. These changes in childbirth practices have been reflected by the changes in the scope of services provided by the Family Planning Association (FPA). The FPA was renamed under its current form in 1950 to provide only birth control services. Currently, the FPA provides a wide range of services from a well women clinic to subfertility counselling. The Hospital Authority only provides public in vitro fertilization (IVF) service in three hospitals and the age limit for the service is 40. The average waiting time is more than two years, which reflects the huge demand for these services.

## Tackling social disadvantage

In many societies, women are socially disadvantaged. Not only are their productive roles as a mother, family member and informal caregiver often overlooked, their efforts in obtaining educational and economic recognition are also often discouraged.

The second of the MDGs, to achieve universal primary education, has had some success. The importance of primary, secondary and tertiary education in promoting gender equality and in empowering women in employment and parliament was given priority in the MDGs [9] together with the need for women to make decisions on childbearing, and in educating men to realign the dynamic roles that men and women play in health.

However, even though female literacy rates have risen globally, male literacy rates remain above female literacy rates (88 per cent versus 79 per cent). In the Asia-Pacific region, Western, Eastern and South Eastern Asia show a gender parity of 0.84, 0.94 and 0.95 respectively, close to the Gender Parity Index (GPI) of 1.00 of developed regions [21]. Of all the MDG regions (East Asia and Pacific, South Asia, Sub-Saharan Africa, Latin America and the Caribbean, Middle East and North Africa, Europe and Central Asia), Southern Asia has the lowest adult literacy rate (62 per cent) with the greatest gender disparity – 73 per cent of all men but only 51 per cent of women had the ability to read and write which equates to a GPI of 0.70. However, there are signs of encouragement with literacy in youth rising to 86 per cent, which improves the GPI to 0.86.

Despite educational developments in reducing discrimination in education and literacy, it is unfortunate that this does not necessarily translate into fairer economic prospects for women. Women often face lower economic prospects compared to their male counterparts [22]. The gender wage gap is the difference between male and female earnings, expressed as a percentage of male earnings and represents the difference between average earnings of male and female employees. Of full-time employees, the gender wage gap still exists in developed countries but is below 12 per cent in New Zealand, Belgium, Poland, Greece and France. However in South-East Asia, the gender wage gap can be as high as 38 per cent, as seen in Korea, and is over 30 per cent in Japan despite legislation to ensure equal pay for equal work regardless of gender. This gender gap is often attributable to gender discrimination with women ending up in lower-paid occupations or due to institutional inertia in promoting women.

In developing countries, improvements in parity may not necessarily correlate to better prospects for girls and women. For example, Kerala, a coastal state in South West India and with women making up 52 per cent of its population, achieved universal primary education, high literacy and high life expectancy for both men and women. However, women remain powerless and poor due to restricted access to economic opportunities, resources and assets, and a lack of political participation [23]. Thus, empowering and supporting women from socially disadvantaged positions into advocacy roles, together with inter-sectoral collaboration and networking, are necessary to impact on health outcomes.

### *Case study 2: tackling social disadvantage – Self Employed Women's Association*

In the 1970s, Ahmedabad was one of the leading industrial cities in India with its wealth of textile mills. At that time, 94 per cent of women had irregular incomes, no job security, lower wages, and exploitation from moneylenders, contractors, policemen and municipal authorities. Ela Bhattt was a lawyer who worked in the legal department of the Textile Labour Association (TLA)'s women's division. Through regular contact with women who did many of the labour-intensive tasks needed in textile production, as well as in other fields of work, she discovered the many challenges that women face on a daily basis. In her pursuit to improve women's wellbeing, she founded the SEWA (Self Employed Women's Association) in 1971 in Gujurat, India.

SEWA is primarily a trade union of informal workers. However, SEWA recognized the need for social and economic upliftment in order to strengthen women's economic statuses, decision-making ability, maternal and child health, and education and housing, on both an individual and a community level to improve health [24] (see Table 39.1).

In SEWA's ethos, the importance of employment, income, nutrition, housing, ownership, leadership, health care, childcare and self-sufficiency are integrated into its programmes. The Health Improvement Index (HII) indicators are shown in Table 39.2 to illustrate SEWA's comprehensive approach to health. SEWA now has over one million members and its activities are multifaceted in empowering women. These include demanding fairness and justice as a trade union, demanding fair pricing as cooperatives, financial stability from tailored insurance and loans from its own cooperative SEWA bank to improve housing with sanitation, as well as curative health, medication subsidies and preventive health programmes. For these women, these measures translate to education and training opportunities that lead to skilled full-time employment and financial planning with available credit and insurance. As a result, women were able to access and afford healthcare

*Table 39.1* Self Employed Women's Association (SEWA) health model

| *Vulnerabilities* | *Risks* | *SEWA empowerment strategy* | | | *Health security* |
|---|---|---|---|---|---|
| | | *Provision of services* | *Individual* | *Institutional* | |
| Poverty<br>Semi-employed status<br>Gender<br>Calamities and violence<br>Life-cycle events | Assets loss<br>Poor health<br>Indebtedness<br>Degraded working and living environments<br>Loss of work and income | Health care<br>Banking<br>Housing and infrastructure<br>Marketing and livelihood promotion | Full employment<br>Leadership<br>Paraprofessionals<br>Self-esteem<br>Self-reliance | Training<br>Organized strength<br>Marketing<br>Advocacy | Access to health care at doorstep<br>Health awareness<br>Better nutrition<br>Improved work and living environment<br>Health insurance |

*Table 39.2* Development of Health Improvement Index (HII) based on SEWA approach and health outcomes

| *Health Improvement Index (HII) indicators for poor women and family (SEWA experience)* |
|---|
| • Access of microcredit (financial security)<br>• Membership of a women's trade organization (solidarity)<br>• Leadership quality (self-confidence)<br>• Full employment and on-the-job training (economic security and self-reliance)<br>• Social networking (community participation)<br>• Access to basic health services and government health programmes at doorstep (reduced friction of distance)<br>• Health insurance of family linked with financial services (freedom from health-related indebtedness)<br>• Access to low-cost medicines and alternate systems of medicine<br>• Access to drinking water and basic sanitation at doorstep (freedom from water-borne disease burden) |

services, build up supportive social networks and remain in employment when faced with challenges to their reproductive and caregiver roles (e.g. childcare, ill health of family member) thus giving women the best opportunity to enhance their mental, physical and social wellbeing.

## Taking a life-course approach

Worldwide, women generally live longer than men (70 years as compared to 67.5 for men) [25]. In the Asia-Pacific region, Japanese women enjoy the longest life expectancy at birth of just over 86 years (86.3 years); compared to Japanese men of 80 years closely followed by Hong Kong women of 86 years and Australia women of 84 years.

The increase in life expectancy is associated with economic development and, whilst developed regions show the greatest advantage, it is the less developed countries that are experiencing the most dramatic changes. It is, however, of concern that in parts of Asia, biological and behavioural advantage of women appears to be lagging [26].

It has been estimated that by 2050, the proportion of those aged 60 years will double to 2 billion worldwide and of those more are likely to be women (especially those aged 80 or older), widowed, living alone and having low incomes [27]. Female deaths at age 60 and over are attributable to non-communicable diseases (NCDs) with ischemic heart disease, cerebrovascular disease and chronic respiratory disease as the leading causes of death. These along with diabetes mellitus cause just under 50 per cent of all female deaths [28]. With the increasing risk of comorbidity with age, women form the majority of this vulnerable group for which social and health resources are likely to become increasingly strained. Additional measures to ensure that women remain healthy and active in elder years have seen the advent of governmental and non-governmental initiatives in the active engagement of the elderly as a community resource and in the improving of physical and mental health.

Whilst governments are preparing for the impact on health services and increasing the need for rehabilitation and long-term care, there has also been a shift in healthcare services and research to encompass a life-course approach in tackling health problems, which is long overdue. The life-course approach looks at the biological and social factors at each stage of the life cycle that contribute to adult health outcomes (see Figure 39.2). For women,

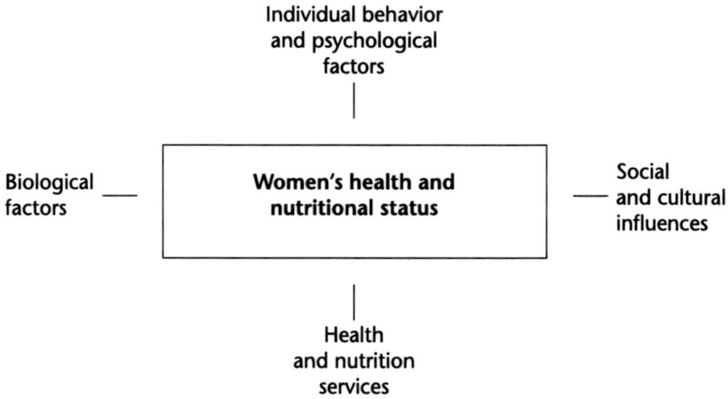


*Figure 39.2* Health and nutrition problems affecting women during the life cycle in developing countries [29]

preconceptual care, antenatal care and postnatal care all set their babies on the road to a healthier life course.

Maternal health contributes to foetal and childhood health, and the later development of chronic diseases, thus prevention of ill health and early interventions are becoming a priority in healthcare services at individual and population levels. For example, in recent years, many countries have recommended the use of human papillomavirus (HPV) immunization in the fight against cervical cancer, with countries, such as the UK and US, adopting national immunization programmes for school-age girls. The impact of HPV immunization in addition to cervical screening in adulthood is yet to be evaluated in the long term but is encouraging in its emphasis on early prevention and intervention. The importance of a life-course approach highlights the need for continuity and seamless care in the transition from childhood to old age, as well as intergenerational health from mother to child (see Figure 39.3).

Challenges exist in establishing mutual shared goals from social and health arenas, and in inter-sectoral collaboration and funding, in order to tackle determinants of women's health throughout the life cycle. For example, tackling HIV/AIDS as the leading cause of death among women of reproductive age globally requires awareness of the vulnerability to HIV infection due to a combination of biological factors and gender-based inequalities, particularly in cultures that limit women's knowledge about HIV and their ability to protect themselves and negotiate safer sex. The most important risk factors for death and disability in this age group in low- and middle-income countries are a lack of contraception and unsafe sex. These result in unwanted pregnancies, unsafe abortions, complications of pregnancy and childbirth, and sexually transmitted infections including HIV. Violence is an additional significant risk to women's sexual and reproductive health and can result in physical harm and other chronic health problems resulting from physical and emotional trauma, such as mental ill health, infertility and, in some cases, even death [9].

Later into midlife, menopause marks the end of the reproductive role for women and the transition into elder years can bring social, physical and mental health challenges. During menopause, many women can experience somatic, psychological and genitourological problems. Of interest, Western cultures appear to experience more somatic symptoms such as flushing and vaginal dryness, whereas Asian cultures generally report low rates of symptoms

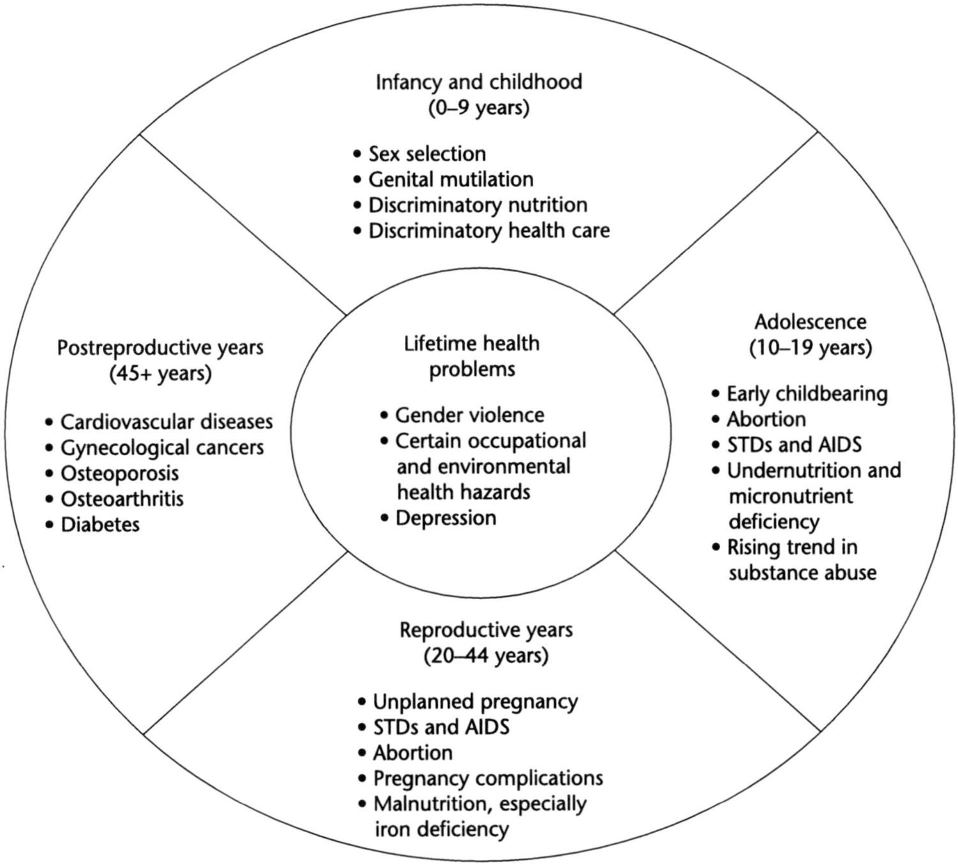


*Figure 39.3* Determinants of women's health and nutritional status through the life cycle [29]

[30], which predominantly appear to be of a physical and psychological nature, such as joint aches and pains, insomnia and irritability [31, 32, 33]. There is some debate as to why this occurs but it is likely to be multifactorial, which includes the social and cultural roles of women, such as positive attitudes about menopause and ageing, as well as biological differences.

Beyond menopause, there are obvious physical changes that threaten women's health. Women's relative cardioprotective state (compared to men's) prior to menopause is mitigated. In addition, the protective role of oestrogen in bone health is also withdrawn and women are at risk of osteoporosis and breast cancer. The rate of depression alone also appears to increase in this age group and continues to increase due to insidious onset of multimorbid conditions.

It is increasingly recognized that despite biological disadvantages, the role of early intervention can affect health outcome in later life (e.g. exercise and smoking cessation in cardiovascular disease, calcium intake in adolescence and young adulthood for bone health, HPV vaccination in cervical cancer). Thus, there is increasing importance to target girls and women earlier in life to improve their health, especially as this could enable them to lead longer, healthier lives. More sex-specific research is needed to reveal sex-specific interventions which may not be evident in large studies in which men are predominant subjects. Efforts such as the Women's Health Initiative [34] and the Million Women Study [35] have done a lot to identify women's health needs and gender, and sex-specific strategies to improve health. Exploring differences in the perception of health and illness across cultures can further impact health-seeking behaviours, treatment and women's physical and emotional wellbeing.

## Ensuring gender and culture sensitive health programmes and services

It is important to recognize that women and men have different needs and strengths, and that these differences should be identified and addressed to rectify the imbalance between the sexes, a process known as gender analysis. Integrating gender analysis in the development of health programmes and services can differentiate the roles of women and men, and inter- and intra-gender power relationships, thus optimizing health and reducing inequality. Several tools attempt to systematically review the differences in condition, welfare, position and status between women and girls versus men and boys in a given population and culture [36–39].

The Harvard Framework was first developed to look at the socio-economic activity of men and women in the community, as well their power and constraints in the access and control of resources [37]. In addition, the often overlooked reproductive role that women play in society can be documented, with gender needs assessed at a practical level, where social gendered roles were unchallenged, and at a strategic level, which seeks to resolve any gender imbalances [36]. These tools help to empower and enhance participation of women [38]. In developing health services for men and women or for women only, such tools can be useful in identifying gendered roles and the health needs of men and women in the community. Culture can also transform gendered roles and defined populations may have fundamental biological differences, such that research developments, health interventions and services in women's health need to be inherently culturally sensitive (e.g. breast cancer screening in Chinese women (see Chapter 36), use of contraception, etc.). Development of gender and culturally sensitive healthcare programmes and services from conceptualization, planning and implementation is key to reducing gender inequality and to improving health for women. Involvement of individuals within the community as 'experts' in identifying, analysing and tackling their own issues can minimize observer bias and can create a more sustainable approach in the development of local health services [39]. Successful health projects that have taken gender and culture as integral to the identification of health needs and in improving health outcomes on a national and local level across Asia-Pacific include those in combating the HIV/AIDS epidemic; such efforts involve the cooperation and participation of men in the community from participatory workshops in addressing violence against women, peer support groups for women and integrating HIV testing in health services [40].

Such is the importance of gender-sensitive strategic efforts that gender mainstreaming has become public policy and is the focus of one of the MDGs. Gender mainstreaming is defined as

> the process of assessing the implications for women and men of any planned action, including legislation, policies or programmes in any area and at all levels. It is a strategy for making the concerns and experiences of women, as well as of men, an integral part of the design, implementation, monitoring and evaluation of policies and programmes in all political, economic and societal spheres so that women and men benefit equally and inequality is not perpetuated. [41]

Positive changes have been seen in the health arena since 2007 when the World Health Organization (WHO) outlined its strategy and action plan [42, 43] across countries to:

- Build capacity for gender analysis and planning;
- Bring gender into the mainstream of WHO's management;
- Promote use of sex-disaggregated data and gender analysis; and
- Establish accountability.

Since then, improvements have been made in sex-aggregated statistics in the Asia-Pacific regions such as China, Indonesia, the Philippines, Vietnam, India, Sri Lanka, Pakistan and Thailand, with reports of aggregated data existing on populations and families, health, education, work, power and decision making, violence against women, the environment and poverty in the Asia-Pacific region [44].

## Providing women's health services

Improving women's health requires healthcare services to be designed with a gender-sensitive perspective from their initiation, with adequate gender and health needs analysis and with the participation of women in implementation at the client and provider level. Such services should aim to be responsive and dynamic to meet individual and community needs, and with the capacity for collaboration across social and health sectors in enhancing continuity of care along the life course. Health services should be culturally sensitive due to influences on gendered roles, norms and behaviours, as well as biological differences in health. Providing education for men alongside women can help redress societal imbalances across gendered roles that impact on health in the community. In addition, advocacy for representative participation of women in academic and political arenas, as well as women's health agendas, can help prioritization and funding of gender-sensitive research and resources for improving women's health.

## Conclusion

Much has been done to improve women's physical health particularly in terms of tackling reproductive health. However, efforts have shown that in order to enhance health, it is necessary to tackle social disadvantages and to view gender as a social determinant of health as a foundation for health needs analysis and for interventional programmes and services that seek to improve emotional, social and physical wellbeing. Such services should be offered earlier in life in order to maximize preventive measures and enhance health outcomes.

## References

1. Beijing Platform for Action, 1995, Chapter IV C. Women and health: 89. [Online]. Available from: http://www.un.org/esa/gopher-data/conf/fwcw/off/a--20.en
2. Framework for the role of gender as a social determinant of health. Final report to the WHO commission on Social Determinants of Health. Women and Gender Equity Knowledge Network, 2007.
3. Report on the safe motherhood technical consultation (18–23 October 1997, Colombo, Sri Lanka). Final report on the program to mark the tenth anniversary of the Safe Motherhood Initiative. Safe Motherhood Inter-Agency Group, 1999. New York: Family Care International.
4. State of the World Population 2004 Report. The Cairo Consensus at Ten: Population, Reproductive Health, and the Global Effort to End Poverty. New York: UNFPA, 2004.

5. State of the World Population 2005 Report. The Promise of Equality, Gender Equity, Reproductive Health and the Millennium Development Goals. New York: UNFPA, 2005.
6. Trends in Maternal Mortality: 1990–2010: WHO, UNICEF, UNFPA and World Bank Estimates. World Health Organization, 2010.
7. United Nations Secretary-General. 'Committing to Action: Achieving the Millennium Development Goals.' Background note by the Secretary General, 2008. [Online]. Available from: http://www.un.org/milleniumgoals/2008highlevel/pdf/committing.pdf
8. The Millennium Development Goals Report 2011. New York, United Nations, 2011. [Online]. Available from: http://www.un.org/millenniumgoals/pdf/(2011_E)%20MDG%20Report%20 2011Book%20LR.pdf
9. The Millennium Development Goals Report 2005. New York: United Nations, 2005.
10. World Health Organization. Women's Health. 2013. [Online]. Available from: http://www.who.int/topics/womens_health/en/
11. HKSAR. Census and Statistics Department. Thematic report: Persons from the Mainland having resided in Hong Kong for less than 7 years, 2012.
12. HKSAR. Home Affairs Department and Immigration Department Statistics on New Arrivals from the mainland. (Third quarter of 2012.)
13. Tsui KL, Chan AY, So FL, Kam CW. Risk factors for injury to married women from domestic violence in Hong Kong. *Hong Kong Medical Journal* 2006; 12(4): 289–293.
14. Hong Kong Family Planning Association. [Online]. Available from: http://www.famplan.org.hk/fpahk/zh/template1.asp?style=template1.asp&content=info/publications/na.asp
15. HKSAR. Department of Health. Maternal Mortality Ratio. 2011. [Online]. Available from: http://www.healthyhk.gov.hk/phisweb/en/healthy_facts/health_indicators/maternal_mortality _ratio/
16. HKSAR. Census and Statistics Department. Babies Born in Hong Kong to Mainland Women, 2011.
17. HKSAR. Census and Statistics Department. Demographic Trends in Hong Kong: 1981–2006. [Online]. Available from: http://www.statistics.gov.hk/pub/B1120017022007XXXXB0200.pdf
18. HKSAR. Judiciary Department. Number of Divorces. 2011. [Online]. Available from: http://www.censtatd.gov.hk/FileManager/EN/Content_1149/T02_05_06_07.xls
19. HKSAR. Judiciary Department. Median Age at First Marriage by Sex. 2011. [Online]. Available from: http://www.censtatd.gov.hk/FileManager/EN/Content_1149/T02_05_06_07.xls
20. Loke AY, Yu, PL, Hayter M. Experiences of sub-fertility among Chinese couples in Hong Kong: a qualitative study. *Journal of Clinical Nursing* 2012; 21(3–4): 504–512.
21. UNESCO Institute for Statistics, Data Centre. Adult Literacy Rate by MDG region. 2008. [Online]. Available from: stats.uis.unesco.org
22. Organization for Economic Co-operation and Development (OECD). Employment and Labour Market Statistics, 2008.
23. India Planning Commission. Chapter 15: Gender and Development, In Kerala Development Report 2008.
24. World Health Organization. Regional Office for South-East Asia. Tackling social and economic determinants of health through women's empowerment: The SEWA case study. 2008.
25. United Nations, Department of Economic and Social Affairs, Population Division (2011). World Population Prospects: the 2010 Revision. [Online]. Available from: http://www.un.org/esa/population/unpop.htm
26. World Health Organization. Women and health. Today's evidence tomorrow's agenda. 2009.
27. Population Division of the Department of Economic and Social Affairs of the United Nations. World Population Ageing 1950–2050. 2002. [Online]. Available from: http://www.un.org/esa/population/publications/worldageing19502050/pdf/preface_web.pdf
28. World Health Organization. Global Burden of Disease. 2004 update. [Online]. Available from: http://www.who.int/healthinfo/global_burden_disease/GBD_report_2004update_full.pdf
29. Tinker A. Determinants of women's health and nutritional status through the life cycle. In A. Tinker, Women's health: the unfinished agenda. *International Journal of Gynaecology and Obstetrics* 2000; 70(1): 149–158.
30. Lock M. Symptom reporting at menopause: A review of cross-cultural findings. *Journal of the British Menopause Society* 2002; 8(4): 132–136.

31. Chim H, Tan BHI, Ang CC, Chew EMD, Chong YS, Saw SM. The prevalence of menopausal symptoms in a community in Singapore. *Maturitas* 2002; 41: 275–282.
32. Haines CJ, Xing SM, Park KH, Holinka CF, Ausmanas MK. Prevalence of menopausal symptoms in different ethnic groups of Asian women and responsiveness to therapy with three doses of conjugated estrogens/medroxyprogesterone acetate. The Pan-Asian Menopause (PAM) Study. *Maturitas* 2005; 52(3–4): 264–276.
33. Ho SC, Chan SG, Yip YB, Chan SY, Sham A. Factors associated with menopausal symptoms reported in Chinese midlife women. *Maturitas* 2003; 44: 149–156.
34. National Institute of Health. Department of Health and Human Services. Women's Health Initiative. [Online]. Available from: http://www.nhlbi.nih.gov/whi/background.htm
35. University of Oxford. Cancer Epidemiology Unit. Million Women Study. [Online]. Available from: http://www.millionwomenstudy.org/
36. Moser C. *Planning and Development. Theory, Practice and Training*. New York: Routledge, 1993.
37. Overholt C, Anderson M, Cloud K, Austin J. *Gender Roles in Development Projects: A Case Book*. West Hartford, CT: Kumarian Press, 1984.
38. Longwe S. Gender awareness: the missing element in the third world development program, In C. March and T. Wallace (eds) *Changing Perception: New Writings on Gender and Development*. Oxford: Oxfam, 1995.
39. Parker, R. *Another Point of View: A Manual on Gender Analysis Training for Grassroots Workers*. New York: UNIFEM, 1993.
40. Gay J, Croce-galis M, Hardee K. *What Works for Women and Girls: Evidence for HIV/AIDS Interventions*. 2nd edition. Washington, DC: Futures Group, Health Policy Project, 2012. [Online]. Available from: www.whatworksforwomen.org
41. United Nations. E/2004/INF/2/Add.2 Resolutions 2004/4. Review of Economic and Social Councils agreed conclusions 1997/2. [Online]. Available from: http://www.un.org/womenwatch/daw/documents/ecosoc2004/eres2004-4Mainstreaming.pdf
42. World Health Organization. Strategy for integrating gender analysis and actions into the work of WHO. WHO Gender Strategy, 2009: 9.
43. World Health Sixtieth World Health Assembly Resolution. WHA60.25. [Online]. Available from: http://apps.who.int/gb/ebwha/pdf_files/WHASSA_WHA60-Rec1/E/reso-60-en.pdf
44. United Nations Statistics Division. The World's Women 2010: Trends and Statistics. Key Findings for Asia and the Pacific. 2010.

# 40
# Developing primary care in China

*Harry Hao-Xiang Wang and Jia-Ji Wang*

## Introduction

Primary care has become of specific interest in China, and the wider and deeper significance of primary care in making healthcare delivery more efficient has increasingly been discussed at a political level. Initiatives to systematically strengthen community-based primary care services are being put at the top of the government agenda. This chapter focuses on describing the past, present and future of primary care development in China in terms of policy, organization and management within the context of China's healthcare reforms. It outlines the historical development of primary care and provides a comprehensive description of the status quo, as well as describing different primary care ownership and management models being implemented in urban areas. Challenges facing primary care in China are discussed and future perspectives are also explored.

## Growth of primary care in China

Primary care, as defined by the World Health Organization (WHO) as 'the first level of contact of individuals, the family and the community with the national health system, bringing health care as close as possible to where people live and work' [1], has experienced several seismic transitions marked by particular features of political, economic and social-cultural changes in China.

### *Phase one: Red Cross Health Stations and barefoot doctors (early 1950s–late 1970s)*

Along with the establishment of the People's Republic of China in 1949, primary care was first established as the cornerstone of China's healthcare system under the centrally planned economy. It had a significant impact and was considered to be an exemplary model for other countries during that era. The national health policy laid heavy emphasis on preventive health services and on mass mobilization health campaigns, aiming to guarantee the coverage of basic health services and the use of cost-effective preventive approaches to deliver health care to the whole population. In major cities, Red Cross Health Stations were set up by neighbourhood committees to address health needs of residents at the community level, raise the public awareness of environmental health, organize activities on hygiene and mobilize campaigns eliminating the 'four pests' (rats, bedbugs, flies and mosquitoes) which were plaguing China [2]. Meanwhile, in rural areas, healthcare stations were set up by Agricultural Production Cooperatives under the Rural Cooperative Medical Scheme (RCMS), together with the 'barefoot doctors' who were responsible for the provision of door-to-door health care services, focusing predominantly on prevention. Patients were referred to healthcare sectors at higher levels by the barefoot doctors based on the severity of the patient's disease or condition. Barefoot doctors played an efficient role in providing equitable access to primary care and public health services for local residents and also led to close doctor–patient relationships. The Red Cross Health Stations and the barefoot doctors received substantial financial subsidy from the government sector and served as the initial point of contact in the health system, which indicated the early commencement of primary care in China [3]. Starting from the early 1980s, some primary-level hospitals and health clinics also functioned as community-based healthcare facilities to address most of the essential health issues. From the early 1950s until the late 1970s, China's primary care contributed to the remarkable progress in the population's health status. Incidence of the major infectious diseases stayed at a very low level and total life expectancy at birth increased from 34.7 years in the 1940s to 67.3 years in 1981 [4, 5] (see Figure 40.1).

### *Phase two: suspension and hibernation (early 1980s–mid-1990s)*

Since the late 1970s and early 1980s when the planned economy ended, the central government significantly withdrew its overall investment in public health and primary care services. In tune with the widespread and rapid economic reforms, a market-oriented healthcare initiative was launched in 1985, which introduced market liberalization and privatization into the healthcare system. Private ownership of healthcare facilities was allowed and encouraged and private clinical practices started to play a role in the health sector [6]. As the financial support from the government to the healthcare system decreased, the economic and social foundations of public first-level hospitals were undermined. Although healthcare services remained public in terms of state-owned ownership, there was still a heavy reliance on user fees and

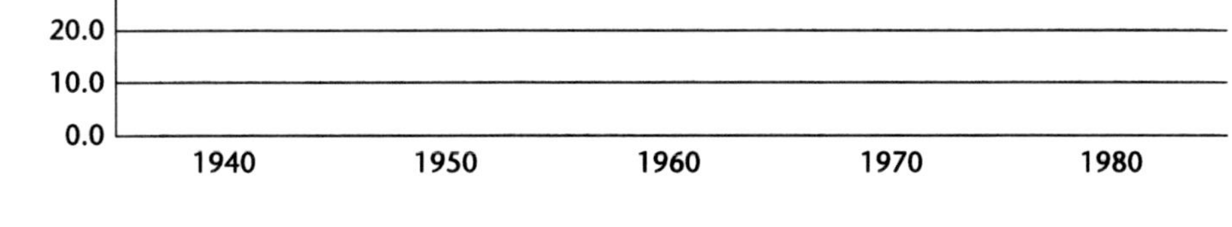


*Figure 40.1* Total life expectancy at birth in China, 1940–1980 [5]

pharmaceutical revenue to survive financially. The need for self-sufficiency in financing gradually led to the irrational prescription of excessive and expensive medications and the provision of unnecessary highly technological diagnostics tests to generate income through maximizing profits from patients. Primary care facilities therefore shifted towards a pattern of providing curative care, which was more profitable, thus largely neglecting the less-profitable health promotion and disease prevention services [7]. A wide scope of basic public health services became fee-for-service items to generate revenue. In rural areas, as the collective way of financing rural health care was abandoned, the prevention-focused Rural Cooperative Medical Scheme (RCMS) was almost dismantled. The barefoot doctors lost their regular source of income and no longer existed. Under-trained fee-for-service village doctors became the source of primary care; however, they made most of their income through drug prescriptions and dispensing activities, and had less incentive to provide preventive healthcare services. In rural areas, it was not unusual for expired and counterfeit pharmaceuticals to be bought at low prices and sold with increased price tags. The term 'primary care' was often associated with low-quality healthcare services, and doctors serving in first-level healthcare facilities were deemed less competent and professional than those working in secondary or tertiary hospitals which emphasized hospital-based, high-tech and speciality care. The progression of primary care was seriously eroded under this market-oriented healthcare reform and therefore led to inadequate preventive care, poor access to quality health care, lack of health insurance coverage and a high level of individual out-of-pocket payments.

### *Phase three: renaissance (early 1997–2003)*

Due to rising public dissatisfaction at the unaffordable health care and inappropriate high demands on hospitals in healthcare delivery, the central government began to explore new ways to fundamentally improve equity in essential health care. The concept of Community Health Service (CHS) was first introduced under this context and referred to as primary care in China.

> The community health care refers to primary-level healthcare services that are efficient, economic, convenient, comprehensive, continuous, and are delivered predominantly by general practitioners as cadre with a focus on primary care. The services emphasize the healthcare needs of women, children, elderly, disabled and patients with chronic diseases. It also integrates preventive, curative and rehabilitative care, aiming at maintaining and improving the health status of the family and the community. It is fundamental and essential to the ultimate goal of achieving basic primary care for all. [8]

This concept was initially piloted into practice in 1996 and since the policy initiative in 1997 [9], the central government started to rebuild the community-based healthcare system to provide preventive and primary care to the communities. In the following years, a series of official documents and guidelines [8, 10–13] were issued to encourage the development of CHS for primary care delivery in urban areas through the establishment of Community Health Centres and Stations (CHCs). Since 1999, the concept of general practice and general practitioners as primary care personnel working in the community was also introduced, deemed as a positive step in the process of primary care reform. In rural areas, a New Rural Cooperative Medical Scheme (NRCMS) was re-established in 2003 to replace the previous insurance scheme for the rural population. The NRCMS was jointly financed by a combined contribution from both central and local governments, as well as from individual households. It aimed to protect rural households from impoverishment due to excessive health expenditure on catastrophic illnesses. However, there was still a rapid increase in health expenditure and inappropriate treatment due to inferior insurance coverage and underpayment for basic primary health care. According to the statistics, 70.3 per cent of the entire population had no medical insurance coverage in 2003 [14], when the massive outbreak of severe acute respiratory syndrome (SARS) further exposed the weakened and dilapidated state of primary care infrastructure and the increasing inequity in the distribution of health care resources in China. This gradually generated the political will to accelerate the reform of primary care.

### *Phase four: booming expansion of primary care (early 2006–present)*

In view of the wider and deeper significance of achieving an equitable primary care system, a series of strategic plans has been announced since early 2006 [15–20] to encourage community-based primary care and further regulate construction standards at national level to establish primary care facilities in terms of ownership, premises, equipment, personnel and management. In early 2009, the Chinese government embarked on a comprehensive healthcare reform programme [21], which stands on four key pillars: healthcare financing, care delivery, drug supply and hospital reforms (see Figure 40.2).

Community-based primary care services are being systematically strengthened as the policy priority to underpin the care delivery pillar in order to provide universally accessible services at affordable prices to China's 1.3 billion population. The 'Healthy China 2020 plan' was also announced at the same time to provide safe, effective, convenient and affordable basic care for citizens by 2020 [22, 23] through an estimated ambitious investment of ¥850 billion (£84bn; €101bn; $135bn) into the healthcare system over the coming years, with the establishment of primary care infrastructures to promote, maintain and improve health as one of the priorities [24]. The importance of CHS is highlighted as the basis and first point of contact for the public health system, aiming to deliver affordable and accessible primary care to increase the public's responsibility for maintaining good health for all, as well as to reduce the burden of the pharmaceutical expenditure on the whole society. The CHCs are being set up in every urban neighbourhood as the main body to provide CHS for people residing in their service area. It is anticipated that CHCs will play an important role in efficiently allocating more appropriate healthcare resources to alleviate overuse of outpatient services at secondary and tertiary hospitals and to curb the unreasonable utilization of large-scale hospitals as convalescent homes. Frequently encountered medical conditions, common minor diseases and chronic illnesses are expected to be addressed at the community level. The national policy [20] also highlighted that for every 30,000 to 100,000 residents there should be a CHC that could be reached by the residents by a 15-minute walk, in order to keep primary care close to home. China has therefore witnessed a great leap in the number of primary care facilities, from 22,656 in 2006 to 32,739 in 2010 in urban areas. In rural areas, the percentage of villages that have established village clinics for primary care delivery gradually increased from 88.1 per cent in 2006 to 92.3 per cent in 2010 [14].

## Primary care under the current health care reform

The rebuilding of a good primary care system is crucially salient as part of China's current healthcare reform, under which the implementation of five key policy components are complementary to the development of the primary care system.

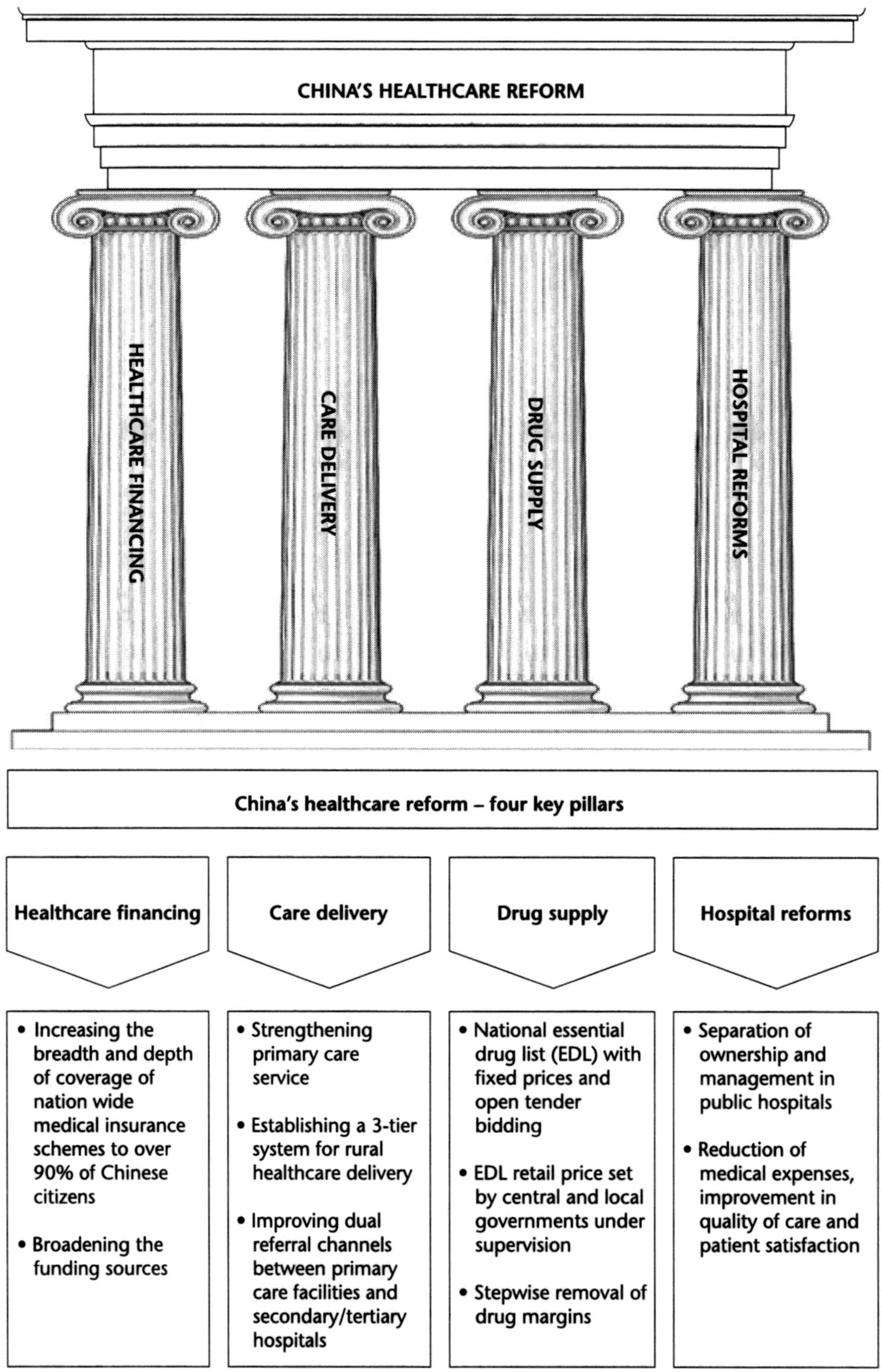


*Figure 40.2* The four key pillars of China's healthcare reform [21]

First, three types of nationwide medical insurance schemes are provided with funding support from both central and local governments, including:

1 Basic medical insurance for the urban population;
2 New Rural Cooperative Medical Scheme (NRCMS) for rural citizens; and
3 Medicaid system for lower socially economic population living in both urban and rural regions.

The basic medical insurance in urban areas will benefit both urban employees and urban residents consisting of children, university students, migrant workers with unstable labour contracts and elderly people who were previously unemployed. The breadth and depth of these medical insurance schemes will be increased to cover more than 90 per cent of the population to improve equity of access to, and utilization of, essential primary care services.

Second, a national essential drug list (EDL) with fixed prices has been launched in order to establish a list of essential medicines that will be manufactured and delivered under government supervision to ensure efficacy, safety and cost-effectiveness. The EDL policy will be incrementally implemented at all primary care facilities at grassroots level in China. It is expected to gradually curb the current increasing dependence on sales of pharmaceuticals at the primary care facilities in which it is common practice to prescribe irrational, unnecessary and expensive medications. All drugs on the list will get a higher reimbursement rate under the insurance scheme.

Third, the public health service systems are being expanded at community-based healthcare facilities rather than at secondary and tertiary hospitals. The CHCs and stations are reinforced throughout urban areas and the enhancement of primary care infrastructure and human resources are emphasized in rural areas to develop a three-tier network at county (county hospital), town (township health centres [THCs]) and village levels (village clinics) for rural populations. Patients are encouraged to consider these primary care facilities as their healthcare gatekeeper to address a wider range of health needs and problems, especially disease prevention and health promotion of chronic medical conditions.

Fourth, a comprehensive package of basic public health (BPH) services are promoted by government investment at both national and local levels to enhance the capacity of disease prevention and health promotion for the general public [25]. The average expenditure per capita from the government on BPH services increased from ¥15 (£1.5; €1.8; $2.4) to ¥25 (£2.4; €3.1; $4.0) in 2011 to ensure an equitable service provision. The BPH services generally contain 11 programmes on six aspects, including:

1 Establishment of healthcare records;
2 Provision of health education;
3 Disease prevention and vaccination;
4 Healthcare management for the elderly (those aged 65 and above), pregnant women, children and patients with hypertension, diabetes or serious mental disorders;
5 Surveillance and control of major infectious diseases, endemic diseases and other public health emergencies; and
6 Sanitation control and healthcare monitoring system [26] (see Table 40.1).

Lastly, pilot reforms of public hospitals are being launched to guard against the tendency of over-commercialization and there are also attempts to clarify the distinct roles of secondary/

*Table 40.1* An overview of the basic public health (BPH) services

| *BPH services* | *Items* |
|---|---|
| Health records | Establishment of health records for urban and rural residents who have resided in the community for more than six months<br>Basic socio-demographic information<br>Regular check-up and health assessment<br>Lifestyle and health condition<br>History of treatment, referral and medication<br>Record on home-visit and follow-up |
| Health education | Provision of health education<br>Healthy lifestyle<br>Screening, disease prevention and treatment<br>Public health emergency and family first-aid<br>Dissemination of health policy documents |
| Vaccination and prevention | Universal childhood immunization<br>Vaccination for specific geographical or environmental risks |
| Health management | Healthcare management for target population including:<br>Elderly (above 65 years old)<br>Pregnant women<br>Children (under 6 years old)<br>Healthcare management for patients with target diseases including:<br>Hypertension<br>Diabetes mellitus<br>Severe mental disorders |
| Disease surveillance and report | Widespread surveillance and control of diseases including:<br>Major infectious diseases<br>Endemic diseases<br>Food poisoning and occupational poisoning<br>Public health emergency and risk assessment |
| Sanitation supervision | Report on food safety<br>Counselling on occupational health<br>Monitoring on drinking water safety<br>Health services in school<br>Supervision on illegal medical practice |

*Source*: [26].

tertiary hospitals and primary care facilities. The 'Separation of Ownership and Management' approach has, however, attracted greater attention to restructuring the managerial hierarchy of the hospitals. Some small-scale hospitals have already been holistically transformed into primary care facilities. Also, dual-direction referral channels between hospitals and CHCs are being explored with the aim that most common and minor illness will be tackled at CHCs whilst more complex problems will be referred to secondary or tertiary hospitals. Such mechanisms will establish a platform to optimize the distribution of healthcare resources and achieve better equity and accessibility.

Moreover, in response to the problem of an insufficient primary care workforce, another arm of the reform is the joint effort between six ministries (National Development and Reform Commission, Ministry of Health, Ministry of Education, Ministry of Finance, Ministry of Human Resources and Social Security) at the national level, which seeks to:

1 Establish general practice (GP) as an independent academic discipline at medical universities;
2 Develop a university-based GP curriculum, clinical rotation and community-based health service programmes for undergraduate-level medical students;
3 Implement a postgraduate-level standardized GP training for fresh medical graduates and in-service training programmes for specialized clinicians to become registered GP practitioners at CHCs; and
4 Provide continuing professional development programmes for primary care professionals including GP practitioners, public health doctors, nurses, pharmacists, care givers, managerial staff, as well as others [27].

Additionally, other attempts have been made to retain the existing primary care workforce, such as the promise of increased remuneration, career promotion prospects and improved working conditions.

Through the rapid and effective policy implementations of these favourable initiatives, it is hoped a smooth way is paved to place primary care as the key and central component of the health services in China.

## Current primary care service delivery

As described, national policy is that primary care facilities are being established as the backbone of the entire health system under China's current healthcare reform. In rural areas, township health centres (THCs) and village clinics are the core primary care providers functioning as community-based coordinating centres together with hospitals and public health institutions. In urban areas, CHCs are the core primary care providers with the main function of providing a six-in-one comprehensive care package [8, 20], including:

1 Disease prevention of major and common infectious diseases, endemic diseases, as well as parasitic diseases;
2 General preventive care and health maintenance for the health status of communities, especially for women, children and the elderly;
3 Diagnosis and treatment of common health problems, basic acute care, as well as dual-direction CHC-hospital referral services;
4 Rehabilitation services and case management of chronic conditions and psychiatric disorders;
5 Health education and promotion of healthy lifestyle; and
6 Counselling services on family planning (see Table 40.2).

Besides clinical treatment, the CHCs are responsible for providing the basic public health (BPH) services package, which receives government subsidies on the basis of the number of population served by the CHCs. Many CHCs also manage community health stations, which provide an even further outreach into the community whereas, in rural areas, THCs and village clinics act similarly to CHCs and the health stations for primary care delivery (see Table 40.3). Services delivered by most primary care providers include both allopathic medicine/Western medicine and traditional Chinese medicine, both subject to industry supervision of the quantity and quality of care by the local health bureau. Basically, healthcare staff, including physicians, are paid a fixed salary plus a floating salary which is largely determined by the total income of the primary care facility in each fiscal period [28]. As the

*Table 40.2* An overview of the six-in-one care package provided by Community Health Services (CHS) facilities

| *Community Health Services (CHS)* | *Items* |
|---|---|
| Prevention | Early diagnosis of community health issues<br>Vaccination and immunization<br>Infectious diseases<br>  Report and surveillance<br>  Prevention of major infectious diseases (tuberculosis/AIDS)<br>  Prevention of common infectious diseases<br>Endemic diseases and parasitic diseases<br>Management of health records<br>Patriotic sanitation initiatives |
| Health protection | Health protection for women, children and elderly people |
| Treatment | Primary medical care of common and frequently occurring diseases<br>Community on-site medical aid<br>Chronic diseases<br>  Screening<br>  Case management of highlighted chronic diseases<br>Psychiatric disorders<br>Referral services between CHCs and hospitals |
| Rehabilitation | Rehabilitation services for disabled and convalescent people<br>Training and guidance on rehabilitation at home and in the community |
| Health education | Dissemination of health knowledge<br>Health management of both individuals and populations<br>Health education for targeted populations and in key public areas<br>Popularization of healthy behaviour and lifestyles |
| Family planning | Counselling services and guidance on family planning<br>Provision of conception control items |

*Source*: [20].

*Table 40.3* The development of primary care facilities between 2005 and 2012 in China

| *Year* | *Community Health Centres and Stations* | *Township Health Centres* | *Village Clinics* | *Total* |
|---|---|---|---|---|
| 2005 | 17,128 | 40,907 | 583,209 | 641,244 |
| 2006 | 22,656 | 39,975 | 609,128 | 671,759 |
| 2007 | 27,069 | 39,876 | 613,855 | 680,800 |
| 2008 | 24,260 | 39,080 | 613,143 | 676,483 |
| 2009 | 27,308 | 38,475 | 632,770 | 698,553 |
| 2010 | 32,739 | 37,836 | 648,424 | 718,999 |
| 2011 | 32,860 | 37,295 | 662,894 | 733,049 |
| 2012 | 33,562 | 37,097 | 653,419 | 724,078 |

*Source*: [14].

*Table 40.4* Total person-time of diagnosis and treatment at primary care facilities between 2005 and 2011 in China

| *Year* | *Community Health Centres and Stations* | *Township Health Centres* | *Village Clinics* | *Total (million person times)* |
|---|---|---|---|---|
| 2005 | 122.2 | 679.2 | 1,234.1 | 2,035.5 |
| 2006 | 176.6 | 700.9 | 1,348.4 | 2,225.9 |
| 2007 | 225.9 | 758.6 | 1,386.8 | 2,371.2 |
| 2008 | 256.7 | 826.8 | 1,368.9 | 2,452.4 |
| 2009 | 377.0 | 876.6 | 1,551.7 | 2,805.3 |
| 2010 | 484.5 | 874.2 | 1,657.0 | 3,015.7 |
| 2011 | 546.5 | 866.5 | 1,792.1 | 3,205.1 |

*Source*: [14].

current healthcare reform does not formulate a rigid 'gatekeeper' system at the policy level, patients are not required to register with any primary care practitioners and any patient can walk in to see a generalist in a primary care facility after paying a fixed one-off registration fee at the clinic reception. The payment for the health visit also covers fees for clinical examination, medical treatment and the cost of pharmaceuticals, which can be the major expenditure. For patients with medical insurance, the fee to be paid is shared between the government and the patient. Also, insured patients have a preferential reimbursement rate if they attend the primary care facilities located near where they live which are often pre-designated by the corresponding medical insurance scheme to encourage the utilization of these grassroots healthcare facilities [29]. See Table 40.4 for total person-time of diagnosis and treatment at primary care facilities between 2005 and 2011 in China.

## Emerging models for primary care in urban areas

Due to the great variations in socio-economical and cultural characteristics in different urban regions, the local establishment and expansion of primary care networks based on CHCs has led to the emergence of different models of ownership and management. The three main models (as shown in Tables 40.5 and 40.6) are:

1 Government-owned and managed CHCs (G-CHCs);
2 Government-owned and hospital-managed CHCs (H-CHCs); and
3 Privately owned and managed CHCs (P-CHCs).

Government-owned and managed CHCs (G-CHCs) are independent of the public hospital system and are directly managed by the local government as non-profit healthcare facilities and are, at the same time, part of the government sector [30]. The services delivered by the G-CHCs are monitored by the local health bureau, which provides professional guidance and regular assessments to ensure quality of services. The typical G-CHC is subject to the Separation of Revenue and Expenditure policy, i.e. the revenue of the CHCs (including fees generated from medical treatment and drug sales) are directly turned in to the local government, whereas the expenditure of the CHC, including premises, equipment, facilities and staff remuneration, are provided from the annual budget from the local government.

*Table 40.5* Three emerging CHC models for primary care delivery in urban areas in China

| | *G-CHCs* | *H-CHCs* | *P-CHCs* |
|---|---|---|---|
| **Ownership and management** | Local government | Public hospitals | Private and social investors |
| **Staff structure** | Clinical physicians, public health doctors, nurses, pharmacists, care givers, managerial staff, etc. | | |
| **Service provided** | Comprehensive care package, including both allopathic/Western medicine and Traditional Chinese Medicine | | |
| **Industry supervision** | Local health bureau | | |
| **Financial support from government** | $$$$$$ | $$ | $ |
| **CHC funding source** |   | 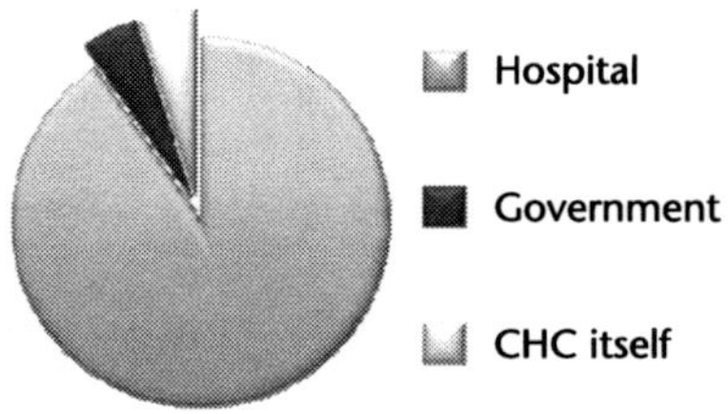  | 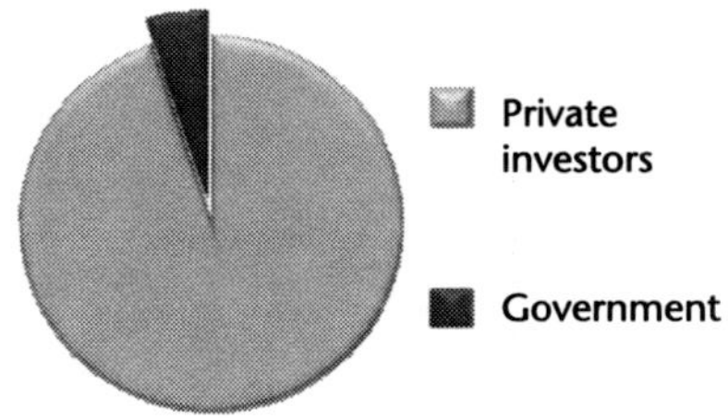  |
| **CHC revenue** | Turned in to the local government | Retained at CHCs | Retained at CHCs |
| **CHC expenditure (incl. staff remuneration)** | Paid from the government budget | Paid from CHC revenue pool | Paid from CHC revenue pool |

*Source*: [31].

*Notes*: CHCs: Community Health Centres
G-CHCs: Government-owned and managed CHCs
H-CHCs: Government-owned and hospital-managed CHCs
P-CHCs: Privately owned and managed CHCs

*Table 40.6* Figures for three emerging CHC models for primary care delivery in urban areas in China (2008)

| | *G-CHCs* | *H-CHCs* | *P-CHCs* |
|---|---|---|---|
| Number | 1,793 | 1,755 | 1,367 |
| Per cent (%) | 36.5 | 35.7 | 27.8 |

*Source*: [44].

*Notes*: CHCs: Community Health Centres
G-CHCs: Government-owned and managed CHCs
H-CHCs: Government-owned and hospital-managed CHCs
P-CHCs: Privately owned and managed CHCs

Government-owned but hospital-managed CHCs (H-CHCs) are owned by the government but managed by the host hospital. Compared with the G-CHCs, the H-CHCs are not part of the government sector and they are financially self-sufficient institutions allowed to make profit. The typical H-CHC functions like an outreach clinic of the host hospital and receives limited subsidies from the government via the host hospital which further allocates funding to the CHC. The host hospital is responsible for the management of the CHC, which includes the provision of healthcare professionals, medical equipment and resources, and the CHC is normally regarded as a department within the hospital.

Privately owned CHCs (P-CHCs) are owned and managed by private organizations which are financially independent. P-CHCs are profit-making organizations which generate their income mainly through the provision of clinical care. Moreover, they also receive limited subsidies from the local government for public health service provision, and the quality of service is supervised by the local health bureau [20].

In sum, these emerging primary care models reflect the extent of government involvement in delivering primary care. In the G-CHC model, there is an overwhelming emphasis on direct provision from the government sector whereas in the H-CHC and P-CHC models, the role of government is largely limited to the layout of the strategic blueprint for primary care delivery and the provision of primary care services is largely left up to hospitals and private organizations which both adopt a more 'for-profit' nature due to their financial self-sufficiency. In addition, the relationship between the ownership and management of primary care organizations and the quality of primary care service provided are of great interest. Some of the preliminary evidence has suggested that the G-CHC model has strengths in reducing social inequality and resulting in better distribution of health resources, probably due to the emphasis on central planning and effective multi-sectoral collaboration [31–33]. Although the P-CHCs have less rigid bureaucratic structures and are more responsive to the grassroots of their locality, the primary care service provided might be inferior due to the lack of government support. It is believed that the plurality of primary care organizational models of service delivery are needed given the diversified local conditions in China; however, the long-term effects of these models on quality of health outcomes remain to be evaluated to ensure that public health goals can be achieved and equal access to high-quality primary care can be accomplished.

## Challenges

The current healthcare policy [21] in China seeks to establish a health system with a strong primary care base in both urban and rural areas. The core problem facing China's current healthcare system is 'the difficulty and high cost of getting medical services' [34], i.e. healthcare resources are dominated by secondary and tertiary healthcare providers which are more expensive and more time-consuming to get access to due to overcrowding. Therefore, the shift of health system development from hospital-based specialist care towards primary care becomes obviously crucial for better allocating limited healthcare resources and to keep the overall healthcare expenditure at a relatively lower level. Although the development of primary care is immutable at the political level and has resulted in some encouraging changes, there are still considerable challenges facing its ambitious progression.

First and foremost, the proposed universal health insurance system for primary care to achieve the goal of health for all requires a huge budget from both the central and local governments, particularly given the increasing ageing population needing more complicated treatment strategies. Although the central government has substantially increased investment, financial support at the local level has not always materialized due to substantial imbalance in socio-economic status between urban and rural areas, and between different regions. In addition, in some parts of western China, local governments have not yet fully recognized the importance of a well-established primary care system for the whole society and have so far failed to afford the investment in primary care facilities as expected due to their insufficient funding capacity [35]. Undeniably, it is a laudable progression on the population coverage rate by the nationwide medical insurance schemes [36] that currently 89 per cent of urban residents and 97 per cent of rural residents are covered as compared with the 2003 figures when only 55 per cent of urban residents and 21 per cent of rural residents had medical insurance coverage. However, the proportion of insurance reimbursement is, on average, only around 30 to 50 per cent and the benefit package is subject to certain predetermined conditions (such as the severity of the medical condition, drug category, whether the healthcare facilities where healthcare expenditures occurred are enlisted in the insurance scheme, employment status and hierarchy and others).

Second, the shortage of well-trained and qualified general practitioners due to a lack of improved medical education and of continuing professional development creates significant barriers. In particular, training standards for primary care in less economically developed areas are sadly lacking [37]. The challenges also come from the limited acceptance and distrust of having a 'gatekeeper' for healthcare at primary care facilities, which are often considered by patients as low-quality service providers due to the widespread and entrenched attitude that generalists serving in these institutions are less competent and professional [38]. The prevailing and embedded custom in which specialists are deemed as the reliable source for addressing health problems inclines patients to bypass the community generalists and to consult specialists directly at outpatient departments particularly in prestigious, large-scale hospitals, regardless of the nature or the severity of their illness [39]. This creates a vicious cycle which undermines the willingness of competent healthcare professionals to work at primary care facilities, therefore contributing to the high staff turnover rate which exists due to inferior remuneration, heavy workload, poor working environment and no promising career opportunities in the primary care setting.

Third, the gatekeeper and referral roles of primary care facilities have not yet been fully recognized and established. According to statistics of patients' initial utilization of healthcare facilities in the first two weeks of illness in urban areas in 2008 [14], more than half (51.7 per cent) of patients would choose secondary or tertiary hospitals for health care, whereas only 35.8 per cent of patients would initially receive medical services at community healthcare facilities, thus reflecting the deficient performance of the gatekeeper function. On the other hand, it is not mandatory for patients to have a prior referral from the primary care generalists to consult specialists at hospitals, whilst hospitals tend to keep patients rather than refer them back to the community due to hospitals being in competition with primary care facilities to maintain a high level of patient volumes for revenue generation. This brings about a fragmented healthcare delivery system and a rigid gatekeeper system is crucial in order to establish an appropriate source of primary care.

Fourth, challenges come from reducing costs but ensuring the quality of primary care is kept at a good level through payment incentives. The reforms of incentive structures for primary care providers are still in the early stages of implementation. It is worth noting that the payment methods would profoundly alter the practice behaviour as it links to the wellbeing of the patients. The single and combined options of various types of provider payment methods, including retrospective payment (such as fee-for-service), aggregated and prospective payment (such as case-based per visit, capitation per person covered, global budget per period) and pay for performance are still being explored through nationwide experiments to find effective and viable incentive systems for provider payment. Moreover, the current performance indicators tend to overemphasize the expenditure and service volume and are less concerned with quality and health outcomes of the population. A rigid regulation system is also crucially needed to avoid providers falsifying reported data for payment-related performance assessment. Further innovations are needed to generate adequate motivation for primary care providers to change from curative care to primary care, and to practice prevention and management of chronic diseases [40, 41].

And lastly, a poor electronic health record (eHR) platform has been identified as a major stumbling block in improving the health outcome for China's population. No universal electronic platform exists for sharing population-based healthcare information and the heavy reliance on paper-based healthcare records is prevailing in the primary care sector. The extent to which primary care physicians are meeting national guideline targets is lacking to inform policy decisions. A standardized data collection procedure and primary care assessment, which are rigorous, objective and evidence-based, will help bring about the wealth of epidemiological data on primary care management available for further analysis which can be used to generate objective evidence. However, software companies in China are less experienced than foreign vendors and most software is designed only for routine administration purposes without a population perspective. A wide range of independent software providers are competing in the market to sell their own products; however, there are no universal guidelines or consistent standards set for software interface and coding exchange between systems. Although some forms of eHR systems have been introduced in a number of primary care facilities, incompatibility with other systems made them less possible to use for data sharing. Challenges facing a widespread adoption of a unified eHR system are huge and successful implementation requires a joint effort involving all stakeholders.

## Future prospects

Recent years have witnessed increasing achievements in primary care development and efforts have gone into consensus for building the primary care infrastructure with sustainable economic and political support; however, these are just the initial steps on the road towards placing primary care as the cornerstone of the healthcare system in China. To improve universal primary care coverage and reduce expenditure on health care, China is also engaged in knowledge exchange, learning from international experiences in primary care service delivery models and about education and training for general practitioners. Lessons on successfully achieving an optimal trade-off between government and market for China's decentralized and commercialized healthcare system are indeed a global issue for other countries undergoing dynamic economic transitions.

A series of recent policies in China are trying to incrementally introduce tiered reimbursement rates to let patients have preferential rates for reimbursement of medical expenditure incurred at CHCs, compared to those at hospitals. Also, an emphasis has been placed on humanitarian qualities through the improved education and training for general practitioners to improve the doctor–patient relationship and restore public respect for primary care professionals. These efforts might help to encourage patients to use CHCs and curb the situation of bypassing primary healthcare facilities because they might want to obtain healthcare services at secondary and tertiary levels [42]. In several cities in the eastern seaboard, particularly in Jiangsu, Zhejiang and Guangdong provinces, general practitioners with good qualifications and professional competence acquire a good local reputation and public acceptance, attracting large numbers of patients at the community level [43].

China is undergoing a huge disease burden transition due to the unprecedented social and environmental changes, which affect the diets and lifestyle of the population, food hygiene, occupational and traffic hazards, and air and water pollution, raising major health concerns. Non-communicable diseases (NCDs) have already become China's number one health threat and this poses a substantial burden on primary care. Cardiovascular disease (CVD), diabetes and chronic kidney disease (CKD) often occur together and share common risk factors and treatments, thus it would be beneficial to have a coordinated and comprehensive approach to detection, treatment and management for such chronic diseases at primary care level. Some ongoing experiments on payment incentive structure such as the introduction of pay-for-performance would greatly help motive primary care providers to deliver more preventive services including health education, health interventions on healthy lifestyle and home visits to address chronic diseases. The concept of enhancing primary care through a longitudinal and coordinated electronic health record platform is envisaged by China, and stepwise progress is being made to provide easily accessible and accurate information on patients' health problems especially for chronic disease management.

There is no doubt that the most salient task of progressing primary care development in China is to improve the quality attributes of primary care in terms of first contact, coordination, continuity, comprehensiveness, as well as family and community centredness, which might help solve the long-standing problem of under-utilization of the primary care facilities as the first point of contact for care, one of the key problems facing the reforms in China. In the long term, the establishment of a well-organized primary care network as the foundation and the first point of contact in the health system requires a multi-sectorial approach. This implies the need for supportive healthcare policies; sustainable financial support from the government; effective care delivery models which cater to the local needs and conditions; a coordinated network of multilevel healthcare facilities; active engagement from the community sector; qualified and skilled primary care workforce; well-designed medical insurance scheme which covers both the residential and floating population; high utilization of, and satisfaction with, the primary care services and an assessment system to ensure better quality of primary care services delivered in divergent areas in China. Given the government's ambitious investment in building up the primary care system, China has an opportunity to again become an exemplary model for primary care in the world once the ongoing reforms achieve their stated goals.

## References

1. *From Alma-Ata to the Year 2000: Reflections at the Midpoint*. Geneva: World Health Organization, 1988.
2. Shapiro J. *Mao's War against Nature: Politics and the Environment in Revolutionary China*. Cambridge: Cambridge University Press, 2001.

3. Yin W, Fu H, An N, Feng X, Yan F, Wang K. The development phase analysis and persistence strategy research of community health services. *Chinese Journal of Hospital Administration* 2004(03): 18–22.
4. Ge Y, Gong S. *Chinese Health Care Reform*. China Development Publishing, 2007.
5. World Bank Databank. World Development Indicators (WDI) and Global Development Finance (GDF), 2012.
6. Hsiao WCL. The Chinese health-care system – lessons for other nations. *Soc Sci Med* 1995; 41(8): 1047–55.
7. Hsiao WCL, Liu YL. Economic reform and health – lessons from China. *New Engl J Med* 1996; 335(6): 430–2.
8. Opinions on development of community health services in the cities. No. 326 document. Division of Primary and Women's Health, Ministry of Health, China, 1999.
9. Decision concerning public health reform and development. State Council. P.R. China, 1997.
10. Decision on establishing basic medical insurance system for urban employees. No. 44 documents. State Council, 1998.
11. Guidance on pharmaceutical and healthcare system reform in urban areas. No. 16 document. State Council, 2000.
12. Guidance on accelerating the community health service development in urban areas. No. 186 document. Ministry of Health, 2002.
13. The implementation scheme of the establishment of national exemplary community health service regions. No. 252 document. Ministry of Health, 2003.
14. *China Health Statistics Yearbook 2012*. Center for Health Statistics and Information, Ministry of Health. P.R. China, 2012.
15. Guidance on development of community health services in the cities. No. 10 document. State Council, 2006.
16. Regulations on community health service organizations in urban areas. No. 239 document. Ministry of Health. P.R. China, 2006.
17. The announcement of the construction standard of community health centres and community health stations in urban areas. No. 240 document. Ministry of Health. P.R. China, 2006.
18. Guidance and opinions on strengthening healthcare professionals cadre for community health service in urban areas. No. 69 document. Ministry of Human Resources and Social Security. P.R. China, 2006.
19. Opinions on promoting the full utilization of community health service among population covered by medical insurance. No. 23 document. Ministry of Labour and Social Security. P.R. China, 2006.
20. Guidelines and opinions on the establishment of community health service facilities in urban areas. No. 96 document. CCP Central Committee, 2006.
21. Opinions on deepening pharmaceutical and healthcare system reform. No. 9 document. State Council, 2009.
22. Chen Z, Gao Q. Moving towards universal medical services with Chinese characteristics. Ministry of Health, 2008.
23. Healthy China Plan 2020. Ministry of Health, 2008.
24. Plan on recent priorities in carrying out the reform of health care system (2009–2011). No. 12 document. State Council, 2009.
25. Notification on disseminating of essential public health service items in Guangdong province. No. 75 document. Guangdong Health Bureau, 2011.
26. Guidelines on Performance of National Basic Public Health Service. Ministry of Health. P.R. China, 2011.
27. A plan for the establishment of a general practitioner led primary-care [in Chinese]. National Development and Reform Commission. State Commission Office for Public Sector Reform, Ministry of Education, Ministry of Finance, Ministry of Human Resources and Social Security, 2011.
28. Staff remuneration. No. 3 document. Ministry of Finance. P.R. China, 2006.
29. Guiding opinions of the State Council about the pilot urban resident basic medical insurance. No. 20 document. State Council. P.R. China, 2007.
30. Accelerating the community health service development in Dongguan. No. 96 document. Dongguan Government, 2007.
31. Wang HHX, Wong SYS, Wong MCS, *et al.* Patients' experiences in different models of community health centers in Southern China. *Ann Fam Med* 2013; 11(6): 517–26.

32. Wong MCS, Wang HHX, Wong SYS, *et al.* Performance comparison among the major healthcare financing systems in six cities of the Pearl River Delta Region, Mainland China. *PLoS One* 2012; 7(9): e46309.
33. Wang HHX, Wong MCS, Wong SYS, *et al.* The impact of cardiovascular multimorbidity on healthcare service utilisation under three primary care organisational models in China. *Int J Cardiol* 2013; 163(Suppl 2): S1–S2.
34. Wagstaff A, Yip W, Lindelow M, Hsiao WC. China's health system and its reform: a review of recent studies. *Health Economics* 2009; 18(Suppl 2): S7–S23.
35. Wang Y, Wang F, Li Y, *et al.* A comparative analysis on implementation and effect of medical insurance policy in community health service stations in the eastern, central and western regions. *Chinese Journal of Health Policy* 2011; 4(6): 17–23.
36. Parry J. Nine in 10 Chinese are covered by medical insurance, but access to treatment remains a problem. *Brit Med J* 2012; 344.
37. Wang JJ, Zhong NS, Zhu AR. Review of the development of family physicians and general practitioners with Chinese characteristics [In Chinese]. Chinese Rural Health Service Administration. 2009; 29(9): 663–5.
38. Wang HHX, Wang JJ, Zhou ZH, Wang XW, Xu L. General practice education and training in southern China: recent development and ongoing challenges under the healthcare reform. *Malaysian Family Physician* 2013; 8(3): 2–10.
39. Parry J. GP based primary care is only just starting to emerge in China. *Brit Med J* 2010; 341.
40. Wang HHX, Wong MCS, Wong SYS, *et al.* The profile of cardiovascular multimorbidity among patients in primary care in southern China: a cross-sectional study. *Int J Cardiol* 2013; 163(Suppl 2): S28.
41. Wang HHX, Wong MCS, Wong SYS, *et al.* Factors associated with cardiovascular multimorbidity among primary care patients in southern China. *Int J Cardiol* 2013; 163(Suppl 2): S8–S9.
42. The Strategic Plan for Developing Community Health Services in Guangdong (2006–2010). No. 75 document. Central Government, 2007.
43. Wang JJ, Liu YH, Wang XW, Chen YM, Lei YX. The exploration and practice in the construction of general practice education system in Guangdong province in China [In Chinese]. *Chinese General Practice* 2006; 9(15): 1228–30.
44. Research on Health Services of Primary Health Care Facilities in China. Ministry of Health, 2008.*

* The long-existing Ministry of Health (MoH) and the National Population and Family Planning Commission (NPFPC) have been recently merged into, and reconstituted as, the National Health and Family Planning Commission (NHFPC) of the People's Republic of China, with effect from 17 March 2013. The NHFPC, after integration, is expected to have better resource allocation. It aims to deepen the current healthcare reform to better improve medical care and public health services, as well as the basic national family planning services for the health and wellbeing of the population in China.

# 41

# Conceptualizing the integration of traditional and complementary medicine in health systems

## Patients, policies, professions and providers

*Vincent C. H. Chung*

### Introduction

The term 'traditional medicine' covers a wide range of therapies and practices which can vary across countries. In some cultures, the term 'complementary medicine' is used interchangeably with traditional medicine. The generic term 'traditional and complementary medicine' (T&CM) is used by the World Health Organization (WHO) to avoid geographical variation [1].[1] T&CM denotes a broad set of healthcare practices that encompass all health systems, modalities and practices, and their accompanying theories and beliefs, other than those intrinsic to the politically dominant health system of a particular society or culture in a given historical period [2]. The use of the phrase 'politically dominant' in this definition denotes that an incompatibility exists between the holistic paradigm of T&CM and the paradigm of bio-medical (conventional) medicine (BM) [3]. Commonly used T&CM are listed in Table 41.1 [4]. Despite their epistemological differences, T&CM has long played a role in many of the world's health systems, alongside BM, and has remained popular to this day [5].

In this chapter, we illustrate how the framework of the four domains of patients, policy makers, professions and providers (4Ps), which are integral to all health systems, may be applied to T&CM by using a case study of Hong Kong, where the integration of traditional Chinese medicine (TCM) started since Hong Kong's reunification with mainland China in 1997.

### Overview of traditional, complementary and alternative medicine

In resource-poor regions like Africa, it is estimated that 80 per cent of the population depends on T&CM for basic health care [6]. Meanwhile, in the West, populations from middle- and

*Table 41.1* List of therapies included as T&CM by the Cochrane Collaboration

1. **Natural products**
   - Aromatherapy
   - Ayurvedic traditional medicine (Ayurveda)
   - Bee products (e.g. honey, pollen, propolis, royal jelly, venom)
   - Diet therapy† (e.g. low fat diets, vegan diets)
   - Dietary supplements (non-herbal)† (e.g. vitamins, hormones, amino acids)
   - Herbal supplements (e.g. echinacea, garlic)
   - Homeopathy
   - Naturopathy
   - Traditional healers and healing practices (e.g. Kampo, Shamanism, Chinese traditional medicine)
2. **Mind and body practices**
   - Alexander technique
   - Biofeedback
   - Distant healing
   - Feldenkrais method
   - Hypnosis
   - Imagery (i.e. visualization techniques)
   - Meditation
   - Morita therapy
   - Qi gong
   - Reiki therapy
   - Relaxation techniques
   - Spiritual healing (e.g. prayer)
3. **Manipulative and body-based practices**
   - Acupressure
   - Acupuncture (e.g. needle acupuncture, electroacupuncture)
   - Chiropractic (i.e. spinal manipulation)
4. **Manipulative and body-based practices (continued)**
   - Craniosacral manipulation
   - Massage
   - Moxibustion
   - Osteopathic manipulation
   - Reflexology
   - Tai chi
   - Therapeutic touch
   - Tui na
   - Yoga
5. **Others**
   - Arts therapy (e.g. dance therapy, drama therapy, music therapy)
   - Balneotherapy
   - Chelation therapy†
   - Colour therapy (i.e. chromotherapy)
   - Electric stimulation therapy† (e.g. transcutaneous electrical nerve stimulation)
   - Electromagnetic therapy†
   - Eye Movement Desensitization and Reprocessing (EMDR)
   - Hydrotherapy
   - Hyperbaric oxygenation†
   - Light therapy† (phototherapy)

- Magnetic field therapy† (e.g. transcranial magnetic stimulation)
- Ozone therapy†
- Play therapy
- Prolotherapy
- Snoezelen
- Speleotherapy
- Ultrasonic therapy†

*Source*: [4].

*Note:* † Depending on the condition being treated, these therapies may also be standard conventional medical treatments.

high-income countries have increasingly turned to T&CM in the past 20 years [7]. Figures for lifetime use of T&CM in Australia and the UK were 47 per cent [8] and 48 per cent [9], respectively, while figures for Canada [10] and Chile [11] reached nearly 70 per cent. In many Asian countries, T&CM is an integral part of the healthcare ecology, in which the usage and practice of T&CM is deeply rooted in the social and cultural fabric of the community [12–16].

Patients being able to choose T&CM as their preferred health modality is a strong bottom-up driver changing the relationship between T&CM and BM, and triggering changes in T&CM policies within health systems. It is postulated that people's demands for T&CM would gradually trigger regulation and assimilation of T&CM practices into the overall health system [17]. In fact, the development of T&CM policy was recognized by the Alma Ata Declaration 30 years ago. Promulgated in the WHO International Conference on Primary Health Care, the declaration emphasized that 'people have the right and duty to participate individually and collectively in the planning and implementation of their care, which includes access to traditional medicine' (Section VII, Point 7) [18]. The WHO has reaffirmed its support for T&CM development with the production of Traditional Medicine Strategy 2002–2005, as well as in the more updated Traditional Medicine Strategy 2014–2023, which specifies goals including:

1 Increasing governmental support for T&CM amongst member states; and
2 Promoting integration of T&CM into member states' national healthcare systems [19].

According to a WHO survey published in 2005, 45 out of 141 responding member states have already issued national policies for T&CM, while 51 were developing relevant policies among the remaining 96 states [20]. Subsequently, in 2008, the Beijing Declaration was disseminated at the WHO Congress on Traditional Medicine. The Declaration regards T&CM policies formulation as a responsibility of governments worldwide and has re-emphasized the importance of including T&CM as part of national health systems amongst member states [21].

Specifically, the WHO Beijing Declaration advocates the following health system actions including:

1 Governments have a responsibility to their people's health needs and should formulate national policies, regulations and standards as part of a comprehensive national health system to ensure appropriate, safe and effective use of traditional medicine;
2 Recognizing the progress of many governments to date in integrating traditional medicine into their national health system, we call on those who have not yet done so, to do so;

3 Governments should establish systems for the qualification, accreditation or licensing of traditional medicine practitioners. Traditional medicine practitioners should upgrade their knowledge and skills based on national requirements; and
4 The communication between conventional and traditional medicine providers should be strengthened and appropriate training programmes should be established for health professionals, medical students and relevant researchers.

These actions recommended by the WHO are key health system responses needed to address the patients' choice for T&CM. It requires response from all major stakeholders in health systems [22]: top-down response from policy makers in recognizing the status of T&CM, changes in the profession to include regulation of T&CM practitioners (T&CMP) and related products, and service providers' input in service redesign that allows for the inclusion of T&CM, including the promotion of inter-professional collaboration between T&CMP and clinicians trained in conventional BM [23].

In addition, the unique historical and health system features of each region/nation would need to contextualize how the four domains of patients, policy makers, professions and providers (4Ps) interact and, subsequently, facilitate or hinder the attainment of the four goals stipulated by the WHO Traditional Medicine Strategy (see Figure 41.1). Using this generic conceptual framework, we can analyse salient issues pertaining to the process and possibly offer health system solutions that foster integration.

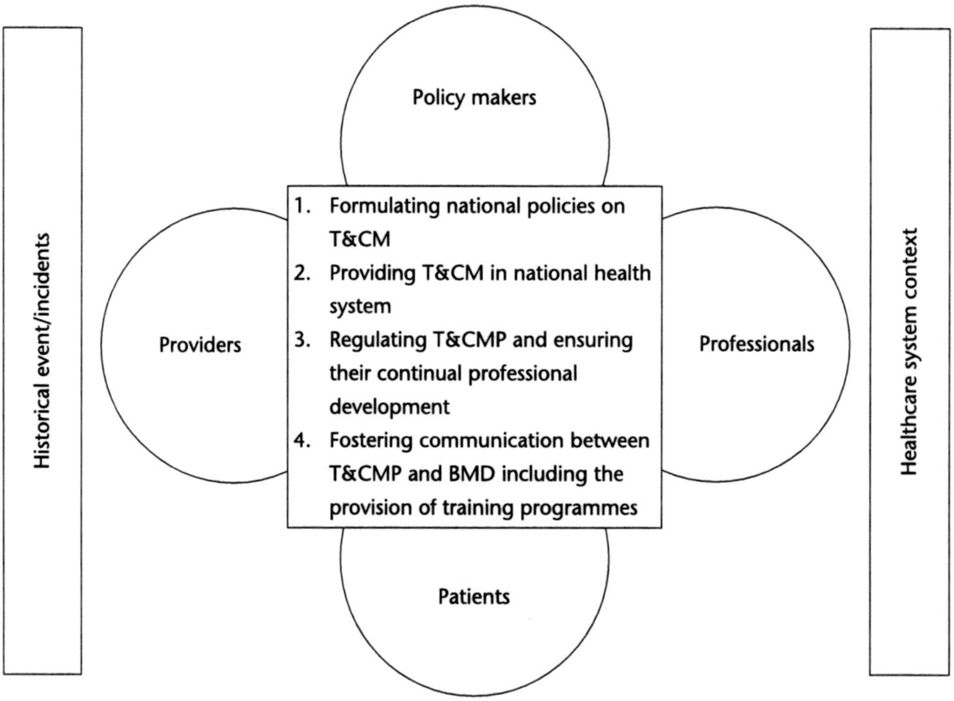


*Figure 41.1* 4Ps framework for analysing health system determinants of integrating T&CM

## Integration of traditional Chinese medicine and biomedicine in Hong Kong: case study using the 4Ps framework

### *Historical and health system context*

Although TCM has been part of the culture in mainland China and Hong Kong for centuries, its official establishment has been varied over the years. It has been officially integrated into the healthcare system in mainland China since 1950 when it was promoted by Mao Zedong and remains a fundamental part of healthcare provision today [24]. In contrast, the status of Hong Kong as a British colony for more than 150 years (1841–1997) led to a different pathway of development. As a former British colony, TCM was part of the informal healthcare provider network in Hong Kong until 1997 when reunification with mainland China led to the formal inclusion of TCM in the healthcare system. Following the Opium Wars, Hong Kong became a British colony in 1841, under the agreement stipulated in the Treaty of Nanking. The local Chinese community, who made up the majority of the Hong Kong population, used TCM as their main form of health care. In the early colonial days, BM mainly served the minority European population and a laissez-faire approach to providing care was adopted towards both TCM and BM by the colonial powers.

The authorities regarded TCM as a form of 'Chinese cultural custom' rather than a formal healthcare modality [25]. The marginal status of TCM was also reflected in legislation relating to health care. The colonial Medical Registration Ordinance specified that only BM doctors (BMD) were subjected to regulation and the practice of TCM was considered to be out of scope [26]. Formal education was not a prerequisite for practice and apprenticeships with relatives or 'masters' were a common education pathway to a TCM career, often supplemented by classroom learning organized by various TCM associations with mixed standards and quality. Sharing clinics between BMD and TCM practitioners (TCMP) was prohibited and TCMP had no rights in issuing death, sick leave or health status assessment certificates. They were also forbidden to use any BM instruments, such as syringes and stethoscopes [27]. Despite its lack of recognition, cultural affinity, geographical proximity to mainland China and easy accessibility contributed in making TCM the preferred choice amongst the Chinese population. The TCM sector remained vibrant until World War II, but in the aftermath, its role was largely displaced by the establishment of a tax-funded BM healthcare system.

### *Policy: from regulation to integration?*

With the reunification of Hong Kong and mainland China on 1 July 1997, the newly established Hong Kong Special Administrative Region (SAR) government was obliged to enact the constitutional law, in which the development of TCM was explicitly stated. This provided a historical opportunity for TCM by establishing its professional identity and status. In his 1997 début policy address, the first Chief Executive of the SAR, Tung Chee-Hwa, announced the government's vision to transform Hong Kong into an 'international TCM centre' [28]. This was followed by an immediate publication of a TCM development consultative document that officially confirmed a formal role for TCM in the healthcare system [29]. Since then, the three major developments in TCM in Hong Kong SAR have been [30]:

1 Formal regulation and registration of TCMP by the Chinese Medicine Council of Hong Kong (CMCHK), a statutory TCM regulation body established under the Chinese Medicine Ordinance;

2 Establishment of full-time undergraduate training of TCMP in three local universities and the implementation of a compulsory Continuing Medical Education (CME) programme for all registered TCMP, under the auspices of the CMCHK; and
3 Introduction of TCM services into the public healthcare system.

Under these new policies, new entrants to the TCM profession must obtain a formal registration from the CMCHK, which requires the passing of a two-part licensing examination with written and clinical components. Currently, only holders of recognized TCM degree(s) are eligible to sit the examination. Since 1998, undergraduate degree programmes have been established in Schools of Chinese Medicine in three public universities: Chinese University of Hong Kong, Hong Kong Baptist University and University of Hong Kong. Regardless of slight differences in structure and emphasis, all three curricula have adopted a lot from TCM universities in mainland China as well as including basic BM taught alongside professional TCM subjects. However, unlike mainland China where graduates are expected to practise both kinds of medicine, Hong Kong TCMP are not allowed to practise BM under the current legislation, which specifies them as clinicians parallel to the BMD. For instance, TCMP are not allowed to order any diagnostics tests and a BMD must be involved in any integrated in-patient treatment.

In 2005, a system of continuing education in Chinese medicine (CME) was launched by the CMCHK as an 'integral component of the registration system'. In order to fulfil their licence revalidation requirement, all registered TCMP must earn 60 CME credits in each of the three-year CME cycles. Those who fail to earn sufficient credits within the three-year period will not be allowed to renew their licences. Around 30 CME programme providers accredited by the CMCHK will be responsible for organizing educational activities. CME learning consists of several components including: attending or giving of lectures, submitting reports on independent studies and publication in TCM journals, with or without peer review requirements [31].

While the establishment of formal regulation and tertiary education have enabled the TCM sector to become professional, these measures alone have failed to link TCMP with BM-trained professionals. TCM services are still mainly provided in a private outpatient setting and even in the 16 TCM clinics located in public BM settings, the two modalities are mostly practised side-by-side as there is no formal procedure for inter-professional referral. Regulation of TCMP and BMD are administered by two separate statutory bodies (Hong Kong Medical Council (HKMC) and CMCHK) and there is no communication platform between the two professions in place. Referral from TCM to BM sector within the public healthcare system is not widely accepted [32]. This professional and systematic compartmentalization of TCM and BM is not aligned with the public's utilization pattern, in which 'double consulting' of both TCMP and BMD is common practice.

### *Patients: coordinating traditional Chinese medicine and biomedicine services responsive to utilization patterns*

The utilization pattern of TCM and BM in Hong Kong clearly indicates the need for bridging the two professions. A large-scale population-based survey conducted in 2005 [33] reported that 16.6 per cent of primary care service users consulted both TCM and BM clinicians in the previous year. These 'double consulters' were more likely to be older, female, patients of chronic non-communicable diseases (NCD) and have higher socio-economic backgrounds. The perceived effectiveness of TCM in treating NCD is characterized by its strengths in:

1 Providing salutogenic (wellbeing enhancing) care;
2 Individualizing treatment to suit different health needs;
3 Delivering thorough therapeutic effects that 'clear the root of the disease'; and
4 Causing few side effects, being generally safer and 'more acceptable to the body' [12].

It is commonly believed that synergistic use of both medicines would yield a better outcome than using either one alone. Holistic advantage would be achieved when the side effects of BM are minimized, whilst the tonic effects of TCM are maximized.

Patients with NCD are more likely to opt for integrated TCM–BM treatment, because they perceive that simultaneous use of both modalities would holistically address their complex therapeutic needs. For example, patients with rheumatoid arthritis may think that BM would provide rapid control of symptoms and better access to laboratory tests that monitor progresses, while TCM would relieve the side effects of BM drugs and provide a tonic effect. This reflected the perceived value of choosing an integrative approach – the lay assumption is that the co-use of TCM and BM would cancel out the weaknesses of both modalities, while retaining their respective strengths [12].

If such utilization patterns are placed within the current policy context of Hong Kong's healthcare system, several questions arise. First, since NCD is an increasingly serious health issue for the elderly in Hong Kong, TCM should be taken into account in the formulation of NCD management strategies. The barriers between TCM and BM professionals result from institutional arrangements which set the professions up in parallel to each other, and also partly due to the lack of inter-professional education, and a lack of exchange of ideas and experience. Increased understanding of the clinical evidence for TCM could facilitate referrals between the two groups, particularly in the management of NCD. In fact, in some cases, BM has little to offer while TCM could improve outcomes (e.g. Chinese herbal medicine for irritable bowel syndrome [34], acupuncture for osteoarthritis of the knee [35]). Equipped with this knowledge, TCM and BM professionals could therefore help their patients in making evidence-based choices in order to optimize their treatment with either TCM or BM.

Another key policy concern is TCM's role within the structure of primary health care (PHC). A PHC system featuring continuity, coordination and comprehensiveness that includes both TCM and BM could potentially enhance the quality and efficiency of chronic care [36]. However, the presence of paradigm differences between these two modalities limits the cross-referral of NCD patients and subsequently hinders the potential synergy [37]. Therefore a policy initiative bringing TCM and BM together under a common primary healthcare system is warranted in order to enhance both the patient's decision-making process and their wellbeing.

### *Professions: towards collaboration between traditional Chinese medicine and biomedicine clinicians*

Implementation of such an initiative would involve an alignment not only of practitioners, but of statutory organizations as well. Currently, the professional standards for TCM and BM are set by two separate statutory councils: the HKMC and CMCHK. The HKMC was founded to assure and promote quality in the medical profession in order to protect patients, foster ethical conduct, and develop and maintain high professional standards. The CMCHK is responsible for implementing regulatory measures for Chinese medicine. The main purpose for regulation of Chinese medicine is to protect public health and consumers' rights and to ensure the professional standard of Chinese medicine practice. A joint partnership between the two regulatory bodies is needed to overcome the ethical, legal and professional barriers that hinder inter-professional collaboration. Mutual recognition of practice would need to be reached to remove barriers such as the inability to formally refer and share patient information [38]. Furthermore, fragmentation of both TCM and BM primary care services presents structural obstacles for collaboration in the care of patients with NCD [39]. In Hong Kong, both TCM and BM outpatient services are dominated by the private sector and hence a top-down initiative for joined-up working is very difficult. There is no infrastructure to facilitate collaboration or information exchange within the PHC system. The proposed development of a universal electronic patient record system would be a potential solution to bring various healthcare service sectors (primary, secondary and tertiary care, private and public sectors, TCM and BM) under a single care coordination platform for common NCD, such as diabetes and hypertension [40].

In Hong Kong, although BMD have positive attitudes towards TCM, due to regulation and cultural affinity, few actual TCM referrals are made given the lack of a formal collaboration policy between TCM and BM within the healthcare system. This structural inhibition is possibly rooted in the historical dominance of BM and failure of services to respond to espoused policy. Amongst Hong Kong BMD, personal consumption and formal education of TCM, rather than use of evidence in decision making, played a stronger role in determining referrals. This implies that inter-professional education is a prerequisite for collaboration between clinicians of TCM and BM. In fact, a recent systematic review has demonstrated that education on T&CM for BMD appears to be effective in improving attitudes, knowledge and skills towards the use of T&CM, particularly when the instructor is trained in both types of medicine [41].

BM education for TCMP is equally important. Local graduates regard the acquisition of BM knowledge as a foundation for the development of integrative medicine. More importantly, patients could be empowered in making informed choices between TCM and BM treatment options [31]. The existing BM education system within the public sector would be ideal for East–West interdisciplinary learning, and its potential benefit could also be extended to BM students who have little knowledge and exposure to TCM practices [42]. In a society that offers both modalities of care in the public system, it makes sense to promote a greater understanding of TCM amongst the whole clinician community. However, education alone is insufficient to strengthen TCMP's linkage with the healthcare system. For instance, in an evaluation of a mental health training programme for Hong Kong TCMP, positive effects on improving TCMP's confidence in diagnosing, managing and referring patients with mental health needs have been noted. However, actual referral to BMD has been minimal due to a lack of referral channels [43]. These observations point to the need to link the two professions at service delivery level.

### *Providers: bridging traditional Chinese medicine and biomedicine services at the organizational level*

While the integration of TCM and BM poses a unique challenge to policy makers and managers at the epistemological level, promoting teamwork between BMD and TCMP at service delivery level, which is responsive to patients' choice, is not impossible. A recent systematic review has summarized organizational strategies for fostering inter-professional collaboration (IPC) between BMD and T&CMP (see Table 41.2). The emergent themes from this synthesis suggest that the nature of the relationship between BMD and T&CMP is similar to those between BMD and allied health professionals. Therefore, interventions for improving collaboration between healthcare teams with different compositions [44] may well be transferable to improve IPC between BMD and T&CMP.

*Table 41.2* Strategies for fostering inter-professional collaboration between conventional medical doctors (BMD) and T&CM practitioners (T&CMP)

| *Strategic areas* | *Key points* |
|---|---|
| 1. Governance | • The need to respond to patients' demand for holistic care, and the need to fill the effectiveness gaps of BM are the main drivers for integration initiatives.<br>• Sufficient funding is essential for building a collaboration-ready T&CMP team and promoting equality for patient access, but securing such funding is a major challenge for central authorities. |
| 2. Leadership | • Clinicians trained both in BM and T&CM are preferred candidates for leading integration.<br>• Leaders may experience less resistance from the management if the participating T&CMP are accredited in their own discipline, covered by liability insurance, and are willing to stay within their defined scope of practice. |
| 3. Support for innovation | • Bridge-building activities, including inter-professional education, mutual practice observation and the creation of communication platforms are beneficial for creating bonding between team members.<br>• Gatekeeping of T&CM services by BMD may elicit a mixed response from T&CMP. Leaders need to reduce this power differential such that T&CMP can be sufficiently empowered for meaningful participation. |
| 4. Connectivity | • BMD is better connected with T&CM modalities that have a lower degree of perceived foreignness – e.g. acupuncture is more accepted than homeopathy.<br>• At clinician level, co-location is critical in fostering trust and also in developing a sense of partnership between BMD and T&CMP.<br>• At an operational level, co-location facilitates efficient referral, feedback, communication, chart-sharing and access to BM testing facilities. |
| 5. Formalization tools | • Included literature highlighted three common types of delegation mechanisms: (i) case-by-case referral, (ii) flexible protocol-based referral and (iii) condition-specific referral protocol.<br>• In the first two delegation mechanisms, the efficacy of the chosen T&CM therapy is usually not assessed. Instead, managers' and BMD's opinions and perceptions on that therapy's safety, as well as the cost and local availability, dominate the decision-making process.<br>• In the third approach, leaders may brand T&CM inclusion as a means for clinical research and this is likely to satisfy sceptics. However, success would often require extra support from experienced researchers. |
| 6. Information exchange | • Shared electronic health records is the preferred mode of information exchange between BMD and T&CMP.<br>• Immediate positive feedback received via record exchange can promote BMD's referral decisions as well as create a stronger trust in T&CMP's competency.<br>• More mature integration programmes usually formalize their evaluation process around outcomes that are recognized both by BMD and T&CMP. |

*Source*: [23].

Recent literature views IPC as a changing process, which posits that 'no single agent has full authority, resources, or expertise to lead the change' required for implementing IPC in health care [45]. From this perspective, even clinicians who are dual-trained in BM and T&CM would not succeed unless a broad coalition of actors, including T&CMP, were mobilized to activate change in healthcare delivery. Power sharing in this 'distributed agency' approach could be a way to build a more balanced IPC model, in which T&CM leaders could possess more negotiating power in protecting T&CM's practice philosophy. Further research must demonstrate how the addition of T&CMP to primary care can improve care quality, reduce costs and, ultimately, benefit patients [46].

## Conclusion: applying the 4Ps framework in formulating development strategies for traditional, complementary and alternative medicine

In this chapter, we have illustrated how the 4Ps framework may be used to identify policy gaps in the processing of integrating T&CM into health systems. To promote progress in integration policy, policy makers need to facilitate consultation and discussion on gaps that are contentious, keeping in mind that these gaps are likely to vary according to the country's health system configuration. Nevertheless, queries on the evidence-based factors of T&CM will certainly be universal in debates on integration policies. While it is well acknowledged that clinical evidence from randomized control trails could be a potential tool for bridging the two paradigms, to balance the demand for both internal and external validities, a wider perspective on evidence could provide a rich toolbox of research methods that will contribute to the evidence-based factors of T&CM. At service and system levels, evidence-based integration process would require results from observational, cost effectiveness and qualitative studies as well. [47]. A broader perspective on evidence may have a significant impact on policy makers' decisions on how to integrate T&CM into health systems and patient centred research should be included as a priority in all integration initiatives.

## Note

1 According to the WHO, traditional medicine is defined as 'the sum total of the knowledge, skills, and practices based on the theories, beliefs, and experiences indigenous to different cultures, whether explicable or not, used in the maintenance of health as well as in the prevention, diagnosis, improvement or treatment of physical and mental illness'; whereas complementary medicine is defined as 'a broad set of health care practices that are not part of that country's own tradition and are not integrated into the dominant health care system' [2]. T&CM merges the two terms, encompassing products, practices and practitioners [1]. The use of the phrase 'not integrated into the dominant health care system' in this definition denotes that an incompatibility exists between the holistic paradigm of T&CM and the paradigm of conventional medicine (CM) [3].

## References

1. The WHO Traditional Medicine Strategy 2014–2023, http://apps.who.int/iris/handle/10665/92455
2. Traditional Medicine: Definations from the WHO, http://www.who.int/medicines/areas/traditional/definitions/en/
3. Quah SR. Traditional healing systems and the ethos of science. *Soc Sci Med.* 2003; 57(10): 1997–2012.
4. Wieland LS, Manheimer E, Berman BM. Development and classification of an operational definition of complementary and alternative medicine for the Cochrane Collaboration. *Altern Ther Health Med.* 2011; 17(2): 50–9.

5. Harris PE, Cooper KL, Relton C, Thomas KJ. Prevalence of complementary and alternative medicine (CAM) use by the general population: a systematic review and update. *Int J Clin Pract*. 2012; 66(10): 924–39.
6. Kasilo OMJ, *et al*. Regional overview: African region. In: Bodeker G, Ong CK, Grundy C, Burford G, Maehira Y. (eds) *WHO Global Altas of Traditional, Complementary and Alternative Medicine: Text Volume*. Kobe, Japan: WHO Center for Health Development, 2005.
7. Harris P, Rees R. The prevalence of complementary and alternative medicine use among the general population: a systematic review of the literature. *Complement Ther Med*. 2000; 8(2): 88–96.
8. MacLennan AH, Wilson DH, Taylor AW. Prevalence and cost of alternative medicine in Australia. *Lancet* 1996 2; 347(9001): 569–73.
9. Thomas KJ, Nicholl JP, Coleman P. Use and expenditure on complementary medicine in England: a population based survey. *Complement Ther Med*. 2001; 9(1): 2–11.
10. Health Canada. Perspectives on Complementary and Alternative Health Care. A Collection of Papers Prepared for Health Canada. 2001.
11. Bodeker G, Burford G. *Traditional, Complementary and Alternative Medicine: Policy and Public Health Perspectives*. London: Imperial College Press, 2007.
12. Chung VC, Ma PH, Lau CH, Wong SY, Yeoh EK, Griffiths SM. Views on traditional Chinese medicine amongst Chinese population: a systematic review of qualitative and quantitative studies. *Health Expect*. 2012; May 31.
13. Ock SM, Choi JY, Cha YS, Lee J, Chun MS, Huh CH, *et al*. The use of complementary and alternative medicine in a general population in South Korea: results from a national survey in 2006. *J Korean Med Sci*. 2009; 24(1): 1–6.
14. Yamashita H, Tsukayama H, Sugishita C. Popularity of complementary and alternative medicine in Japan: a telephone survey. *Complement Ther Med*. 2002; 10(2): 84–93.
15. Siti ZM, Tahir A, Farah AI, Fazlin SM, Sondi S, Azman AH, *et al*. Use of traditional and complementary medicine in Malaysia: a baseline study. *Complement Ther Med*. 2009; 17(5–6): 292–9.
16. Lim MK, Sadarangani P, Chan HL, Heng JY. Complementary and alternative medicine use in multiracial Singapore. *Complement Ther Med*. 2005; 13(1): 16–24.
17. Leckridge B. The future of complementary and alternative medicine – models of integration. *J Altern Complement Med*. 2004; 10(2): 413–16.
18. The WHO Alma Ata Declaration, http://www.who.int/hrp/NPH/docs/declaration_almaata.pdf
19. The WHO Traditional Medicine Strategy 2002–5, http://whqlibdoc.who.int/hq/2002/who_edm_trm_2002.1.pdf
20. National Policy on Traditional Medicine and Regulation of Herbal Medicines – Reports of a WHO Global Survey, http://apps.who.int/medicinedocs/pdf/s7916e/s7916e.pdf
21. The WHO Beijing Declaration, http://www.who.int/medicines/areas/traditional/congress/beijing_declaration/en/
22. Bosch-Capblanch X, Lavis JN, Lewin S, Atun R, Røttingen JA, Dröschel D, *et al*. Guidance for evidence-informed policies about health systems: rationale for and challenges of guidance development. *PLoS Med*. 2012; 9(3): e1001185.
23. Chung VC, Ma PH, Hong LC, Griffiths SM. Organizational determinants of interprofessional collaboration in integrative health care: systematic review of qualitative studies. *PLoS One*. 2012; 7(11): e50022.
24. Xu J, Yang Y. Traditional Chinese medicine in the Chinese health care system. *Health Policy*. 2009; 90(2–3): 133–9.
25. Topley M. Chinese and Western medicine in Hong Kong: some social and cultural determinants of variation, interaction and change. In: Kleinman A, Kunstadter P, Alex ER, Gales JL. (eds) *Medicine in Chinese Cultures: Comparative Studies of Health Care in Chinese and Other Societies*. Washington, DC: US Government Printing Office, 1975.
26. Lee RPL. Chinese and Western health care systems: professional stratification in a modernizing society. In: King AYC, Lee RPL. (eds) *Social Life and Development in Hong Kong*. Hong Kong: Chinese University Press, 1981.
27. Xie YG. *History of Traditional Chinese Medicine in Hong Kong* (in Chinese). Hong Kong: San Lian Book Shop, 1998.
28. Chief Executive of the Hong Kong SAR. Policy Address 1997: Building Hong Kong for a New Era. 1997; 2006(Sep/27).

29. Health W, Food Bureau, the Hospital Authority. The future direction for the development of traditional Chinese medicine services in the public sector. 2005 June 13(CB(2)1748/04-05(05)).
30. Griffiths S, Chung V. Development and regulation of traditional Chinese medicine practitioners in Hong Kong. *Perspect Public Health*. 2009; 129(2): 64–7.
31. Chung VC, Law MP, Wong SY, Mercer SW, Griffiths SM. Postgraduate education for Chinese medicine practitioners: a Hong Kong perspective. *BMC Med Educ*. 2009; 9: 10.
32. Dixion A, Peckham S, Ho PY. Informing UK policy development on the regulation of CAM practitioners: lessons from Hong Kong? *Social Policy & Administration*. 2007; 41(7): 711–28.
33. Chung VCh, Lau CH, Yeoh EK, Griffiths SM. Age, chronic non-communicable disease and choice of traditional Chinese and Western medicine outpatient services in a Chinese population. *BMC Health Serv Res*. 2009; 9: 207.
34. Bensoussan A, Talley NJ, Hing M, Menzies R, Guo A, Ngu M. Treatment of irritable bowel syndrome with Chinese herbal medicine: a randomized controlled trial. *JAMA*. 1998; 280(18): 1585–9.
35. Witt C, Brinkhaus B, Jena S, Linde K, Streng A, Wagenpfeil S, *et al*. Acupuncture in patients with osteoarthritis of the knee: a randomised trial. *Lancet*. 2005; 366(9480): 136–43.
36. Rothman AA, Wagner EH. Chronic illness management: what is the role of primary care? *Ann Intern Med*. 2003; 138(3): 256–61.
37. Fan R, Holliday I. Which medicine? Whose standard? Critical reflections on medical integration in China. *J Med Ethics*. 2007; 33(8): 454–61.
38. The Hong Kong Hospital Authority Chinese Medicine Information System.
39. Li DKT, Griffiths S, Wong AHS, Yeoh EK. The primary care system and health insurance in Hong Kong. *Hong Kong Practitioner*. 2008; 30(1): 38–42.
40. Greenhalgh T. *Primary Health Care: Theory and Practice*. Malden, MA: Blackwell/BMJ Books, 2007.
41. Quartey NK, Ma PH, Chung VC, Griffiths SM. Complementary and alternative medicine education for medical profession: systematic review. *Evid Based Complement Alternat Med*. 2012; 2012: 656812.
42. Schwarz S, Messerschmidt H, Volzke H, Hoffmann W, Lucht M, Doren M. Use of complementary medicinal therapies in West Pomerania: a population-based study. *Climacteric*. 2008; 11(2): 124–34.
43. Lam TP, Mak KY, Goldberg D, Lam KF, Sun KS. Western mental health training for Traditional Chinese Medicine practitioners. *Acta Psychiatr Scand*. 2012; 126(6): 440–7.
44. Buljac-Samardzic M, Dekker-van Doorn CM, van Wijngaarden JD, van Wijk KP. Interventions to improve team effectiveness: a systematic review. *Health Policy*. 2010; 94(3): 183–95.
45. Chreim S, Williams BE, Janz L, Dastmalchian A. Change agency in a primary health care context: the case of distributed leadership. *Health Care Manage Rev*. 2010; 35(2): 187–99.
46. Bosch M, Faber MJ, Cruijsberg J, Voerman GE, Leatherman S, Grol RP, *et al*. Review article: effectiveness of patient care teams and the role of clinical expertise and coordination: a literature review. *Med Care Res Rev*. 2009; 66(6 Suppl): 5S–35S.
47. Walach H, Falkenberg T, Fønnebø V, Lewith G, Jonas WB. Circular instead of hierarchical: methodological principles for the evaluation of complex interventions. *BMC Med Res Methodol*. 2006; 6: 29.

# 42
# Health systems in Asia
## Achievements and challenges

*Eng Kiong Yeoh, Patsy Y. K. Chau and Carrie H. K. Yam*

## Introduction

Growth and development in Asian economies have received global attention in recent decades. The dramatic rise of Japan as an economic powerhouse in the decades after the Second World War was followed by impressive economic developments in the four Asian tigers – South Korea, Taiwan, Singapore and Hong Kong – between the 1960s and 1990s, and the more recent spectacular progress that has been made in the world's most populous nations, China and India. Economic developments have since permeated the whole of Asia. Gross national income (GNI) per capita has increased across the continent and there are now 34 out of 40 jurisdictions classified as high- or middle-income countries, with GNI per capita of US$1,036 or more [1]. Equally dramatic have been the social developments and the achievements made in improving the health of populations in Asia. In tandem with the global experience life expectancy has improved substantially in the past 40 years, resulting mainly from the reductions in mortalities in children and women [2]. Improvements in socio-economic conditions, availability of safe water and better sanitation, better disease control programmes, investments in health systems and improvements in health services have all contributed to the improvements in life expectancy. However, economic progress has also brought new problems and challenges for health and health systems. Changing disease patterns arising from changing lifestyles and demographic transitions, and rising expectations of a more educated and affluent population, are emerging issues which pose challenges for health systems.

## Context

The discussion of the achievements and challenges of health systems in Asia has to be made in the context of their heterogeneity. The countries and jurisdictions in Asia vary considerably in size, socio-economic and political development, historical legacies and ethnic origins. The very diverse health systems evident in each of the jurisdictions have taken root from historical designs, organization and provision, and have evolved over time, influenced and shaped by socio-economic developments and defined by systems of health stewardship and governance.

In almost all the jurisdictions rapid economic growth and development is a recent phenomenon and individually countries are at varying stages of development. Japan, South Korea, Taiwan, Singapore and Hong Kong had an early start in economic development and have GNI per capita similar to that of high-income economies, in contrast to Afghanistan, Bangladesh, Cambodia, Korea DPR, Myanmar and Nepal, in which economic development is at an early stage with GNI per capita of low-income economies. Much of the initial focus of the health systems was in developing key public health programmes, improving sanitation, providing safe water, and preventing and controlling epidemics of infectious diseases. Community health centres, public health clinics and basic medical services were developed – with substantial investments – when the economy grew, and there was rapid expansion of hospitals with the capacity of providing technologically advanced and complex care. The financing of health care came predominantly from taxes and general government revenue and from private sources, mainly in the form of household out-of-pocket expenditure.

Contributions from philanthropic sources and development aid were also sources of revenue for health, accounting for varying proportions in different countries. Developments in health insurance were a much later feature in the evolution of the health systems and were a reflection of the broader socio-economic developments, with private health insurance developing alongside the growth of the insurance industry and public forms of health insurance with other forms of social insurance. The different countries and jurisdictions in Asia also vary considerably in their demographic profiles and epidemiologic patterns.

## Achievements of health systems in Asia

The achievements made in Asia have been in (i) improvement in health with longer life expectancy and substantially lower infant and maternal mortality rates across all the countries, and (ii) greater health expenditure and investments and improvements in the health system infrastructure.

### *Life expectancy*

According to World Bank World Development Indicators [3], average life expectancy at birth in the Asia-Pacific regions increased from 50.9 years to 71.2 years over the period 1960–2011 (see Figure 42.1). The improvement of life expectancy was generally correlated ($r = 0.76$, $p < 0.001$) with the level of income of the countries. After 1980, the difference in the life expectancy between different income group countries was steady up to 2011. The jurisdictions in eastern Asia or in the category of high-income countries have higher life expectancy at birth than other jurisdictions in the Asia-Pacific regions (see Figure 42.2). The corresponding mortality rate during the same period fell from 16.5/1,000 persons to 6.6/1,000 [3].

### *Infant mortality rates*

In the three decades from 1980 to 2010, infant mortality rates (IMRs) have declined dramatically throughout the whole of Asia, falling by as much as 82.5 per cent to two deaths per 1,000 live births in Singapore (see Table 42.1). Even in Afghanistan, the country with the highest IMR, the decline during these decades was 58 per cent. Average IMRs for the Asia-Pacific regions fell from 68.8 per 1,000 live births in 1980 to 24.7 in 2011. The three most important predictors of infant mortality are sanitation, availability of safe water and literacy rates [4].

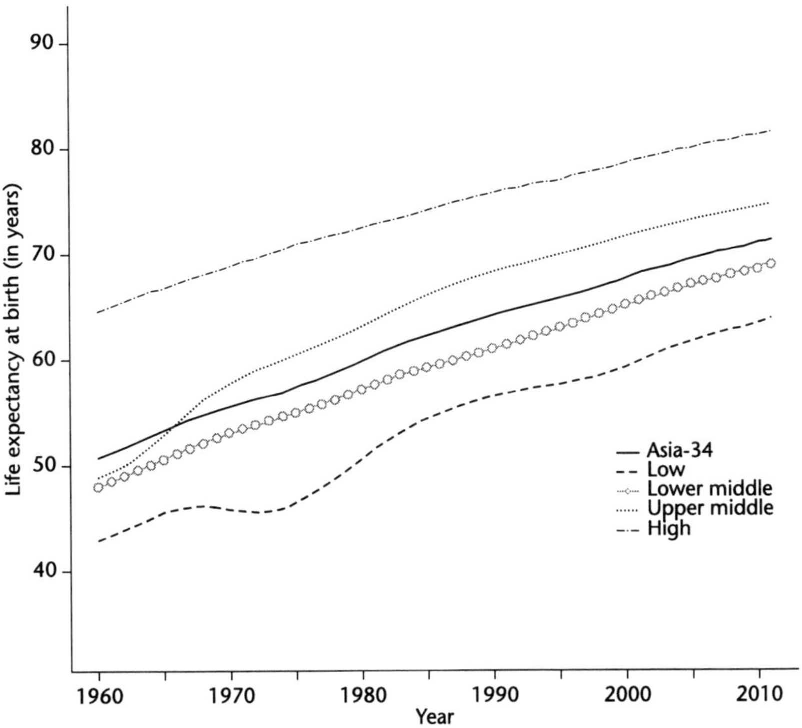


*Figure 42.1* Trends in life expectancy at birth by different income groups in Asia-Pacific regions, 1960–2011 [3]

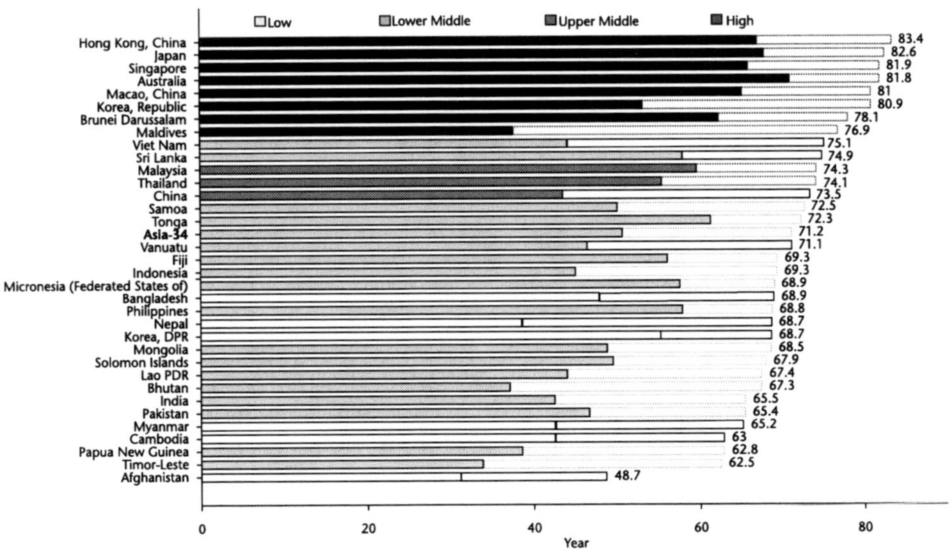


*Figure 42.2* Life expectancy at birth in Asia-Pacific regions, 1960 and 2011 [3]

*Table 42.1* Infant mortality rate per 1,000 live births, 1980 and change to 2011

| | *1980* | *Change from 1980 to 2011 (%)* |
|---|---|---|
| ***Low-income group*** | **129.8** | **–63.9** |
| Afghanistan | 173.0 | –58.0 |
| Bangladesh | 130.1 | –71.8 |
| Cambodia | 119.9 | –69.8 |
| Myanmar | 95.1 | –49.6 |
| Nepal | 130.9 | –70.2 |
| ***Lower middle-income group*** | **70.9** | **–59.4** |
| Bhutan | 134.4 | –68.8 |
| Fiji | 31.6 | –55.4 |
| India | 101.9 | –53.7 |
| Indonesia | 75.7 | –67.2 |
| Kiribati | 82.4 | –54.2 |
| Lao PDR | 128.1 | –73.6 |
| Marshall Islands | 53.4 | –58.6 |
| Micronesia (Federated States of) | 48.7 | –31.2 |
| Mongolia | 100.6 | –74.7 |
| Pakistan | 110.7 | –46.5 |
| Papua New Guinea | 79.5 | –43.6 |
| Philippines | 52.6 | –61.6 |
| Solomon Islands | 47.1 | –60.9 |
| Sri Lanka | 36.6 | –71.3 |
| Tonga | 26.2 | –49.6 |
| Vanuatu | 49.9 | –77.2 |
| Viet Nam | 45.5 | –62.0 |
| ***Upper middle-income group*** | **57.9** | **–74.9** |
| China | 47.9 | –73.7 |
| Malaysia | 25.9 | –78.4 |
| Maldives | 113.9 | –91.9 |
| Thailand | 50.2 | –78.9 |
| Tuvalu | 51.8 | –51.5 |
| ***High-income group*** | **11.5** | **–68.0** |
| Australia | 10.9 | –62.4 |
| Brunei Darussalam | 12.3 | –54.5 |
| Japan | 7.4 | –67.6 |
| Korea, Republic | 15.3 | –73.2 |
| Singapore | 11.4 | –82.5 |
| ***Asia-32*** | **68.8** | **–63.9** |

In addition to developing programmes to provide access to clean water and installation of sanitation facilities, developing nations have also invested in the infrastructure required for essential public health programmes. From 1990 to 2010 the percentage of the population in the Asia-Pacific regions who had access to improved water sources increased from 77.2 per cent to 87.7 per cent (see Figure 42.3). In the same period, access to improved sanitation improved from 58.7 per cent amongst the populations in the Asia-Pacific regions to 71.4 per cent.

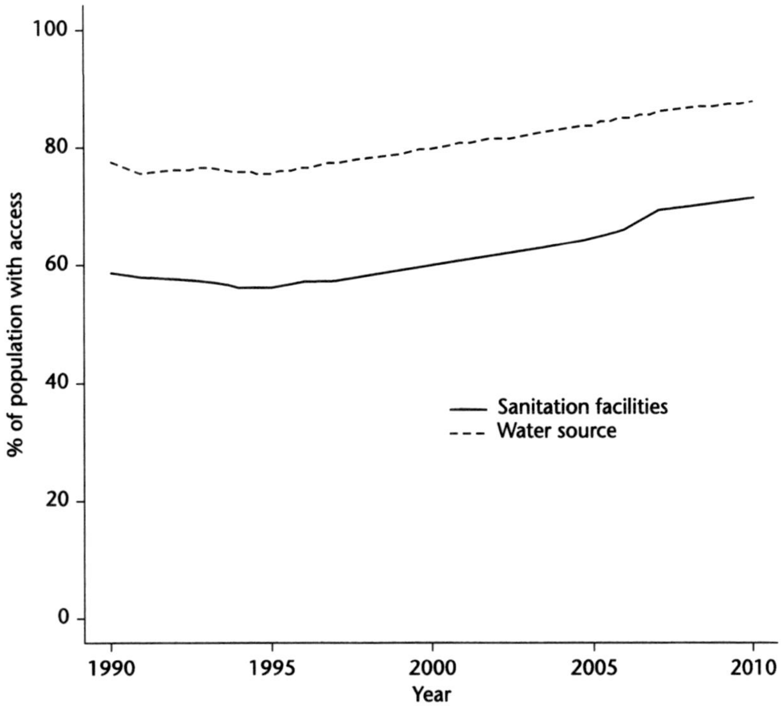


*Figure 42.3* Trends in accessibility of sanitation facilities and water source from 1990 to 2010 [3]

One notable public health programme was the initiative in the 1970s of the expanded programme of immunization (EPI) for vaccine-preventable diseases by low- and middle-income countries in collaboration with the World Health Organization (WHO), the United Nations Children's Fund (UNICEF), and other agencies and donors. It has taken up to two decades for many countries to scale up the programmes to reach the desired 80 per cent coverage. Data from the WHO for Asia-Pacific regions for immunization coverage of major childhood vaccines from 1980 to 2005 show coverage rates of Bacilli Calmette-Guerin (BCG) rising from less than 20 per cent in 1980 to reach almost 80 per cent in the late 1990s (see Figure 42.4). The low-income countries – approximately – reached the coverage rates of the lower middle-income groups and the upper middle-income countries approximated to the level of high-income countries after the implementation of the immunization programmes. The coverage for measles shows a similar improvement from a low single digit number of 1 per cent in a few countries in 1980 rising to over 80 per cent on average by 1992. The coverage rate for diphtheria, pertussis (whooping cough) and tetanus (DPT) also showed significant improvements from 38.7 per cent in 1980 to 89.1 per cent in 2011 [3].

A second notable example of the achievements was the investment in, and provision of, antenatal care for pregnant women. The WHO Global Health Observatory Data Repository [5] shows that in 2010, 85 per cent of pregnant women in the Asia-Pacific Region received at least one antenatal visit with trained health workers. There is, however, significant variation amongst the different countries, with rates of 100 per cent amongst the high-income

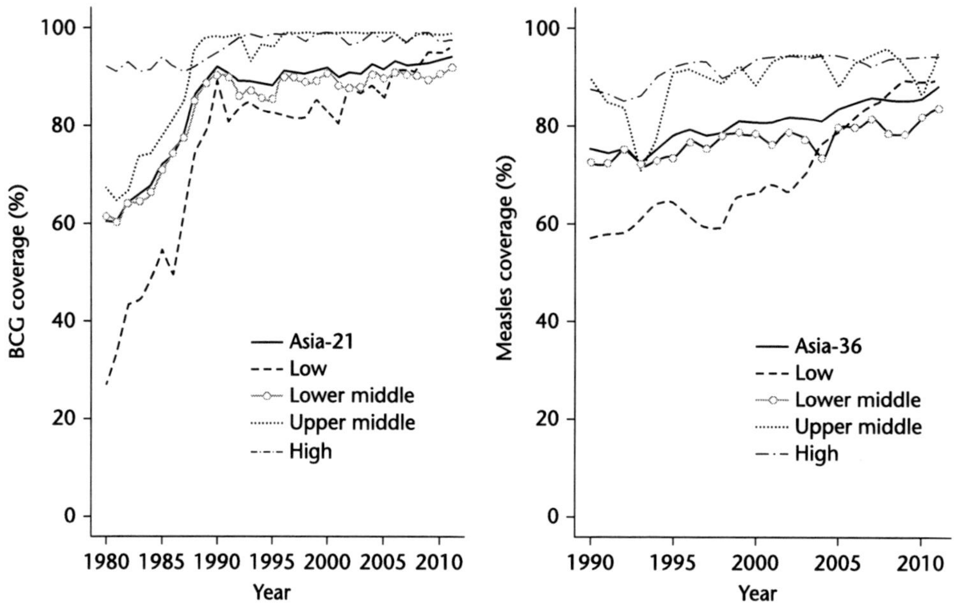


*Figure 42.4* Trends in BCG and measles immunization coverage among 1 year olds [5]

countries and rates between 54 and 89 per cent in low-income countries, Korea DPR being an exception with a rate of 100 per cent.

## *Maternal mortality rate*

In parallel with the decline in IMRs, maternal mortality has also been reduced in Asian and Pacific countries, due to improvements in women's health, education, family planning and better antenatal care. Between 1990 and 2010, the average maternal mortality ratio (MMR) across 32 Asian-Pacific countries was reduced to 262 deaths per 100,000 live births from 393 deaths (see Figure 42.5). Variations were seen in the region, following a general trend of lower rates in the high-income countries, intermediate rates in upper middle-income countries and higher rates in lower middle- and low-income countries, although there were exceptions. Exceptionally low MMRs were observed in the Republic of Korea, Australia, New Zealand and Singapore; and high ratios in Bhutan, Afghanistan and Lao PDR.

# Health expenditure and investments in health system infrastructure

## *Health expenditure*

With economic development and progress, governments tend to invest more in health services. In the ten-year period from 2000 to 2010, per capita health spending in real terms was 5.6 per cent per year in Asia, higher than the 3.6 per cent seen in OECD countries [6]. In Asian jurisdictions, based on the World Bank WDI Database [3], there is a correlation between total health expenditure per capita and GDP per capita (see Figure 42.6). Health

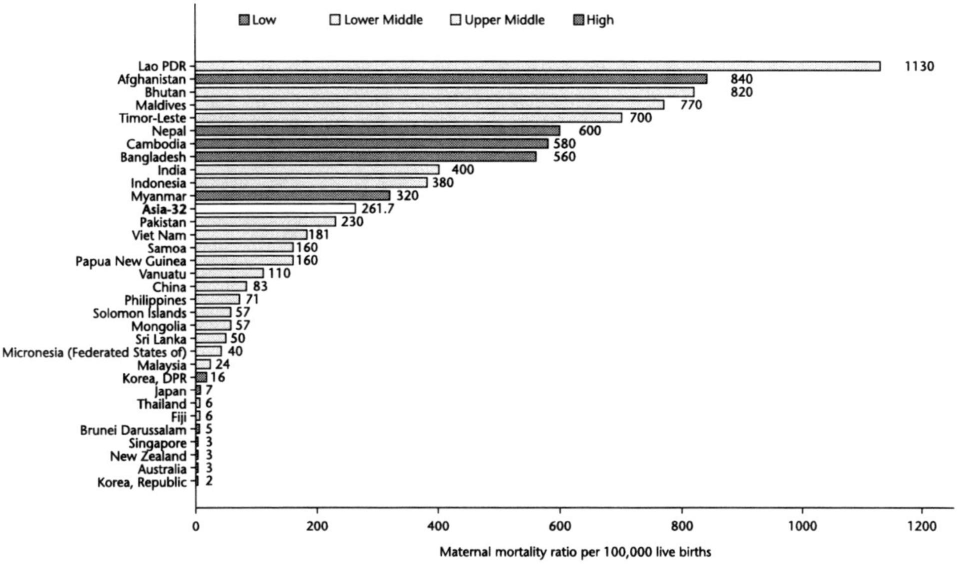


*Figure 42.5* Difference in maternal mortality ratio per 100,000 live births between 1990 and 2010 [3]

expenditure as a share of GDP was also observed to increase with per capita GDP in the Asia-Pacific regions, which parallels the experience in OECD countries [6]. In the past decade, growth in health expenditure in most Asian countries has exceeded economic growth with only two countries, Pakistan and Brunei Darussalam, showing a slight decline of the growth rate as compared to the GDP growth rate.

## *Investments in health system infrastructure*

Reflecting the growth in health expenditure, substantial investments in healthcare facilities, equipment, commodities and health professionals have been made throughout Asian health systems. However, the number of hospital beds per 1,000 population in 22 Asian countries is 3.6, still far lower than the average of 4.9 in OECD countries [6]. Significant variations are seen between countries, with Japan having the highest with 13 beds per 1,000 population, and Bangladesh and Philippines having the lowest with less than 0.6 per 1,000 population.

Significant progress has also been made in many Asian health systems in training health professionals required for access to high-quality health services, although the number of doctors, nurses and other health professionals per capita in the continent are significantly lower than the OECD average (3.1 for doctors and 8.7 for nurses) [3, 6]. However, there is considerable variation in the number of health professionals per capita between countries. Notably Korea DPR has 3.3 doctors per 1,000 population, equalling the average of 3.1 in OECD (see Figure 42.7). This rate can be attributed to the governments' policy and priority to support training of health professionals. The lowest numbers are observed in Cambodia, Lao PDR, Solomon Islands, Nepal and Papua New Guinea of 0.2 or less, and these are the countries that also have low levels of health expenditure. A similar variation is seen in the

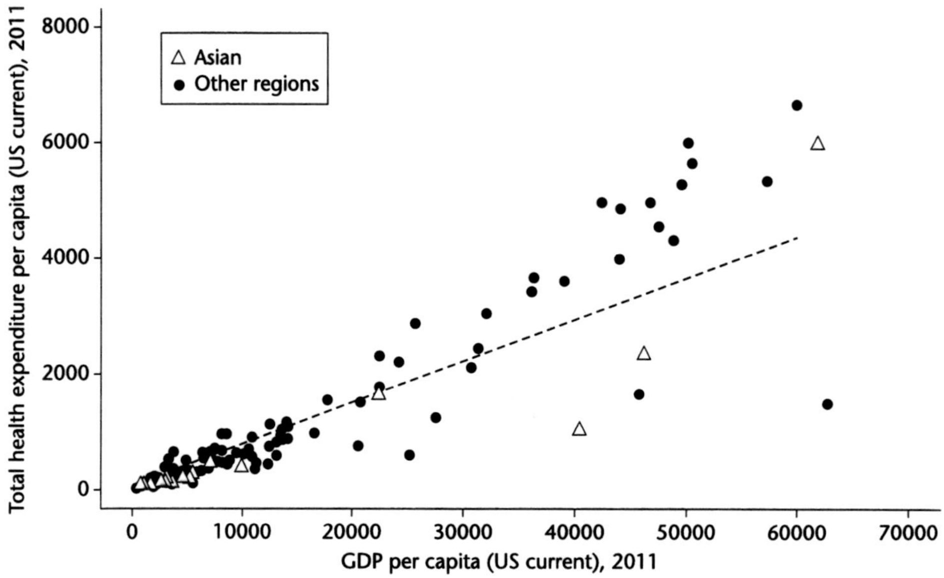


*Figure 42.6* Health expenditure versus gross domestic product per capita, 2011 [3]

number of nurses per capita, with Japan having the highest health expenditure as a proportion of GDP with 4.1 per 1,000 population, paralleling the Asia-35 average of 3.8, and Bangladesh and Bhutan having the lowest numbers of 0.4 or less (see Figure 42.8).

Countries that made an earlier start in socio-economic development also initiated organization transformations of their health systems. Japan and South Korea have well-established social health insurance systems which provide universal health coverage for their populations and protection against the cost of catastrophic illness. Taiwan (see Chapter 43) brought in a National Health Insurance (NHI) system in 1995, which has improved access of the poor to health care and resulted in a more equitable system [7]. Thailand also embarked on a social insurance system in 2001 which now covers 75 per cent of the population [8]. In recognition of the undesirable effects on the market reforms in China (see Chapter 40) on affordability and access to health care, the government has embarked on a comprehensive strategy of health reforms which includes the enhancement of social health insurance [9]. The Philippines (see Chapter 44) has also committed to improve coverage through a social health insurance system. Singapore (see Chapter 46) has taken a different route, opting for a three-pillar model of health financing: Medisave, Medishield and Medifund, which emphasizes individual responsibility for health expenses. The three-pillar model was developed in stages, beginning with the introduction of the Medisave system of individual personal accounts for healthcare expenditure in 1984, subsequently supported by Medishield in 1990, a voluntary insurance system which protects against the cost of catastrophic illness, and finally by Medifund in 1993, which supplements healthcare expenditure for the poor who do not have sufficient financial means [10]. Organizational reform has also been initiated in Asia, notably the corporatization of all public hospitals in Singapore and Hong Kong to improve the responsiveness and efficiency of health services [11].

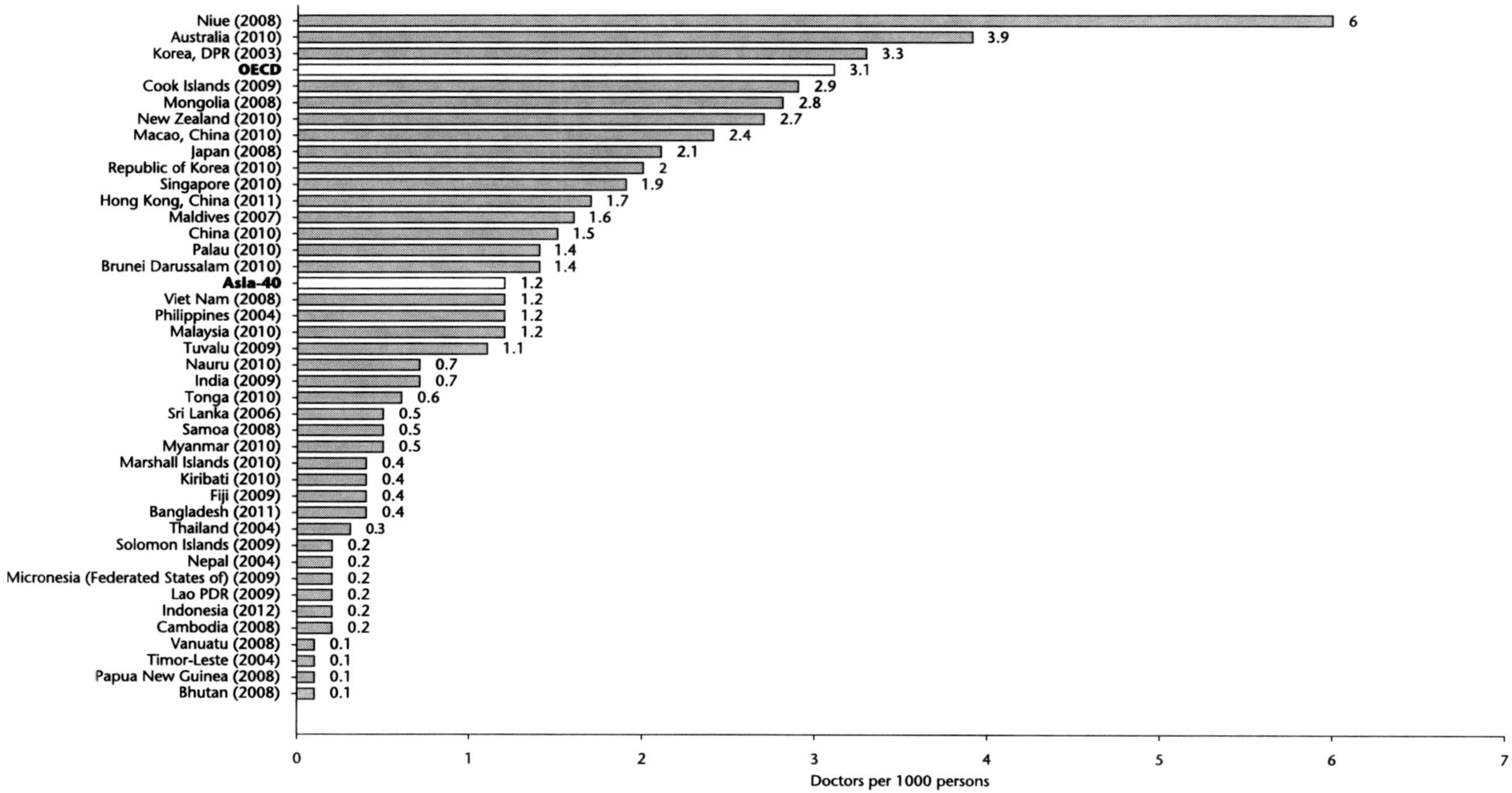


*Figure 42.7* Doctors per 1,000 persons in Asia-Pacific regions [5]

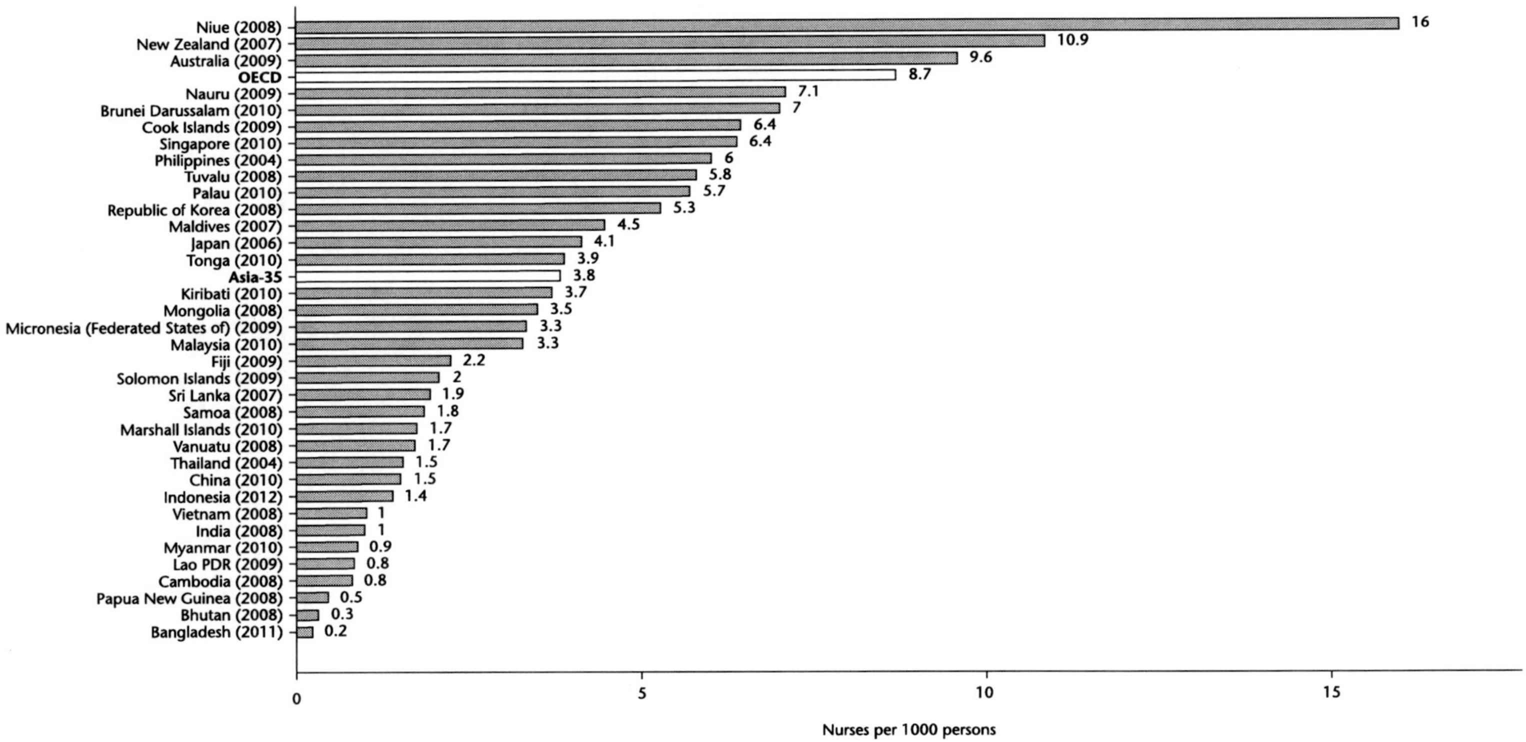


*Figure 42.8* Nurses per 1,000 persons in Asia-Pacific regions [5]

## Challenges

The rapid economic growth and socio-political developments, and the achievements of health systems in Asia in improving health of populations and life expectancy, have also created a number of major challenges for the health systems in their ongoing agenda to enable better access to health care, address inequities, improve quality and enhance efficiency in health service delivery.

### *Demographic and epidemiological transition*

Environmental degradation has been associated with economic growth in many Asian countries. In 2004, the WHO estimated that 242 and 124 people per million die each year from ambient air pollution (see Chapter 22) in Western Pacific and South-East Asian regions, respectively [12]. Other pollutants and toxins in water, food and soil all contribute to the rising burden of non-communicable diseases (NCDs) which are often chronic in their course. Changing lifestyles associated with economic development, notably lower levels of physical activity and increasing consumption of food rich in fats (saturated fats in particular) and high in calories and sugars are also contributing to the increasing prevalence of NCDs. Deaths from NCDs are the commonest causes of death in Asia, accounting for two-thirds of deaths across 20 Asian countries [6]. In high-income economies, NCDs are responsible for approximately 80 per cent of all deaths. Even in the low-income countries, they account for a range of 28.9 to 50.9 per cent of all mortality [5].

With the gains in life expectancy across all Asian countries, over 50 per cent of the world's ageing population, aged 65 and above, are living in 18 Asian jurisdictions [13]. The demographic transition is also contributing to the chronic disease burden.

### *Health expenditure*

Despite the substantial increases in health expenditure in Asian economies, total health expenditure as a share of GDP in Asia is, on average, half of that in OECD countries. The proportion of GDP allocated to health in Asian countries was 4.5 per cent on average, compared to 9.5 per cent in OECD countries [6]. Japan was the only country with an allocation of 9.5 per cent of GDP, matching the OECD average. Of greater significance, the public share of total health expenditure was 46.6 per cent in 2010, rising only marginally from 44.4 per cent in 2000 [6].On average, in OECD countries, the public share of total health expenditure was 72.2 per cent. In Asia only the economies with social insurance systems, Japan and Thailand, and the smaller economies of the Solomon Islands and Brunei Darussalam, match the public spending levels as a percentage of total health expenditure at the levels in OECD countries [6]. Even in South Korea and Taiwan, with established social insurance systems, the public share was below the levels in OECD countries, due to the higher levels of co-payments [6, 7]. Correspondingly, private expenditure accounts for 53.4 per cent of total health expenditure in Asian countries, with household out-of-pocket payments accounting for most of this and a very much smaller contribution from private prepaid plans and non-profit institutions [6]. Private prepaid plans contributed to 10 per cent or more of private health spending only in five countries: Thailand, Malaysia, Singapore, the Philippines and Fiji. The high levels of out-of-pocket payments for health care have adverse effects on the utilization of health services, particularly for the poorer populations [14]. In a study of 11 Asian countries, a close association was found between the overall out-of-pocket payments and the extent to which households encounter financial catastrophe and impoverishment as a result of expenditure for health care [15]. It is estimated that 150 million households are faced with financial catastrophe each year because of expenditure for health care; about 105 million of these households are in Asia [16]. The WHO has advocated systems of prepayment and pooling for financing health care, to protect against financial catastrophe and improve equity in financial contributions [17]. The two mechanisms of healthcare financing that can potentially provide universal coverage are social health insurance and tax-based financing. High levels of co-payments and too much exclusion in social insurance schemes and excessive user fees and informal payments in tax-based systems pose important financial barriers to access. None of the major economies in Asia that rely on tax-based financing systems spend sufficiently to provide a comprehensive range of primary, secondary and tertiary services as seen in the United Kingdom National Health Service.

The *challenge* for health systems in Asia is how to establish the mechanism to scale up healthcare expenditure in both tax-based and social health insurance systems to appropriate levels in order to ensure universal coverage of good quality health care, which adequately protects against the cost of catastrophic illness and is equitable. The relative proportions of contributions from the public sector and private sector, in particular out-of-pocket household expenses, need to be carefully gauged.

### Investments in health system infrastructure

Public health expenditure in the majority of the countries in Asia is financed from tax revenues and, other than the smaller economies, none of the larger ones with tax-based systems spend levels close to those of OECD countries. The consequence of this lower allocation of public resources is either an under-provision in the public sector, with a greater reliance on the private sector or high out-of-pocket expenses, or both. The under-investments also have an effect on the quality and types of services. Poorer households bear the brunt of the inequity in health care utilization.

Under-investments in healthcare services also present another form of inequity, often between urban and rural populations. The more economically endowed urban populations usually have better access, especially from entrepreneurial private providers. Public provision, particularly of specialist and hospital care, also tends to favour urban populations.

The organization of the healthcare delivery system is problematic in these tax-based systems which are inadequately resourced, as 'dual systems' of public and private health care with limited or no co-ordination between them. Patients use either or both systems and in the absence of a single 'payer', there is limited scope to 'channel' patients to share clinical information. In these systems, when a patient chooses to switch seeking health care from the public to the private sector or vice versa, the succeeding physician may not have access to the information of the investigations and clinical management plan initiated and therapeutic responses that followed in the antecedent consultation. This would lead to duplication in clinical investigations and could result in overlap of clinical approaches and/or gaps in clinical management. The duplication and gaps in clinical management would adversely affect the quality of health care and impact on the efficiency of the healthcare system. Problems of coordinating duplication and fragmentation of, and gaps in, care potentially affect quality and adversely impact efficiency. Problems of coordinating primary and ambulatory care, with more specialized secondary and tertiary hospital care, are evident in economies such as Malaysia, Hong Kong and Singapore, where over 80 per cent of hospital services are provided by the public sector and the bulk of primary care is in the private sector. The challenge of coordination is even more daunting in the context of the epidemiological transition evolving in Asia, where chronic NCDs have become the major cause of mortality, and populations living with one or more chronic illness will have to be cared for in coherent and coordinated systems of health care over their lifetimes. Health systems will have even more daunting issues of coordination with social, community and family care, as the burden of chronic disease and disability grows. Regulation of the private healthcare market is required to ensure efficiency, protect consumers, whilst also assuring quality and transparency. Unfortunately, low-income countries that depend largely on private sources for financing their health systems also have the greatest need of regulation, but conversely also have the least capacity to design and implement effective regulations of the private healthcare market [18].

The under-investment in the infrastructure of health systems is reflected in the lower numbers of health professionals per capita, with only 1.2 doctors per 1,000 population and 3.8 nurses per 1,000 population on average of the Asia-Pacific regions (see Figures 42.7 and 42.8). Higher income countries tend to have higher per capita numbers of health professionals and low-income countries low levels, although there are exceptions. Mal-distribution of health professionals between countries is also evident. In a review of human resources for health in Southeast Asia, there was no shortage of training of health workers overall for the region, but there was a mal-distribution, with five low-income countries having the greatest deficit. All countries had a mal-distribution of health professionals within their own territories, with understaffing in rural areas. Weak coordination was also observed between production and employment capacities [19]. Emigration of the health workforce from the lower income countries to higher income countries outside the region is also occurring, further depleting the already stretched workforce in these countries. The emigration may either be temporary to take up financially and professionally rewarding employment or permanent for residency or citizenship of the designated countries. The usual destinations include the USA, Canada, Australia, UK and Middle East. Singapore (see Chapter 46), Thailand (see Chapter 45) and Malaysia (see Chapter 46) attract many international patients creating problems of health professionals moving from the public to the private sector. Malaysia and Singapore also need to import health professionals to meet the demand of medical tourism, whereas the Philippines and Indonesia are main exporters of doctors and nurses.

## Conclusion

In the last four decades, health systems in Asia have made impressive inroads in developing the infrastructure required to meet the needs of their populations. Significant investments, reflected by the growth in health expenditure, have been accompanied by outstanding achievements in the health of populations. However daunting challenges remain, including (i) scaling up the investments in health care to ensure universal health care, which is affordable, sustainable, equitable, accessible and of good quality, and (ii) the use by governments of policy instruments that engage the private sector to provide health care which contributes to health system goals. Good health governance and effective stewardship by governments will be crucial to meet the challenges outlined in this chapter.

## References

1. The World Bank. Data – How we classify countries. World Bank list of economies July 2012. 30 June 2013. Available from: http://data.worldbank.org/about/country-classifications

2. Wang, H., *et al.*, Age-specific and sex-specific mortality in 187 countries, 1970–2010: a systematic analysis for the Global Burden of Disease Study 2010. *The Lancet* 2012. 380(9859): 2071–94.
3. The World Bank. The World Bank Data. 30 June 2013. Available from: http://data.worldbank.org/
4. Hertz, E., J.R. Hebert, and J. Landon, Social and environmental factors and life expectancy, infant mortality, and maternal mortality rates: results of a cross-national comparison. *Social Science & Medicine* 1994. 39(1): 105–14.
5. World Health Organization. Global Health Observatory Data Repository. 30 June 2013. Available from: http://apps.who.int/gho/data/view.main
6. OECD/WHO, Health at a Glance: Aisa/Pacific 2012. 2012.
7. Chiang, T.L., Taiwan's 1995 health care reform. *Health Policy* 1997. 39: 225–39.
8. Thailand's Universal Coverage Scheme: Achievements and Challenges. An independent assessment of the first 10 years (2001–2010). 2012: Nothaburi, Thailand.
9. Barber, S.L. and L. Yao, World Health Report 2010 Background Paper No. 37 – Health Insurance Systems in China: A Briefing Note. 2010: Geneva.
10. Lim, M., Transforming Singapore health care: public–private partnership. *Ann Acad Med Singapore* 2005. 34(7): 461–7.
11. Preker, A.S. and A. Harding, *Innovations in Health Service Delivery: The Corporatization of Public Hospitals*. 2003: World Bank Publications.
12. World Health Organization. Quantifying environmental health impacts – Global estimates of burden of disease caused by the environment and occupational risks – Table: Attributable mortality by risk factor and WHO subregion, 2004. 30 June 2013. Available from: http://www.who.int/quantifying_ehimpacts/global/en/
13. Yeoh, E.K., Trends in the Private Health Sector and Challenges for Health System Goals in Asia, in Knowledge Event on: Engaging the Private Sector to Achieve Health System Goals – Private Hospitals and the Private Sector as Partners for Universal Health Care Coverage: Policies, Strategies and Tools. 2013: Hong Kong.
14. Kwon, S., *et al.*, Direct household payments for health services in Asia and the Pacific. 2012, Asia Pacific Observatory on Health Systems and Policies.
15. van Doorslaer, E., *et al.*, Effect of payments for health care on poverty estimates in 11 countries in Asia: an analysis of household survey data. *The Lancet* 2006. 368(9544): 1357–64.
16. Kwon, S., Health care financing in Asia: key issues and challenges. *Asia-Pacific Journal of Public Health* 2011. 23(5): 651–61.
17. World Health Organization, The World Health Report 2010 – Health Systems Financing: The path to universal coverage. 2010: Geneva.
18. Ensor, T. and P. Palmer, *The Oversight and Regulation of Non-state Health Care Providers: A Rapid Review in Selected Middle and High Income Countries*. 2009: Oxford Policy Management.
19. Churnrurtai, K., *et al.*, Human resources for health in Southeast Asia: shortages, distributional challenges, and international trade in health services. *The Lancet* 2011. 377: 769–81.

# 43

# Health care financing in Taiwan

*Tung-liang Chiang*

## Introduction

Today, the right to health care in Taiwan is no longer considered one's own responsibility, as was the case half a century ago. Following a phase of rapid economic transition and industrialization, together with an epidemiological shift, universal health insurance was inaugurated as a response to a dynamic mix of socio-cultural, economic and political factors. Almost two decades after its inauguration, Taiwan's National Health Insurance (NHI) is now one of the most received public policies. It not only provides equitable access for all citizens to healthcare providers practising in Taiwan and its surrounding islands, but also protects citizens against impoverishment as a result of out-of-pocket payments for health care.

This chapter begins by illustrating the general contextual framework leading up to the introduction of the NHI, which includes a descriptive portrait of the historical and political development associated with Taiwan's healthcare system and mechanisms of health financing. This is followed by a review of the NHI's main features and achievements, which provides the grounds for an analysis of trends for national health expenditures, as well as the associated reforms undertaken in line with the quest for the NHI's financial sustainability. Finally, the chapter concludes with an unfinished agenda.

## The road to National Health Insurance

Not as solitary as it appears geographically, Taiwan has gone through numerous remarkable external influences throughout its political and socio-cultural history [1]. Taiwan is an island nation with a population of over 23 million, encompassing an entire area of over 36,000 square kilometres and possessing a gross national product of US$20,690 in 2011 (US$1 = NT$30.37 in 2011). Its geographically nearby neighbours are the People's Republic of China (PRC), Japan and the Philippines.

As unique as its evolutionary story may be, Taiwan's modern health system is like any type of reform that has occurred in history, where the major underlying force was very much political rather than about social welfare or healthcare needs. It was indeed greatly involved with the government and politics in nature. A number of ruling influences have contributed to shaping Taiwan into the country it is today. It experienced imperialist colonization and was ruled under different forces before reaching to democratic reforms promulgated by former president Chiang Ching-kuo in the late 1980s.

## *A laissez-faire approach under political power transfers*

Taiwan was initially inhabited by an indigenous Taiwanese population until Dutch colonization in the seventeenth century. After 38 years of ruling, the imperialist Dutch were defeated by Koxinga and his troops in 1662, who aimed to transform Taiwan into a military base by restoring the Ming Dynasty. However, the Qing Dynasty subsequently took over Taiwan in 1683 and it was 200 years later when it ceded the island to Japan in 1895. Imperial Japan governed Taiwan from 1895 to 1945 as a part of their expansion southward, a period during which they introduced public health administration and a public hospital system across the island to help control the spread of infectious diseases [2].

Because of the long period of Chinese influence, healthcare delivery in Taiwan had been predominated by Traditional Chinese Medicine (TCM), without any formal education programmes or licensing systems. Yet, under Japanese reign, this soon began to change and the change has since been deep-rooted in Taiwan's current healthcare system. It includes the establishment of school education and a licensing system for healthcare professionals, the dominance of Western medicine over TCM, a combination of prescribing and dispensing drugs, and the development of close-system hospitals with large outpatient departments [3].

The Republic of China (ROC) government was established in 1912 during a time of instability and turmoil. At the end of World War II in 1945, Japan surrendered Taiwan to ROC military forces (led by the Kuomintang or the KMT party), on behalf of the allies. Although Western medicine continued expanding and set firm grounds in the delivery of healthcare services, the delivery system was still overlooked by the new government as it made strong efforts to improve public health using measures such as mass vaccination and malaria control.

Following the Chinese civil war, the Communist Party of China took full control of mainland China and founded the PRC in 1949, when the ROC government under the KMT withdrew to Taiwan and Chiang Kai-shek declared martial law. The ROC relocated its government to Taiwan, and its jurisdiction became limited to Taiwan and its surrounding islands. In 1971, the PRC assumed China's seat at the United Nations, which the ROC originally occupied. Thus, the ROC has gradually moved to the outer fringes of the international community as most countries switched recognition to the PRC. Meanwhile, the Department of Health (DoH) was established by the Taiwanese government under the Executive Yuan in the same year, pushing for the government's imminent active involvement in healthcare reforms [4].

## *Developing the healthcare delivery system*

By the 1970s, with a decrease in death rates, the health of people in Taiwan had significantly improved. From 1952 to 1970, the crude death rates declined from 9.9 per cent to 4.9 per cent, the infant mortality rate reduced from 45 per cent to 16.9 per cent, and life expectancy at birth increased from 57 and 61 years to 66 and 71 years for males and females, respectively (see Table 43.1). This demographic shift was accompanied by an epidemiologic transition of the disease pattern: non-communicable diseases (NCDs), such as cancer, stroke, heart diseases,

*Table 43.1* Basic and healthcare indicators: Taiwan, 1960–2010

| | *1960* | *1970* | *1980* | *1990* | *2000* | *2010* |
|---|---|---|---|---|---|---|
| ***Basic indicators*** | | | | | | |
| • Population (millions) | 10.7 | 14.7 | 17.8 | 20.2 | 22.2 | 23.2 |
| • Per capital GNP (US$) | 154 | 389 | 2,344 | 7954 | 14,216 | 19,175 |
| • Crude death rate (1/1,000) | 6.8 | 4.9 | 4.8 | 5.2 | 5.7 | 6.6 |
| • Infant mortality (1/1,000) | 35.0 | 16.9 | 9.8 | 5.3 | 5.8 | 4.2 |
| • Life expectancy (years) | | | | | | |
| • Male | 61.8 | 66.1 | 69.6 | 71.3 | 72.6 | 76.2 |
| • Female | 67.1 | 71.2 | 74.5 | 76.8 | 78.3 | 82.7 |
| • % of population aged 65+ | 2.5 | 3.0 | 4.3 | 6.2 | 8.6 | 10.7 |
| ***Healthcare resources*** | | | | | | |
| • Physicians per 1,000 persons | 0.5 | 0.4 | 0.7 | 1.0 | 1.3 | 1.7 |
| • Hospital beds per 1,000 persons | 0.7* | 2.4** | 3.2*** | 4.1 | 5.1 | 6.9 |
| • % of public hospital beds | 71.3* | 60.8** | 53.3*** | 42.7 | 35.1 | 34.0 |
| ***Healthcare financing*** | | | | | | |
| • % of population insured | 6.3 | 7.9 | 16.0 | 47.3 | 96.5 | 99.6 |
| • Per capita health spending (US$) | na | na | 78 | 330 | 669 | 1,217 |
| • Health spending as % of GDP | na | na | 3.3 | 4.2 | 5.5 | 6.6 |
| • % of public health spending | na | na | 31.3 | 50.8 | 60.0 | 56.8 |

*Sources*: [8, 19, 28, 29].

*Notes*: * 1961; **1971; *** 1982; na = not available.

hypertension and diabetes mellitus, already replaced communicable diseases, such as malaria, gastroenteritis and tuberculosis, as major causes of death [5].

Economically, the exceptionally high growth rate gained Taiwan the reputation of being one of the four highly developed economies, or the 'Four Asian Tigers', along with Singapore, Hong Kong and South Korea. The rapid economic development and industrialization facilitated Taiwan's economy in a transition from agricultural to industrial, from import-oriented to export-oriented and from relative poverty to prosperity. Hence, with the combination of the excelling economy, an epidemiological shift to chronic diseases and an increasing ageing population, people's demand for health care drastically escalated in spite of the overall improved population health [4].

At the time, Taiwan's health policies were devoted primarily to meet rising healthcare demands by expanding the supply of healthcare professionals and healthcare facilities. By the early 1970s, Taiwan was facing a national shortage of physicians, with a declining density from 0.45 physicians per 1,000 population in the 1950s to 0.41 per 1,000 in the 1970s (see Table 43.1). The most attractive solution was to expand the medical student enrolment by launching more medical schools, augmenting class sizes of existing medical schools and initiating new postgraduate programmes [6]. The goal was to achieve one physician per 1,000 population. As well as that, hospital capacity was concomitantly targeted to increase to up to four hospital beds per 1,000 population. In addition to governmental endeavours, this was partly mobilized by the private sector, which benefited from the growing economy and was capable of investing in hospitals and construction of large-scale medical facilities.

Along with the growth of healthcare resources, the government took further actions to tackle the geographical mal-distribution of physicians and hospitals. First, the Group Practice Centers (GPCs) programme was initiated in 1983 to improve the access to physicians for people who live in under-served areas [7]. To promote the programme, the DoH strategically subsidized teaching hospitals for staffing with GPC physicians and rewarded GPC physicians by allowing them to keep 80 per cent of their net profits [7]. Public-sponsored medical graduates were additionally assigned to practise in GPCs annually for a consistent influx of medical staff. Then, in 1985, the DoH took a great leap to implement the Medical Care Network programme, dividing Taiwan into 17 medical care regions. Under the programme, a development fund was set up to encourage the private sector to build small hospitals in under-served areas. Meanwhile, the DoH was authorized to prohibit the construction of new hospitals with more than 100 beds or prohibit hospital expansion projects in the saturated regions [8].

## *Moving toward universal health coverage*

By 1990, Taiwan had achieved the objectives of one physician and four hospital beds per 1,000 population. Yet, without removing financial barriers, the growth of healthcare resources simply does not guarantee universal access to health care. Regrettably, the Taiwanese government had been overlooking the issue of universal health coverage. Public hospitals and health stations charged health services as if they were private providers (see Table 43.2).

In 1986, for the first time, the government declared the goal of 'health insurance for all' to protect against its legitimacy crisis [4]. Prior to the policy announcement, there were three social health insurance schemes: Labor Insurance (LI), Government Employees' Insurance (GEI) and Farmers' Health Insurance (FHI), covering less than 25 per cent of the total population in Taiwan [3, 9].

The LI was the first and largest social insurance promulgated together with the passing of the Labor Insurance Act in 1956. By the 1980s, the LI already extended its coverage to workers aged 15 to 60; the dependents of the workers, however, were not eligible. The Labor Insurance Act required that all employers – employing five or more workers – be the insured unit on their workers' behalf. The participation was also compulsory for labour union members who were self-employed.

The GEI was introduced in 1958 as a fringe benefit of government employees. During the 1980s, its coverage was extended to active and retired public servants and their spouses and parents, as well as to active and retired employees of private schools and their spouses. Only for active public servants, however, was enrolment compulsory.

The FHI started off as a pilot programme in 1985 and became mandatory in 1989 as a result of strong political pressure. It covered all members of farmers' associations on a compulsory basis, and those aged 15 and over and spending more than 15 hours per week in farming on a voluntary basis.

All three social health insurance schemes were employment-oriented. Non-working individuals, such as children, the elderly, the unemployed and housewives, could not easily access health care. Moreover, participation of the LI for employed workers in companies and manufacturers with fewer than five people was voluntary, and since most businesses in Taiwan were small, many workers, therefore, did not have health insurance coverage. In other words, the uninsured population was more likely to be the one in greater need of healthcare services, but less capable of sustaining economic independence.

*Table 43.2* Major historical events and healthcare reform policies in Taiwan, 1945–2013

| *Year* | *Event* |
|---|---|
| 1949 | The Kuomintang (KMT) retreated to Taiwan and declared Martial Law |
| 1950 | Labor Insurance (LI) established |
| 1958 | Government Employees' Insurance (GEI) established |
| 1965 | Malaria eradication achieved |
| 1971 | Department of Health (DoH), Executive Yuan, established |
| 1983 | Group Practice Centers (GPCs) programme implemented |
| 1985 | Medical Care Network programme implemented |
| | Farmers' Health Insurance (FHI) pilot programme implemented |
| 1986 | The goal for 'health insurance for all' declared |
| | The Democratic Progressive Party (DPP) established |
| 1987 | Martial Law lifted |
| 1988 | The National Health Insurance Planning Task Force formed |
| 1989 | Mandatory FHI implemented |
| 1992 | First full election of Legislative Yuan members |
| 1994 | The NHI Act passed by the Legislative Yuan |
| 1995 | NHI programme fully implemented (premium rate: 4.25%) |
| 1996 | First general presidential election |
| 1998 | Dental global budget phased in |
| 1999 | Co-payment applied for prescription drugs (NT$100 cap per prescription) |
| 2000 | Chinese medicine global budget phased in |
| 2001 | Primary care global budget phased in |
| | Pay-for-performance mechanism introduced |
| 2002 | Hospital global budget phased in (global budget system fully implemented) |
| | Premium rate raised from 4.25% to 4.55% |
| 2004 | Taiwan-RVS for physician services phased in |
| 2010 | Premium rate raised from 4.55% to 5.17% |
| | Taiwan-DRGs phased in |
| 2011 | Capitation pilot programmes implemented |
| 2013 | Second-generation NHI programme implemented |

Then, opportunity came knocking when Taiwan undertook drastic political reforms between 1986 and 1992 [3, 4]. In 1986, Taiwan's first opposition party, the Democratic Progressive Party (DPP) was officially formed, followed by the lift of the Emergency Decree Law (a martial law) in 1987, and the first full election of the Legislative Yuan (congress members) in 1992. As a result, the KMT was shifting towards the competing position rather than being the dominating political force.

In order to consolidate political power, the KMT was no longer passive and set to develop the National Health Insurance (NHI). In 1988, the government had assembled a task force composed of Taiwanese public health scholars to draft blueprints for the NHI. Two years later, after a preliminary NHI plan was submitted to the Cabinet, another task force was created to plan the details and prepare for implementation. Before the second full election of the Legislative Yuan in December 1995 and a presidential election in March 1996, the KMT mobilized its legislators to pass the NHI Law on 19 July 1994. The Executive Yuan further ordered the Bureau of National Health Insurance (NHI Bureau) to fully implement the NHI by March 1995.

## The NHI's main features and achievements

Learning from the past and from abroad, Taiwan's NHI has clearly identified three objectives: to provide equal access to adequate health care for all citizens, to control healthcare costs at a socially affordable level (macro-economic efficiency) and to promote efficient use of healthcare resources (micro-economic efficiency) [10]. With reference to these objectives, in this section, we will describe the main features of Taiwan's NHI and its achievement.

### *Main features of Taiwan's NHI*

In order to achieve its three objectives, Taiwan's NHI has been implemented with the following major strategies: universal coverage, payroll tax financing, comprehensive benefits, public single payer and national global budget [4].

#### Universal coverage

Regardless of age, sex, family income and health status, it is compulsory for all Taiwanese citizens to take part in the NHI. The current coverage rate is almost 100 per cent, and even includes soldiers and prisoners. There are certain individuals who lose their enrolment status over outstanding NHI premium payments. However, the Supreme Court ruled in 2002 that no one in Taiwan could be denied access to care because of a lack of the ability to pay the premium.

#### Payroll tax financing

By nature, Taiwan's NHI is a social health insurance scheme financed mainly by premiums in the form of payroll tax with heavy governmental subsidy. In 2010, the total premium collected was NT$437 billion, with a contribution rate of 38 per cent, 36 per cent and 26 per cent from employees, employers and the government, respectively [11]. The employee has to pay the premium for himself/herself, plus for up to three dependents, while the employer pays for the worker plus 0.7 dependents to avoid the possibility of discrimination against workers with large families. To ease the financial burden on the low socio-economic groups, the government has instituted variable premium subsidy and waiver programmes. For example, the government pays 40 per cent of the contribution for the self-employed, 70 per cent for farmers and 100 per cent for low-income families.

#### Comprehensive benefits

With political consideration rather than economic, the benefits of Taiwan's NHI are uniform and comprehensive, including ambulatory care, inpatient care, emergency care, prescription drugs, X-ray and laboratory tests, rehabilitation, mental illness treatment, dental care, TCM and home care. The patient is completely free to choose healthcare providers and there is no rationing of care in Taiwan.

However, moderate cost sharing has been advocated to reduce moral hazard. The patient has to pay a basic co-insurance rate of 20 per cent for primary care and 10 per cent for inpatient care, and an extra co-insurance rate of 10–30 per cent for heavy users seeking primary care from the hospital without referral [12]. Nevertheless, the law requires a cap on out-of-pocket cost sharing to prevent low-income families and patients with major diseases from adverse health effects.

### Public single payer

The NHI Bureau is the only agency responsible for the operation of the NHI. In order to increase administrative efficiency and to exercise the monopsony power of a single payer, the NHI Bureau has consolidated all existing social health insurance schemes and set up six regional offices to process enrolment and review claims [4]. The administrative cost of Taiwan's NHI is less than 2 per cent of the total NHI payments [13]. Meanwhile, the NHI Bureau enters contracts with both private and public providers in Taiwan, appreciating the importance of 'money follows the patient' in the pursuit of efficiency. Currently, the NHI engages with 100 per cent of the hospitals and more than 90 per cent of the clinics in Taiwan [12].

### National global budget

To achieve macro-economic efficiency, the NHI Planning Task Force recommended a national global budget system in 1990. However, the NHI Bureau did not carry out global budgeting immediately after the inauguration of the NHI. It had been phased-in starting from the dental sector in 1998 and ending with the hospital sector in 2002. Operationally, the global budget should be decided three months before each new fiscal year by the Negotiation Committee on Health Care Expenditure, which consists of representatives of providers, consumers, employers, scholars or experts and the government.

Under the global budget system, there are diversified methods of paying for health care. Fee-for-service with a uniform fee schedule has been the prevailing method in Taiwan. The law requires the NHI Bureau to work with providers to develop the uniform fee schedule, which defines how much is to be reimbursed for what kind of services [4]. Yet, the method of fee-for-service has always been criticized for giving providers a perverse incentive to deliver unnecessary services. Thus, the NHI Bureau has continued to undertake payment reforms.

## *Achievements of the NHI*

It is almost 18 years since the inauguration of Taiwan's NHI so what has it achieved? Overall, Taiwan's NHI has performed well in closing the gap in access to health and protecting care, and removing financial risk from catastrophic health spending.

### Access to health care

Actual or realized access to health care can be evaluated through various utilization rates. In order to examine the effects of Taiwan's NHI on healthcare utilization, Cheng and Chiang [14] followed a cohort sample of 1,211 adults over a nine-month period after the inauguration. They found that among those who were hitherto uninsured, the probability of using physician services and hospital care increased by 69 per cent and 145 per cent, respectively. Thus, Taiwan's NHI brought the hitherto uninsured up to a par with those who previously had social health insurance. Presently, the admission rate is about 120 per 1,000 people and on average each person visits 15 times per year, of which 12 are physician visits [15].

It also seems that low socio-economic groups have benefited more from the NHI. For example, the ratio of NHI payments to NHI premiums for the bottom 20 per cent of households was 1.75 in 1998, compared with 1.16 and 0.96 for the middle 20 per cent and top

20 per cent of households, respectively [16]. Also, the low socio-economic group might receive better health care since it is able to spend more money on health care after the introduction of Taiwan's NHI. However, in terms of household health expenses, the middle social class has benefited the most. Between 1994 and 1998, the growth rate of household health expenses for the middle 20 per cent of households was 64.5 per cent, compared with 24.5 per cent and 33.5 per cent for the bottom 20 per cent and top 20 per cent of households, respectively [16].

### Financial risk protection

Taiwan's NHI has substantially contributed to reducing direct out-of-pocket payments for health care. Currently, direct payments represent about one-third of the total health expenditures, falling from more than two-thirds in 1980. Consequently, less than 3 per cent of the population in Taiwan currently experiences catastrophic health spending (i.e. out-of-pocket expenditure constitutes more than 40 per cent of household disposable incomes after deducting expenses for food each year) [16]. This figure is comparable to that of Western welfare states.

Reducing economic hardship has the most significant influence on the low socio-economic groups because this group is more likely to suffer catastrophic health spending. For example, healthcare expenses as percentages of household disposable incomes largely increased from 5.1 per cent for the top 20 per cent of households to 14.0 per cent for the bottom 20 per cent of households in 1998 [16]. Meanwhile, the low socio-economic groups have trivial savings. In 1988, the ratio of household savings to disposable incomes largely shrank from 38.8 per cent for the top 20 per cent of households to 7.0 per cent for the bottom 20 per cent of households [16].

Fortunately, low socio-economic groups receive disproportionate payments from the NHI. For example, the NHI payments as percentages of household healthcare expenses increased from 65.1 per cent for the top 20 per cent of households to 76 per cent for the bottom 20 per cent of households in 1998. As a result, the proportion of the NHI payments exceeding household savings substantially increased from 8.7 per cent for the top 20 per cent of households to 57.1 per cent for the bottom 20 per cent of households in the same year [16].

### Public satisfaction

Immediately after its inauguration, the proportion of adults aged 20 and above who were satisfied with the NHI was as low as 30 per cent, as a consequence of implementation chaos [4]. However, with it successfully removing financial risks and barriers to access, the NHI is currently the most popular public policy in Taiwan – the public satisfaction rate is more than 80 per cent [12]. Besides this, the success story of Taiwan's NHI has become internationally well known [17].

## The quest for financial sustainability

There are always challenges ahead. The ultimate challenge for Taiwan's NHI is its financial sustainability. This is extremely critical in a country like Taiwan where, for the first time in history, negative economic growth has been experienced twice in the past decade and an ageing society is imminent in the next decade. In this section, we will first examine the trends for national health expenditures in Taiwan and then review recent healthcare reforms undertaken by the NHI to tackle the financial crisis and to improve the efficient use of healthcare resources.

## *Trends for national health expenditures*

The expansion of social health insurance schemes, particularly through the introduction of the NHI, has had a significant impact on trends for national health expenditures in Taiwan, including how much money is being spent on health care, where the money comes from and where money goes.

### National health spending

National health expenditures in Taiwan have risen rapidly in the past decades [13, 18]. Between 1980 and 2010, the national health expenditures increased from NT$49 billion (US$1.36 billion) to NT$887 billion (US$29.21 billion), with a growth rate of 10.1 per cent per year. Adjusting for the size of the population, per capita health expenditures increased from NT$2,805 to NT$38,323 during the same period.

Because national health expenditures have increased faster than economic growth, the health-spending share of the GDP increased from 4.3 per cent in 1980 to 6.5 per cent in 2010. Compared with OECD countries, Taiwan has a much lower percentage of GDP spent on health care, partly due to better economic development in the last century. Between 1980 and 2000, the growth rate of Taiwan's GDP reached 9.8 per cent per year [19]. Yet, economic growth has slowed down to 3.5 per cent per year in the first decade of the new century.

### Source of funds

The mix of financing sources for health care in Taiwan has also changed significantly. The public share of health spending went up from 31.3 per cent in 1980 to 60.0 per cent in 2000, and then slightly declined to 56.8 per cent in 2010. The most important explanation for this remarkable shift is the expansion of social health insurance schemes in the late 1980s and early 1990s. The proportion of the insured population increased from 16.0 per cent in 1980 to 47.3 per cent in 1990, and to more than 95 per cent in 1996, one year after the inauguration of NHI [4].

The only statistical data available are for recent trends in out-of-pocket payments in Taiwan [13]. Between 1996 and 2010, household direct payments increased from NT$112 billion (US$4.07 billion) to NT$321 billion (US$10.57 billion), representing a growth rate of 7.8 per cent per year. Because the household direct payments rose faster than the national health expenditures, the out-of-pocket share of national health expenditures increased rapidly from 26.4 per cent to 36.2 per cent during the same period, reaching to the ceiling suggested by the World Health Organization for low- and middle-income countries [20]. It is a serious warning sign of augmenting financial catastrophe and impoverishment.

### Spending by sector

National health expenditures in Taiwan have gone primarily to personal healthcare services provided by hospitals and clinics. Between 1996 and 2010, personal healthcare expenditures increased from NT$3,641 billion (US$132 billion) to NT$7,695 billion (US$253 billion), with the share of national health expenditures slightly increasing from 81.7 per cent to

86.8 per cent [13]. Other allocation categories of national health expenditures include public health efforts, general administration, capital formation and xenopayments.

The trends for payments vary amongst different healthcare sectors [13]. Hospitals are always the recipients of the largest share of personal healthcare expenditures, maintaining at about the 60 per cent level. This is followed by physician clinics whose share declined substantially from 22.6 per cent to 17.0 per cent between 1996 and 2010, followed by the dental clinics' share increasing from 9.9 per cent to 12.2 per cent and Chinese-medicine clinics declining from 3.5 per cent to 3.2 per cent. In addition, pharmaceutical expenditures as percentages of personal healthcare expenditures increased from 21.8 per cent to 28.9 per cent during the same period.

### *Decomposition of national health expenditures*

To examine the factors accounting for the trends for national health expenditures, we decompose growth in nominal health expenditures into general economic inflation, excess healthcare inflation, population growth, and the increase in volume and intensity of services [21, 22, 23], as shown in Table 43.3.

#### Nominal and real growth

Between 1980 and 2010, on average, the nominal growth rate of national health expenditures was 10.1 per cent per year. Adjusting for healthcare price inflation of 2.6 per cent, the real growth rate of national expenditures was 7.3 per cent per year. Further adjusting for population growth of 0.9 per cent, volume–intensity of services per person grew an average of 6.3 per cent per year. Healthcare prices, on average, increased annually by 1.1 per cent, faster than general economic inflation did.

Yet, national health expenditures do not increase constantly and may greatly fluctuate. For example, national health expenditures increased by more than 10 per cent per year in the late 1980s and early 1990s, which was in part due to the rapid expansion of social health insurance schemes. However, since the introduction of the NHI, both nominal and real growth rates have been slowing down substantially. In the 2000s, on average, national health expenditures grew by 4.4 per cent each year, and healthcare inflation accounted for about half of the growth.

#### Volume–intensity increase

Volume and intensity of services per capita is the residual of decomposition. Notably, volume–intensity in Taiwan increased an average of 1.6 per cent per year in the 2000s, which is much lower than 9.0 per cent in the 1980s and 8.5 per cent in the 1990s. In addition to the expansion of health insurance coverage as aforementioned, income, population ageing and the capacity of the healthcare system all have a bearing on the growth of volume–intensity.

Income, as measured by the GDP per capita, has repeatedly shown to be one of the major determinants of national health expenditures. Unfortunately, since the late 1990s, Taiwan's economic development has attenuated substantially and encountered severe economic crises. Accordingly, national health expenditures have increased at a much slower pace. This is critical for the low socio-economic groups, whose disposable incomes have increased only slightly in the last decade. Between 2000 and 2010, the health expenses of the bottom 20 per cent of households grew only by 1.3 per cent per year, and the health expenses ratio of the top

*Table 43.3* Decomposition of health expenditure increases into price, population and volume–intensity increase in Taiwan, 1980–2010

| *Year* | *Share of health expenditure in GDP, first year* | *Annual compound rate of growth, 1980–2010* | | | | | | | *Share of health expenditure in GDP, last year* |
|---|---|---|---|---|---|---|---|---|---|
| | | *National health expenditure growth* | *Healthcare price deflator* | *Of which GDP deflator* | *Of which excess healthcare inflation* | *Real expenditure growth* | *Of which population growth* | *Of which per capita volume–intensity growth* | |
| | *(1)* | *(2)* | *(3)* | *(4)* | *(5)* | *(6)* | *(7)* | *(8)* | *(9)* |
| 1980–1985 | 3.3 | 14.8 | 4.6 | 3.7 | 0.8 | 9.8 | 1.6 | 8.1 | 4.0 |
| 1985–1990 | 4.0 | 12.9 | 1.6 | 2.4 | −0.7 | 11.0 | 1.1 | 9.8 | 4.2 |
| 1990–1995 | 4.2 | 15.4 | 2.8 | 2.9 | −0.1 | 12.2 | 0.9 | 11.2 | 5.3 |
| 1995–2000 | 5.3 | 8.3 | 2.4 | 2.1 | 1.6 | 5.7 | 0.8 | 4.8 | 5.8 |
| 2000–2005 | 5.8 | 3.8 | 2.4 | −0.5 | 2.9 | 1.4 | 0.5 | 0.9 | 6.1 |
| 2005–2010 | 6.1 | 5.0 | 2.1 | −1.0 | 3.1 | 2.8 | 0.4 | 2.5 | 6.6 |
| 1980–1990 | 3.3 | 13.8 | 3.1 | 3.0 | 0.0 | 10.4 | 1.3 | 9.0 | 4.2 |
| 1990–2000 | 4.2 | 12.3 | 2.6 | 1.9 | 0.7 | 9.5 | 0.9 | 8.5 | 5.8 |
| 2000–2010 | 5.8 | 4.4 | 2.2 | −0.7 | 3.0 | 2.1 | 0.5 | 1.6 | 6.6 |
| 1980–2010 | 3.3 | 10.1 | 2.6 | 1.6 | 1.1 | 7.3 | 0.9 | 6.3 | 6.6 |

*Source*: Calculated by author using data from [13, 19, 30].

20 per cent of households to bottom 20 per cent of households increased from 1.6 to 2.1 times (data calculated by author) [23].

The effect of population ageing on volume–intensity in Taiwan has been steadily increasing from 1.2 per cent in the 1980s to 1.4 per cent in the 1990s, and to 1.6 per cent in the 2000s (data calculated by author). As the proportion of the population aged 65 years and above will increase from 10.7 per cent in 2010 to 16.1 per cent in 2020 [24], its effect on volume–intensity will increase by 2.1 per cent each year (data calculated by author).

In response to increased demands and capital investments, the capacity of the healthcare system in Taiwan has been greatly expanded after the introduction of the NHI, particularly for the hospital industry. Between 1990 and 2010, the number of hospital beds per 1,000 people increased from 4.1 to 6.9 (see Table 43.1). What is alarming is the withering of small and middle-sized hospitals, together with the substantial growth of large hospitals. For instance, the number of medical centres increased from 13 to 23 between 1994 and 2000 [25]. Health services provided by large hospitals tend to be more intensive and costly. When people are more likely to seek care from large hospitals in the absence of a gatekeeper system and low cost sharing, it adds fuel to the fire. It was estimated that these 'upgrading effects' contributed to more than 50 per cent of the growth in total NHI payments between 1996 and 2000 [22]. The upgrading effects to date have been levelled off, but the NHI has continued to suffer the financial burden resulting from the distorted medical ecology.

## *Recent healthcare reforms*

With the rapid rise of healthcare expenditures, Taiwan's NHI began experiencing financial deficits as early as 1998. To meet this financial challenge, the NHI Bureau has undertaken a series of actions to increase revenues and improve health system performance.

### Financial reforms

Measures to increase NHI revenues can be grouped into the following: to raise the ceiling of premium base, to increase premium rate and to broaden the sources of premiums, and most of them are under DoH's authority. For example, the ceiling of the NHI premium base has been increased now to NT$182,000 (US$5,993) [15] from NT$53,000 (US$1,944) in 1995 [26]. The DoH is also authorized to adjust the premium rate within a range of 5 per cent, but it always becomes a political issue. In 2002, for the first time, the premium rate was raised from 4.25 per cent to 4.55 per cent at the price of the resignation of a Health Minister. In 2010, the premium rate was raised again to 5.17 per cent, with a promise to return to 4.91 per cent if the amendment of the second-generation NHI reform was passed in the Legislative Yuan.

The DoH began drafting the second-generation NHI reform proposal in 2001. Five years later, a reform package was submitted to the Executive Yuan for review. This legislative amendment proposed to change the NHI premium contribution from a payroll tax base to a household income base, thereby broadening the sources of premiums. However, due to its controversy, the draft legislative amendment never made it to the first reading. Since then, the DoH took no further action until 2009 when Professor C.L. Yaung was appointed as the Minister of Health. Minister Yaung advocated the amendment forcefully and a new NHI amendment was passed in January 2011. Yet, the final version of amendment, effective on 1 January 1 2013, is substantially different from the original household income-based proposal. Instead, it approves the collection of extra 2 per cent supplementary premiums from income sources including part-time jobs, professional practice, rents, interests, bonuses and capital gains. Besides this, a supervisory board of the NHI has been appointed to be in charge of reviewing the benefit and premium policies.

### Performance improvement

Improving the performance of the healthcare system is equally as important as increasing revenues for the financial sustainability of Taiwan's NHI. Accordingly, Taiwan's NHI has continued reforming its benefit designs and payment methods to achieve a high-performing healthcare system.

Cost sharing is one of the common strategies in benefit reforms. Yet, before the 1995 healthcare reform, social health insurance enrolees seldom paid directly for health care received except for registration fees. In the beginning, the NHI adopted a moderate cost-sharing policy, which seemed to have limited effects on healthcare utilization. Later, the DoH added extra cost sharing for prescription drugs, non-referral outpatient care and heavy users, but few of them generated significant performance improvement [27].

Since its inauguration, Taiwan's NHI has taken many initiatives in payment reforms. As aforementioned, the NHI has fully implemented the national global budget system as a macro-management strategy to control healthcare spending. It started with case payment for normal deliveries and caesarean sections in 1995 for hospital payment reform. By 2003, a total of 54 procedures were reimbursed by using the case payment method. In 2010, the NHI Bureau began to phase in a diagnosis-related groups system (Taiwan-DRGs) after six years of preparation. Yet, regrettably, its full implementation date has been extended without any specific deadline since 2011.

Physician payment reform started with the implementation of a regressive sliding scale for reasonable outpatient loading in the inauguration year. In 2001, the NHI experimented with the method of pay-for-performance for five diseases, but only seven diseases are on the current list, including asthma, breast cancer, early chronic kidney disease, diabetes, hepatitis carrier, schizophrenia and tuberculosis. Between 2004 and 2006, aiming for a fair payment system for physician services, the NHI phased in a relative value resources-based system (Taiwan-RVS). In 2011, the NHI further experimented with a risk-adjusted capitation project in seven study sites in pursuit of efficient healthcare delivery.

## Conclusion: an unfinished reform agenda

Over the last century, Taiwan's healthcare financing has evolved from a laissez-faire approach to universal coverage. The NHI not only closes the rich and poor gap in access to health care by removing financial barriers, but also helps to break the shackles of poverty through the risk-pooling mechanism of social insurance. Today, most people in Taiwan are very happy with the NHI. Yet, there is no free lunch. We have also witnessed the rapid escalation of healthcare costs along with the expansion of health insurance coverage. Accordingly, how to achieve and maintain the financing sustainability of the NHI has become the ultimate challenge for Taiwan, an ageing, technologically blessed society in an era of economic downturn.

What is more important is that everything is connected to everything else. As an unintended consequence, the success of the NHI has contributed significantly to the deteriorating of Taiwan's medical ecology. Medical centres and regional hospitals have increased at an incredible pace – people have continued overusing physician and hospital services, disregarding all kinds of financial and payment reforms. The message is clear: Taiwan's NHI has an unfinished reform agenda and future reforms should focus on the healthcare system, not just on healthcare financing.

## Acknowledgements

This chapter was completed when the author was a Visiting Professor at The Chinese University of Hong Kong in 2013 for which he acknowledges the hospitality of the CUHK Research Institute for the Humanities.

## References

1. Department of Information, Executive Yuan. *The Republic of China Yearbook 2012*, Taipei: Executive Yuan. Available from: http://www.ey.gov.tw/2012yearbook/index.html [Accessed 14 January 2013].
2. Chiang, T.L. Health care delivery in Taiwan: progress and problems. *Journal of National Public Health Association (ROC)* 1998; 8: 75–90 (in Chinese).
3. Lu, J.F.R. and Chiang, T.L. Evolution of Taiwan's health care system. *Health Economics, Policy and Law* 2011; 6: 85–107.
4. Chiang, T.L. Taiwan's 1995 health care reform. *Health Policy* 1997; 39: 225–39.
5. Chiang T.L. Mortality in Taiwan since 1951. *Journal of National Public Health Association (ROC)* 1987; 7(2): 53–64 (in Chinese).
6. Chiang, T.L. Physician manpower policy in Taiwan, 1945–1994. *Taiwan Journal of Public Health* 1995; 14: 383–91 (in Chinese).
7. Chiang, T.L., Yaung, C.L. and Lew-Ting, C.Y. The impact of group practice centers on access to health care. *Taiwan Journal of Public Health* 1991; 10: 260–8 (in Chinese).
8. Chiang, T.L. *Health Care Policy in Taiwan*, 3rd edn, Taipei: Chu Liu Book Co, 2007: 73–6 (in Chinese).
9. Chiang, T.L. Health care financing in Taiwan: issues and directions. *Taiwan Journal of Public Health* 1992; 11: 20–31 (in Chinese).
10. Council for Economic Planning and Development. The Report of National Health Insurance Plan (the CEPD Report), Taipei: Council for Economic Planning and Development, 1990.
11. Department of Health, Executive Yuan. Health Statistics in Taiwan 2010. 2012 Available at: http://www.doh.gov.tw/CHT2006/DM/DM2_2.aspx?now_fod_list_no=12183&class_no=440&level_no=2 [Accessed 14 January 2013].
12. Bureau of National Health Insurance. A Synopsis to the National Health Insurance, Taipei: Bureau of National Health Insurance, 2012. Available at: http://www.nhi.gov.tw/webdata/webdata.aspx?menu=17&menu_id=659&webdata_id=2891&WD_ID=897 [Accessed 14 January 2013].
13. Department of Health, Executive Yuan. Taiwan National Health Expenditure 2011. 2012. Available at: http://www.doh.gov.tw/CHT2006/DM/DM2_2.aspx?now_fod_list_no=12486&class_no=440& level_no=2 [Accessed 14 January 2013].
14. Cheng, S.H. and Chiang, T.L. The effect of universal health insurance on health care utilization. *Journal of the American Medical Association* 1997; 278: 89–93.
15. Bureau of National Health Insurance. National Health Insurance Annual Statistics 2010, Taipei: Bureau of National Health Insurance, 2011. Available at: http://www.nhi.gov.tw/webdata/webdata.aspx?menu=17&menu_id=1023&WD_ID=1043&webdata_id=4004 [Accessed 14 January 2013].
16. Chiang, T.L. *Essays on National Health Insurance in Taiwan*, 2nd edn, Taipei: National Taiwan University Press, 2008: i, 109–11 (in Chinese).
17. Public Broadcasting Service. Frontline. Sick around the world. Available at: http://www.pbs.org/wgbh/pages/frontline/sickaroundtheworld/ [Accessed 14 January 2013].
18. Lin, S.S. National health expenditure in Taiwan: its financing and allocation, Final report submitted to the Taiwan Department of Health, Executive Yuan, 1993 (in Chinese).
19. Council for Economic Planning and Development. *Taiwan Statistical Data Book 2012*, Taipei: CEPD, 2012. Available at: http://www.cepd. gov.tw/encontent/m1.aspx?sNo=0001453 [Accessed 14 January 2013].

20. World Health Organization. *The World Health Report 2010 – Health Systems Financing: The Path to Universal Coverage*, Geneva: World Health Organization, 2010.
21. Schieber, G.J. and Poullier, J.P. Overview of international comparisons of health care expenditure. *Health Care Financing Review* (December Special Issue) 1989: 1–7.
22. Chiang, T.L. Analysis on trends for healthcare expenditures in Taiwan. *Taiwan Journal of Public Health* 2002; 21: 157–63 (in Chinese).
23. Wen, Y.P., Huang, S.M. and Chiang, T.L. An analysis of the growth of healthcare expenditure in Taiwan: healthcare inflation, volume-intensity, and equity. *Taiwan Journal of Public Health* 2012; 31: 1–10 (in Chinese).
24. Council for Economic Planning and Development. Population Projection for R.O.C. (Taiwan): 2012–2060, Taipei: CEPD, 2013. Available at: http://www.cepd.gov.tw/encontent/m1.aspx?sNo=0001457 [Accessed 14 January 2013].
25. Chiang, T.L. Two principles for sustainably financing the National Health Insurance. *United Daily*, 22 January 2013 (in Chinese).
26. Bureau of National Health Insurance. National Health Insurance Annual Statistics 1995, Taipei: Bureau of National Health Insurance. 1996. Available at: http://www.doh.gov.tw/CHT2006/DM/DM2_2.aspx?now_fod_list_no=9653&class_no=440&level_no=2 [Accessed 14 January 2013].
27. Lee, Y.C., Yang, M.C., Huang, Y.T., Liu, C.H. and Chen, S.B. Impacts of cost containment strategies on pharmaceutical expenditures of the National Health Insurance in Taiwan, 1996–2003. *Pharmacoeconomics* 2006; 24: 891–902.
28. Department of Health, Executive Yuan. Health and Vital Statistics, Volume I. General Health Statistics, 1985, Taipei: Department of Health, Executive Yuan, R.O.C., 1986.
29. Department of Health, Executive Yuan. Statistics of Causes of Death 2011, Taipei: Department of Health, Executive Yuan, R.O.C., 2012.
30. Directorate-General of Budget, Accounting and Statistics, Executive Yuan. National Income of the Republic of China 2012, Taipei: DGBAS, Executive Yuan, R.O.C., 2012.

# 44

# The challenge of managing health human resources

## A case study on the Philippines

*Maria Elena Baltazar Herrera*

> At the heart of each and every health system, the workforce is central to advancing health . . . Health service providers are the personification of a system's core values – they heal and care for people, ease pain and suffering, prevent disease and mitigate risk – the human link that connects knowledge to health action.
>
> *(World Health Organization 2006 [1])*

### Introduction

The World Health Organization (WHO) defines Health Human Resources (HHR) or the 'health workforces' as 'all people engaged in actions whose primary intent is to enhance health' [1]. With healthcare facilities, healthcare workers (HCWs) are the primary channel for the delivery of health care. Global experience shows that a well-performing workforce can improve immunization coverage; outreach of primary care; infant, child and maternal survival; and other disease outcomes [1].

The WHO considers human resources as one of the six building blocks of a health system [2]. 'Alternative health system frameworks' (i.e. Evans's markets; Hurst's OECD's flow of funds and payments; Frenk's actors and their interactions; Cassels's institutional components; Murray and Frenks's systems performance; Hsiao *et al.*'s control knobs; Mills *et al.*'s strengthening capacity to improve performance; Atun and Menabde's system dynamics), particularly that of Anand and Bärnighausen [3], give more weight to HHR and place it at the centre of the system, recognizing that it cannot be isolated from other system components since 'most functions of a health system are either directly undertaken by, or depend for their implementation on, the health worker' [3].

A 'well-performing' workforce is evaluated by both quantity and quality dimensions. This means that a country's HCWs should be available in sufficient numbers, be fairly distributed, and be competent, responsive and productive [2]. It is this variation in size, composition and distribution – critical supply factors – that countries attempt to manage in order to respond effectively and efficiently to the demand for healthcare services. Size and composition are a function of inflow and outflow, both influenced by factors such as education and training, and migration and movement to other sectors. Distribution, on the other hand, is primarily influenced by a country's incentive scheme [3, 4].

In order to understand the challenges involved in managing HHR, it is important to understand the challenges within the health system itself. In terms of health policy agenda, most countries, including the Philippines, are committed to the achievement of universal health care (UHC). In the 2010 World Health Report, the WHO explains that UHC has three critical dimensions: who is covered, what services are covered and how much of the cost is covered. UHC calls for equity of access and financial risk protection to ensure that 'everyone in the population has access to appropriate promotive, preventive, curative and rehabilitative health care when they need it and at an affordable cost' [5]. The most difficult challenge lies in reaching marginalized populations, especially those in remote and isolated areas.

Demographic trends also exert pressure on a country's health system. In most of the developed world, life expectancies are increasing and birth rates are slowing. The result is a greying population with ever-increasing demands for health care. In these countries, the need for HCWs is not only for primary and curative care, but also increasingly for assisted living and palliative end-of-life care. These demands often cannot be met by local supply and the relatively high wages in these countries encourage the immigration of HCWs.

This worldwide trend is reflected in varying degrees in Asian countries, where population growth is slowing [6]. To a large extent, these lower birth and death rates are explained by economic development in the region [6, 7]. Asian economies have proven relatively resilient and economic growth is reflected in improved health outcomes. Economic development has also translated into an improvement in educational outcomes with the result that many of the developing countries in Asia are now producing HCWs capable of practising on a global stage. Ironically, this improvement in production of qualified HCWs has increased the likelihood of migration towards more affluent societies. The pressure is particularly difficult for the nations in the middle as their healthcare systems attract patients from less developed nations further displacing the marginalized local populations.

Morbidity patterns, too, are changing. Increased global commerce, which increases global travel, has radically increased the likelihood of disease outbreaks crossing national boundaries. Changes in disease patterns and other health risks (pollution and climate change, increases in the occurrence of lifestyle diseases, demand for elderly care) are emerging [6, 7] as well.

To boost the responsiveness of the health system to these demand trends, the service delivery machinery has to be primed. While this calls for a system-wide approach, the focus of this chapter is to illustrate the dynamics between supply (i.e. size, distribution and composition) and demand for health human resources using the Philippines as a case study. The chapter delves into the resulting challenges to the Philippine health system and how the Philippines attempts to address these challenges through innovative programmes. While there are five major categories of professionals that are recognized internationally (i.e. doctors, nurses, midwives, dentists and physical therapists), the focus of this chapter will be on doctors and nurses.

## Background on the Philippines

Similar to other countries in the region, the Philippines faces many challenges in managing its health human resources. The mobilization and deployment of physical and human resources across the 7,107 islands of the Philippines poses great challenges. Philippine demographic trends also parallel that of the region. As of 2010, the population stands at 92.3 million, making the Philippines the twelfth most populous in the world. Since 2000, the annual population growth rate has been approximately 1.9 per cent. Compared to the

*Table 44.1* Total fertility rates of ASEAN member states and Japan (%)

| *Year* | *1960* | *1970* | *1980* | *1990* | *2000* | *2010* |
|---|---|---|---|---|---|---|
| Cambodia | 6.3 | 5.9 | 5.9 | 5.7 | 3.8 | 2.6 |
| Indonesia | 5.7 | 5.5 | 4.4 | 3.1 | 2.5 | 2.1 |
| Japan | 2 | 2.1 | 1.8 | 1.6 | 1.3 | 1.4 |
| Laos | 6 | 6 | 6.3 | 6.2 | 4.2 | 2.8 |
| Malaysia | 6.3 | 4.9 | 3.8 | 3.5 | 3.1 | 2.6 |
| Myanmar | 6.1 | 6.1 | 4.6 | 3.5 | 2.4 | 2 |
| Philippines | 7.2 | 6.3 | 5.1 | 4.3 | 3.8 | 3.1 |
| Singapore | 5.5 | 3 | 1.8 | 1.8 | 1.6 | 1.3 |
| Thailand | 6.2 | 5.6 | 3.4 | 2.1 | 1.7 | 1.6 |
| Vietnam | 7.1 | 7.4 | 5.4 | 3.6 | 2 | 1.8 |

*Source*: [8].

1960 population, however, the 2010 population grew annually by 2.5 per cent. While the country's total fertility rate has been decreasing over the years, Table 44.1 shows that it remains the highest among ASEAN member states [8]. Moreover, the country continues to have a relatively young population, although population pyramids show a narrowing base (see Tables 44.2–44.4). There are also signs of an ageing population:

- In the past 40 years, the proportion of population in the older age group has increased more rapidly (see Table 44.3);
- Median age continues to increase but is lower relative to other ASEAN countries (see Table 44.4);
- Life expectancies for both sexes are increasing (see Table 44.5); and

*Table 44.2* Percentage distribution of Philippine population by age group

| *Age group* | *1970* | *1975* | *1980* | *1990* | *1995* | *2000* | *2007* | *2010* |
|---|---|---|---|---|---|---|---|---|
| 0–4 | 15.9 | 15.4 | 15.8 | 14 | 13.6 | 12.6 | 11.9 | 11.1 |
| 5–9 | 16.1 | 15 | 13.8 | 13.3 | 13 | 12.7 | 12 | 11.2 |
| 10–14 | 13.7 | 13.5 | 12.4 | 12.3 | 11.7 | 11.7 | 11.5 | 11 |
| 15–19 | 11.1 | 11.8 | 10.9 | 11 | 10.9 | 10.5 | 10.5 | 10.5 |
| 20–24 | 8.6 | 9.1 | 9.6 | 9.5 | 9.1 | 9.2 | 8.8 | 9.1 |
| 25–29 | 6.7 | 7.1 | 8 | 8.2 | 8.4 | 7.9 | 8.1 | 8 |
| 30–34 | 5.6 | 5.5 | 6.2 | 6.9 | 7.1 | 7.2 | 7 | 7.3 |
| 35–39 | 5.2 | 5.3 | 5 | 5.8 | 6.3 | 6.4 | 6.6 | 6.5 |
| 40–44 | 4 | 4.1 | 4.3 | 4.5 | 5 | 5.4 | 5.6 | 5.9 |
| 45–49 | 3.5 | 3.5 | 3.5 | 3.7 | 4 | 4.4 | 4.8 | 5.1 |
| 50–54 | 2.8 | 2.7 | 2.9 | 3.1 | 3 | 3.4 | 3.9 | 4.2 |
| 55–59 | 2.2 | 2.2 | 2.3 | 2.4 | 2.5 | 2.5 | 2.9 | 3.2 |
| 60–64 | 1.7 | 1.9 | 1.9 | 1.9 | 1.9 | 2.1 | 2.1 | 2.4 |
| 65–69 | 1.1 | 1.2 | 1.5 | 1.3 | 1.4 | 1.5 | 1.6 | 1.6 |
| 70–74 | 0.8 | 0.9 | 0.9 | 0.9 | 1 | 1 | 1.2 | 1.2 |
| 75–79 | 0.4 | 0.3 | 0.6 | 0.6 | 0.6 | 0.7 | 0.7 | 0.8 |
| 80 and over | 0.7 | 0.5 | 0.4 | 0.5 | 0.6 | 0.6 | 0.7 | 0.7 |

*Source*: [8].

*Table 44.3* Philippine population by broad age group

| *Age group* | *1970* | *1975* | *1980* | *1990* | *1995* | *2000* | *2007* | *2010* | *Growth rate * (1970–2010)* |
|---|---|---|---|---|---|---|---|---|---|
| 0–14 | 16,757,313 | 18,493,255 | 20,181,547 | 23,993,713 | 26,296,206 | 28,313,897 | 31,381,020 | 30,717,524 | **1.5** |
| 15–64 | 18,864,652 | 22,375,237 | 26,220,572 | 34,505,317 | 39,905,635 | 45,257,770 | 53,251,374 | 57,374,256 | **2.8** |
| 65–over | 1,062,521 | 1,202,168 | 1,636,341 | 2,060,086 | 2,414,695 | 2,932,410 | 3,664,221 | 4,004,125 | **3.4** |
| ***Total*** | **36,684,486** | **42,070,660** | **48,038,460** | **60,559,116** | **68,616,536** | **76,504,077** | **88,304,615** | **92,095,905** | **2.3** |

*Source*: [8].

*Note*: *Computed as compounded annual growth rate.

*Table 44.4* Median age of ASEAN member states in years

| *Year* | *Philippines* | *Thailand* | *Viet Nam* | *Malaysia* | *Indonesia* | *Singapore* | *Cambodia* | *Myanmar* | *Lao PDR* |
|---|---|---|---|---|---|---|---|---|---|
| 1960 | 17 | 18 | 22 | 18 | 20 | 19 | 19 | 21 | 19 |
| 1970 | 17 | 18 | 18 | 17 | 19 | 20 | 18 | 19 | 19 |
| 1980 | 18 | 20 | 18 | 20 | 19 | 24 | 18 | 20 | 18 |
| 1990 | 19 | 25 | 20 | 21 | 22 | 29 | 18 | 21 | 18 |
| 1995 | 20 | 27 | 21 | 22 | 23 | 32 | 17 | 23 | 18 |
| 2000 | 21 | 30 | 23 | 24 | 25 | 35 | 18 | 25 | 18 |
| 2005 | 22 | 31 | 26 | 25 | 26 | 38 | 20 | 26 | 19 |
| 2010 | 23 | 33 | 29 | 26 | 28 | 41 | 22 | 28 | 21 |
| 2030 | 29 | 39 | 37 | 33 | 35 | 48 | 29 | 35 | 27 |
| 2050 | 35 | 41 | 42 | 38 | 41 | 54 | 35 | 40 | 33 |

*Source*: [8].

*Table 44.5* Life expectancy at birth by sex

| *Year* | *2000* | *2001* | *2002* | *2003* | *2004* | *2005* |
|---|---|---|---|---|---|---|
| Male | 66.3 | 66.6 | 66.9 | 67.2 | 67.5 | 67.8 |
| Female | 71.6 | 71.9 | 72.2 | 72.5 | 72.8 | 72.5 |

*Source*: [62].

- Old-age dependency ratio has increased from 5.6 per cent in 1970 to 7.0 per cent in 2010, which means that more working people now have to support a single retiree [8].

While the quality of life is generally improving, there are pressing health issues that must be addressed. First, the Millennium Development Goals are due in 2015, but the country is lagging behind considerably in some of the health MDGs – neonatal deaths are keeping infant mortality high; the country is likely to miss its target for maternal deaths, with the MMR remaining high at 221 deaths per 100,000 live births as of 2011; and the number of HIV cases reported per month has spiked in the past 25 years. In effect, what the country has is a 'double burden' of diseases, with both communicable and non-communicable diseases (NCDs) occupying the country's top morbidities [9, 10].

From a macroeconomic point of view, chronic poverty continues to be a pressing concern. As of 2009, individual poverty incidence is estimated to fall within 25.6 to 27.3 per cent, with the highest incidence occurring among vulnerable sectors (i.e. fishermen, farmers, children, informal sector and women) and specific regions (i.e. CARAGA at 47.8 per cent, Region V at 45.1 per cent, Region IX at 43.1 per cent and ARMM at 42.8 per cent) (see Figure 44.1a–b) [11]. As of 2012, the unemployment rate and underemployment rate stood at 7 per cent and 22.7 per cent, respectively, signifying that a significant number of people in the labour force are still in search of more productive occupations.

## The Philippines health human resources situation

### *Stocks and trends in production capacity and employment*

Estimating the stock of health human resources in the Philippines can be quite challenging. In the absence of a comprehensive registry or database that can guarantee their numbers and distribution,[1] researchers rely on multiple sources to provide a reliable estimate. At a national level, the Philippines is faring well relative to neighbours in Southeast Asia. In terms of density of doctors, nurses and midwives per 1,000 population, the Philippines showed the highest density at 7.3. At least one recent study reported no critical shortage (below 2.28 per 1,000 population) according to WHO standards [12].

The Philippine HHR situation is characterized by both scarcity and excess. On the one hand, there is an oversupply of nurses – this is driven by increasing global demand and a relatively low local absorptive capacity. On the other hand, there is an underproduction in other categories of other health professionals, such as doctors [13, 14, 15]. To illustrate the point, the Philippines produces 78 nurses per 100,000 population and only 4 doctors per 100,000 population [12]. Since the late 1990s, the country's production of doctors has been rather stagnant at roughly 2,500 doctors annually. The total supply is, of course, depleted by retirement, death and emigration. Since 2005, the number of doctors accredited by the national

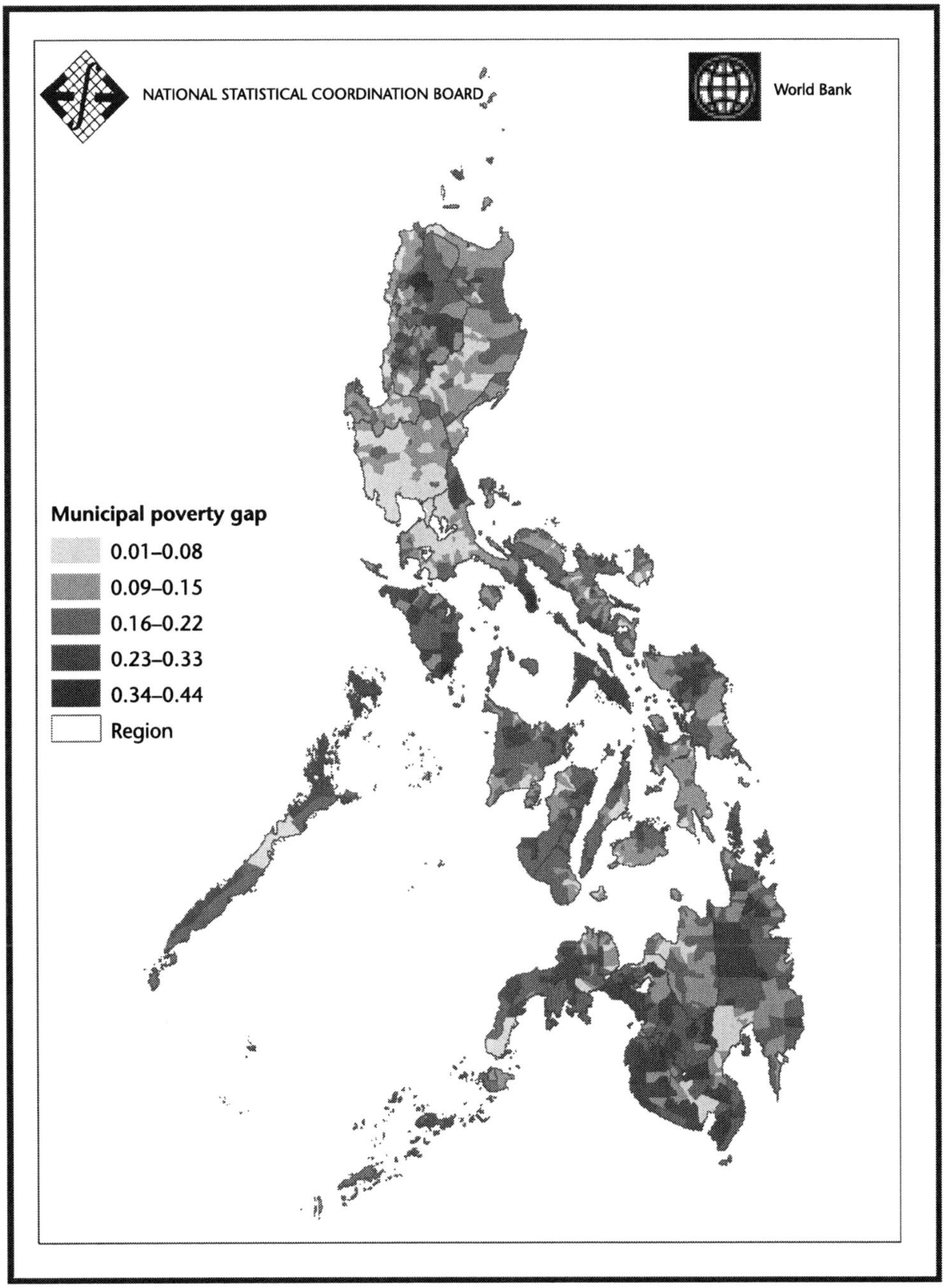


*Figure 44.1a* Philippines poverty gap [61]

(*Continued overleaf*)

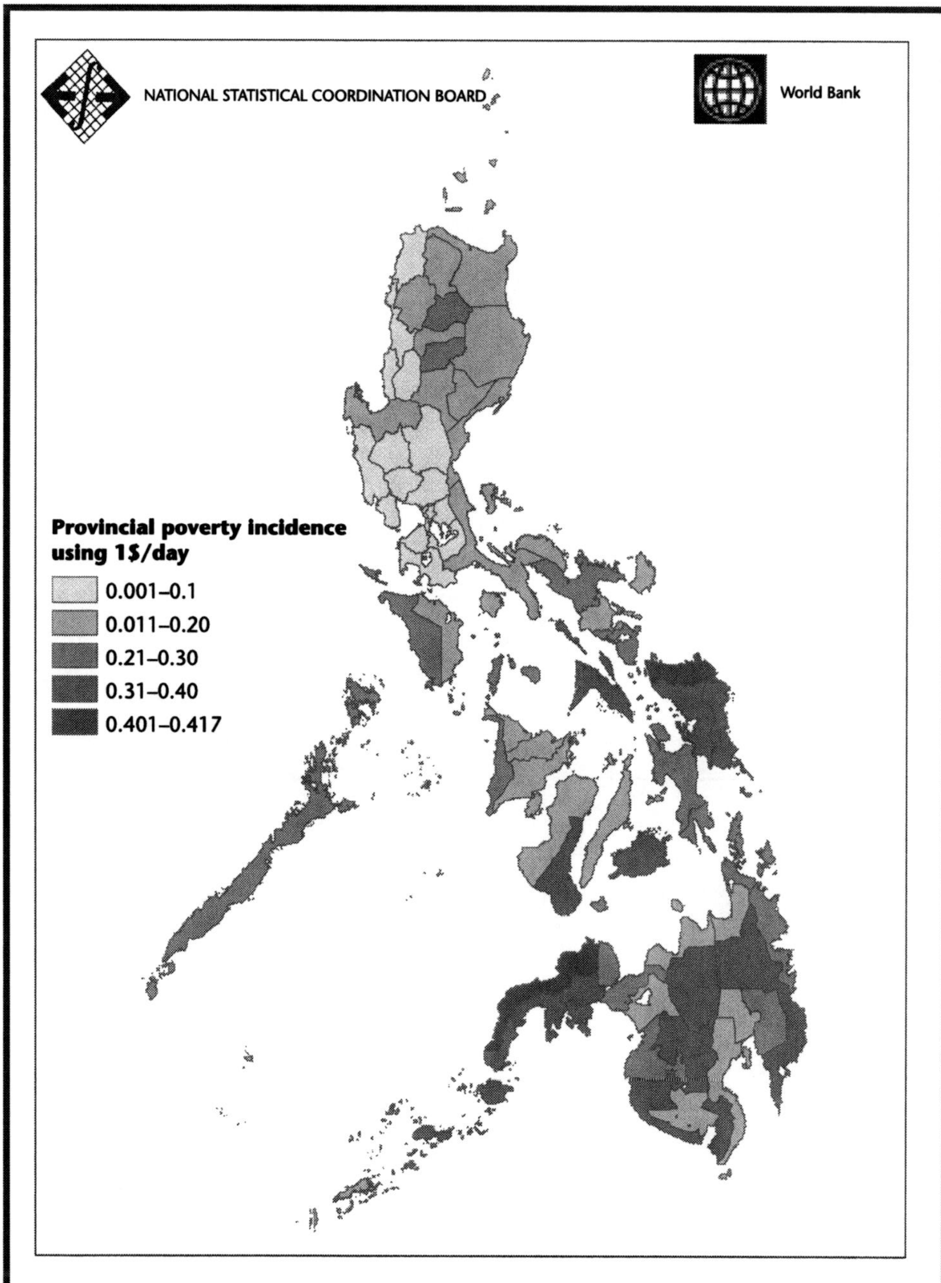


*Figure 44.1b* Continued

social health insurance organization, the Philippine Health Insurance Corporation (PhilHealth or PHIC), and those in the Department of Health's (DOH) National Database on Human Resources for Health Information System (NDHRHIS), which approximate the number of doctors that are actively practising in the country, has ranged from 20,000 to 26,000. Comparing these numbers to the Philippine HRH projected requirement of at least 30,000 doctors beginning 2005 [16] leads to an estimated resource gap of roughly 10,000–20,000 doctors in the country (see Tables 44.6–44.8).

In stark contrast, the country has indeed turned into a nursing market that produces a large supply of nurses for global consumption [17]. In response to overseas demand, enrolments in Bachelors Nursing degrees started increasing rapidly from 2001. By 2009, total graduates reached 140,000 (see Table 44.9 and Figure 44.2). Both the government and private sector were quick to

*Table 44.6* Population growth and growth in the production of nurses and doctors

| *Year* | *Population* | *Percentage change in population* | *Graduates (doctors)* | *Percentage change in doctors* | *Graduates (nurses)* | *Percentage change in nurses* |
|---|---|---|---|---|---|---|
| 2000 | 77,309,965 | – | 2,542 | – | 5,672 | – |
| 2001 | 78,964,389 | 2.14 | 2,345 | (7.75) | 4,409 | (22.27) |
| 2002 | 80,630,416 | 2.11 | 2,732 | 16.50 | 5,425 | 23.04 |
| 2003 | 82,293,990 | 2.06 | 2,812 | 2.93 | 8,477 | 56.26 |
| 2004 | 83,936,698 | 2.00 | 2,420 | (13.94) | 13,120 | 54.77 |
| 2005 | 85,546,427 | 1.92 | 2,745 | 13.43 | 34,582 | 163.58 |
| 2006 | 87,116,275 | 1.84 | 2,892 | 5.36 | 57,457 | 66.15 |
| 2007 | 88,652,631 | 1.76 | 2,058 | (28.84) | 79,149 | 37.75 |
| 2008 | 90,173,139 | 1.72 | 1,732 | (15.84) | 94,863 | 19.85 |
| 2009 | 91,703,090 | 1.70 | No data | No data | 140,330 | 47.93 |
| 2010 | 93,260,798 | 1.70 | No data | No data | 96,936 | (30.92) |

*Sources*: [56, 57].

*Table 44.7* Number of PhilHealth-accredited professionals

| *Health professional* | *2005* | *2006* | *2007* | *2008* | *2009* | *2010* | *2011* |
|---|---|---|---|---|---|---|---|
| ***Doctors (MS + GP)*** | **20,843** | **21,049** | **20,664** | **25,999** | **23,001** | **21,903** | **23,474** |
| Medical Specialist | 10,357 | 10,455 | 10,491 | 13,678 | 11,092 | 11,286 | 12,701 |
| General Practitioner | 10,486 | 10,594 | 10,173 | 12,321 | 11,909 | 10,617 | 10,773 |
| Dentist | 218 | 238 | 208 | 266 | 195 | 184 | 201 |
| Midwife | 87 | 141 | 147 | 313 | 355 | 357 | 522 |

*Source*: [23].

*Table 44.8* Workforce projections for various health professional groups

| *Group* | *2005* | *2010* | *2015* | *2020* | *2025* | *2030* |
|---|---|---|---|---|---|---|
| Doctors | 30,525 | 33,277 | 36,289 | 39,586 | 43,196 | 47,151 |
| Nurses | 170,423 | 185,788 | 202,603 | 221,010 | 241,166 | 263,244 |

*Source*: [16].

*Table 44.9* Number of enrolees and graduates of Medicine and BS Nursing from 1998 to 2011

| *School year* | *Doctors* | | | *School year* | *Nurses* | | |
|---|---|---|---|---|---|---|---|
| | *Enrolees* | *Graduates* | *Percentage graduates* | | *Enrolees* | *Graduates* | *Percentage graduates* |
| 1998–1999 | 13,201 | 2,312 | 17.51 | 1998–1999 | 27,396 | 8,822 | 32.20 |
| 1999–2000 | 14,556 | 2,542 | 17.46 | 1999–2000 | 25,463 | 5,672 | 22.28 |
| 2000–2001 | 15,185 | 2,345 | 15.44 | 2000–2001 | 29,046 | 4,409 | 15.18 |
| 2001–2002 | 13,925 | 2,732 | 19.62 | 2001–2002 | 49,874 | 5,425 | 10.88 |
| 2002–2003 | 15,229 | 2,812 | 18.46 | 2002–2003 | 92,842 | 8,477 | 9.13 |
| 2003–2004 | 11,511 | 2,420 | 21.02 | 2003–2004 | 175,720 | 13,120 | 7.47 |
| 2004–2005 | 11,286 | 2,745 | 24.32 | 2004–2005 | 261,563 | 34,582 | 13.22 |
| 2005–2006 | 10,735 | 2,892 | 26.94 | 2005–2006 | 385,974 | 57,457 | 14.89 |
| 2006–2007 | 10,769 | 2,058 | 19.11 | 2006–2007 | 452,793 | 79,149 | 17.48 |
| 2007–2008 | 8,767 | 1,732 | 19.76 | 2007–2008 | 418,106 | 94,863 | 22.69 |
| | | | | 2008–2009 | 413,680 | 140,330 | 33.92 |
| | | | | 2009–2010 | 342,614 | 96,936 | 28.29 |
| | | | | 2010–2011 | 254,938 | – | – |
| ***Total*** | **125,164** | **24,590** | | ***Total*** | **2,930,009** | **549,242** | **18.75** |

*Source*: [56].

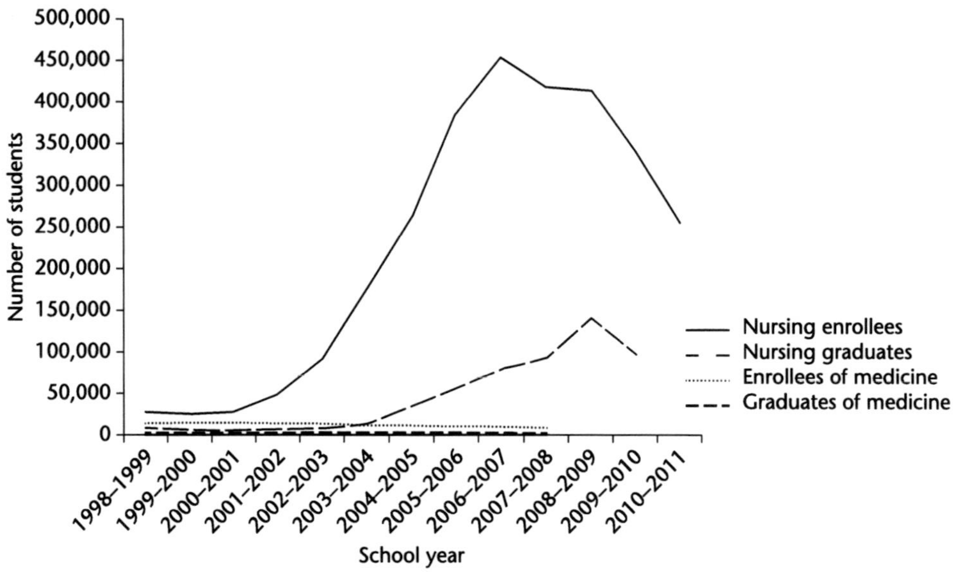


*Figure 44.2* Trends in enrolment and graduation of nurses and doctors [56]

respond to the demand and 28 new nursing schools (18 private and 10 public) were opened (see Table 44.10). Currently, the Philippines is second only to Indonesia in having the highest number of nursing institutions/schools in Southeast Asia (i.e. 517 versus 682 schools) [12].

The DOH-NDRHIS data, however, registers only 36,500 nurses across all regions raising the question of where the remaining nursing graduates are. In 2008 alone, around 400,000

*Table 44.10* Increase in number of nursing schools from 2006 to 2008

| *Region* | *AY 2006–2007* | | *AY 2007–2008* | | *Percentage change in no. of schools (gov't)* | *Percentage change in no. of schools (private)* |
|---|---|---|---|---|---|---|
| | *Government* | *Private* | *Government* | *Private* | | |
| NCR | 7 | 85 | 7 | 89 | 0.00 | 4.71 |
| CAR | 3 | 12 | 3 | 13 | 0.00 | 8.33 |
| I – Ilocos Region | 6 | 23 | 6 | 24 | 0.00 | 4.35 |
| II – Cagayan Valley | 2 | 14 | 2 | 14 | 0.00 | 0.00 |
| III – Central Luzon | 11 | 36 | 14 | 40 | 27.27 | 11.11 |
| IVA – CALABARZON | 7 | 52 | 8 | 53 | 14.29 | 1.92 |
| IVB – MIMAROPA | 2 | 5 | 2 | 6 | 0.00 | 20.00 |
| V – Bicol Region | 5 | 20 | 5 | 20 | 0.00 | 0.00 |
| VI – Western Visayas | 2 | 18 | 2 | 18 | 0.00 | 0.00 |
| VII – Central Visayas | 4 | 29 | 8 | 28 | 100.00 | –3.45 |
| VIII – Eastern Visayas | 4 | 12 | 4 | 12 | 0.00 | 0.00 |
| IX – Zamboanga Peninsula | 2 | 12 | 3 | 12 | 50.00 | 0.00 |
| X – Northern Mindanao | 4 | 17 | 4 | 17 | 0.00 | 0.00 |
| XI – Davao Region | 0 | 19 | 1 | 21 | 100.00 | 10.53 |
| XII – SOCCSKSARGEN | 1 | 11 | 1 | 16 | 0.00 | 45.45 |
| CARAGA | 0 | 7 | 0 | 7 | 0.00 | 0.00 |
| ARMM | 0 | 6 | 0 | 6 | 0.00 | 0.00 |
| ***Total*** | **60** | **378** | **70** | **396** | **16.67** | **4.76** |

*Source*: [56].

licensed nurses were not gainfully employed [18]. There was clearly a gap between absorptive capacity and production capacity, and problems arise when production is not in sync with recruitment and employment.

In the Philippines, government recruitment is stalled by rigid processes and structures. As a result of population increases, the need is continually increasing. However, the creation of permanent positions available in government cannot be adjusted easily [9, 15]. On the other hand, the education sector has morphed into machinery that focuses on production. What has developed is a 'market-driven, export-led production of nurses and doctors that seeks to respond to international demand' [12]. While in the 1950s, state universities had a monopoly over nursing education, the situation changed drastically when global demand peaked in the 1990s. This prompted the enterprising private sector to respond aggressively by expanding nursing programmes (i.e. a mushrooming or proliferation of nursing schools took place) in an attempt to maximize profit. There wasn't necessarily appropriate consideration for quality of education and students' subsequent employment opportunities. Since teaching and training resources could not keep up with the volume of students, the quality of teaching, supervision and student competency were compromised [12]. Figure 44.3 illustrates this decline in quality, as reflected by the significant decrease in the average passing rates for the Board of Nursing licensure exam from 1992 to 2011 [19].

Figure 44.2 and Table 44.9 show the apparent disparity between the number of nursing enrolees and graduates. Only 19 per cent actually graduate and this number is further reduced

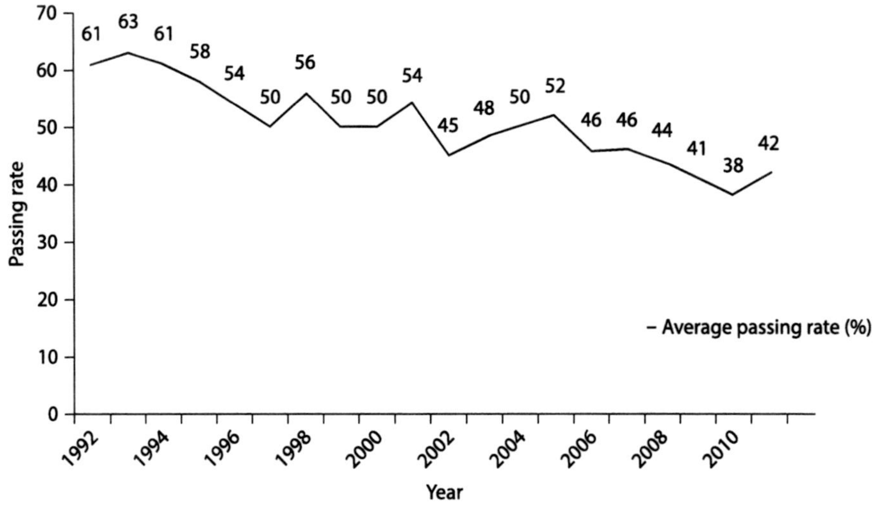


*Figure 44.3* Average passing rate for Board of Nursing licensure exam, 1992–2011 [19]

by those who do not pass the licensure exam. Since 2011, the Commission on Higher Education (CHED) has already closed down about 700 programmes in the Philippines due to poor quality of education. They are anticipating phasing out more if quality standards are not met [20].

Unable to find gainful employment and practise their nursing profession domestically, nursing graduates end up engaging in what Villagomeza [21] calls 'interprofessional migration' from nursing to other non-health professions. Given the skill sets that they have acquired during their undergraduate education (i.e. adaptability to night shift routines, fluency in English, service orientation, people skills), Business Process Outsourcing Organizations (BPOs), especially those engaged in health-related services, find these fresh graduates very suitable for hiring. As business process outsourcing is now a very lucrative industry in the Philippines, these graduates are compensated well, thereby having no more incentive to revert to nursing [17].

## *Inequitable distribution of health human resources*

Mirroring the experience of other countries in Southeast Asia, the inequitable distribution of health human resources is a long-running problem in the Philippines [12, 15]. Table 44.11 shows the distribution of HHR per region and sector. Consistent with the literature [13, 15], more physicians continue to practise in the private sector. The trend for nurses was slightly reversed in 2012, which may be attributed to the mass hiring of nurses by the DOH and the Philippine Health Insurance Corporation (PhilHealth) for their RNHeals and PhilHealth CARES (Customer Assistance, Relations and Empowerment Staff) programmes, which aim to deploy more than 20,000 nurses to improve service delivery in communities [22, 23].

Even though the country seems to be doing well on an aggregate level, the geographic distribution of HHR (see Table 44.11, and Figures 44.4 and 44.5) paints a quite different picture. The National Capital Region and two nearby regions, Regions III and IV-A, host almost half of the total number of doctors and nurses in the country, as of December 2012, and the poorest regions in Mindanao (ARMM and CARAGA) have less than 3 per cent of these health professionals.

*Table 44.11* Distribution of doctors and nurses per region and sector, December 2012

| *Region* | *Doctor* | | *Nurse* | |
|---|---|---|---|---|
| | *Private* | *Public* | *Private* | *Public* |
| NCR | 4,234 | 4,305 | 3,880 | 5,577 |
| CAR | 330 | 466 | 528 | 822 |
| I – Ilocos Region | 720 | 703 | 1,138 | 1,161 |
| II – Cagayan Valley | 321 | 458 | 620 | 742 |
| III – Central Luzon | 1,602 | 955 | 2,060 | 1,456 |
| IVA – CALABARZON | 1,745 | 513 | 2,864 | 754 |
| IVB – MIMAROPA | 127 | 287 | 145 | 616 |
| V – Bicol Region | 310 | 456 | 390 | 910 |
| VI – Western Visayas | 505 | 509 | 1,085 | 821 |
| VII – Central Visayas | 466 | 633 | 1,751 | 983 |
| VIII – Eastern Visayas | 259 | 450 | 330 | 838 |
| IX – Zamboanga Peninsula | 182 | 377 | 637 | 875 |
| X – Northern Mindanao | 353 | 540 | 846 | 1,057 |
| XI – Davao Region | 488 | 219 | 635 | 349 |
| XII – SOCCSKSARGEN | 460 | 324 | 1,055 | 624 |
| CARAGA | 128 | 292 | 256 | 674 |
| ARMM | 0 | 59 | 0 | 69 |
| ***Total*** | **12,230** | **11,546** | **18,220** | **18,328** |
| Overall | | 23,776 | | 36,548 |

*Source*: [58].

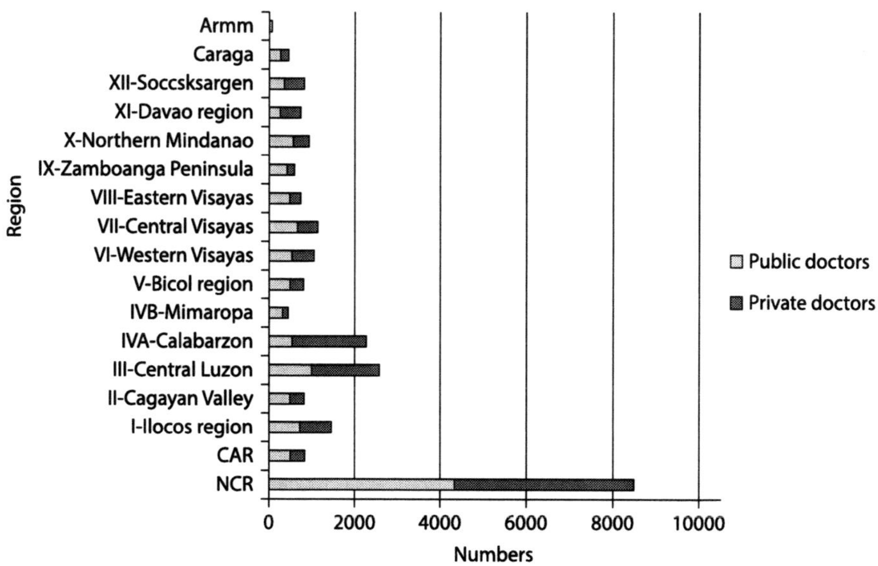


*Figure 44.4* Distribution of doctors per region, December 2012 [58]

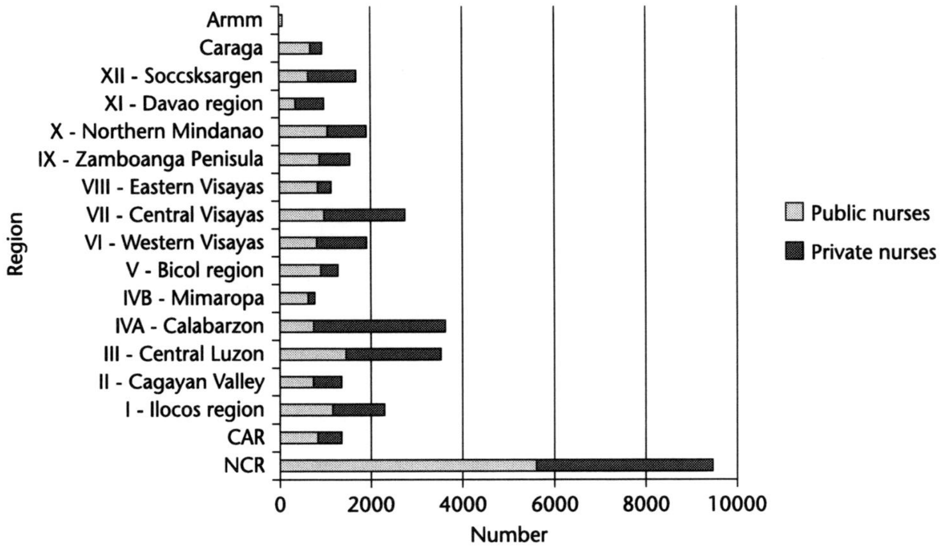


*Figure 44.5* Distribution of nurses per region, December 2012 [58]

Table 44.12 shows the urban–rural divide, with public nurses being the exception. Private/public doctors and private nurses tend to be highly concentrated in urban centres.[2] Many factors contribute to this inclination to practise in urban centres, but the most influential of them are economic incentives, including higher salaries and wages, professional career and development opportunities, and higher living standards [12, 15]. In the Mindanao areas that are affected by active conflict (e.g. ARMM), physical safety is the primary concern of workers.

In the Philippines, salaries for government employees are standardized by law and fixed according to salary grades (SG). Government physicians start at SG18 (i.e. for residency training and local government posts), medical specialists at SG22–24, hospital chiefs at SG25–27 and top-level officials at SG27–30.[3] With these salary grades (see Table 44.13), monthly income ranges from PhP 31,000 (USD 756) to PhP 85,000 (USD 2,073). In addition to this basic salary, government doctors can obtain an 'authority to (private) practise' from

*Table 44.12* Urban–rural distribution of doctors and nurses, 2012

| *Urban/ rural* | *Doctors* | | | | *Total in per cent* | *Nurses* | | | | *Total in per cent* |
|---|---|---|---|---|---|---|---|---|---|---|
| | *Private* | | *Public* | | | *Private* | | *Public* | | |
| | *No.* | *Per cent* | *No.* | *Per cent* | | *No.* | *Per cent* | *No.* | *Per cent* | |
| Urban* | 8,535 | 69.79 | 6,625 | 57.38 | 63.76 | 11,190 | 61.42 | 9,119 | 49.75 | 55.57 |
| Rural** | 3,695 | 30.21 | 4,921 | 42.62 | 36.24 | 7,030 | 38.58 | 9,209 | 50.25 | 44.43 |

*Source*: [58].

*Notes*: * Urban – NCR, Regions III, IVA, VII, XI.
** Rural – CAR, I, II, IVB, V, VI, VIII, IX, X, XII, CARAGA, ARMM.

*Table 44.13* Base pay per salary grade, April 2012

| *Professional* | *Salary grade* | *Step 1 (Min)* | | *Step 8 (Max)* | |
|---|---|---|---|---|---|
| | | *In PhP* | *In USD** | *In PhP* | *In USD** |
| **Nurses** | **11** | 18,549 | 452 | 19,887 | 485 |
| | **12** | 19,940 | 486 | 21,379 | 521 |
| | **15** | 24,887 | 607 | 26,868 | 655 |
| | **18** | 31,351 | 765 | 33,846 | 826 |
| | **19** | 33,859 | 826 | 36,554 | 892 |
| | **20** | 36,567 | 892 | 39,478 | 963 |
| | **21** | 39,493 | 963 | 42,636 | 1,040 |
| | **22** | 42,652 | 1,040 | 46,047 | 1,123 |
| | **23** | 46,064 | 1,124 | 49,731 | 1,213 |
| **Doctors** | **24** | 49,750 | 1,213 | 53,709 | 1,310 |
| | **25** | 53,730 | 1,310 | 58,006 | 1,415 |
| | **26** | 58,028 | 1,415 | 62,646 | 1,528 |
| | **27** | 62,670 | 1,529 | 67,658 | 1,650 |
| | **28** | 67,684 | 1,651 | 73,071 | 1,782 |
| | **29** | 73,099 | 1,783 | 78,916 | 1,925 |
| | **30** | 78,946 | 1,926 | 85,320 | 2,081 |

*Source*: [59].

*Note*: * Exchange rate: USD 1: PhP 41.

their employer so this can become an additional source of income [14]. For private practitioners, monthly income depends heavily on the volume of patients seen since most doctors act as consultants[4] and are therefore not salaried by the hospitals (unless they fulfil administrative duties). Higher professional fees come with seniority or experience, a higher degree of specialization and character of local demand (with both numbers and relative ability to pay being higher in urban centres). At a minimum, monthly income ranges from PhP 50,000/ USD 1,219 for general practitioners to PhP 100,000/USD 2,439 for specialists. They are also entitled to receive fees from social and private insurers [14].

Salaries of nurses are significantly lower than those for physicians. While the Nursing Law of 2002 mandates that starting salaries of government nurses be pegged at SG15, which is equivalent to about PhP 25,000/USD 610 (see Table 44.13), budget and other constraints have resulted in this provision not being strictly implemented and nurses receive only rates for SG11–SG12, which is about PhP 6,000/USD 146 lower than what is required. Nurses in the private sector, on the other hand, receive even lower compensation. Those practising in small private hospitals can receive salaries as low as PhP 4,000/USD 100 to PhP 5,000/USD 122 per month [14]. Low compensation has been a source of extreme dissatisfaction among nurses, driving them to other countries in search of better remuneration and even to the streets to rally [24].

## *Migration of health human resources*

In 2003, it was estimated that a staggering 85 per cent or more than 300,000 of the country's nurses choose to work abroad [9, 17, 25]. Figure 44.6 shows the fluctuating nature of nurse

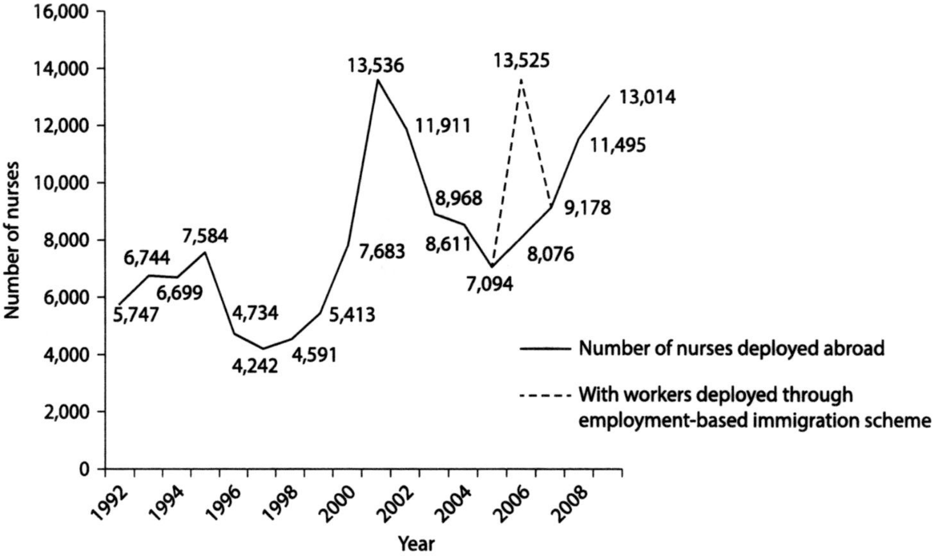


*Figure 44.6* Number of nurses deployed abroad, 1992–2009 [60]

migration, with a rapid increase in the number of nurses deployed abroad starting in the late 1990s, reaching peaks in 2001 at 13,536, 2006 at 13,525 and 2009 at 13,014. Although several downtrends can be observed – the most recent ones being attributed to the global recession, stricter migration regulations and stiff competition from other countries also in the business of exporting nurses – rapid increases are expected from 2011 onwards [17]. Filipino nurses continue to have a competitive edge in the market due to their high performance, fluency in speaking the English language, service orientation and caring nature [17, 26].

Tables 44.14 and 44.15 show that this massive emigration can be either permanent or temporary in nature. While two out of three doctors migrate permanently, around 80 per cent of nurses tend to migrate temporarily, with the Middle East, UK and Singapore as their primary destinations. The top three destinations for permanent migration are

*Table 44.14* Number of deployed Filipino nurses by top destination countries, new hires, 2004–2010

| *Country* | *2004* | *2005* | *2006* | *2007* | *2008* | *2009* | *2010* |
|---|---|---|---|---|---|---|---|
| ***All destinations*** | **8,879** | **7,768** | **8,528** | **9,004** | **12,618** | **13,465** | **12,431** |
| Saudi Arabia | 5,926 | 4,886 | 5,753 | 6,633 | 8,848 | 9,965 | 8,771 |
| Singapore | 166 | 149 | 86 | 276 | 667 | 745 | 723 |
| United Arab Emirates | 250 | 703 | 796 | 616 | 435 | 572 | 478 |
| Libya | 10 | 23 | 158 | 66 | 104 | 276 | 417 |
| Kuwait | 408 | 193 | 354 | 393 | 458 | 423 | 409 |
| United Kingdom | 800 | 546 | 145 | 38 | 27 | 51 | 66 |
| Qatar | 318 | 133 | 141 | 214 | 245 | 133 | 294 |
| Taiwan | 6 | 357 | 273 | 174 | 231 | 202 | 252 |
| Jordan | 120 | 2 | 38 | 27 | 51 | 66 | 112 |
| Bahrain | 46 | 38 | 67 | 24 | 63 | 55 | 93 |

*Source*: [27].

*Table 44.15* Distribution of health professionals by type of migration, 1997–2008

| *Health professional* | *1997* | *1998* | *1999* | *2000* | *2001* | *2002* | *2003* | *2004* | *2005* | *2006* | *2007* | *2008* | *Total* | *Percent* |
|---|---|---|---|---|---|---|---|---|---|---|---|---|---|---|
| ***Doctors*** | | | | | | | | | | | | | | |
| Temporary | 60 | 55 | 59 | 27 | 61 | 129 | 112 | 91 | 97 | 169 | 164 | 214 | 1,238 | 33.66 |
| Permanent | – | 128 | 65 | 158 | 179 | 204 | 237 | 295 | 275 | 358 | 286 | 255 | 2,440 | 66.34 |
| ***Nurses*** | | | | | | | | | | | | | | |
| Temporary | 4,242 | 4,591 | 5,413 | 7,683 | 13,536 | 11,866 | 8,968 | 8,611 | 10,718 | 8,076 | 8,429 | 11,495 | 103,628 | 80.90 |
| Permanent | 438 | 321 | 370 | 1,231 | 1,575 | 2,248 | 2,245 | 3,988 | 3,827 | 5,953 | 1,267 | 1,009 | 24,472 | 19.10 |

*Source*: [15].

the USA, Canada and Australia – developed countries that are considered favourable for residence [15, 27]. This massive outflow of human resources raises a red flag that cannot be ignored – why is it that so many Filipino doctors and nurses migrate overseas? Analogous to the determinants of domestic distribution, a mix of 'push' and 'pull' factors are said to account for this. As rational economic agents that seek to maximize their economic gains, factors related to work and professional development are the most significant drivers of migration [28].

Aside from being a 'job-scarce environment' (for example, the low absorptive capacity to hire nurses), poor working conditions are said to push nurses out of the country. Nurses are overworked given their high patient load and long duty hours, but continue to be undercompensated. The salary differential is quite astounding – as of 2006, medical doctors earning a monthly average of USD 342.16 in the Philippines can earn six times more (USD 2,614.22) in foreign countries. Nurses being paid only USD 168.76 per month in the Philippines can earn up to USD 342.47–718.39 [14, 29] and even USD 3,000–5,000, according to some anecdotes [24]. It is not surprising that the substantially higher salary levels pull health human resources out of the country in large numbers.

A few years ago, the phenomenon of Filipino nurse medics (i.e. doctors training to practise as nurses) – another form of interprofessional migration – has caught the attention of many. Although actual numbers remain unavailable, estimates say that the number of nurse medics has grown from 2,000 in 2001 to about 9,000–11,000 in 2009. In addition to economic and work-related factors, a more interesting mix of push–pull factors was noted to result in this behaviour. One factor is immigration-related – it is said that it is easier to get a visa as a nurse than as a doctor. At that time, there was also an impending threat brought about by the proposed malpractice law and compulsory malpractice insurance for doctors in the Philippines [21, 28].

One of the enabling elements to this movement of persons within Southeast Asia is the ASEAN Framework Agreement on Services signed in 1995. The agreement aims to enhance cooperation within the region and progressively liberalize trade in services in order to boost its efficiency and global competitiveness. Cooperation[5] is geared toward improving production capacity, while trade liberalization facilitates and streamlines the acquisition of productive inputs to service production and delivery [30, 31, 32]. The same agreement provides for a system of 'mutual recognition', such that member states 'may recognise the education or experience obtained, requirements met, or licenses or certifications granted in another Member State, for the purpose of licensing or certification of service suppliers'.

In 2006, a mutual recognition agreement (MRA) for nursing services was signed, followed by another MRA for medical practitioners in 2008. Both MRAs aim to facilitate and promote the mobility of persons, exchange of information and expertise, adoption of best practices and access to capacity building/training opportunities [30, 31, 32]. As in any mutual agreement, the implementation of these MRAs is met with many obstacles, most of which stem from the diversity of the member states in terms of education and training, regulation, professional practices, and culture and norms, among other factors. The required work experience (three years for nurses and five years for doctors) also proves to be difficult to comply with [12] and creates a vacuum for skilled personnel for the countries of origin, who have invested in the training of these workers.

## Moving forward: implications on health human resource management

Globalization is a fact of life. All countries, including the Philippines, need to find an appropriate approach to global market integration. The movement of health human resources is one of the most tangible manifestations of the country's contribution to the world economy. This movement, however, is a double-edged sword. While it is indeed beneficial for the Philippine economy's growth and resilience, and has undoubtedly helped improve the lives of migrant workers and their families, it does create gaps in the national health system that cannot be left unaddressed.

Over the years, the Philippines has developed many innovations and solutions to help the country cope with these health human resource gaps and issues. A common theme is that these solutions do not resist global demand, but rather create competitive alternatives to keep human resources in the country in order to address local needs.

## *Government-initiated mass hiring and mobilization of health human resources: Doctors to the Barrio (DTTB) Programme and other parallel programmes*

Beginning with the Doctors to the Barrio[6] (DTTB) programme, the DOH has spearheaded programmes that aim to deploy health professionals to the poorest and most remote areas of the country that for the longest time have been unreached and underserved by the health system (referred to as 'doctorless' and single-doctor communities). Three other programmes that parallel the DTTB are the Leaders for Health Programme, also for doctors, and the RNHeals and PhilHealth CARES programmes for nurses.

### Doctors to the Barrio (DTTB) Programme

The DTTB programme was launched in 1993 to address the shortage of doctors in 271 poor and far-flung municipalities in the Philippines that registered the highest morbidity and mortality rates due to disease and poor health conditions [33]. The programme was implemented at a critical time when the Local Government Code of 1991 was just being implemented and the country was transitioning to a devolved health system wherein service delivery, including management of health workers, became the responsibility of local politicians who lacked the needed competencies to manage health systems. These changes damaged the morale of health staff and led to massive resignations. Relative to urban areas, local government units (LGUs) from rural areas could not offer incentives that were attractive enough to bring in doctors. The combination of these factors led to the shortage and decline in health outcomes [34].

The DTTB programme deploys doctors in batches, twice or thrice annually, to underserved rural communities. For a minimum of two years, these doctors assume the role of municipal health officers (MHO) in the community and are essentially responsible for running their entire local health system (i.e. policy and programme implementation, resource management and development, service delivery and management of information systems, among others). Given the enormity of the task at hand, a good financial and incentive package had to be designed. As regular SG24 employees of the national DOH, they received healthy salaries and a full set of employee benefits (e.g. employee compensation, social security and health insurance benefits, clothing, subsistence, and a laundry and hazard allowance), and were also given priority status if they decided to pursue further studies, including a Master's degree or clinical residency programmes [34]. The programme was eventually expanded to factor in population growth – more than one doctor was deployed per municipality and those on study leave had to be covered. To augment the existing incentive package, Continuing Medical Education (CME), was offered to the DTTBs [34]. CME covers courses that intend to upgrade the skills of doctors. The Certificate Course in eHealth and telemedicine offered to the twenty-ninth batch of deployed doctors, for instance, is a six-month blended learning course interspersed with intensive face-to-face activities and field practice and mentoring. This teaches doctors how to use telemedicine applications, including telereferrals, which link doctors in the poorest municipalities (i.e. bottom fifth and sixth class municipalities) and geographically isolated and disadvantaged areas to specialists in the Philippine General Hospital when they encounter difficult-to-handle cases [35]. Through a partnership between the DOH and the Development Academy of the Philippines, the most recent batches are allowed to credit their CMEs for a Master's degree in Public Management with a major in Health Systems and Development [34]. Deployment is now implemented annually to accommodate this development.

The DTTB programme became vulnerable to the rapid out-migration of doctors in the country, especially in 2005. It was a good thing that the media took notice of the programme, portraying DTTB doctors as heroes who needed everyone's support. This led to an increase in application rates and political backing for the programme, including support for doctors' equipment and medical scholarships that were tied to mandatory deployment and service in rural areas [34, 36, 37].

As of November 2012, the DOH has deployed 29 batches of doctors, mobilizing 553 physicians to serve in 390 municipalities across the country since the programme started. The most recent batch was the largest with 114 recruits (92 deployed as of November). Concerns have been raised, however, on the recent change in the DOH's employment practice for this last batch whose doctors were hired as contractual employees, rather than being given regular positions. While the expected salary is generally higher, these doctors are no longer entitled to receive the full set of benefits mandated by the implementing rules and regulations of the DTTB programme [38, 39]. The effect of this shift in employment practice is yet to be observed.

The biggest issue that currently faces the DTTB programme is the retention of doctors. Monitoring shows that out of the 452 doctors who participated in the programme from 1993 to 2011, only 81 (18 per cent) chose to stay in their posts and be absorbed by the LGU permanently as their own employee. A study conducted by Leonardia *et al.* [34] shows that the factor that influences retention the most is local government support that provides an enabling environment for doctors to manage their local health systems effectively. Skewed politics and lack of support can be demoralizing to doctors [40]. Moreover, 'where LGU support is lacking, personal security, the availability of drugs, medical supplies, health program funds and even the provision of DTTB benefits become problematic' [34].

## Leaders for Health Programme (LHP)

In recognition of the reality that an LGU's prioritization of health is indeed vital for local health systems to run effectively, the Leaders for Health Programme (LHP) was created. LHP is a product of a tripartite agreement between the DOH, the Ateneo Graduate School of Business and Pfizer Philippines Foundation. Similar to the DTTB, the programme also fields volunteer doctors for two years, but provides a more in-depth pre-service and on-service support for these doctors [41]. The programme offers a two-pronged approach to build local health system capacity [41]:

1 As part of a Master's degree programme in Health Care Management, innovative learning approaches, including classroom and online interactions, are used to train volunteer doctors. Support in the form of retreats, incentives and performance-based recognitions continues to be given once they are onsite; and

2 An important innovation that was introduced by the programme is the capacity building of 'local health leaders', including the volunteer doctor assuming the role of a municipal health officer, the municipal mayor and local community leaders. This team is brought together to collaborate in developing and implementing a 'comprehensive and systemic approach' to address the community's health issues.

The LHP recognizes that indeed, doctors are not silver bullets and they cannot act alone in order to make a health system work. Local government and community support are of utmost importance.

With respect to the concern of retention of the DTTBs, the following recommendations can be derived from the study of Leonardia *et al.* [34] and lessons from the LHP:

1 Provide continuing support from the DOH, especially in terms of education and training. It has been noted that support diminishes once doctors are absorbed by the LGUs. This is actually a critical phase because it is at this point when doctors become more vulnerable to local politics and governance issues;
2 Ensure availability of adequate supplies and equipment at the local level to enable the delivery of quality care;
3 Provide a more adequate compensation package. While DTTBs are fairly compensated during the first two years that they are contracted by the programme, it has been noted that they suffer from salary downgrades upon absorption in LGUs, especially in poorer municipalities. Considering that most doctors have families to support, this is a critical issue that must be addressed. Total remuneration solutions must include benefits, not simply cash compensation; and
4 Develop capacity-building programmes that involve key people in communities to complement the pool of health human resources in the area.

## RNHeals and PhilHealth CARES programmes

The Registered Nurses for Health Enhancement and Local Service (RNHeals) Programme of the DOH and PhilHealth Customer Assistance Relations and Empowerment Staff (PhilHealth CARES) address the recruitment and deployment of nurses.

The primary intention of RNHeals is capacity building of nurses. They are deployed as pre-service trainees to support service delivery in hospital and community settings (i.e. rural health units). They receive a monthly allowance of PhP 8,000 (USD 200) with health and social security benefits. More than 30,000 (see Table 44.16) nurses have been deployed to municipalities, cities and DOH hospitals across the country since the programme's implementation in 2011, and about 22,500 nurses were expected to be deployed in January 2013 [22, 42].

PhilHealth CARES was launched by the Philippine Health Insurance Corporation in 2012, deploying an initial batch of 530 registered nurses to all accredited Level 3 and 4 hospitals and Level 1 and 2 government hospitals on a rotation basis. CARES nurses respond to basic member and stakeholder enquiries, with the primary intention of improving their knowledge and utilization of insurance benefits. These nurses were hired as SG15 project-based contractors receiving a salary of PhP 15,500 (USD 388) per month with a PhP 300 (USD 7) communication allowance [23].

While these programmes are yet to be assessed, their transitory nature and continuing sustainability raises concerns [9]. The relatively short contract duration of one year has been

*Table 44.16* RNHeals deployment

| *Batch* | *Deployment schedule* | *Number of deployed nurses* | *Areas served* |
|---|---|---|---|
| 1 | Feb. 2011 | 9,518 | 1,235 municipalities |
| 2 | Oct. 2011 | 11,283 | 70 DOH hospitals, 1,500 municipalities and cities |
| 3 | Mar. 2012 | 10,000 | 1,491 municipalities and 143 cities |
| 4 | Jan. 2013 | 22,500 | 70 DOH hospitals, 1,491 municipalities, 143 cities, 13 districts of Metro Manila |

*Source*: [42].

criticized as too short to allow effective integration into their respective settings and produce expected outputs. For PhilHealth CARES specifically, initial feedback suggests that training quality must be improved before deploying these nurses. Their knowledge of fine points in membership and benefits that can be applied on a case-to-case basis is critical for their functioning as customer empowerment staff.

As a training programme, the DOH must recognize that one of the advantages that their RNHeals nurses can acquire is context-specific knowledge – an in-depth understanding of the systems and dynamics in the communities to which they were assigned and how these contribute to/undermine the achievement of desired health outcomes. This understanding can only be fully leveraged if these nurses are eventually retained and integrated into these settings. This issue of uprooting trained/skilled professionals from the settings where they are beginning to integrate mimics the problem that countries face with the mutual recognition agreements for nursing services and medical practitioners. Since work experience is required, it means that individual countries have to give up skilled staff especially from rural areas where experienced workers are scarce and hence difficult to replace.

## *EntrepreNurse: generating employment and achieving public health objectives*

In response to the oversupply and unemployment of many licensed nurses in the country, EntrepreNurse was launched in 2010 by the Philippine Department of Labour and Employment (DOLE), in collaboration with the DOH, Board of Nursing – Professional Regulation Commission (BON-PRC), PhilHealth, the University of the Philippines College of Nursing (UPCN), the Philippine Nurses Association (PNA) and other local institutions. EntrepreNurse is an innovation that marries both employment and public health objectives. It encourages nurse entrepreneurship 'by giving opportunities to unemployed licensed nurses to create cooperatives servicing health care needs of the rural poor communities' [43, 44].

The process begins when a group of nurses get together to organize themselves as a cooperative and formally register under the Cooperatives Development Authority (CDA). In close coordination with the local community and government units, the registered cooperative will prepare a business proposal and design that takes into consideration both the actual needs of the community as well as business viability. This proposal will then be marketed and presented to DOLE, the LGU and other potential donors to secure specific funding for the initiative. Currently, DOLE has budgeted about PhP 300,000 to PhP 500,000 (USD 7,500 to USD 12,500) for the start-up capital of promising cooperatives [44, 45, 46].

Cooperatives are expected to serve as the focal point of service delivery. Upon establishment of nursing clinics, they can explore various forms of entrepreneurship (i.e. facility management, outsourcing of service delivery, etc.) and services to be offered. This could include primary and home healthcare services, diagnostic services, emergency medical services and community-based pharmacies. Cooperatives would then deploy nurses to poor and underserved communities (one nurse per month per village) as health educators and service providers. They would be paid on a per-visit basis at no less than PhP 1,000/USD 25 per visit by the LGU, PhilHealth/HMO or the patient if he/she has the capacity to pay. With grant money from DOLE for five cooperatives, the programme is now being pilot-tested in five provinces in Mindanao [17, 43, 44, 45].

The success and sustainability of the cooperatives rely heavily on how well they are managed. The training of nurses in management and business practices is deemed critical [45]. Moreover, nurses should learn to take advantage of available funding streams, including reimbursements from PhilHealth, which have been found to fuel facility enhancement even in resource-scarce environments. In essence, money really flows into the facility as a function of the volume of PhilHealth members they cater to. The first step in accessing this stream is to ensure that their facilities are accredited or contracted by PhilHealth to service their pool of members [47].

### *Medical tourism and foreign retirement in the Philippines*

Medical tourism started gaining ground in the Philippines in the 1970s when the government started establishing speciality hospitals such as the Philippine Heart Center, the National Kidney Transplant Institute and the Lung Center of the Philippines, with the vision of making the Philippines the medical centre of Asia [48]. In recent years, the thrust to develop medical tourism has begun to originate not from the health sector but from other government branches, such as the Office of the President and Department of Tourism. In 2004, the president mandated agencies to pursue strategies for expanding exports in three sectors, including health and wellness. This gave way to the establishment of the Philippine Medical Tourism Program (PMTP), a private–public partnership programme, and an enabling legal scaffold, Republic Act No. 9593 or the Tourism Act of 2009, which aims to develop and promote the country as a centre for medical tourism [48]. In 2010, this was followed by an act that aims to institute a 'comprehensive and holistic mechanism for the promotion of medical tourism in the country' [49], but the bill has not yet been legislated to date, possibly due to prioritization of policies in the country. There are some (understandable) concerns about the possible negative effect of unbridled medical tourism on the availability of services to citizens.

While the PMTP's target is to establish an enabling environment that would allow the country to earn annual revenues of least USD 2 billion from the booming global medical tourism market (estimated to be at USD 40 billion in 2010 and projected to grow rapidly to USD 70 billion by 2013), a 2011 study showed that there was a 'failure to sustain and effectively capitalize on the momentum of the PMTP' [50] leading to lost opportunities for the country. Data on the exact counts of medical tourists in the country continue to be lacking (as there is no clear data gathering mechanism), but there is a report that the Philippines catered to 250,000 non-resident patients in 2006, generating revenue of USD 350 million, 14 per cent of the Asian market at the time [51]. Another source showed that the number of medical tourists was 100,000 in 2010 [48].

Longer waiting times, inadequate supply and limited coverage, and expensive healthcare costs are what push these tourists out of their home countries in search of high-quality medical services offered at lower costs. These factors as well as ageing populations and the current economic/financial crisis in many countries are driving individual retirees and their governments to search for countries where the elderly population can settle [12, 50, 52, 53].

Currently, Singapore, Malaysia and Thailand are the top destinations for those seeking health care in Southeast Asia. These countries have invested heavily in the necessary infrastructure and a policy and incentive framework that would attract tourists from all over the world. Nonetheless, the Philippines is considered to be an emerging competitor and it is highly probable that it will catch up if it 'puts in place [an] attractive investment environment that will enable the country to expand its healthcare infrastructure, more open and liberal travel arrangements for medical tourists and better and more extensive international marketing promotions programs' [52], and establishes a quality health management system that is built around predictability, accountability and consistency [54].

In the Philippines, private medical centres and joint ventures are seen to drive medical tourism. As a guarantee of quality and adherence to global standards, international accreditation and international partnerships are being pursued. There are currently 38 Joint Commission International (JCI)-accredited hospitals in Southeast Asia, three of which (i.e. St Luke's Medical Center and the Medical City in Metro Manila, and Chong Hua in Cebu City) are in the Philippines. Other internationally accredited hospitals in the Philippines include Makati Medical Center and the Asian Hospital, an affiliate of Thailand's Bumrungrad Hospital [12, 48, 51]. In terms of wellness treatments and alternative medicine, The Farm at San Benito, a venture run by foreign investors in the province of Batangas, is gaining international recognition.

Based on comparative cost analysis, the Philippines is said to have a competitive advantage in the following service segments [49, 50, 51]:

1 Elective surgery (cardiovascular care, joint replacement, eye care, kidney transplants);
2 Aesthetic services (dermatologic, plastic and reconstructive surgery, and dental care); and
3 Wellness treatments and alternative medicine (including spas, executive check-ups and diagnostic procedures, and alternative therapies, such as stem cell or regenerative medicine).

The country's target market is unique in the sense that in addition to foreign nationals, demand for these services is also strong among Filipino immigrants. The movement of Filipinos across the globe is expected to drive both demand and supply [49, 50, 51].

In terms of retirement, the Retirement and Healthcare Coalition (RHC) was formed in 2007 by the European, American, Japanese and Korean Chambers of Commerce. In view of the above-mentioned trends and pressures, this group is proactively negotiating with the Department of Tourism and the Philippine Retirement Authority to create an environment that is conducive to foreign retirement in the Philippines. More and more, negotiations are beginning to bring in private sector partners and the academic sector to foster such an enabling environment in the country [55].

Indeed, medical tourism and foreign retirement create many opportunities and challenges for the country. It can be argued that the creation of international demand within national borders helps confine and retain health human resources within the country (versus the stock depletion brought about by migration). Moreover, social justice and ethical recruitment can be fostered through mutually beneficial bilateral/multilateral agreements. Such agreements can be used as a platform to drive investments aimed at building infrastructure, enhancing workforce capacity through training, transferring technologies and knowledge, and strengthening accreditation and quality standards [9, 12].

There are, however, dangers that the country must bear in mind. For one, benefits of medical tourism are likely to be concentrated in economic centres where the level of health care is already high, thereby aggravating the inequity in workforce distribution that already exists. It may also increase prices in the long run, as tourism shifts the health sector's priority beyond necessary to 'high-end and technology-intensive healthcare'. Implementation of mutual agreements and fulfilment of commitments may also prove to be challenging [12].

Former Secretary of Health, Jaime Galvez-Tan, called 2012 the 'golden year for health' in the Philippines due to the abundance of resources made available to the health sector. From 9.4 billion in 2006 (0.91 per cent of GAA), the health budget rose to 50.4 billion pesos (2.5 per cent of GAA). The passage of the Sin Tax Bill is also expected to generate more revenue for the universal healthcare agenda. Indeed, this is an opportunity for the country to address the challenges and invest in its human health resources [9].

## Conclusion and future directions

The Philippines, with its 7,107 islands and relatively high levels of poverty, faces many health challenges. The country has a mixed provider system and the private sector is a very important part of the provider ecosystem. Both demand-based as well as supply-based solutions are used in the health sector. Demand-based solutions address affordability challenges. However, the geographic and social challenges result in great variability between communities with rural areas, especially those with active conflict, being particularly vulnerable. The devolved system also means that local healthcare availability is greatly affected by local government situations and agendas. These necessitate approaches that address the supply side. On the supply side, even with the granularity of health physical infrastructure requirements successfully addressed, the availability of skilled healthcare workers would constitute a continuing challenge. The quantity and quality of local demand, as well as the resource constraints of local government units, are challenges to addressing healthcare worker availability. This is aggravated not only by competing opportunities in Philippine urban settings but also by international demand and opportunities.

The Philippine educational system produces healthcare workers who enjoy a high level of international demand not only for their technical capabilities but also for their language capabilities and perceived warm and caring approach to care. Owing to a vibrant private education sector, the Philippines has responded quite quickly to international demand. Historically, this has resulted in pockets of oversupply (e.g. nursing graduates). The local response to challenges of managing the availability of healthcare workers is multi-sectoral, involving both the public sector, as well as the private sector. More recently, initiatives have included the use of mobile technology in order to connect local health workers in remote and underserved areas to specialists in urban areas. This is expected to continue. Given the country's commitments to ASEAN initiatives, as well as its strong leanings toward democratic and free market principles, its approach has been, and is expected to be, responsive to international market situations. This essential balance of ensuring free markets while addressing local needs, especially of marginalized populations, will continue to be both the Philippine approach and its challenge.

## Notes

1 Note that registration does not equate to practice. There are many instances when professionals remain 'registered' in the country, although they are practising overseas [9, 15].

2 In 2000, the NSO released a report detailing the level of urbanization per region. Regions considered as 'urban centres' include those regions that were more than 40 per cent urbanized at that time. This group includes Metro Manila and nearby regions, Metro Cebu and Metro Davao.

3 For referencing purposes, note that the highest salary grade is SG33, given to the President of the Philippines. Government physicians' salary grades are at the higher end of the spectrum, which means that they are already at an advantage compared to other civil service employees.
4 Consultants are not formally employed by the hospital, but they are allowed to practise and use the facilities and resources of the hospital.
5 Cooperation cuts across the following areas: improving infrastructural facilities; joint production, marketing and purchasing arrangements; research and development; and exchange of information [30, 31, 32].
6 A *barrio* is a small district of a town, similar to the notion of a village. In the Philippines, it connotes more of a rural setting that is distant from development.

## References

1. World Health Organization. *The World Health Report 2006: Working Together for Health*, WHO, Geneva, 2006.
2. World Health Organization. Everybody's Business: Strengthening Health Systems to Improve Health Outcomes. WHO's Framework for Action, WHO, Geneva, 2007.
3. Anand, S. and Bärnighausen, T. Health workers at the core of the health system: framework and research issues. *Health Policy* 2011, doi: 10.1016/j.healthpol.2011.10.012:3.
4. Kabene, S., Orchard, C., Howard, J., Soriano, M., Leduc, R. The importance of human resources management in health care: a global context. *Human Resources for Health* 2006; 4: 20.
5. World Health Organization. Achieving Universal Health Coverage: Developing the Health Financing System, Technical Briefs for Policy-Makers Number 1, WHO, Geneva, 2005.
6. Asian Development Bank. Population and Human Resource Trends and Challenges, Key Indicators of Developing Asian and Pacific Countries 2002, Asian Development Bank, Manila, 2002: 1–37.
7. United Nations. *Statistical Yearbook for Asia and the Pacific 2008*, UN Economic and Social Commission for Asia and the Pacific (ESCAP), 2008.
8. National Statistical Coordination Board. Beyond the Numbers: Understanding Changes in the Philippine Population. 2012. Available from: http://www.nscb.gov.ph/beyondthenumbers/2012/11162012_jrga_popn.asp [Accessed 25 January 2013].
9. Galvez-Tan, J. Who will heal us now? Realizing universal health care amidst unavailable and under-utilized health human resources. The Secretary's Cup Health Talk Series. Asian Institute of Management, Makati, 2013.
10. Herrera, M. and Yu, A. Evaluation of the social safety net for health in the Philippines: a benefit delivery approach. 2009 (unpublished paper).
11. National Statistical Coordination Board. 2009 Philippine Poverty Statistics. 2011.
12. Kanchanachitra, C., Lindelow, M., Johnston, T., Hanvoravongchai, P., Lorenzo, F., Huong, N., Wilopo, S., dela Rosa, J. Human resources for health in Southeast Asia: shortages, distributional challenges, and international trade in health services. *Lancet* 2011; 377: 769–81.
13. Domingo, E. Reforms in the health human resource sector in the context of universal health care. *Acta Medica Philippina* 2010; 44(4): 43–57.
14. Institute of Health Policy and Development Studies (IHPDS). Philippines: Mobility of Health Professionals. University of the Philippines National Institutes of Health, Manila, Philippines, 2012.
15. World Health Organization. The Philippines Health System Review, Health Systems in Transition, Vol. 1, No. 2. WHO Regional Office for the Western Pacific, Manila, Philippines, 2011.
16. Lorenzo, F. The Philippine HRH Master Plan (2005–2030). First GHWA Conference. Uganda, 2008.
17. Asian Institute of Management. Nursing Markets: Creating the Philippines as the Nursing Education Capital of the World, Case Study No. AIM-3-10-0047-CS. Asian Institute of Management, Makati City, 2010.
18. Tan, K. POEA eyes apprenticeship to address oversupply of nurses. GMA News. 2008. Available from: http://www.gmanetwork.com/news/story/120914/pinoyabroad/poea-eyes-apprenticeship-to-address-oversupply-of-nurses [Accessed 26 January 2013].
19. Professional Regulation Commission (PRC) records. 2011.
20. Pazzibugan, D. CHEd to close down more nursing programs in 2013. *Philippine Daily Inquirer*. 2012. Available from: http://newsinfo.inquirer.net/314211/ched-to-close-down-more-nursing-programs-in-2013 [Accessed 1 February 2013].

21. Villagomeza, L. Shifting paradigms: the development of nursing identity in foreign-educated physicians retrained as nurses practicing in the United States. Unpublished graduate dissertation. University of South Florida, 2009.
22. Department of Health. RN Heals Project for Registered Nurses and Midwives. 2011. Available from: http://www.doh.gov.ph/node/7565.html [Accessed 1 February 2013].
23. Philippine Health Insurance Corporation. PhilHealth Deploys CARES. 2012. Available from: http://www.philhealth.gov.ph/news/2012/deploys_cares.html [Accessed 29 January 2013].
24. Mindanao Examiner. Philippine nurses cry over low pay. 2008. Available from: http://www.mindanaoexaminer.com/news.php?news_id=20080725020927 [Accessed 31 January 2013].
25. Aiken, L., Buchan, J., Sochalski, J., Nichols, B., Powell, M. Trends in international nurse migration. *Health Affairs* 2004; 23(3): 69–77.
26. Heyes, A. The economics of vocation or why is a badly paid nurse a good nurse? Discussion Paper No. 4. Royal Holloway University of London, 2003.
27. Philippine Overseas Employment Administration. *Overseas Employment Statistics 2010*. Available from: http://www.poea.gov.ph/stats/2010_Stats.pdf [Accessed 25 January 2013].
28. Lorenzo, F., Galvez-Tan, J., Icamina, K., Javier, L. Nurse migration from a source country perspective: Philippine country case study. *Health Services Research* 2007; 42(3–2): 1406–18.
29. Department of Labor and Employment (DOLE) Records. 2006.
30. Association of Southeast Asian Nations. ASEAN Mutual Recognition Arrangement on Medical Practitioners. 2012. Available from: http://www.asean.org/communities/asean-economic-community/item/asean-mutual-recognition-arrangement-on-medical-practitioners-2 [Accessed 18 January 2013].
31. Association of Southeast Asian Nations. ASEAN Framework Arrangement on Services. 2012. Available from: http://www.asean.org/communities/asean-economic-community/item/asean-framework-agreement-on-services [Accessed 18 January 2013].
32. Association of Southeast Asian Nations. ASEAN Mutual Recognition Arrangement on Nursing Services. 2012. Available from: http://www.asean.org/communities/asean-economic-community/item/asean-mutual-recognition-arrangement-on-nursing-services [Accessed 18 January 2013].
33. Department of Health. HSR Management in the DOH Program. 2012. Available from: https://www.google.com/url?sa=t&rct=j&q=&esrc=s&source=web&cd=1&cad=rja&ved=0CC4QFjAA&url=http%3A%2F%2Fregion11.healthresearch.ph%2Findex.php%3Foption%3Dcom_phocadownload%26view%3Dcategory%26download%3D49%3Apriority-project-description%26id%3D30%3Ahealth-systems-research-management-in-the-doh-program&ei=zpcQUf_4D6a9iAeZqYHgBg&usg=AFQjCNGiTxAbCrVM5VipFPkHj-UYDd0MJg&bvm=bv.41867550,d.aGc [Accessed 1 February 2013].
34. Leonardia, J., Prytherch, H., Ronquillo, K., Nodora, R., Ruppel, A. Assessment of factors influencing retention in the Philippine National Rural Physician Deployment Program. *BMC Health Services Research* 2012; 12: 411.
35. UP National Telehealth Center. 70 New Doctors Trained on Telemedicine before Barrio Work. 2011. Available from: http://one.telehealth.ph/beta/2011/10/28/70-new-doctors-trained-on-telemedicine-before-barrio-work/ [Accessed 2 February 2013].
36. Department of Health. Message of Secretary Francisco T. Duque III During the Luncheon Meeting with the First Gentleman Mikey Arroyo, the Medical Scholars, and the Doctors to the Barrios. 2006. Available from: http://www.doh.gov.ph/system/files/doctors_0.pdf [Accessed 1 February 2013].
37. Philippine Daily Inquirer. First Gentleman sends doctors to the barrios. 2010. Available from: http://lifestyle.inquirer.net/artsandbooks/artsandbooks/view/20100621-276665/First-Gentleman-sends-doctors-to-the-barrios [Accessed 1 February 2013].
38. Philippine Daily Inquirer. Give doctors dignity they deserve. 2012. Available from: http://opinion.inquirer.net/42787/give-doctors-dignity-they-deserve [Accessed 1 February 2013].
39. Philippine Information Agency. Ona: no more doctorless municipalities by year end. 2012. Available from: http://www.pia.gov.ph/news.index.php?article=2401352269165 [Accessed 1 February 2013].
40. Philippine Center for Investigative Journalism. Health politics demoralizes doctors. 2005. Available from: http://pcij.org/stories/health-politics-demoralizes-doctors/ [Accessed 1 February 2013].
41. Center for Health Market Innovations. Leaders for Health Program. 2012. Available from: http://healthmarketinnovations.org/program/leaders-health-program [Accessed 25 January 2013].

42. Sunstar Manila. Over 22K nurses set for deployment nationwide. 2013. Available from: http://www.sunstar.com.ph/manila/local-news/2013/01/12/over-22k-nurses-set-deployment-nationwide-262544 [Accessed 2 February 2013].
43. Center for Health Market Innovations. EntrepreNurse. 2012. Available from: http://healthmarketinnovations.org/program/entreprenurse [Accessed 25 January 2013].
44. Department of Labor and Employment. Project EntrepreNurse: Introducing the Concept of Nurse Entrepreneurship among Unemployed Nurses to Achieve Public Health Objectives. 2010. Available from: http://healthmarketinnovations.org/sites/healthmarketinnovations.org/files/entreprenurse_brochure_0.doc [Accessed 28 January 2013].
45. Dimaya, R., McEwen, M., Curry, L., Bradley, E. Managing health worker migration: a qualitative study of the Philippine response to nurse brain drain. *Human Resources for Health* 2012; 10(47): 1–8.
46. Zaldivar, J. Project EntrepreNurse Launched. 2010. Available from: htpp://projectentreprenurse.blogspot.com/search/label/Project%20EntrepreNURSE [Accessed 1 February 2012].
47. Banzon, E. Universal health care in Zamboanga and Tawi-Tawi. *Business Mirror.* 2012. Available from: http://www.businessmirror.com.ph/index.php/news/opinion/1540-universal-healthcare-in-zamboanga-and-tawi-tawi [Accessed 26 January 2013].
48. Hodges, J., Kimball, A., Turner, L. Medical tourism in Southeast Asia: opportunities and challenges. In *Risks and Challenges in Medical Tourism*, ABC-CLIO, Santa Barbara, CA, 2012.
49. Philippine Senate Bill No. 959. An Act Instituting a Comprehensive and Holistic Mechanism for the Promotion of Medical Tourism in the Country and for Other Purposes. Available from: http://www.senate.gov.ph/lisdata/84096962!.pdf [Accessed 2 February 2013].
50. Healthcore. Executive Summary: The Philippine Medical Tourism Compendium 2011 (Facts, Figures & Strategies). 2011. Available from: http://www.healthcore.com.ph/pdf/Philippine%20Medical%20Tourism%20Compedium%202011.pdf [Accessed 2 February 2013].
51. Porter, M., De Vera, M., Huang, B., Khan, O., Qin, Z., Tan, A. Medical Tourism in the Philippines. Microeconomics of Competitiveness: Firms, Clusters and Economic Development. 2008. Available from: http://www.isc.hbs.edu/pdf/Student_Projects/Philippine_Medical_Tourism_2008.pdf [Accessed 2 February 2013].
52. Manila Bulletin. Medical tourism earnings reach $1.3B. 2011. Available from: http://mb.com.ph/node/340732/medical-touri#.URAncqU4uSo [Accessed 3 February 2013].
53. Sunstar Cebu. RP urged to improve healthcare tourism. 2012. Available from: http://www.sunstar.com.ph/cebu/local-news/2012/03/04/rp-urged-improve-healthcare-tourism-209382 [Accessed 2 February 2013].
54. Vergara, J.M. Patient Safety. Retirement and Healthcare Seminar. Cebu, Philippines, 2012.
55. Retirement and Health Care Coalition International. The RHC. 2012. Available from: http://www.rhc.com.ph/about-us-the-rhc/ [Accessed 3 February 2013].
56. Institute of Health Policy and Development Studies (IHPDS). *Philippines: Mobility of Health Professionals*, University of the Philippines National Institutes of Health, Manila, Philippines, 2012.
57. World Bank Statistics. Population, total. 2012. Available from: http://data.worldbank.org/indicator/SP.POP.TOTL [Accessed 25 January 2013].
58. Department of Health. The National Database of Selected Human Resources for Health (NDHRHIS). 2012. Available from: http://www.hhrdb.doh.gov.ph/ndhrhis/ [Accessed 28 January 2013].
59. Office of the President of the Philippines. Executive Order No. 76 s. 2012, 'Implementation of the Fourth Tranche of the Modified Salary Schedule for Civilian Personnel and Base Pay Schedule for Military and Uniformed Personnel in the Government'. 2012. Available from: http://www.gov.ph/2012/04/30/executive-order-no-76-s-2012/ [Accessed 25 January 2013].
60. Philippine Overseas Employment Administration (POEA) records. 2009.
61. National Statistical Coordination Board and World Bank. Estimation of Local Poverty in the Philippines. 2005. Available from: http://www.nscb.gov.ph/poverty/sae/NSCB_LocalPoverty Philippines.pdf [Accessed 28 February 2013].
62. National Statistical Coordination Board. Philippine Minimum National Social Data Set: Life Expectancy at Birth by Sex. 2012. Available from: http://www.nscb.gov.ph/stats/mnsds/mnsds_life.asp [Accessed 25 January 2013].

# 45

# Medical tourism in Thailand

*Siripen Supakankunti*

## Introduction

The healthcare industry in Thailand has grown domestically due to the changes in key health determinants such as socio-economic and political development, demography and migration, biomedical technology advancement, and health seeking behaviour and lifestyle changes during the past decades. The data from the National Economic and Social Development Board (NESDB) show the country's increasing total health expenditures. The increasing trend is also observed in both public and private sectors. In addition to an increase in domestic demand, medical tourism has been emerging globally and has boosted the international demand for healthcare services attracting people from all around the world. Sizeable opportunities in the healthcare sector are predicted for Southeast Asia, including Thailand. However, this imposes many problems regarding the impacts of the Medical Hub policy, and its consequences, in both positive and negative lights. Various studies have shown the existence of these problems, with many supporting the promotion of medical tourism and also many disagreeing with this policy. The Thai health system is quite complex, involves many stakeholders and has a long history of development.

## Thailand's economic background

Thailand is classified as an upper middle-income country with a population of over 69 million. Historically, the country was an agriculture-based economy in the eighteenth and nineteenth centuries making inroads into the modernization of all fields; embracing industrialization and liberal capitalism; and adopting all technologies with scientific orientation. Ethnically, the country is quite homogeneous: 95 per cent are Thai and Buddhists, 4.5 per cent are Muslims and around 0.5 per cent are from hill tribes. The population growth rate has been less than 1 per cent annually since 2005 due to a very successful family planning campaign of the past three decades. In 2005, the country's population average age was 30.1 years, with 23.1 per cent of the population in the age group of 14 years and under, 10.9 per cent in the elderly (60 years and over) group and the rest (around two-thirds of the entire population) is aged between 15 and 59 years old. It is projected that, by 2025, the age composition of the country will change quite dramatically – the working population will constitute 62.1 per cent of the population, children 18 per cent and the elderly 19 per cent [1]. Clearly, it is anticipated that Thailand will go through a rapid demographic transition towards a society with an ageing population with serious health consequences. See Table 45.1 for figures of life expectancy at birth in Thailand.

The last three to four decades have seen a dramatic change in the country's politics and economic status as Western imperial powers have withdrawn their influence and support for the local administrative regimes of small and middle-income countries. Thailand has transformed itself from a subsistence agrarian society into a rapidly industrializing one. By 1990, the country was experiencing sustained economic growth, averaging 7 per cent per year, due to a thriving export-oriented industry. Economic progress has been accompanied by significant achievements in health development. Reductions in population growth and the infant mortality rate, along with improvements in life expectancy, have contributed to Thailand's rapid demographic transition (see Table 45.2). The Expanded Program of Immunization (EPI) successfully led to a decreasing incidence of a number of infectious diseases, such as malaria and TB. At the same time, the incidence of non-communicable, chronic and degenerative diseases is rising [2].

*Table 45.1* Life expectancy at birth in Thailand, by gender

| *Year* | *Male* | *Female* |
|---|---|---|
| 1964–1965 | 55.9 | 62.0 |
| 1974–1976 | 58.0 | 63.8 |
| 1985–1986 | 63.8 | 68.9 |
| 1990–1995 | 68.6 | 73.4 |
| 1995–1996 | 69.9 | 74.9 |
| 1995–2000 | 69.4 | 74.1 |
| 2000–2005 | 70.2 | 74.7 |
| 2005–2010 | 71.0 | 75.4 |
| 2010–2015 | 71.6 | 75.9 |
| 2015–2020 | 72.2 | 76.5 |

*Source*: [18].

*Table 45.2* Economic and health indicators, Thailand, 1970–2010

| *Indicators* | *1970*[a] | *1980* | *1990* | *1999* | *2010* |
|---|---|---|---|---|---|
| GDP per capita (US$)[b] | 325 | 563 | 1,543 | 1,950 | 4,873 |
| Population growth (%) | 3.0 | 1.8 | 0.7 | 1.2 | 0.6 |
| Life expectancy (M/F) | 58.0/63.8 | 62.6/68.1 | 65.9/70.6 | 67.4/71.8 | 71.2/76.1 |
| Adult mortality rate (M/F) | 264.7/190.0 | 251/150.3 | 197.9/105.5 | 259.2/125.4 | 199.7/99.8 |
| Under 5 mortality rate | 87.9 | 49.2 | 23.3 | 14.5 | 8.9 |

*Sources*: [1, 18–22].

*Notes*: a GDP per capita and life expectancy under the 1970 column are from 1975.
b The GDP per capita is converted into USD using the current-year exchange rate.

The country's economy is highly dependent on exports, with exports accounting for 71 per cent of the country's gross domestic product (GDP) in 2010 [3]. Thailand's GDP was worth USD (Purchasing Power Parity – PPP) 591 billion in 2010, with per capita GDP reaching USD (PPP) 8,554 and USD 4,873 [3]. Over the period 1961 to 2010, GDP growth was 6.4 per cent on average [3]. In 2009, however, GDP contracted by 2.3 per cent due to the global financial crisis which, together with domestic political uncertainties, had an impact on the growth rate of international patients seeking medical treatment in Thailand.

## Health care and health insurance systems in Thailand

### *Health care system*

In the field of health, Thailand has striven vigorously to attain the most advanced scientific medicine by investing heavily (through financial resources mobilized internally and externally) in hospitals, medical schools and medical education. Such heavy investment has greatly assisted the country in promoting the efficacy of medical services provided to the public. However, there has been a trade-off between efficacy of medical care and services, and their accessibility and equal distribution. It is undeniable a historical analysis will show that the country's health policy has not been exclusively defined by the health needs of the people, but has been subject to realignment with the country's other priority needs, such as national security, economic development and social investment, amongst others.

Therefore, for a country with a land size of 512,000 square kilometres, the challenge of providing adequate medical or healthcare services to people dispersed widely throughout the 76 administrative units (called 'provinces') with an annual budget of roughly USD 20 billion, is quite daunting. The distribution of the population throughout the country adds to this picture as more than one-quarter of the population are concentrated in the north-eastern plain of non-fertile land of the country and, by income statistics, are the poorest (see Tables 45.3 and 45.4).

Historically, the healthcare system in Thailand relied on varied traditional time-honoured healing techniques, empirically tested but beyond scientific verification. This has now been replaced by current scientific-based medical technology. Scientific-based medicine and traditional medicine used to peacefully coexist with acceptance of both modalities empirically tested through their efficacy when used by the general public. However, scientific-based medicine edged out traditional medicine with the promulgation of the Physician License Act in 1936, two years after the nationalization of all hospitals in the country. At the same time, donations to hospitals were made tax-exempt. In 1942, the first health authority in Thailand, the Ministry of Health, was established, leading to the institutionalization of scientific medicine. It was only in 1985 that traditional medicine was again reinstated as alternative medicine and an Office for Indigenous Medicine headed by a scientific medical doctor was established to reconcile it back into the field of mainstream healthcare services. During the period prior to and after World War II, due to acute scarcity of the government's budget, legislature and regulation were passed to enable hospitals to take user fees from the public who were seeking services and could afford to pay, and to keep the revenue to finance their hospital operations. To encourage doctors to provide services to complement the public health services, private practice by medical doctors was also made income tax exempt. Despite private practice gaining official recognition and being established as the mainstream health services, the powerful Thailand Medical Association was established as a peer-group

*Table 45.3* GDP per capita and population data for the provinces of Thailand

| *North-eastern region* | *45,766* | *22,652* |
|---|---|---|
| *Province* | *GDP per capita* | *Population (thousands)* |
| 1. Loei | 56,304 | 656 |
| 2. Nong Bua Lamphu | 33,912 | 529 |
| 3. Udon Thani | 48,747 | 1,610 |
| 4. Nongkhai | 40,900 | 964 |
| 5. Sakon Nakhon | 39,859 | 1,141 |
| 6. Nakhon Phanom | 36,077 | 743 |
| 7. Chaiyaphum | 43,435 | 1,189 |
| 8. Khon Kaen | 76,385 | 1,876 |
| 9. Kalasin | 44,393 | 1,000 |
| 10. Mukdahan | 44,340 | 340 |
| 11. Maha Sarakham | 39,178 | 1,021 |
| 12. Roiet | 41,091 | 1,350 |
| 13. Yasothon | 35,787 | 612 |
| 14. Amnat Charoen | 34,006 | 395 |
| 15. Nakhon Ratchasima | 56,877 | 2,790 |
| 16. Buriram | 38,034 | 1,633 |
| 17. Surin | 38,260 | 1,431 |
| 18. Sisaket | 34,326 | 1,523 |
| 19. Ubon Ratchathani | 42,567 | 1,849 |

*Source*: [23].

*Note*: The 15 provinces with the lowest GDP per capita are all located in north-eastern region of Thailand.

*Table 45.4* GDP per capita by regions, 2008

| *Region* | *GDP per capita** | *Population (thousands)* |
|---|---|---|
| Bangkok and vicinity | 329,885 | 11,443 |
| Central region | 228,016 | 3,019 |
| Eastern region | 309,985 | 4,497 |
| Northern region | 70,105 | 12,086 |
| North-eastern region | 45,766 | 22,652 |
| Southern region | 93,616 | 9,143 |
| Western region | 106,048 | 3,642 |
| All of Thailand | 136,511 | 66,482 |

*Source*: [24].

*Notes*: * Real GDP in Thai Baht.
Not updated for 2009.

regulating body. Since its establishment, very few foreign medical graduates have applied or received a practising licence due to many reasons, including language barriers.

In the past, health care in Thailand was delivered by a wide range of providers. Local populations could seek health services from health centres in their communities, but these were not staffed by medical doctors and were poorly funded. Hospitals were mostly publicly funded and were concentrated in the capital and provincial towns. Medical school hospitals were very much sought after by the majority of the public as they were sophisticated, but mostly concentrated around the capital with a few in remote provinces. In the early days, there were only a handful of small private hospitals dispersed throughout the country. Private clinics were operated by government doctors out of office hours after their day's work at public hospitals, providing a limited service and acting mainly as extended outpatient clinics for doctors in the hospitals in which they were employed. Despite this array of health establishments, healthcare services and resources still fell short of public needs due to both inadequacy and mis-distribution of health resources. As the economy progressed and people were financially better off, public dissatisfaction of availability, and accessibility to, health service intensified [4].

Today, the healthcare system in Thailand, triggered by lack of access, consists of many levels of service, from private clinics or public health centres, to regional or university hospitals, which may provide tertiary care. A unique characteristic of the Thai health system is the government's consistent investment in the health infrastructure of health facilities and medical education. In 2009, healthcare spending was 4.3 per cent of GDP, a high 76 per cent of which was government expenditure (see Table 45.5). The figure amounted to USD 345 per capita, much higher than the USD 145 average of other low- and middle-income countries [5]. Over a period of 45 years (1960–2006), the government has developed National Health Plans to serve as guidelines for health investment with a view to improve the health delivery system in the country. Health facilities have expanded and been upgraded to such a degree that there is now one primary health centre per 5,000 people and at least one hospital, typically with ten to sixty beds, in each district (see Table 45.6). The production of human resources has been given high priority. The Ministry of Public Health (MoPH) has educated its own nurses since 1961, partly as a response to the scaling-up of public facilities, and has enforced a law that requires all health professionals to serve in remote areas for three years after graduation, thereby easing the accessibility gap of health services between urban and rural areas. Table 45.7 shows changes in the ratio of the population to a selected group of healthcare providers over time.

Nevertheless, the availability of medical facilities and personnel varies significantly across regions in Thailand. In 2007, 5 medical schools, 14 specialized hospitals and 68 public health centres served Bangkok, while 6 medical schools, 25 regional hospitals, 47 specialized hospitals and 70 general hospitals served the rest of the country.

## *The health insurance system*

Prior to the recent initiation of the universal coverage scheme in October 2001, Thailand's population was covered by several government programmes. The four main ones were: the Low Income Card Scheme (LICS), the Civil Servant Medical Benefit Scheme (CSMBS), the Social Security Scheme (SSS) and the Voluntary Health Card Scheme (VHCS). As late as 1991, government investment and promotion of these health insurance programmes was very low – as much as 67 per cent of the Thai population was not covered by any scheme. However, over the next decade, health insurance became increasingly important to both the government and the people.

The current health insurance system in Thailand is largely shaped by the introduction of the universal coverage scheme (UCS) in 2001 and is composed of some of the same schemes that preceded it, including SSS, CSMBS, Car Insurance (CAI) and Workmen Compensation Fund (WCF), as well as private health insurance. Universal health coverage, commonly

*Table 45.5* Health expenditure

| *Member state* | *Per capita health expenditures[a]* | | | | | | | | *Gross national income per capita[c] (PPP int. $)* | | | | | | | | | |
|---|---|---|---|---|---|---|---|---|---|---|---|---|---|---|---|---|---|---|
| | *Per capita total expenditure on health at average exchange rate (US$)* | | *Per capita total expenditure on health[b] (PPP int. $)* | | *Per capita government expenditure on health at average exchange rate (US$)* | | *Per capita government expenditure on health[b] (PPP int. $)* | | | | | *MDG 1 Population living on <$1 (PPP int. $) a day[d] (%)* | *Per capita total expenditure on health / gross national income per capita (PPP i nt. $) (%)* | | *Per capita government expenditure on health / gross national income per capita (PPP int. $) (%)* | | *Per capita private expenditure on health / gross national income per capita (PPP int. $) (%)* | |
| | *2000* | *2008* | *2000* | *2008* | *2000* | *2008* | *2000* | *2008* | *1990* | *2000* | *2009* | *2000–2008* | *2000* | *2008/2009* | *2000* | *2008/2009* | *2000* | *2008/2009* |
| Brazil | 265 | 721 | 494 | 875 | 107 | 317 | 199 | 385 | 5,050 | 6,830 | 10,200 | 5.2 | 7.23 | 8.58 | 2.91 | 3.77 | 4.32 | 4.80 |
| Chile | 324 | 762 | 613 | 1,088 | 169 | 335 | 319 | 479 | 4,430 | 8,880 | 13,440 | <2.0 | 6.90 | 8.10 | 3.59 | 3.56 | 3.31 | 4.53 |
| Colombia | 161 | 317 | 382 | 517 | 130 | 266 | 309 | 434 | 4,180 | 5,730 | 8,600 | 16.0 | 6.67 | 6.01 | 5.39 | 5.05 | 1.27 | 0.97 |
| Costa Rica | 265 | 618 | 461 | 1,059 | 203 | 413 | 354 | 708 | 4,340 | 6,630 | 10,930 | 2.0 | 6.95 | 9.69 | 5.34 | 6.48 | 1.61 | 3.21 |
| Germany | 2,366 | 4,720 | 2,667 | 3,922 | 1,888 | 3,523 | 2,128 | 2,927 | 18,590 | 25,700 | 36,780 | . . . | 10.38 | 10.66 | 8.28 | 7.96 | 2.10 | 2.71 |
| Japan | 2,827 | 3,190 | 1,969 | 2,817 | 2,298 | 2,568 | 1,600 | 2,268 | 19,160 | 25,950 | 33,470 | . . . | 7.59 | 8.42 | 6.17 | 6.78 | 1.42 | 1.64 |
| Malaysia | 128 | 353 | 304 | 621 | 67 | 156 | 159 | 274 | 4,590 | 8,370 | 13,710 | <2.0 | 3.63 | 4.53 | 1.90 | 2.00 | 1.73 | 2.53 |
| Republic of Korea | 543 | 1,245 | 824 | 1,806 | 247 | 671 | 375 | 974 | 8,180 | 17,130 | 27,310 | . . . | 4.81 | 6.61 | 2.19 | 3.57 | 2.62 | 3.05 |
| Singapore | 648 | 1,404 | 937 | 1,833 | 291 | 479 | 421 | 625 | 17,650 | 32,900 | 49,780 | . . . | 2.85 | 3.68 | 1.28 | 1.26 | 1.57 | 2.43 |
| Sweden | 2,277 | 4,858 | 2,284 | 3,622 | 1,933 | 3,794 | 1,939 | 2,829 | 19,070 | 27,730 | 38,590 | . . . | 8.24 | 9.39 | 6.99 | 7.33 | 1.24 | 2.05 |
| Thailand | 67 | 164 | 165 | 328 | 38 | 122 | 92 | 244 | 2,820 | 4,860 | 7,640 | <2.0 | 3.40 | 4.29 | 1.89 | 3.19 | 1.50 | 1.10 |
| ***Income group*** | | | | | | | | | | | | | | | | | | |

| | | | | | | | | | | | | | | | | | | |
|---|---|---|---|---|---|---|---|---|---|---|---|---|---|---|---|---|---|---|
| Low income | 13 | 32 | 37 | 74 | 5 | 13 | 14 | 30 | 689 | 843 | 1,457 | 51.4 | 4.39 | 5.08 | 1.66 | 2.06 | 2.73 | 3.02 |
| Lower middle income | 37 | 99 | 95 | 197 | 14 | 45 | 35 | 88 | 1,137 | 2,078 | 4,696 | 26.9 | 4.57 | 4.20 | 1.68 | 1.87 | 2.89 | 2.32 |
| Upper middle income | 216 | 570 | 438 | 830 | 115 | 326 | 236 | 479 | 5,535 | 7,053 | 12,447 | 5.2 | 6.21 | 6.67 | 3.35 | 3.85 | 2.86 | 2.82 |
| High income | 2,650 | 4,590 | 2,740 | 4,246 | 1,572 | 2,854 | 1,626 | 2,589 | 17,712 | 26,907 | 36,708 | . . . | 10.18 | 11.57 | 6.04 | 7.05 | 4.14 | 4.51 |

*Source*: [26, 27].

*Notes*: a. All the indicators shown are measured as financing agents except 'external resources for health', which are measured as a financing source. The regional, income and global figures are calculated using Purchasing Power Parity (PPP) terms. When the number is smaller than 0.05%, the percentage may appear as zero. For per capita expenditure indicators, this is represented as <1. In countries where the fiscal year begins in July, expenditure data have been allocated to the later calendar year (for example, 2008 data will cover the fiscal year 2007–08) unless otherwise stated for the country. Absolute values of expenditures are expressed in nominal terms (current prices). National currency unit per US$ is calculated using the average exchange rates for the year. For 2008, the use of yearly average exchange rates (compared to year-end exchange rates) may not fully represent the impact of the global financial crisis. *Source*: [25].

b. A PPP series resulting from the 2005 International Comparison Project (ICP), estimated by the World Bank, has been used. In countries where this is not available, PPPs are estimated by WHO.

c. PPP int. **$** = Purchasing Power Parity at international dollar rate. The income-group figures relate only to WHO member states and therefore may differ from those reported in the World Development Indicators Database. *Source*: [26].

d. These figures reflect the World Bank default poverty line.

*Table 45.6* Health facilities in the public sector, 2007

| *Administrative level* | *Health facility* | *Number* | *Coverage (%)* |
|---|---|---|---|
| Bangkok Metropolis | Medical school hospitals | 5 | |
| | General hospitals | 26 | |
| | MoPH | 4 | |
| | Royal Thai Police | 1 | |
| | Ministry of Justice | 4 | |
| | Ministry of Defence | 5 | |
| | BMA | 8 | |
| | State enterprises | 4 | |
| | Specialized hospitals/institutions | 14 | |
| | Public health centres/branches | 68/77 | All districts under BMA |
| Regional level and branches | Medical school hospitals | 6 | |
| | Regional hospitals | 25 | |
| | Specialized hospitals | 47 | |
| | Health promotion hospitals | 12 | |
| | Psychiatric hospitals | 13 | |
| | Neurological hospitals | 1 | |
| | Rajprachasamasai Institute | 1 | |
| | Bamrasnaradura Institute | 1 | |
| | Chest Disease Institute | 1 | |
| | Cancer prevention and control centres | 6 | |
| | Drug dependence treatment centres | 5 | |
| | Metta Pracharak Hospital | 1 | |
| | Centre for elderly care | 1 | |
| | Dermatology Centre | 1 | |
| | Dental Institute | 1 | |
| | Sirindhorn National Medical Rehabilitation Centre | 1 | |
| | Thanyarak Institute | 1 | |
| | Maha Vajiralongkorn Centre at Thanyaburi | 1 | |
| Provincial level (75 provinces) | General hospitals, under MoPH | 70 | 100 |
| | Military hospitals under the Ministry of Defence | 59 | |
| | Hospital under the Royal Thai Police | 1 | |
| 796 districts 81 minor districts | Community hospitals (Mar. 2007) | 730 | 91.70 |
| | Branch hospital | 1 | |
| | Municipal health centres (Oct. 2003) | 214 | |
| 7,255 subdistricts 74,435 villages | Health centres (2006) | 9,762 | 100 |
| | Community health posts | 311 | |
| | Community PHC centres (2003) | | |
| | Rural | 66,223 | 89.00 |
| | Urban | 31,085 | |

*Source*: [1].

*Table 45.7* Ratios of population to healthcare providers in Thailand, 1999–2005

| *Population/provider ratio* | *1999* | *2001* | *2003* | *2005* |
|---|---|---|---|---|
| Population/doctors | 3,395 | 3,277 | 3,476 | 3,182 |
| Population/dentists | 15,295 | 14,384 | 17,182 | 14,901 |
| Population/pharmacists | 10,158 | 9,054 | 8,807 | 7,847 |
| Population/professional nurses | 905 | 796 | 687 | 613 |
| Population/technical nurses | 1,952 | 2,080 | 2,625 | 3,910 |

*Source*: [1].

known as the '30-baht scheme', is the most recent and quite possibly the most ambitious undertaking by the government. Replacing LICS and VHCS, and complementing the CSMBS and SSS, the UCS guarantees health care at any public facility to every otherwise uninsured person, regardless of their income. Previous problems with the LICS and the VHCS that involved the misidentification of low-income cards and a relatively high premium of voluntary health cards are limited under the UCS. Originally, the co-payment for each visit was 30 baht (approximately USD 1 at the current exchange rate) and the very poor were exempted. There is no co-payment at present but the current administration, headed by Prime Minister Yingluck Shinawatra, has plans to bring it back. The UCS is financed through the government's budget. In 2002, one year after the implementation of the scheme, approximately 45 million people were covered, accounting for over 70 per cent of the population [6]. See Table 45.8 for a comparison between the main health insurance schemes in Thailand.

*Table 45.8* Comparison of main health insurance schemes in Thailand

| *Characteristics* | *UCS* | *CSMBS* | *SSS* |
|---|---|---|---|
| Beneficiaries | Social welfare | Fringe benefit | Compulsory |
| Covered population | People not covered by CSMBS and SSS | Government employees and their dependents | Private employees in the formal sector in a firm with more than one worker |
| Source of funds | General tax | General tax | Tripartite, 1.5% of payroll from the employee, the employer and the government each |
| Financing body | National Health Security Office (NHSO) | Ministry of Finance | Social Security Office |
| Payment mechanism | Capitation for OP and DRG for IP | Fee-for-service for OP and DRG for IP | Risk-adjusted capitation |
| Co-payment | No co-payment at the present but with plans to switch back to 30 baht per visit | Co-payment for IP at any hospital. IP in private hospitals are limited only for life-threatening care | Co-payment for maternity and emergency services if beyond the predetermined ceiling |
| Capitation rate (2005 figure) | 1,308 baht | 3,980 baht (approximately) | 1,500 baht |

*Source*: [28].

## Multilateral and regional trade negotiations

### Multilateral trade negotiations

The General Agreement on Trade in Services (GATS) resulted from the Uruguay Round of multilateral trade negotiations, and came into force in 1995. It is aimed at establishing a system of international trade rules based on the principle of non-discrimination. The basic obligations under the GATS are either of general or specific nature. Key components of the general obligations, which apply to all members and services sectors, are the most-favoured-nation (MFN) treatment, as well as transparency. Specific commitments exist for market access and national treatment in specific sectors. Since member countries are free to determine coverage and content of specific commitments, these mostly reflect national policy objectives and constraints. Each World Trade Organization (WTO) member is required to have a Schedule of Specific Commitments, which consists of horizontal sections that apply to all sectors listed in the schedule and sector-specific sections that only apply to a specific sector [7].

The GATS includes a category on Health and Social Services, which in turn includes hospital services. Medical and dental services and the services provided by nurses, midwives, physiotherapists and para-medical personnel are categorized separately as 'Professional Services'. So far, few commitments – to enhance professional movement and investment across countries – have been made in the area of health services, including from Thailand [7].

### Regional trade negotiations

The most important regional trade agreement for trade in services is the 1995 ASEAN Framework Agreement on Services (AFAS). Under the GATS-plus principle, ASEAN member states schedule commitments under AFAS that go beyond their GATS commitments or offer new sectors that have not been scheduled under GATS, as in the case of Thailand. The Protocol to Implement the 8th Package of Commitments under the AFAS was signed in 2010. The health sector is one of the identified priority areas under AFAS and a Healthcare Services Sectoral Working Group was subsequently set up. In 2006, a Mutual Recognition Agreement (MRA) was signed on nursing services and, in 2009, in line with the ASEAN Economic Community (AEC) Blueprint, another was signed on medical practitioners and dental practitioners. The first MRA took two years to negotiate, the main barriers being different standards of curriculum and educational institutes, different professional definitions and scopes of practice, different levels of education to enter into professional education programmes, different standards of regulatory systems and licences to practise, differences in continuing education and training, professional conservatism and protectionism, language barriers and cultural sensitivity [8]. The MRA do not really facilitate the movement of natural persons since 'doctors, dentists and nurses from the original countries still need to comply with the requirements of the domestic laws and regulations of host countries which may include, for example, permanent residence and licensing examinations in the local language'. The AEC Blueprint also stipulates that under Mode 3, foreign (ASEAN) equity participation of not less than 51 per cent by 2008 and 70 per cent by 2010 for the four priority services sectors; not less than 49 per cent by 2008, 51 per cent by 2010 and 70 per cent by 2013 for logistics services; and not less than 49 per cent by 2008, 51 per cent by 2010 and 70 per cent by 2015 for other service sectors, should be allowed [9].

Thailand is committed through the ASEAN Free Trade Agreement (AFTA) and other regional trade agreements, such as ASEAN–China FTA (2002), ASEAN–India FTA (2003), ASEAN–Korea FTA (2003), Bay of Bengal Initiative for Multi-Sectoral Technical and Economic Cooperation (BIMSTEC) FTA (2004), ASEAN–Japan FTA (2008) and ASEAN–Australia–New Zealand FTA (2009).

### *Bilateral FTA negotiations*

Thailand has entered into bilateral free trade agreements with several countries, namely Laos (limited, 1991), Bahrain (as a stepping stone toward an FTA with the Gulf Cooperation Council (GCC) countries, 2002), China (agriculture, 2003), India (2003), Peru (2003), Australia (2004), New Zealand (2005) and Japan (2007). Thailand's pace of FTA negotiations has somewhat slowed down since 2006 in light of the political tensions.

With the shift from multilateral negotiations to bilateral trade negotiations, the structure of trade negotiations was again reformed. A Committee on International Trade Policy, which includes the ministers of the ministries of Finance, Foreign Affairs, Agriculture and Cooperatives and Industry, in addition to the Secretary-General of the National Economic and Social Development Board, was appointed by the prime minister in 2003. The Committee on International Trade Policy can appoint chief negotiators for the teams negotiating with each country, as well as sub-committees and working groups. While the MoPH is not a member of the Committee on International Trade Policy, it is invited to join meetings that deal with health-related issues.

In addition, since preparations for FTA services and investment negotiation positions involve country and sector preparations, the MoPH emerged as the focal point in sector preparations with relevance for the health sector, with the Bureau of Policy and Strategy being the central secretariat. To *inter alia* assess the implications of trade liberalization policies on the Thai health sector, the MoPH established the Committee on Trade in Health and Social Services in 2004. Besides government agencies, stakeholders from other sectors are also involved [10].

## Thai medical hub policy

### *Overview of tourism in Thailand*

The tourism industry is considered to be a crucial economic system of the world. It is accepted that growth of tourism in almost all countries has quickly become the main industry in international trade. In many countries, tourism is the major industry important to stimulate economic growth. The Thai tourism industry is now one of the most important economic sectors of the country. The revenue from foreign tourists reached 6 per cent of the national income in 2010. Although this revenue amounts to only 10 per cent of the value of exports of goods, the revenue is still important because the tourism industry utilizes the resources in the country and gives back to the Thai people. Income from tourism increased continuously from 367,380.36 million baht in the year 2005 to 585,961.80 million baht in the year 2010 [11], and the number of tourists travelling to Thailand between 2001 and 2010 has been increasing annually. The revenue from tourism is likely to increase even further in coming years.

## *Overview of medical tourism in Thailand*

Thailand has been an attractive tourist destination for decades. Many tourists visit frequently for business and leisure, and if they are or fall ill, they are able to receive treatment in Thai hospitals and are satisfied with the quality of medical care. The numbers have grown and now groups of foreigners fly directly to Thailand to receive medical care. In the wake of the 1997 Asian economic crisis, bed occupancy in most private hospitals significantly declined, prompting high-end private hospitals, which invested substantially during the economic boom, to seek out medical tourists from abroad (e.g. Japan, Europe and the Middle East). The Export Promotion Department of Ministry of Commerce recognized the high reputation of Thai medicine, and in order to stimulate economic growth during the economic crisis in 1997, the Ministry of Commerce collaborated with various agencies, such as the Ministry of Foreign Affairs, the Tourism Authority of Thailand, the Institute of Thai Enterprises Development, the Thai Chamber of Commerce and the Association of Private Hospitals, to promote health tourism (medical tourism) to patients from upper- and high-income countries, and also to attract retired people to the country. Since then, every Thai government has announced various policy measures to promote medical tourism in order to generate revenue for the country.

The major factors of success in medical tourism are the quality of medical services, low cost of obtaining services of similar/acceptable quality, price certainty through fixed package prices offered by medical facilities, the well-developed tourism industry and other supporting industries (e.g. low cost of travelling, accommodation and food for a companion, as well as other tourism activities, attractions and entertainment), excellent hospitality and low entry barriers. Thailand originally focused on tourism-related areas such as spas, traditional massages, herbal treatments and other kinds of alternative medicine. However, in recent years private hospitals have discovered niche markets in elective medical procedures, such as plastic surgery.

Figure 45.1 shows that Thailand had 60.31 per cent and Singapore has 14.74 per cent of the market share from medical tourism in Asia classified by number of tourists, highlighting that Thailand is the destination for many medical tourists. However, Figure 45.2 shows that the share of the revenue was only 30.23 per cent, compared with 47.55 per cent for Singapore [12].

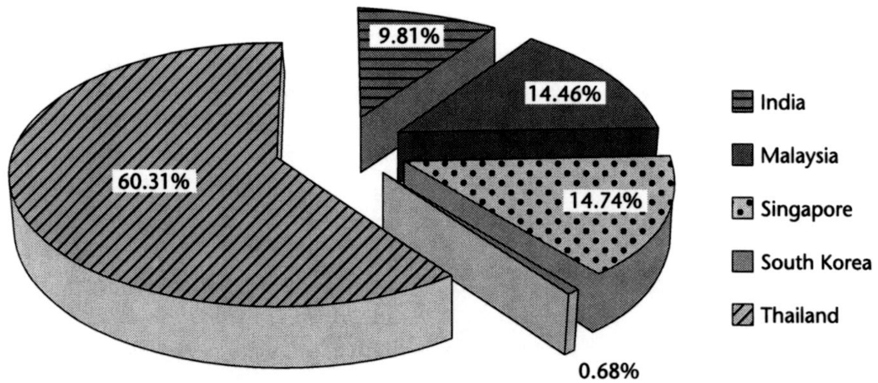


*Figure 45.1* Share of the tourism market-oriented medical classification based on the number of service users [16]

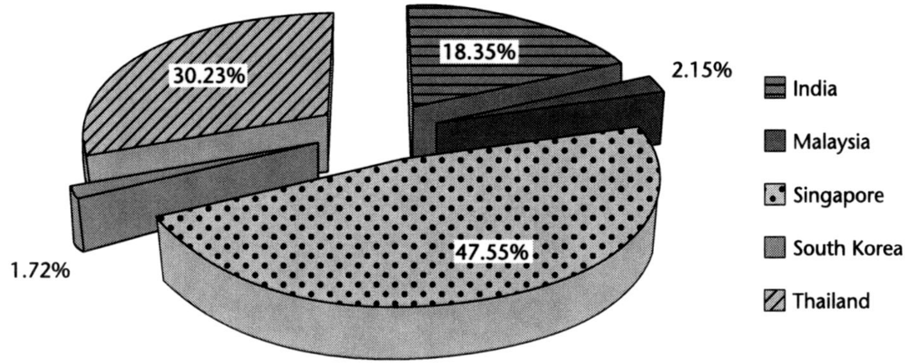


*Figure 45.2* Share of the tourism market-oriented medical service by revenue [16]

## *Definition and development of the medical hub of Thailand*

The definition of the medical hub is unclear. However, expert opinions agree that it signifies a centre of health-oriented tourism (medical tourism), which consists of three main service areas, namely medical services business, health promotion services, and health and wellness products (e.g. Thai herbs). With the standards of excellence in medical services and medical technical aspects at present, the country is known as Thai medical hub and one of the best in Asia. The 'Medical Hub' or 'Centre of Excellence' policies require Thailand to become a 'Centre of Medical Research' and a 'Centre of Medical Education and Training'. The number of foreign patients receiving medical care in the country each year increased up to 1.37 million people in 2007 and 1.36 million people in 2008 by approximately 20 per cent coming from countries in Europe, and only about 20 per cent coming from other places in Central Asia and East Asia. Foreign patients make up 23.7 per cent of the patients in the private hospitals. These foreign patients can be divided into three groups, namely people working in Thailand and the nearby countries (50 per cent), foreigners who fly directly for treatment (27.6 per cent) and tourists who suffer from illnesses or get into accidents whilst travelling (22.2 per cent). Forty-five private hospitals are the major providers and the three highest ranked are in Bangkok. There are also some university hospitals and public hospitals which are located in the tourists' destination provinces.

## *Policy for the centre of excellent health care of Asia*

There are currently two operational government policies for medical tourism: an ad hoc Committee of the Prime Minister, which focuses on the development of the country as a centre for international health (medical hub) and the committee for developing the centre for international health. The Ministry of Public Health continues to support strategic planning for the development of the international health centre (2010–2014), which is now taking shape, and consists of four main themes: medical services, health promotion services, medical services plan of Thai herbal medicine and alternative health products. There are three main strategic plans: improving the competitiveness of the health service business, health system development for higher quality health services, and world-class standards and promoting marketing and PR activities. The medical hub strategy in general is aimed at developing Thailand into a first-class destination for medical tourists. To provide world-class services, standards for hospital accreditation in Thailand have been set and international standards, such as the International Organization for Standardization (ISO) and Joint Commission

International (JCI), introduced. In addition, a controversial medical malpractice law is being discussed to strengthen the rights of patients.

However, one of the remaining major problems is policy incoherence, which results in continued competition for medical professionals caused by the competing demands of the universal coverage policy and the medical hub policy, and the potential worsening of problems of the internal brain drain and competition between the revenue earned by private sectors at the expense of the public sector.

For the past ten years, Thailand, like many other countries, has sought to become an explicit 'Medical Hub'. The number of international patients was 1.4 million in 2009, including general tourists and foreigners who work or live in Thailand as shown in Figure 45.3, with medical tourists accounting for an estimated 30 per cent [13], reflecting that Thailand has become a leading destination for medical tourists from almost all continents. However, the growth rate of the number of international patients decreased during the past couple of years due to Thailand's political problems and the global financial crisis as mentioned above. Trade in health services was estimated to be worth 63,822 million baht in 2008, of which 62 per cent was accounted for by medical services and 27 per cent by health promotion [14].

Despite the problems with the medical hub policy, Thailand remains highly competitive with other countries on medical hub strategies (see Table 45.9). Thailand's main advantages are its high quality medical professionals and a hospitable and service-minded culture. In addition, the costs of medical treatments are reasonable. Besides that, since Thailand has traditionally been a major tourism destination worldwide, its strengths are tourism-related medical treatment and wellness packages. Hence, the general tourism infrastructure like hotels, shopping malls and restaurants is also an important component of the hospital supply chain for international patients and supports Thailand in becoming a leading medical hub in Asia. However, there are several weaknesses as discussed above. To develop Thailand into a first-class destination for medical tourists and provide world-class services, a SWOT analysis was carried out in order to identify the Strengths, Weaknesses, Opportunities and Threats of the medical hub of Thailand [10]. The results of the SWOT analysis are shown in Table 45.10.

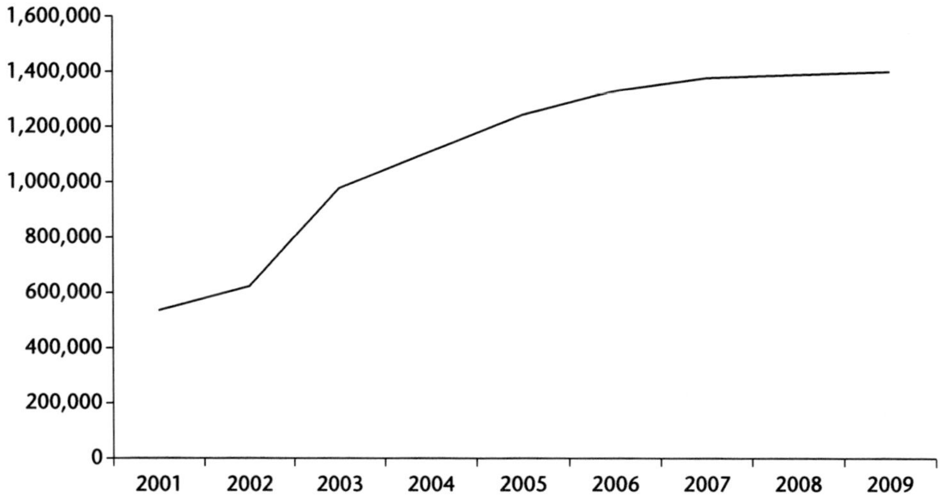


*Figure 45.3* Number of foreign patients treated in Thailand, 2001–2009 [17]

*Table 45.9* Competitive advantage of health facilities in Asian countries providing healthcare services to foreign patients

| *Competitive advantage* | *Thailand* | *Singapore* | *India* | *Malaysia* |
|---|---|---|---|---|
| Service and hospitality | ***** | ** | * | * |
| High-technological hardware | ** | **** | ** | * |
| HR quality | **** | **** | ** | ** |
| International accredited hospital | ** | ** | – | * |
| Pre-emptive move | ** | *** | * | * |
| Synergy/strategic partner | * | ** | * | * |
| Accessibility/market channel | ** | *** | * | ** |
| Reasonable cost | **** | * | **** | *** |

*Source*: [10].

*Table 45.10* SWOT analysis

| | |
|---|---|
| ***Strengths***<br>• High-quality medical professional workforce<br>• Hospitality and service minded<br>• Low cost of medical treatments<br>• State of the art medical equipment<br>• High quality and standard of medical care<br>• Variety of services and continuous new product and service development<br>• Good physical infrastructure (hospitals, research centres, educational institutions, tourism sites, transportation, etc.)<br>• Large private hospitals run by experienced management teams<br>• Thai medicines, massage and herbal products | ***Opportunities***<br>• Increased contribution of medical tourism to economic growth<br>• Increased competitive pressures (which may help improve medical infrastructure and increase the quality of medical professionals further)<br>• Demographic change, rising prevalence of chronic diseases and cost escalation in developed countries<br>• Trend toward health and wellness tourism and use of herbal medicine and traditional treatment alternatives<br>• Strong local demand for cosmetic surgical procedures |
| ***Weaknesses***<br>• Production and distribution of human resources<br>• Possible negative impact of medical tourism on (i) internal brain drain, (ii) equitable access to quality health services for Thai people and (iii) medical expenses for self-paying Thai patients<br>• Lack of foreign language skills<br>• Intense competition among domestic and regional hospitals<br>• Few strategic partnerships<br>• Policy incoherence and lack of cooperation among key stakeholders<br>• Weak medical malpractice law<br>• Most medical equipment and medicines are imported<br>• High energy dependence<br>• Political instability<br>• Lack of funding, especially for SMEs | ***Threats***<br>• Intense competition among domestic and international medical and tourism providers triggering consolidation of the sector<br>• Emergence of new players such as Malaysia<br>• Demographic change in Thailand<br>• No clear dominance in technological or basic research<br>• Lack of support from the population and prevalence of inequities<br>• European sovereign debt crisis |

*Source*: [10].

## Roles of policies, regulations and institutional support

Enhancing the strengths and opportunities and mitigating weaknesses and threats, the SWOT analysis suggests further actions in government policy. Investing in modern medical technology, especially high-tech medical equipment, as well as establishing a clear dominance in technological or basic research and providing funding for new entrepreneurial ideas, will make Thailand a leading destination for medical tourists subject to favourable external factors.

In addition, pull factors, such as the low cost of obtaining services of similar/acceptable quality, price certainty through fixed package prices offered by medical facilities and well-developed tourism industry and other supporting industries, should be strengthened further. The Office of International Healthcare Centre has been created underneath the Department of Health Service Support, MoPH, which is responsible for the strategic plan for the medical hub policy. Most importantly, however, is the identification of government agencies involved so that a dialogue and cooperation among all stakeholders can be encouraged [10].

For the national policy to further develop Thailand as a medical hub in the region, government policies should be more comprehensive, that is, have a more precise explicit framework and promote Thai medicine with international quality standards, but with price rates cheaper than in the other countries. Therefore, the relevant authority must have a clear operational plan. The government should also improve public health systems within the country to provide higher quality of care benchmarked with international standards and ensure a strong public, as well as private, system, which will require cooperation from the private sector. This means the development of tourism needs to be more creative and to increase its 'added value' by creating a tourism-oriented medical industry from the supply chain that already exists, starting from the production planning process to the services produced. Each process in every activity must add value creating a value chain.

To address the problem of the shortage of medical professionals, government support for training medical professionals to ensure sufficient supply is needed as it will improve the distribution of health services. This is because the health system is a labour-intensive system and workforce problems will affect the overall health system. Cooperation is needed between the Ministry of Education and administrative organizations to provide scholarships to children in the districts and provinces. As well as that, the retirement age of doctors could be prolonged as another tactic of addressing this problem. A related problem is that medical education is largely publicly subsidized, while private hospitals who are recruiting medical graduates from the same pool of graduates, hardly share the costs of producing them. Bonding and offering financial incentives have been employed to prevent the internal brain drain from rural public hospitals to urban private hospitals, and, more generally, from rural to urban areas, and this approach could be strengthened. Given the excess capacity in the private sector, attempts should be made to harness the existing private sector better to achieve health system goals by implementing various strategies, such as contracting to a fuller extent, which in turn would require a move towards a regulatory framework that is more supportive of public–private partnerships. In addition, a non-prohibitive special tax on revenue earned from medical tourism could be imposed as *inter alia* discussed in Pachanee [15].

## References


1. MoPH. *Thailand Health Profile 2005–2007*. Bangkok: Ministry of Public Health, Bureau of Policy and Strategy, 2008. Available from: http://www.moph.go.th/ops/thp/index.php?option=com_content&task=view&id=6&emid=2&lang=en
2. Kachondham, Y, Chunharas, S. At the Crossroads: Challenges for Thailand's Health Development. *Health Policy and Planning* 1993; 8(3): 208–16.
3. World Bank. World Development Indicators. Available from: http://data.worldbank.org/country. [Accessed 24 February 2012].
4. Khumthong, CN, Supakankunti, S. The National MediAid Plan: A Stride to Attain 'Health for All' with Decentralisation. Chulalongkorn Discussion Paper, 2003.
5. Patcharanarumol, W, Tangcharoensathien, V, Limwattananon, S, Panichkriangkai, W, Pachanee, P, Poungkantha, W, Gilson, L, Mills, A. Why and How Did Thailand Achieve Good Health at Low Cost? 2010. Available from: http://ghlc.lshtm.ac.uk/
6. Supakankunti, S, Witvorapong, N. Health Care in Thailand. 2012.
7. WTO. Understanding the WTO – Services: Rules for Growth and Investment. 2011. Available from: http://www.wto.org
8. Pachanee, C, Wibulpolprasert, S. Incoherent Policies on Universal Coverage of Health Insurance and Promotion of International Trade in Health Services in Thailand. *Health Policy and Planning* 2006; 21(4): 310–18.
9. ASEAN. Requirements for International Trade in Services Thailand. 2008. Available from http://www.asean.or g/22517.zip
10. Supakankunti, S, Herberholz, C. Transforming the ASEAN Economic Community (AEC) into a Global Services Hub: Enhancing the Competitiveness of the Health Services Sector in Thailand. In ERIA Research Project Report 2011, No. 1 Developing ASEAN Economic Community (AEC) into a Global Service Hub, 2012: 147–72.
11. Klongdee, S. Factors Determining the Demand and Competitiveness of Medical Tourism in Thailand. Master's Thesis, Faculty of Economics, Chulalongkorn University MoPH, 2011.
12. MoPH. Health Policy in Thailand. Ministry of Public Health, Bureau of Policy and Strategy. 2009.
13. NaRanong, A, NaRanong, V. The Effects of Medical Tourism: Thailand's Experience. *Bulletin of the World Health Organization* 2011; 89: 336–44.
14. MoPH. (n.d.). Trade in Health Services in the ASEAN Regions: Thailand Opportunity.
15. Pachanee, C. Implications on Public Health from Mode 2 Trade in Health Services: Empirical Evidence [A Case of Thailand]. Paper presented at the Workshop on the Movement of Patients across International Borders – Emerging Challenges and Opportunities for Health Care Systems, 24–25 February 2009, Kobe, Japan. Online. 2009. Available from: http://ihppthaigov.net/publication/attachresearch/ 181/chapter1.pdf
16. The Tourism Authority of Thailand. Information Infrastructure Investments for Businesses in the Tourism Industry Project.
17. MoPH. Department of Export Promotion, Ministry of Commerce. 2009. Available from: http://www.thailandmedicaltourismcluster.org [Accessed 24 February 2012].
18. Thailand Health Profile, 1999–2000. Available from: http://www.moph.go.th/ops/thp/index.php?option=com_content&task=view&id=8&Itemid=2
19. Bank of Thailand. Statistics. Available from: http://www.bot.or.th/Thai/Statistics/Pages/index1.aspx
20. Central Intelligence Agency. (n.d.). *World Factbook*. Available from: https://www.cia.gov/library/publications/the-world-factbook/geos/th.html [Accessed 15 September 2012].
21. Thailand Health Profile 2001–2004. Available from: http://www.moph.go.th/ops/thp/index.php?option=com_content&task=view&id=7&Itemid=2
22. Bureau of Policy and Strategy. Report: Macroeconomics and Health Framework for Investing in Health – Thailand. A document distributed by the Bureau of Policy and Strategy, the Ministry of Public Health, the Royal Thai Government, 2005.
23. Thai Websites. GDP Per Capita and Population Data for the Provinces of Thailand. Available from: http://www.thaiwebsites.com/provinces-GDP.asp
24. Office of the National Economic and Social Development Board (NESDB).
25. WHO National Health Accounts (NHA). Country health information. Geneva, World Health Organization, February 2010. Available from: http://www.who.int/nha/country/en/

26. World Bank. World Development Indicators Database. Washington, DC, World Bank. December 2010 update. Available from: http://www.worldbank.org/data
27. World Health Organization. *World Health Statistics 2011.* Available from: http://www.who.int/whosis/whostat/2011/en/index.html
28. Supakankunti, S, Pradithavanij, PA. Preliminary Study of Hospital Transition in Health System Reform in Thailand. Country Reports for the ANHSS Knowledge Event, 2010.

## Bibliography

Department of Trade Negotiations (2010). Health Services. A document distributed by the Department of Trade Negotiations, the Ministry of Commerce, the Royal Thai Government.

Hempisut, P., Pachanee, C., Pitayarangsarit, S., Wibulpolprasert, S. (2004). International Service Trade and its Implications for Human Resources for Health: A Case Study of Thailand. Online. Retrieved from: http://www.human-resources-health.com/content/pdf/1478-4491-2-10.pdf

Janjaroen, W.S. and Supakankunti, S. (1998). International Trade in Health Services in the Millennium: the Case of Thailand. Bangkok College of Public Health, Chulalongkorn University. Available online at: http://www.who.int/trade/en/THpart3chap8.pdf

Janjaroen, W.S., Pinitpuvadol, S., Pongpanich, S., Samrongthong, R., Sitthi-amorn, C., Supakankunti, S., *et al.* (1999). Preliminary Study on Trade Liberalization in Health Services Sector: Its Consequences on Social and Health Care System in Thailand.

Janjaroen, W.S., Pongpanich, S., Supakankunti, S. (2007). Socio-economic Impacts of Trade Agreements on Health Services and Health Systems in Thailand. Bangkok: Centre for Health Economics, Chulalongkorn University.

NHSO. (2011). *Annual Report 2010.* Bangkok: National Health Security Office.

Pachanee, C., and Wibulpolprasert, S. (2004). Policy Coherence between Health Related Trade and Health System Development: Case Study of Thailand. Trade and Health – Compilation of Presentations made at the Inter-regional Workshop, New Delhi. WHO.

PReMA. (2010). *PReMA Handbook 2010/2011.* Bangkok: Pharmaceutical Research and Manufacturers' Association.

Sakunphanit, T. (2006). Universal Health Care Coverage through Pluralistic Approaches: Experience from Thailand. ILO.

SET Market Analysis and Reporting Tool. (n.d.). Online. Retrieved from: http://www.setsmart.com/ism /login.jsp

SSO. (2010). Annual Report 2009. Online. Retrieved from: http://www.sso.go.th/wpr/eng/annual-report. html

Supakankunti, S. (1999). Future Prospects of Voluntary Health Insurance in Thailand. *Health Policy and Planning* 15(1): 85–94.

Supakankunti, S. (2001). Determinants of Demand for Health Card in Thailand. HNP Discussion Paper. Online. Retrieved from: http://siteresources.worldbank.org/HEALTHNUTRITIONAND POPULATION/Resources/281627-1095698140167/Supakankunti-DeterminantsofDemand-whole.pdf

Supakankunti, S. (2003). Impact of Universal Coverage – Challenges for the Future. Paper presented in the conference on Asia Healthcare & Insurance 2003 organized by IBC ASIA (S) PTE Ltd., Bangkok, Thailand, 26–27 June 2003.

Supakankunti, S. (2003). Thai Health System in Transition: The Challenge of the Mutual Responsibilities. Paper presented at the Regional Workshop & Conference on Health Care Environment and Patient's Rights. Asia Foundation in Taipei, Taiwan, 6–7 November 2003. Also presented at the National University of Singapore, Joint Workshop between Department of Economics, National University of Singapore and the Faculty of Economics, Chulalongkorn University, Thailand, 12 December 2003.

Supakankunti, S. (2003). Thai Universal Health Insurance Scheme in Transition: Challenges for the Future. Paper presented at iHEA, San Francisco, USA, 2003.

Supakankunti, S., Herberholz, C. (2011). Trade in Health Services – Harnessing the Benefits and Avoiding the Pitfalls: The Case of Thailand. Research report.

Supakankunti, S. and Janjaroen W.S. (1998). Health Services Systems and the Consequences from the General Agreement on Trade in Services (GATS). Paper presented at the conference: A

Macroeconomic Core of Open Economy for Progressive Industrialization and Development in Asia in the new Millennium, organized jointly by Chulalongkorn University and American Committee on Asian Economics Studies, Bangkok, Thailand, 16–18 December 1998.
Suppradit, T. (2010). Thailand: Medical Hub Update 2010. Cluster of International Affairs, Private Hospital Association.
UN ESCAP. (2009). Medical Travel in Asia and the Pacific – Challenges and Opportunities. Bangkok: United Nations Economic and Social Commission for Asia and the Pacific.

# 46

# Comparative health systems in Asia

*Kai Hong Phua and Mary Lai Lin Wong*

## Introduction

In the World Health Report 2000, the World Health Organization (WHO) asserts that a large part of the variation in the health statuses of countries can be attributed to differences in health system performance. In particular, differences in health system performance explain the marked variation even amongst countries with similar incomes and expenditures. Asia spans two WHO regions of South-East Asia and the Western Pacific, and accounts for 60 per cent of the world's population. It encompasses more than 20 nations. Some have health systems that rank amongst the world's best, and yet others have difficulty providing the basics of safe drinking water and modern sanitation. With populations ageing at an ever-increasing rate, non-communicable diseases (NCDs) have, or will soon, overtake communicable diseases as the main cause of disability and premature mortality. Neuropsychiatric disorders, cardiovascular diseases and malignant neoplasms are responsible for the bulk of the burden of the NCDs. The burden of communicable diseases also remains significant. Many of the less developed countries operate in a 'worst-case scenario', facing a double burden of communicable and non-communicable diseases, with threats of new emerging infectious diseases. Poverty is a major cause of health inequalities in Asia, along with often poverty-related factors such as access to basic health care and education. Given such conditions, what should be the role of health systems towards the improvement of public health in Asia? Comparisons of health systems in the many diverse countries of Asia are challenging, since they are currently classified under different regional groupings for political and economic cooperation, including health matters which are divided under the WHO South-East Asia and Western Pacific Regional Offices (see Table 46.1). This chapter will examine the main determinants and common criteria for comparing health systems performance to achieve better public health.

## Definition of a health system

As defined by the WHO, a health system 'includes the resources, actors and institutions related to all the activities whose primary purpose is to promote, restore or maintain health' [1]. Within these boundaries is the professional delivery of personal medical attention,

*Table 46.1* Regional groupings of Asian countries

| | *ASEAN* | *WHO** | *UNESCAP* | *APEC* | *East Asia Summit* | *ASEAN Regional Forum* |
|---|---|---|---|---|---|---|
| Bangladesh | | S | √ | | | |
| Bhutan | | S | √ | | | |
| Brunei | √ | W | √ | √ | √ | √ |
| Cambodia | √ | W | √ | | √ | √ |
| China | | W | √ | √ | √ | √ |
| India | | S | √ | | √ | √ |
| Indonesia | √ | S | √ | √ | √ | √ |
| Japan | | W | √ | √ | √ | √ |
| Lao PDR | √ | W | √ | | √ | √ |
| Malaysia | √ | W | √ | √ | √ | √ |
| Mongolia | | W | √ | | | |
| Myanmar | √ | S | √ | | √ | √ |
| Nepal | | S | √ | | | |
| Pakistan | | S | √ | | | |
| Philippines | √ | W | √ | √ | √ | √ |
| Singapore | √ | W | √ | √ | √ | √ |
| Sri Lanka | | S | √ | | | √ |
| South Korea | | W | √ | √ | √ | √ |
| Thailand | √ | S | √ | √ | √ | √ |
| Timor-Leste | | S | √ | | | √ |
| Vietnam | √ | W | √ | √ | √ | √ |

*Notes*: * S – WHO South-East Asia Region, W – WHO Western Pacific Region
ASEAN – Association of Southeast Asian Nations
WHO – World Health Organization
UNESCAP – United Nations Economic and Social Commission for Asia and the Pacific
APEC – Asia-Pacific Economic Cooperation

traditional healing and use of medication, including self-medication. Other components of the system are health-enhancing activities such as public health, and occupational and environmental safety. Education, despite the fact that it has a beneficial but secondary effect on health, is outside the system but, in contrast, health education has the primary goal of enhancing health and is, therefore, within the health system [2]. This has a lot in common with other definitions of health systems. For example, the definition proposed by Roemer [3] is that it is 'a combination of resources, organizations, financing and management that culminate in the delivery of health services to the population'. The notable difference is the concept of 'health activity', which, in the WHO definition, is used in a more all-encompassing sense and is not restricted to formal health services.

Working on the premise that the health status of a population is largely determined by the performance of the health system that serves it, the next question is: How do we assess a health system's performance? Frameworks that have been proposed for measuring health system performance fall into two groups [2]: lists of desirable attributes of health systems and a reliance on available indices to construct performance measures, which often replicates their inadequacies. The problem with the first group is that such lists are often lengthy and the attributes often overlap. Using a third approach, the WHO builds from first principles by initially articulating the goals of health systems.

*Table 46.2* Health system goals in relation to components for assessment

| | *Average level* | *Distribution* |
|---|---|---|
| Health improvement | √ | √ |
| Responsiveness to expectations | √ | √ |
| Fairness in financial contribution | – | √ |

*Source*: [2].

According to the WHO framework, the primary goal of health systems is to improve health. This should be self-evident given the definition of health systems used above. The other goals of health systems are common to all social systems: responsiveness of the system to the legitimate expectations of the population and fairness in the financial contribution required to make the system work. Each of these goals is assessed on the average level of attainment and the nature of distribution, or, in other words, the levels of goodness and fairness. Financing is the exception in that only distribution is assessed, there being no intrinsically good or bad level of financing (see Table 46.2).

Furthermore, these indicators of attainment (what has been achieved) are translated into indicators of performance (what should be achieved). The level of attainment for each indicator is compared to what can be demanded from a health system, given the resources available. This is done by defining the upper and lower boundaries of attainment for different levels of health expenditure and availability of human capital (as reflected in the average years of schooling in the adult population). Moving towards the upper boundary indicates improvements in performance, whereas the reverse holds true when moving towards the lower boundary.

These concepts proposed by the WHO are not entirely new. The concept of performance corresponds to the macroeconomic definition of efficiency – the outcomes of a system relative to the total system costs. In this case, the notion of performance does not explicitly incorporate microeconomic notions of cost-effectiveness and avoiding waste, although these process-related measures are determinants of macroeconomic efficiency [4]. In addition, distribution and fairness correspond to concepts of equality and equity, with equality referring to the reduction in differences between groups, and equity carrying with it the additional notions of ethical values and social justice [5].

## Determinants of a health system's performance

The functions of a health system will be examined below as essential roles for financing, provision, regulation and stewardship, in order to identify the key issues influencing performance in Asian health systems.

### *Financing*

The purpose of health financing is to increase the availability of funds for the provision of health services. High-income countries, with 16 per cent of the world's population, accounted for 89 per cent of the total health expenditure, or slightly more than $2 trillion. In these countries, the goal has generally shifted from generating funds to cost containment [4]. In contrast, many low- and middle-income countries face the problem of generating sufficient funds simply for the provision of a minimal package of health services. Of the total global spending on health, low- and middle-income countries, with 84 per cent of the world's population, accounted for only 11 per cent of this spending [6]. There are basic mechanisms of fund generation: out-of-pocket payments (user fees), voluntary insurance rated by income or risks, donations from non-government organizations, compulsory insurance (social insurance that is community- or population-rated), general taxes, earmarked taxes and transfers from donor agencies [7]. The first three are private sources of revenue, whereas the last four are public ones.

In low-income countries, the ability to generate funds from public sources is limited. There are a number of reasons for this, including large rural populations who are poor, a small formal employment sector, too few large and easy-to-tax enterprises and a weak tax administration capacity. The choice of mechanism has a direct impact on one of the key goals of health systems, which is fair financing. Each mechanism performs differently with respect to horizontal and vertical equity. General taxation achieves horizontal equity but taxes are generally related only to income. Income tax is the most progressive form of revenue generation when income tax rates are higher at higher income brackets [8]. Compulsory insurance is horizontally equitable but tends to be regressive. This is because contributions are usually subject to a ceiling. Voluntary insurance rated by risk (as seen in most private health insurance schemes) has similar characteristics. Its regressivity is due to the disproportionate burden of disease borne by the poor.

It has been said that out-of-pocket payments are the most difficult to make progressive. Income-based exemptions are one way of reducing the risk of regressivity, but have proven difficult to manage [9]. In China, the collapse of rural insurance in the 1980s resulted in an increase in the importance of out-of-pocket payments from 24 per cent to 36 per cent of health financing. The effect was that, as one commentator put it, 'access to health care is largely based on the patient's ability to pay, and many cannot afford care' [10]. The higher the proportion of out-of-pocket payments, the greater the financial burden will be on poor people.

However, proponents of co-payments argue that they are a way of moderating demand and containing costs [11]. The theory behind this is that other mechanisms of fund generation, for example when health insurance is combined with fee-for-service payment, cause serious 'moral hazards' as neither provider nor patient is concerned about costs. Most of the individual patient's healthcare burden may fall heavily on the household, and therefore family members can strengthen traditional support mechanisms for health care based on their savings, especially in old age. This principle of pooling individual and family savings to cover intergenerational transfers is implemented in Singapore's Medisave system [12]. With rising medical costs and population ageing, it is also intended to provide a demand-side personal responsibility to manage healthcare consumption. Third-party payments create the illusion of a free service at the point of consumption; in other words, the 'proverbial free lunch'. This phenomenon is also known as the 'buffet syndrome', where people tend to take more food than needed thereby contributing to wastage (as they pay a fixed amount of money for unlimited consumption like the case of unmanaged indemnity insurance).

## Provision

Provision of health services refers to the combination of inputs into a production process that takes place in a particular organizational setting, leading to the delivery of a series of interventions. Health services may be personal or non-personal. Personal health services are consumed directly by the individual and include most of what is commonly viewed as 'health care'. These include most of the preventive, curative or diagnostic interventions administered by doctors and health workers in the setting of a clinic or a hospital. Non-personal health services include interventions applied to population groups, such as health education, and also to their environments, including the management of sanitation and provision of safe drinking water.

One of the most important considerations in the provision of health services is in the choice of interventions. This revolves around the concept of economic efficiency: maximizing the use of available resources in order to achieve the desired outcomes. As mentioned earlier, this is one of the determinants of macroeconomic efficiency or performance. There are two types of microeconomic efficiency – allocative efficiency and technical efficiency. Allocative efficiency, or cost-effectiveness, is what we hope to achieve in our choice of intervention – we should devote resources to the mix of interventions that produces the most health gains. Failure to do so, misallocation of resources, has been identified as one of the major problems in health systems in addition to lack of productive efficiency.

Differences in outcomes for any intervention do occur from system to system. This can be due to differences in the incidence or prevalence of disease, the varying probability of death from disease, the cost of inputs and implementation processes. However, differences in cost-effectiveness between interventions are often much larger than the uncertainty in estimates. In spending public resources on interventions, cost-effectiveness is never the only justification. Other social and humane concerns should also be taken into account, such as assisting individuals and their families with catastrophic illness and offering protection for the poor.

It should be noted that in Asia, 'modern' medical interventions have a relatively short history compared to many traditional systems of medicine. Throughout the region, there are as many different systems as there are cultures, some of which have existed for millennia. But the common feature in Asian countries is the degree of utilization of traditional interventions. This is often in the context of medical pluralism – the use of multiple forms of health care. China is one of the leading countries in Asia in the integration of traditional medicine (TM) into its national health system. In terms of volume, hospitals practising traditional Chinese medicine (TCM) treat 200 million outpatients and 3 million inpatients annually. Most general hospitals also have TM departments where they treat 20 per cent of outpatients daily. This integration was directed by health officials trained in modern medicine, with the aim of harmonization with modern medicine through a science-based approach [13].

In many countries, traditional health functions are parallel with the national health system rather than integrated with it. Partially due to lack of a strong central control mechanism, many regulatory issues involving licensing of practitioners, standardization and prescription of drugs have emerged as points of contention. This has even resulted in mass demonstrations and strikes in Korea throughout the 1990s. In such situations where reactions to attempts at government regulation have been unfavourable, self-regulation may be a viable option. Malaysia has recently adopted this approach, with the establishment of a council, under which organizations representing Malay, Chinese and Indian traditional health systems undertake a process of internal regulation, including accreditation and registration of practitioners. In Singapore, the Ministry of Health has recommended that TCM bodies develop an internal regulatory framework. Despite some problems in bringing about integration on a national scale, there have been a number of successes on a project level [14]. A WHO study found that volunteers for traditional healers in Thailand performed better than other volunteers. Villagers were also more confident about having someone they already knew draw blood and administer treatment. In Bangladesh, a project to train midwifes to work with traditional birth attendants helped to lower maternal mortality rates (MMR) by 60 per cent over ten years.

## Regulation

In most other Asian countries, TM providers are part of the private sector. Many of the issues relating to the role of TM are also relevant in analyses of the public–private mix in national health systems. As with TM, regulation of the private sector as a whole is a problem in most Asian countries. The regulatory framework is especially weak in less-developed countries. This has led to problems of unqualified and unlicensed practitioners using Western practices and prescription drugs. Patients treated by private practitioners may receive inappropriate and inadequate courses of therapy, with patients spending more than they need to. Private practitioners seldom offer services of a public health or preventive nature, including services such as immunization, and they tend to over-prescribe (especially antibiotics and injections).

The overall pattern is one whereby individuals most able to benefit from an intervention select those provider types with the lowest technical quality/efficacy because there is a perception that they are of better quality or because of ease of access. The paradoxical outcome is one of access to services with little positive impact, or even negative impact, on health. Thus, the problem in most low-income countries in Asia does not seem to be primarily one of access – spending on personal ambulatory care services accounts for 55 per cent and 72 per cent of total health spending, respectively in India and Bangladesh. As a share of household out-of-pocket expenditure on health, the figures are even more striking – in excess of 60 per cent and 90 per cent respectively [15].

With regards to the public–private mix, the focus of governments on improving access through direct provision of services should therefore be shifted to improving the performance of the sizeable private sector. Public health authorities need to play a guiding role in providing public-oriented rather than profit-oriented leadership in health systems [16]. There is, therefore, a need for health reforms in less-developed countries in which private sector providers are brought into the public health sector framework in different forms of public–private participation. This may be achieved largely by improving regulation, but also through organizing, financing, and educational activities targeted at both healthcare consumers and providers [17].

In the more developed countries in Asia, there has been a similar push towards increased regulation of the private sector, albeit from the perspective of cost containment. A past Ministerial Committee on Health Policy in Singapore published a White Paper with the conclusion that in spite of Singapore's strong belief in, and commitment to, a free market, 'market forces alone will not suffice to hold down medical costs to the minimum. The health care system is an example of market failure. The government has to intervene directly to structure and regulate the health system' [18].

## Stewardship

The fourth and final function of a health system is stewardship. It occupies a special place as it involves oversight of all other functions and makes the attainment of each health system goal possible. In its 2000 World Health Report, the WHO states that the stewardship of health systems is a government responsibility [1]. Three different aspects of stewardship have been described [2]:

1 Setting, implementing and monitoring the rules for the health system;
2 Assuring a level playing field for all parties in the system; and
3 Defining strategic directions for the system.

In turn, these three aspects have been divided into sub-functions, namely overall system design, performance assessment, consumer protection, priority setting, regulation and inter-sectoral advocacy. Some of these sub-functions have been discussed, including performance assessment in relation to goal attainment in Asian health systems, consumer protection in health financing, priority setting in the context of the cost-effectiveness of interventions and regulation of health service providers. The last sub-function on the list, inter-sectoral advocacy, is the promotion of related activities, which are not part of the health system but have a significant secondary health-enhancing effect. This often involves collaboration with other social systems.

Conceptually, the premise of stewardship is that it is possible to create a system that is not only efficient but is also good. Stewardship has been defined as 'the willingness to be accountable for the well-being of the larger organization by operating in the service rather than in the control of those around us' [19]. As stewardship encompasses notions of trust and ethical behaviour, and because of the need for stewardship to transcend economic concerns, it is clear that the profit-oriented private sector cannot fulfil this role. Saltman *et al.* [20] go further, describing stewardship as 'a function of governments responsible for the welfare of populations and concerned about the trust and legitimacy with which its activities are viewed by the general public'. These ideas may find a receptive audience in Asian countries. The concept of stewardship bears a strong resemblance to Confucian ideals of morality and government, and the need for those who govern to be principled and virtuous. China, Japan, Singapore, Taiwan and Korea are clear examples of societies with a strong Confucian basis.

## Comparative health systems

According to Roemer, a health system is the combination of resources, organization, financing and management that culminate in the delivery of health services to the population [3]. Most national health systems do show varying degrees of complexity and coherence. No two health systems are alike as health systems are always changing and evolving whether in their structural form or in their organization. A health system can be defined as a 'societal mechanism which transforms generalized resources or inputs into specialized outputs in the form of health services aimed at the health problems of the society' [21]. Medical care systems are one element or subsystem within society which seeks to ensure the health of its members. This subsystem interacts with other subsystems to carry out society's goals. If defined as a purposeful process in which health care resources are organized and financed, health services in all modern societies have developed into recognizable relationships that can be described as a healthcare system [22].

In planning health systems, the interactions both within the system and with other systems cannot be ignored. Whether the health system is perceived as a combination of various health resources to improve the health of the population as in the early definitions, or in the societal view as a social mechanism to deliver health services to the society as in the latter definitions, health systems are seen as a complex interaction of multiple variables to produce health or to meet healthcare needs.

There are many ways of looking at health, although how they are managed will deliver different results. According to Roemer, every health system has components which are definite although the characteristics of each component may vary greatly. Therefore, in order to appropriately evaluate any health system, it must have boundaries set by well-defined objectives which the system hopes to achieve. Phua classifies health systems by categorizing them according to the level of development of their respective economies: developed, high performing, newly industrializing, transitional and developing [23]. His theories generalize regional health systems at different stages of socio-economic development of individual countries by a typology of common issues, challenges and responses. This classification allows for longitudinal development and criteria for evaluation in terms of efficiency, equity, quality and sustainability. Phua's classification is quite similar to the World Bank's classification of countries by income or the gross national product (GNP) per capita. Asian countries can be grouped according to their levels of socio-economic development, and their health systems could be analysed and compared within this context. Thus, the stages of demographic and epidemiological transitions could be related to socio-economic changes that influence the driving forces for health sector reforms, including delivery and financing systems. A World Bank publication categorized health financing systems into those of high-, middle- and low-income countries, and offered policy options for reforms that fit their needs and contexts [24]. However, looking at this from an economic status standpoint is not sufficient as policy makers do not always make decisions based on the economic conditions of the country alone, but take into account other factors, such as the political climate, and cultural and societal values.

## *Health system reform*

Every country has different forms of health systems deriving from their peculiar historical, social, cultural, economic and political contexts, and many of these systems are experiencing various stages of reform as they evolve. In any health system, the main function is to provide or deliver health services to its defined population. The questions lie in whether such health services provided are acceptable, effective and affordable for the population concerned. Policy makers and providers are required to make certain decisions and choices pertaining to the functions of the system, such as what services to provide, what level of skills and training are required for its personnel, what arrangements are to be made among the quantity and quality of providers, which target groups are to be given priority, what proportion of allocation is for public services provided, how to organize the provision in the most efficient way, what sort of incentives should be given for the providers, as well as others. Thus, organizing a health system is very complex and getting the right balance is important for the system to function and to deliver its services so that it will give the most impact to the population at large. Any changes or improvements made, whether organizational or structural, in the delivery of services, financing and distribution of resources will lead to reforming the health system. Healthcare reform has been described as a 'global epidemic' as it consists of very complex policy choices [25]. In a more macro-perspective, the reason for reform in the health sector could be due to market failure and thus the need for government intervention.

In 1987, the World Bank led a global health reform when it released a publication entitled *Financing Health Services in Developing Countries: An Agenda for Reform*, which proposed four changes: imposing user fees at government facilities, introducing social insurance or other risk coverage systems, using non-governmental resources more effectively, and decentralizing planning, budgeting and purchasing of government health services [26]. The intention of this reform was to shift government expenditures to cater for the poor and reduce subsidies for the rich, thus increasing the role of the market in the health sector. Following this publication, the Bank came out with another document entitled the *World Development Report: Investing in Health* [27] in 1993, which outlined a more comprehensive agenda for health reform with a three-pronged approach: fostering an economic environment to enable households to improve their own health, redirecting government spending from specialized care towards cost-effective programmes, and promoting greater diversity and competition in health financing and delivery of health services.

The World Bank approaches health system reform from a macro-perspective although the policy context or the factors affecting the health system is similar to that of WHO. It focuses on the pursuit of macroeconomic policies that emphasize the reduction of poverty. The policy process is looking at the health systems and their problems, and tackling them accordingly within the confines of the country's economic status and income which is determined by what the government is able and willing to spend on health care. The main problems identified are misallocation, inequity, efficiency and exploding costs. The World Bank recommends that governments should finance public health measures and nationally defined packages of essential health services only [28]. The remaining clinical services are discretionary and should be financed privately or by social insurance.

An alternative approach to the World Bank's essential package is its proposed comprehensive package which identifies the injustices in the current healthcare system and then goes on to make the necessary modifications to achieve that change. The policy process created must ensure acceptable decisions are made [29]. According to Chernichovsky, private and competitive provision of care may be unrealistic in many developing areas because of scarcity of real resources, mainly human resources and health needs. He suggests that developing countries should strengthen what is probably the most fundamental initial systemic asset they have – public finance [30]. This is the case as most developing countries have healthcare systems that are tax financed and they may not be sustainable. Some tax-based systems inherited from the British colonial legacy have generally worked well in Hong Kong, Malaysia, Singapore and Sri Lanka. Yuen suggests that the way forward is to fine-tune the existing system rather than to replace it with other systems, which are known to have higher transaction costs and more serious supply-side moral hazards [31].

According to Berman, the essence of reform is 'sustained, purposeful change to improve the efficiency, equity and effectiveness of the health sector' [32]. His definition implies sustained, purposeful and fundamental changes and that reform should be based on a holistic view of the health sector [33]. The government is in the best position to manage this change. The role of the government is important not only to ensure that the health system operates at its optimal level for greater efficiency, but also to ensure accessibility and quality of health services to its population. Studies have shown that emphasis on outcomes rather than process have not supported sustainable reforms or achieved the government's goal of improving health and ensuring equity for the citizens of the country, and there is a need to identify the most critical processes, build and manage these processes in a systematic way, and monitor and evaluate the results [34]. Governments need to have the organizational and institutional capacity to undertake these policy processes [34, 35]. Besides building capacity to implement change, a rational policy development should explicitly consider multiple goals for the health sector [36].

Policies and strategies are changing to meet these new demands – some systems are more successful than others, and many others are learning from someone else's failures or experiences. Whatever the reform, health systems are expected to perform and to contribute to the better health of the entire population. There is no universal system for all, neither is there a perfect system. According to Collins *et al.*, it is important to understand the policy context, which comes in many different perspectives, such as demographic and epidemiological changes, processes of social and economic change, economic and financial policies, politics and political regimes, ideologies, public policies and the public sector, and external factors. These policy contexts are linked with an overall understanding of the policy process. While governments are facing major problems in policy-making for health sector reforms, the main problem lies with the lack of internal policy-making capacity [37].

## *Health system performance*

Kawabata [38] states that health systems in all countries, no matter how wealthy or poor, can improve their performance. What is important is to identify internal and external factors that are responsible for a health system's merits and shortcomings. Each system is judged according to the resources at its disposal. Besides resources, health systems are also judged by health outcomes in relation to inputs, but such assessment does not tell much about achievements in relation to its potential or what is expected from the system. According to the WHO, comparing actual attainment with potential would show how far from its own frontier of maximum performance is each country's health system [39]. Health systems that can achieve more with the same resources are considered to have made improvements in performance.

The WHO has since come out with a common conceptual framework for health systems' performance assessment, which lays down the empirical basis for assessing and comparing national health systems. The result was the 2000 World Health Report, which reported for the first time an index of national health systems' performance for achieving three overall goals: good health, responsiveness to the expectations of the population and fairness in financial contribution. The WHO assesses each health system by ranking them based on the attainment of goals and performance in the measure of disability-adjusted life expectancy, health equality in terms of child survival, responsiveness level, responsiveness in distribution, fairness of financial distribution, performance on the level of health and, finally, the overall health system performance, which is the composite measure of achievement of the other measures.

The WHO's approach was very different to the World Bank's reform agenda which assumed that economic growth was a condition for good health and vice versa, and that the private sector was in a better position than the government in the financing and provision of health care. The WHO, on the other hand, focused on goals' attainment and performance of the system, whether private or public. An assessment of the capacity and the performance of a health system was a necessary precondition for any reform in the system. The WHO provided an initial platform for such an option which would need further refinement over time.

The goal of improving health for all was also very general and population expectations could differ from one culture to another. Fairness in financial contribution primarily examined the financial contribution of the household to the financing of the health system, which is purely based on what the population could afford. What is a fair financial contribution really depends on the type of financing system in the health sector. How much the household contributes may not accurately be measured by this component. Some countries are rooted in welfare whereas others may prefer more cost-sharing and risk-pooling systems. Comparing such measures among member countries with different financing schemes does not give a fair and just measurement.

Performance is a relative concept and health systems are never held accountable for past mistakes or given credit for past success [40] unless they are assessed over a longer period to include what has been achieved over many years. There is still a choice which policy makers of different countries have to make and this should be measured against individually set goals and not universally arranged goals. There should not be 'a one-size-fits-all' standardized advice for all countries [41]. Each society makes its own choices and the country concerned has its own policy choices which seem to be the best, given the constraints the health system is facing. Therefore, developing a categorization or measures of key factors that will affect the health system must be thoroughly debated and accepted by all stakeholders concerned.

When assessing which of the key functions of the health system have fallen short of their potential, the questions often lie with the planning, management and operation of the health system. Many health systems have fallen short due to a lack of an appropriate and balanced mix of resources; poorly structured, organized and managed systems; and the usual inadequate funding. Many health systems have undergone much reform and are experiencing continuous change to deal with the ever-changing healthcare needs, and demands and expectations which could be partly driven by economic, political, technological and, simply, ideological forces. Therefore, the criteria presented by the WHO are not exhaustive as many other factors can equally influence the system besides the three goals mentioned. Even common goals may be interpreted differently for various reasons and have to be defined properly, incorporating the heterogeneity of the countries. Factors, such as the local environment, values and culture, and the historical, political, cultural and socio-economic contexts – which over a long time have moulded the health system – cannot be ignored. Past development efforts and the current conditions will have to be examined thoroughly before any comparison and ranking of different countries can be made.

Despite the criticisms that have been brought forth, the World Health Report 2000 has succeeded in stimulating governments to be more aware and accountable for their health systems. Policy makers, civil society and the research community are beginning to seriously consider measurements of performance and focus more on the achievements of health systems. Since the report, the WHO has initiated a series of technical and regional consultations involving scientists and policy makers, and the establishment of a scientific peer review group overseen by an external advisory group that has shown the transparency, objectiveness and thoroughness of the WHO to bring health system performance to the attention of policy makers [42]. What is really needed by the countries concerned is not just a comparison of each other's health systems' performance, but also a process to monitor the status of health goals in relation to resources spent [43]. What policy makers are looking for is practical guidance on how they can reform their health systems so that they will perform better [44]. The countries concerned can then use this platform to share their experiences with each other and improve on their own goals, measurements and performance. The initiative taken by the WHO to bring together the member countries to debate and review the methodology of assessment, both at the conceptual and operational levels, was a good start for the improvement of health system performance.

## Concepts of equity and efficiency in health systems

Inequalities are rising in many countries, especially in transitional and emerging economies that are experiencing rapid growth and they are finding it difficult to implement and sustain equitable policies. Inequity creates social gaps in health and health care which are unacceptable both in the developing as well as in the newly industrialized countries of Asia. These imbalances can be serious for poorer countries especially in terms of distribution of human and physical resources, as well as quality care which can widen the gap of inequity and inefficiency of the system. At the same time, efficiency cannot be divorced from issues of distribution and equity [45]. These two issues are faced by healthcare systems throughout the world in their distribution of healthcare resources. Most healthcare reforms, whether in developed or developing countries, must consider the advantages of equity and efficiency in public as well as private health care [46]. These two goals, more often than not, are in conflict rather than being complementary.

## *Equity in health systems*

Equity, in simple terms, means fairness. It means reducing unfair disparities as well as meeting acceptable standards. Equity is defined as a principle governing distributive functions designed to reduce or offset socially unjust inequalities, and is applied to evaluate the distribution of financial resources and the use of health services [47]. Equity in health care requires equity in the way healthcare resources are allocated, the way health services are received and the way health services are paid for. There are many definitions of equity in health care, such as equality of utilization, distribution according to need, equality of access, equality in health, as well as others. According to Culyer [48], the most dominant one is equality in health, but according to Mooney [49], the most commonly adopted is equal access for equal need. For example, Culyer defines equity in health care as encompassing equality of utilization, distribution according to need, equality of access and equality in health, which are all mutually incompatible [48]. Others include equal access for equal need [49], equity in terms of outcomes and ability to pay [50].

The different definitions and the varying levels of importance placed on them show that the issue of equity cannot be applied as a one-for-all. What is deemed fair or equitable by one person may not be seen as fair or equitable by another, as everyone is driven by different values and represents different moral positions [50]. Equality of access means providing an equal availability and an equal opportunity to use health services for all. Equal access allows for an individual's preferences for the consumption of health care and whether the individual chooses to consume or not is entirely up to her or him, but the health services are made available and accessible should he or she require them [51]. Although this equity is not tied to need but aims to ensure equality of access for all, allocation of funds and resources for health care are distributed geographically according to the need in different populations in order to maintain equality of access to all who have the same needs.

According to Gutman, the principle of equal access demands that every person who shares the same type and degree of health needs to be given an equally effective chance of receiving the appropriate treatment of equal quality [52]. Unequal access is the outcome of unequal distribution of healthcare resources. Despite the vast literature on the notion of equity of access existing, little agreement has been reached on what exactly the notion ought to mean [53]. Equity, in essence, is a policy that is being promoted to narrow socio-economic gaps, whether it is between different socio-economic groups or between different geographical areas through the distribution of healthcare resources. Therefore, it is not surprising why equity is one of the key objectives in most healthcare systems. The market system does not promote equity and will always result in unequal distribution of healthcare resources since equity has something to do with fairness and justice as opposed to profits and value for money. Economic recession and weak economic performance can also threaten equity.

There are two types of equity: horizontal and vertical. The notion of horizontal equity is that people in similar situations should be treated similarly and placing individuals to be treated differently is undesirable [54]. It refers to needs that are relatively the same, such as degrees of sickness. If two individuals have the same condition then *ceteris paribus* they should both be treated equally [55] and this implies equal effectiveness [56]. In practice, although two individuals may have the same problem and be given the same treatment, their outcomes may differ. According to Musgrove, where costs are equal, horizontal equity and cost-effectiveness are perfectly compatible [56].

Vertical equity, on the other hand, is about meeting different needs. It involves the unequal treatment of individuals that have different health conditions [57]. It does not imply a policy objective of equalizing health and wellbeing across groups or individuals, but it entails the treatment of different groups differently, yet equitably, based on the set of values adopted [58]. It means preferential treatment for people with worse problems [59] or unequal but equitable treatment of those who have different problems [60]. According to Jack, vertical equity is really an efficiency argument for the allocation of resources as it wishes to distribute wellbeing from those who have more of it to those with less [61]. These two types of equity can be applied either geographically or across socio-economic groups or classes.

Mooney *et al.* [62] have illustrated a few approaches to what constitutes equity. The common one is the basic needs approach. The notion behind this approach is the right to minimum health care. This approach wishes to address the issue of allocating resources to disadvantaged groups. Another approach is the 'communitarian claims' or the 'claims approach'. Claims are 'reasons' supported by the notion of duty and why one group should be allocated more resources than another. It focuses on vertical equity in the allocation of health service resources [63]. This approach is open to a wider set of values and value judgement is required. It also promotes a greater degree of transparency in the use of values in resource allocation decisions. Both of these approaches give the justification of why resources are allocated more to certain groups than to others.

Equity can be easily assessed and evaluated through the geographical distribution of healthcare resources, for example, the distribution of human resources, hospital beds, immunization coverage, and others. According to Ellencweig, a descriptive evaluation of equity consists of comparisons of the availability of health-related resources among smaller areas within the country or among different nations [64]. One way of assessing distribution is by analysing the budget allocation and expenditure. The breakdown of the budgets allocated and the actual expenditure for different geographical areas will clearly show whether any disparity exists and how much policy for an equitable distribution of resources has been achieved for the different states, regions, rural–urban mix and for different health programmes. Data, such as distribution of health facilities per population by region; state, urban or rural ratio of different categories of health human resources per population; health expenditure per capita; percentage of capital and operational budget allocated to the different states according to economic status; and some health output and outcome data by states, will be important to show the geographical distribution of health resources and expenditure.

The government fiscal capacity of many Asian countries is low and social health insurance for the employed sector is absent or small, restricting the mobilization of additional resources from payroll contributions. Financing health care in most developing countries greatly relies on out-of-pocket payments, with most donors focusing on specific diseases or interventions rather than the broader health system.

Besides assessing equity through the distribution of healthcare resources, there is also evidence of income-related inequalities that relate to inequalities in health. A study done in Asia on income-related inequalities in self-assessed health showed that across these countries, there is a strong association between inequalities in health and inequalities in income [65]. There is a growing concern about the effects of healthcare financing arrangements on the distribution of income, as well as on the catastrophic effects of healthcare on household incomes in many transitional economies in Asia [66]. There are a number of measurements on equity of financing health care, one of which is the Kakwani Index to measure progressivity of the health financing system. Evidence from a study of international comparison of financing mixes [66] shows that, generally, out-of-pocket payments are apparently becoming more regressive, taxes are a progressive means of raising revenue and private insurance is regressive. However, evidence shows that such conclusions vary depending on the degree of out-of-pocket payments and for which income groups of the population the financing methods are applied. Sometimes a regressive effect is offset by progressive changes elsewhere.

### *Efficiency in health systems*

Unlike equity, the whole concept of efficiency in health care is about making the right decision with whatever limited resources are available, and to produce healthcare goods and services that will give the maximum value to improving the health of the population in relation to the costs of producing them. It is making the money invested work where costs of producing any given output are minimized and the satisfaction derived from the utility of the healthcare services are maximized. In any healthcare system, a large amount of money is invested for the provision of health services, and the question that is often asked is whether the allocation of resources has been efficient or wasteful. According to Mehrota *et al.*, inefficiency occurs when more resources than necessary are used to produce the services that are currently provided or when there is an oversupply of technology or when money is spent on acute care rather than public health, which may produce more in terms of longevity and quality of life [67].

The simple notion of efficiency is analogous to the economist's concept of productivity or the accountant's concept of value for money [68]. According to WHO, in economic terms, performance is a measure of efficiency [69]. Health systems that have made improvements in performance are systems that can achieve more with the same resources or achieved the desired outcomes with given available resources. Although there are two types of efficiency – allocative efficiency and technical efficiency – some authors have divided this into three other areas, also including social efficiency which is the achievement of maximizing the total value of outputs produced [70], meaning that benefits will be maximized with the available resources. Allocative efficiency is about maximizing health within the constrained resources [71]. Health is maximized through attaining the right mix of outputs with the given resources. The principle behind this is the principal of optimality. Allocative inefficiency may occur if the system produces too many or too few of certain services relative to health improvements. There is no point spending a lot of money on treatment of cases for which health improvements or survival are remote or on technical procedures rather than proven preventive activities, for example, health education.

Technical efficiency is where the costs of producing a given output are minimized, or where the output is maximized for a given cost. It refers to the effective use of resources in producing outputs. It addresses the system performance, and can be quantified as the ratio of inputs to outputs. It is producing output at the least cost. Inputs are expressed either in monetary or physical terms, for example, level of healthcare expenditure measures as a percentage of GNP. Where output is concerned, it involves both intermediate and final outputs. They are normally expressed through a variety of indicators, for example, mortality indices, morbidity measures or utilization levels.

Sometimes a distinction needs to be made between final output and intermediate output, as the measurement of output may be indirect rather than direct. Inefficiency occurs when care is not managed in a way that maximizes potential productivity [72]. This is not about whether the activity is worth carrying out at all but rather about which activity will cost the least. Cost efficiency refers to the minimum level of economic resources required to produce a desired level of outputs. Cost-effectiveness is one approach to determine technical efficiency. Improved technical efficiency would mean a lower unit cost than what is current within the objectives being maximized, for example, costs per patient care.

In order to have an efficient healthcare system, supply-side measures must be implemented judiciously because, by their nature, they require government intervention for allocative efficiency and technical efficiency to be achieved [73]. Even if an allocationally efficient set of interventions is produced by the health system, its organization must assure technical efficiency by looking at the issues of productivity and quality. There are a number of strategies to improve efficiency, which the government can apply, such as streamlining of capital investment, regulation of improper use of high-cost technologies and revision of incentives for healthcare providers [73]. The use of telemedicine also has the potential of significant economic advantages on the basis of more efficient use of resources [74, 75]. There has always been a presumption that resource allocation that is controlled and directed by the government is less efficient than privately run health care whose priority is profit maximization. Any organization or system that is not efficient in its production will result in unnecessary high costs and wastefulness. Such a system is not sustainable nor is it desirable no matter how benevolent the organization is in the long run, whether it is government-controlled or privately run.

Efficiency analysis is centrally concerned with measuring the competence with which inputs are converted into valued outputs. The measurement of an organization's technical efficiency is to produce the production possibility frontier. The measure of allocative efficiency is purchasing the right mix of inputs or producing the right mix of outputs (i.e. an optimal mix of inputs and outputs) [76].

Basically, the issues and problems faced by most healthcare systems can be summed up in three main aspects: poor planning, problems with rising costs and financing, and issues of how effective, efficient and equitable healthcare resources are distributed and used. According to Frenk, holding national wealth and health expenditures constant, performance depends on the degree of efficiency and equity with which healthcare resources are deployed [77]. Different actors in the health system favour different criteria in this process. Efficiency is usually not favoured by society, the politicians and the policy makers, as opposed to the other equally important criterion: equity or fairness [78]. The pursuits of these two criteria will necessary involve some trade-offs as both of these goals are not compatible.

## Health expenditure and resource allocation issues in health systems

According to the WHO, healthcare expenditure has risen worldwide, and this increase has prompted every government to look for more sustainable health-financing arrangements [79]. World trends have shown that total health spending increases from around 23 per cent of GDP in low-income (< US$1,000 per capita) countries to typically 89 per cent in high-income (> US$7,000) ones [80]. Roemer states that as expenditures for health services as a percentage of GNP have been rising throughout the world, the share of health spending derived from governmental sources has also been increasing [81]. By examining the health expenditure of each health system, the achievement of a health system's performance in relation to the resources at its disposal is measured. A study done by the WHO on the performance level of health (in terms of disability-adjusted life expectancy) relative to health expenditure per capita of 191 member states in 1999, showed that higher health expenditure is associated with better health outcomes [82], which does not necessarily mean one is the direct cause of the other but only that they are correlated.

According to Griffin, inevitably the speed of success and the characteristic of government intervention in the health of the population boils down to the question of policy and how countries choose to spend their health resources [83]. Health expenditure is a good indicator to show how efficient and equitable a public health system is. The WHO has recommended that for developing countries, health expenditure should be 5 per cent of the GNP. However, other research has shown that the level of expenditure on health has more to do with the level of national income than with the degree of state involvement in health care [84, 90]. Some research has even stated that the relationship between GDP and health spending is unhelpful and almost certainly misleading for health policy development [85]. Many researchers have also argued that spending more on healthcare services does not necessarily lead to an improved health status [86, 87, 88, 89].

The arguments above have to be considered in light of how resources are distributed to achieve the best outcomes. Health expenditure needs to be targeted to achieve these goals and therefore policy and planning and the allocation of resources are processes to determine public health system performance. Improving targeting to the poor involves not simply rearranging the public subsidies, but also addressing the constraints that prevent the poor from accessing these services [90]. In addition, the attainment of an improved health status may not necessarily be accorded to whether the government spends more or less on the health sector. It is more appropriate to look at the process than the final outcome in assessing the performance of the health system. Should any gap exist, resources can then be allocated accordingly to correct the inequity and inefficiency.

A study on public health spending in poor countries [90] concludes that public spending on curative health care favours mostly the better off rather than the poor. The review showed that most curative health subsidies are not particularly well targeted to the poor and this problem cannot be solved simply by adjusting the subsidy allocations. Constraints that prevent the poor from taking advantage of these services must also be addressed, such as income, service quality, access, direct-user charges and gender, if the public subsidies are to be effective in reaching the poor. One way to improve targeting is reallocating public subsidies towards services used primarily by the poor. Expenditure reallocation would improve targeting only if it led to a significant increase in the use of such services by the poor. Monekosso [91] has come out with three types of health expenditure models:

1 Public and private expenditure are almost equal;
2 Low public expenditure (< 15 per cent) with high private expenditure; and
3 High public expenditure (> 70 per cent) but low private expenditure.

Malaysia happens to fall under the first category based on the 2002 Malaysian National Health Accounts Report where the public–private health expenditure is 56 per cent public and 44 per cent private [92]. If government spending is relatively high, the government may have to find means to reduce its share as it may displace private spending [93]. On the other hand, if government spending is low, it must set its priorities to solve the serious problems first with the available resources and allocate its resources wisely. For those whose expenditure falls in the middle, the decision will be more complex as to where to spend and how much to spend. Abel-Smith and Mach [94] suggest that studies of expenditures and sources of finance in the health sector should be an integral part of the national planning process. The importance of health expenditure as part of a bigger master plan cannot be taken lightly as it serves as a guide to the government to appropriate the right resources should any gaps exist. The master plan of all financial and material resources will normally involve data stretching far outside the ministry of health budget into the budgets of other government departments, compulsory health insurance agencies, industry, voluntary bodies and the private sector. But, in reality, such data may not be readily available, especially for those outside the public sector.

Problems may arise when policy objectives are vague or data on resource allocation are unobtainable for various reasons, as this will hamper a detailed study. Griffin suggests that a 'health map' laying out priorities for public spending will be useful because once the public health problems are known, it will be easy to quantitatively determine which methods would be most appropriate economically and how to establish priorities among competing needs [95]. Governments in developing countries are promoting equity to ensure health services are affordable and accessible to the poor as an essential goal to protect them from ill health and any catastrophic health expenditure. Yet, at the same time, governments are also implementing cost-containment measures to control rising costs, such as cost sharing by patients [95], introducing medical savings accounts to wean off dependence on the state [96] and improving health system performance through using healthcare resources efficiently [97].

The rising cost of health care is putting a heavy burden not only on governments but also on individuals and on communities. Decisions on resource allocation and distribution will promote and reinforce the principles adopted for the health system. There are a number of resource allocation methods. The historical incrementalist type of budgeting and resource allocation method has been slow in redressing inequities in the distribution of scarce healthcare resources. A study has shown that regions with high levels of deprivation and a relatively greater need for healthcare resources are getting less than their fair share [98]. Therefore, improved and new methods have been developed and implemented. Such changes are inevitable if the health system aims to be responsive to the health needs of the population.

## Conclusion

Throughout the world, governments are reassessing their role in health service delivery. They are doing so in response to common problems with public sector service delivery including inefficiency, poor quality and responsiveness to users, waste and, sometimes, fraud and corruption. To reach their goal of improving performance, health policy makers are applying a variety of organizational and management reforms. These reforms share the characteristics of maintaining predominant public financing, as well as public ownership, while simultaneously adopting best practices from the private sector, such as more performance-oriented organizational and management structures, stronger incentives and exposure to increased consumer pressures.

In an effort to improve equity, efficiency and responsiveness, many health systems in Asia have experimented with devolution and decentralization, and varying degrees of public–private participation, especially in the context of rapid socio-economic development and population ageing. It is fertile ground to validate and document the processes and experiences through health systems research. But it is also high time that the evidence of comparative lessons and best practices in Asia be shared and debated to inform global health and public policy.

## References


1. *The World Health Report 2000: Health Systems – Improving Performance*. Geneva: World Health Organization, 2000.
2. Murray CJL, Frenk J. A Framework for Assessing the Performance of Health Systems. *Bulletin of the World Health Organization*, 2000; 78(6): 717–731.
3. Roemer MI. *National Health Systems of the World*. New York: Oxford University Press, 1991.
4. Merson MH, Black RE, Mills AJ. *International Public Health: Diseases, Programs, Systems, and Policies*. Gaithersburg, MD: Aspen Publishers, 2001.
5. Gwatkin DR. Health Inequalities and the Health of the Poor: What Do We Know? What Can We Do? *Bulletin of the World Health Organization*, 2000; 78(1): 3–18.
6. Schieber G, Maeda A. Health Care Financing and Delivery in Developing Countries. *Health Affairs*, 1999; 18(3): 193–205.
7. Murray CJL, Frenk J. A Framework for Assessing the Performance of Health Systems. *Bulletin of the World Health Organization*, 2000; 78(6): 717–731.
8. Doorslaer E, Wagstaff A, Rutten F. *Equity in the Finance and Delivery of Health Care: An International Perspective*. CEC Health Services Research Series. Oxford: Oxford University Press, 1993.
9. Creese A, Kutzin J. Lessons from Cost Recovery in Health. Forum on Health Sector Reform, Discussion Paper No. 2. Geneva: World Health Organization, 1995.
10. Hsiao W, Liu Y. Economic Reform and Health Lessons from China. *New England Journal of Medicine*, 1996; 335: 430–432.
11. Akin J, Birdsall N, Ferranti D. *Financing Health Services in Developing Countries: An Agenda for Reform*. Washington, DC: World Bank, 1987.
12. Phua KH. Saving for Health. *World Health Forum*, 1987; 8: 38–41.
13. Bodeker G. Lessons on Integration from the Developing World's Experience. *British Medical Journal*, 2001; 322: 164–167.
14. World Bank. *World Development Report 1993: Investing in Health*. New York: Oxford University Press for the World Bank, 1993.
15. Berman P. Organization of Ambulatory Care Provision: A Critical Determinant of Health System Performance in Developing Countries. *Bulletin of the World Health Organization*, 2000; 78(6): 791–802.
16. McPake B, Mills A. What Can We Learn from International Comparisons of Health Systems and Health System Reform? *Bulletin of the World Health Organization*, 2000; 78(6): 811–820.
17. Musgrove P. *Public and Private Roles in Health: Theory and Financing Patterns*. Washington, DC: World Bank, 1996.
18. Singapore. Affordable Health Care: A White Paper. Singapore: Ministry of Health, 1993.
19. Block P. *Stewardship – Choosing Service over Self-interest*. San Francisco, CA: Berrett-Koehler Publishers, 1993.
20. Saltman RB, Ferroussier-Davis O. The Concept of Stewardship in Health Policy. *Bulletin of the World Health Organization*, 2000; 78(6): 732–739.
21. Ellencweig A. *Analysing Health Systems*. Oxford: Oxford University Press, 1992, pp. 67, 1621.
22. Phua KH. Health Systems, in Phoon WO and Chen PCY (eds) *Textbook of Community Medicine in South-East Asia*. Chichester: John Wiley, 1986: 305–312.
23. Phua KH, Chew AH. Towards a Comparative Analysis of Health Systems Reforms in the Asia-Pacific Region. *Asia Pacific Journal of Public Health*, 2002; 14(1): 9–16.
24. Gottret P, Schieber G. *Health Financing Revisited: A Practitioners Guide*. Washington, DC: World Bank, 2006.
25. Maynard A, Bloor K. Health Care Reform: Informing Difficult Choices. *International Journal of Health Planning and Management*, 1995; 10(4): 247–264.
26. Akin, *et al*. World Bank, 1987.
27. World Bank, 1993, p. 36.
28. The World Bank estimates the minimum package would need about one physician per 10,000 population, between two and four nurses per physician and one district hospital bed per 1,000 population.
29. Jayasinghe KSA, De Silva D, Mendis N, Lie RK. Ethics of Resource Allocation in Developing Countries: The Case of Sri Lanka. *Social Science & Medicine*, 1998; 47(10): 1619–1625.
30. Chernichovsky D. What Can Developing Economies Learn from Health System Reforms of Developed Countries? *Health Policy*, 1995; 32(1–3): 79–91.

31. Yuen PP. Health Care Financing in Hong Kong. *International Journal of Health Planning and Management*, 1999; 14(1): 3–18.
32. Berman P. Paper presented at the Conference on Health Sector Reform in Developing Countries: Issues for the 1990s. Durham, NH, September, 1993.
33. Berman P. Health Sector Reform. *Health Policy*, 1995; 32(1–3): 13–28.
34. Oyaya CO, Rifkin SB. Health Sector Reforms in Kenya. *Health Policy* 2003; 64: 113–127.
35. Olsen IT, Sustainability of Health Care. *Health Policy and Planning* 1998; 13(3): 287–295.
36. Hammer JS, Berman P. Ends and Means in Public Health Policy in Developing Countries. *Health Policy*, 1995; 32(1–3): 29–45.
37. Collins C, Green A, Hunter D. Health Sector Reform and the Interpretation of Policy Context. *Health Policy*, 1999; 47(1): 69–83.
38. Kawabata K. A New Look at Health Systems. *Bulletin of the World Health Organization*, 2000; 78(6): 716.
39. WHO, 2000, p. 41
40. Murray CJL, Frenk J. A Framework for Assessing the Performance of Health Systems. *Bulletin of the World Health Organization*, 2000; 78(6): 717–728.
41. Feachem RGA. Health Systems: More Evidence, More Debate. *Bulletin of the World Health Organization*, 2000; 78(6): 715.
42. Brundtland GH, Frenk J, Murray CJL. WHO Assessment of Health Systems Performance. *Lancet*, 2003; 361(9375): 2155.
43. Wibulpolprasert S, Tangcharoensathien V. Health Systems Performance – What's Next? *Bulletin of the World Health Organization*, 2001; 79(6): 489.
44. Kawabata K. A New Look at Health Systems. *Bulletin of the World Health Organization*, 2000; 78(6): 716.
45. McGuire A, Henderson J, Mooney G. *The Economics of Health Care: An Introductory Text*. London: Routledge & Keegan Paul, 1988, p. 74.
46. Broomberg J. Managing the Health Care Market in Developing Countries. *Health Policy and Planning*, 1994; 9(3): 237–251.
47. Almeida C, Travassos C, Porto S, Labra ME. Health Sector Reform in Brazil. *International Journal of Health Services*, 2000; 30(1): 129–162.
48. Culyer AJ, Wagstaff A. Equity and Equality in Health and Health Care. *Journal of Health Economics*, 1993; 12(4): 431–457.
49. Mooney G, Jan S, Wiseman V. Staking a Claim for Claims. *Social Science and Medicine*, 2002; 54(11): 1657–1667.
50. Ke Xu. Catastrophic Health Expenditure. *Lancet*, 2003; 362(9388): 997.
51. Mooney G. *Key Issues in Health Economics*. New York: Harvester Wheatsheaf, 1994, p. 82.
52. Gutman AS. For and Against Equal Access to Health Care, in Bayer R, Caplan AL, Daniels N. (eds) *In Search of Equity*. New York: Springer, 1983, p. 44.
53. Oliver A, Mossialos E. Equity of Access to Health Care. *Journal of Epidemiology and Community Health*, 2004; 58(8): 655–658.
54. Jack W. Public Spending on Health Care. *Health Policy*, 2000; 53(1): 61–67.
55. McGuire A, Henderson J, Mooney G. *The Economics of Health Care: An Introductory Text*. London: Routledge & Keegan Paul, 1988, p. 56.
56. Musgrove P. Public Spending on Health Care. *Health Policy*, 1999; 47(3): 207–223.
57. McGuire A, Henderson J, Mooney G. *The Economics of Health Care: An Introductory Text*. London: Routledge & Keegan Paul, 1988, p. 55.
58. Mooney G, Jan S, Wiseman V. Staking a Claim for Claims. *Social Science and Medicine*, 2002; 54(11): 1657–1667.
59. Musgrove P. Public Spending on Health Care. *Health Policy*, 1999; 47(3): 207–223.
60. Mooney G, Jan S. Vertical Equity. *Health Policy*, 1997; 39(1): 79–87.
61. Jack W. Public Spending on Health Care. *Health Policy*, 2000; 53(1): 61–67.
62. Mooney G, Jan S, Wiseman V. Staking a Claim for Claims. *Social Science and Medicine*, 2002; 54(11): 1657–1667.
63. Mooney G, Jan S. Vertical Equity. *Health Policy*, 1997; 39(1): 79–87.
64. Ellencweig A. *Analysing Health Systems*. Oxford: Oxford University Press, 1992, p. 120.
65. O'Donnell O, van Doorslaer E, Rannan-Eliya RP, *et al.* Who Pays for Health Care in Asia? *Journal of Health Economics*, 2008; 27: 460–475.

66. Van Doorslaer E, O'Donnell O, Rannan-Eliya RP, *et al.* Catastrophic Payment for Health Care in Asia. *Health Economics*, 2007; 16: 1159–1184.
67. Mehrota A, Dudley RA, Luft HS. What's Behind the Health Expenditure Trends? *Annual Review of Public Health*, 2003; 24: 385–412.
68. Jacob R, Smith PC, Street A. *Measuring Efficiency in Health Care: Analytic Techniques and Health Policy.* Cambridge: Cambridge University Press, 2006, p. 2.
69. WHO, 2000, p. 41.
70. McGuire A, Henderson J, Mooney G. *The Economics of Health Care: An Introductory Text.* London: Routledge & Keegan Paul, 1988, p. 77.
71. Aday LA, *et al. Evaluating the Health Care System*, 2nd edn. Chicago, IL: Health Administration Press, 1998, p. 108.
72. Ibid., p. 110.
73. Tangcharoensathien V, Lertiendumrong J. Health System Performance. *Lancet*, 2000; 356(1001): S31.
74. Kontodimopoulos N, Nanos P, Niakas D. Balancing Efficiency of Health Services and Equity of Access in Remote Areas in Greece. *Health Policy*, 2006; 76(1): 49–57.
75. Yusof K, Neoh KH, Hashim MA, Ibrahim I. Role of Teleconsultation in Moving the Healthcare System Forward. *Asia Pacific Journal of Public Health*, 2002; 14(1): 29–34.
76. Jacob R, Smith PC, Street A. *Measuring Efficiency in Health Care: Analytic Techniques and Health Policy.* Cambridge: Cambridge University Press, 2006, p. 4.
77. Frenk J. Dimensions of Health System Reform. *Health Policy*, 1994; 27(1): 19–34.
78. Kontodimopoulos N, Nanos P, Niakas D. Balancing Efficiency of Health Services and Equity of Access in Remote Areas in Greece. *Health Policy*, 2006; 76(1): 49–57.
79. WHO, 2000, p. 95.
80. Musgrove P, Zeramdini R, Carrin G. Basic Patterns in National Health Expenditure. *Bulletin of the World Health Organization*, 2002; 80(2): 134–141.
81. Roemer MI. Health Care Costs and Financing in World Perspective. *Yale Journal of Biology and Medicine*, 1991; 64(5): 435–441.
82. WHO, 2000, p. 43.
83. Griffin C. *Health Care in Asia: A Comparative Study of Cost and Financing.* Washington, DC: World Bank, 1992, p. 44.
84. Hunter DJ. The Privatization of Public Provision. *Lancet*, 1983; 321(8336): 1264–1268.
85. Kanavos P, Mossialos E. International Comparisons of Health Care Expenditures. *Journal of Health Service Research and Policy*, 1999; 4(2): 122–126.
86. Hunter DJ. The Privatization of Public Provision. *Lancet*, 1983; 321(8336): 1264–1268.
87. Tangcharoensathien V, Lertiendumrong J. Health System Performance. *Lancet*, 2000; 356(1001): S31.
88. Retzlaff-Roberts D, Chang CF, Rubin RM. Technical Efficiency in the Use of Health Care Resources. *Health Policy*, 2004; 69(1): 55–72.
89. Carr-Hill RA. Efficiency and Equity Implications of the Health Care Reforms. *Social Science and Medicine*, 1994; 39(9): 1189–1201.
90. Castro-Leal F, Dayton J, Demery L, Mehra K. Public Health Spending in Africa. *Bulletin of the World Health Organization*, 2000; 78(1): 66–74.
91. Monekosso GL, Economics Health Care and Health Status, in Griffiths A, Bankowski Z. (eds) *Economics and Health Policy.* XIIIth CIOMS Round Table Conference. Council for International Organizations of Medical Sciences and the Sandoz Institute for Health and Socio-Economic Studies. Geneva: World Health Organization, 1980, pp. 40–44.
92. *MNHA Project – Health Expenditure Report (1997–2002)*, Ministry of Health, Malaysia, 2006, p. 12.
93. Griffin C. *Health Care in Asia: A Comparative Study of Cost and Financing.* Washington, DC: World Bank, 1992, p. 53.
94. Abel-Smith B, Mach EP. *Planning the Finances of the Health Sector: A Manual for Developing Countries.* Geneva: World Health Organization, 1983, p. 14.
95. Griffin C. *Health Care in Asia: A Comparative Study of Cost and Financing.* Washington, DC: World Bank, 1992, p. 154.
96. Lim MK. Shifting the Burden of Health Care Finance. *Health Policy*, 2004; 69(1): 83–92.
97. Evan DB, Tandon A, Murray CJ, Lauer JA. Comparative Efficiency of National Health Systems. *British Medical Journal*, 2001; 323(7308): 307–310.
98. Van Doorslaer E. *et al. Health Economics*, 2007.

# Part VII
# Future challenges

# 47
# Looking to the future

*Siân M. Griffiths, Jin Ling Tang and Eng Kiong Yeoh*

In constructing this *Handbook of Global Public Health in Asia* we have sought to provide a perspective on the major health challenges from a variety of angles. As we said at the beginning, we did not aim to be a comprehensive textbook but to show how diverse and dynamic the public health issues and responses in the most rapidly transitioning part of the world are. Asia is made up of high-, low- and middle-income countries, of huge urban conurbations and remote rural areas. It faces the threats of emerging disease, of environmental as well as physical disaster and a growing tide of non-communicable diseases (NCDs).

## A global public health perspective

Throughout the book we have based our approach on the WHO definition that public health refers to all organized measures (whether public or private) to prevent disease, promote health and prolong life among the population as a whole. This includes activities that aim to provide conditions in which people can be healthy and that focus on entire populations, not on individual patients or diseases [1]. Thus, we emphasize that public health is concerned with the total system and not only the eradication of a particular disease. The structure of the book follows the three domains model [2] for public health practice used in the UK to support the public health workforce. The fundamental tenet is that global population health will only improve if not only the factors relevant to individuals but also those that impact on populations are addressed. This will include concern to address poverty and inequity. The term global public health recognizes that, as a result of globalization, forces that affect public health can and do come from outside state boundaries, and that responding to public health issues now requires attention to cross-border health risks, including access to dangerous products and environmental change [1].

The sixteenth-century poet John Donne [3] wrote the immortal lines that 'No man is an Island, entire of itself; every man is a piece of the Continent, a part of the main'; and later in the poem 'any man's death diminishes me, because I am involved in Mankind'.

These words carry with them the key sentiment of global public health – the essential interconnection and impact of all global policies be they trade, business, scientific research or humanitarian response [4], reflected more recently by William Foege [5] when he observed

'People are beginning to understand there is nothing in the world so remote that it can't impact you as a person.' In a more recent debate in the *Lancet*, Fried and other US public health leaders [6] defined the tenets of global public health as:

- Dedication to better health for all, with attention to the needs of vulnerable populations;
- Translation of knowledge in practice, not limited by political boundaries;
- A scientific approach to health promotion and disease prevention medicine and clinical care remain essential pillars;
- Commitment to an integrated, multidisciplinary, prevention-oriented approach in the community and clinics;
- Multilevel systems-based interventions; and
- Comprehensive frameworks for financing and structuring health policies and services.

Underpinning these tenets is the essential principle that public health is a public good, benefiting all members of every society and it is these tenets that we seek to reflect. Achieving good health, as is clear from the pages of this collection of writings, is a broad and diverse concept requiring both in-depth vertical programmatic approaches, such as those for tackling malaria, HIV and TB, as well as horizontal integrated perspectives, be they at government level, such as Health in All Policies [7] or locally based community development programmes. To illustrate their breadth, these are just some of the campaigns in which public health workers may be involved:

**Campaigns involving public health workers**

Vaccination and control of infectious diseases
Motor-vehicle safety
Safer workplaces
Safer and healthier foods
Safe drinking water
Healthier mothers and babies and access to family planning
Decline in deaths from coronary heart disease and stroke
Recognition of tobacco use as a health hazard.

*Source*: [1].

The new global public health perspective requires broader engagement by health organizations and all countries for the objectives of health equity, access and coverage. It also requires engagement of the health services. We know that improving health is one of the best ways to fight poverty, yet, as Julio Frenk comments, too often the health system is seen as something in the abstract, not as an integral part of the fabric of societies. Discussions of health need to be a central part of social, political and ethical life. Thus one of the biggest challenges for health reform remains what Frenk describes as the false dilemmas – the idea that leaders must choose between individual health and population health, between prevention and treatment, or between fighting poverty and providing health care – that can separate what should be an integrated, holistic system [8].

## Poverty and health are closely interrelated

Another key theme across the pages of this volume is that poverty and poor health are inextricably linked. Better health is both a fundamental human right and a sound social investment. Thus within healthy public policy, there needs to be an explicit concern for health and equity in all areas of policy and an accountability for the health impact of these policies. The development of healthy public policy requires not only an investment of resources by government – linking economic, social and health policies – but also a foundation built on the basic principles of social justice to ensure health promotion and healthy lives.

Health is not just a cost, it is an investment; although health expenditure may be regarded as an economic burden, the real cost to society are the direct and indirect costs linked to ill health. Strategies to reduce poverty are essential for improving health opportunity. Addressing the root causes of poverty whilst promoting greater equity are key strategic objectives underpinning the work of the WHO Commission on Social Determinants of Health [9], which advocates strategic action across four main dimensions – political, economic, social and cultural.

One focus for strategic action is identifying the priorities for the next iteration of the Millennium Development Goals, the international commitment to reduce poverty. There are many contenders, not only those areas where, despite progress, targets were missed, but a wide range of new competing topics including ensuring a life-course approach to the battle against NCDs, peace as a prerequisite for health and the inclusion of the neglected diseases of poverty, which pose massive health burdens but have low profiles.

## Looking forward: some global health challenges

**Global health challenges**

Emerging infections
Climate change and environmental sustainability
Non-communicable diseases
Ageing population
Migration
Cost of health services
Innovations and new technology
Peace and stability
Well-trained public health professionals.

The future of health of Asian countries will continue to be affected by the rapid transition they are going through. Whilst in the past infectious diseases were a major threat, there are growing concerns with the epidemic of NCDs accompanying increasing affluence and globalized lifestyles. But continued vigilance and surveillance remain essential as new infections emerge. In 2013 we have seen new variants of flu emerge – H7N7, H7N9 amongst them. No one is sure of their potential impact – or of that of MERS – but memories of SARS are acute in Asia, particularly in those countries affected by the 2003 outbreak. They know only too well of the devastating impact on wider society wreaked by the epidemic – its social and economic costs, as well as the morbidity and mortality. This underlines the importance of understanding interrelationships between emerging patterns of infectious diseases and environmental changes and living conditions, described in several chapters in this book.

Others have described the growing threat of NCDs. These diseases are a long-standing, progressive and a costly threat to healthy populations. Diseases such as diabetes not only are associated with the problems of diminished functional capacity, increased physical and psychosocial morbidity, comorbidities and complications, but also lead to higher utilization of health services and higher medical costs, as well as opportunity costs that are associated with self-care and disability and shorter life expectancy. And the challenge is complicated not only by the growing number of patients with multi-morbidity, but by the increasing longevity of many Asian populations. Just as economies are in transition so too are living conditions, lifestyles and patterns of behaviour. Global corporates fight for a share of the market irrespective of health impact and sugary, salty products are promoted openly in the media. Alcohol has become a major trading commodity in Hong Kong, with increased sales a cause for celebration not anxiety about their potential health harms. Tobacco companies are succeeding in selling more tobacco, at times supported by national governments.

Older people are particularly affected as their expectations of support from their families has to change. As younger people migrate to cities to find better paid work, many older people are left behind in the rural areas, often caring for their grandchildren (see Figure 47.1).

In cities, particularly those that are wealthy such as Hong Kong, Beijing and Shanghai, the cost of housing is escalating and people are forced to live in smaller, expensive spaces with no room for elderly dependants. And with increasing longevity, the burden of chronic diseases, including dementia, on health services is growing. As described in this book, the costs of health care and pensions are significant challenges to governments even in affluent developed

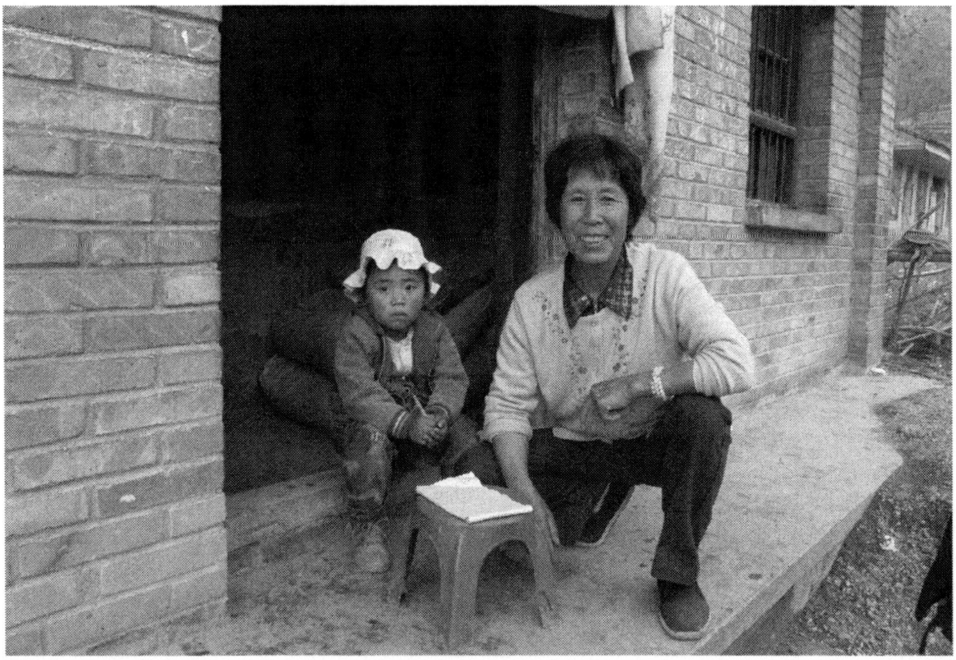

*Figure 47.1* Grandmother and granddaughter in rural Gansu

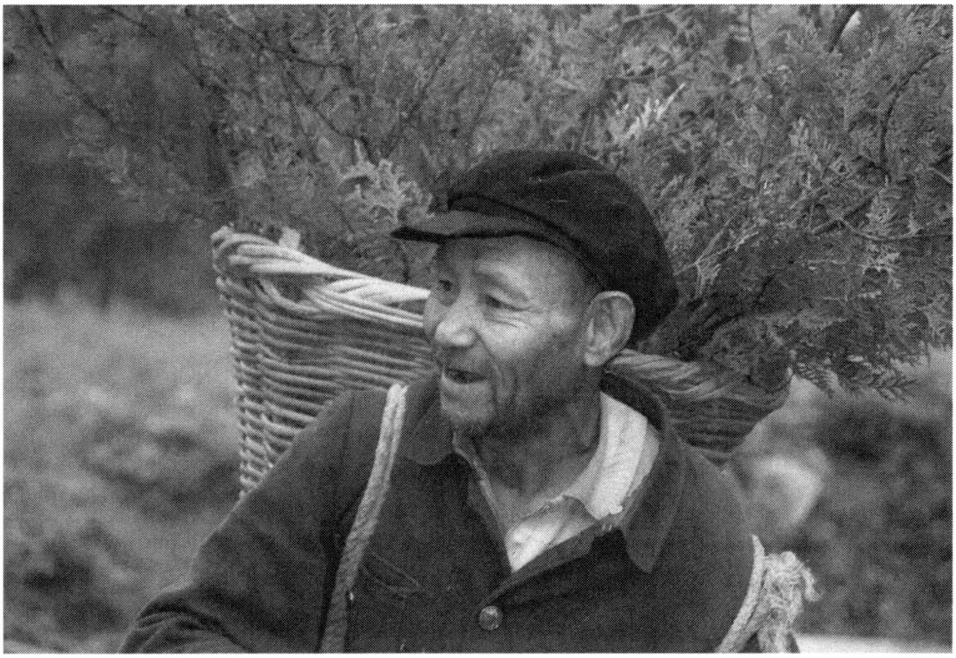

*Figure 47.2* Older man carrying saplings in the mountains

societies. Healthcare costs are also affected not just by the increasing populations they care for but by the range of innovations and new technologies that are emerging – not least the developments of genetics and personalized medicine.

There is an emerging and new social order which impacts on all levels of society creating new threats to health, as well as the opportunities, related to increasing affluence.

In the face of such challenges, professionals with skills to work at the community/population level are needed. They are needed at community level, linked to primary care provision to promote healthy practices and behaviours to ensure that populations stay healthy. They are needed at policy level to ensure health is a political consideration in all policies that are developed. They are needed within the health services to ensure prevention is part of every patient's care, every doctor's practice, every healthcare worker's concern. They are needed in NGOs to share their skills and within local government to protect health in the local environment. They are needed within global organizations. Asia, like many other regions of the world, is facing severe shortages, skews in skill-mix and inequitable distribution of health workers. Adequate investment is needed to educate more and better public health professionals for the twenty-first century capable of mobilizing knowledge and other resources necessary to achieve equitable 'patient and population-centred' health systems.

This is a tall order, but one we must rise to if we wish to see the health of our population at its optimum. We hope this book contributes not only to the education of future generations of public health workers but to greater understanding by a wider range of readers of the challenges we face in ensuring global public health particularly in Asia.

## References


1. World Health Organization. Trade, Foreign Policy, Diplomacy and Health. *Public Health*. Available from: http://www.who.int/trade/glossary/story076/en/index.html
2. Griffiths S, Jewell JA, Donnelly P. Public Health in Practice: The Three Domains of Public Health. *Public Health* 2005; 119: 907–13.
3. Donne J. 'No Man is an Island'. Available from: http://www.goodreads.com/author/quotes/77318.John_Donne
4. DeCock KM, Simone PM, Davison V, Slutsker L. The New Global Health. *Emerging Infectious Disease* 2013; 19(8): 1192–7.
5. Foege HW. Global Health Champions. Available from: http://www.pbs.org/wgbh/rxforsurvival/series/champions/william_h_foege.html
6. Fried LP, Bentley ME, Buekens P, Burke D, Frenk JJ, Klag MJ, Spencer HC. Global health is public health. *Lancet* 2010; 375(9714): 535–7.
7. European Portal for Action on Health Inequalities. Health in All Policies (HiAP). Available from: http://www.health-inequalities.eu/HEALTHEQUITY/EN/policies/health_in_all_policies/
8. The coming transformation in global health: a conversation with Crisp, Frenk and Farmer. February 28, 2013, Harvard Medical School and the Harvard School of Public Health. Available from: http://www.globalhealthdelivery.org/blog/2013/03/enabling-change-in-health-systems/
9. World Health Organization. Closing the Gap in a Generation: Health Equity through Action on the Social Determinants of Health. Commission on Social Determinants of Health Final Report. Available from: http://whqlibdoc.who.int/publications/2008/9789241563703_eng.pdf

# Index